SURGICAL-ORTHODONTIC
TREATMENT

SURGICAL-ORTHODONTIC
TREATMENT

WILLIAM R. PROFFIT, D.D.S., Ph.D.

Professor and Chairman
Department of Orthodontics
The University of North Carolina at Chapel Hill
School of Dentistry
Chapel Hill, North Carolina

RAYMOND P. WHITE, Jr., D.D.S., Ph.D.

Professor
Department of Oral and Maxillofacial Surgery
The University of North Carolina at Chapel Hill
School of Dentistry
Chapel Hill, North Carolina

With 2053 illustrations

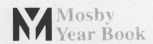

Mosby
Year Book

St. Louis   Baltimore   Boston   Chicago   London   Philadelphia   Sydney   Toronto

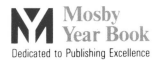
Mosby
Year Book
Dedicated to Publishing Excellence

Editor Robert W. Reinhardt
Developmental Editor Maureen Slaten
Assistant Editor Cynthia E. Lilly
Project Manager Patricia Gayle May
Production Donna L. Walls
Manuscript Editor Donna L. Walls
Design Candace F. Conner

Printed in the United States of America

Mosby–Year Book, Inc.
11830 Westline Industrial Drive, St. Louis, Missouri 63146   RK529.P76   1990

Library of Congress Cataloging-in-Publication Data

Proffit, William R.
    Surgical-orthodontic treatment / William R. Proffit, Raymond P.
White, Jr.
      p.   cm.
    Includes index.
    ISBN 0-8016-5291-X
    1. Teeth—Abnormalities—Surgery. 2. Jaws—Abnormalities—
Surgery. 3. Face—Abnormalities—Surgery. 4. Orthodontics,
Corrective. I. White, Raymond P., 1927-   . II. Title.
    [DNLM: 1. Face—surgery. 2. Jaw Abnormalities—surgery.
3. Orthodontics, Corrective. 4. Surgery, Oral.   WU 101.5 P964s]
RK529.P76 1990
617.5′22—dc20
DNLM/DLC
for Library of Congress   90-6147
                                   CIP

C/W/W 9 8 7 6 5 4 3 2 1

Contributors

PETER M. SINCLAIR, D.D.S., M.S.D.

Associate Professor
Department of Orthodontics
The University of North Carolina at Chapel Hill
School of Dentistry
Chapel Hill, North Carolina

BILL C. TERRY, D.D.S.

Professor
Department of Oral and Maxillofacial Surgery
The University of North Carolina at Chapel Hill
School of Dentistry
Chapel Hill, North Carolina

MYRON R. TUCKER, D.D.S.

Associate Professor
Department of Oral and Maxillofacial Surgery
The University of North Carolina at Chapel Hill
School of Dentistry
Chapel Hill, North Carolina

TIMOTHY A. TURVEY, D.D.S.

Professor
Department of Oral and Maxillofacial Surgery
The University of North Carolina at Chapel Hill
School of Dentistry
Chapel Hill, North Carolina

with a special chapter by

H. ASUMAN KIYAK, Ph.D.

Professor
Department of Oral and Maxillofacial Surgery
University of Washington
School of Dentistry
Seattle, Washington

REBECCA BELL, D.D.S., M.S.D.

Private Practice in Orthodontics
Anchorage, Alaska

Preface

We have been privileged to be a part of the evolution of surgical-orthodontic treatment over the past 3 decades. Increasing sophistication in diagnosis and planning, improvements in orthodontic mechanics and techniques, and significant advances in anesthesia and orthognathic surgery have allowed patients with the most complex problems the option of treatment to correct their skeletal jaw deformity and align their teeth. The total treatment time for the majority of patients can be less than 2 years, and improved function and esthetics can be expected. The treatment of patients with dentofacial deformity is a major emphasis in the training of future orthodontists and oral and maxillofacial surgeons. Significant numbers of patients are being treated in university centers and in community practices across the United States and throughout the world.

The treatment of patients with dentofacial deformity must be interdisciplinary. The orthodontist and surgeon are always involved, frequently assisted by the general dentist, the peridontist, and the prosthodontist. Orthodontists and oral and maxillofacial surgeons in clinical practice have the expertise to provide treatment in their respective fields to patients with complex dentofacial problems. But interdisciplinary treatment is demanding, requiring an interaction among all involved over an extended timeframe. Orthodontists and surgeons are trained in different environments, have different expertise, and look at the same problems with a different perspective. Despite the best efforts, communication can be garbled or incomplete. The primary goals of this text are to enhance communication between the orthodontist and the surgeon and foster an understanding of the complex diagnosis and treatment among other dental specialists who may participate for the benefit of the patient.

The book is divided into four major sections. In the first section (Chapters 1 to 3), the indications for surgical-orthodontic treatment are discussed, and background information on the physical and psychosocial development of patients with dentofacial deformity is provided. This includes a review of the psychologic response to treatment, summarizing recent important research data on this important subject.

The second section (Chapters 4 to 6) details the diagnostic and treatment planning approaches effective in surgical-orthodontic treatment. This section is based on the application of the problem-oriented approach. It includes an in-depth discussion of indications for diagnostic procedures and a detailed description of the steps in planning treatment.

The third section of the text (Chapters 7 to 11) describes and illustrates the orthognathic surgical procedures commonly performed today, including a discussion of current surgical principles and the application of rigid internal fixation techniques.

The final and longest section (Chapters 12 to 19) discusses the clinical problems for which patients seek treatment. The emphasis is on the options available to both the orthodontist and the surgeon for effective treatment of the problem within the most reasonable timeframe, indicating where other dental specialists might contribute, and on the interaction among the clinicians that is necessary for optimal treatment results.

Much of the data presented here for physiologic adaptation and stability after treatment was derived from studies supported by NIH grant DE-05215 from the National Institute of Dental Research. We are grateful for their continuing support. The research data base at the University of North Carolina was organized by Dr. Ceib Phillips, and the availability of data is due to her statistical expertise and excellent laboratory support from Debora Price and Kyle Harrison. In addition, major support for the studies of psychologic responses to treatment was provided by NIDR grant DE-05744 to the University of Washington.

We thank Nancy Arellano for typing and patiently organizing the manuscript and illustrations, Ramona Hutton-Howe for photographic services, Peter Bedick and Marian Blackburn for art work, Drs. William Brown and Peter Lee for invaluable assistance in preparing and organizing the case reports, and Dr. Arden Hegvedt for a critical review and proofreading of the text. In many ways, the work represents the efforts of a larger team than the authors themselves.

Although this text does not discuss every possible diagnostic approach, surgical technique, or clinical problem that might arise, we have attempted to cover the spectrum of dentofacial deformity, avoiding both significant omissions and unnecessary redundancy. Above all, our objective has been to make the book a practical, useful reference for clinical practice. We hope we have achieved our goals.

William R. Proffit
Raymond P. White, Jr.

Contents

SURGICAL-ORTHODONTIC
TREATMENT

THE SPECTRUM OF DENTOFACIAL DEFORMITY

CHAPTER 1

The Need for Surgical-Orthodontic Treatment

William R. Proffit
Raymond P. White, Jr.

Indications for surgical-orthodontic treatment
Prevalence of dentofacial deformity
Development of combined orthodontic and surgical treatment

INDICATIONS FOR SURGICAL-ORTHODONTIC TREATMENT

In our society, if teeth are noticeably irregular or protruding or if there is an obvious jaw deformity, people seek orthodontic treatment to improve both jaw function and facial esthetics. Recently, the more severe problems that might require a combination of surgery and orthodontics have been termed *dentofacial deformities*, to distinguish them from the less severe malocclusions that are treatable by orthodontics alone. Even for a dentofacial deformity, treatment is elective—no one dies from uncorrected orthodontic problems, with the exception of occasional suicides in which depression related to facial appearance may have played a role—but it can be very important in the quality of life and life adjustment.

The patient's physical health can be affected by a dentofacial deformity in several ways. If the problem is severe enough, mastication can be impaired, with an impact on digestion and general health. Most patients maintain adequate nutrition but learn to avoid certain foods that they simply cannot handle. Despite the marvelous adaptations that are possible in speech, tooth and jaw malposition can cause speech problems. It is more difficult to maintain good oral hygiene if the teeth are markedly protruding and irregular, and pa-

tients who resent their teeth are less motivated to do so—thus susceptibility to both caries and periodontal disease may be increased. There is some evidence that temporomandibular (TM) joint pain and dysfunction are more likely to develop in some types of jaw deformities.

As the National Research Council (NRC) noted in its report on the effect of these problems,[1] the psychosocial impact of a dentofacial deformity is usually more important than the related physical problems. This is not to say that the physical impact is unimportant— the physical effects are both real and important—but rather that an individual's entire life adjustment and role in life can be altered by the psychosocial effects. Both self-image and the image of others are very much affected by facial and dental appearance.[2,3] It is not a trivial handicap to have a long face and an anterior open bite in a society where the caricature of mental retardation is just that appearance. The greater the deviation from normal appearance, the greater this handicap becomes. The NRC report suggests that approximately 5% of the population has an orthodontic problem of such significance that it should be considered handicapping. It is patients like this who often need a combination of surgery and orthodontics to correct the deformity.

The simplest answer to the question, "Who is a candidate for surgery in addition to orthodontics?" is that surgery will be needed if there is a severe skeletal or very severe dentoalveolar problem, too severe to correct by orthodontics alone. The answer to the logical second question, "What makes a problem too severe for orthodontics alone?" is more subtle and is the focus of the discussion that follows.

If the jaw relationship is correct, crowded and mala-

A

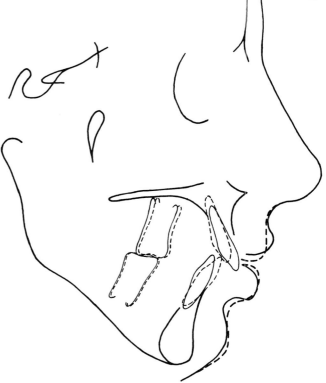

B

C

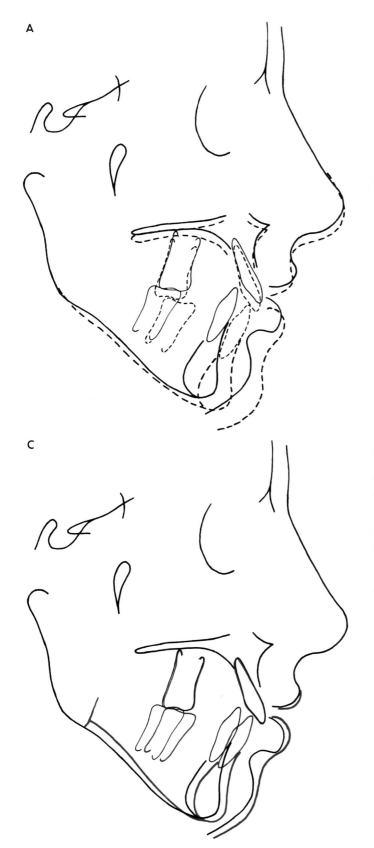

Fig. 1-1. There are three possible treatments for correction of a dentofacial deformity, as illustrated in these cephalometric tracings of potential treatment results for a patient with excessive incisor overjet resulting from mandibular deficiency. **A,** Tooth movement coupled with growth modification. Here the cephalometric prediction shows the possible result of treatment in a growing individual, with restraint of the normal downward and forward movement of the upper jaw and excellent forward growth of the lower jaw. Such a result would require both beginning treatment before the adolescent growth spurt and cooperation from the patient. **B,** Orthodontic tooth movement to camouflage the underlying jaw relationship without changing it. As this cephalometric prediction for a nongrowing patient shows, the upper teeth can be moved back and the lowers forward, but there are limits both in the amount of tooth movement possible and in the potential esthetic effect of this treatment. **C,** Surgical repositioning of the jaw or jaws, as in this prediction of the result of surgical mandibular advancement. If there is no growth remaining, this is the only way to correct the jaw discrepancy underlying the protruding upper incisors.

ligned teeth nearly always can be corrected by orthodontic tooth movement. However, there are limits to how far a tooth can be moved, and these limits become important when bite relationships must be changed to correct crossbite, deep bite, open bite, or incisor protrusion. A jaw discrepancy is usually involved in a severe malocclusion, and in broad terms, only three possible treatments exist (Fig. 1-1): (1) modification of growth, (2) camouflage (displacing the teeth to obtain proper function despite the jaw deformity), which produces a dental compensation for the skeletal discrepancy, or (3) surgical repositioning of the jaws and/or dentoalveolar segments to obtain proper positioning.

Growth modification, insofar as it is possible, is the ideal approach. Orthodontic treatment of the type now often called *dentofacial orthopedics* can alter the expression of growth and improve jaw problems, at least to some extent (how much remains highly controversial). However, a current consensus exists on two important points: (1) the pattern of growth can be modified in a favorable way for at least some patients, and (2) the extent is rather limited; that is, the upper and lower jaws can be induced to grow a few millimeters more or less than would have occurred without treatment, but they will not undergo major transformations.

Even when the aim of orthodontic treatment is growth modification, the treatment inevitably also displaces the teeth in the direction of correcting the occlusal relationship. This tooth movement, which can be termed *dental compensation for skeletal discrepancy*, prevents a total skeletal correction and introduces an element of camouflage. For example, the ideal way to correct a Class II malocclusion resulting from an underdeveloped lower jaw is to stimulate the mandible to grow forward, but when this treatment is attempted, it is difficult to prevent some forward movement of the lower teeth on the mandibular base and backward movement of the upper teeth relative to the maxilla. If the amount and direction of jaw growth are favorable, there will be less dental compensation than if growth is unfavorable.

If there is no growth at all in a patient with a jaw discrepancy, the only possibility for orthodontic treatment alone is camouflage by displacement of teeth relative to the jaws. Extraction of some teeth to allow enough movement of the others will probably be required. The resulting dental compensation may produce reasonably normal dental occlusion, but as with a growing patient, the result is satisfactory only if facial esthetics as well as tooth relationships are acceptable. Major tooth movements may correct the dental occlusion without improving facial esthetics, or even make facial esthetics worse. In such a case, the result is not satisfactory even if the dental occlusion is perfect.

Once growth has stopped, surgery is the only way to correct, rather than compensate for and camouflage, a jaw discrepancy. The more dental compensation is present, the less the surgeon can correct the jaw relationship without producing malocclusion. This is true whether the compensation occurred naturally or was introduced by orthodontic treatment, and it explains why "reverse orthodontics," deliberately making the occlusion worse initially, is often necessary in prepar-

ing for jaw surgery. If the tooth relationships are not the limiting factor, it is nevertheless true that there are limits on how far the jaws can be moved surgically, but these limits are larger than the limits of camouflage and growth modification.

The "envelope of discrepancy"[4] graphically illustrates the current concepts of how much change can be produced by the various treatments (Fig. 1-2). The inner circle indicates the limits to orthodontic tooth movement (camouflage) alone; the middle circle, tooth movement combined with growth modification; and the outer circle, surgical correction. The exact dimensions of the envelope for each of the three treatments can be debated. Good data support some of the limits shown in Fig. 1-2; other limits, for which research data are not now available, are based on our clinical judgment.

The precise dimensions of the envelope are much less important than the concept. It is obvious that greater change can be produced in a growing child by a combination of growth modification and tooth movement than could be produced in a nongrowing individual by tooth movement alone. In an adult, camouflage of a jaw deformity must be produced strictly by tooth movement. Therefore, all other things being equal, it should be possible to treat with orthodontics alone a deformity in a child that could not be corrected without surgery in an older individual.

The answer to our question, "What makes a problem too severe for orthodontics alone?" now becomes clearer. A problem in a child is too severe for orthodontic treatment alone if it cannot be corrected by a combination of growth modification and camouflage. In an older individual, if the jaw discrepancy is too great to compensate for and camouflage by tooth movement alone, surgery is the only way to obtain a reasonable result.

The concept presented above states explicitly that correcting the occlusal relationships of the teeth is not an adequate description of successful treatment. Occlusion is important, but satisfactory facial esthetics must accompany it. We explore this concept further by reviewing three patients.

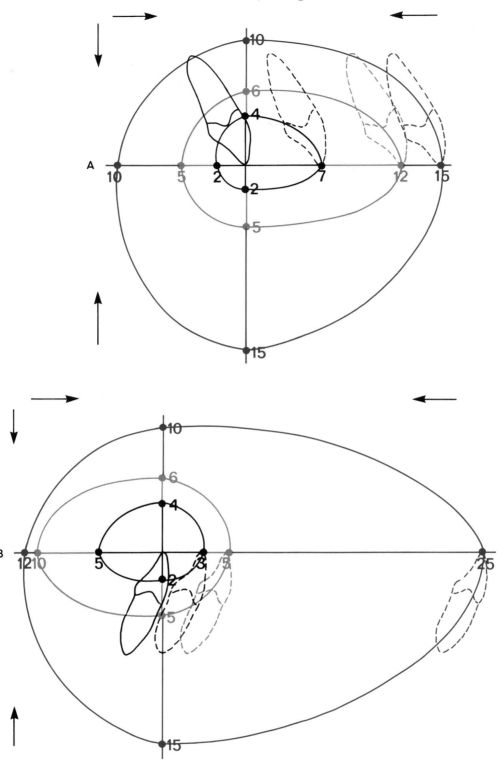

Fig. 1-2. The envelope of discrepancy, showing the amount of change in all three planes of space that could be produced by orthodontic tooth movement alone (the inner circle of each diagram); orthodontic tooth movement combined with growth modification in a growing child (the middle circle); and orthognathic surgery (the outer circle). Note that the possibilities of each treatment are not symmetric with regard to the planes of space. For example, greater tooth movement is possible anteroposteriorly than vertically, growth modification is more effective in mandibular deficiency than in mandibular excess, and surgery to move the lower jaw back has greater potential than surgery to advance it.

Case 1 (Figs. 1-3 to 1-9)

D.S., age 14 years, 10 months, appeared quite mature physically when she first sought orthodontic consultation. Her chief complaint was her "crooked front teeth," which were apparent when she smiled. There was no significant medical or dental history, dental or soft-tissue pathology, or problems of jaw function. She had a classic Class II, division 2 malocclusion with a moderate anterior deep bite, and cephalometric analysis revealed mandibular deficiency (see Chapter 4 for a discussion of the cephalometric analysis approach).

D.S. and her parents were told that there were two treatment possibilities: (1) orthodontic treatment with extraction of the upper premolars, which would resolve the problem of malaligned upper incisors and give her good dental occlusion but would require excellent coop-

eration during treatment, including wearing headgear as needed to control posterior anchorage; or (2) surgical-orthodontic treatment with advancement of the mandible. She was told that a good result functionally and esthetically could be achieved either way, provided that she was willing to cooperate fully with the orthodontic plan. She opted for the orthodontic treatment.

After the maxillary first premolars were extracted, a complete fixed orthodontic appliance was placed, including a maxillary transpalatal lingual arch to reinforce anchorage. The appliance was removed at age 16 years, 7 months after 21 months of active treatment. A positioner was used for 3 months. Final records were obtained and retainers were placed at age 16 years, 10 months.

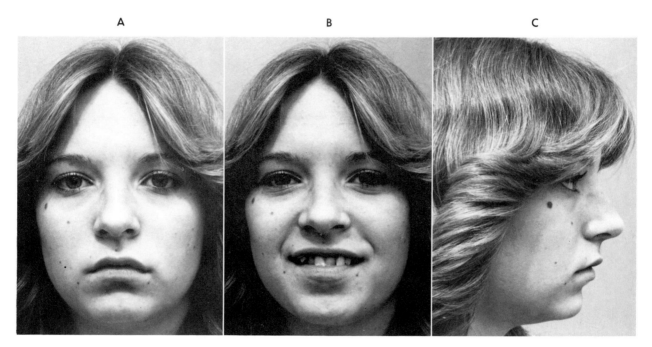

A   B   C

Fig. 1-3. Patient D.S., age 14 years, 10 months, before treatment. Her chief complaint was the appearance of her maxillary anterior teeth. From her degree of maturity, further growth was considered unlikely. On close examination of the profile, mandibular deficiency can be observed, but it is not obvious and is not a problem to the patient.

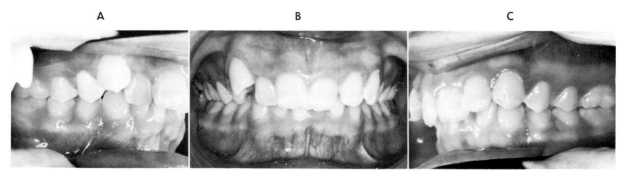

A   B   C

Fig. 1-4. Patient D.S., intraoral views. There is a classic Class II, division 2 malocclusion, with a deep bite anteriorly.

For this patient, the camouflage approach was judged to be entirely satisfactory. Good occlusal relationships and function were obtained, and facial esthetics were excellent. The key to successful treatment was the control of maxillary posterior anchorage, so that the upper incisors could be retracted and intruded slightly and the roots torqued to proper inclination.

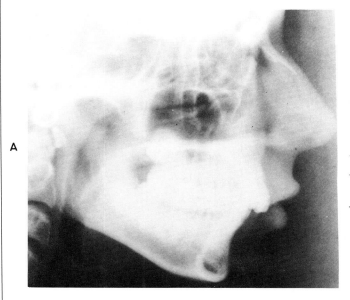
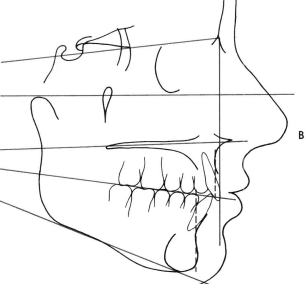

Fig. 1-5. Patient D.S., cephalometric radiograph and tracing before treatment. The radiograph was taken in natural head position (NHP), as were all for this book (see Chapter 4). Note that the true horizontal line is close to but not quite coincident with the Frankfort plane. The maxilla is well related to the cranium, but the mandible is deficient. At her level of maturity, growth modification is not possible—the only orthodontic treatment possibility is camouflage.

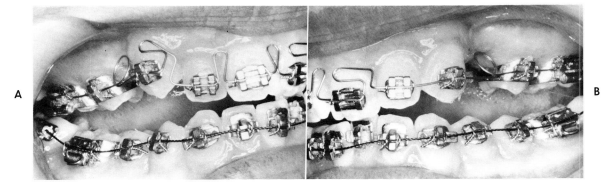

Fig. 1-6. Patient D.S. To carry out camouflage orthodontic treatment, maxillary first premolars have been extracted, and a maxillary transpalatal lingual arch has been placed to augment anchorage. Note the use of loops in 14-mil (.014-inch) wire to begin retraction of the maxillary canines.

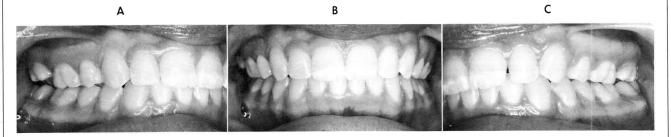

Fig. 1-7. Patient D.S., posttreatment occlusion. Active treatment time was 21 months.

Continued.

Case 1—cont'd.

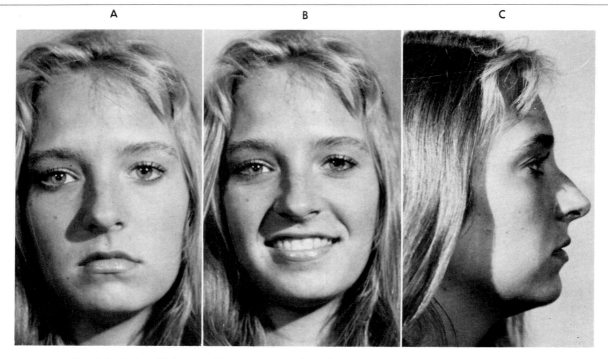

A   B   C

Fig. 1-8. Patient D.S., age 16 years, 7 months, after treatment. The mandibular deficiency has not been corrected but has been camouflaged successfully; that is, both dental occlusion and facial esthetics are satisfactory. The residual mandibular deficiency is not apparent and the patient is quite satisfied with the esthetic result.

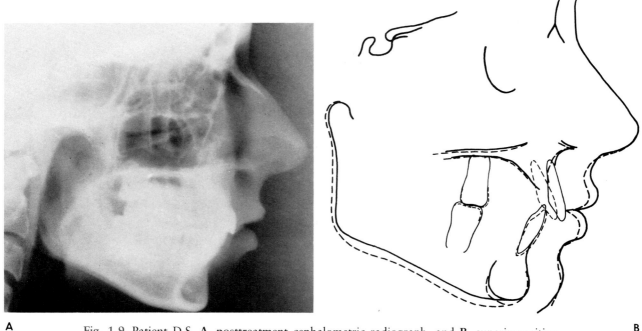

A   B

Fig. 1-9. Patient D.S. **A,** posttreatment cephalometric radiograph, and **B,** superimposition tracing. Note the good anchorage control in the maxillary posterior segments. There was slight elongation of the posterior teeth, resulting in a slight downward and backward rotation of the mandible during treatment, which made the mandibular deficiency marginally worse but did not affect the success of the treatment.

Case 2 (Figs. 1-10 to 1-15)

L.H., age 45 years, 5 months and a teacher, sought surgical-orthodontic consultation 5 years after completion of orthodontic treatment to correct her Class III malocclusion when she learned from one of her students that jaw surgery was planned for the student's similar problem. Although her occlusion was good, she was not satisfied with the orthodontic treatment result because "my chin still protrudes." The facial photographs and cephalo-metric analysis documented maxillary deficiency, with a short anterior face height that resulted in the mandible rotating up and forward to accentuate its prominence.

Before surgical treatment to improve jaw relationships by moving the maxilla forward and somewhat downward could be carried out, preparatory orthodontic treatment to remove the dental compensation introduced by the previous orthodontics was necessary. For this patient,

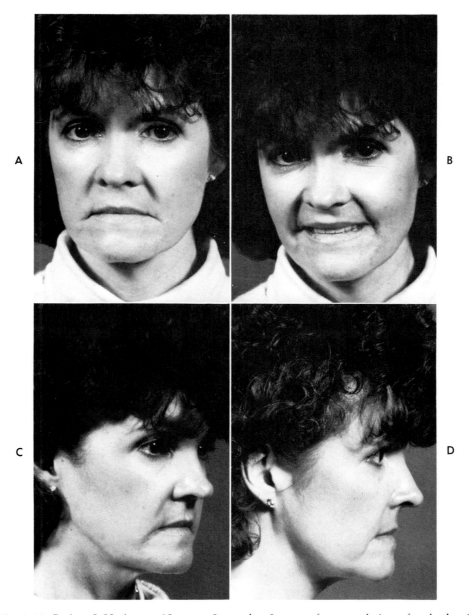

Fig. 1-10. Patient L.H. At age 45 years, 5 months, 5 years after completion of orthodontic treatment for a skeletal Class III malocclusion, she sought further treatment because she was dissatisfied with the continuing prominence of her chin, which was her chief complaint at the time of her original treatment.

Continued.

Case 2—cont'd.

as for many individuals with jaw discrepancies, the orthodontic treatment to prepare the patient for surgical correction was just the opposite of what would be needed for orthodontic treatment only. During the orthodontics-only treatment, she wore Class III elastics. In preparation for surgery, Class II elastics were used to recreate the reverse overjet.

A LeFort I osteotomy was used to move the maxilla downward and forward, and rigid internal fixation was employed for stabilization. The result was essentially the same occlusion she had presurgically, but with a better relationship between the jaws and between the teeth of each jaw and their supporting bone. She was pleased with the esthetic improvement.

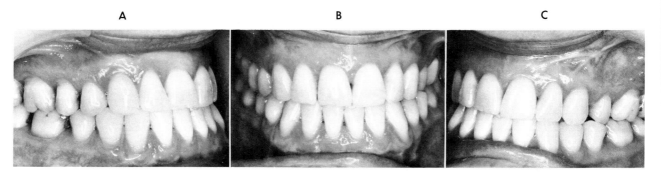

Fig. 1-11. Patient L.H., intraoral views before the surgical-orthodontic treatment. With the use of Class III elastics to produce dental compensation, the previous orthodontic treatment had resulted in good occlusion.

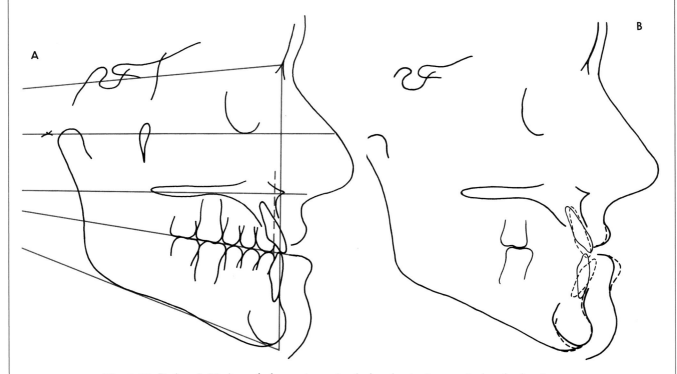

Fig. 1-12. Patient L.H. **A,** cephalometric tracing before beginning surgical-orthodontic treatment. **B,** Superimposition showing the result of the presurgical orthodontics in which Class II elastics were used to recreate the reverse overjet that had existed before the orthodontics-only treatment. Note the upright position of the lower incisors and proclined position of the upper incisors after the original orthodontic treatment. It was necessary to establish reverse overjet before surgery to obtain good tooth-jaw relationships postsurgically.

Case 2—cont'd.

In this case, the initial attempt at camouflage of the malocclusion must be considered to have failed because of the patient's dissatisfaction with the esthetic result. As a general rule, Class III malocclusion is more difficult to camouflage than is Class II. When the lower incisors are retracted with Class III elastics, the chin often becomes more, rather than less, prominent.

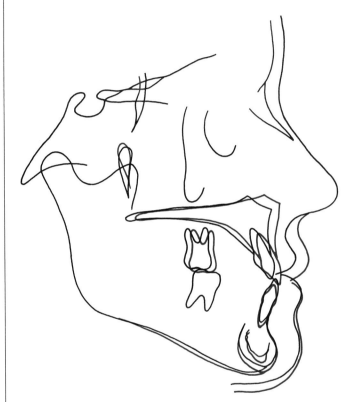

Fig. 1-13. Patient L.H. After 8 months of presurgical orthodontic preparation, a LeFort I osteotomy was used to move the maxilla forward and slightly downward. This cephalometric superimposition shows the changes from immediately before surgery to after completion of treatment.

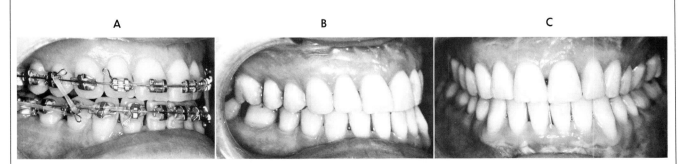

Fig. 1-14. Patient L.H. **A,** Use of vertical elastics for settling of the occlusion during postsurgical orthodontic treatment. **B** and **C,** Posttreatment occlusal relationships.

Continued.

Case 2—cont'd.

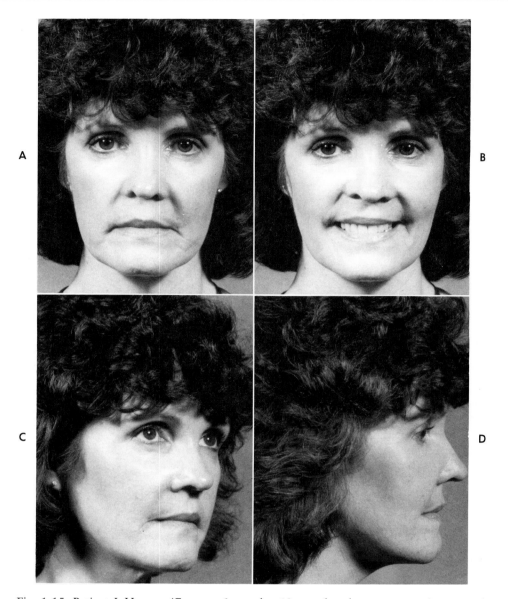

Fig. 1-15. Patient L.H., age 47 years, 6 months, 12 months after surgery and 15 months after orthodontic appliances were removed, at the point retention was discontinued. The occlusion was stable, and she was pleased with the esthetic result.

Case 3 (Figs. 1-16 to 1-23)

V.F., age 24 years, 4 months and a graduate student, sought treatment because of the appearance of her anterior teeth. She had wanted orthodontic treatment previously and now felt that it would be better to correct these problems before entering her career as a university faculty member. There were no medical or dental problems, but she did have clicking of both TM joints without pain.

The casts showed a half cusp Class II relationship of the posterior teeth, with a Class II, division 2 appearance of the incisors and an extreme anterior deep bite. Clinical examination of facial appearance suggested and cephalometric analysis confirmed that her anterior face height was short and that moderate mandibular deficiency existed. Both the upper and lower incisors were somewhat retrusive relative to the nose and chin, respectively.

V.F. was told that it would be possible to correct the alignment of her teeth and give her good dental occlusion with orthodontic treatment alone. This would involve extraction of the upper first and lower second premolars and extensive use of interarch elastics. However, this would leave her teeth positioned less prominently in her face than their ideal position, so the facial esthetics would be less than optimal. The alternative would be to align the teeth in each arch without extraction, and then use mandibular surgery to advance the mandible and rotate it downward anteriorly. Although satisfactory dental alignment and occlusion could be produced either way, facial esthetics might not be acceptable with orthodontics alone, so the surgical-orthodontic approach was recommended.

A   B   C

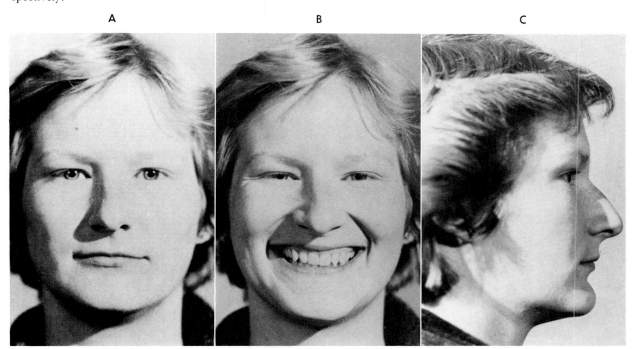

Fig. 1-16. Patient V.F., age 24 years, 4 months, before treatment. She was concerned generally about the appearance of her teeth, which she had always wanted to have corrected. At the time of the initial consultation, she had not thought about the possibility of jaw surgery.

A   B   C

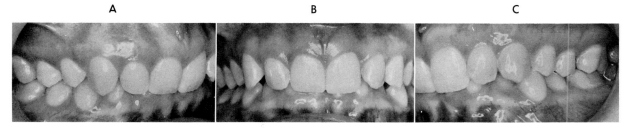

Fig. 1-17. Patient V.F., pretreatment intraoral views. Note the half cusp Class II relationship in the buccal segments and the extreme overbite anteriorly.

Continued.

Case 3—cont'd.

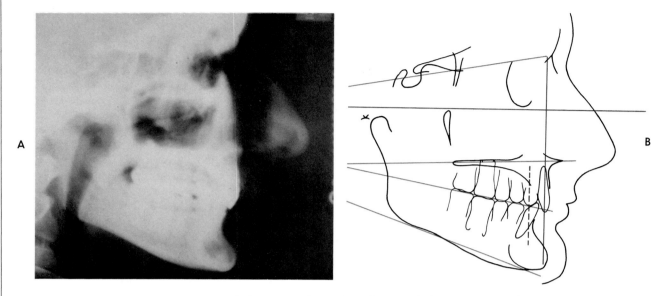

Fig. 1-18. Patient V.F., cephalometric radiograph and tracing before treatment. The relative retrusion of both upper and lower incisors can be seen. There is a moderate anteroposterior mandibular deficiency, with a short anterior face height and a prominent chin button relative to the lower lip.

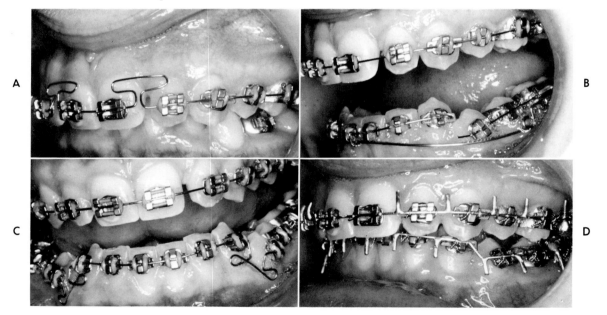

Fig. 1-19. Patient V.F., stages in presurgical orthodontic treatment. **A,** Initial appliance placement. Because of the deep overbite, only the upper arch was banded initially, and loops in round wire were used to create overjet by tipping the crowns forward and torquing the roots back simultaneously. **B,** In the lower arch, an auxiliary depressing arch was applied to the lower incisors to tip them forward and slightly intrude the central incisors so that the increase in face height at surgery would not be too great (note the segmentation of the base arch, to facilitate intrusion). **C,** Later in the presurgical orthodontic preparation, a continuous 14-mil arch wire with loops was employed to slightly extrude the premolars. **D,** Presurgical stabilizing arch wires in place. Note that the lower arch has not been completely leveled so that elongation of canines and premolars can be done postsurgically, thereby increasing face height. Orthodontic preparation for surgery required 7 months.

Case 3—cont'd.

After thinking about it for 3 months and talking with other patients who had had surgical-orthodontic treatment, she opted for surgery. The presurgical orthodontics involved aligning the teeth, without completely leveling the lower arch until after surgery. Slight depression of the lower incisors was desired, but most of the leveling would be accomplished by elongating the canines and premolars postsurgically. Treatment began in October, then a bilateral sagittal-split–ramus osteotomy was performed the following May; orthodontic treatment resumed in August, after 8 weeks of maxillomandibular fixation and 2 weeks of function into the splint that was used during fixation, and appliances were removed in October. A positioner was worn for 1 month, and retention began in November, just as she left for a position at another university. Follow-up records were obtained 3 years after surgery when she returned to Chapel Hill for a visit.

In this case, the result provided both excellent function and esthetics, and the patient was very pleased with her decision to have surgery. The TM joint clicking disappeared soon after orthodontic treatment began and has not reappeared. The esthetic improvement resulted from greater prominence of the teeth, to which both tooth movement and the rotation of the mandible contributed, and to the increase in face height to more normal values.

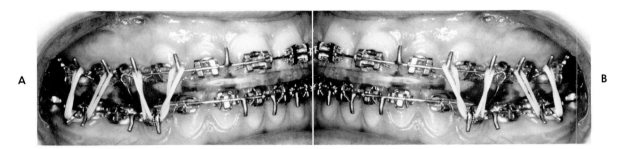

Fig. 1-20. Patient V.F. After release of intermaxillary fixation, she was allowed to function into the surgical splint, with light guiding elastics, before the beginning of postsurgical orthodontics. Note that the splint is tied to the upper arch wire with a ligature that wraps around it in the premolar regions.

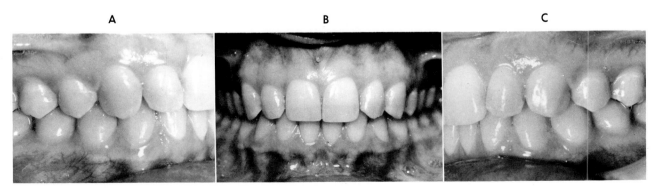

Fig. 1-21. Patient V.F., intraoral views 3 years after surgery and 18 months after discontinuation of retention. Occlusal relationships were excellent, and the TM joint clicking apparent before surgery had disappeared.

Continued.

Case 3—cont'd.

A   B   C

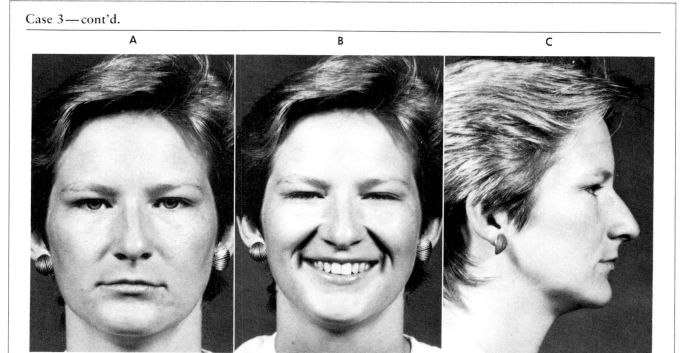

Fig. 1-22. Patient V.F., age 27 years, 11 months, 3 years after surgery. She was quite pleased with the result of treatment.

A   B   C

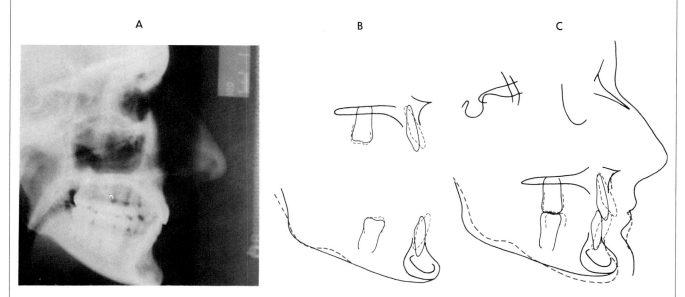

Fig. 1-23. Patient V.F., **A,** Posttreatment cephalometric film. **B** and **C,** Cephalometric superimpositions showing treatment effects. The pretreatment tracing is black, and the posttreatment tracing is red. Note that the lower incisor was advanced about half the total distance by tipping it forward orthodontically, and advanced the rest of the distance as a consequence of the rotation of the mandible at surgery. Because of the change in the mandibular plane angle, the incisor moved forward at surgery but the chin moved almost straight down.

For many patients, camouflage can be an entirely satisfactory method of treatment, as it was for D.S. However, even if excellent occlusion is achieved, the treatment is not satisfactory if the patient cannot accept the facial esthetics. The decision as to whether to treat a patient with orthodontics alone, or to use combined surgical-orthodontic treatment even though satisfactory dental occlusion could be obtained without surgery, often can be made only by considering esthetics as carefully as dental relationships. It is significant that in both of the surgical cases presented above, the problem had a major vertical component. Anteroposterior dental compensation is easier to achieve with orthodontic treatment, and more successful as camouflage, than is vertical compensation. These considerations are examined in detail in the Chapters 4 to 6 on diagnosis and treatment planning and in Chapters 12 to 19 on the treatment of specific types of problems.

PREVALENCE OF DENTOFACIAL DEFORMITY

There are two problems in estimating the prevalence of dentofacial deformities severe enough to warrant surgical correction. First, almost no data exist for the prevalence of facial characteristics, so it is necessary to infer the presence of jaw deformities from data on dental occlusal relationships. Second, the best American data for dental occlusion[5,6] are now more than 20 years old, so any recent population changes cannot be documented. In addition, the existing data are for children and youths almost exclusively, whereas most patients who are candidates for surgical-orthodontic treatment have completed their growth and are adults. Nevertheless, it is possible to gain some feel for the magnitude of dentofacial deformity problems from a survey of the present data.[7] Better data for wider age groups will be forthcoming soon from the 1988-1990 National Health and Nutrition Estimates Study (NHANES III), now being carried out by the U.S. National Center for Health Statistics.

Table 1-1 summarizes our present knowledge of occlusal characteristics and the skeletal proportions that presumably underlie them. Moving from these data to the number of patients who need surgical-orthodontic treatment requires a series of assumptions, and so must be done with a recognition of the possibility of error.

Consider first the condition currently most likely to require surgical treatment, a deficiency of the lower jaw (cases 1 and 3 above). From Table 1-1, it can be seen that approximately 10% of 12- to 17-year-old youths (in the 1960s) had 7 mm or more of anterior overjet. This measurement is highly correlated with the presence of a skeletal Class II malocclusion, which in turn is known to result from mandibular deficiency in most patients[8] (but mandibular deficiency does not guarantee excess overjet, as Figs. 1-4 and 1-17 show).

TABLE 1-1 Malocclusion types in U.S. youths (ages 12 to 17)

Problem	Percent of population		
	White	Black	Total
Alignment			
Severe crowding (TPI displacement score 8 or higher)	27.1	20.9	26.2
Width discrepancies			
Lingual crossbite—three or more teeth (Narrow maxilla/wide mandible?)	2.8	3.9	3.0
Buccal crossbite—three or more teeth (Wide maxilla/narrow mandible?)	0.4	0.2	0.3
Anteroposterior discrepancies			
Overjet 7 mm or more (Class II?)	10.0	5.5	8.0
Reverse overjet 2 mm or more (Class III?)	0.6	0.5	0.6
Vertical discrepancies			
Open bite 4 mm or more (Long face?)	0.3	3.4	0.6
Overbite 6 mm or more (Short face?)	11.7	1.4	10.3

Data from Kelly JE and Harvey C: An assessment of the teeth of youths 12-17 years, DHEW Pub No (HRA) 77-1644, Washington, DC, 1977, National Center for Health Statistics.

How many of these individuals have such severe mandibular deficiency that surgical advancement would be required to correct it?

Grainger's Treatment Priority Index (TPI)[9] was the epidemiologic index in the U.S. Public Health Service (USPHS) studies of the 1960s from which the data in Table 1-1 are taken. Overjet is one component in calculating the total TPI score. From the standard interpretation of TPI scores, about 5% of the population is said to have such severe malocclusion that the condition can be considered handicapping. Perhaps it is a reasonable assumption that only the worst 5% of those with 7 mm or more of overjet have such severe underlying problems that surgical treatment would be required—the other 95% presumably could be treated by some combination of growth modification and orthodontic camouflage. Only 10% of the total population has severe overjet, but the handicapped group drawn from the total population almost certainly contains a higher percentage of individuals with excessive overjet and jaw deformity; thus the estimate that only the

TABLE 1-2 Estimated prevalence of mandibular deficiency severe enough to indicate surgery		
Parameter	Percentage*	Number†
Prevalence of skeletal Class II malocclusion	10	22,500,000
Appropriate age for treatment (neither too young nor too old)	65	14,625,000
Severe enough to warrant surgery	5	731,250
Mandibular advancement	70	510,000
Maxillary setback	10	67,500
Both	20	145,000
New patients added to population yearly‡	0.5	21,250

*Of the number for the line above; first line is based on Table 1-1.
†At 225,000,000 U.S. population.
‡At 4,250,000 live births per year.

TABLE 1-3 Estimated prevalence of Class III problems severe enough to indicate surgery		
Parameter	Percentage	Number
Prevalence of Class III malocclusion (Table 1-1)	0.6	1,350,000
Appropriate age for surgical treatment	65	877,500
Severe enough to warrant surgery (need mandibular setback and/or maxillary advancement)	33	290,000
Mandibular setback	45	130,000
Maxillary advancement	35	101,000
Both	20	58,000
New patients added to population yearly	0.2	8,500

worst 5% of those with severe overjet would need surgery is probably conservative. However, even with this conservative estimate, we calculate that there are currently about 700,000 individuals in the United States with mandibular deficiency so severe that surgery would be required to correct it, and about 21,000 new individuals with deformity of this severity are being added to the population per year (Table 1-2).

The presence of a skeletal Class III malocclusion (see Figs 1-10 to 1-12) can be estimated from reverse overjet in somewhat the same way. For mandibular prognathism, however, neither growth modification nor orthodontic camouflage is as successful as it is with mandibular deficiency. A conservative assumption is that two-thirds of those with 3 mm or more of reverse overjet can be managed orthodontically, whereas a third are affected severely enough to require surgical advancement of the maxilla, setback of the mandible, or both. Based on this (Table 1-3), it appears that there are currently nearly 300,000 individuals in the United States who would need surgery to correct their Class III malocclusion, with 8500 new potential surgical patients being added each year.

Currently, there simply is not enough information to do more than make an educated guess as to what the proportions for maxillary versus mandibular surgery would be in this Class III group. Our guess is shown in Table 1-3. Until the 1970s, a surgical mandibular setback was almost always used to correct a Class III malocclusion, but this resulted more from lack of familiarity with maxillary advancement than from good data to demonstrate that the problem was truly a mandibu-

lar one. The number of patients whose Class III problems are treated with maxillary surgery has increased dramatically in the last decade, as a more objective evaluation of the deformity rather than the technical difficulty of surgical correction has determined the type of operation.

The long-face pattern of deformity is probably third in frequency among conditions requiring surgery for treatment. It is particuarly difficult to calculate the prevalence of this problem from data on dental occlusal relationships. Approximately two-thirds of patients with excessive anterior face height have an anterior open bite, but a third do not. One approach is simply to assume that a 3-mm or more anterior open bite reflects a skeletal problem, hoping that the false negatives (long face but no open bite) will balance out the false positives (open bite but normal face height). Although prolonged and difficult orthodontic treatment is required, the long-face condition can be treated by growth modification. However, a long face is very difficult to camouflage after growth has been completed. If one assumes that the worst 25% of the long-face group would require surgery for correction, there are 220,000 surgical candidates in the United States, and over 6000 are added to the population yearly (Table 1-4).

Other problems exist that require orthognathic surgery for satisfactory treatment, but no data exist to allow a further subdivision of prevalence by patient types. Most patients fall into one of the major categories described above—patients with a short-face pattern, for instance, usually also have a mandibular deficiency, and narrow maxillas are found most often in those with a long-face pattern.

The number of individuals who require surgical treatment for satisfactory correction of their dentofa-

TABLE 1-4 Estimated prevalence of patients with long-face pattern severe enough to indicate surgery

Parameter	Percentage	Number
Prevalence of severe anterior open bite	0.6	1,350,000
Appropriate age for treatment	65	877,500
Severe enough to warrant surgery (need superior repositioning of maxilla)	25	220,000
New patients added to population yearly	0.15	6,375

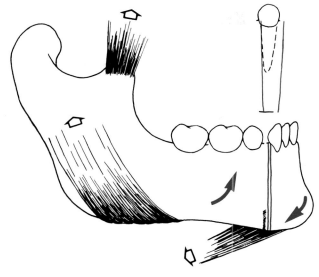

Fig. 1-24. During the first half of the twentieth century, the body ostectomy shown diagrammatically here was used frequently for correction of mandibular prognathism. Because the muscle pull postsurgically tends to rotate the posterior segment up and the anterior segment down, relapse into open bite is a problem. Surgeons were concerned that the precious-metal orthodontic appliances available at that time were not rigid enough to stabilize the segments during healing. Rigid arch bars (fracture splints) like those shown in Fig. 1-25 were preferred.

cial deformities comes as a surprise to many people. Perhaps the point is that even if the numbers shown here are overstated, it is clear that a dentofacial deformity severe enough to warrant surgical intervention is a highly prevalent problem. As combined orthodontic and surgical treatment has become available in recent years, the demand for that treatment has increased tremendously. There is every reason to believe this trend will continue until the number of those who would benefit from treatment more closely approximates the number receiving it.

DEVELOPMENT OF COMBINED ORTHODONTIC AND SURGICAL TREATMENT

Before the 1960s, surgical correction of a jaw deformity was almost exclusively reserved for patients with mandibular prognathism. In that era, the surgical treatment was done either without the patient ever having orthodontic treatment, after orthodontic appliances had been removed, or, occasionally, before any orthodontics was begun. Part of the reason for this approach was a lack of appreciation for the improvement that could be obtained by coordinating the two types of treatment more carefully. A major additional stumbling block was the unwillingness of the surgeon or orthodontist to use the orthodontic appliance for post-surgical stabilization.

Previously, when a body ostectomy was used to set the mandible back, as was usually the case until mid-century (Fig. 1-24), stabilizing the jaw segments was a major problem. With this operation, the anterior segment tends to tilt downward anteriorly and create an open bite during healing. A rigid bar spanning the ostectomy site was necessary to control this problem. The orthodontic appliances of that time were made of precious metal, and many patients, even those treated with the edgewise appliance, did not have bands on all the teeth. The combination of delicate arch wires and relatively long spans between attachments meant that the orthodontic appliance lacked the rigidity needed at surgery, and the surgeons understandably preferred fracture arch bars (Fig. 1-25).

As steel arch wires replaced gold and as full-banded orthodontic-appliance therapy became more commonplace, the ramus osteotomy for prognathism began to supercede the body ostectomy. The result was decreased stress during the surgical phase of treatment on an orthodontic appliance that had shorter interbracket spans and greater rigidity and therefore could withstand the stress better. With experience, surgeons came to appreciate that the edgewise appliance with full-dimension steel rectangular wires (Fig. 1-26) could give excellent control, better than that obtained with the heavier but less precise arch bars. Having the orthodontic appliance in place at the time of surgery also meant that it was possible to do some orthodontics before surgery and the remainder afterward, rather than doing everything in advance or, the less frequent previous alternative, doing all the orthodontics afterward. It quickly became apparent that a certain degree of finishing orthodontics was beneficial for all surgery patients. This allowed the orthodontist to bring the teeth into an excellent final occlusion and also provided bet-

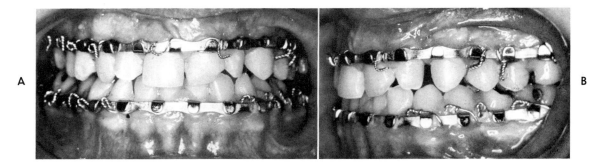

Fig. 1-25. Arch bars of the type shown here were once used routinely and can still be used for stabilization after orthognathic surgery, but unless the orthodontic appliance is present at surgery, postsurgical finishing is extremely difficult and is usually not attempted, resulting in a compromised occlusion. In contemporary orthognathic surgery, this method is rarely used.

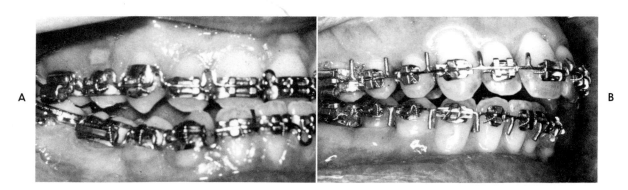

Fig. 1-26. A, Orthodontic stabilizing arch wires as used in the mid-1960s. The wire is 21.5 × 28 mil blue Elgiloy in a 22-slot appliance, to give maximum rigidity. Bent-in hooks are used for attaching wires or elastics for maxillomandibular fixation. **B,** Orthodontic stabilizing arch wires used in the 1980s. The wire is 17 × 25 mil steel, with soldered hooks, in a bonded 18-slot appliance. With modern surgical techniques, this lighter appliance is perfectly adequate for stabilization.

ter control over minor relapse tendencies, which could be compensated by slightly repositioning the teeth.

The more perfect the occlusal relationships that can be achieved in the operating room, the more precisely the surgeon can position the jaws, and vice versa. Unless the teeth interdigitate extremely well at the time of surgery, some additional way to hold the jaws in position is needed. The introduction of the occlusal wafer splint (see Fig. 1-20) to provide positive indexing between the teeth in the operating room was an important step in allowing surgery to occur before orthodontic detailing of the occlusion was completed. The splint, which is made to fit the jaw position established from model surgery, provides a more positive seating of the teeth in the operating room than can be obtained without it in all but the most perfect occlusions.

Using splints, it was possible to experiment with surgery earlier in the course of orthodontic treatment than otherwise would have been possible. The observation

was that much of the orthodontic tooth movement, particularly leveling of the dental arches, could be accomplished much more quickly and easily after surgery because repositioning the jaws had removed occlusal interferences. Consequently, the improved efficiency of the orthodontic treatment reduced the total treatment time significantly. At present, it is now routine to treat even the most complex surgical-orthodontic patients in less time (typically 15 to 18 months) than is required for most orthodontics-only patients (Table 1-5). The proper timing of surgery (i.e., the proper decisions about what orthodontics should be done before versus after surgery) is a major factor in controlling the duration of treatment.

During the 1980s, internal fixation with bone plates and screws (rigid internal fixation [RIF]) (Fig. 1-27) largely replaced maxillomandibular (intermaxillary) and wire fixation. Patients greatly prefer not having their jaws wired together when this can be avoided,

TABLE 1-5 Time estimates for surgical-orthodontic treatment

Stage of treatment	Time required	Comment
1. Presurgical orthodontics	2 to 12 months	Varies with difficulty of alignment
2. Surgery/hospitalization	2 to 6 days	Typically 3 to 4 days
3. Under surgeon's care before beginning postsurgical orthodontics	3 to 8 weeks	Reduced with rigid fixation (3 to 5 weeks) as compared with maxillomandibular fixation (5 to 8 weeks)
4. Postsurgical orthodontics	3 to 6 months	Over 6 months indicates a problem or inadequate preparation

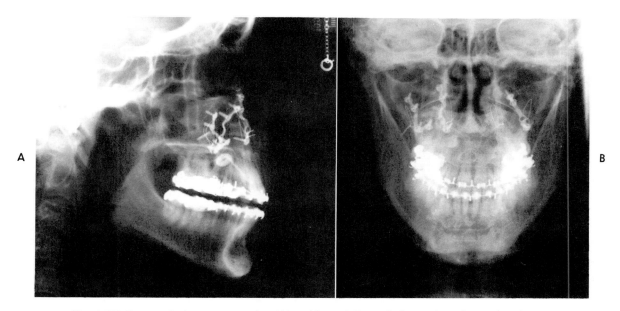

Fig. 1-27. Postsurgical posteroanterior (**A**) and lateral (**B**) cephalometric radiographs of L.H. (Figs. 1-10 to 1-15), showing the use of bone plates and screws for rigid internal fixation. This reduces or eliminates the need for maxillomandibular fixation, greatly increasing patient comfort and the acceptance of orthognathic surgery.

and RIF makes this possible. The interaction between orthodontist and surgeon is affected by the change in fixation techniques, and it is fair to say that the impact of RIF still has not been totally evaluated. Fewer restrictions on the patient during the healing period do not necessarily produce faster and better healing or more stability, and the newer approach probably makes the orthodontist's work more difficult, just as it does the surgeon's work. However, the advantage perceived by the patient is so great that RIF has already become the standard procedure. Its use makes the proper sequencing of orthodontics and surgery more important than ever.

The goal of presurgical orthodontics is to align the teeth of each arch over their own jaw and produce compatible arch forms, so that at the time of surgery there are no obstacles to putting the jaws in the proper position. It is not necessary to have perfect transverse compatibility of the arches, but experience has shown that the teeth should be within a half cusp of their final transverse position so that postsurgical occlusion does not lock them into a crossbite. When the maxilla is moved forward or back, excessively protruding or retroclined incisors would obviously cause a problem in positioning the jaw (see Figs. 1-12, 1-18, and 1-27). The orthodontic treatment to put the incisors in the correct position usually involves removing dental compensation, which means that the dental relationships temporarily become worse.

Before surgery, the orthodontist must establish not only the anteroposterior and transverse position, but also the vertical position of the teeth. For instance, in patients who will have only a mandibular ramus osteotomy, the vertical position of the incisor teeth deter-

A   B

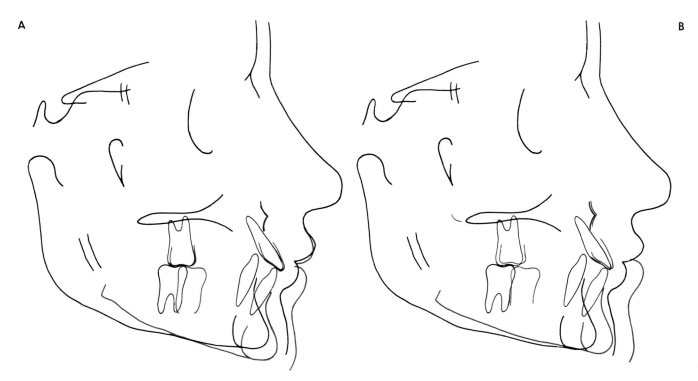

Fig. 1-28. Because the incisors must be placed in occlusion at surgery, their vertical position determines the change in face height that will be produced. In this patient with mandibular deficiency and elongated lower incisors, note the difference in the predicted result of surgical advancement with the incisors in their initial position at the time of surgery (**A**) as compared with the result with the incisors depressed before the advancement is done (**B**). Presurgical orthodontics to intrude the incisors obviously would be important for this patient. However, if an increase in face height were desired in a patient with short-face pattern (as in V.F., Figs. 1-16 to 1-23), it would be equally important to keep from depressing the incisors too much before surgery. This is an important point in planning the orthodontic phase of treatment.

mines the postsurgical face height (Fig. 1-28). This, in turn, will determine whether leveling an excessive curve of Spee should be done by intrusion of incisors or elongation of premolars, and whether the leveling should be done presurgically or postsurgically (see Fig. 1-19).

Inadequate orthodontic preparation can jeopardize the quality of the surgical result, whereas excessive preparation can significantly and unnecessarily lengthen the overall treatment time, resulting in patient frustration and poor compliance. Integrating the orthodontic and surgical treatment so that the surgery is done at the optimal time is important.

For the average patient, experience has shown that 3 to 6 months of postsurgical orthodontic treament is required to produce optimal results with the greatest overall treatment efficiency. It is almost impossible to complete the treatment and remove the orthodontic appliance with less than 3 months of postsurgical finishing treatment, without risking loss of control of the inevitable postsurgical changes. Conversely, postsurgical orthodontics should usually be completed in 6 months.

To the patient, the surgery and its accompanying hospitalization represent a high point of treatment, and psychologically it may be difficult for the patient to tolerate more than 6 months of postsurgical orthodontic treatment. For this reason, in current therapy, the amount of presurgical orthodontics is the major variable in treatment time. The surgery and its subsequent period for healing, and the postsurgical orthodontics, should be much more constant in duration (see Table 1-5).

Before making the diagnosis and beginning treatment planning for patients with a dentofacial deformity, it is important to understand where the patient is coming from, in both the historical and psychologic senses of that phrase. The remaining chapters in this introductory section focus on the etiology of the physical deformity (Chapter 2) and its psychosocial impact (Chapter 3). Their goals are to provide the background for understanding a patient's developmental history and his or her reasons for seeking treatment in terms of goals, motives, and potential reactions to the changes that accompany treatment.

REFERENCES

1. Morris AL, et al: Handicapping orthodontic conditions, Washington, DC, 1975, National Academy of Sciences.
2. McGregor FC: Social and psychological implications of dentofacial disfigurement, Angle Orthod 40:231-233, 1970.
3. Jenny J: A social perspective on need and demand for orthodontic treatment, Int Dent J 25:248-256, 1975.
4. Proffit WR, Ackerman JL: A systematic approach to orthodontic diagnosis and treatment planning. In Graber TM, and Swain BF, editors: Current orthodontic concepts and techniques, ed 3, St. Louis, 1985, The CV Mosby Co.
5. Kelly JE, Sanchez M, Van Kirk LE: An assessment of the occlusion of the teeth of children 6-11 years, DHEW Pub No (HRA) 74-1612, Washington, DC, 1973, National Center for Health Statistics.
6. Kelly JE, Harvey C: An assesment of the teeth of youths 12-17 years, DHEW Pub No (HRA) 77-1644, Washington, DC, 1977, National Center for Health Statistics.
7. McLain JB, Proffit WR: Oral health status in the United States: prevalence of malocclusion, J Dent Educ 49:386-396, 1985.
8. McNamara JA: Components of Class II malocclusion in children 8-10 years of age, Angle Orthod 51:177-202, 1981.
9. Grainger RM: The orthodontic treatment priority index, DHEW Pub No 100, Series 2, No 25, Washington, DC, 1967, National Center for Health Statistics.

CHAPTER 2

Etiologic Factors in the Development of Dentofacial Deformity

William R. Proffit

Dentofacial deformity is a developmental problem. Occasionally the deformity is due to a single specific cause, but much more frequently it results from a complex interaction among multiple factors that influence growth and development (Fig. 2-1). For most patients, it is difficult or impossible to describe a specific etiologic cause. In an adult, the etiologic factors that caused the problem to develop during growth may no longer have an effect even if they are still present. And yet, some thought must be given to etiology when treatment is planned because this is a major factor in estimating the stability of results, particularly in children but also in adults.

In this chapter, we assume that the reader has a reasonable knowledge of facial growth and suggest refer-

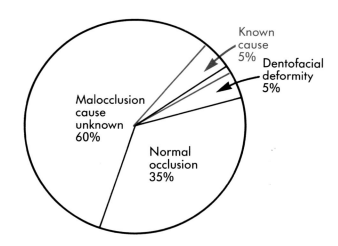

Fig. 2-1. When the entire population is viewed broadly, only about a third have normal occlusion. Sixty percent have mild to severe malocclusion, and about 5% have a problem of such severity that it would fall into the dentofacial deformity category and potentially require surgical-orthodontic treatment. Only a small proportion of patients with malocclusion have their problem because of a known specific cause, and this also is true for the more severely affected patients with dentofacial deformity, who will require surgical-orthodontic treatment. In both groups of patients, a complex interaction between heredity and environment (function) usually is involved in the etiology.

TABLE 2-1 Soft-tissue changes from surgical-orthodontic treatment

Unit	Site(s)	Mechanism	Determinant
Cranial vault	Sutures	Intramembraneous bone formation in response to suture separation	Growth of brain (intracranial pressure)
Cranial base	Synchondroses	Endochondral ossification	Intrinsic stimulus (? influenced also by growth of brain)
Maxilla	Sutures	Intramembraneous bone formation in response to suture separation	Pull by soft-tissue growth and/or nasal septum
	Passive forward carry	Push from cranial base	Cranial base growth
Mandible	Condyle	Endochondral ossification	Pull by soft tissues (? which)
	Surfaces	Intramembraneous bone formation/resorption (remodeling)	Pull by soft tissues (? which)
	Passive carry (can be forward or backward)	Relocation of temporal fossa	?

ence to standard sources[1,2] for more details. Current concepts of facial growth are very briefly summarized in Table 2-1. The review that follows is oriented strongly toward understanding both how disturbances in facial development arise and the role of early surgical intervention in the treatment of these problems.

The etiologic factors for dentofacial deformity severe enough to require surgical-orthodontic treatment can be divided into three major groups: (1) known specific causes, (2) hereditary factors, and (3) environmental influences. Each of these major groups is discussed separately below, and then a perspective on the interaction of heredity and environment in the development of surgical-orthodontic problems follows.

SPECIFIC CAUSES

The known specific causes of dentofacial deformity fall into two major groups: (1) facial syndromes and congenital defects, whose etiology clearly is prenatal; and (2) postnatal growth disturbances of known origin, including the effects of trauma.

Facial Syndromes and Congenital Anomalies

The syndromes and anomalies that compose most of the known specific causes of dentofacial deformities usually also produce cranial and other defects.[3] These extremely complex conditions, fortunately, are relatively rare, but they are observed in up to 5% of patients who seek surgical-orthodontic treatment.[4] The focus of this book is not on these craniofacial problems. Instead it is on the majority of potential surgical-orthodontic patients whose problems, even if quite severe, are limited to the jaws and teeth. Nevertheless, an understanding of the way in which craniofacial syndromes arise is a necessary background for dealing with these unfortunate individuals. It also provides

some insight into the less severely affected majority of patients who in some instances may represent minor forms of the recognized anomalies.

The developmental aspects and early treatment stages of conditions with a particular impact on the face and jaws are briefly discussed below, and orthognathic clinical treatment at older ages is reviewed in Chapters 15 and 18. For details of the overall management of these unfortunate individuals, see texts on craniofacial anomalies.[5]

Much has been learned in the 1980s about the embryology and teratology of craniofacial malformations. In a recent overview of abnormal craniofacial development, Johnston and Bronsky[6] identified five principal stages: (1) germ layer formation and the initial organization of craniofacial structures; (2) neural tube formation and the initial formation of the oropharynx; (3) origins, migrations, and interactions of cell populations (in which neural crest cells and their derivatives are particularly important); (4) formation of organ systems (e.g., pharyngeal arches, primary and secondary palates); and (5) final differentiation of tissues (e.g, skeletal, muscular, nervous). Almost all the tissues of the face and anterior neck, including the muscular and skeletal elements derived from mesoderm elsewhere in the body, are of ectodermal origin. Most develop from neural crest cells that migrate downward beside the neural tube and laterally under the surface ectoderm. After the crest cells have completed their migration, facial growth is dominated by regional growth centers as the organ systems are formed and the final differentiation of tissues occurs.

From this perspective, abnormal development in some craniofacial anomalies can be traced all the way back to the first stage in some instances, as in the fetal alcohol syndrome and related defects. More frequently, the problems appear to arise in the third stage (e.g., thalidomide and isotretinoin teratology, hemifacial microsomia, mandibulofacial dysostosis). For cleft defects, the expression of achondroplastic growth, and the craniosynostosis syndromes, they may arise as late as the fourth and fifth stages.

Fetal Alcohol Syndrome and Related Problems

Deficiencies of midline tissue of the neural plate very early in embryonic development give rise to a series of malformations collectively known as the holoprosencephalies, which are characterized by a failure of the first three ventricles of the brain to separate. The olfactory placodes, which are partly derived from the anterior neural plates, are too close together, and this causes deficient development of the median nasal prominences. The result is a spectrum of facial deformities ranging from total absence of the nose and related structures to an intact but moderately underdeveloped midface. Exposure to high levels of ethanol at early stages of fetal develoment produces fetal alcohol syndrome (FAS), which now is recognized as one of the holoprosencephalies. It is a mild version of more serious defects like arhinencephaly.[7-9] FAS may or may not be more prevalent now than it was in previous years, but it occurs with distressing freq-

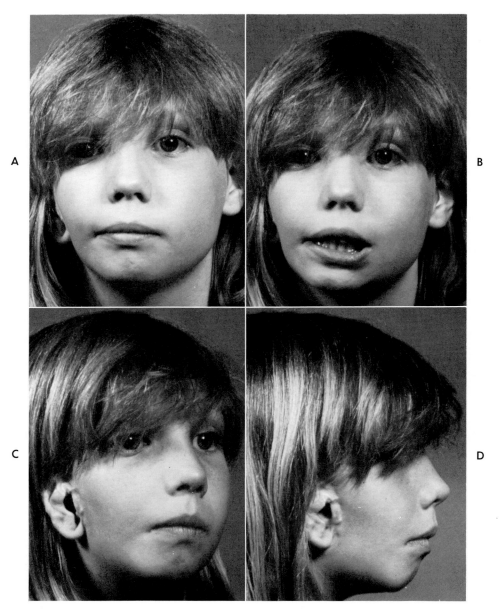

Fig. 2-2. Patient C.R., a 12-year-old girl with hemifacial microsomia. Note the underdevelopment of the right side of the face.

uency, and clinicians should recognize the possibility that it contributes to maxillary and midface deficiency.

Abnormalities of Neural Crest Origin and Migration

Retinoic Acid and Thalidomide Teratology. In the 1970s, exposure to thalidomide caused major congenital defects, including facial abnormalities, in thousands of children and focused attention on drug-induced teratogenic effects. More recently, severe craniofacial malformations in children exposed in utero to high levels of the vitamin A analogue isotretinoin (Accutane) have been reported.[10] The affected children have a characteristic facial malformation characterized by mandibular underdevelopment, cleft palate, and brain abnormalities, including cerebellar defects. They also have thymic deficiency and cardiovascular anomalies. Webster and colleagues[11] have shown that isotretinoin directly interferes with the development of cranial neural crest cells, and a subsequent deficiency of tissues derived from these cells explains the malformation pattern, including the thymus and cardiovascular changes. The marked similarities between the facial malformations produced by isotretinoin and those associated with thalidomide make it likely that both drugs produce defects in the formation and/or migration of neural crest cells.

Hemifacial Microsomia. Hemifacial microsomia is a congenital defect characterized by a lack of tissue on the affected side of the face, usually in the area of the mandibular ramus and external ear (Figs. 2-2 to 2-4).

Rarely, both sides of the face are affected, but the condition is usually unilateral and always asymmetric even if both sides are involved.[12,13]

Experimental work by Poswillo in the 1970s, following up an earlier suggestion by Keith that hemorrhage and tissue necrosis might be involved in the development of hemifacial microsomia, provided an attractive theory for its etiology.[14,15] In humans, the stapedial artery forms a temporary blood supply to the area of the developing ear and mandibular ramus between approximately the 33rd and 40th days of gestation. As development proceeds, the maxillary artery takes over the supply to this area, and the outer part of the stapedial artery atrophies and seals off. Poswillo suggested that hemorrhage from the stapedial artery caused tissue necrosis in this area, which led to the facial defects associated with hemifacial microsomia.

More recent work, however, has cast doubt on this hypothesis, and it now appears that hemifacial microsomia is another example of problems arising mostly from early loss of neural crest cells.[6,16] The association of the facial defects of hemifacial microsomia with additional defects elsewhere has been recognized for many years, and patients with major additional anomalies often are classified as having a different syndrome (e.g., Goldenhar's syndrome, oculoauricular-vertebral syndrome). On careful examination, a high percentage of hemifacial microsomia patients are found to have cardiovascular and/or limb anomalies. There is a high incidence of cleft palate (reports range from 6% to 22%), and 5% to 6% have renal anomalies. The experimental studies with isotretinoin indicate this spec-

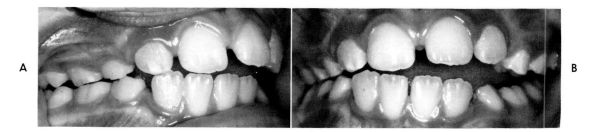

Fig. 2-3. Patient C.R., occlusal relationships. Note the open bite on the normal left side.

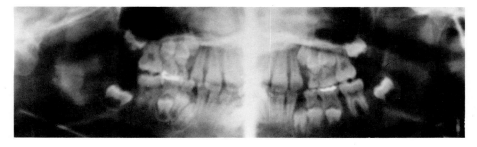

Fig. 2-4. Patient C.R., panoramic radiograph. Note the deficient ramus and condylar process on the right side. See Chapter 15 for a report of treatment for this patient.

trum of defects can be produced by early loss of crest cells.[17] In most countries, thalidomide was used for nausea associated with pregnancy. Therefore the drug was not given before the critical period for facial development had passed. In Germany, however, it was used as a nonprescription antidepressant, and the early exposure of embryos produced a wide range of craniofacial malformations, including both ear/jaw malformations similar to hemifacial microsomia in children with other defects as well and facial patterns resembling mandibulofacial dysostosis. This suggests that the variations in naturally occurring hemifacial microsomia result from differing expressions of the same basic defect, early loss of neural crest cells, rather than heterogeneity within the syndrome group. Although focal hemorrhage at a later time may be involved in some cases, it is unlikely to be the primary defect.

Treatment of hemifacial microsomia is limited by the amount of missing tissue in the involved area.[18] If the condition is quite mild, the child may respond to functional appliance therapy alone with no necessity for surgery. In the more severe cases, treatment generally involves two or more stages of surgical intervention and extensive orthodontic treatment. Treatment for hemifacial microsomia is discussed in some detail in Chapter 15.

Mandibulofacial Dysostosis. Mandibulofacial dysostosis (Treacher Collins' syndrome) is another disorder of missing facial tissue (Figs. 2-5 to 2-7). It differs from hemifacial microsomia in that it is always expressed bilaterally (though one side may be more affected) and in the pattern of the facial defects. The characteristics of the condition are deficiencies in the lateral orbital rim and zygomatic area in addition to absent or rudimentary mandibular condyles, short mandibular ramus, severe antegonial notching, and retrogenia.[19] The shape of the mandible, with a marked downward displacement of the symphysis, seems to be characteristic.[20] Down-turned palpebral fissures, coloboma, missing eyelashes, aberrant facial hair over the malar area, and ear deformities are likely to be present.[21] Deformities of the nasomaxillary region, choanal atresia, and supralaryngeal stenosis may be present. Some of the masticatory musculature is missing, and the suprahyoid musculature and the stylomandibular and sphenomandibular ligaments may be affected.

It was recognized in the early 1970s, before thalidomide and isotretinoin had provided human examples, that loss of neural crest cells in experimental animals could produce facial defects analagous to mandibulofacial dysostosis, and Poswillo suggested then that this was probably the cause of the human malformation.[22] The experience with thalidomide, however, suggests that the critical time for inducing a deformity pattern such as mandibulofacial dysostosis is later than the time at which crest cells originate and migrate initially. Sulik and coworkers[23] have recently presented evidence that excessive cell death in the trigeminal gan-

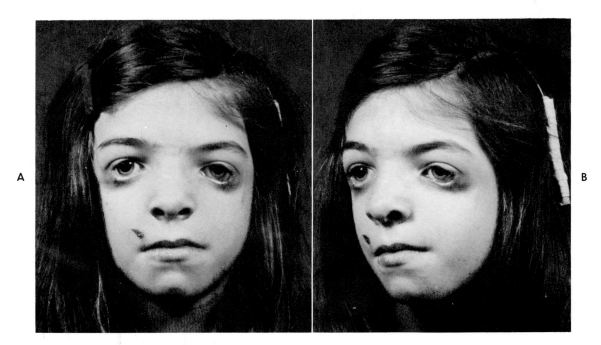

Fig. 2-5. Patient T.F., a 12-year-old girl with mandibulofacial dysostosis (Treacher Collins' syndrome). **A,** Full-face and **B,** three-quarter facial views. Note the reasonably symmetric deficiencies in the lateral orbital margins that extend into the mandibular area.

A   B   C

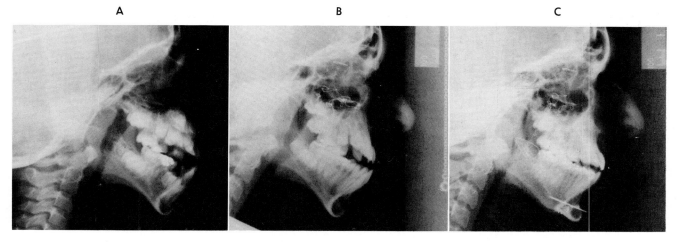

Fig. 2-6. Cephalometric radiographs of patient T.F. **A,** Age 8. **B,** Age 14, after initial grafts to the zygomatic area and orthodontic treatment to align the teeth in preparation for orthognathic surgery. In this case, mandibular growth was more normal than was maxillary growth, leading to a Class III rather than the more common Class II malocclusion seen in this syndrome. **C,** Age 16, after surgery to augment the lateral orbital rims and zygoma, set the mandible back, and augment the chin.

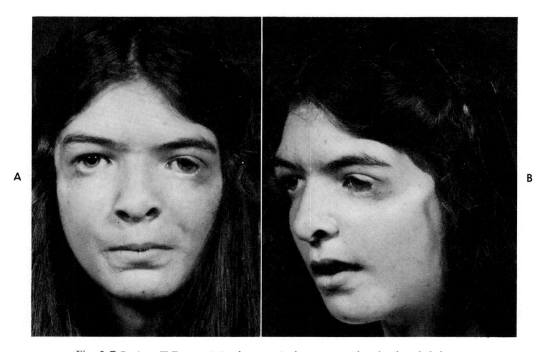

Fig. 2-7. Patient T.F., age 16, after surgical treatment for the facial deformity.

glion, which secondarily affects neural crest–derived cells, is more likely to be the primary cause of this deformity. This bilateral loss of cells appears to be responsible for secondary defects in tissues derived from crest cells, particularly the zygomatic bones, but also the external and middle ears and the mandible. Deficiencies in the posterior part of the maxillary prominence appear to account for the high incidence of clefts of the soft palate in mandibulofacial dysostosis patients.[24] This revised view of the primary defect makes it easier to understand why the defects in mandibulofacial dysostosis are more symmetric than are those in hemifacial microsomia and clarifies the relationship between the two conditions.

Treatment of mandibulofacial dysostosis depends on surgical reconstruction of the deficient areas. The growth pattern is unfavorable for orthodontic treatment alone; that is, growth modification treatment is ineffective.[25] Orbital and zygomatic reconstruction usually is undertaken at approximately 8 years of age by onlay bone grafting. Surgery to reposition the jaws and chin is delayed until approximately age 14, after the adolescent growth spurt and eruption of the canine teeth. Treatment for these patients is discussed in Chapter 15.

Facial Clefting Syndromes

The most prevalent congenital defect of dentofacial development is clefting of the lip and/or palate, which occurs in approximately 0.1% of births in the United States. In addition to these obvious clefts, Tessier[26] has described 14 additional facial clefting possibilities that involve failure of developmental processes to totally fuse even though the epithelium is intact. Although most of these clefts occur very rarely, they can help explain complex and frequently quite severe facial deformities. In essence, this classification describes as clefts what other investigators have called areas of tissue deficiency, but often it can be seen at surgery that skeletal elements surrounding the orbits and extending into the cranium and nose failed to fuse. These more extensive clefts may or may not involve the lip and palate.

The way in which clefts of the lip and palate develop has been clarified considerably in recent years as the morphogenetic movements of the involved tissues have become better understood. For example, three recent findings are worth a brief comment:

1. The first step in development of the primary palate is a curling forward of the lateral edge of the olfactory placode, which initiates the development of the lateral nasal process and positions it so that contact with the median nasal process is possible. Interference with this movement can lead to clefting of the primary palate. Maternal cigarette smoking now has been shown to be a major factor in the etiology of cleft lip and palate.[27] The mechanism is thought to be hypoxia-induced failure of the movement of the lateral nasal process.[28]
2. A genetic predisposition to clefting has been recognized for many years. Recent studies suggest that about a third of cleft lip and palate cases are due to a single recessive gene, which offers possibilities for determining the molecular nature of the defect.[29,30] The effect may be on the relative size of the processes that form the lip, so that a cleft can result from the combination of only slightly small processes and slightly increased width dimensions of the face.[31]
3. Closure of the secondary palate depends on removal of the tongue from between the palatal shelves, and a relatively large tongue in the af-

fected twin of a monozygotic pair discordant for cleft palate seems to be a frequent finding.[32] It is clear now that almost all cases of isolated cleft palate are related to problems in tongue removal, shelf elevation, and contact of the shelves at the proper time.

Recent advances in understanding the etiology of cleft lip and palate are reviewed more completely by Johnston and Bronsky.[6]

Two aspects of the treatment of patients with cleft lip and palate are particularly related to combined surgical-orthodontic management: (1) alveolar bone grafts to stabilize the dental arch, and (2) surgical repositioning of the maxilla and/or mandible after growth is essentially complete. The overall management of cleft patients is reviewed briefly, and these aspects of treatment are covered in detail in Chapter 18.

Achondroplasia

Failure of the primary growth cartilages of the limbs and cranial base to grow properly creates the rare (in humans) condition of achondroplasia. Achondroplasia is an autosomal dominant trait, so it is highly prevalent in affected families, but it also appears sporadically in other kindreds because of spontaneous mutations.

Part of the normal mechanism for forward growth of the midface is the lengthening of the anterior cranial base to which it is attached, which in turn is caused by proliferation of cartilage at the sphenoccipital, intersphenoidal, and sphenoethmoidal synchondroses. In achondroplasia, growth is diminished at these synchondroses just as it is in the epiphyseal plates of the long bones. The results are very short arms and legs and a characteristic midface deficiency that is most accentuated at the bridge of the nose (Fig. 2-8). Interestingly, the anterior cranial base is of approximately normal length but the posterior cranial base is extremely short; that is, the sphenoccipital synchondrosis is affected much more than is the sphenoethmoidal.[33]

Correction of the Class III malocclusion and midface deficiency in achondroplasia ideally is accomplished by a LeFort III osteotomy to move the entire midface forward (Fig. 2-8, *C* and *D*). Unfortunately, no analagous surgical procedure exists to deal with the limb deficiencies, although progress has been made recently toward lengthening the short limbs.[34]

Premature Fusion of Cranial and Facial Sutures: The Craniosynostosis Syndromes

The flat bones of the cranial vault develop from mesenchymal condensations over the developing brain. They grow primarily by apposition of bone at their edges, which later become the cranial sutures, and secondarily by surface remodeling. As with the other membrane bones of the head, continuing separation at the sutures is important for growth. The increase in

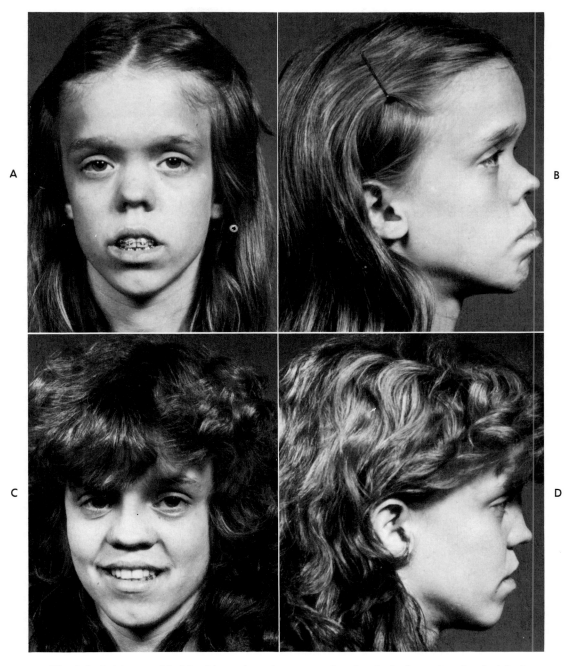

Fig. 2-8. A 14-year-old girl with moderately severe achondroplasia (hypochondroplasia). **A** and **B,** Before surgery. Note the deficiency of the midface, which is related to decreased anterior projection because of the lack of cartilage growth in the cranial base and perhaps in the nasal septum. Growth of the mandible, where cartilaginous proliferation is secondary rather than primary, is normal. **C** and **D,** Facial appearance after LeFort III osteotomy for midface advancement.

cranial size that occurs in individuals with increased intracranial pressure (hydrocephalus) clearly illustrates the stimulus to apposition of new bone from separation of the sutures by pressure from the expanding brain (Fig. 2-9).

Premature fusion of midsagittal or posterior cranial sutures can produce deformities of head shape without affecting the face. For example, in scaphocephaly (Fig. 2-10), the cranium is long and narrow as a result of premature closure of the sagittal suture. Unilateral fusion along the coronal suture ring (plagiocephaly) has the potential to produce facial deformity as well as cranial asymmetry (Fig. 2-11). Depending on the location and extent of the premature fusion, either a pure vertical discrepancy of the orbits or a transverse asymmetry with or without increased separation of the orbits may occur.[35] When plagiocephaly is detected during infancy, the fused sutures can be released surgically and the forehead and orbits reconstructed, possibly resulting in symmetric facial development (Figs. 2-12 and 2-13).[36,37]

Abnormalities of the cranial base also are found in patients with premature fusion of cranial sutures, particularly in those with plagiocephaly and the syndromes discussed below. Whether the suture fusion leads to cranial base malformations, the classical view suggested by Virchow many years ago, or whether primary cranial base malformations secondarily produce premature suture fusion, as Moss suggested more recently,[38] remains controversial. Recent experiments in animals have shown that suture fusion sometimes occurs before any cranial base abnormalities can be seen and that fusing the coronal suture with an adhesive can produce a secondary cranial base deformity.[39] It thus appears that the suture fusion can be the primary defect in some situations—which does not mean that it is in all. The good response to early release of the fused cranial suture in plagiocephaly implies that the suture fusion is the primary problem in most of these patients, whereas the poor response to similar surgery in patients with Crouzon's or Apert's syndromes can be taken as further evidence for primary cranial base involvement in these problems.

Crouzon's syndrome (Figs. 2-14 to 2-16) is characterized by a symmetric maxillary deficiency that affects the infraorbital area. It results from premature (prenatal) fusion of the posterior and superior sutures of the maxilla along the wall of the orbit.[40] The orbits are extremely shallow, which is the major reason that the eyes protrude and often are widely separated. The premature fusion often extends into the cranium. Three-fourths of these patients have synostosis of the coronal, sagittal, and/or lambdoidal sutures. The anterior cranial base is short, and a primary defect in the synchondroses is considered likely.[41]

Release of prematurely fused cranial sutures in these

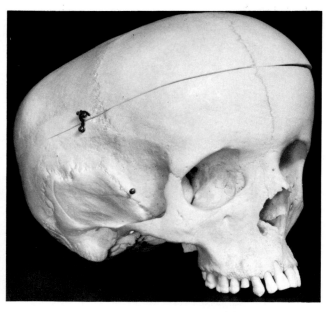

Fig. 2-9. The skull of an individual with hydrocephalus who, judging from the stage of dental development, died in his early teens. Note the tremendously enlarged cranium. In millimeter measurements, the distance from nasion to anterior nasal spine is essentially normal, whereas cranial length and breadth are almost twice the normal size. The cranial sutures are patent but not widened. As typically is the case in hydrocephalus, increased intracranial pressure has tended to separate the flat bones of the cranial vault at their sutures, which stimulates the formation of new bone in those areas. The result is an increase in the size of all the membrane bones of the cranial vault. (Courtesy Dr. T.A. Turvey.)

patients may be indicated for other reasons, but it does not correct the maxillary deformity. Release of the sphenozygomatic suture and the sutures of the cranial base has been advocated, but access to these sutures is difficult and release does not seem to result in subsequent normal growth.[42] Depending on the severity of the condition, treatment involves orthodontic treatment for the Class III malocclusion and/or frontal and midface advancement via a LeFort III osteotomy after growth is essentially complete.[43]

Apert's syndrome (Figs. 2-17 and 2-18) also results from fusion of multiple facial and cranial sutures and early fusion of the synchondroses of the cranial base. Thus these patients are somewhat similar in appearance to patients with Crouzon's syndrome. The distinction is primarily on the basis of syndactyly occurring in Apert's syndrome, but also on the fact that the metopic suture and anterior fontanel are characteristically open at birth and during infancy in such patients, so that pronounced frontal bossing and a high steep forehead appear. The maxilla is always retrognathic and may be hypoplastic. As in Crouzon's syndrome, surgical release of sutures leads to rapid refusion of the osteot-

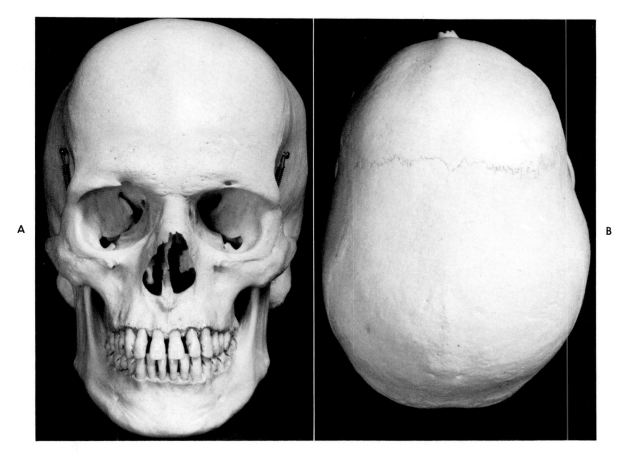

Fig. 2-10. The skull of an individual with scaphocephaly. **A,** Front view and **B,** superior view. Note the absence of the mid-sagittal suture and the extremely narrow width of the cranium. In compensation for its inability to grow laterally, the brain and the braincase have become abnormally long anteroposteriorly. (Courtesy Dr. T.A. Turvey.)

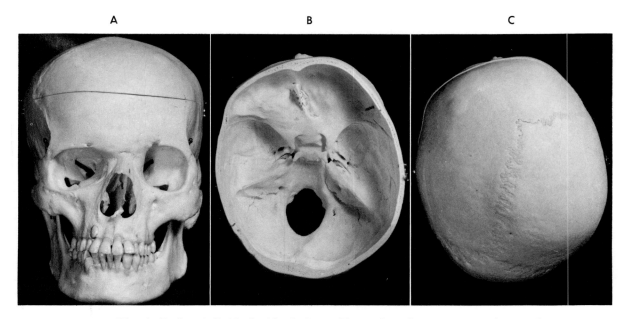

Fig. 2-11. The skull of an individual with plagiocepahly resulting from premature fusion of the coronal suture ring on the left side. **A,** Anterior view, **B,** view of the cranial base with the cranium removed, and **C,** view of the cranium from above (note that the left coronal suture is fused). The cranial vault is a three-dimensional structure, and the coronal suture extends inferiorly along the side and beneath the developing brain. Note in **B** that the asymmetry affects the anterior cranial base, which twisted laterally as it grew anteriorly. This helps explain the effects on the orbits and the nasomaxillary complex. The mandible also is skewed laterally. (Courtesy Dr. T.A. Turvey.)

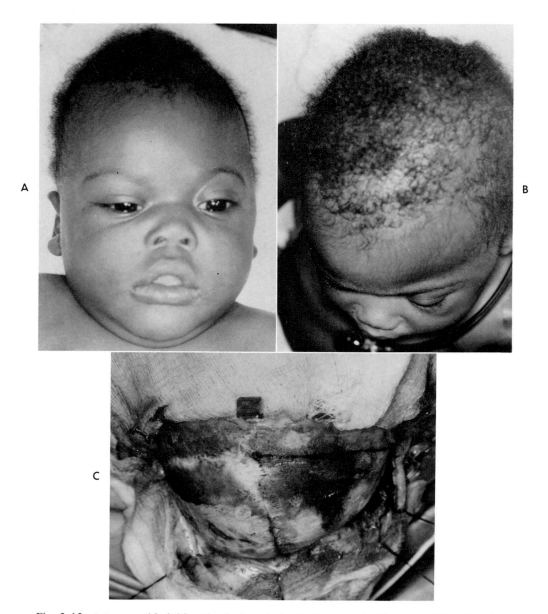

Fig. 2-12. A 1-year-old child with plagiocephaly. **A,** Anterior facial view and **B,** view from above. Note the flattening of the left side of the forehead and the vertical asymmetry in the position of the eyes and eyebrows. **C,** View at surgery, with a forehead flap reflected. The unilaterally fused suture on the left has been marked. The patent suture on the right can readily be seen. Bone was removed from the fused area during the operation, releasing the premature synostosis.

omy sites, with little or no effect on the long-term growth pattern.[44]

Although cranial base distortions apparently can arise from primary fusion of cranial sutures, as discussed above for plagiocephaly, there is good evidence for primary involvement of the cartilaginous cranial base in Apert's and Crouzon's syndromes.[41,45] In both syndromes, there is a progressive synostosis of sutures in the cranium and face, and also progressive calcification of the cervical spine and often of the bones in the hands and feet. A biochemical defect related to calcifi-

cation may turn out to be the cause of all these problems.[46]

Various other craniosynostosis syndromes have been described, which for the purposes of this brief discussion can be treated as variants of the conditions described above. Tessier, who developed most of the modern procedures for craniofacial reconstruction in these severely affected patients, has recently reviewed his approach to surgical treatment in patients with craniosynostosis, providing an excellent summary of the subject.[35]

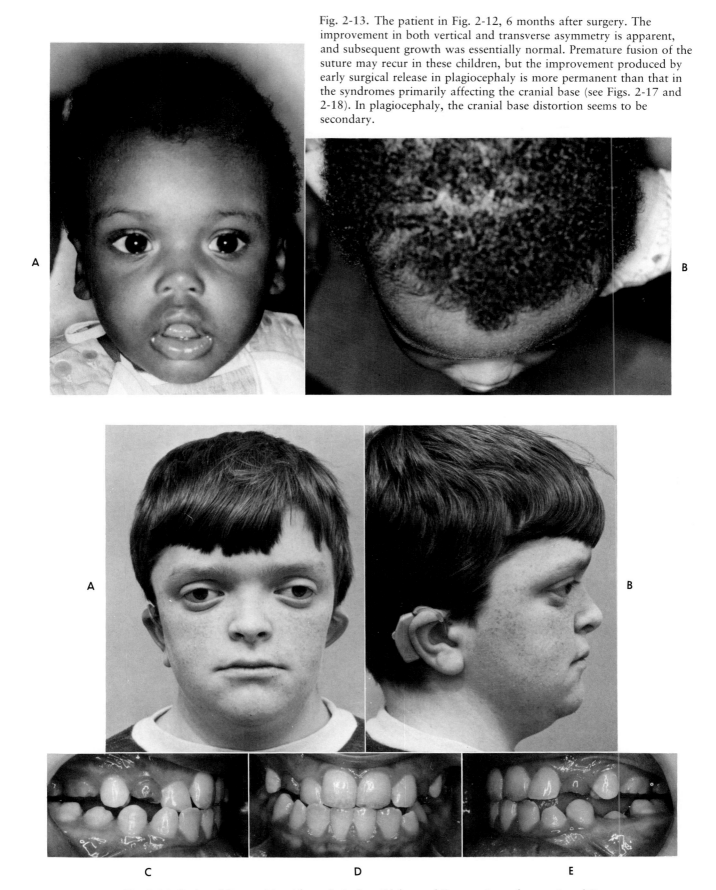

Fig. 2-13. The patient in Fig. 2-12, 6 months after surgery. The improvement in both vertical and transverse asymmetry is apparent, and subsequent growth was essentially normal. Premature fusion of the suture may recur in these children, but the improvement produced by early surgical release in plagiocephaly is more permanent than that in the syndromes primarily affecting the cranial base (see Figs. 2-17 and 2-18). In plagiocephaly, the cranial base distortion seems to be secondary.

Fig. 2-14. Patient S.J., age 14, with a relatively mild form of Crouzon's syndrome. A and B, Facial appearance. C, D, and E, Intraoral views. Note the hypertelorism and the deficient projection of the midface. The dental occlusion is just on the verge of anterior crossbite.

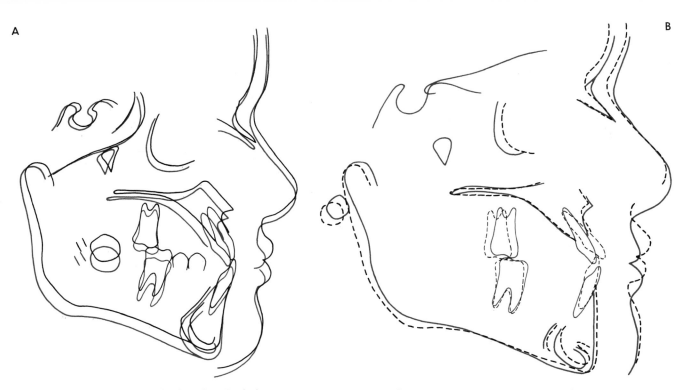

Fig. 2-15. Patient S.J. Cephalometric superimpositions showing (**A**) age 9 years, 11 months *(black)* to 16 years *(red)* with no treatment, and (**B**) age 16 years to 17 years, 10 months *(dashed black)* during orthodontic treatment. He and the family did not desire surgical treatment for the hypertelorism and midface deficiency, and the relatively moderate malocclusion was treatable with orthodontics alone.

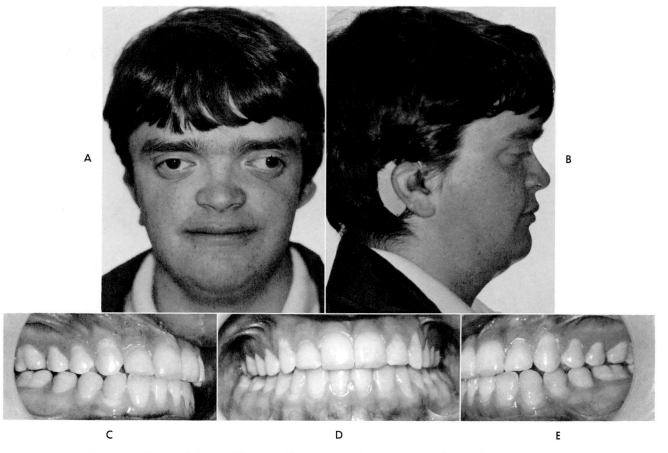

Fig. 2-16. Patient S.J., age 17 years, 10 months at the conclusion of orthodontic treatment. **A** and **B**, Facial appearance. **C**, **D**, and **E**, Intraoral views.

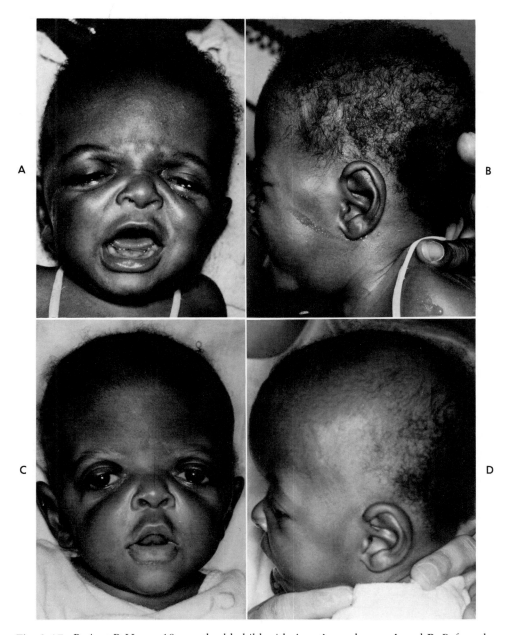

Fig. 2-17. Patient R.H., an 18-month-old child with Apert's syndrome. A and B, Before the initial surgery to release the fused coronal sutures. C and D, Three months later. The short-term improvement is apparent, but growth in an abnormal pattern continued, unlike the normal growth response in the infant with plagiocephaly shown in Fig. 2-13.

Postnatal Growth Disturbances of Known Origin
Trauma

General Principles. Traumatic injuries occurring before growth is complete have the potential to create a steadily worsening deformity by interfering with the displacement of the cranial and facial bones that occurs during normal growth. Effects on skeletal growth from trauma are not so much caused by the trauma itself as by the resulting scarring within the soft tissues that restricts further growth.

The effect of postnatal trauma in producing a dentofacial deformity can be understood best with the current theories of facial growth as a background. The maxilla normally grows downward and forward because of a combination of push from behind by the lengthening cranial base (which is largely complete after age 2 or thereabouts) and pull from anteriorly positioned tissue elements. The mandible seems to be almost entirely pulled forward by the soft tissue matrix in which it is embedded. In a growing child, trauma

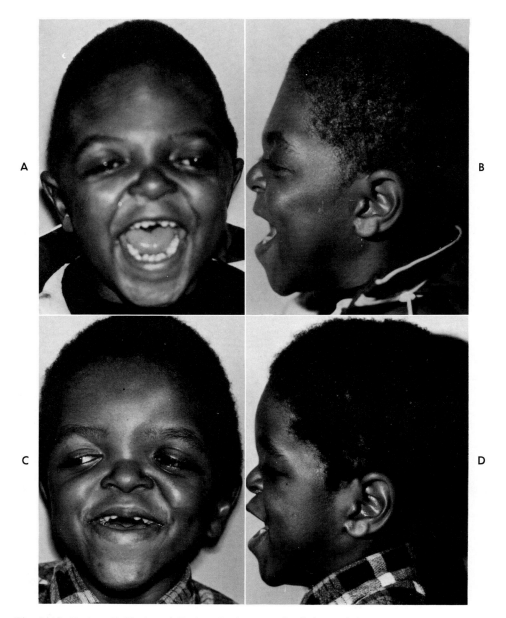

Fig. 2-18. Patient R.H. **A** and **B**, Age 8, showing the failure of the initial suture release to produce normal facial proportions. **C** and **D**, Age 9, 8 months after a second surgical procedure to advance the midface and again release fused sutures. With this surgery also, the result was disappointing. Primary involvement of the cranial base in this syndrome seems to be a major limiting factor in the effectiveness of early surgical intervention.

that interferes with this forward pull, either by decreasing its magnitude or by creating areas of scarring to inhibit it, would distort subsequent growth and could thereby create a progressively worsening deformity.

Mechanical restriction on growth that occurs before birth is not usually thought of as trauma, but the effects are instructive because they mimic the restriction that scar tissue can create later on normal growth. For example, in rare instances, a limb presses against the midface during fetal life, and the result is a characteristic depression of that area. Because the normal forward

pull should be present when the pressure is released after birth, one would predict that the deformity would at least stabilize and probably improve. This is in fact what happens.

Prenatal mechanical restriction on growth of the mandible is uncommon but occurs in Pierre Robin syndrome. The problem arises because the head is flexed tightly against the chest, preventing the mandible from growing forward normally. This can occur for any of several reasons—for instance, a decreased volume of amniotic fluid. The result is an extremely small mandible at birth. In this condition, a cleft of the palate usually is present because the restriction on mandibular displacement forces the tongue upward and prevents normal closure of the palatal shelves. The reduced volume of the oral cavity often leads to respiratory problems at birth, and it may be necessary to suture the tongue forward temporarily.[47]

If the deformity at birth were entirely caused by a prenatal mechanical restriction on mandibular growth that was not present postnatally, one would predict normal growth after birth. There might even be enough downward and forward carry of the mandible by the normal soft tissues to eventually produce a normal mandible, despite the severity of the problem at birth. In fact, exactly this favorable outcome does occur for some children with Pierre Robin syndrome.[48] Others, unfortunately, do not experience enough postnatal growth to make up for the defect, perhaps because of either a lack of intrinsic growth potential or a continuing mechanical restriction in a damaged TM joint (Fig. 2-19).

Maxillary Trauma. One possible source for the forward pull that contributes to maxillary growth is proliferation of cartilage in the nasal septum. In transplant experiments to test whether it has intrinsic growth potential and therefore could serve as a "pacemaker" for maxillary growth as Scott[49] suggested, this cartilage does grow. The growth is highly variable, however, sometimes almost not occurring at all and occasionally occurring reasonably well.[50] The independent growth potential appears to be about half or less that of epiphyseal plate cartilage. The cartilages of the cranial base and nose mature more rapidly than those of the limbs, and so have less growth potential at almost any postnatal age despite their similar embryonic origin. This may explain some of the difference in growth potentials, but the nasal cartilage appears to be intrinsically somewhat less able to grow on its own than are the limb cartilages.

Another way to test the importance of a structure for normal growth is to observe the effect of removing it. In experimental animals, there is no question as to what happens when the cartilage of the nasal septum is removed. There is a dramatic decrease in forward growth of the midface.[51] To some investigators, this indicates that the intrinsic growth potential of the nasal cartilage is important in creating forward growth.[52] To others, the effect simply results from a mechanical collapse of the snout in long-snouted animals that are not particularly analogous to primates and humans.[53]

Injury to the nasal septum in childhood has been shown to reduce downward and forward growth of the maxilla.[54] Removal of the nasal septum in humans is quite rare, but it has been done occasionally following severe injuries in children. As Fig. 2-20 illustrates, midface deficiency may occur in humans as well as in animals if the cartilage is absent. This does not mean that the only or even the major stimulus to growth of the

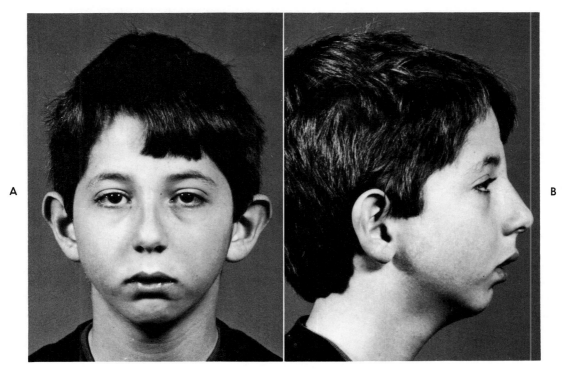

Fig. 2-19. Patient M.H., age 9 years, 3 months, who was noted at birth to have a very small mandible and a cleft palate and was diagnosed as having Pierre Robin syndrome. Note the persistence of severe mandibular deficiency despite considerable postnatal growth of the mandible.

A   C   E

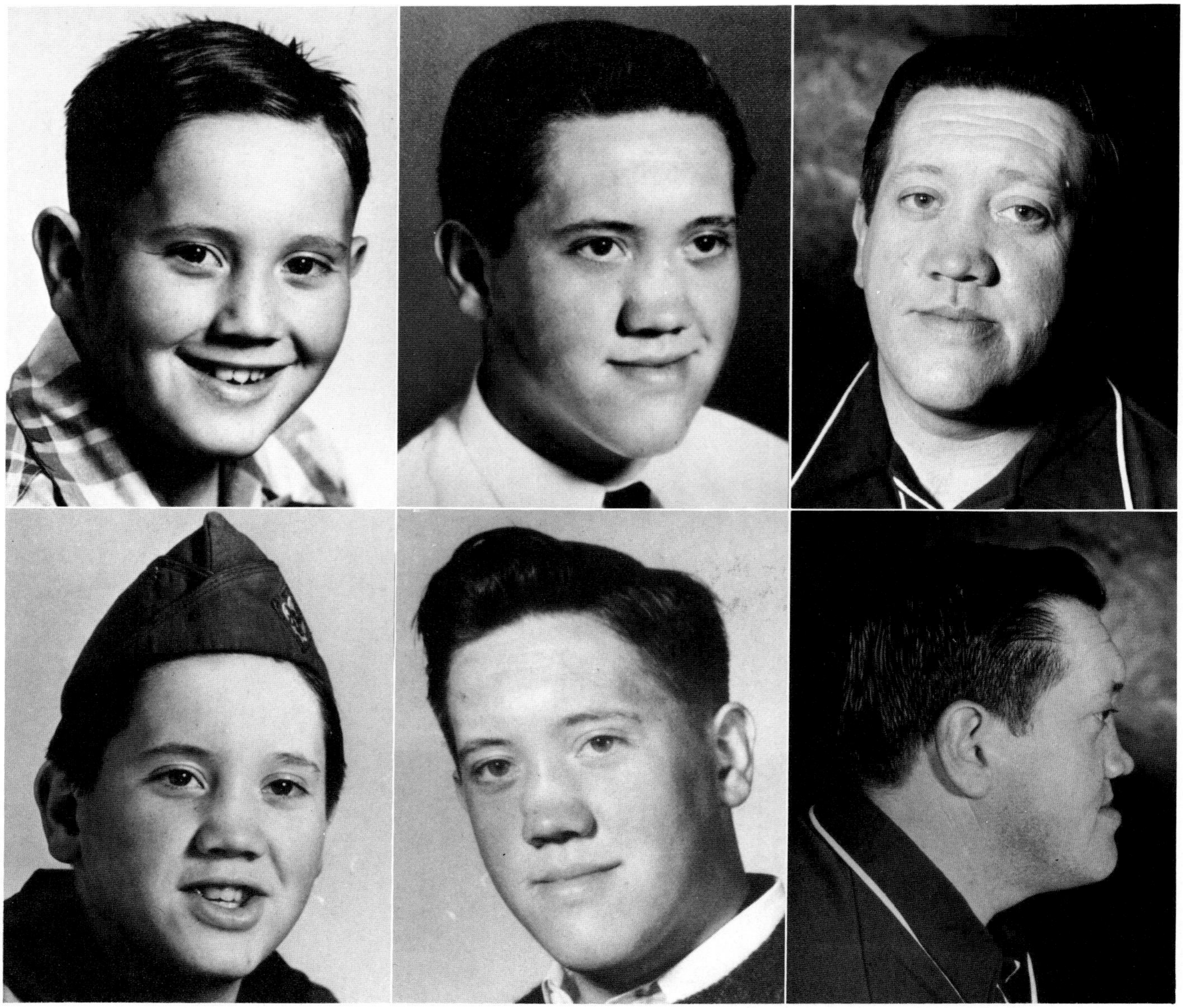

B   D   F

Fig. 2-20. A patient whose nasal septum was removed following an accident in childhood. **A,** Age 7, before the accident. **B,** Age 10, 1 year after removal of all nasal septum cartilage after his bicycle collided with a tree. **C,** Age 15. **D,** Age 19. **E** and **F,** Age 31, when he sought surgical-orthodontic consultation. The lack of midface projection is striking.

maxilla and associated structures is the cartilage of the nasal septum, but it does appear that the septum makes a contribution.

The other potential sources of a forward pull on the maxilla are pressures created by function and/or growth of the soft tissues that surround and envelop it. If the growth of the soft tissues in which the maxilla is embedded is a major stimulus to its bony development, as it seems to be, we simply do not know at present

what controls the soft-tissue growth. However, viewing maxillary growth as being strongly influenced by the soft tissues around it does explain the effect of trauma to lateral areas. Scarring from trauma would diminish the normal pull and/or restrict the response.

Trauma to the maxilla that is severe enough to cause scarring across the posterior and superior sutures fortunately is rare but does occur (Fig. 2-21). When this happens, the growth defect is nearly always unilateral,

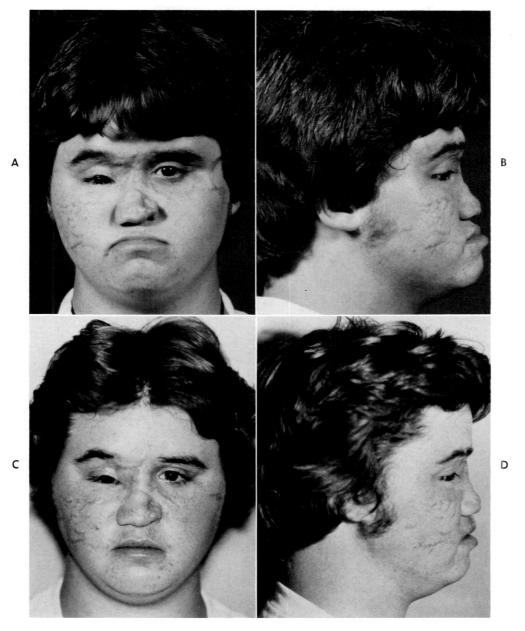

Fig. 2-21. Patient R.D., a 16-year-old male with maxillary deficiency secondary to trauma occurring to the maxilla in an automobile accident in early childhood. **A** and **B,** Facial appearance before surgical treatment. Following the injury, the maxillary deficiency became steadily worse because scarring interfered with the normal downward and forward growth of the maxilla. The appearance of mandibular prognathism largely results from deficient vertical development of the maxilla and overclosure. **C** and **D,** Facial appearance 1 year after surgery to move the maxilla down and forward and reconstruct the nasion area with Silastic.

concentrated on the side where the greatest scarring occurred. The benefits of reconstructive surgery at an early age must be balanced against the realization that the surgery itself inevitably will introduce further scarring and restrictions on growth. Whenever possible, it is better to defer surgical intervention in maxillary trauma cases until growth is essentially complete. When this is not possible and surgery must be carried out before the adolescent growth spurt, partial relapse is likely because of continuing distorted growth, and further surgery often is necessary.

Mandibular Trauma. There are three major sites of growth for the mandible: (1) the mandibular condyle, where proliferating cartilage at the base of the fibrocartilage layer covering the articular surface is replaced by bone, (2) the surfaces of the ramus, where extensive remodeling includes major apposition of bone on the posterior and outer surfaces and resorption on anterior and inner surfaces, and (3) the alveolar process, where new bone is added as the teeth erupt. Less evident but significant remodeling of the mandible also occurs in other locations.

Although the mandibular condyle is only one site of growth, and not nearly as large a one as the surfaces of the ramus and alveolar ridge, the presence of cartilage at the condyle has attracted a disproportionate amount of attention. One possible mechanism for mandibular growth would be a proliferation of cartilage at the condyle pushing the mandible downward and forward, with growth at the other sites then occurring secondarily in response to this forward push. Another possibility is that the mandible is pulled downward and forward by soft-tissue growth around it. Then growth at the condyle, like the remodeling of the ramus and growth at the other sites, would be considered a secondary reaction.

Although the cartilage-push theory of mandibular growth was widely accepted until the 1960s, neither laboratory experiments nor the available experiments of nature with human subjects support this concept. The cartilage of the mandibular condyle is a late secondary cartilage, arising considerably after the primary cartilage of the chondrocranium and the early secondary cartilage of the nasal septum. It first appears as a mesenchymal condensation at some distance from the developing body of the mandible and joins the main part of the mandible relatively late in development. When this cartilage is transplanted or placed into culture, it shows little independent growth potential and produces only about 25% of the growth pressure that epiphyseal plate cartilage produces.[55] In experimental animals, extirpation of the condyle and its associated cartilage has led to varying results. In some circumstances, there has been little or no effect on growth, whereas in others, growth deficits have been observed. In humans, the neck of the mandibular condyle is

relatively fragile and can easily be fractured by a blow against the body of the mandible on the opposite side. When this occurs, the lateral pterygoid muscle tends to displace the condylar fragment, and the displaced fragment then resorbs and is lost. Therefore an early condylar fracture can result in loss of the condylar cartilage. Based on the forward-push theory of mandibular growth, one would expect this to be a devastating injury in terms of its effect on subsequent mandibular growth, and this concept was included in many oral surgery texts until relatively recently.

In the 1960s, in an effort to observe the effects of open versus closed reduction of condylar fractures in monkeys and to create jaw discrepancies that then could be corrected by experimental surgery, Walker deliberately produced condylar fractures in young monkeys. He observed, not the expected progressive mandibular deficiency, but a continuation of essentially normal growth.[56] When some of these animals were subsequently sacrificed and examined histologically, it was clear that not only had the condylar process regenerated totally after the fracture, but a new layer of cartilage had also formed on the articular surface that appeared essentially identical to the original cartilage.

Several years later, two reports of the effect of early condylar fractures in humans appeared, both based on Scandinavian data.[57,58] Both these studies showed that, in humans as well as in animals, there is the potential for a lost condyle to regenerate without any adverse effect on growth (Fig. 2-22). However, perfect regeneration was not observed in the human sample. Instead, approximately 25% of the patients did have growth disturbances following the condylar fractures.

The normal growth that usually follows loss of the condylar cartilage can be explained readily on the basis of a forward-pull theory of growth, and the growth restriction that occurs in some individuals also can be explained by this theory. Even if the condylar process has been damaged, the body of the mandible can be displaced normally by growth of the soft tissues around it. In this circumstance, normal growth will occur and the condyle will regenerate. If, in the aftermath of an injury, scarring around the TM joint prevents soft-tissue growth from carrying the mandible downward and forward normally, a growth deficit will occur. This does not result from any loss of cartilage, but rather from a restriction on free translation of the mandible after the injury. Therefore the extent of scarring is the determining factor in whether a growth deficit occurs after loss of the condylar process in a child.

This concept is highly relevant to the management of condylar fractures in children. It suggests, and clinical experience supports, the idea that open reduction of such a fracture would do more harm than good. There would be little, if any, gain from surgically repositioning the condylar fragment, and the scarring inevitably

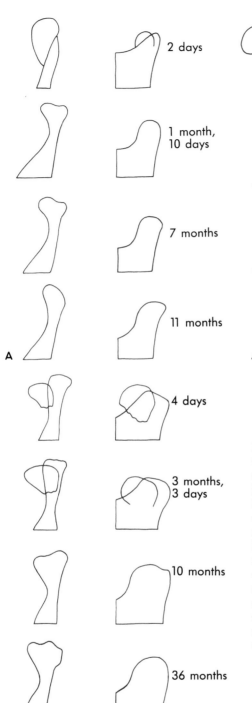

Fig. 2-22. Contour drawings of oblique frontal (Townes views) (left) and panoramic radiographs from children who suffered a condylar fracture. The length of time since the injury is given alongside each tracing. **A,** A high fracture in a boy age 8 years, 1 month at the time of injury. Remodeling and regeneration resulted in normal condylar form after 11 months. **B,** A low fracture in a girl age 9 years, 5 months. Extensive remodeling produced a normal condylar form 30 months later. **C,** A high fracture with displacement of the condylar fragment in a girl age 17 years, 2 months. Remodeling continued over a 3-year period, but the contours were still irregular and regeneration would be considered only partial at the end of that time. (Redrawn from Lund K: Mandibular growth and remodelling processes after mandibular fractures, Acta Odont Scand 32[Suppl 64], 1974.)

produced by surgical intervention would have the potential to inhibit future growth. Clinical experience suggests that if the condyle and its investing periosteum are removed surgically, there is an even greater chance of a subsequent deformity developing. However, the key difference seems to be the extent of the surgery, not the loss of specialized tissues at the condyle.

During opening, the mandible first rotates, then translates downward and forward as the condyle moves out of the temporal fossa onto the articular eminence. A diminution in normal growth would be expected to accompany a restriction on normal translation of the condyle, even if hinge movement were unaffected. Therefore it is possible to speak of a "functional ankylosis" of the mandible.[40] A mandible affected in this way would be able to function because of its rotation on a hinge and limited translation; it would be ankylosed and therefore growth-deficient because of the restriction on normal translation. Unimpeded translation, not function as such, seems to be the key for normal jaw growth.

Occasionally, total resorption of a condylar process occurs after trauma. It is interesting that even in this circumstance, normal growth and function can con-tinue if soft-tissue restrictions do not interfere with the downward and forward translation of the mandibular body. Consider the case of patient D.M. (Figs. 2-23 to 2-26). Although the condylar process almost certainly was lost at age 2, mandibular growth continued quite normally until interference at the coronoid process developed several years later. Conversely, when a restriction on growth did develop at age 8, it rapidly became

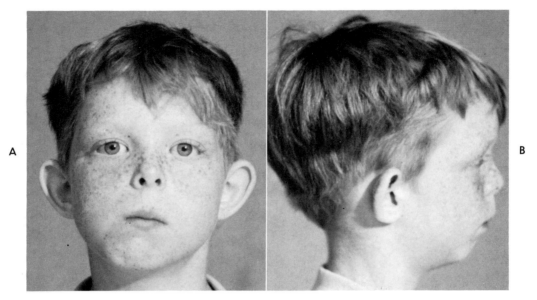

Fig. 2-23. D.M., a 9-year-old boy with an obvious facial asymmetry that had developed during the past year. He had been injured in a fall from a moving car at age 2, but had been noted only to have cuts and abrasions at that time. The mandibular asymmetry developed after age 8.

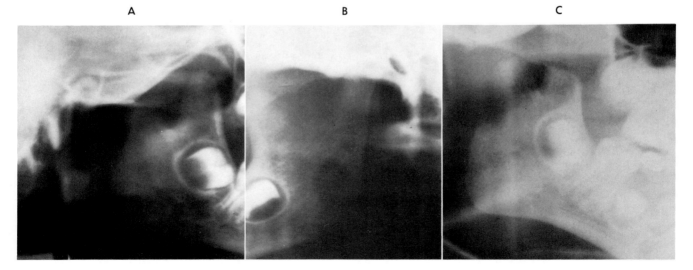

Fig. 2-24. Patient D.M. **A,** Panoramic view of the right ramus at age 9, showing the missing condylar process and elongated coronoid process. **B,** Panoramic view of the normal left side. A tentative diagnosis of ankylosis at the coronoid process was made. **C,** Panoramic view after surgery at age 9 to release the coronoid on the right side. Movement of the mandible immediately became possible.

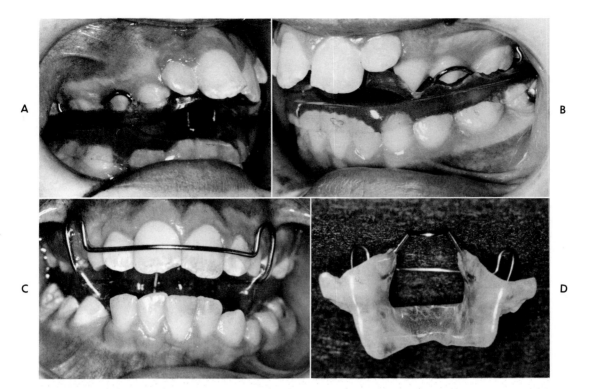

Fig. 2-25. Patient D.M. After surgery, although it was possible for him to move the jaw, the patient was very reluctant to do so. **A,** A split-plate appliance was made with a jackscrew to move the upper plate laterally relative to the lower, so that the jaw could be gradually forced toward the midline. The lower plate was moved laterally two turns (0.5 mm) per day. After 3 weeks, the jaw was in the midline, but he could not advance it to normal occlusion without again deviating to the left. **B,** A second split-plate appliance, shown here after its use was completed, was used to bring the mandible to the midline from an advanced position, which required another month. **C,** At that point a modified bionator was made to hold the normal position. **D,** The bionator differed from the conventional only in that the lingual flange was made longer on the left side to help prevent the mandible from deviating on opening.

progressively worse, and surgical treatment to release the ankylosis was then required.

Our experience at the Dentofacial Clinic at the University of North Carolina (UNC) is that an old condylar injury is the most frequent cause of mandibular asymmetry in children.[59] Most of the condylar fractures that eventually led to growth deficits were undiagnosed at the time, sometimes because of the child's minimal response to the injury and sometimes because the jaw fracture was missed in the presence of other, more severe, injuries. It is important to keep in mind that when an asymmetry develops because of restricted movement, it is likely to become progressively worse as growth continues. The greater the inhibition of translation, the more progressive will be the deformity. Treatment should focus on getting the jaw to move freely, which usually requires surgery to release restrictions. Then a functional appliance can be used postsurgically to guide subsequent growth and maintain as much freedom of movement as possible.[60,61]

Muscle Disturbances

Muscular activity can affect jaw growth in two ways: (1) the formation of bone at the point of muscle attachments depends on the muscle, and (2) the musculature is part of the total soft-tissue complex whose growth provides a major part of the normal forward carry of the jaws during growth.

Loss of one of the mandibular elevator muscles can occur from unknown causes in utero (perhaps related to hemifacial microsomia, but the defect in that condition is more than just muscle), as the result of an injury at birth, or from accidental denervation at a later time. When this happens, one would expect a deficiency in growth of the maxilla and mandible on the affected side, involving all three planes of space but most noticeable vertically (Fig. 2-27). The bone at the angle of the mandible forms in response to the muscle attached to it, so there would be an obvious bony deficiency in this area. Stimulation of any remaining viable nerve-

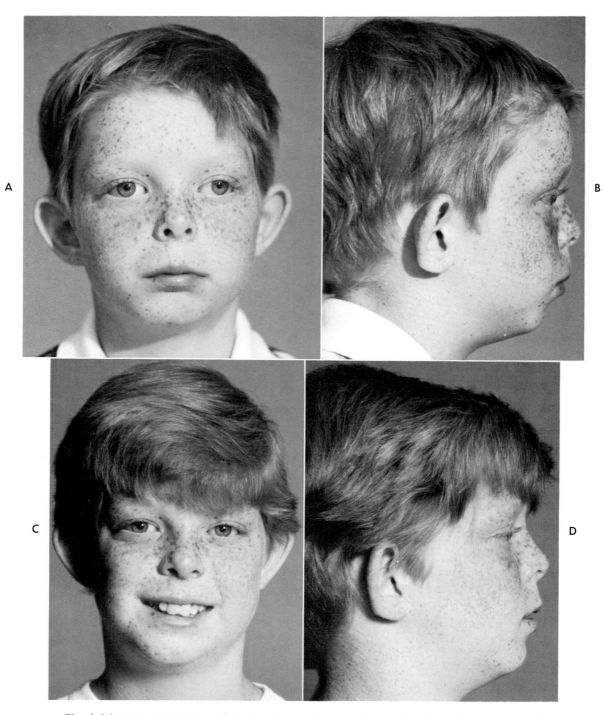

Fig. 2-26. Patient D.M. **A** and **B,** Age 9 years, 11 months, at the point when postsurgical functional appliance treatment was discontinued. **C** and **D,** Two years later. After doing very well for that period, the facial asymmetry began to worsen again, and functional appliance therapy was reinstated. Radiographs showed that the coronoid process was again elongating, and reankylosis in this area presumably was again the cause of the growth distortion. Further surgery probably will be required in the future but will be delayed as long as possible.

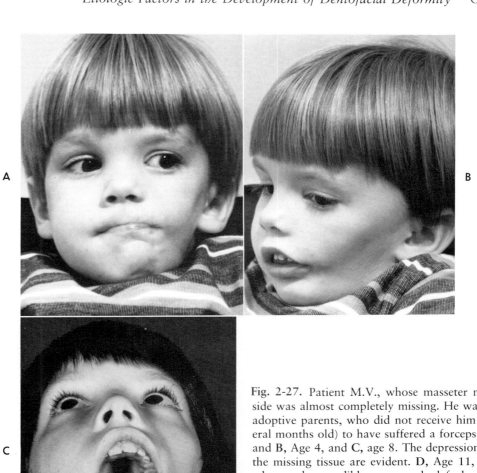

Fig. 2-27. Patient M.V., whose masseter muscle on the left side was almost completely missing. He was reported (by his adoptive parents, who did not receive him until he was several months old) to have suffered a forceps injury at birth. **A** and **B,** Age 4, and **C,** age 8. The depression in the cheek and the missing tissue are evident. **D,** Age 11, before surgery to advance the mandible more on the left than on the right side to correct the gradually worsening asymmetry. **E,** Age 11, 3 months after surgery.

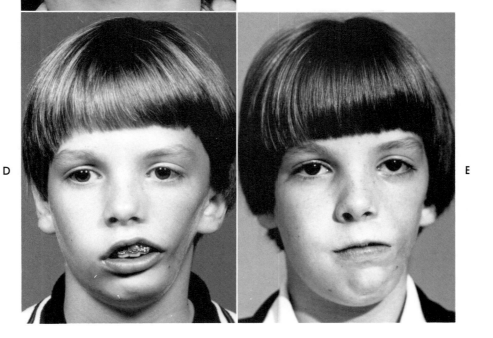

muscle unit may partially overcome the growth deficit. The only other potential therapeutic approach is repositioning muscle from another location, usually by transposing part of the temporal muscle down into the cheek.[62] It also is possible to fill out the deficient soft-tissue contour by placing a free graft of fatty tissue,[63,64] which can improve the appearance caused by the asymmetry but of course does not replace the muscle function.

Mechanical restriction on growth from aberrant muscle activity is most evident in muscular torticollis, a twisting of the head caused by excessive tonic contraction of the neck muscles on one side (primarily the sternocleidomastoid). The condition usually is treated early in life by distal tenotomy of the sternocleidomas-

toid, ideally during the first year but satisfactorily up to 5 years of age.[65] More extensive surgery or selective denervation may be required in older children.[66] Although surgical treatment minimizes its effect on growth, torticollis still can result in considerable facial asymmetry because the altered head posture affects mandibular posture. Ultimately, deposition of bone at the areas of muscle attachment and asymmetric eruption of teeth lead to an asymmetry that affects the mandible more than the maxilla, but involves both jaws (Figs. 2-28 to 2-30).

If asymmetry resulting from torticollis does begin to develop during childhood despite surgical treatment of the muscle problem, functional-appliance therapy may help to control it. Reconstructive surgery should be de-

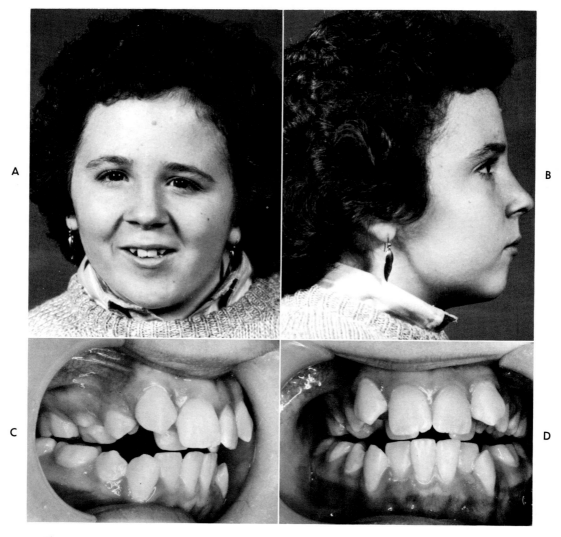

Fig. 2-28. Patient C.W., age 15 years, 7 months. In this patient, torticollis was recognized at an early age and corrected surgically, but a noticeable facial asymmetry developed. The deviation of the mandible is reflected in the dentition despite some compensation of incisor position. The severe crowding was unrelated to the torticollis. **A** and **B**, Facial views before treatment. **C** and **D**, Intraoral views.

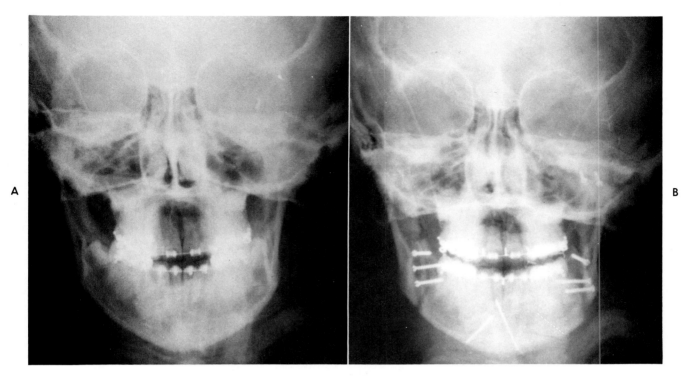

Fig. 2-29. Patient C.W. **A,** PA cephalogram before surgery. **B,** PA ceph after surgery. Surgical treatment consisted of a cartilage graft to the left zygoma, bilateral sagittal split of the mandibular ramus to bring the mandible to the right, and an inferior border osteotomy to bring the chin to the right.

ferred until the end of the growth period. At that point it is usually possible to produce a stable correction of the jaw deformity because the jaw muscles are not affected directly and the deformity was produced by indirect effects on repositioning of the mandible during growth. By the same token, jaw surgery will do nothing about the underlying neck deformity, and head posture will continue to be altered even if a symmetric jaw position can be achieved.

A decrease in tonic muscle activity—the opposite of the asymmetric increase in muscle tone that occurs in torticollis—occurs in muscular dystrophy, various muscle weakness syndromes, and some forms of cerebral palsy. In children with these diseases, multiple muscle groups are affected, usually symmetrically. This decrease in muscle activity also affects facial growth.[67,68] The usual result is excessive vertical growth of the maxilla and excessive eruption of the posterior teeth (Figs. 2-31 and 2-32). The mandible rotates downward and backward, and there is a severe anterior open bite.

The problem develops because of altered mandibular posture, so in theory orthodontic treatment to prevent eruption of posterior teeth and maintain the postural position of the mandible (e.g., a vertical-pull chin cup) should serve to control the unfavorable growth pattern. In practice, this treatment places almost impossible demands on the patient because it would have to continue throughout growth. Although surgery to reposition the jaws can improve the situation, postsurgical relapse is likely, particularly when additional growth occurs. In severe cases, two stages of surgical treatment, the first in midchildhood and the second in late adolescence, usually are needed. Orthodontic growth modification is used after the first surgery to help maintain the correction as long as possible.

Condylar Hyperplasia

In acromegaly, which is caused by an anterior pituitary tumor that secretes growth hormone, excessive growth at the condyles occurs in some, but not all, patients. Growth of hands, feet, brow ridges, and the mandible in an adult are the characteristic signs of acromegaly (Fig. 2-33), but rarely do all occur in the same patient. Proliferation of the condylar cartilage usually occurs, but it is difficult to be sure whether this is the cause of renewed mandibular growth or if it merely accompanies it. When mandibular overgrowth does occur, it is bilateral but may not be perfectly symmetric. The excessive growth stops when the tumor is removed or irradiated, but the skeletal deformity persists and often requires orthognathic surgery.[69,70]

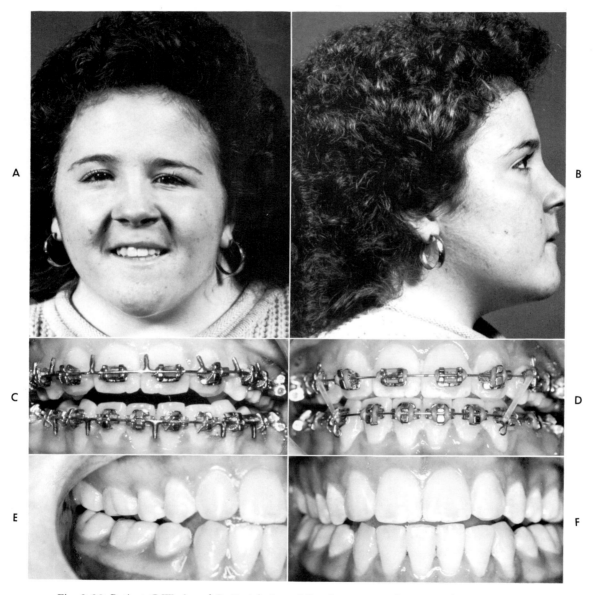

Fig. 2-30. Patient C.W. **A** and **B,** Facial views following surgery. **C,** Intraoral views immediately before surgery. **D,** Intraoral view during postsurgical finishing. **E** and **F,** Intraoral views 1 year after completion of treatment. The maxillary lateral incisors and mandibular first premolars were extracted during the orthodontic phase of treatment.

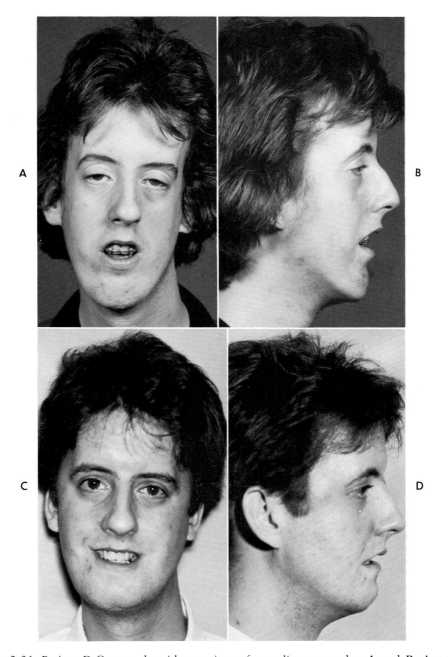

Fig. 2-31. Patient D.G., a male with a variant of nemaline myopathy. **A** and **B,** Age 16 years, 5 months, facial appearance before treatment. The extreme long face is apparent. **C** and **D,** Age 20 years, 2 months, facial appearance following surgery at age 16 to elevate the maxilla and at age 19 to shorten and recontour the chin. In patients of this type, continued growth following surgical correction can cause marked relapse.

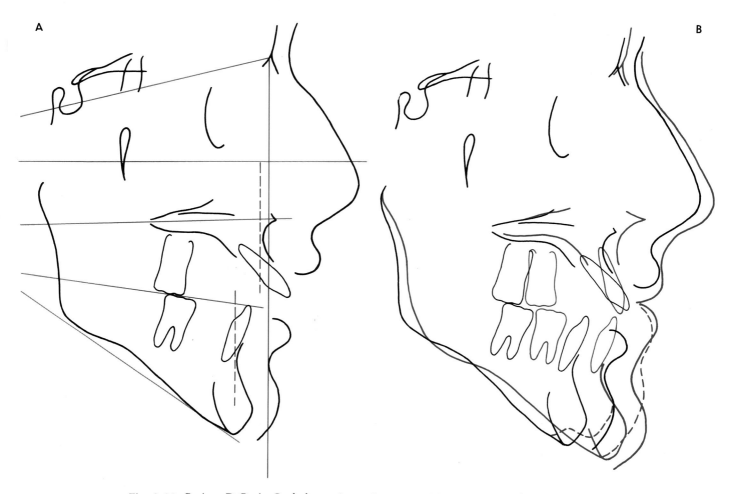

Fig. 2-32. Patient D.G. **A,** Cephalometric tracing at age 12 years, 9 months. Note the extreme elongation of the face and downward-backward rotation of the mandible. **B,** Superimposition showing the change produced by a combination of growth, orthodontic treatment with premolar extractions, and surgery to elevate the maxilla *(in red)* and subsequently recontour the chin *(in dashed red)*.

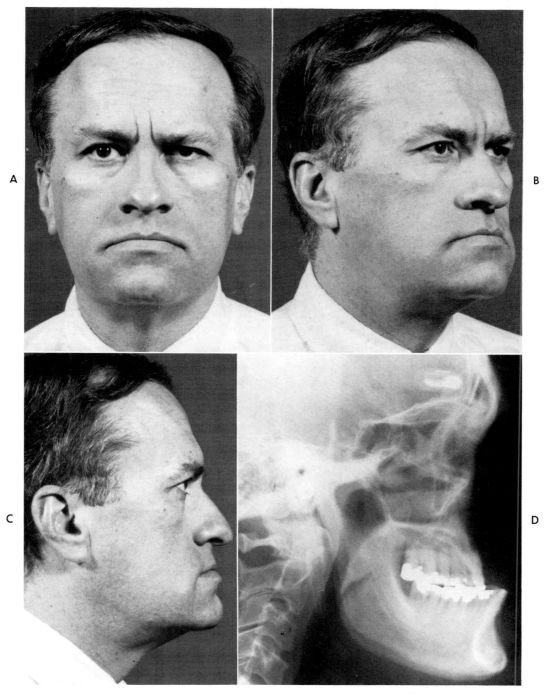

Fig. 2-33. A 45-year-old male with acromegaly, which was diagnosed 3 years previously after he went to his dentist because his lower jaw had come forward. Subsequently, he underwent trans-sphenoidal hypophysectomy, but he noticed that the jaw continued to grow, and growth hormone levels remained high. The hypophyseal area was then irradiated, hormone levels dropped, and mandibular growth ceased. **A, B,** and **C,** Facial appearance is typical of acromegaly. Note the loose soft tissue, increased supraorbital ridges and prominence of the zygomatic arches, and mandibular prominence. **D,** The enlargement of the sella turcica and loss of definition of its bony outline can be noted on the cephalometric radiograph along with the considerable overgrowth of the mandible, which remains as a legacy of the disease that can be corrected by orthognathic surgery if desired.

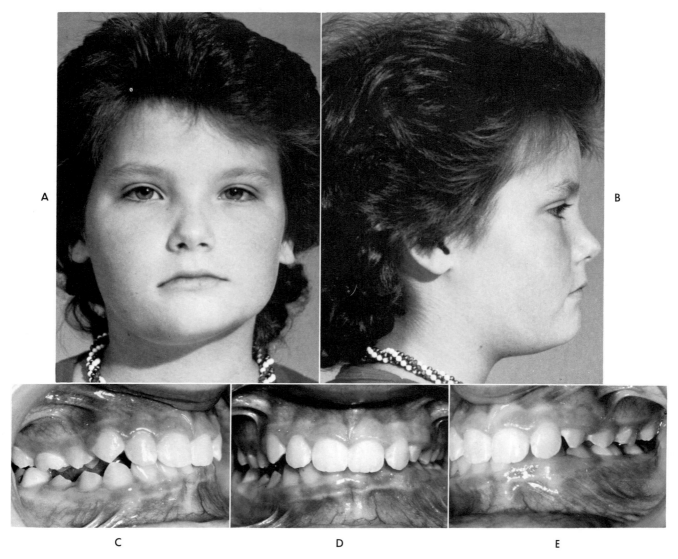

Fig. 2-34. Patient R.H. **A** and **B**, Facial appearance at age 10, when her facial asymmetry was first noticed. It had developed rapidly during the previous year. **C**, **D**, and **E**, Dental occlusal relationships at that time.

In some metabolically normal individuals, unilateral excessive growth of the mandible creates a facial asymmetry. This is the opposite of the asymmetry discussed above that results from growth restriction on one side and that occurs in younger children. Traditionally, excessive growth of this type has been called *condylar hyperplasia*, a descriptive term that implies a primary role for the mandibular condyle in the development of this condition. Because the excessive growth may affect other parts of the mandible and sometimes may be more prominent away from the condyle, this is not necessarily an accurate description. Obwegeser and Makek[71] have recently described several variants of the condition based on the part of the mandible that is most affected and the vertical versus horizontal components of the resulting deformity. They differentiate hemimandibular hyperplasia, hemimandibular elongation, and hybrid forms of the two, emphasizing that tissues other than those at the condyle are involved.

In some individuals the condition is accompanied by a tremendous increase in the size of the condyle itself (Figs. 2-34 to 2-36), whereas in others the condyle increases in size little if any, but the condylar neck increases in length. It is conceivable that in the "enlarged condyle" type of the condition, an inappropriate response of the condylar cartilage (to growth hormone or other normal stimuli) is the primary defect. In acromegaly, the condyles show variable responses to the in-

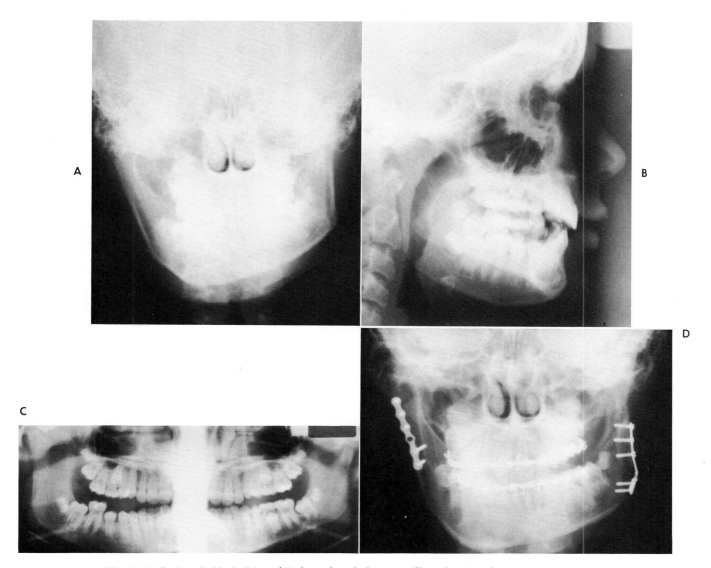

Fig. 2-35. Patient R.H. **A,** PA and **B,** lateral cephalometric films showing the excessive mandibular growth on the right side. **C,** The enlarged right condyle can be seen clearly on the panoramic film. After a ^{99}Tc bone scan confirmed that active growth was continuing at the right condyle, a condylectomy and reconstruction with a costochondral graft were planned. **D,** PA cephalometric film following surgery. A sagittal-split osteotomy was done on the left side so that the cant of the mandible could be leveled. Postsurgically, a hybrid functional appliance (see Chapter 17 for more details) was used to bring the teeth into occlusion.

creased levels of growth hormone, so tissue responsiveness can be an important variable. In the "elongated neck" forms of unilateral excessive growth, the activity of the condylar cartilage is less dramatic, and it may be that the condylar area is merely adapting to a different stimulus that carries the mandible downward and forward on the affected side.

Unilateral excessive mandibular growth is primarily a problem of individuals in the 15- to 25-year-old age range, although it occurs rarely as early as age 10 or as late as age 40. The condition usually is self-limiting, but the extent of growth can vary widely. The elongated neck form of the deformity seems more likely to stop growing spontaneously. For this reason and also because condylar function is less impaired, this variant is more likely to be treatable with ramus surgery than is the enlarged condyle version, which frequently requires condylectomy because of a combination of continued excess growth and interference with function.

Treatment for these problems is discussed in more detail in Chapter 17.

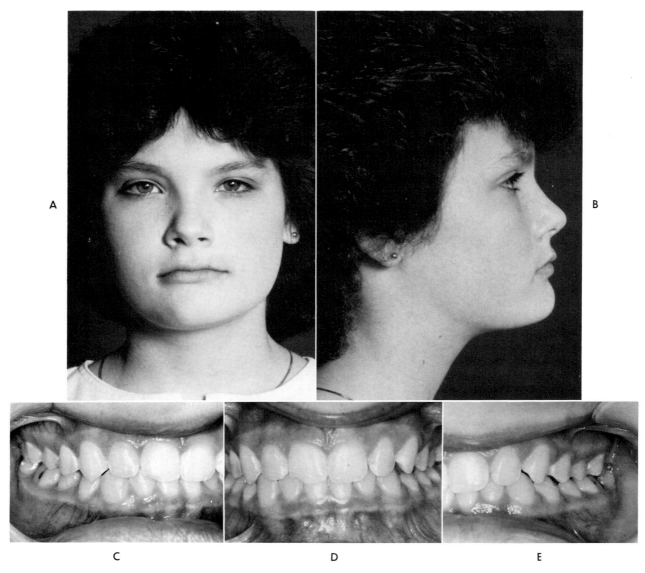

Fig. 2-36. Patient R.H. **A** and **B,** Facial appearance and **C, D,** and **E,** dental occlusion at age 14, 3½ years after the initial surgery. Removal of bone from the inferior border of the right mandible to correct the residual canting of the mandible was suggested but not accepted—the patient and her parents were pleased with the result.

INHERITED TENDENCIES

The extent to which dentofacial deformity can be inherited has been vigorously debated for at least a century. There is no doubt that certain types of deformities run in families. The classic example is the mandibular prognathism in the German royal family that was prevalent enough to become known as the Hapsburg jaw. This can be traced through many generations, in which it always was expressed. In many other jaw deformities as well, it is often obvious from examining the parents that a patient's problem represents an extension of a tendency apparent in previous generations. Even individuals with a deformity severe enough to re-

quire surgery usually have a considerable resemblance to other family members.

At one time, it was widely believed that most jaw discrepancies were caused by ill-assorted facial features that resulted from crosses between different racial and ethnic groups. Malocclusion is much more common now than it was in primitive human populations.[72] It seemed logical that one effect of increased intermarriage among previously isolated population subgroups would be an increased number of individuals requiring orthodontic or orthodontic-surgical treatment. This concept was reinforced by the interpretation of breeding experiments in dogs,[73] in which it was shown that

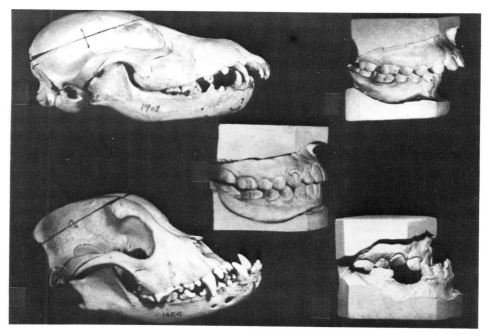

Fig. 2-37. In breeding experiments with dogs in the 1930s, Professor Stockard demonstrated that severe malocclusions could be developed by crossing morphologically different breeds. His analogy to human malocclusion was a powerful influence in replacing the prevailing belief of the 1920s that improper jaw function caused malocclusion with the concept that malocclusion was largely an inherited problem. (From Stockard CR, Johnston AL: Genetic and endocrinic basis for differences in form and behavior, Philadelphia, 1941, The Wistar Institute of Anatomy and Biology.)

crossing different breeds could result in striking dentofacial deformities, particularly a mandibular prognathism that resembled the human variety (Fig. 2-37). Only much later was it realized that many of these deformities were caused by variable expressions of achondroplasia, a common genetic trait in many breeds of dogs. In dogs, the gene has partial penetrance and so may or may not produce variations in jaw size. In humans, achondroplasia is rare but is an autosomal dominant trait. Therefore the breeding experiments with dogs are misleading.

A careful study of the prevalence of malocclusion in Hawaii, which has experienced probably the greatest interracial mixing of any locale, has shown that interracial crosses do not produce a major increase in malocclusion and that severe dentofacial problems do not occur in any greater proportion than in other populations.[74] Instead, the Hawaiian data show a modest additive effect; that is, in a cross between Orientals with a degree of mandibular prognathism and Europeans with mandibular retrognathism and dental crowding, the offspring have about the same incidence of each problem as did the parent populations. The occurrence of quite severe problems, as might occur if a child inherited a small upper jaw and a large lower one, is not increased.

The classic way to determine to what extent a characteristic is determined by inheritance as opposed to environmental influences is to compare monozygotic with dizygotic twins. If it is assumed that twins who have been brought up together have experienced the same environment, greater variability in dizygotic twin pairs would be caused by hereditary factors. This provides a way to calculate heritability, the proportion of the variability in a given characteristic that is caused by heredity versus environment.

Studies of this type are limited in several ways, principally by difficulties in obtaining the necessary numbers of twin pairs for study, but also by problems in establishing zygosity and in confirming that the environments were in fact the same for both members of a twin pair. Lundstrom[75] has shown that the skeletal overjet (i.e., the A-B difference projected to the occlusal plane) has a considerably stronger inherited component than the dental overjet. Dental overjet provides an excellent illustration of one of the problems of twin studies. Thumb or finger sucking is a known environmental influence on this characteristic. This can become a confounding variable if dizygotic twins behave differently from monozygotic pairs in this regard, as apparently is the case. If this source of difference in variability is taken into account, the influence of heredity is reduced.

Corrucini, Potter, and coworkers[76,77] suggest that with the proper corrections, the hereditability of overjet is almost zero, a conclusion that most other workers in the field find extreme.

The hereditability of facial proportions and characteristics has not been studied extensively in twin samples because of the difficulty of obtaining satisfactory material, particularly the cephalometric radiographs that would be required. Lundstrom[78] found that the hereditability of vertical facial dimensions (0.26) was not as strong as that for horizontal dimensions (0.62). Intuitively, this seems reasonable, given the ease with which environmental influences could cause rotation of the mandible, but the sample was relatively small.

The other classic method of estimating the influence of heredity is to study family members, observing similarities and differences in father-child, mother-child, and sibling pairs. For most cephalometric skeletal measurements, correlation coefficients for parent-child pairs are about 0.5.[79] For dental characteristics, the correlation coefficients are lower, ranging from a maximum of 0.4 to 0.5 for overjet to a minimum of 0.15 for overbite.[80]

The influence of inherited tendencies seems to be particularly strong for mandibular prognathism. A typical finding is that a third of a group of children who presented with severe Class III malocclusion had a parent with the same problem, and a sixth had an affected sibling.[81] Data of this type do not exist for other types of dentofacial deformities, but a reasonably strong inherited component almost surely is present.

With the exception of mandibular prognathism, a reasonable current assumption might be that 50% of the variation in facial skeletal characteristics is caused by inherited factors (and therefore 50% is environmental), whereas dental variations are more environmentally determined. Thus it seems unlikely that severe dentofacial deformities can be explained largely, or even to a major extent, by inheritance alone. Conversely, an unacceptable deformity rather than an acceptable deviation from the ideal is most likely to occur when environmental influences or other effects accentuate a preexisting hereditary tendency.

ENVIRONMENTAL INFLUENCES
The Importance of Posture in Controlling Soft-Tissue Pressures

Environmental influences on dentofacial development include obvious external influences such as trauma. But more importantly, this category includes the group of etiologic factors related to function. The effects of specific causes of deformities may be considered experiments of nature that provide insight into the more usual cases where no dramatic single event caused a growth problem. Many examples (see Figs. 2-21 to 2-32) make it obvious that there is an interaction

between form and function, but exactly how function affects form during growth has proved difficult to elucidate. Recent research has at least partially clarified the situation. The form-function interaction includes both the effects of active movement and the subtle but long-lasting effects of the soft tissues on the developing skeletal and dental structures. For dentofacial development, the influences of the soft tissues at rest (postural activity) are more important than the effects of muscle contraction and jaw movements. To say it another way, how you posture your lips, tongue, and jaw is more important as an influence on the pattern of growth than how you move them.

Several lines of evidence from both animal and human studies support this concept. When functional stresses on a bone are increased (e.g., as when an individual who has been sedentary goes on an exercise program), bone density increases, but the external contours of the bone show little change. The reverse is true during a period of inactivity such as bed rest: skeletal demineralization occurs without much change in the shape of the bones.

The erupting teeth carry alveolar bone with them, and so forces against the teeth can shape the dental arches and the alveolar processes of the maxilla and mandible. Experiments with the response of teeth demonstrate that pressure against them must be maintained for 4 to 6 hours to initiate bone remodeling and tooth movements.[82,83] For habits like thumb or finger sucking that can affect the shape of the dental arches, the intensity of the habit (i.e., the amount of force placed against the teeth) is less important than its duration in hours per day.

Tongue habits, particularly tongue-thrust swallowing, have been blamed for many instances of protrusion of incisors and anterior open bite. In this situation also, it now seems clear that the postural position of the tongue at rest, rather than where the tongue tip is placed during function, is the important factor in determining the position of the teeth.[84,85] The forces against the teeth that are generated during chewing, swallowing, or even speaking are more than heavy enough to produce tooth movement. However, during these functions, the force is not maintained long enough to have an appreciable effect. Even repeated activities such as the tongue contacts made during swallowing or speaking do not total anything near the multiple hours of pressure required to produce an effect.

In contrast, both bone and teeth are sensitive to more subtle but long-lasting neuromuscular and soft-tissue influences. Light forces of long duration are produced by contraction of skeletal muscles during the maintenance of posture, and these can affect both skeletal development and the path of tooth eruption.

Most bones can be viewed as consisting of a core to which muscular or other functional processes are at-

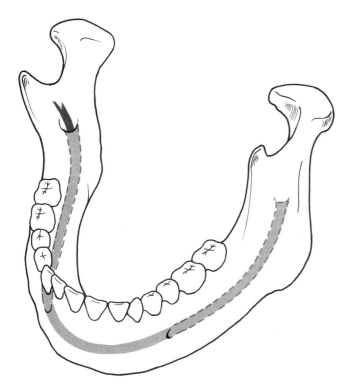

Fig. 2-38. Diagrammatic representation of the mandible as a core *(red)* with functional processes. In this concept, the function of processes such as the gonial angle, coronoid process, mylohyoid ridge, and genial tubercles is attachment of the muscles. The condylar process functions to attach the mandible to the skull, the alveolar process to support the teeth, and the chin to brace the mandible against lateral stresses. The "functional paradigm" for mandibular growth suggests that movement of the core (presumably related to growth of the soft tissues around it) leads to adaptive changes in the functional processes. This would apply equally to normal and aberrant growth.

tached. The mandible is a particularly clear example (Fig. 2-38). Its core consists of the bone that immediately surrounds the inferior alveolar nerve and vessels. To this bone are attached small bony projections for attachment of the small muscles of the suprahyoid complex and major bony processes for attachment of the mandibular elevator muscles. The coronoid process serves as a point of attachment for the temporalis muscle, and the gonial angle region serves for attachment of the medial pterygoid and masseter muscles. The shape of both these areas is extremely sensitive to the position and probably to the postural activity of these powerful muscles. When the elevator muscles are small and relatively underdeveloped, the coronoid process is small, the mandibular ramus tends to be short, and the distance from the lingula (where the inferior alveolar neurovascular bundle enters the mandible) to the gonial angle is small. When the elevator muscles are large

and well developed, coronoid size and ramus length are greater and more bone forms in the gonial-angle area to serve as an attachment for the muscles.

Two extreme situations, which are specific causes of dentofacial deformities in the muscle-disturbances category discussed above, offer excellent illustrations of the importance of the muscle attachment in the shape of the mandible. In the rare condition of masseteric hypertrophy, bone can actually project out horizontally from the angle of the mandible, forming a shelf for additional muscle attachment (Fig. 2-39). The response of the bone seems to be more to the mass of the muscle and the need for a point of attachment than just to the increased stress. In muscular dystrophy or similar syndromes that affect the elevator muscles, the ramus is short and the gonial angle is underdeveloped (see Fig. 2-31).

The dependence of bone on muscle attachment at the gonial angle also is clearly illustrated in the patient's response to orthognathic surgery that involves detachment of the elevator muscles. When muscles are detached, they shorten and eventually reattach at a new location that reflects the shortening. After a mandibular osteotomy, there is nearly always loss of bone in the gonial-angle area (Fig. 2-40), not because of the surgical trauma or where the bone was placed postsurgically, but because the bone remodels when the muscles are detached. If the muscle attachment moves to a new location, the uncovered bone that served only as a muscle attachment resorbs and is lost. Because muscle attachments can migrate across the surface of a bone even if the muscle was not surgically detached, remodeling and changes in contour can accompany treatment that did not surgically reposition the muscle but only changed its function and thereby point of attachment.

The soft tissues of the lips, cheek, and tongue exert pressure against the teeth and alveolar processes while the tissues are at rest as well as when they are moving in function. Although these "resting pressures" (which really are mostly postural pressures) are small, in the range of 5 to 15 gm,[84] they are large enough to cause tooth movement and remodeling of the alveolar process. To some extent, the teeth occupy a position of balance between opposing pressures of the tongue and lips, but the balance is not a precise one. In some locations, resting tongue pressure is greater than lip pressure, whereas in others it is smaller. The stability of the teeth under these circumstances probably is explained by stabilizing forces generated within the periodontal ligament by the same mechanism that produces eruption of the teeth.[83] Nonetheless, when the difference between tongue and lip pressure becomes great enough, tooth movement is inevitable.

Many experiments in nature exist to demonstrate this fact. As an example, scarring of the lip results from the electrical burn produced when a small child bites

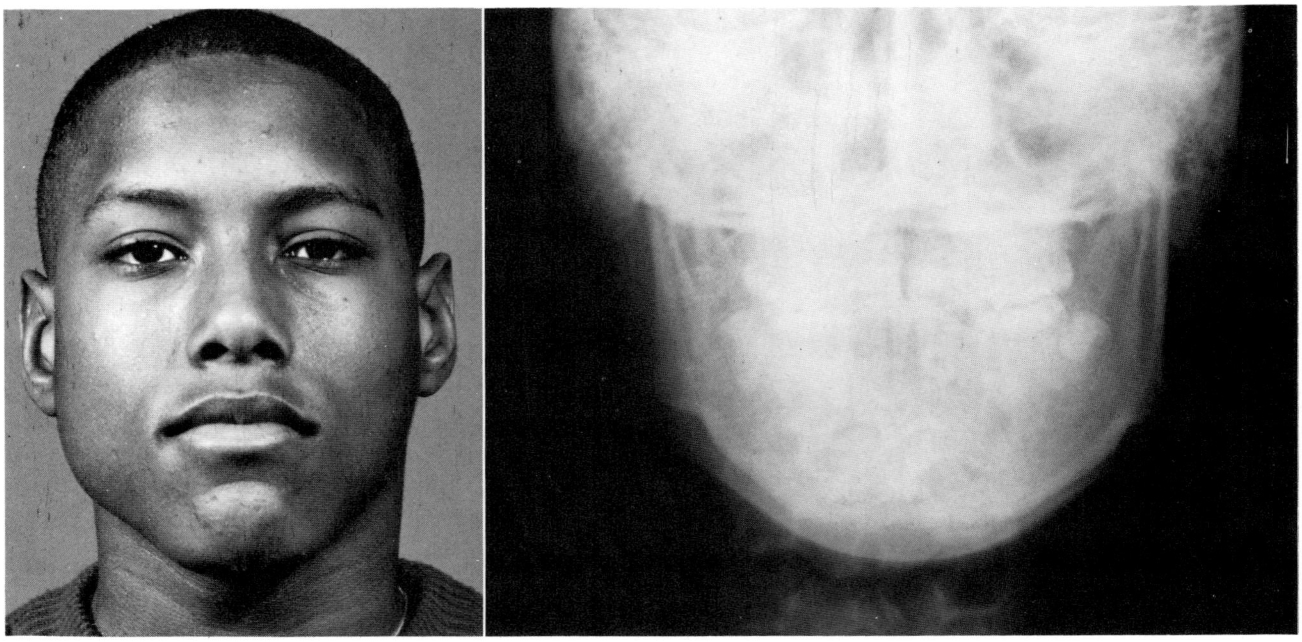

Fig. 2-39. A patient with masseteric hypertrophy. **A,** On clinical examination, the swollen appearance in the region of the masseter muscles is apparent. **B,** In the PA cephalometric film, proliferation of bone at the angles of the mandible can be seen. The increased muscle mass stimulates bone formation at its point of attachment.

into an electric cord. The resulting scar contracture distorts the shape of the dental arch and alveolar process in the vicinity of the injury. Also, loss of cheek tissue from an infection or trauma leads to a distortion and expansion of the dental arch. Similarly, congenital absence of part of the tongue or surgical excision of tongue tissue later in life leads to a characteristic collapse in the adjacent dental arch, and the change in tongue posture produced from a paralytic stroke causes tooth movement and arch distortion (Fig. 2-41).

During growth, distortions of the dental arch and an alteration in the pattern of jaw development can be produced by the same mechanisms, operating slowly and more subtly than in the examples above. Although tongue-thrust swallowing per se is not an important in-

fluence, an altered posture of the tongue can change both the postural position of the mandible and the position of the teeth in all three planes of space. For example, if the tongue is carried very low in the floor of

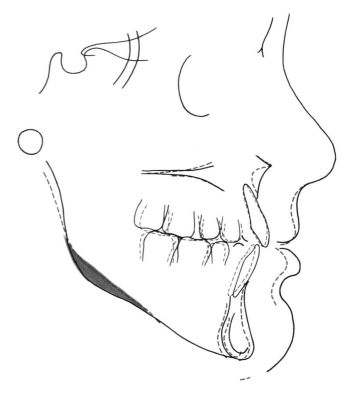

Fig. 2-40. Cephalometric superimposition immediately after surgery to elevate the maxilla and advance the mandible *(in red)*, and 9 months later when orthodontic appliances were removed. For this patient, there was moderate relapse. Note the remodeling of bone in the area of the gonial angle. The length of the ramus has decreased because the elevator muscles shortened after they were detached during the surgery and then reattached at a higher level along the ramus. The bone that no longer served as an area of muscle attachment resorbed and was lost. Ultimately, the location of the muscle attachment determines the surface contour of a muscular functional process, no matter where the bone was put at surgery.

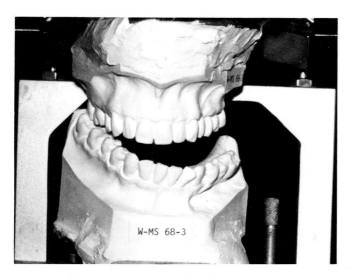

Fig. 2-41. Dental casts showing the effects of tongue pressure in a patient whose tongue rested against the mandibular left posterior teeth following a paralytic stroke. Before the stroke, the occlusion was normal. Constant light pressure from soft tissues, just as from an orthodontic appliance, can move teeth—the key is not so much the pressure magnitude as its duration. (Courtesy Dr. T.R. Wallen. Reproduced from Proffit WR: Contemporary orthodontics, St. Louis, 1986, The CV Mosby CO.)

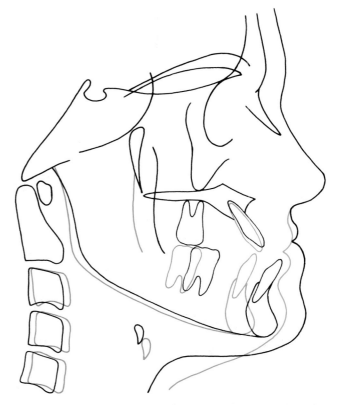

Fig. 2-42. Cephalometric superimposition showing the changes associated with surgery to move the mandible back. Note that although the mandible moved posteriorly, the hyoid bone (and therefore the base of the tongue in which it is embedded) moved downward and slightly forward, thus protecting the pharyngeal airway dimensions. This movement also can be seen in the altered contour of the submandibular soft-tissue outline.

the mouth, it is likely that the mandibular dental arch will be unusually wide and the maxillary arch transversely narrow. Depending on where the tongue tip is placed, either the upper or the lower incisors may be relatively displaced forward. An enlarged tongue can expand the dental arch to the point that there is generalized spacing, and there is also a possibility that the mandible will be postured forward. The tongue's location most of the time, not what it does when it is in motion, is the key to its influence on development.

Tongue posture is not a learned phenomenon. Instead, it is influenced by respiratory needs and several other complex feedback mechanisms. Although speech therapists have considerable success in teaching adaptive movements for the formation of speech sounds, it is another matter to teach a different tongue posture. The success of "myofunctional therapy" in producing changes in posture and thereby improving the pattern of dentofacial development is much less impressive than the improvements in speech that somewhat similar therapy can produce.[85]

The condylar process of the mandible also can be viewed as a functional process (see Fig. 2-38). The condyle serves to maintain an attachment between the mandibular body and the temporal bone, and within limits it responds to forward displacement by growing upward and backward. A constant forward posture therefore has some potential to stimulate growth in this area. Conceivably, one result of an enlarged tongue or

a tongue that is postured downward and forward could be a forward posture of the mandible that would cause the bone to grow larger than normal, perhaps to the point of developing mandibular prognathism. Conversely, if the mandible did grow anomalously large for some other reason, a forward tongue posture would be expected to accompany it because the base of the tongue is attached to the mandible, which makes it difficult to distinguish cause and effect.

It is difficult to be sure whether a tongue is truly enlarged or merely postured forward. Theoretically, a prognathic mandible could result from a large tongue, but it seems unlikely that this is often the cause of the skeletal problem. One piece of evidence suggesting that the tongue did not cause the problem initially for most patients is that when the mandible is repositioned surgically, tongue posture adapts to the new jaw position (Fig. 2-42). It is almost never necessary for the surgeon to reduce the size of the tongue when the size of the jaw is reduced. Occasionally a failure of adaptation is seen, and in those patients the tongue posture may have been a contributing factor in the etiology.

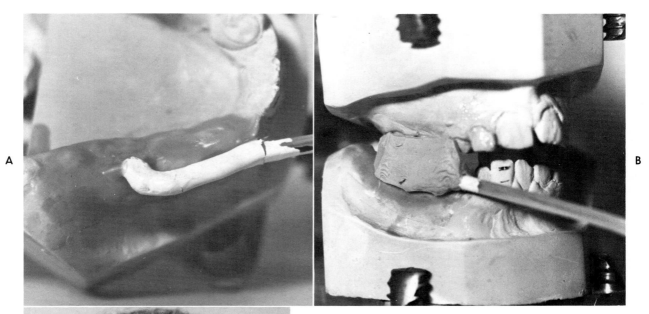

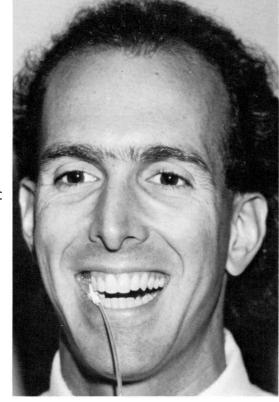

Fig. 2-43. **A,** A 6 mm quartz crystal bite-force transducer mounted on the mesiobuccal cusp of the lower molar of a presurgical patient before recording occlusal force. Undercuts and the occlusal surface of other teeth are waxed out, and composite resin is used to fill any voids between the transducer surface and the tooth. **B,** The transducer is mounted in a silicone rubber carrier, which ensures that it will be in the proper place between the teeth when the patient bites down. **C,** The transducer in place in the mouth.

Biting Force and Jaw Morphology

One characteristic of patients with the long-face condition is that the posterior teeth erupt further than normal. Conversely, in short-face patients, the teeth are infra-erupted. It is possible that how much the teeth erupt is determined by the growth pattern that also determines how much the upper and lower jaws are sep-

arated. Conversely, jaw posture is strongly influenced by the position of the teeth, so it also is possible that whatever controls the amount of eruption could determine whether the mandible rotates down and back, as in the long-face condition, or up and forward, as in the short-face condition. It seems obvious that biting force, which opposes eruption, should be involved in its control. Is it possible that differences in muscle strength, and therefore in biting force, are involved in the etiology of long- and short-face problems?

Biting force varies depending on what is being chewed, where along the dental arch the force is measured (e.g., it is heavier on the molars than the incisors), and several other variables that can be difficult to control experimentally.[86] In contemporary studies, the force of occlusal contact usually is measured with electronic devices placed between the teeth (Fig. 2-43) and is evaluated under three circumstances: (1) maximum effort ("bite as hard as you can without hurting yourself"), (2) simulated chewing ("bite as if you were chewing a piece of steak"), and (3) swallowing ("take a sip of water and swallow it"). It was noted some years ago that long-face individuals have lower, and short-face persons higher, maximum force than those with normal facial dimensions. More thorough recent stud-

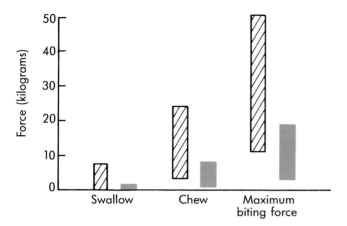

Fig. 2-44. Comparison of occlusal force at 2.5 mm molar separation in normal-face *(in black)* and long-face *(in red)* adults. Note that the normal subjects have much greater occlusal force during swallowing and chewing as well at maximum biting force. The differences are highly significant statistically. (From Proffit WR, Fields HW, Nixon WL: Occlusal forces in normal and long face adults, J Dent Res 62:566-571, 1983.)

ies have shown that the difference between long-face and normal-face patients is highly significant statistically and that occlusal forces are different under all three conditions (Fig. 2-44).[87]

This association between facial morphology and occlusal force does not prove a cause-and-effect relationship, of course. There are three possibilities: (1) the muscular weakness and low occlusal forces may allow the teeth to erupt too much and cause a downward and backward mandibular rotation; (2) excessive eruption of the teeth may cause the mandible to rotate downward and backward, putting the muscles at a mechanical disadvantage that reduces occlusal force; or (3) the long-face pattern and the drecrease in occlusal force are both caused by something else and are not necessarily closely related. In the rare muscular weakness syndromes discussed above, there is a downward and backward rotation of the mandible associated with excessive eruption of the posterior teeth, but this is almost a caricature of the more usual long-face condition, not just an extension of it. If there was evidence of decreased occlusal forces in children who were showing the long-face pattern of growth, argument for a possibly causative relationship would be strengthened.

It is possible to identify a long-face pattern in children before puberty. Measurement of occlusal forces in this group produces a surprising result: there are no differences between children with long faces and normal faces, nor between either group of children and adults with long faces.[88] All three groups have forces far below those of normal adults (Fig. 2-45). Therefore

it appears that the occlusal-force differences arise at puberty, when the normal group gains masticatory muscle strength and the long-face group does not. Because the long-face growth pattern can be identified before the occlusal-force differences appear, it seems more likely that the different biting force is an effect rather than a cause of the condition.

One explananation of the effect of jaw deformities on biting force would be that the aberrant growth pattern changes the geometry of the jaw lever system and therefore would affect the output of the musculature.[89] In theory, surgery to move the maxilla upward would improve the mechanical advantage of the masseter and temporalis muscles; therefore biting force would increase. Moving the mandible forward would put the dentition further from the muscles, causing biting force to decrease.

In fact, surprisingly large changes in occlusal force under all three measurement conditions occur following orthognathic surgery (Fig. 2-46 and Table 2-2).[90] Following superior repositioning of the maxilla, most, but not all, patients have an increase in force, and the changes are much larger than can be explained by the different geometry after surgery. After mandibular advancement, force is as likely to increase as to decrease, and although the mean change for a group of patients is near zero, the large changes in individuals (both increases and decreases) are striking. When the mandible is set back, changes in both directions also occur. There seems to be no relationship between the occlusal-force changes and the stability of the surgical result.

These findings suggest that the force exerted by the masticatory muscles is not a major environmental factor in the etiology of most dentofacial problems. The effect of muscular dystrophy and related syndromes shows that there can be definite effects on growth if the musculature is abnormal, but in the absence of syndromes of this type, the form-function interaction seems to be more an effect of form on function than the other way around. Currently there is no reason to believe that how hard a patient bites is a major determinant of his or her facial vertical dimensions.

Respiratory Influences

Breathing through the mouth rather than through the nose has been blamed for many problems in humans, from altered dentofacial development all the way to mental illness and assorted degenerative diseases. The link to anything other than changes in the pattern of physical growth is entirely unsupported, but it is possible to document a relationship between facial development and oral versus nasal breathing. The important question is not whether there is a relationship—there is—but the extent to which mouthbreathing can cause dentofacial deformities.

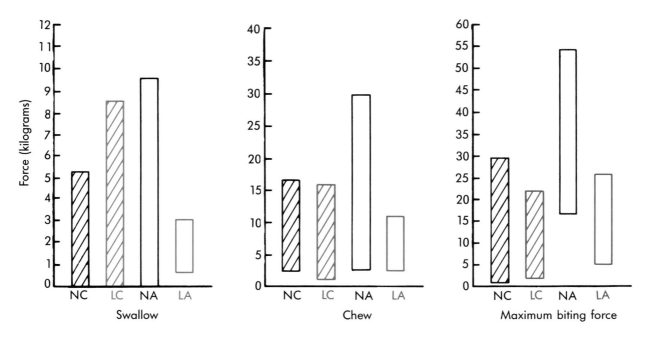

Occlusal force (6 mm opening)

Fig. 2-45. Comparison of occlusal force at 6 mm molar separation in normal-face children (*NC*, black crosshatch), long-face children (*LC*, red crosshatch), normal adults (*NA*, black) and long-face adults (*LA*, red). Values for both groups of children and long-face adults are similar, whereas values for normal adults are significantly higher. The implication is that the differences in occlusal force in adults result from failure of the long-face group to gain strength during adolescence, not to the long-face condition per se. (From Proffit WR, Fields HW: Occlusal forces in normal and long face children, J Dent Res 62:571-574, 1983.)

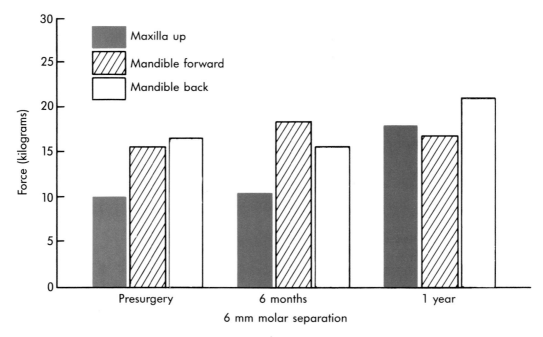

6 mm molar separation

Fig. 2-46. Changes in maximum biting force (MBF) following surgery to superiorly reposition the maxilla, advance the mandible, and set back the mandible. In each surgical group, there was a considerable increase in MBF between 6 and 12 months. Although on the average MBF was greater at 1 year following surgery than before surgery in all groups, there was large individual variation—see Table 2-2. (From Proffit WR, Turvey T, Fields H, et al: The effect of orthognathic surgery on occlusal force, J Oral Maxillofac Surg 47:457-463, 1989.)

TABLE 2-2 Percent of sample with changes in maximum biting force after orthognathic surgery

Type of surgery	MBF ↑ >20%	MBF ± 20%	MBF ↓ >20%
Maxilla up	65%	20%	15%
Mandible forward	32%	32%	36%
Mandible back	29%	42%	29%

Two lines of evidence support a link between oral respiration and the development of facial disharmonies, the first based on animal experiments, the second on observation of humans. In experiments with monkeys, Harvold and colleagues[91] showed that totally blocking the nares led to various moderate-to-severe malocclusions. Because the lower jaw was postured forward, the deformity almost always included a component of mandibular prognathism along with various displacements of the teeth. Interestingly, anterior open bite was not a prominent finding in Harvold's results. These primates do not adapt to mouthbreathing as readily as humans or in exactly the same way, so the experiments can be criticized as potentially misleading, but they do show the potential effect of respiratory adaptation.

Total nasal obstruction of the type produced in experimental animals is extremely rare in humans, but case reports make it clear that when this does occur, the pattern of facial growth is altered. In human juveniles who develop total obstruction, there is a severe downward and backward rotation of the mandible, and subsequent growth produces a long-face deformity (Fig. 2-47).[92,93] In both humans and animals, the mechanism of altered development is also reasonably clear: adapting to total mouthbreathing forces a change in head and jaw posture. This in turn changes the jaw relationship as the mandible rotates to a new position. It also alters the pattern of forces on the teeth, which allows eruption in some areas and impedes it in others and displaces teeth transversely and anteroposteriorly as they erupt.

Because total nasal obstruction in humans is so rare, the important clinical question is whether partial nasal obstruction, of the type that occurs occasionally for a short time in everyone and chronically in some children, can lead to a similar pattern of deformity. The question is difficult to answer, primarily because it is difficult to quantify the extent of mouth-breathing. This is expressed best as the nasal/oral ratio; that is, as the percentage of total airflow that passes through the nose versus the mouth. Observers often assume that when the lips are separated, an individual is breathing through the mouth. In fact, it is perfectly possible to

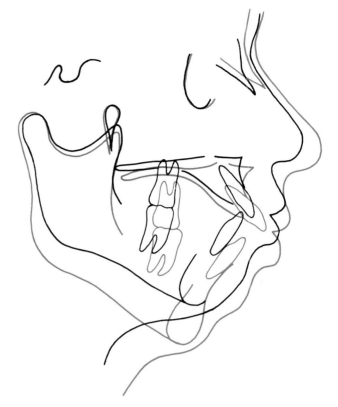

Fig. 2-47. Cephalometric superimposition showing the effect of total nasal obstruction produced by a pharyngeal-flap operation that sealed off the nose posteriorly. From age 12 years *(black outline)* to age 16 years, 9 months, *(red outline)* the mandible rotated downward and backward as the patient grew significantly. (Redrawn from McNamara JA: Influence of respiratory pattern on craniofacial growth, Angle Orthod 51:269-300, 1981.)

have 100% nasal breathing when the lips are apart. The necessary seal to prevent airflow through the mouth is then obtained by placing the tongue against the roof of the mouth. Nor can mouth-breathing be ascertained by simple clinical tests such as looking for condensate on a mirror beneath the nostrils or for movement of cotton wisps in the nasal air stream. Errors by clinicians in assessing respiratory mode occur frequently.[94] To be certain of the nasal/oral ratio, special instrumentation that measures nasal and oral airflow simultaneously must be employed.[95,96]

As one would expect, the nasal/oral ratio changes as physical effort and airflow increase. Normal individuals switch to partial oral breathing at airflows above 40 to 45 L/min, which is about half the total airflow at maximum exertion.[97] At rest, minimum airflow is 20 to 25 L/min. This can easily be supplied by the nose alone, but transition to partial oral breathing also normally can occur during heavy mental concentration or normal conversation.

It seems reasonable to assume that individuals who require surgical removal of hypertrophied adenoids would have a degree of nasal obstruction, and Linder-Aronson demonstrated a tendency toward lengthening of anterior face height in children who were scheduled for tonsillectomy and adenoidectomy in Stockholm.[98] Further studies showed that face height and mandibular plane angle in the children who had their adenoids removed tended to return toward the mean of the control group of children who did not require surgical treatment, although the surgery group never came back totally to the mean of the control group.[92] The differences in face height and mandibular plane angle at all stages were statistically significant and undoubtedly real, but their magnitude was not large. The adenoidectomy group on the average had a 3-degree greater mandibular plane angle and approximately 3 mm additional face height as compared with the control group. It seems reasonable that the more severe the obstruction, the greater might be the change. There also is some evidence to support this from studies of children with cleft palates who underwent pharyngeal flap surgery, which obstructs the nasal airway.[99] But the lack of quantitative information as to the amount of obstruction does not allow this conclusion.

Another indirect way to evaluate whether a patient is mouth-breathing is to measure the resistance to nasal airflow, which can be calculated from the pressure drop across the nasal cavity at measured rates of airflow. Using this technique, Turvey and colleagues[100] showed that in a sample of 50 patients with long-face pattern, 11 had moderately elevated nasal resistance and 6 had very high resistance, whereas the remaining two-thirds were normal. These data were taken from patients before surgery, after growth was complete, and so do not indicate the situation during growth. Furthermore, nasal resistance measures what the patient could do, not what he or she does. It is possible that some individuals in the study with normal nasal resistance nevertheless were mouth-breathers. However, the data do suggest that mouth-breathing is not a necessary concomitant of the long-face condition.

Data from quantitative studies of the nasal/oral ratio remain scanty because the necessary instrumentation was developed only recently and is available at only a few centers. In a study of children with normal and long faces using the quantitative nasal/oral approach, Fields and colleagues[101] found no statistically significant relationship between the nasal/oral ratio and cephalometric indicators of vertical facial proportions. On the average, long-face children had a slightly higher nasal/oral ratio, and a slightly larger number of these children had ratios below 50:50 (Fig. 2-48). These data seem quite compatible with the previous observation that individuals who breathe predominantly through the mouth are over-represented in a long-face population. Yet, most individuals developing the long-face pattern have normal respiration. It appears that respi-

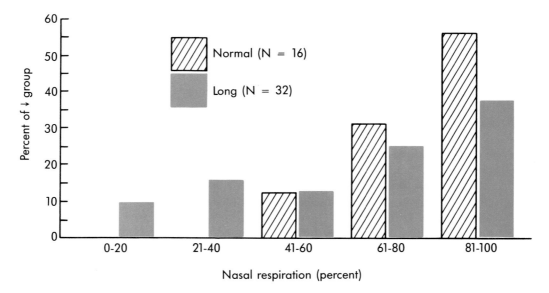

Fig. 2-48. Comparison of the percentage of nasal respiration in long-face versus normal-face adolescents. About a third of the long-face group have less than 50% nasal respiration, whereas none of the normal-face group have such. But most of the long-face group, like the normal-face group, are predominantly nasal breathers. The data suggest that impaired nasal respiration may contribute to the development of the long-face condition but is not the sole or even the major cause. (From Fields HW, Warren DW, Black BK: Relationships between dentofacial morphology and respiratory variables in adolescents, Am J Orthod Dentofac Orthop [in press].)

ratory obstruction can lead to the long-face pattern of deformity, but this is not the usual cause and may not even be a predisposing factor for many individuals with this particular problem.

SUMMARY AND OVERVIEW: WHAT CAUSES DENTOFACIAL DEFORMITY?

From the discussion above, it is apparent that, in a few cases, the etiology of a dentofacial deformity can be confidently ascribed to a specific cause. In most cases, a complex interaction between environmental influences on growth, cellular and tissue responses to growth-promoting agents, and hereditary susceptibility is involved in the etiology. Perhaps this is a complex way of saying that we still have little idea exactly how or why most of these problems develop. To the extent that environmental influences are involved, there is hope of identifying and overcoming these so as to decrease the number of individuals who will require surgical treatment in the future.

One important factor that must be kept in mind is the tendency of a growth pattern, once established, to be maintained thereafter. Since the classic description of this by Brodie[102] in the early days of cephalometrics, there have been many chances to observe that significant changes in growth pattern occur occasionally but are rare. Some patients develop a dentofacial deformity as a result of a change in pattern. Most show the signs of their growth problem at an early age and continue to grow thereafter in a way that leads to a gradual worsening of the problem. It is difficult to believe that genetic control has nothing to do with this, particularly when similar, if less severe, conditions usually can be observed in parents and siblings. The pattern of growth also is a factor in the timing of surgical intervention. If a disproportion is corrected early, it is quite likely to recur because of further growth in the same pattern than led to the problem in the first place. One might hope that treatment to change function to a normal pattern would result in normal growth proportions thereafter, but this hope rarely is realized.

So far as we currently know, all environmental influences eventually affect the pattern of dentofacial development by altering the postural position of the jaws, lips, and tongue. This affects the path of tooth eruption and alveolar development and also changes the jaw relationship itself. A direct effect on the neuromuscular system, as in the muscular weakness syndromes, or a necessary neuromuscular adaptation, as in obligatory mouth-breathing, would produce similar effects on growth.

In some cases, condylar hyperplasia being the best example, the etiology of a deformity may lie in an altered response of cells to normal growth stimuli. The extent to which this mechanism is involved in other types of deformities is totally unknown, but the possi-

bility exists. Inappropriate expression of growth in response to apparently normal stimuli may lead to excessive growth in condylar hyperplasia, but it could also lead to deficient growth and to other types of deformities. A relative resistance to growth hormone by elements within the mandibular elevator muscles, for instance, could lead to some types of mandibular deficiency. There is simply no information as to how this occurs, if indeed it does.

So how does a dentofacial deformity develop in the absence of some specific cause? Consider a mandibular deficiency severe enough to require mandibular advancement. It seems likely that such problems are seen primarily in individuals who were genetically programmed toward a small mandible and in whom some other etiologic factor also came into play. An insult to growth that would have produced only a moderate and orthodontically treatable problem in an individual with good mandibular growth potential can put the patient outside the range of orthodontic correction if the growth potential was diminished already by hereditary factors. The same is true for patients with other types of dentofacial deformities. In short, in the patients in whom there is no obvious specific cause for the growth problem, a combination of inherited tendencies and some environmental determinant probably is required to produce a deviation from normal growth severe enough to require surgery and orthodontics. At this point, we know much less than we should about the environmental factors and how they interact with the genetic control mechanisms.

All in all, our knowledge of the etiology of dentofacial deformities must be acknowledged as remarkably incomplete. The ideal way to treat these problems is by modifying growth as it occurs, keeping it within the normal pattern, and controlling deleterious environmental influences—which is difficult, of course, when the environmental factors are mostly unknown. Among the limitations of current surgical therapy is its minimal effect on the pattern of growth, which means that it must be directed at correcting deviant growth after it has occurred, rather than redirecting it while the problem is developing. As more becomes known in the future about controlling deviant growth, it is likely that earlier treatment to intercept the development of a deformity will become more effective and corrective treatment at a later age will be less necessary.

REFERENCES

1. Enlow D: Handbook of facial growth, ed 2, Philadelphia, 1982, WB Saunders Co.
2. Ranly DM: A synopsis of craniofacial growth, New York, 1980, Appleton-Century-Crofts.
3. Gorlin RJ, Pindborg JJ, Cohen MM: Syndromes of the head and neck, ed 2, New York, 1990, McGraw-Hill.

4. Proffit WR, Phillips C: Who seeks surgical-orthodontic treatment? Int J Adult Orthod Orthognath Surg [in press].

5. McCarthy J, editor: Plastic surgery, Philadelphia, 1990, WB Saunders Co.

6. Johnston MC, Bronsky PT: Abnormal craniofacial development: an overview, J Craniofac Genet Dev Biol [in press].

7. Sulik KK, Johnston MC: Sequence of developmental changes following ethanol exposure in mice: craniofacial features of the fetal alcohol syndrome (FAS), Am J Anat 166:257-262, 1983.

8. Sulik KK: Craniofacial embryogenesis and dysmorphogenesis. In Siebert JR, Cohen MM, Jr, Sulik KK, et al, editors: The holoprosencephalies: an atlas and overview, New York, in press, Wylie-Liss.

9. Webster WS, Ritchie HE: The teratogenic effects of alcohol and isotretinoin on craniofacial development: an anaylsis of animal models, Dev Biol [in press].

10. Lammar EJ, Chen DT, Hoar RM: Retinoic acid embryopathy, New Engl J Med 313:837-841, 1985.

11. Webster WS, Johnston MC, Lammer EJ, Sulik KK: Isotretinoin embryopathy and the cranial neural crest: an in vivo and in vitro study, J Craniofac Genet Dev Biol 6:211-222, 1986.

12. Ross RB: Lateral facial dysplasia (first and second branchial arch syndrome, hemifacial microsomia), Birth Defects 11(7):51-59, 1975.

13. Whitaker LA, Schut L, Rosen HM: Congenital craniofacial asymmetry: early treatment, Scand J Plast Reconstr Surg Hand Surg 15:227-233, 1981.

14. Poswillo DE: The pathogenesis of the first and second branchial arch syndrome, Oral Surg Oral Med Oral Pathol 35:302-328, 1975.

15. Poswillo DE; Hemorrhage in development of the face, Birth Defects, Original Article Series XI:61-81, 1975.

16. Johnston MC: Embryology of the head and neck. In McCarthy J, editor: Plastic surgery, Philadelphia, 1990, WB Saunders Co.

17. Sulik KK, Cook CS, Webster WS: Teratogens and craniofacial malformations: relationships to cell death, Development 103(suppl):213-219, 1988.

18. Vargervik K, Osterhut DK, Farias M: Factors affecting long-term results in hemifacial microsomia, Cleft Palate J 23(Suppl 1):53-68, 1986.

19. Marsh JL, Celin SE, Vannier MW, et al: The skeletal anatomy of mandibulofacial dysotosis (Treacher Collins syndrome), Plast Reconstr Surg 78:460-470, 1986.

20. Grayson BH, Bookstein FL, McCarthy JG: The mandible in mandibulofacial dysostosis: a cephalometric study, Am J Orthod Dentofacial Orthop 89:393-398, 1986.

21. Herring SW, Rowlatt UF, Pruzansky S: Anatomical abnormalities in mandibulofacial dysostosis, Am J Med Genet 3:225-259, 1979.

22. Poswillo D: Otomandibular deformity: pathogenesis as a guide to reconstruction, J Maxillofac Surg 2:64-72, 1974.

23. Sulik KK, Johnston MC, Smiley SJ, et al: Mandibulofacial dysostosis (Treacher Collins syndrome): a new proposal for its pathogenesis, Am J Med Genet 27:359-372, 1987.

24. Sulik DD, Smiley SJ, Turvey TA, et al: Pathogenesis involving the secondary palate and mandibulofacial dysostosis and related syndromes, Cleft Palate J 26:209-216, 1989.

25. Bjork A, Skieller V: Contrasting mandibular growth and facial development in long face syndrome, juvenile rheumatoid polyarthritis and mandibulofacial dysostosis, J Craniofac Genet Dev Biol Suppl 1:127-138, 1985.

26. Tessier P: Anatomical classification of facial, craniofacial and latero-facial clefts, J Maxillofac Surg 4:69-92, 1976.

27. Khoury MK, Weinstein A Parry S, et al: Maternal cigarette smoking and oral clefts: a population based study, Am J Public Health 77:623-625, 1987.

28. Bronsky PT, Johnston MC, Sulik KK: Morphogenesis of hypoxia-induced cleft lip in CL/Fr mice, J Craniofac Genet Dev Biol Suppl 2:128-133, 1986.

29. Chung CS, Bixler D, Watanabe T, et al: Segregation analysis of cleft lip with or without cleft palate: a comparison of Danish and Japanese data, Am J Human Genet 39:603-611, 1986.

30. Ardinger JJ, Beutow KH, Bell GI, et al: Association of genetic variation of the transforming growth factor-alpha gene with cleft lip and palate, Am J Hum Genet 45:348-355, 1989.

31. Johnston MC, Hunter WS: Cleft lip and/or palate in twins: evidence for two major cleft lip groups, Teratology 39:461-462, 1989.

32. Johnston MC, Hunter WS, Niswander JD: Facial morphology in twins discordant for clefts of the lip and palate: a pilot study [in preparation].

33. Cohen MM, Jr, Walker GF, Phillips C: A morphometric analysis of the craniofacial configuration in achondroplasia, J Craniofac Genet Dev Biol Suppl 1:139-166, 1985.

34. DeBastiani G, Aldeghiri R, Brivio LR, et al: Chondrodiatasis-controlled symmetrical distraction of the epiphyseal plate. Limb lengthening in children. J Bone Joint Surg [Br] 68:550-556, 1986.

35. Tessier P: Craniofacial surgery in syndromic craniosynostosis. In Cohen MM, Jr, editor: Craniosynostosis: diagnosis, evaluation and management, New York, 1986, Raven Press.

36. Kreiborg S, Moller E, Bjork A: Skeletal and functional craniofacial adaptations in plagiocephaly, J Craniofac Genet Dev Biol Supp 1:199-210, 1985.

37. Friede JF, Lilja J, Laurizen C, et al: Skull morphology after early craniotomy in patients with premature synostosis of the coronal suture, Cleft Palate J Suppl 1:1-8, 1986.

38. Moss ML: Functional anatomy of cranial synostosis, Childs Brain 1:22-33, 1975.

39. Persson KM, Roy WA, Persing JA, et al: Craniofacial growth following experimental craniosynostosis and craniectomy in rabbits, J Neurosug 50:187-197, 1979.

40. Kreiborg S: Crouzon syndrome: a clinical and roentgenographic study, Scand J Plast Reconstr Surg Hand Surg Suppl 18, 1981.

41. Kreiborg S: Craniofacial growth in craniosynostosis. In Cohen MM, Jr, editor: Craniosynostosis: diagnosis, evaluation and management, New York, 1986, Raven Press.

42. Rune B, Selvik G, Kreiborg S, et al: Motion of bones and volume changes in the neurocranium after craniectomy in Crouzon's disease: a roentgen stereometric study, J Neurosurg 50:494-498, 1979.
43. Raulo Y, Tessier P: Fronto-facial advancement for Crouzon's and Apert's syndromes, Scand J Plast Reconstr Surg Hand Surg 15:245-250, 1981.
44. Kreiborg S, Pruzansky S: Craniofacial growth in patients with premature craniosynostosis, Scand J Plast Reconstr Surg Hand Surg 15:171-186, 1981.
45. Stewart RE, Dixon G, Cohen A: The pathogenesis of premature craniosynostosis in acrocephalosyndactyly (Apert's syndrome), Plast Reconstr Surg 59:699-707, 1977.
46. Cohen MM, Jr: Craniosynostosis: diagnosis, evaluation and management, New York, 1986, Raven Press.
47. Randall P: The Robin anomalad: micrognathia and glossoptosis with airway obstruction. In Converse JM, editor: Reconstructive plastic surgery, Philadelphia, 1977, WB Saunders Co.
48. Pruzansky S: Not all dwarfed mandibles are alike. Birth Defects 5:122-127, 1972.
49. Scott JH: Dento-facial development and growth, Oxford, 1967, Pergamon Press.
50. Kvinnsland S: Autogenous transplantation of the nasal septum cartilage in the rat, Arch Oral Biol 19:767-770, 1974.
51. Sarnat BG: The postnatal maxillary-nasal-orbital complex: some considerations in experimental surgery. In McNamara JA, editor: Factors affecting growth of the midface, Ann Arbor, 1976, University of Michigan.
52. Johnston LE: The functional matrix hypothesis: reflections in a jaundiced eye. In McNamara JA, editor: Factors affecting the growth of the midface, Ann Arbor, 1976, University of Michigan.
53. Moss ML: The role of the nasal septal cartilage in midfacial growth. In NcNamara JA, editor: Factors affecting the growth of the midface, Ann Arbor, University of Michigan, 1976.
54. Rock WP, Brain DJ: The effects of nasal trauma during childhood upon growth of the nose and midface, Br J Orthod 10:38-41, 1983.
55. Copray JCVM, Jansen HWB, Duterloo HS: Growth and growth pressure of mandibular condylar cartilage and some primary cartilages of the rat in vitro, Am J Orthod Dentofacial Orthop 90:19-28, 1986.
56. Walker RV: Traumatic mandibular condyle dislocations: effect on growth in the Macaca rhesus monkey, Am J Surg 100:850-863, 1960.
57. Gilhuus-Moe O: Fractures of the mandibular condyle in the growth period, Stockholm, 1969, Scandinavian University Books (Universtatsforlaget).
58. Lund K: Mandibular growth and remodelling processes after mandibular fractures, Acta Odontol Scand 32(suppl 64), 1974.
59. Proffit WR, Vig KWL, Turvey TA: Early fracture of the mandiblar condyle: frequently an unsuspected cause of growth disturbances, Am J Orthod 78:1-24, 1980.
60. Vig PS, Vig KWL: Hybrid appliances: a components approach to dentofacial orthopedics, Am J Orthod 90:273-285, 1986.
61. Hotz RP: Functional jaw orthopedics in treatment of condylar fractures, Am J Orthod 73:365-377, 1978.
62. Clodius L, Harii K: Surgical therapy for facial paralysis. In Serafin D, Georgiade NG, editors: Pediatric plastic surgery, St. Louis, 1984, The CV Mosby Co.
63. Wells JH, Edgerton MT: Correction of severe hemifacial atrophy with a dermis-free fat flap from the lower abdomen, Plast Reconstr Surg 59:223-228, 1977.
64. Hemmer KM, Marsh JL, Clement RW: Pediatric facial free flaps, J Reconstr Microsurg 3:221-229, 1987.
65. Tse P, Cheng J, Chow Y, et al: Surgery for neglected congenital torticollis, Acta Orthop Scand 58:270-272, 1987.
66. Lee EH, Kang YK, Bose K: Surgical correction of muscular torticollis in the older child, J Pediatr Orthop 6:585-589, 1986.
67. Gavit E, Bornstein N, Lieberman M, et al: The stomatognathic system in myotonic dystrophy, Eur J Orthod 9:160-164, 1987.
68. Proffit WR, Gamble JW, Christensen RL: Myopathy with severe anterior open bite, Am J Orthod 54:101-111, 1968.
69. Brennan MD, Jackson IT, Keller EE, et al: Multidisciplinary management of acromegaly, J Am Med Assn 253:682-683, 1985.
70. Tornes K, Gilhuus-Moe O: Correction of jaw deformities subsequent to treatment for acromegaly, Int J Oral Maxillofac Surg 15:446-450, 1986.
71. Obwegeser HL, Makek MS: Hemimandibular hypertrophy, hemimandibular elongation, J Maxillofac Surg 14:183-208, 1986.
72. Wolpoff WH: Paleoanthropology, New York, 1980, Alfred A Knopf, Inc.
73. Stockard CR, Johnson AL: Genetic and endocrine basis for differences in form and behavior, Philadelphia, 1941, Wistar Institute.
74. Chung CS, Niswander JD, Runck DW, et al: Genetic and epidemiologic studies of oral characteristics in Hawaii's schoolschildren. II. Malocclusion. Am J Human Genet 23:471-495, 1971.
75. Lundstrom A: A twin study of postnormal occlusion, Trans Europ Ortho Soc pp. 43-56, 1963.
76. Corrucini RS, Potter RHY: Genetic analysis of occlusal variation in twins, Am J Orthod 78:140-154, 1980.
77. Potter RHY, Corrucini RS, Green LJ: Variance of occlusal traits in twins, J Craniofac Genet Develop Biol 1:217-227, 1981.
78. Lundstrom A: Nature versus nuture in dentofacial variation, Europ J Orthod 6:77-91, 1984.
79. Saunders SR, Popvich F, Thompson GW: A family study of craniofacial dimensions in the Burlington Growth Centre sample, Am J Orthod 78:394-403, 1980.
80. Harris EF, Smith RJ: A study of occlusion and arch widths in families, Am J Orthod 78:155-163, 1980.
81. Litton SF, Ackerman LV, Isaacson RJ, et al: A genetic study of Class III malocclusion, Am J Orthod 58:565-577, 1970.
82. Davidovitch Z, Shanfield JL: Cyclic nucleotide levels in alveolar bone of orthodontically treated cats, Arch Oral Biol 20:567-574, 1975.

83. Proffit WR: Equilibrium theory revisited, Angle Orthod 48:175-186, 1978.
84. Proffit WR: Muscle pressures and tooth position: findings from studies of North American whites and Australian Aborigines. Angle Orthod 45:1-11, 1974.
85. Proffit WR, Mason RM: Myofunctional therapy for tongue thrusting: background and recommendations, J Am Dent Assoc 90:403-411, 1975.
86. Fields HW, Proffit WR, Case JC, et al: Variables affecting measurement of vertical occlusal force, J Dent Res 65:135-138, 1986.
87. Proffit WR, Fields HW, Nixon WL: Occlusal forces in normal and long face adults, J Dent Res 62:566-571, 1983.
88. Proffit WR, Fields HW: Occlusal forces in normal and long face children, J Dent Res 62:571-574, 1983.
89. Throckmorton GS: Biomechanics of differences in lower facial height, Am J Orthod 77:418-421, 1980.
90. Proffit WR, Turvey T, Fields H, et al: The effect of orthognathic surgery on occlusal force, J Oral Maxillofac Surg 47:457-463, 1989.
91. Harvold EP, Tomer BS, Vargervik K, et al: Primate experiments on oral respiration, Am J Orthod 79:359-372, 1981.
92. Linder-Aronson S: Nasorespiratory function and craniofacial growth. In McNamara JA, editor: Nasorespiratory function and craniofacial growth, Ann Arbor, 1979, University of Michigan.
93. McNamara JA: Influence of respiratory pattern on craniofacial growth, Angle Orthod 51:269-300, 1981.
94. Spalding PM, Vig PS: Respiration characteristics in subjects diagnosed as having nasal obstruction, J Oral and Maxillofac Surg 46:189-195, 1988.
95. Keall CL, Vig PS: An improved technique for the simultaneous measurement of nasal and oral respiration, Am J Orthod Dentofacial Orthop 91:207-212, 1987.
96. Warren DW, Hinton VA, Hairfield WM: Measurement of nasal and oral respiration using inductive plethysmography, Am J Orthod Dentofacial Orthop 89:480-484, 1986.
97. Niinimaa V, Cole P, Mintz S, et al: Oronasal distribution of respiratory airflow, Resp Physiol 43:69-75, 1981.
98. Linder-Aronson S: Adenoids: their effect on mode of breathing and nasal airflow and their relationship to characteristics of the facial skeleton and the dentition, Acta Odontol Scand Suppl 265, 1970.
99. 99. Long RE, McNamara JA: Facial growth following pharyngeal flap surgery: skeletal assessment on serial lateral cephalometric radiographs. Am J Orthod 87:187-196, 1985.
100. Turvey TA, Hall DJ, Warren DW: Alterations in nasal airway resistance following superior repositioning of the maxilla, Am J Orthod 85:109-114, 1984.
101. Fields HW, Warren DW, Black BK: Relationships between dentofacial morphology and respiratory variables in adolescents, Am J Orthod Dentofac Orthop [in press].
102. Brodie AG: On the growth pattern of the human head from the third month to the eighth year of life, Am J Anat 68:209-262, 1941.

CHAPTER 3

Psychosocial Considerations in Surgery and Orthodontics

H. Asuman Kiyak
Rebecca Bell

Orthognathic surgery changes more than the physical features and oral functioning of patients. The treatment has a significant effect on the patient's psychologic well-being and on the reactions of society to the individual. In this chapter, we focus on the psychosocial meanings of facial appearance, self-reported motives for orthodontics and surgery, the effect of surgery on patients' adaptive responses, and the short- and long-term psychologic adjustments to changes in function and appearance.

PSYCHOSOCIAL IMPLICATIONS OF FACIAL DEFORMITIES

Meanings of the Face

Appearance is a major concern of many people who seek surgical-orthodontic treatment. This is not surprising, considering the extensive literature on the relationship between appearance and social acceptance.[1-3] The face is the area of one's body that produces the greatest concern regarding physical attractiveness; it is the individual's focal point and the source of vocal and emotional communications with others. In a survey of over 1000 adults, Berscheid and colleagues found that people who were satisfied with their facial features expressed greater self-confidence.[4] The area of greatest dissatisfaction for subjects in this large sample was the appearance of their teeth.

As Macgregor has noted in describing patients' motives to change their facial appearance, the face and its individual features symbolize significant aspects of the self.[5] Indeed, personality characteristics have been attributed to facial features by the general public, although no studies support this notion. Attractive adults and children are evaluated as more successful and more intelligent than are unattractive persons and are viewed as more socially skilled.[6-9] Performance ratings of attractive female workers are more favorable than ratings of women described as unattractive.[10] Attractiveness also elicits more aid from other people, and this effect has been observed in children as young as 3 years of age.[11,12]

Evidence is growing that social responses may influence an individual's self-concept, not only in terms of perceived attractiveness but also in defining oneself as confident and socially skilled. In this process, a self-fulfilling prophecy may be perpetuated; an individual is rewarded by parents, peers, teachers, and supervisors for attractiveness, thereby enhancing self-esteem and social skills. This heightened level of self-esteem helps the individual in establishing and maintaining successful interpersonal relationships. Conversely, an unattractive person, perceived as less intelligent, socially awkward, and a poor student or worker, will gradually come to see himself or herself in this manner.[6]

Psychosocial Characteristics of Patients with Facial Deformities

People with craniofacial deformities are particularly likely to internalize the negative reactions of others. A study comparing the self-concept of children with cleft lip and palate to children without these conditions found a significantly lower self-concept in the former group.[13] Both boys and girls from age 8 to 18 with cleft lip and palate expressed poorer self-concept than did children without this affliction, but this is an especially serious problem for young girls.[14] Pertschuk and Whitaker found children with craniofacial anomalies (e.g., hemifacial microsomia and craniofacial dysostosis) to be more introverted and neurotic and to express a poorer self-concept than do normal children.[2] Children with these anomalies were described by parents as more hyperactive and by teachers as more difficult in the classroom. Differences by age and type of craniofacial anomaly were not predictors of the children's maladjustment. Behavorial problems also were cited more often by parents of children aged 2 to 12 with cleft lip and palate and were exacerbated in children with associated congenital malformations such as Pierre Robin syndrome and neuromotor dysfunction.[15]

In response to concerns for the social adjustment of individuals with major craniofacial deformities, a trend exists toward surgery at a younger age. Early intervention can prevent social rejection by family members and peers and promote development of higher self-esteem. Recent trends in surgical treatment of children with Down's syndrome are another example of interventions to improve social and self-acceptance.[16] The goal of surgery in these patients is to produce a more "normal" face by improving facial proportions and correcting open bite. Strauss and colleagues, using photographs, obtained ratings from 227 adolescents comparing the attractiveness, intelligence, and social acceptance of children with Down's syndrome before undergoing surgery to children who had no abnormalities.[17] Significant differences were found: the children with

Down's syndrome were rated as being less intelligent, less attractive, and less socially acceptable. Postoperative ratings of these same children were significantly more positive in all three domains, and the improvement in facial appearance was correlated with the intelligence rating.

A study by Arndt and colleagues of 22 children aged 8 to 17 who were undergoing surgery for Crouzon's syndrome and other moderate to severe craniofacial deformities revealed significant improvements in self-esteem and self-assessments of facial appearance.[18] Parents reported decreased self-consciousness in their children following surgery, as well as increased motivation in school and more confidence when meeting strangers. These findings offer hope to people undergoing surgery for craniofacial deformities regardless of age. Correction of the deformity can improve the individual's psychosocial well-being. Even in less extreme conditions such as severe malocclusion, researchers have found a preference for normal occlusion, both by individuals rating their own attractiveness and observers rating others.[19-22] Using photos of children in which the same faces had either normal occlusion or malocclusion, Shaw found that faces with normal occlusion were rated as more attractive, intelligent, and desirable as friends. Both adults and children gave similar responses.[21] In a study by Helm and colleagues, unfavorable self-perceptions of facial appearance were expressed more often by young adults with extreme overjet, deep bite, or crowding.[20] Concerns with overall body image were expressed more often by women (42%) than by men (27%) and were much more frequent among respondents with a malocclusion. These individuals also recalled incidents of teasing by peers when they were children seven times more frequently than did respondents who had normal occlusion. Teasing was experienced most frequently by persons with extreme overjet.

Researchers and policy makers have recommended that a handicapping orthodontic condition (i.e., dentofacial deformity) should be treated if the disfigurement or functional defect is likely to be an obstacle to the individual's psychologic and physical well-being.[23,24] A seriously handicapping orthodontic condition was defined by the NRC committee as one that "severely compromises a person's physical or emotional health."[25] Physical compromise is defined as serious problems with breathing, speaking, or eating, especially if accompanied by tissue destruction. Emotional health includes others' reactions to the individual in a way that influences self-esteem. As early as 1960, Meyer and colleagues found that patients with facial abnormalities look to surgery as a way of improving not only their appearance, but also their self-esteem and their self-deprecating attitudes.[26] Indeed, Crowell and colleagues reported that patients undergoing surgery for dentofacial malrelations were more satisfied with the effects of surgery on their personality and appearance than with improvements in their oral function.[27] Most of these patients reported positive life changes as a result of surgery. Similar results were obtained by Hutton in his survey of 32 patients who had undergone surgery for mandibular prognathism.[28] Almost unanimous agreement emerged on improved appearance (90%), and 50% reported improvements in their personality. Unfortunately, the author did not measure specific personality traits in this study.

In summary, research in the areas of self-esteem and attractiveness indicates that the face is a major source of one's psychologic identity. Individuals are often judged by others on the basis of facial attractiveness; attractive people are perceived to be more successful and intelligent. Such feedback from society plays an important role in the development of an individual's self-concept and self-confidence. To the extent that a person is rewarded for being attractive, confidence and self-esteem are heightened. For people with dentofacial deformities, self-esteem may be impaired because of teasing and criticism by others. When peers, teachers, and family members convey the message that the individual is not attractive, intelligent, or socially acceptable, the effect on the individual is compounded. However, after correction of the deformity, others' evaluations improve and the individual's self-esteem rises.

Orthognathic surgery differs from surgery for congenital anomalies in that the changes in appearance are less dramatic and improvements in occlusion, mastication, speech, and TM joint function are likely to be major reasons for treatment. Nevertheless, patients undergoing orthognathic surgery usually want and expect esthetic changes. They must adapt not only to changes in their oral function, but also to changes in their perceived appearance and interactions with others. In this chapter, we review patients' motives for and expectations from treatment, reactions to surgery and its outcomes, and adaptations to the changes in facial features and oral function as well as to other people's responses to their new appearance. The effect of deciding against surgery when it has been recommended by specialists is examined. Much of the information has been derived from our own research on the psychologic characteristics of patients undergoing orthognathic surgery or conventional orthodontics.

PSYCHOSOCIAL STUDIES OF PATIENTS WITH DENTOFACIAL DEFORMITIES
The First Study

Kiyak and colleagues have completed two prospective (longitudinal) studies of psychologic factors in which patients completed questionnaires that measured specific psychologic predictors and outcomes associated with surgery and its sequelae. The second study also examined patients who elected conventional orthodontics alone after considering orthognathic surgery.

The first study was undertaken in 1978 to examine systematically patients' motives for seeking orthognathic surgery, the effect of this procedure on people with diverse needs, and patients' satisfaction with treatment outcomes. At that time, no longitudinal observations of patients undergoing orthognathic surgery had yet been reported. Even in the plastic-surgery literature, much of the data came from clinical observations and psychologic measures that were administered retrospectively, but not at a specified period after surgery. In one study, questionnaires were administered 16 weeks to 16 years following surgery.[28]

The first study explored patients' motives for surgery, personality characteristics before and after surgery, and satisfaction with outcomes. Open-ended questions were asked to determine patients' attitudes toward their orthodontic and surgical treatment. Cooperation of patients in completing the 6 questionnaires over a 26-month period was excellent (see Table 3-1 for timeline and sample sizes). Questionnaires were self-administered so that patients could respond in private. At the last presurgical clinic visit, generally within 1 week before surgery, the first questionnaire was given directly to each patient by a member of the research team, who explained the study and the forms. Patients were asked to complete and return this questionnaire *before* undergoing surgery; those which were returned postsurgically were not included in the study. The second questionnaire also was delivered personally to patients on the second postoperative day while they were still in the hospital and then collected before they left the hospital, ensuring a high response rate (72 of the original 74 patients [97%]). With the objective of determining adaptation to maxillomandibular fixation, the third questionnaire was given to patients 2 to 4 weeks later and resulted in an 88% response rate. To assess return to jaw functioning, the fourth questionnaire was mailed to patients 8 to 10 weeks after release from maxillomandibular fixation. Only 2 of the 63 respondents to the third questionnaire failed to return this form (82% of the original sample). A fifth package was mailed to respondents 9 months after surgery, resulting in a 74% response rate.

The final questionnaire sought to assess long-term effects of surgery and orthodontics and was completed 2 years after the patient's surgery date. Even with the drop in participation (N = 50), a 33% attrition rate over 2 years is better than that achieved by most longitudinal studies. The patients who returned the final questionnaires were compared with those who did not complete the study. No significant differences emerged in the distribution of the two groups on relevant study variables, including age, sex, treatment need, functional complaints, motives at entry to the study, and

TABLE 3-1 Questionnaire administration in two longitudinal studies

	Presurgery		Surgery	Postsurgery						
	6 to 12 months presurgery	1 week presurgery	1 day	2 to 4 weeks	6 weeks	4 months	6 months	9 months	24 months
Study 1 Age: 22 ± 7.45	N =	T_1 74		T_2 72	T_3 63		T_4 61		T_5 55	T_6 50
Study 2 Surgery Age: 26 ± 8.5	T_1 N = 122	T_2 103		T_3 112		T_4 112		T_5 112	T_6 109
Orthodontics Age: 24.5 ± 5.2	N = 33	*		32		*		30	30
No treatment Age: 30 ± 4.3	N = 33	*		31		*		29	29

*Questionnaires were not administered to comparison-group patients at T_2 and T_4.

satisfaction immediately after surgery, suggesting that the patients who completed the 24-month assessment were representative of the complete sample of surgery patients.[29]

Because so little research on psychologic factors associated with orthognathic surgery was available before this study, specific hypotheses were not tested. Instead, variables and measures representing psychologic concepts of interest were selected on the basis of several research questions. These focused on motives for treatment, oral function, social adjustment before and after treatment, self-esteem and body image during each treatment phase, extroversion initially and 2 years later, neuroticism, locus of control, and satisfaction with the outcome. No standardized measures existed for most variables; most of the scales were pretested and expanded with open-ended questions. For personality dimensions such as neuroticism, extroversion-introversion, locus of control, and self-esteem, tests that had been standardized with similar populations were used.

The Second Study

The second longitudinal study attempted to examine in greater detail the variables that emerged as significant predictors of long-term outcomes. The study included an evaluation of patients' expectations of functional, social, and esthetic changes; perceptions of facial esthetics; and treatment outcomes, including social integration and depression. In addition, the effect of orthognathic surgery was measured by comparing patients who underwent surgery and orthodontics with those who were recommended to have both but elected orthodontics alone.

In the second study, 6 questionnaires were administered before and up to 24 months after surgery to a new group of 122 patients who underwent surgery between 1981 and 1983 (see Table 3-1). In an attempt to examine patients' personalities and treatment expectations well before surgery, the first questionnaire was administered 6 to 12 months before their anticipated surgery date. The second questionnaire was given to patients during their final presurgical appointment, within 1 week of surgery (as with the first questionnaire in the first study). The third questionnaire was administered to all surgery patients on the day after surgery (as with the second questionnaire in the first study). The fourth questionnaire was mailed to patients just before the wires holding their teeth together were removed to assess patients' experience with fixation (all patients were in maxillomandibular fixation for both of these studies). The fifth and sixth questionnaires were designed to measure long-term outcomes; the fifth was mailed 6 months after surgery (versus 9 months in the first study), and the sixth was a 24-month follow-up questionnaire, similar to the final questionnaire in the first study.

Two comparison groups were included in the second study. In addition to understanding the effect of surgery, we were interested in the effects of conventional orthodontics alone for patients who chose that course. A total of 33 such persons, referred from the same orthodontic practices involved with the surgery patients, were available for this comparison study. Another 33 patients, who were referred for surgery and orthodontics but decided against any treatment, volunteered to participate in the other comparison group. These respondents were matched with surgery patients to establish a similar baseline of knowledge about surgical procedures among all patients in the study. Comparison-group respondents received questionnaires at the same times as their matched surgery patients, except for the second and fourth questionnaires, which were specifically focused on changes associated with surgery. As Table 3-1 shows, the largest sample consisted of surgical patients in the second study (N = 122). Attrition was quite small from presurgery to 24 months postsurgery, despite the fact that some 24-month follow-up questionnaires were sent out up to 36 months after our first contact with the patients. Thus 89% of the original surgery sample completed the fifth questionnaire, and 94.5% returned the sixth. Similarly, 91% of the orthodontics-only group and 88% of the no-treatment sample returned their final questionnaires.

The patients completing these two studies were typical of those in the United States who undergo orthognathic surgery. The majority (65%) were females aged 20 to 29 years. Note in Table 3-1 that patients rejecting all treatment in this sample were significantly older. No national data exist to indicate whether older patients referred for treatment are indeed more likely to decide against surgery and orthodontics. It may be that older patients are more concerned about the risk/benefit issues of surgery than are younger patients, whose parents are often more involved with the decision. The most common surgical procedures in the second study were mandibular advancement (47%), combined mandibular advancement and maxillary intrusion (22%), and maxillary advancement (15%).

The major findings from both studies are presented below. A series of research publications provides greater detail about the measures used and results obtained.[29-37]

PATIENTS BEFORE SURGERY
Motives for Treatment

Patients' motives for surgical correction of a facial deformity have been discussed widely in the plastic surgery and orthognathic surgery literature. In the first study, we examined patients' motives before surgery for the combined orthodontic and surgical procedures they were undergoing, using a checklist developed in pilot studies and asking respondents to indicate other motives that were not included in the checklist.[30] A significant proportion of both females (53%) and males (41%) indicated that esthetic factors or a desire to improve their appearance played a major role in their decision (Table 3-2). A greater proportion stated that improved appearance was an important or moderately important motive in the studies by Laufer and colleagues (89%), Flanary and colleagues (78%), and Jacobson (76%).[38-40] However, esthetic motives were less important in a study of 67 patients in Switzerland,

Parameter	Male (N = 29)		Female (N = 45)	
Professional advice				
Orthodontist	24	83%	34	76%
Family dentist	12	41%	17	38%
Other	5	17%	1	2%
Desire esthetic changes	12	41%	13	53%
Functional problems				
Mastication	12	41%	13	29%
Speech	4	14%	1	2%
TM joint	1	3%	7	16%
Social: family, friends	12	41%	24	53%

TABLE 3-2 **Motives for surgery**

where 30% of the females and 10% of the males primarily desired improved appearance.[41] The differences may result from different cultural values, third-party payment procedures for surgery, or differences in patients' willingness to admit that esthetics played an important role in their decisions. The most frequently mentioned reason for seeking surgery was a professional's advice, most often that of an orthodontist (83% and 76% respectively among men and women). General dentists also served as major sources of advice; 41% of women and 38% of men noted their influence.

These figures are higher than those of Ouelette[42]; 36% of his sample reported that their dentist or physician was the key deciding factor for undergoing treatment. Dental professionals have a powerful influence in helping patients make the decision to undergo treatment. When the patient's perception of need for treatment is reinforced by the dentist's judgment, the patient is more likely to undergo orthodontics and surgery.

It is clear that a desire for functional change is an incentive for many surgical-orthodontic patients. In our sample, 41% of male patients reported problems with mastication and 14% with speech. Comparable rates for females were 29% and 2%, respectively. Laufer and colleagues found that 40% of their patients reported improved chewing as a motive for treatment and 41% desired improved speech.[38] Olson and Laskin reported that 39% expected only better jaw function as a result of treatment, whereas another 44% expected both a functional improvement and greater attractiveness.[43] Not surprisingly, TM joint problems were more often cited by females than by males in our study (16% versus 3.4% reported this problem).

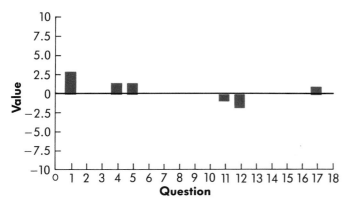

Questions	Score
1. Less difficulty with chewing	3
2. Stop jaw from clicking	0
3. Eat foods unable to eat now	0
4. Better fit of upper/lower teeth	1.5
5. General health improvement	1.5
6. Possible pain after surgery	0
7. Better smile	0
8. Improved profile, jaw and chin	0
9. Straight teeth	0
10. Cost of surgery	0
11. Lost time from work/school	0.8
12. Chance of unsuccessful surgery	1.9
13. Be able to speak clearer	0
14. Less self-conscious	0
15. Perform better in job/school	0
16. Advice of family/friends	0
17. Advice of dentist/orthodontist	0.9
18. Know of someone else's surgery	0

Fig. 3-1. The SEU items are based on interviews with orthognathic-surgery patients, orthodontists, and oral-maxillofacial surgeons. Using a 10-point scale, patients are asked to indicate the importance of each item in the list below the figure and whether they consider it positive (prosurgery), negative (antisurgery), or neutral. The results can be shown graphically as illustrated here for an actual (and not very enthusiastic) patient.

A Scale to Assess Patients' Motives

Patients who decide to undergo surgery may have a different set of motives for treatment or attribute greater importance to such factors as esthetics and social acceptance than do patients who decide against surgery. To test this hypothesis, we developed a measure of patient expectancies, an instrument based on the theory of decision making known as the Subjective Expected Utility (SEU) model. This theory assumes that an individual's likelihood of choosing a particular mode of behavior is determined by the weight he or she attributes to a series of values associated with that behavior; that is, subjective utilities that the individual expects from making that decision. The model has been found to predict with considerable accuracy people's decisions to bear children, to retire, and to seek preventive medical care.[44-46]

TABLE 3-3 Major influences on treatment decisions

Treatment/no treatment		Surgery/no surgery	
Parameter	Value	Parameter	Value
Cost	.86	Cost	.55
Dentist/orthodontist	.38	Family/friends	.49
Straight teeth	.31	Speak clearly	.48
Profile/chin	.26	Chewing/biting	.30
Family/friends	.18	Better occlusion	.28
		Others's surgery	.16

The SEU approach first establishes a series of values associated with a specific decision, both in favor of and opposed to the decision (e.g., the decision to seek preventive dental care is influenced by the cost of dental care—a negative value—versus the advantage of healthy teeth—a positive value). These are established through interviews with experts or peers who have made similar decisions. Once established, the scale can be used by having individuals in that decision situation assign weights and scores to each value in the listing. The scale developed for surgical-orthodontics is illustrated in Fig. 3-1. It was based on a hierarchy of values garnered from open-ended comments by patients in our first study. Six categories of values associated with undergoing or not undergoing surgery were organized within the larger three categories. Each of these categories in turn consisted of three motives for and against surgery. This scale was found to discriminate among the patients who chose surgical-orthodontic treatment, orthodontics only, or rejected all treatment (Table 3-3). In particular, only five items (cost, family or friends' advice, the advice of a dental professional, appearance of teeth, and appearance of profile) were necessary to predict with 80% accuracy whether a patient would choose treatment (surgical and/or orthodontics) or no treatment.

Six items could correctly classify 67% of surgery versus no-surgery cases (cost, family or friends' advice, ability to speak better, ability to chew or bite better, improved occlusion, and knowledge of others' surgery). Note that cost and the advice of family or friends predicted both the overall decision for treatment and the decision to undergo surgery. Thus patients who make a decision in favor of conventional orthodontics or orthognathic surgery have received support in this decision from friends and/or family and perceive the costs of treatment to be manageable. Our findings with the SEU suggest that the decision to seek surgical correction is influenced by functional reasons such as improved speech, chewing, biting, and occlusion. Conversely, the decision to reject surgery and un-

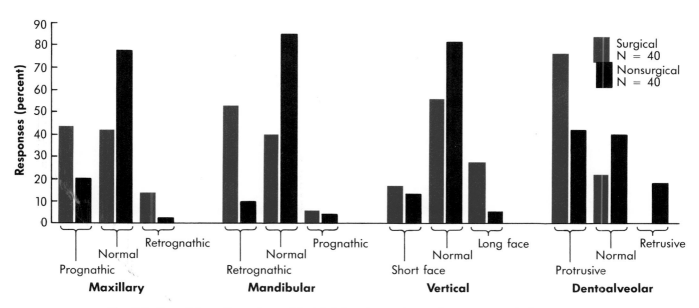

Fig. 3-2. For all four dimensions of facial deformity, patients who accept surgical treatment view themselves as less normal than do those who opt for no treatment or orthodontics only—but there are surprisingly small differences between the groups on cephalometric analysis.

dergo conventional orthodontics seems to be based more on a desire for improved esthetics.

Self-Perceptions of Facial Profile

In an attempt to determine if the severity of the problem (perceived or objective) may explain differences in patients' decisions to undergo surgery, we examined self-ratings; ratings by laypersons, orthodontists, and surgeons; and cephalometric measures of 40 patients in the orthognathic surgery group and of 40 in the orthodontics-only or no-treatment groups. These patients were randomly selected from the total sample of 188 patients in the larger study.

A rating sheet with a series of profile drawings of vertical (short face to long face), maxillary and mandibular (deficient to excessive), and dentoalveolar (retrusive to protrusive) relationships was used to score the severity of the dentofacial problems for each patient. Profile and full-face photographs were used. No information on the patients' decisons regarding treatment was given to the raters. The same four rating scales were used by patients to evaluate their own profiles, but they were not provided with photos of themselves. The results, described in detail by Bell and colleagues,[59] are presented briefly in this chapter.

In comparison with the two nonsurgical groups (who are presented together in Fig. 3-2 because they did not differ significantly), patients who had opted for surgery were significantly less likely to perceive themselves to be in the normal range. On the vertical dimension, most patients rated themselves as normal. However, surgery patients were more likely than the other two groups to rate themselves with long faces and open bites. More viewed themselves in the maxillary prognathic and mandibular retrognathic range than patients who had decided against surgery. They were also more likely to perceive a dentoalveolar protrusion than were the nonsurgical respondents. Indeed, almost 75% of surgery patients rated themselves as protrusive, compared with 45% of nonsurgical patients.

Despite these differences in self-ratings, the groups did not differ significantly in most cephalometric measures corresponding to these dimensions (i.e., SNA, SNB, percent nasal height, Steiner's S-plane, and Ricketts' esthetic plane). Patients who had decided to undergo surgical correction exhibited a mean ANB angle of 5.8 degrees and an A-N-pogonion angle of 9.8 degrees. Patients who had decided against surgery or any treatment had significantly lower mean ANB angles (4.0 degrees) and A-N-pogonion angles (7.4 degrees).

In comparing self-ratings with those of laypersons and dental professionals who were familiar with patients' treatment decisions, we found low but significant correlations among the four groups. Laypersons were more likely to rate all patients in the normal range than were patients themselves. Their ratings were more highly correlated with dental professionals' ratings than with patients' self-ratings. Not surprisingly, correlations between orthodontists' and oral surgeons' ratings were higher than any other pairs of ratings (r = .90 to .97), suggesting similarities in diagnostic perspectives. In addition, professionals' ratings on these four dimensions were more significantly associated

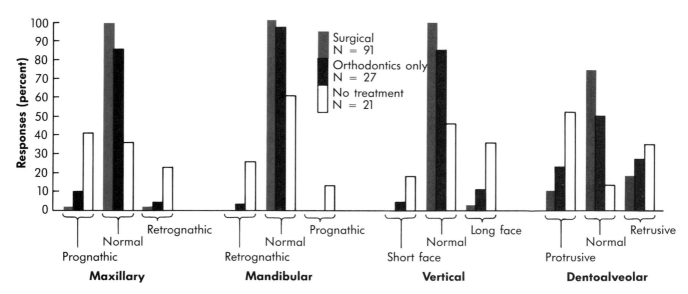

Fig. 3-3. At the 24-month follow-up assessment, nearly all the surgery patients rated themselves as normal on the maxillary, mandibular, and vertical scales, and 75% did so on the dentoalveolar scale, a dramatic improvement (compare with Fig. 3-2). Orthodontics-only patients also rated themselves improved on all scales, but the improvement was not as great.

with the cephalometric assessments of these patients than were the ratings by patients or laypersons.

A subsequent analysis of self-ratings 24 months later by all patients remaining in the study (Fig. 3-3) revealed significant improvements on all four dimensions for surgery patients.[37] Self-assessments by surgery patients were much more likely at 24 months to fall within the normal range than were nonsurgical patients' ratings (see Fig. 3-6). Study participants who had decided against any treatment were least likely to perceive their profiles in the normal range and most likely to rate their profiles in the extreme. It is noteworthy that a greater proportion of orthodontics-only patients judged their profiles to be in the normal range after their treatment was completed than they had 2 to 3 years earlier. The greatest improvements occurred for this group on the mandibular, maxillary, and dentoalveolar dimensions. Most continued to rate themselves as normal on the vertical scale.

These findings indicate that surgical patients experience the greatest improvement in their subjective assessments of facial profiles. Orthodontics alone can also result in improved self-evaluations, but to a lesser extent than the combined procedure. There are two possible explanations for the greater esthetic improvement reported by the surgical patients as compared with the orthodontics-only group. One is that they really do have more changes, which often is the case. The other is that surgical patients have an exaggerated negative assessment of their appearance. Indeed, it may be this extreme perception of their dentofacial disharmony that motivates them to seek surgery, whereas

others who see themselves in the more normal range do not perceive a need for surgery. The latter group may opt for orthodontics only, or no treatment as in this sample. The results are consistent with the findings of Lewis and colleagues among children seeking orthodontic treatment.[60] In comparing children with malocclusion to children with normal occlusion in their preference for photographs of various occlusal situations, these researchers found that the children with malocclusion were more negative about occlusal relationships that resembled their own.

Sex Differences

Another area of interest is sex differences in motives for and satisfaction with surgery. In particular, esthetic improvement has been suggested as a major goal of women undergoing orthognathic surgery. This is not surprising because the psychoanalytic literature is replete with descriptions of the importance of facial attractiveness for women. Deutsch has stated that "narcissism is a specific and differentiating trait of femininity."[48] Horney suggests that physical attractiveness assumes a greater role for women who are unable to form satisfactory relationships with men than for those who do.[49] Such women attribute this failure to a real or imaginary defect. Broverman and colleagues have found experimental evidence that women place relatively greater importance on physical attractiveness.[50] Differential attention to their own physical features is illustrated by Kurtz' finding that women can more easily distinguish what they like and dislike about their bodies than can men of the same age, who give only global self-descriptions.[51] Because of the growing acceptance of cosmetic surgery among men, men and women may be more similar in their views today in the attention they give to physical attractiveness.

Cosmetic-Surgery Patients

Whether the surgery is for a severe or mild deformity, often it is assumed that women seeking surgery to alter facial appearance are more neurotic, more narcissistic, and more difficult to satisfy than are men in the same situation. However, studies of personality and motivational differences have produced disparate results. One limitation is that many of these studies focus only on females or on males. For example, Meyer and colleagues conducted psychiatric interviews with 30 women seeking rhinoplasty and found that fully half could be given a psychiatric diagnosis, particularly as having neurotic, obsessive, or schizoid tendencies.[26] Others were classified as obsessive personalities. Unfortunately, the researchers did not compare these women with men seeking similar surgery.

Webb and colleagues interviewed 43 women seeking face-lifts.[52] Most of the women had low self-esteem, rigid attitudes, and high expectations of improved appearance. In a series of studies conducted at Johns Hopkins University, Edgerton and Knorr found that 72% of the patients seeking cosmetic surgery could be given a psychiatric diagnosis.[53] Depression, low self-esteem, and hysterical traits were observed in 60%. Contrary to popular beliefs, men seeking rhinoplasty were described as having more psychologic disturbances than women in the same group, although several cases of personality disorders were found among women. These conclusions have been supported by Edgell.[54] However, in one of the few systematic investigations (using standardized personality scales) of patients undergoing cosmetic surgery, Shipley and colleagues found results that contradict many of these clinical observations.[55] They concluded that women seeking breast augmentation were just as psychologically stable as women who were satisfied with their physical features. The only significant difference was their greater concern with physical attractiveness and dress. Using a series of personality traits, Reich found that most females who sought cosmetic surgery had normal personality characteristics.[56] He suggests that this may reflect the increased acceptance of esthetic surgery today. Note that the studies conducted by Edgerton and Knorr[53] and by Edgell[54] are almost 20 years old; those by Shipley and colleagues[55] and Reich[56] are more recent.

Another area of research concerns sex differences in motives for cosmetic surgery. Schultz-Coulon reported that men seeking rhinoplasty gave an equal number of functional and appearance motives, whereas for women, reasons of appearance prevailed.[57] Hay found

that married women thought cosmetic surgery would give them a new start on life, whereas men more often believed it would improve their career prospects.[58] These findings support the traditional sex role stereotypes of women as more concerned with appearance and men with achievement. Unfortunately, little systematic research exists to refute these assertions.

Orthognathic-Surgery Patients

In comparing some personality characteristics of male and female patients before orthognathic surgery, we found that although the women had higher scores on measures of neuroticism, both men and women scored within the normal range, notably better than the cosmetic-surgery population. Women in our sample gave less positive self-evaluations than did men on the facial body-image measure, with greater variation across items describing the face, as did the cosmetic-surgery patients reported by Kurtz.[51] However, males and females in the orthognathic group did not differ on extroversion, self-esteem, and overall body-image scores at the presurgical assessment.[30] A comparison of males and females 2 years after surgery revealed no significant differences on any of these variables; indeed, females experienced significantly greater improvement in facial body image following surgery than did male patients.[29]

Sex differences were not significant in postsurgical satisfaction or in self-reports of pain. However, two personality variables appeared to moderate these effects. Men who were more introverted reported more postoperative pain than those who were extroverted. Among women, the discriminating variable appeared to be neuroticism. The higher her score on the neuroticism scale, the more likely was a woman to report pain immediately after surgery, but these differences did not last beyond the first few days after surgery.

RESPONSE TO TREATMENT
Functional Outcomes

Patients generally adapted well to the physical and psychologic changes that they had experienced. Orthodontic treatment was completed for 44% of the sample by 9 months and for all patients by 24 months. Self-reports revealed considerable satisfaction in all areas of oral function (Table 3-4). At 9 months, nearly all the respondents indicated that their occlusion was improved. Only 7% thought it was worse, and this dropped to 5% at 24 months. Similarly, 75% of those with presurgery TM joint problems reported improvement, but at 9 months, 25% reported more problems in this area than before surgery. By 24 months, however, only 2% of the sample reported TM joint difficulties, as opposed to 35% presurgically.

Some degree of paresthesia persisted in 49% of the patients at the final follow-up session, mostly in the

---

TABLE 3-4 Functional problems before and after surgery

Problem	Percent of patients reporting problem		
	Before surgery N = 74	9 months after surgery N = 55	2 years after surgery N = 50
Occlusion	84.6	7.1	5.1
Mastication	50.0	10.5	12.0
TM joint	35.0	24.6	2.0
Maxillary sinus	14.0	25.0	18.9

TABLE 3-5 Surgery-related problems 2 days to 2 years after surgery

Problem	Percent of patients reporting problem		
	Immediately after surgery N = 74	9 months after surgery N = 55	2 years after surgery N = 50
Paresthesia	90.1	58.0	49.0
Pain	81.2	7.4	16.7
Scars	15.0	16.5	17.5

---

chin and lower-lip region (Table 3-5). Reports of pain had diminished by 9 months, such that only 7% described continuing pain or discomfort. It is surprising that there was a noticeable increase in the proportion reporting facial pain at the 24 month follow-up session, from 7.4% at 9 months to 16.7% at 24 months.

One objective of the 24-month follow-up session was to examine the patients' views of their nutritional status in more detail.[62] Mastication had improved for 56% of the patients by 9 months and for 88% by 24 months, but 10.5% reported more problems than before surgery in this area at the 9-month follow-up session. At the 24-month assessment, 79% reported better eating habits, an increased variety of foods consumed, and other general nutritional improvements. Despite these improvements, 30% indicated some problems in this area, including difficulty with mouth opening, biting, and chewing. Patients who expressed nutritional problems were significantly less satisfied with the results of surgery than were patients who reported only improvements at the final assessment.

Despite lingering problems for some people, most patients reported very high satisfaction with the outcomes; 84% rated their satisfaction levels as moderate to high. At the 9-month follow-up assessment, 92% said they would recommend the surgery to others. This level of satisfaction remained through the final assessment and is consistent with the findings of Rittersma and colleagues in the Netherlands.[61] In their sample of patients who were interviewed at least 1 year after surgery, 94% expressed satisfaction and 87% would recommend the surgery to others. It may be that cognitive dissonance is operating here; that is, after undergoing such a major surgery and its orthodontic sequelae, surgical patients feel the need to justify their experience by expressing high satisfaction.

The Relationship of Personality Characteristics to Reported Outcomes

The personality dimensions of neuroticism and locus of control affect the outcomes reported by patients.[31] Using Eysenck's Personality Inventory,[47] we found that neuroticism (the potential for one's emotions to shift suddenly and often erratically) was significantly correlated with satisfaction in the early postoperative period. The higher the neuroticism score, the more a patient complained about eating and speech just after surgery. Reports of pain and swelling were also more widespread among patients with neurotic tendencies. Similarly, the more external a patient's locus of control (i.e., the greater the belief that his or her fate is controlled by powerful others), the more likely was that individual to report eating and speech difficulties after surgery.

Overall satisfaction immediately after surgery was better predicted by a patient's expectations of pain and paresthesia than by locus of control or neuroticism (Table 3-6). Patients who reported less pain and numbness than they expected, and those with lower neuroticism scores, were more satisfied with surgical outcomes

TABLE 3-6 Predictors of postoperative satisfaction

Parameter	Immediately after surgery	9 months after surgery
Pain experienced versus expected	$p < .02$	NS
Paresthesia experienced versus expected	$p < .05$	NS
Neuroticism score	$p < .05$	NS
Locus of control score	NS	NS

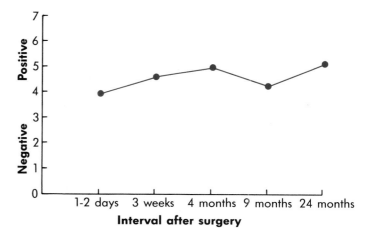

Fig. 3-4. Overall satisfaction with the outcomes is generally high at all postsurgical assessments. In the first study, we observed a statistically significant improvement from the immediate postoperative stage to 2 years later, with a slight decline at 9 months.

than those who had anticipated less pain and numbness and were more neurotic. These effects did not persist beyond the first few weeks after surgery.

Although neuroticism emerged as a significant predictor of several short-term outcomes, it did not affect satisfaction in the long term. A neurotic personality style does not necessarily indicate a problem patient. These individuals may be more sensitized to negative stimuli during their early recovery period, but they are no more likely than other patients to express long-term dissatisfaction or to complain of surgical sequelae.

The image of the chronically dissatisfied patient does not follow from our findings. Indeed, in our 9-month and 24-month follow-up assessments, we found no significant differences in complaints by personality type.[29-31]

Satisfaction with Treatment and Its Components

Both of the studies included longitudinal analyses of overall satisfaction; overall body image, profile, and facial body image; and overall self-esteem and components of self-esteem. Complete data on these variables were available for 46 patients (62% of the total) in the first study and for 83 surgery patients (68%) in the second study. Although there were interesting patterns of change, these measures were more stable than in plastic-surgery patients.[5]

Overall Satisfaction

Significant changes in overall satisfaction ocurred as patients progressed through the postsurgical period (Fig. 3-4). Overall satisfaction steadily improved from the immediate postsurgery period to 4 months, but showed a decline at the 9-month assessment.

Self-Esteem

In the area of self-esteem (the individual's assessment of his or her own self-worth), we found high scores before and up to 4 months after surgery, a decline at 9 months, and an improvement again at 24 months (Fig. 3-5). The 24-month scores were not significantly differ-

ent from presurgical levels. This was true for overall self-esteem and its three components: self-concept vis-a-vis social interactions, family relations, and feelings about oneself (i.e., satisfaction with one's level of self-control, intelligence, and ability to manage problems). The finding that self-esteem remains high during the first 4 months after surgery has been supported by subsequent research by Auerbach and colleagues.[63] It is noteworthy that patients undergoing surgical orthodontics express self-esteem levels in the moderately high range, not unlike the general population on which this scale was first developed. Unlike people with major

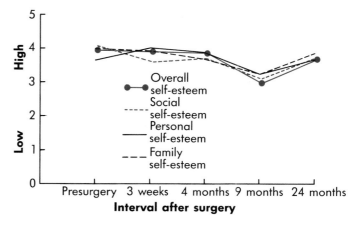

Fig. 3-5. Overall self-esteem is generally in the high-neutral range for surgical patients. The first study revealed a decline in self-esteem at the 9-month follow-up assessment, with a return to moderately high levels at 2 years. The curves for the components of self-esteem (personal, family, and social self-esteem) were very similar.

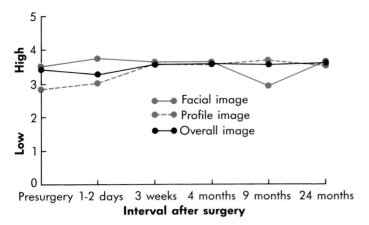

Fig. 3-6. Overall body image *(in red)* was found to be in the moderate range throughout the course of treatment. Its variations from pre- to postsurgery are not statistically significant. Facial body image *(in black)* is generally high in surgical patients and shows a slight improvement up to 4 months after surgery. Note the significant drop at 9 months and recovery at 24 months. The decline occurred in patients whose orthodontics had not yet been completed. Profile body image *(in dashed black)* was generally lower than facial or overall image. Although this improved over treatment, the changes were not statistically significant.

dentofacial deformities described in the beginning of this chapter, it appears that patients seeking orthoganthic surgery generally have a high evaluation of their self-worth.

Body Image

Body image is defined as the individual's self-concept of his or her physical features. It develops over time, influenced by one's own awareness and feedback from others. The higher the score on a body-image scale, the more attractive an individual feels. Overall body image remained relatively steady through the course of treatment in our studies, but profile image, which had been most negative of all aspects of body image presurgically, improved at 3 weeks after surgery and stabilized at a higher level. It is noteworthy that self-assessed facial image showed a sharp decline at 9 months and improved again by 24 months. Neither the profile assessment nor the overall body-image assessment showed such a decline; instead both remained high after the increase at 3 weeks. This difference may reflect a critical period in the process of integrating new facial features into an individual's evaluations of his or her facial appearance during the first 9 months after surgery (Fig. 3-6).

The Effects of Postsurgical Orthodontics

To determine whether the decline in satisfaction and facial image at 9 months could be attributed to respon-

dents who were still wearing orthodontic appliances at this time, we examined longitudinal patterns in the areas of satisfaction, body image, and self-esteem for those still under orthodontic therapy separately from those who had already completed their treatment. Those who were still in orthodontics showed significant declines in overall satisfaction and self-esteem, as well as in the three components of self-esteem. In contrast, respondents who had had their orthodontic appliances removed showed a significant increase in satisfaction. Only on the personal dimension of self-esteem, the component that defines the individual's feelings about himself/herself as an individual rather than as a member of a social network, was there a decline at 9 months for patients who were out of orthodontic treatment.

The finding of a "slump" in psychologic well-being at the 9-month assessment offers a warning for practitioners working with orthognathic-surgery patients. By this time, most patients have recovered fully from the surgery and are experiencing improved oral function and better nutritional patterns than before surgery. But a sense of incompleteness, or a lack of closure in their treatment, arises if their active orthodontic treatment is not finished in a reasonable time. The clear distinction in interpersonal well-being between those whose orthodontic appliances have been removed and those who are still in bands suggests that wearing retainers is less of a problem than wearing major orthodontic appliances. Both orthodontists and oral surgeons must repeatedly warn these patients that postsurgical orthodontic treatment is necessary and that it proceeds more slowly than surgery. However, completing the treatment as soon after surgery as possible should be the goal.

Comparison of Orthognathic-Surgery Patients with Orthodontics-Only and No-Treatment Patients

Body image was assessed again at all measurements in our second study, which included patients who opted for orthodontic treatment only or rejected any treatment. In addition to using the approach developed for the first study, we developed a parallel measure indicating the relative importance of each body part. Because the two scores were correlated, we report only the results of the first measure.

As Figs. 3-7 and 3-8 illustrate, average scores on the body-image scale were at about the mid-point of the scale for all groups. Despite this, both overall body image and facial image were lowest at the initial assessment for surgery patients and then improved over the 24-month follow-up period. Orthodontics-only patients also showed some improvement, but less than did the surgical patients. The no-treatment patients experienced a slight improvement, then a decline by the

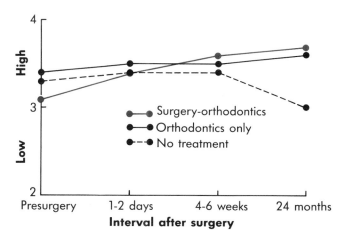

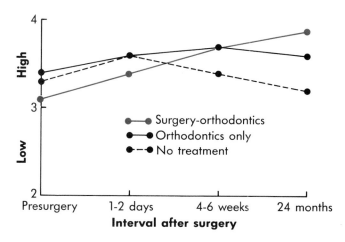

Fig. 3-7. Overall body-image scores for surgical-orthodontic, orthodontics only, and no-treatment patients. In the second study, surgery patients initially expressed a lower body image than did nonsurgical and no-treatment patients. However, they showed a significant improvement over the next 2 years, whereas the body image declined when all treatment was declined. Patients who received conventional orthodontic treatment retained a moderately high body image over 24 months.

Fig. 3-8. Facial body-image scores for surgical-orthodontic, orthodontics only, and no-treatment patients. As with overall body image, facial body image was lowest initially for surgery patients and then significantly improved, so that it was highest after 24 months. The changes for orthodontics-only and no-treatment patients were not statistically significant.

end of our interviews. In contrast to our findings in the first study,[29,31] body image remained high at the intermediate (6 months) point for the two treatment groups. However, we did not assess patients at 9 months in the second study. The "slump" observed in the first study among those still in orthodontic bands at 9 months may be a phenomenon that develops later than 6 months after surgery.

It is noteworthy that patients who decided against any treatment reported a significantly different pattern of body image than did surgical patients. Although they were highest initially on both facial and overall body image, they expressed much lower levels 2 years later than did either treatment group, lower even than their initial body image. This suggests caution in advising patients about surgery; although the practitioner cannot ethically force patients to undergo treatment, it appears that people who should have surgery but reject any treatment fare badly in the long run. Their self-image deteriorates as they realize that they have not changed physically. In extreme cases, it may even be useful to suggest psychologic counseling for such patients who reject orthodontic or surgical treatment.

Pretreatment Needs and Posttreatment Outcomes

The presence or absence of problems with oral function, types of surgery, or specific motives had no effect on patient satisfaction, body image, and self-esteem and cannot predict a patient's likelihood of successful or unsuccessful postsurgical adaptation. Patients with several functional problems before surgery were just as

likely to be satisfied with outcomes, even if surgery did not improve these functions. Similarly, respondents who underwent extensive surgery for correction of both maxillary and mandibular conditions were just as likely to report a willingness to undergo surgery again as those who underwent mandibular surgery alone. Patients who reported multiple problems of pain, paresthesia, and oral function (TM joint and occlusion) at 9 and 24 months were compared with those who did not have such complaints, including those with only 1 or 2 problems at the long-term assessment. No significant differences emerged in satisfaction, desire to undergo surgery again, overall self-esteem, overall body image, or any components of these last two personality variables.

Satisfaction was influenced by difficulties in eating (e.g., opening the mouth, chewing, avoiding certain foods) in patients whose problems in this area continued or emerged after surgery. That is, people who reported problems with mouth opening or eating after surgery were less likely to report satisfaction up to 2 years after completing treatment. Satisfaction also was less when the patient perceived the esthetic changes to be less positive than expected.

It is noteworthy that patients react more negatively to less-than-adequate esthetic or nutritional changes than to problems with persistent pain and paresthesia following surgery. In discussions with patients before treatment, greater emphasis needs to be placed on the range of esthetic and oral functional outcomes of surgery and the possibility that these changes may not fulfill patients' expectations. Research by Robinson and Merav on thoracic patients[64] and a report by Lewis on

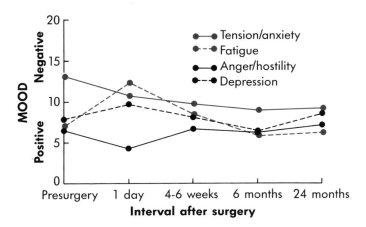

Fig. 3-9. Mood-state scores for surgical-orthodontic patients (N = 72). Surgical patients had high levels of tension and anxiety just before surgery, with a steady and significant decline to moderately low levels by 24 months. Contrary to our hypotheses, depression rose to its highest level just after surgery but remained quite low throughout the postsurgical course.

plastic-surgery patients[65] reveals the importance of repeating key issues with patients several times before initiating treatment and reiterating the possibility of less-than-ideal outcomes.

Transient Emotional Reactions to Surgery

Another objective of our research has been to examine the effect of surgery on patients' self-reported mood states, particularly depression. In the first study, emotional well-being was not measured systematically, but several patients spontaneously described experiences of depression and feeling alone and ignored by family and friends, especially at the intermediate postsurgical stages.[29,31] For these reasons, we selected a standardized test of emotional well-being, known as the Profile of Mood States (POMS), for use in the subsequent study.[66] The instrument represents six moods: depression-dejection, tension-anxiety, anger-hostility, confusion, fatigue, and vigor. It was administered just before surgery and at all postsurgical periods.[34]

Analysis of POMS scores from just before surgery to 2 years after surgery revealed significant changes (Fig. 3-9). The greatest shifts occurred just after surgery. Anticipatory anxiety was demonstrated by high scores on the tension-anxiety dimension at the presurgical measurement, which were greatest just before surgery and most positive at the 6-month follow-up assessment. Depression scores were highest just after surgery and steadily decreased at the 4- to 6-week and 6-month assessments. Although changes for the total group were not statistically significant, there were several patients with a dramatic rise in depression scores at various periods postsurgically. A perusal of their questionnaire responses at each measurement period revealed the following:

- Patients who reported higher-than-average depression at a given measurement period scored in the upper quartile of the neuroticism scale for this sample.
- The same patients reported higher expectations for improvement in oral function and interpersonal relations than did other patients.
- These patients were experiencing other major life events at the same time that they reported the dramatic increase in their depression levels.

These findings for individual cases were borne out by a series of correlations between POMS scores and personality variables. Depression, tension, anger, and confusion were directly correlated with neuroticism at all measurement periods, suggesting that the more neurotic a surgical patient, the more labile his or her emotions. Furthermore, satisfaction with surgical outcomes at all postoperative stages was greatest among patients with low scores on depression, anger, tension, confusion, and fatigue measures; that is, among patients experiencing the fewest emotional problems. Surgical patients experiencing negative moods at the immediate postsurgery, 4- to 6-week, and 6-month assessments were also more likely to report greater pain, surgical discomfort, and problems with function and interpersonal relations.

These correlations do not indicate a direction of causality. Persistent pain or problems with oral and social functioning following surgery may cause negative emotional states; it is equally likely that negative moods may heighten a patient's perception of pain or problems with oral and social functioning. The practitioner is warned to examine both directions of causality in patients who display anger or depression and complain about postsurgical problems and to forewarn patients about depression as a potential short-term complication of surgery.

A clinical psychologic study by Stewart and Sexton of six patients who reported postoperative depression provides some insights into reasons for such a reaction.[67] Drugs used for pain and anxiety management (e.g., meperidine [Demerol] and diazepam [Valium]) may produce unanticipated depressive moods. In addition, the change in diet that is necessary for up to 6 weeks following surgery may influence patients' moods. Even though a high-protein, high-calorie diet is prescribed, many patients emphasize the liquid intake but avoid the necessary calories, some because they view this period as an opportunity to lose weight. Those experiencing rapid weight loss during the recovery phase may be at greater risk for depression. Stewart and Sexton provide evidence that weight loss is associated with increased secretion of cortisol and increased corticotropin-releasing factor, which can produce sev-

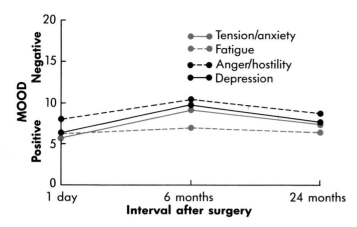

Fig. 3-10. Mood-state scores for orthodontics-only patients (N = 26). Patients undergoing orthodontics-only treatment experienced significant negative changes in mood states at the 6-month assessment (which was 12 to 18 months after orthodontics began because the timing was matched to a surgery patient). The scores improved at 24 months, when orthodontics usually had been completed.

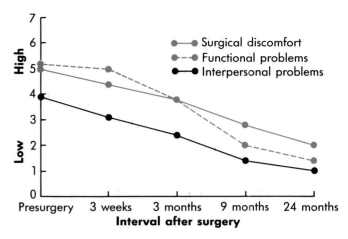

Fig. 3-11. Surgical-orthodontic patients: changes in expectations and experiences. In comparing patients' expectations from surgery with their postoperative experiences, we found that expectations matched the actual experience well for most patients, and that, as we expected, reports became less negative over time.

eral physiologic and behavorial symptoms of depression.

One of the most striking findings in mood states was the difference between orthognathic-surgery patients and those who underwent orthodontics alone (compare Fig. 3-9 with Fig. 3-10). Surgical patients expressed a more postive mood, less fatigue, more vigor, less depression, and less tension at 6 months than at the immediate postsurgical assessments. In contrast, orthodontics-only patients reported greater depression, tension-anxiety, and anger-hostility at the later assessment.

To determine whether patients who were still in orthodontic appliances were responsible for this effect, we compared 3 groups of orthodontic patients at the 6-month follow-up assessment: 12 were still in bands, 13 were out of bands but in retainers, and the remainder were wearing a splint. Although no statistically significant differences emerged across the subgroups, the direction of differences was consistent. Orthodontics-only patients who were still wearing bands expressed the greatest depression, tension-anxiety, confusion, and anger-hostility at this 6-month assessment, whereas those who were out of bands had the most positive scores on these dimensions of moods, but still not as positive as those who had surgery.

Orthodontic treatment, independent of surgery, is associated with emotional shifts that are at least partially alleviated by debanding. The patient may not feel totally free of treatment after debanding because he or she must continue to wear retainers indefinitely, but this is equally true for those who have surgery. As patients who were referred for surgery but instead chose

orthodontics alone approach the end of treatment, it becomes more obvious that orthodontic treatment alone is insufficient to correct the existing malrelation between the upper and lower jaws. These patients may have finally realized that by deciding against surgery, they were settling for a less-than-optimal solution.

Patients' Expectations versus Outcomes

The first study revealed that patients' expectations before surgery significantly predicted satisfaction with the outcomes. To measure more systematically what expectations patients had and to what extent these were fulfilled, we developed a questionnaire to indicate how much discomfort the respondent expected. At each postoperative assessment, patients were asked to rate how much discomfort they were actually experiencing. The results of our pre- and postsurgical comparisons are described in detail in a recent publication.[36] A brief summary of these findings is presented here.

Factor analyses at all measurement periods revealed three major dimensions: (1) oral function (e.g., eating, swallowing, speaking), (2) postsurgical discomfort (e.g., numbness, swelling), and (3) interpersonal relations (e.g., being out in public, feeling depressed or blue). Changes from presurgery to 2 years after surgery on each dimension were analyzed and are presented in Fig. 3-11.

We found no significant differences from presurgery to immediate postsurgery, suggesting that the surgery patients as a group were generally well informed and realistic about what to expect from the procedure. The areas with the greatest expectations of discomfort were functional problems and surgical discomfort. Patients expected and experienced far fewer problems in the area of interpersonal relations. Patients were most accurate in their expectations regarding the first few days following their surgery. Their experiences during maxillomandibular fixation and later were less stressful than anticipated.

Individual patients had expectations that were inconsistent with their experiences at the early postsurgical stages. A difference between what the patient expected and what he or she experienced predicted dissatisfaction and mood disturbance immediately after surgery and at the 2-year follow-up assessment. In addition, patients who were described as "vigilant copers," those expecting moderate to high numbers of problems, had lower mood scores and expressed greater dissatisfaction than patients described as "avoidant copers," those expecting few problems.

Our results suggest that patients with a pessimistic outlook toward their surgery seek to confirm their expectations by reporting more problems with the surgery and by indicating dissatisfaction with the outcomes of surgery. This is consistent with the theory of self-fulfilling prophecies; the more people expect problems to occur with a given experience, the more they will subsequently find such problems. Furthermore, correlational tests at each postsurgical assessment revealed a significant association between problems in a given area and overall satisfaction at the immediate and intermediate postoperative periods. However, at the 24-month follow-up assessment, these correlations were no longer significant. Mood state was the only area that reflected patients' dissatisfaction at this final assessment. Patients who continued to experience problems with oral function and interpersonal relations, though few in number, had more negative scores on the measures of depression, anger, hostility, tension and anxiety.

The finding that vigilant copers fared worse after surgery than did avoiders suggests that vigilance may result in unnecessary anxiety and, as George and Scott[68] and George and colleagues[69] reported, may serve as a self-fulfilling prophecy. Despite their unusually high concern and focus on potential problems associated with surgery, vigilant copers in this group were not necessarily more informed about the surgery than were avoiders. Vigilant copers may tend to be more anxious individuals or express more situational anxiety in a stressful situation such as surgery. The avoidant copers, on the other hand, may not necessarily have been denying the threatening aspects of surgery, but instead may have been quite realistic about the risks associated with these surgical outcomes.

Perhaps the definition of "unrealistic expectations" should be modified for this type of surgery; it may be that the individual who expects serious problems from surgery is more unrealistic than one who expects few problems. The patient with a heightened anticipation or anxiety that exceeds the actual level of problems usually associated with orthognathic surgery may report dissatisfaction later because of a discrepancy between expectations and outcomes. This is consistent with the conclusions of Cohen and Roth[70] and Miller and Mangan.[71] Nevertheless, it is crucial to prepare patients thoroughly for the procedures they will undergo. Without attributing a negative value to the experiences or describing them as problems, the orthodontist and oral surgeon must inform patients about each stage of the surgical process. Our results and those of Olson and Laskin[43] suggest that patients want to be informed about the treatment but do not necessarily want the information to be described as "risks" or "problems."

The results of these studies raise an important dilemma for the orthodontist and oral surgeon. Facts about the duration of pain, paresthesia, hospital stay, recall appointments, and methods of enhancing one's oral functions after surgery must be emphasized. Current doctrines of informed consent often are interpreted as requiring that the patient be told about all possible risks of surgery, resulting in undue anxiety in many patients. But to what extent should potentially serious but statistically improbable events be emphasized in favor of the many positive outcomes of treatment? The dilemma between creating a well-informed versus a fearful patient will continue to be a critical issue for the practitioner so long as concerns about informed consent and malpractice overshadow the personal needs of patients. See Chapter 6 for a further discussion of this issue.

APPLICATION OF RESEARCH FINDINGS TO PATIENT MANAGEMENT
Summary of Research Findings

The results of our longitudinal studies and the work of others suggest that patients undergoing orthognathic surgery nearly always are within the psychologically normal range in self-esteem, body image, neuroticism, and mood states. As a group, they are more emotionally stable and have a higher self-esteem than people who seek plastic surgery. Their greatest concern before treatment appears to be self-consciousness regarding their facial body image, but functional problems also are important to nearly all of those who want esthetic improvement and are the most important for a significant minority. Patients who choose surgical correction for a dentofacial deformity tend to regard their dentofacial deformity as more severe than do those patients with similar problems who have decided against surgical treatment and are undergoing orthodontics only. Nevertheless, the orthodontics only group may experience greater changes in their emotional state during the course of treatment. Orthodontics-only patients report more negative emotions during the later stages of their treatment than do surgical patients, a finding one would not expect from orthodontic patients for whom surgery was never recommended.

Most patients adjust quite rapidly to the changes brought about by orthognathic surgery. Females with a tendency toward neuroticism and introverted males are more likely to report problems with immediate postoperative pain. Patients of either sex who tend toward neuroticism and an external locus of control report more problems with eating and speech in the immediate postoperative period. Major changes in facial appearance appear to be readily integrated into the individual's self-concept and to fulfill the patient's goals of improved appearance. Contrary to the literature on cosmetic surgery, most patients undergoing orthognathic surgery readily accept changes in appearance and are satisfied with the esthetic effects. Besides esthetics, patients generally seek treatment for functional problems, including difficulties with mastication, food selection, speech, and the TM joint. Their expectations are generally fulfilled within 24 months following surgery.

Although 85% to 90% of the patients undergoing surgical-orthodontic treatment eventually indicate that they are satisfied with the treatment and would recommend it to others, the percentage of patients who are satisfied soon after surgery is much lower. In the short term, postsurgical discomfort and functional problems are causes of dissatisfaction to the extent that they were not anticipated—but patients who anticipated high levels of discomfort are more likely to report dissatisfaction. Personality traits, particularly the degree of neuroticism, have an effect on short-term satisfaction but not on the long-term outcome. If postsurgical orthodontic treatment has not been completed by 9 months, patients who have less positive mood states are more likely to express dissatisfaction. In the long term, poorer esthetic results than the patient expected seem to be the main cause of dissatisfaction.

Recommendations for Interaction with Patients

Our findings point up the importance of determining what each patient expects from treatment. Nearly every patient has both functional and esthetic concerns, but all variations in emphasis are present in a typical patient population. If a patient focuses on jaw function, he or she nearly always reports improvement and satisfaction, even if there is paresthesia or limitation of range of motion after surgery. If he or she focuses on esthetics, the likelihood of a satisfactory outcome is better than it is with patients who seek purely cosmetic surgery, but the chance of dissatisfaction is greater. For this reason, we suggest that the functional improvements from treatment should be emphasized in consultations with surgical-orthodontic patients, rather than

making esthetic improvement the only reason for treatment. A patient who deep down inside is unsure about the esthetic changes nevertheless can accept the treatment result as satisfactory if he or she can see a functional improvement.

It is important to consider the patients' motives for treatment, counsel them realistically about achieving their expectations, and continue working with them long after surgery to help them adjust to the changes they are bound to experience. The results point to the need for systematic selection of patients, preparation for surgical treatment, and careful psychologic management throughout the course of surgical and orthodontic treatment. The hithertofore neglected patient who decides to select orthodontics only, even though surgery has been recommended, may in fact require as much attention and support from the dental team as does a patient who undergoes orthognathic surgery.

Rittersma and colleagues have emphasized the importance of rapport-building and consistency in communications with patients, preferably by the same practitioners who initiate, carry out, and complete all phases of treatment.[61] This could prevent postoperative surprises and the perception that patients have not been adequately prepared, as was found in Rittersma's study and a similar retrospective study by Flanary and colleagues.[39] In a recently completed longitudinal study of 55 orthognathic-surgery patients, Holman found that 35% of the patients complained about a lack of information about their treatment and inattention from and poor rapport with their dental team up to 6 months following surgery.[73] Every effort must be made to rectify this situation in the future. Holman's study also points to the importance of emotional support from significant others to enhance the patient's adaptation and satisfaction with surgical outcomes in the first few months after surgery. It is important to involve key family members and/or friends in treatment decisions from the beginning.

Our results support the importance of providing greater psychosocial support and encouragement for the patient with a neurotic personality style, especially in the early stages of treatment. Both the surgical-orthodontic team and the patient's family must provide this support. Neurotic patients can indeed benefit from combined surgical and orthodontic therapy, but their treatment will require greater understanding and patience from all those involved.

Our research in this field has taken us into the realm of testing alternative modes of patient preparation. The feasibility and effectiveness of individual consultation with a psychologist, patient support groups, and patient education materials are being tested among both surgical and orthodontics-only patients. Individual consultation with a psychologist can be quite useful for patients who have special problems, but it is not prac-

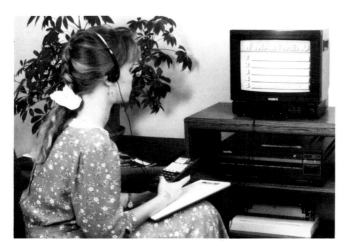

Fig. 3-12. Patient education using an interactive videodisc requires a videodisc player with a computer interface (usually built into the player) so that the patient can choose from the menu of items on the disc. This is the most flexible approach to presentation of educational materials yet devised.

tical or necessary for most of those who seek surgical-orthodontic treatment. Better guidelines for selecting patients who need this referral are needed, and with continuing experience we hope to be able to provide these in the future. Interaction with other patients who are undergoing similar treatment seems to be quite helpful. At the stage when patients are deciding whether to accept a recommendation for surgery, they often ask if it is possible to talk with others who have had this treatment, and the treatment team should make every effort to make this possible. Presurgical patients find it useful to hear "testimonials" from other patients about their surgical experience.

Patient education materials offer at least two major advantages. The information is provided in a standard way so that no important points are omitted, and the patient can review it repeatedly to gain a better understanding of the process. Booklets and video tapes have been used successfully. The most recent innovation in this area (Fig. 3-12) is the interactive videodisc. A commercially available program for orthognathic surgery patients, produced by the Videodiscovery Company of Seattle, allows some flexibility in the presentation. Potential complications, pain, paresthesia, diet, oral hygiene, and recovery are presented in a "menu" format. This makes it possible for patients and family members to select the topics that are of greatest interest to them, see them in order of personal priority, and test their understanding by taking an interactive quiz on each topic. Evaluations of the videodisc have shown that it enhances understanding of the surgery and its sequelae and the role of family and friends during the recovery process; it also serves as a springboard for more indepth discussions with the oral surgeon before surgery.

A series of suggestions and comments for interaction with the patient and others is provided in Table 3-7. Further research is needed to provide a better understanding of the factors that influence psychologic outcomes at each stage of treatment. We hope to develop even more effective methods to assist patients to make the best decision regarding treatment vis-a-vis their expectations and potential outcomes and to help them understand their treatment, thereby easing the stress associated with surgical-orthodontic treatment.

REFERENCES

1. Pertschuk MJ, Whitaker LA: Psychosocial considerations in craniofacial deformity, Clin Plast Surg 14:20, 1987.
2. Pertschuk MJ, Whitaker LA: Social and psychological effects of craniofacial malformations in childhood, Clin Plast Surg 9:297-306, 1982.
3. Pertschuk MJ, Whitaker LA: Psychosocial adjustment and craniofacial malformations in childhood, Plast Reconstr Surg 75:177-182, 1985.
4. Berscheid E, Walster E, Bohrnstedt G: Body image, Psychology Today 7:119-131, 1973.
5. Macgregor FC: Social and psychological implications of dentofacial disfigurement, Angle Orthod 40:231-233, 1970.
6. Adams GR: Physical attractiveness research: toward a developmental social psychology of beauty, Hum Dev 20:217-230, 1977.
7. Adams GR: Racial membership and physical attractiveness effects on preschool teachers' expectations, Child Study J 8:29, 1978.
8. Dion KK, Berscheid E, Walster E: What is beautiful is good, J Pers Soc Psychol 24:285, 1972.
9. Goldman W, Lewis P: Beautiful is good: evidence that the physically attractive are more socially skillful, J Exp Psychol: General 13:125, 1977.
10. Landy D, Sigall H: Beauty is talent: task evaluation as a function of the performer's physical attractiveness, J Pers Soc Psychol 29:299, 1974.
11. Brundage LE, Derlega VJ, Cash TF: The effects of physical attractiveness and need for approval on self-disclosure, Personality Soc Psychol Bull 3:63-66, 1977.
12. Dion KK: Young children's stereotyping of facial attractiveness, Dev Psychol 9:183, 1973.
13. Jones JE: Self-concept and parental evaluation of peer relationships in cleft lip and palate children, Pediatr Dent 6:132-138, 1984.
14. Tobiasen JM: Psychosocial correlates of congenital facial clefts: a conceptualization and model, Cleft Palate J 21:3, 1984.
15. Tobiasen JM, Levy J, Carpenter MA, et al: Type of facial cleft, associated congenital malformations, and parents' ratings of school and conduct problems, Cleft Palate J 24:209-215, 1987.
16. Strauss RP, Mintzher Y, Feuerstein R, et al: Down syndrome oral-facial surgery: effects on peer social perceptions, Inter Assoc Dent Res March, 1987 (abs).

TABLE 3-7 Psychosocial considerations in clinical interaction

Treatment stage	Steps in psychologic management
A. Initial assessment	1. Explore motives for treatment and expectations from treatment in detail. Why treatment? Why now instead of last or next year? 2. Consider using an auxiliary with a warm personality to do at least part of the interview. Patients often are intimidated by the doctor and may not reveal their true concerns. 3. Be careful not to create unrealistic expectations—it is better not to discuss the specifics of treatment procedures before the diagnostic workup has been completed, but a broad outline including the possibility of surgery should be presented.
B. Orthodontic consultation	1. The spouse or a family member/close friend should attend if at all possible—but be careful about invasion of privacy. 2. Begin with a discussion of the patient's problems; be sure doctor and patient agree as to what is most important; then describe how the problems might be solved, beginning with the most important problem and presenting the alternatives (see Table 6-1). 3. Encourage—indeed, insist on—an early appointment with the surgeon if surgical treatment may be needed.
C. Surgical consultation	1. Review patient's records with same general approach as the orthodontist, emphasizing the problems and their possible solutions. 2. Discuss the functional and esthetic benefits of surgery, in that order. It is better to tell patients they will have functional benefits and esthetic changes than the reverse. Functional changes nearly always are appreciated, esthetic changes may not be. 3. Provide more detail about the surgical experience, to the extent the patient has questions, but keep the discussion relatively general. Many details can wait until just before surgery. 4. Consider using patient education materials at this stage, such as booklets, video cassettes, and videodisc. 5. Offer now to help with insurance preauthorization.
D. Presurgical treatment	1. Evaluate the patient's personality characteristics and psychologic stability in more detail. Focus on: neuroticism, degree of external locus of control, introversion in males, mood states (particularly depression and current major life events), and tendency for patient to be a "vigilant coper."
E. Immediate presurgery	1. Review the planned surgery in detail, but take the patient's psychologic profile into account. Patients who expect the worst are more likely to experience it. 2. Discuss with family members and close friends the importance of their psychologic and emotional support postsurgically. Be sure the "significant other" is prepared for changes in the patient's facial appearance so that they do not express shock or dismay.
F. Immediate postsurgery	1. Expect a period of mood swings and negative emotions, which usually peak at about 2 weeks. Reassure the patient and family/friends that these emotions are very normal and will soon disappear. 2. A visit from the orthodontist, and perhaps flowers or a "care package" of easy-to-eat foods keeps the patient from feeling forgotten.
G. Postsurgical orthodontics	1. Negative emotions and mood swings are more likely to be seen by the orthodontist in patients who return for finishing orthodontics more quickly and in older patients. Reassurance and psychologic support may be needed. 2. Remember that a decrease in satisfaction and facial body image occurs if active treatment takes more than 6 months postsurgically. If treatment has not been completed by this time, progress should be reviewed with the patient and an anticipated completion date discussed.

17. Strauss RP, Mintzker Y, Feuerstein R, et al: Social perceptions of the effects of Down syndrome facial surgery: a school-based study of ratings by normal adolescents, Plast Reconstr Surg 81:841-851, 1988.
18. Arndt EM, Travis F, Lefebvre AN, et al: Beauty and the eye of the beholder: social consequences and personal adjustments for facial patterns, Brit J Plast Surg 39:81-84, 1986.
19. Gochman DS: The measurement and development of dentally relevant motives, J Public Health Dent 35:160-164, 1975.
20. Helm S, Kreiborg S, Solow B: Psychosocial implications of malocclusion: a 15 year follow-up study in 30-year-old Danes, Am J Orthod 87:110-118, 1985.
21. Shaw WC: The influence of children's dentofacial appearance on their social attractiveness as judged by peers and lay adults, Am J Orthod 79:399-415, 1981.

22. Tedesco LA, Albino JE: Psychosocial meanings of facial appearance, Inter Assoc Dent Res June, 1986 (abs).
23. Baldwin DC, Barnes ML, Baldwin MA, et al: Social and cultural variables in the decision for orthodontic treatment, Inter Assoc Dent Res March, 1967 (abs).
24. McCann MC: Malocclusion as a handicap, Angle Orthod 37:320-322, 1967.
25. Morris AL, et al: Seriously handicapping orthodontic conditions, Washington, DC, 1976, National Academy of Sciences.
26. Meyer E, Jacobson WE, Edgerton MT, et al: Motivational patterns in patients seeking elective plastic surgery, Psychosom Med 22:193-201, 1960.
27. Crowell NT, Sazima MJ, Elder ST: Survey of patients' attitudes after surgical correction of prognathism: study of 33 patients, J Oral Surg 28:818-822, 1970.
28. Hutton C: Patients' evaluation of surgical correction of prognathism: survey of 32 patients, J Oral Surg 25:255-258, 1967.
29. Kiyak HA, Hohl T, West RA, et al: Psychologic changes in orthognathic surgery patients: a 24-month follow-up, J Oral Maxillofac Surg 42:506-512, 1984.
30. Kiyak HA, Hohl T, Sherrick P, et al: Sex differences in motives for and outcomes of orthognathic surgery, J Oral Surg 39:757-764, 1981.
31. Kiyak HA, McNeill RW, West RA, et al: Predicting patient responses to orthognathic surgery, J Oral Surg 40:150-156, 1982.
32. Kiyak HA, West RA, Hohl T, et al: The psychological impact of orthognathic surgery: a 9-month follow-up, Am J Orthod 81:404-412, 1982.
33. Kiyak HA, Beach LR: Development of a decision making aid in orthodontics and surgery, Inter Assoc Dent Res March, 1983 (abs).
34. Kiyak HA, McNeill RW, West RA: The emotional impact of orthognathic surgery and conventional orthodontics, Am J Orthod 88:224-234, 1985.
35. Kiyak HA, McNeill RW, West RA, et al: Personality characteristics as predictors and sequelae of surgical and conventional orthodontics, Am J Orthod 89:383-392, 1986.
36. Kiyak HA, Vitaliano PP, Crinean J: Patients' expectations as predictors of orthognathic surgery outcomes, Health Psychol 7:251-268, 1988.
37. Kiyak HA, Zeitler DL: Self-assessment of profile and body image among orthognathic surgery patients before and two years after surgery, J Oral Maxillofac Surg 46:365-371, 1988.
38. Laufer D, Glick D, Gutman D, Sharon A: Patient motivation and response to surgical correction of prognathism, Oral Surg 41:309, 1976.
39. Flanary CM, Barnwell GM, Alexander JM: Patient perceptions of orthognathic surgery, Am J Orthod 88:137-145, 1985.
40. Jacobson A: The influence of children's dentofacial appearance on their social attractiveness as judged by peers and lay adults, Am J Orthod 79:399-415, 1981.
41. Pepersack WJ, Chausse JM: Long-term follow-up of the sagittal splitting technique for correction of mandibular prognathism, J Oral Maxillofac Surg 6:117-140, 1978.
42. Ouelette PL: Psychological ramifications of facial change in relation to orthodontic treatment and orthognathic surgery, J Oral Surg 36:787-790, 1978.
43. Olson RE, Laskin DM: Expectations of patients from orthognathic surgery, J Oral Surg 38:283, 1980.
44. Beach LR, Campbell FL, Townes BD: Subjective expected utility and the prediction of birth-planning decisions, Organizational Behav Hum Perform 24:18-28, 1979.
45. Prothero J, Beach LR: Retirement decisions: expectation, intention and action, J Appl Soc Psychol 14:162-174, 1984.
46. Beach LR, Barnes V: Approximate measurement in a multivariate utility context, Organizational Behav Hum Peform 32:417-424, 1983.
47. Eysenck HJ, Eysenck SBG: Eysenck personality inventory manual, San Diego, 1968, Educational and Industrial Testing Service.
48. Deutsch H: The psychology of women, vol 1, New York, 1944, Grune & Stratton, Inc.
49. Horney K: Feminine psychology, New York, 1967, WW Norton & Co, Inc.
50. Broverman IK, Clarkson FE, Rosenkrantz PS, et al: Sex-role stereotypes and clinical judgments of mental health. In Bardwick JM, editor: Readings on the psychology of women, New York, 1972, Harper & Row, Publishers, Inc.
51. Kurtz R: Sex differences and variations in body attitudes, J Consult Clin Psychol 33:625-629, 1969.
52. Webb WL, Slaughter R, Meyer E: Mechanisms of psychosocial adjustment in patients seeking "face-lift" operation, Psychosom Med 27:183, 1965.
53. Edgerton MT, Knorr NJ: Motivational patterns of patients seeking cosmetic (esthetic) surgery, Plast Reconstr Surg 48:551-557, 1971.
54. Edgell PG: A psychiatrist joins a surgery of appearance symposium: a personal point of view, J Otolaryngol 2:72-77, 1973.
55. Shipley RH, O'Donnell JM, Bader KF: Personality characteristics of women seeking breast augmentation—comparison to small-busted and average-busted controls, Plast Reconstr Surg 50:369-376, 1977.
56. Reich J: Factors influencing patient satisfaction with the results of esthetic plastic surgery, Plast Reconstr Surg 55:5-13, 1975.
57. Schultz-Coulon HJ: Rhinoplasty—mainly aesthetic or functional operation? Laryngol Rhinol Otol (Stuttg) 56:233-243, 1977.
58. Hay GD: Dysmorphobia, Br J Psychiatry 116:399-406, 1970.
59. Bell R, Kiyak HA, Joondeph DR, et al: Perceptions of facial profile and their influence on the decision to undergo orthognathic surgery, Am J Orthod 88:323-332, 1985.
60. Lewis EA, Fox RN, Albino JE, et al: Accuracy of self-perception of occlusal state, Inter Assoc Dent Res March, 1979 (abs).
61. Rittersma J, Casparie AF, Reerink E: Patient information and patient preparation in orthognathic surgery: a medical audit study, J Oral Maxillofac Surg 8:206-209, 1980.

62. Trask G: The impact of nutritional changes following orthognathic surgery. Report submitted to Biomedical Research Support Grant Summer Fellowship Committee, University of Washington, September, 1981.

63. Auerbach SM, Meredith J, Alexander JM, et al: Psychological factors in adjustment to orthognathic surgery, J Oral Maxillofac Surg 42:435-440, 1984.

64. Robinson G, Merav A: Informed consent, recall by patients tested postoperatively, Ann Thorac Surg 22:209-212, 1976.

65. Lewis CM: Dissatisfaction among women with thunder thighs undergoing closed aspirative lipoplasty, Aesthetic Plast Surg 11:187-191, 1987.

66. Lorr M, McNair DM: Manual for the profile of mood states, San Diego, 1971, Educational and Industrial Testing Service.

67. Stewart TD, Sexton J: Depression: a possible complication of orthognathic surgery, J Oral Maxillofac Surg 45:847-851, 1987.

68. George J, Scott D: The effects of psychological factors on recovery from surgery, J Am Dent Assoc 105:251-257, 1982.

69. George J, Scott D, Turner S, et al: The effects of psychological factors and physical trauma on recovery from oral surgery, J Behav Med 3:291-310, 1980.

70. Cohen LJ, Roth S: Coping with abortion, J Human Stress 10:140-145, 1984.

71. Miller S, Mangan CE: Interacting effects of information and coping style in adapting to gynecological stress: when should the doctor tell all? J Pers Soc Psychol 45:223-236, 1983.

72. Johnston M: Pre-operative emotional states and post-operative recovery, Adv Psychosom Med 15:1-22, 1986.

73. Holman A: Evaluation of patient reactions to orthognathic surgery and treatment results utilizing an adaptive task framework. Ph.D. dissertation submitted to the California School of Professional Psychology, June, 1987.

DIAGNOSTIC AND TREATMENT PLANNING APPROACHES

Is there a difference in diagnosis and treatment planning between conventional and surgical orthodontics? Should there be? If so, what? For diagnosis, there is no difference. The object of the diagnostic process is to find out the truth about the patient, and the truth has nothing to do with the treatment approach. The diagnosis should not be—indeed, must not be—influenced by premature thoughts about the treatment that ultimately will be offered. Conversely, the object of treatment planning is not truth, but wisdom—planning the treatment that will maximize the benefit to the patient. This requires the application of judgment, and the impact of various possible treatment procedures must be considered. Planning treatment for combined orthodontics and surgery requires predicting the potential results of alternative procedures in a way that often goes beyond what is possible or necessary in forecasting orthodontics.

The problem-oriented approach to diagnosis and treatment planning that was introduced into medicine in the 1960s has proved extremely helpful in orthodontics and orthognathic surgery. The problem-oriented sequence for surgical-orthodontic patients is outlined in the figure on page 94. In this scheme, diagnosis begins with the establishment of a data base of information about the patient. Three distinct types of information are gathered from an interview, clinical examination, and analysis of diagnostic records to compose the data base. Then the process of classification is used to systematically delineate the patient's problems. The resulting problem list is the diagnosis.

Malocclusion and dentofacial deformities are caused by deviations from normal growth and development, not by disease. An important aspect of diagnosis is differentiating developmental problems from problems resulting from acute or chronic pathologic processes. The developmental problems are treated by orthodontics and/or orthognathic surgery, the pathologic problems by other means. For this reason, it is necessary to develop two problem lists, one for pathology, the other for developmental problems. Patients with pathology (e.g., high blood pressure, diabetes, periodontal disease) can have surgical-orthodontic treatment, but the disease processes must be brought under control first.

The first step in using the list of developmental problems to produce a treatment plan is placing these problems in priority order. Deciding what is most important for an individual patient should be based on a judicious combination of the patient's concerns and the clinician's best judgment. It would be foolish to ignore the patient's chief complaint in deciding what is most important, but patients often do not completely understand their problems and may require some education and guidance from the doctor. It is important to realize that the same problem list pri-

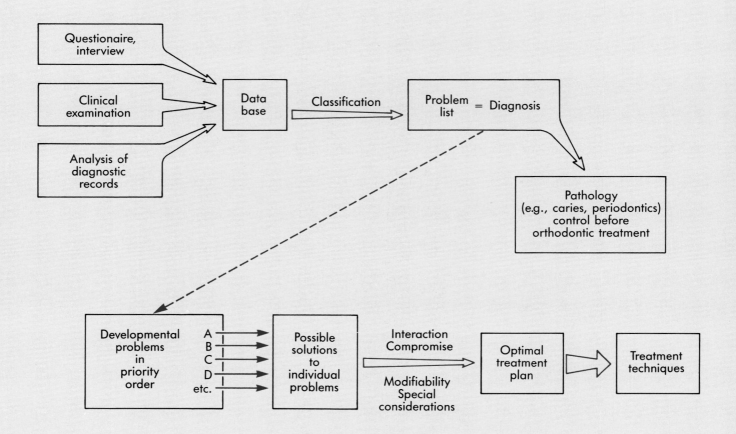

oritized differently can result in different treatment plans, so this is an extremely important step. Unless priorities are considered carefully, the clinician's biases can distort the process of maximizing benefit to the patient. If a patient whose major concern is protruding front teeth consults an oral surgeon who focuses instead on the deficient lower jaw, surgery to advance the mandible may become a more prominent part of the treatment plan than is really warranted. Conversely, if a patient whose major concern is a deficient lower jaw consults an orthodontist who focuses on protruding front teeth, an undue emphasis on overjet rather than jaw position may lead to downplaying the need for surgery. Keeping an open mind and focusing on the importance of the problem, rather than how it might be treated, is critical at this stage. The more problems a patient has, the more complex it is to plan treatment.

The next step in the treatment planning process is to consider the possible solutions to the patient's problems, taking the most important one first and considering each problem as if it were the only one the patient had. Solutions at this stage still should be in general terms (e.g., "move maxillary incisors upward"). Incisors could be moved upward surgically or orthodontically and by a variety of surgical or orthodontic techniques. The solution to the problem is moving them. Exactly how that is to be done is not deduced until the next stage. When the possible solutions for each problem have been assembled, it usually becomes apparent that one or more solutions to the most important problem also solve other problems. Other possible solutions to the most important problem often do not solve secondary problems and may in fact make them worse. All other things being equal, the preferred solution would solve more than the primary problem. It may not be possible to solve all the problems, and then solutions to the most important problems would be preferred.

This also is the point at which cost-benefit (with cost taken in a broader sense than just money) and risk-benefit factors should be considered. Solutions that provide the most benefit for the least cost and risk obviously are better. If these practical considerations are introduced too soon, they can distort the broad overview of possibilities, but if they are not considered at all, the goal of maximizing benefit to the patient cannot be realized. At this final stage in the development of the treatment plan, it also becomes apparent whether some aspects of the total treatment would be done better surgically or orthodontically, and when that has been decided, the surgeon and orthodontist can consider the techniques each will use.

Although the scheme may seem complex and cumbersome when it is described in detail, in practice one can move through the various steps quickly. The method simply becomes a systematic procedure, somewhat analogous to the checklist used by pilots before take-off, to ensure that nothing important has been overlooked and that unwarranted assumptions have not been made. In reasonably simple and straightforward cases, the clinician can proceed through these steps so quickly and automatically that the background organization of the thought process is almost inapparent. In more complex cases, consciously sticking to the steps can be a considerable timesaver ultimately because of the way it forces sequential decisions in the correct order. In the chapters that follow, the overall scheme of Fig. II-1 is the basis of organization. The focus of Chapter 4 is the acquisition of the data base and the steps in abstracting a problem list from it. In Chapters 5 and 6, the steps in planning treatment are discussed and the sequencing of orthodontic and surgical treatment is explored in some detail.

CHAPTER 4

The Search for Truth: Diagnosis

William R. Proffit

The acquisition of a data base of pertinent information is the first step in the diagnosis of any patient (Fig. 4-1). The data base can be divided into three major parts: (1) interview data, from written and oral questions of the patient, (2) clinical examination data, and (3) data from analysis of diagnostic records.

INTERVIEW DATA: THE FIRST COMPONENT OF THE DATA BASE

Data from the interview is of three major types: (1) the patient's chief complaint, (2) information related to the patient's social-psychologic status; that is, the patient's motivation for and expectations of treatment, and (3) information related to the patient's physical status; that is, the medical-dental history and related findings.

The Patient's Chief Complaint

The first goal of the interview is to establish the patient's major reason for seeking treatment, which is the chief complaint. It often is necessary to ask a series of leading questions to gain a clear understanding, but the object is to discover exactly what the patient objects to about the present situation.

Patients who seek surgical-orthodontic treatment—more correctly, those who seek treatment whose developmental problems are severe enough to require surgery, as many in the beginning have no idea that they might need it—fall into two broad groups.

The first group, who typically range in age between the late teens and early forties, are concerned generally about the appearance and function of their face and teeth. Although the initial complaint may focus on a specific aspect of appearance (e.g., the protrusion of the upper incisors), further discussion makes it clear that what these patients want is a general improvement. These individuals want treatment to overcome a feeling of inferiority or insecurity related to their dental and facial appearance, improve their oral function, and increase their chances of a more successful life and lifestyle in the future. A typical comment might be "I have known for years that my protruding teeth need to be

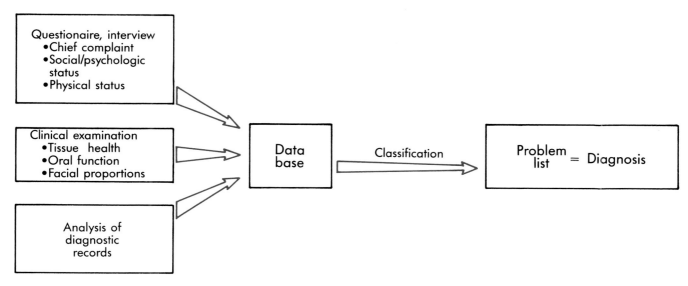

Fig. 4-1. Diagnosis begins with the establishment of a data base. The first step is the collection of data from questions to the patient, covering the patient's chief complaint, motivation for and expectations of treatment, and medical-dental history and related findings. This is followed by a clinical evaluation, at which the necessary diagnostic records are obtained. Later, the analysis of the records completes the data base.

fixed, and now finally I have everything arranged so I can do it."

The second group, who most often are between ages 35 and 55 but may be younger or older, are concerned about a specific health-related problem, usually having to do with potential or actual loss of teeth. They have periodontal disease or broken-down teeth from caries and have learned that, unless their bad bite can be corrected, it may not be possible to save their teeth and/or replace those already missing. A typical comment might be "My dentist tells me that my deep bite is destroying my front teeth, and if I lose them he won't be able to make a replacement."

Although it is fair to say that the first group is more concerned about esthetics and the second about dental function, this is not the exclusive focus in either case. The younger group, whose chief complaint is an appearance that may compromise their chances of getting ahead in the world, nevertheless expect to improve dental function and to reduce the chance of developing dental disease in the future. The older group, whose complaint is the possible loss of what they already have, may be concerned about esthetics only secondarily, but appearance cannot be ignored because of that fact. The chief complaint gives considerable insight into what is most important, however, and that information is vital for the rest of the diagnostic and treatment planning process.

Social-Psychologic Status

The information sought in the area of social-psychologic status is an extension of the chief complaint. It

can be summarized as the answers to two questions: (1) Why are you seeking treatment, and why now as opposed to some other time? and (2) What do you expect as a result of treatment? Although these questions explore related areas, they are not the same, and a more thorough evaluation is done if motivation and expectation are considered separately. The following discussion focuses on information that is directly relevant to the data base for diagnosis and treatment planning. Chapter 3 contains a detailed discussion of social and psychologic factors in surgical-orthodontic patients.

Motivation

In broad terms, motivation can be considered internal or external. Internal motivation comes from within the individual. He or she has decided "I want treatment for my own satisfaction, to meet my own needs" and seeks treatment on that basis. External motivation is primarily at the instigation of someone else. The externally motivated patient seeks treatment because, in the classic situation for a child brought to the orthodontist, "My mother wants me to have this treatment" or for some adults, "My husband really wants me to get these protruding teeth fixed." Often it is difficult to divide the motivation so neatly. For example, a patient who may have wanted treatment for his or her own reasons for some time may be seeking it now because a new spouse agrees and encourages it, or an individual who never thought about seeking treatment until someone else suggested it comes to realize that he or she really does need it.

It is important to ask enough questions to thoroughly explore motivation because a patient whose motivation is primarily external presents an increased risk for treatment in at least two ways: (1) cooperation with treatment and tolerance of treatment procedures both are likely to be poorer than with internally motivated individuals, and (2) there is an increased risk that the patient will be unhappy with the changes produced by treatment, even if the individual who wanted treatment in the first place is pleased. Internal motivation is best; a mixture of external and internal motivation is satisfactory, particularly if the internal component predominates; and purely external motivation is a danger signal that should be recognized during the diagnostic evaluation.

Expectation

Much of a patient's motivation is related to his or her expectations from treatment. If you did not expect some improvement as a result of treatment, your motivation to have it would be limited. Nevertheless, the source of motivation and what one expects from treatment are different and should be explored separately. It is entirely realistic for patients to expect better alignment and function of the teeth and jaws as a result of orthodontic or orthodontic-surgical treatment. It also is entirely realistic to expect a change in dental and facial appearance that will lead to an esthetic improvement. Other expectations may not be realistic at all.

One of the significant differences between adolescents and older patients is the increasingly complex expectations of the older individuals. For an adolescent or young adult, it often is enough that the treatment will make them potentially healthier and happier in the future, without great specificity. For an older patient the expectations frequently are quite specific. Sometimes these are realistic, as in expecting an asymmetric chin to be brought to the midline. Sometimes they are much less realistic, as in expecting to look 10 years younger. Sometimes they are totally unrealistic, as in the patient who expected that if her prominent chin was corrected, the impending breakup of her marriage would be averted.

There are several possible effects of a dentofacial deformity on personality[1] (Fig. 4-2). These range from the development of exceptional personality characteristics that might be considered overcompensation for the deformity, to no effect at all, to personality inadequacies in which the deformity is used as a shield for other shortcomings, to a total loss of reality in which entirely

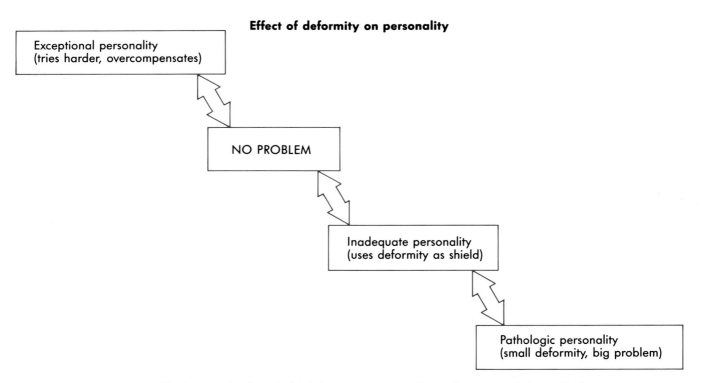

Fig. 4-2. The impact of a dentofacial deformity on personality varies greatly. A few individuals overcompensate for the deformity, developing exceptional personality characteristics; the majority take the deformity in stride, so that there is little or no effect on personality; others use the deformity as a shield for other shortcomings, and so have some degree of personality inadequacy; and a few are out of touch with reality, so that entirely inappropriate problems are blamed on the deformity. Evaluating where a patient is on this spectrum is important diagnostically.

inappropriate problems are blamed on the deformity. One of the best ways to tell where on the spectrum a potential patient is located is to explore in depth what he or she expects as a result of treatment. The more realistic the expectation, the less the chance of personality disorders related to the deformity, and vice-versa. It is much better to decline to treat a patient because his or her expectations are bizarre than to proceed with treatment and then have to deal with an unhappy and disappointed individual later.

The patient's expectations should be carefully recorded for future reference in planning treatment. Meeting a patient's realistic needs is of primary importance when treatment options are considered. Too often in interdisciplinary treatment of complex problems, the wishes of the patient are overlooked.

Physical Status: Medical-Dental History and Related Findings

The object of this phase of inquiry concerning the medical-dental history is to obtain the answers to two broad questions: (1) What is the patient's present condition and how did it get that way? and (2) What, if anything, may change in the near future that would affect the course of orthodontic or surgical-orthodontic treatment? The questions are phrased in this way to emphasize not only the present findings but also an important point that surgeons and orthodontists sometimes overlook, the patient's developmental status. What the patient is at present and the likelihood of future change are affected by pathologic conditions if they are present, but also by the stage of growth and development. Both must be evaluated to ascertain the patient's physical status.

Medical-Dental History

The patient's medical and dental history initially is reviewed from a questionnaire that the patient fills out at the initial registration. These data are used to focus follow-up questions when the doctor first sees the patient. Because the purpose of the printed questionnaire is to streamline the direct interview that will follow, many forms are satisfactory. The only requirement is that the coverage be thorough so that no important area is overlooked. The implications of positive findings are discussed in Chapter 5.

Evaluation of Physical Growth Status

An important consideration for most potential surgical-orthodontic patients is whether growth has declined to the very slow levels that are characteristic of adults,[2] or whether significant postadolescent growth is continuing. Questions about recent growth can help establish the situation. In females, the onset of menses is a valuable marker for the end of the adolescent growth spurt, and so not only whether menstruation has begun but also when, if this was recent, is important. Clearly,

a pattern of recent weight and height increases in younger patients indicates that significant growth is continuing.

Although questions can provide useful information, some aspects of the physical growth status must be determined from clinical examination. It may be valuable to verify the reported height and weight. A hand-wrist radiograph to more precisely establish developmental status may be indicated if there is a considerable discrepancy between the patient's chronologic age and apparent developmental status. In an immature-looking 17-year-old male with mandibular prognathism, for example, a hand-wrist film to obtain skeletal age might be helpful. Interpretation of these films is discussed below.

Implications of Medical Problems

An important reason for recognizing congenital syndromes (the major ones were reviewed briefly in Chapter 2; Gorlin and colleagues[3] provide a comprehensive review) is that affected individuals often have an unusual pattern of growth. It should be kept in mind that an immature patient with facial proportions that are outside the range of normal variation may exhibit further growth that also is not in the expected pattern. The response to orthodontic and surgical treatment also may be unusual. It often is wise to refer such patients for evaluation by the craniofacial anomalies team now available at most major university medical centers (a directory is available from the American Cleft Palate Association, 1218 Grandview Avenue, Pittsburg, PA 15271).

Because continued change is the one constant in life, the question really is not whether things will change in the future for a potential patient, but whether changes will occur that could affect surgical-orthodontic treatment. Growth certainly could do that and therefore must be anticipated. Changes resulting from progression of disease also could have an effect. Patients with medical problems can have surgical-orthodontic treatment, but only if the medical problems are under control.

For surgical-orthodontic patients, chronic conditions rather than acute diseases are of greatest concern. Acute problems, presumably, can be corrected before surgical-orthodontic treatment is undertaken, but chronic conditions will continue to be present, and their potential effect must be considered carefully. The relationship of various medical diagnoses to treatment planning is discussed in Chapter 5.

CLINICAL EXAMINATION DATA: THE SECOND COMPONENT OF THE DATA BASE

One of the purposes of the clinical examination is to determine what radiographs and other diagnostic records should be taken. The minimum set of records for an orthodontic evaluation includes panoramic and lateral cephalometric radiographs, dental casts, and photographs. We recommend that the panoramic dental film be taken for all patients immediately, at the first visit, so that it is available during the initial clinical examination. The discussion that follows is based in part on the availability of this initial screening radiograph. Without it, the clinical examination is more difficult, and appropriately ordering other radiographs may not be possible.

Information from the clinical examination can be divided into three broad areas: (1) health of the hard and soft tissues, (2) oral function, including TM joint evaluation, and (3) facial proportions/esthetics. Data are obtained in each of these areas during the examination, and a decision must be made as to what diagnostic records are needed for a more detailed later analysis. Appropriate diagnostic records are discussed below relative to each area of the clinical examination. Procedures for obtaining the records, with particular emphasis on radiographic technique, are described later in this chapter.

Health of Hard and Soft Tissues
Dental Examination

Clinical and radiographic examination for dental caries or other dental pathology is not different for surgical-orthodontic patients, but the radiographic evaluation has changed in recent years, reflecting both the decline in dental pathology resulting from widespread fluoridation and concerns about radiation hygiene. Posterior bite-wing radiographs no longer are recommended routinely for recall patients who are not at high risk for caries. In an adolescent or young adult patient with a history of regular dental care, no previous caries experience, no obvious pathology on the panoramic radiograph, and a history of exposure to optimal fluoridation, a panoramic film is sufficient for dental evaluation. There is no reason even to take additional bite-wing radiographs to check for interproximal caries because the chance that a significant lesion would be discovered is small. If the patient has had previous caries experience or has obvious caries clinically, bite-wing radiographs should be ordered, and if deep caries are noted, supplemental periapical films of the involved teeth may be indicated.[4]

Because the midlines often are not visualized well on panoramic films, midline periapical radiographs may be needed to obtain a clear image of this area but should be ordered only if there is a specific reason for doing so. The presence of a maxillary midline diastema greater than 2 mm is such an indication (Fig. 4-3).

Periodontal Health

Periodontal breakdown and pocketing must be evaluated in potential surgical-orthodontic patients in the same way that it is in other patients, by periodontal probing and detailed observation. There is no reason to believe that surgical-orthodontic patients are any different in their susceptibility to periodontal disease than are other adults. Conversely, the prevalence of periodontal problems goes up sharply with increasing age, and the possibility of unsuspected periodontal breakdown must be kept in mind for any adult patient. The best current data suggest that 12% to 15% of patients

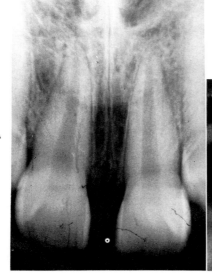
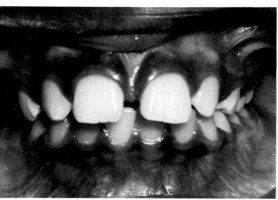

Fig. 4-3. **A** and **B**, A midline periapical radiograph is needed to supplement the panoramic film when a midline diastema is greater than 2 mm. The presence of a midline supernumerary tooth or other anomaly must be ruled out, and the contour of the bony defect in the midline needs to be evaluated in planning treatment. As a general rule, the more apparent the bony notch, as seen here in the radiograph, the greater the difficulty of keeping the diastema closed after treatment.

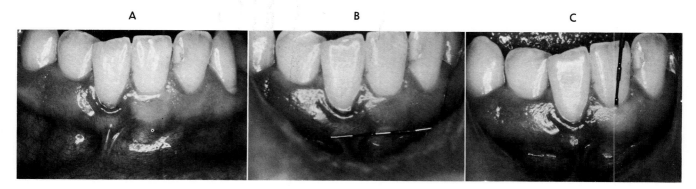

Fig. 4-4. The adequacy or inadequacy of the attached gingiva can be evaluated in several ways. For this patient, the area around the mandibular central incisors is suspect. **A,** Note the tension created by frenum pull near the right central incisor. **B,** The edge of the periodontal probe can be used in the "wrinkle test" to find the edge of the keratinized tissue, which here is about 3 mm below the gingival margin. **C,** The periodontal probe is used to determine how much of the keratinized tissue is attached; that is, the distance between the tip of the probe at the depth of the sulcus and the margin of the keratinized tissue is established. This is the amount of keratinized tissue that is available to resist the stresses of treatment. (**A-C** courtesy Dr. John Moriarty.)

over age 30 have evidence of at least locally severe periodontal problems.[5] Periodontal disease is now known to occur in bursts of activity.[6] There is not yet any radiographic evidence of bone loss at the stage of rapid breakdown—that appears only during the recovery phase, and so radiographs serve more to indicate what has happened than what is currently happening.

The best indication of the presence of active periodontal disease is bleeding on gentle probing.[7] If there is no bleeding on probing, one can be almost 100% certain that there is no active disease. However, bleeding indicates the presence of disease in only about 33% of the patients in whom it is observed. Because periodontal problems are most likely to occur on the distal edge of the molar teeth, the best initial periodontal exam is to gently wipe a thin periodontal probe through the gingival sulcus in these areas and observe whether bleeding occurs. If it does, a more detailed examination should follow. Obviously, it is important to establish whether periodontal pocketing exists.

When periodontal breakdown around posterior teeth is noted on the panoramic film or from probing, bitewing radiographs definitely are indicated, and selected periapical films of areas with breakdown also may be needed.[4] Periodontal destruction around anterior teeth dictates the need for periapical films in this region.

It also is important to note the adequacy of the attached gingiva (Fig. 4-4) because the gingiva can be affected by tooth movement and by vestibular incisions for orthognathic surgery. In the aftermath of such incisions, scar contraction associated with healing creates a pull against the gingiva that can convert a marginally adequate gingival attachment into an inadequate one, leading to loss of attachment and stripping away of the gingival tissues. In some instances, gingival grafts to create additional attached gingiva may be needed before surgical-orthodontic treatment in areas that would not have required grafts if orthognathic surgery were not planned. Preparatory periodontal treatment of this type is discussed in detail in Chapter 6.

In addition to appropriate dental radiographs to supplement the panoramic film, if any are needed, intraoral photographs to document the initial condition of the hard and soft tissues should be a routine part of diagnostic records. The suggested photographic technique is discussed later in the chapter.

Oral Function

Patients with severe discrepancies in the size and position of their jaws and the position of their teeth often have difficulty in oral function. Mastication can be impaired, and certain foods may be difficult to incise and chew. Commonly, patients cannot eat pizza or sandwiches. Cheek and lip biting often occurs during mastication. Careful questioning will reveal the extent to which patients modify their eating patterns.

Speech may also be affected by jaw deformity. If the patient cannot bring the tongue and lips into the proper position, it may not be possible to produce a particular sound properly. However, the degree of adaptation of the neuromuscular system in this regard is remarkable. For example, patients with very severe lip incompetence, to the extent that the lips cannot be brought into contact at all, often make the bilabial sounds (/b/, /m/, /p/) via tongue-lip contact. Speech difficulties therefore are less frequent than might be expected. Lisping, the most common articulation error, may be caused by irregular anterior teeth. The possible

TABLE 4-1 Speech problems potentially related to dentofacial deformity

Speech difficulty	Affected sound	Dentofacial problem
Distortion of labiodental fricatives	/f/, /v/	Mandibular prognathism
Distortion of linguodental fricatives	/th/, /sh/, /ch/	Severe open bite
Lisp	/s/, /z/	Severe open bite
Difficulty to say	/t/, /d/	Lingually positioned or irregular upper incisors

relationships between other types of speech difficulties and dentofacial deformities are summarized in Table 4-1.

It is doubtful that diagnostic tests of function that can be carried out in the orthodontic or surgical office, besides careful observation of the patient, are useful for most patients. Some such procedures have been proposed, primarily by advocates of myofunctional therapy who assume that tongue and lip function are major causes of the anatomic problem in the first place. That assumption is largely incorrect (see Chapter 2 for a review). Measuring lip strength or how hard the patient can push with the tongue therefore adds little or nothing to the diagnostic evaluation. It is true that neuromuscular adaptation to the changes that would be created by surgical-orthodontic treatment is important. Part of the clinical evaluation should be a check on whether the patient has normal coordination and movements. If not, as in an individual with cerebral palsy or other types of gross incoordination, it may be impossible to obtain a stable correction of the deformity because of failure of adaptation. If the patient's neuromuscular status is in doubt, referral for a thorough medical evaluation is wise.

Jaw function is much more than TM joint function, but functional adaptation or aberration can lead to joint problems. The relationship of TM joint problems to severe malocclusion and dentofacial deformities is complex but important. Although there is some evidence that patients with specific types of malocclusion may have increased susceptibility to TM joint problems, the increased risk seems relatively small.[8,9] In general terms, potential surgical-orthodontic patients are remarkably similar to patients with normal facial proportions in the prevalence of TM joint problems.[10] Nevertheless, patients must be treated as individuals, not abstracts or averages, and it is important to evaluate TM joint function.

The form that we recommend for recording a routine clinical examination of jaw function is shown in the box below. This screening method, developed for use in the Pain Clinic at the University of North Carolina by Dr. T.A. Lundeen, consists of items usually included in more elaborate TM joint exams that correlate strongly with the presence of significant problems. Patients who do not have positive findings on a screening evaluation of this type are unlikely to have significant TM joint problems. For these individuals, TM joint radiographs and other special diagnostic procedures are not indicated. Dental casts, oriented to document the occlusal relationship, are the minimum diagnostic record.

It is more difficult to know what additional steps in evaluation should be taken for those who have positive findings. Joint pain and joint sounds should be noted, as should areas of muscle tenderness from more thorough palpation. Radiographs of the joint are likely to be needed in many individuals, but exactly which radiograph should be ordered depends on what is suspected, based on the clinical examination.

In many instances of positive TM joint findings, it may be difficult to obtain a clear indication of the current jaw position with the muscles relaxed without placing a "diagnostic splint"[11] for a short while to overcome muscle spasticity that guides the jaw to an assumed position. Such a splint, worn for a week or so before cephalometric radiographs and dental-cast recordings are made, can give a clearer picture of jaw relationships than could be obtained otherwise. This approach can be particularly helpful when articulator-mounted casts are needed to ascertain a true relaxed position in the presence of severe deflective contacts of the teeth.

An overview of TM joint imaging techniques and a perspective on the need for articulator mounting of casts are provided below in the section on diagnostic

---

Screening Exam for Jaw Function (TM joint)

Jaw function/TM joint
  complaint now: [ ] No [ ] Yes
  If yes, specify: _____
History of pain: [ ] No [ ] Yes _____ duration
History of sounds: [ ] No [ ] Yes _____ duration
TM joint tenderness
  to palpation: [ ] No [ ] Yes [ ] Right
                                        [ ] Left
Muscle tenderness to palpation: [ ] No [ ] Yes
  If yes, where? _____
Range of Motion: Maximum opening _____ mm
                   Right excursion _____ mm
                   Left excursion _____ mm
                   Protrusion _____ mm

records. Chapter 19 has a more detailed presentation of evaluation procedures for patients who have jaw deformities and also a major problem with TM pain and dysfunction.

Facial Proportions/Esthetics

The evaluation of facial esthetics is notoriously subjective and difficult. There is no single esthetic ideal. A facial appearance considered highly esthetic by one individual or group may be judged less so by another, and general opinions about esthetics change over time. There are fashions in facial esthetics as in everything else.

However, there is no doubt that impaired dental and facial esthetics can be an important problem for patients with dentofacial deformities, and the extent and severity of the esthetic problem must be addressed in the diagnostic evaluation. This difficulty can be alleviated by applying a principle known to artists at least since it was pointed out by Durer in the 17th century, and probably longer than that: disproportionate human faces are unesthetic, whereas proportionate features are acceptable if not always beautiful. Therefore evaluating faces can be made less subjective and more precise by replacing esthetics with proportions and noting disproportions as problems.

The best recent studies of facial proportions are those of Farkas,[12,13] whose extensive cross-sectional anthropometric measurements of Canadians of northern European origin provided the data for Tables 4-2 and 4-3. Measuring the height and width of the face requires appropriate calipers (Fig. 4-5) but can be done quickly and easily. Suggested measurements, keyed to Table 4-2, are illustrated in Fig. 4-6.

Note that some of the measurements in Table 4-2 could be made on a cephalometric film, but others could not. There is no substitute for recording the facial width measurements clinically, as opposed to waiting for the cephalometric analysis, and it is preferable to record clinically even the vertical measurements that could be taken from the lateral cephalometric film because the soft-tissue as well as hard-tissue distances can be important.

The proportional relationship of height and width, more than the absolute value of either, establishes the overall facial type. A patient with a long lower-face height and anterior open bite may or may not have a disproportionately long face—that depends on the width of the face. In a well-proportioned face, the ratio of bizygomatic width to face height is 0.88 for males and 0.86 for females. The face should taper somewhat: the ratio of bigonial to bizygomatic width should be

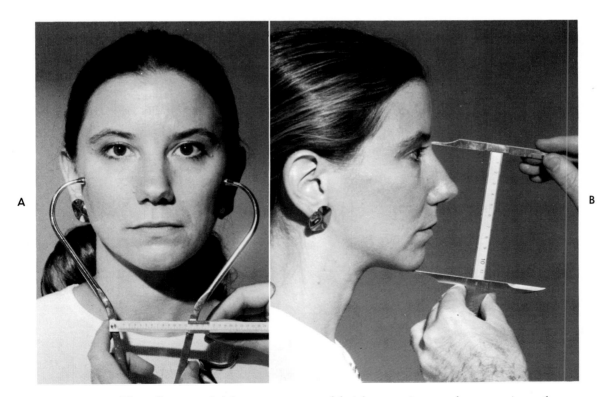

Fig. 4-5. The calipers needed for measurement of facial proportions are larger versions of the instruments often used by dentists. **A,** The bow caliper, illustrated here in measurement of bizygomatic width (zy-zy), is particularly useful in measurements across the face or head. **B,** The straight caliper, which resembles a large Boley gauge, is used for shorter distances or points that the tips can easily reach, as in this nasion-gnathion (n-gn) measurement.

TABLE 4-2 Facial anthropometric measurements (young adults)

Parameter	Male	Female
1. Zygomatic width (zy-zy) (mm)	137 (4.3)	130 (5.3)
2. Gonial width (go-go)	97 (5.8)	91 (5.9)
3. Intercanthal distance	33 (2.7)	32 (2.4)
4. Pupil-midfacial distance	33 (2.0)	31 (1.8)
5. Nasal base width	35 (2.6)	31 (1.9)
6. Mouth width	53 (3.3)	50 (3.2)
7. Face height (N-gn)	121 (6.8)	112 (5.2)
8. Lower face height (subnasale-gn)	72 (6.0)	66 (4.5)
9. Upper lip vermillion	8.9 (1.5)	8.4 (1.3)
10. Lower lip vermillion	10.4 (1.9)	9.7 (1.6)
11. Nasolabial angle (degrees)	99 (8.0)	99 (8.7)
12. Nasofrontal angle (degrees)	131 (8.1)	134 (1.8)

Measurements are illustrated in Fig. 4-6.
Standard deviation is in parenthesis.
Data from Farkas LG: Anthropometry of the head and face in medicine, New York, 1981, Elsevier Science Publishing Co, Inc.

about 0.70. Other proportions that may be clinically useful are given in Table 4-3.

Differences in facial types and body types obviously must be taken into account when these facial proportions are assessed, and variations from the average ratios certainly are compatible with good facial esthetics. However, an important point in planning treatment is to avoid treatment that would change the ratios in the wrong direction while correcting an occlusal prob-lem—for example, a mandibular setback in a patient with a Class III malocclusion whose gonial angles already are broad relative to the bizygomatic width.

From the frontal view, it is particularly important to evaluate the transverse symmetry of the face. For the assessment of symmetry, it can be helpful to divide the face as shown in Fig. 4-7. Note that the nose, center of the lips, and middle of the chin should fall along a true vertical line. The base of the nose should be approximately the same width as the inter-innercanthal distance, the width of the mouth should approximate the distance between the inner margins of the iris of the eye, and the width of the orbits should approximate the bigonial width of the mandible.

The major indication for ordering a PA cephalometric film is significant asymmetry. This radiograph is not needed routinely.

The relationship of the dental midlines to the skeletal midlines must be recorded during the clinical examination. Deviation of the skeletal and dental midlines from the midfacial axis must also be noted. If a PA film is not taken, this information cannot be obtained later from diagnostic records. Even with a PA film, the clinical data are needed.

In the vertical plane of space, the height of the midface, from the supraorbital ridges to the base of the nose, should equal the height of the lower face, which extends from the base of the nose to the undersurface of the chin. Within the lower face, the mouth should be about a third of the way between the base of the nose and the chin. Vertical proportions, as Fig. 4-8 illustrates, can be assessed equally well from the frontal or lateral view. The lateral cephalometric film, which is needed routinely as part of the diagnostic records, can be used later to confirm and extend this clinical judgment.

From the lateral view, it is important to check for

TABLE 4-3 Facial indices (young adults)

Index	Measurements	Male	Female
Facial	n-gn/zy-zy	88.5 (5.1)	86.2 (4.6)
Mandible-face width	go-go/zy-zy	70.8 (3.8)	70.1 (4.2)
Upper face	n-sto-/zy-zy	54.0 (3.1)	52.4 (3.1)
Mandible width—face height	go-go/n-gn	80.3 (6.8)	81.7 (6.0)
Mandibular	sto-gn/go-go	51.8 (6.2)	49.8 (4.8)
Mouth-face width	ch-ch × 100/zy-zy	38.9 (2.5)	38.4 (2.5)
Lower face—face height	sn-gn/n-gn	59.2 (2.7)	58.6 (2.9)
Mandible-face height	sto-gn/n-gn	41.2 (2.3)	40.4 (2.1)
Mandible-upper face height	sto-ng/n-sto	67.7 (5.3)	66.5 (4.5)
Mandible-lower face height	sto-ng/sn-gn	69.6 (2.7)	69.1 (2.8)
Chin-face height	sl-gn × 100/sn-gn	25.0 (2.4)	25.4 (1.9)

Standard deviation is in parenthesis.
From Farkas LG, Munro JR: Anthropometric facial proportions in medicine, Springfield, Ill, 1987, Charles C Thomas, Publisher.

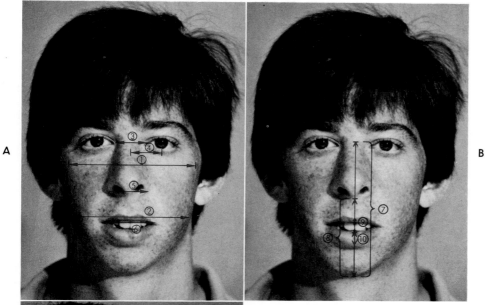

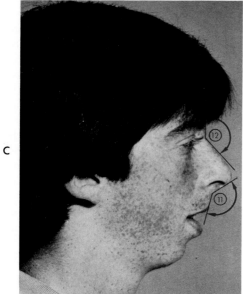

Fig. 4-6. Commonly employed facial anthropometric measurements (numbers are keyed to Table 4-2).

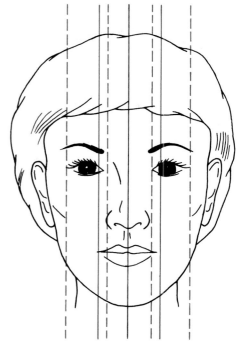

Fig. 4-7. Vertical lines are used to establish the horizontal symmetry and proportions of the face. Bilateral structures should be placed symmetrically. In addition, note that the width of the nose should be approximately the same as the inner-intercanthal distance, the width of the mouth should be the same as the distance between the inner margins of the iris of the eyes, and the width of the mandible at the gonial angles should be approximately the same as the width of the orbits.

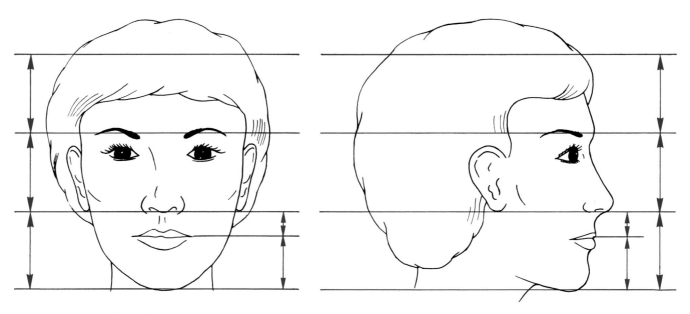

Fig. 4-8. Horizontal lines are used to establish the vertical proportions of the face. Classically, the ideal face has been divided into approximately equal thirds, as illustrated here. Within the lower face, the mouth should be a third of the way between the base of the nose and the chin. Farkas' data (see Tables 4-3 and 4-4) suggest that the modern lower face may be slightly longer than this, but the classic proportions are still a good starting point for clinical examination.

profile convexity or concavity, which indicates a jaw disproportion. In some ways, describing the analysis of profile relationships is harder than doing it, so careful definition of terms is important to avoid confusion. Profile divergence, convexity, and concavity are illustrated in Figs. 4-9 through 4-11. We use divergence (Figs. 4-9 and 4-10) in the same way as does Hellman.[14] Concavity and convexity, illustrated in Fig. 4-11, are defined similarly to some but not all previous authors.

The ideal profile line is straight (neither convex nor concave) and vertical (not divergent). Some Caucasians and a few members of other racial groups have a posteriorly divergent profile. This simply means that a line from the bridge of the nose through the base of the nose and the chin is straight or nearly so, but slopes posteriorly relative to the true vertical line. Most people of all races have a relatively straight profile; that is, the profile line is not only straight but also approximates the true vertical line. A few Caucasians and many blacks and Orientals have an anteriorly divergent profile in which the profile line is straight or nearly so but slopes anteriorly relative to the true vertical line.

If the profile line is approximately straight, without excess concavity or convexity, divergence is of no consequence. It does not indicate a dentofacial deformity and, in and of itself, is not a problem. By the same token, if the profile line is excessively convex or concave, a jaw disproportion exists. Which jaw is at fault can be determined at least grossly by evaluating its promi-

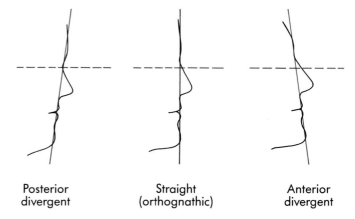

Posterior divergent   Straight (orthognathic)   Anterior divergent

Fig. 4-9. When the patient is in natural head position (NHP); that is, with his or her own visual axis level, the profile line most often is approximately vertical but may slope backward (posterior divergence, in Hellman's terminology) or forward (anterior divergence). Profile divergence, in and of itself, is not a problem because it is quite compatible with both normal function (including normal dental occlusion) and good esthetics. Posterior divergence in a well-proportioned individual is most likely in Caucasians of northern European background but may occur in other racial or ethnic groups. Anterior divergence is seen occasionally in Caucasians but frequently in blacks and Orientals.

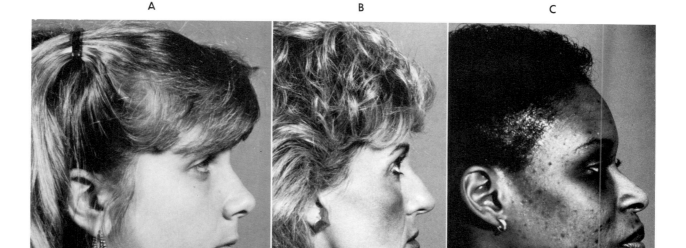

Fig. 4-10. **A,** A female of Scandinavian descent with a posteriorly divergent profile. She has only minimal overjet and no complaints about facial esthetics. **B,** A female with an anteriorly divergent profile, producing a strong chin but with normal occlusion and acceptable esthetics. **C,** A female with a more accentuated anterior divergence (which is not uncommon among both blacks and Orientals), again with normal occlusion and acceptable esthetics.

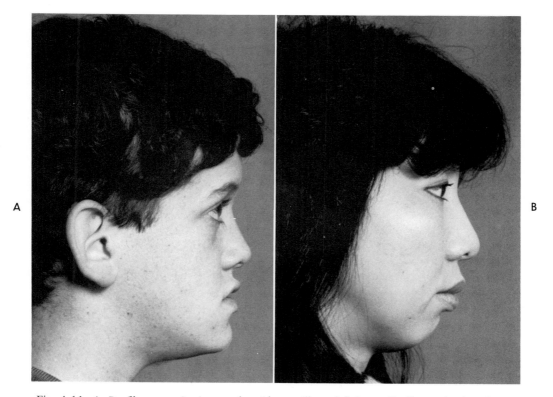

Fig. 4-11. **A,** Profile concavity in a male with maxillary deficiency. **B,** Convexity in a Japanese female with mandibular deficiency. Profile concavity or convexity is established by comparing the inclination of a line from the nasal bridge (nasion) to the base of the nose (subnasale) with a line from subnasale to the chin (pogonion). In a well-proportioned face, the line should be nearly straight—the norm is mild convexity. Excessive convexity or concavity reflects skeletal Class II or Class III malocclusion. Which jaw is at fault is determined by comparing the position of each jaw to a true vertical line that passes through the forehead area; this process may require cephalometric analysis for precision. The presence of convexity or concavity in itself does not indicate which jaw is at fault, only that there is a disproportion.

nence relative to the forehead and the true vertical line. For example, if the profile is concave and the maxilla is behind the true vertical line but the mandible is on or in front of it (Fig. 4-12), the patient almost surely has a maxillary deficiency. If the profile is concave but the maxilla is on the true vertical while the mandible is forward from it, then mandibular excess is the more likely problem.

In the section below on cephalometric analysis, a highly analagous approach to the cephalometric film is advocated. That is not coincidence. The diagnostician should be able to detect from an evaluation of the facial profile much of the information on facial proportions that will be contained in the cephalometric radiograph. The cephalometric film is used to confirm the clinical impression and make it more precise rather than provide the information anew.

TECHNIQUES FOR OBTAINING DIAGNOSTIC RECORDS
Photographs

Although judgments of the health and function of oral tissues and of esthetics should be made primarily from the clinical examination, extraoral and intraoral photographs are an essential part of the diagnostic records. Their main purpose is to document the condition at the beginning of treatment, but they also are useful during the final synthesis of the diagnostic information into a problem list and in planning treatment.

We recommend a minimum of four extraoral photographs (see Figs. 4-39 and 4-43): (1) full face with lips relaxed, (2) full face smile, (3) 45-degree oblique, and (4) profile. If there is significant asymmetry, both the left and right sides should be photographed, otherwise one oblique view and one profile is satisfactory.

Because in a busy practice there is always the temptation to examine the face superficially during the clinical evaluation and then rely on the photographs when all the information is pulled together later, the limitations of these photographs must be recognized. Even the best set of still photographs may not show such things as asymmetries in lip elevation during function, the relationship of dental to skeletal midlines, or the clinical appearance of asymmetry, which often is subtly but noticeably different in three-dimensional real life than in a two-dimensional photograph. The facial photographs are important, but they cannot supplant a careful clinical evaluation.

The intraoral photographs also are a record of the pretreatment condition, documenting what was evaluated primarily on clinical examination. Five standard intraoral photographs are suggested: right, center, and left views with the teeth in occlusion, and maxillary and mandibular occlusal views (see Figs. 4-40 and 4-44). The photographs should document the soft as well as hard tissues to the extent that this is possible. Max-

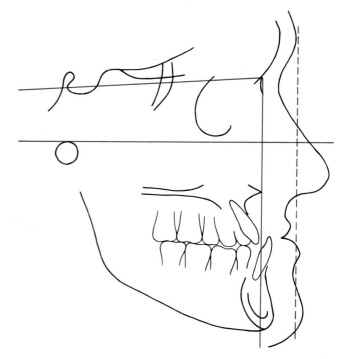

Fig. 4-12. In a patient with profile convexity or concavity, the source of the disproportion can be established by comparing the position of each jaw to a true vertical line (perpendicular to true horizontal) from the forehead across the face. This can be done mentally during clinical examination of the patient and more precisely later using a cephalometric tracing as shown here. Both a soft-tissue line from the forehead (analogous to the clinical examination) and a hard-tissue line from nasion (the usual cephalometric reference line) show that this individual has components of both maxillary deficiency and mandibular excess; that is, the maxilla is behind the reference line and the mandible is in front of it.

imum retraction of the cheeks and lips is needed for the photographs. If there is a special soft-tissue problem area (e.g., a mandibular anterior region with no attached gingiva), an additional photograph of this region should be taken.

Radiographic Technique: Rare-Earth Screens and High-Speed Film to Reduce Radiation

Intensifying screens in the film cassette traditionally have been used in making cephalometric and panoramic radiographs to provide an acceptable image with reduced radiation. The standard technique of the early 1980s called for calcium tungstate screens and medium-speed films adapted to their characteristics. More recently it has become possible to use intensifying screens in which rare-earth compounds (usually containing lanthanum or gadolinium) replace the calcium tungstate. When these screens are coupled with faster films to take full advantage of their capabilities, a dramatic decrease in the amount of radiation neces-

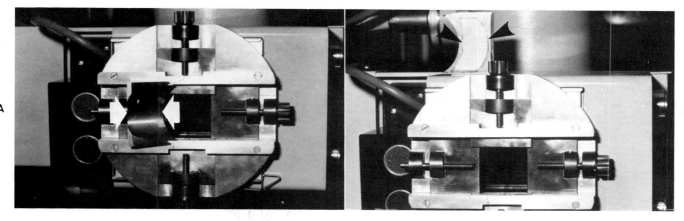

Fig. 4-13. A rare-earth filter supplementing the aluminum filtration typically used in cephalometric radiography can both reduce the patient's radiation exposure and improve the soft-tissue image. The rare-earth filter is most conveniently placed behind the aluminum filter. **A,** The collimator of a cephalometric unit, showing the aluminum wedge. **B,** The aluminum wedge removed and reversed, showing the rare-earth filter attached behind it. (From Tyndall DA, Matteson SR, Soltmann RE, et al: Exposure reduction in cephalometric radiography: a comprehensive approach, Am J Orthod Dentofacial Orthop 93:400-412, 1988.)

sary for panoramic and cephalometric radiographs, on the order of 80%, can be achieved.[15] In modern practice, this technologic improvement should be employed.

To obtain an image of the soft-tissue profile on a cephalometric radiograph as well as the image of the underlying hard tissues, it is necessary to either reduce the radiation passing through the soft tissue or partially block the intensifying screen in that area. In the cephalometric technique of less radiation-concious times, the second method was commonly employed (e.g., by placing a light-absorbing dye in the front edge of the screen to reduce its output). In terms of radiation exposure, it obviously would be preferable to reduce the radiation. This can be done now by placing a rare-earth filter in the anterior portion of the radiograph beam, supplementing the aluminum filtration normally employed to absorb low-energy radiation (Fig. 4-13). The additional decrease in overall radiation exposure to the anterior facial tissues is significant (90%),[16] and the soft-tissue image is at least as good as with the older approach, often better.

Natural Head Position in Cephalometrics

The standard cephalometric headholder was adapted from headholders originally devised by anatomists to position skulls from ancient burial mounds or other archaeologic sources. A convention held at Frankfort in Germany in 1886 adopted a standard position: the ear canals were placed level to orient the head transversely, and a plane forward from the upper portion of the ear canals to the lower border of the orbit (afterward called the *Frankfort plane*) was used to orient the skull

vertically. Experience has confirmed the anatomists' view that this provides the best approximation of how the head would have been oriented during life.

Each living individual has a characteristic head posture, the natural head position (NHP), which is determined physiologically rather than anatomically. It is based on sensory data from the labyrinths of the inner ear and is modified by visual inputs. Although the NHP for most individuals closely approximates the posture produced by orienting the head with the Frankfort plane level, it is not surprising that there are differences for some individuals. Nor, on reflection, should a common clinical observation be surprising: the greater the deviation from normal anatomy, the greater the chance that the NHP differs from the Frankfort orientation.

This means that patients with dentofacial deformities are particularly likely to have a NHP that differs from the Frankfort positioning. Therefore it is especially useful to obtain their cephalometric radiographs in their NHP. For routine orthodontic patients, it probably makes little or no difference whether the NHP or the Frankfort position is used, but for the patients with dentofacial deformities who may need surgical-orthodontic treatment, the difference can be important diagnostically.

NHP varies slightly depending on the technique and is 1 to 2 degrees different between sitting and standing for most individuals.[17] For research, it is important to precisely specify the technique, and usually the standing NHP is preferred. For diagnostic purposes, the small differences between the techniques for NHP are less important than the possibility of finding a major

Fig. 4-14. **A,** NHP cephalometric films are obtained most conveniently using a mirror opposite the headholder so that the patient's head position can be established by gently manipulating the head while the patient looks into his or her own eyes. The chain hanging from the headholder, which is in the midsagittal plane just in front of the patient's nose, serves two purposes. First, it gives a way to establish the midsagittal plane when the headholder cannot be used. **B,** Second, its image on the film establishes a true vertical line for reference. With the patient in his or her NHP, the true horizontal is perpendicular to the image of the chain.

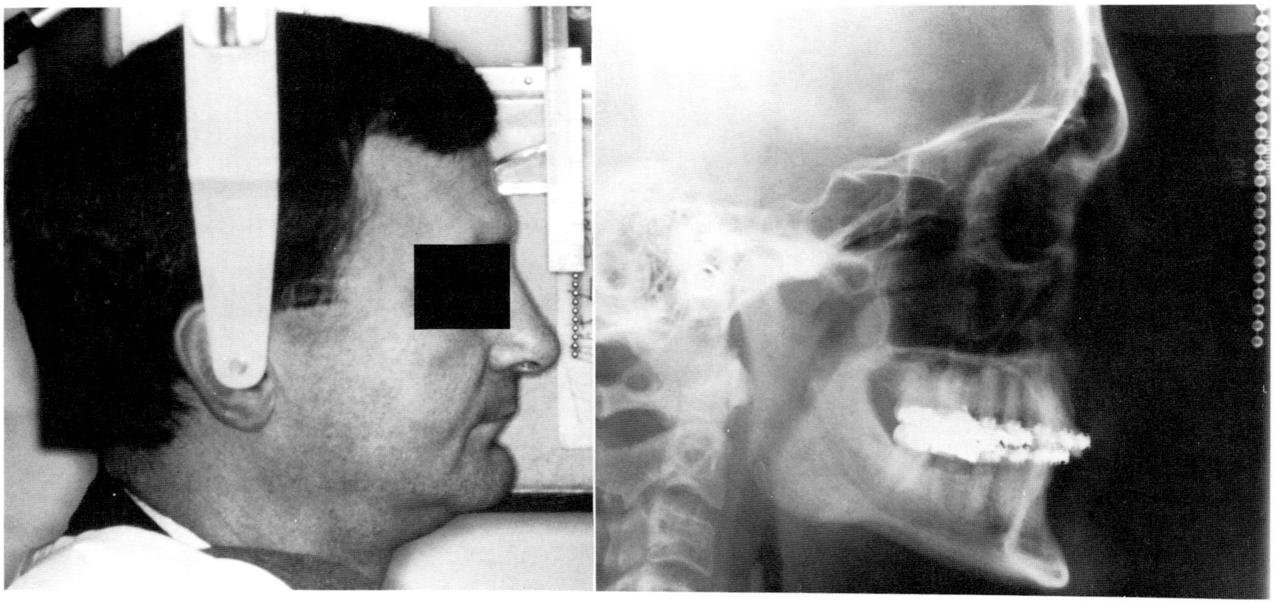

discrepancy between the Frankfort position and the NHP.[18] The following simplified technique is recommended for diagnosis:

1. Use a sitting or standing position, whichever is more convenient.
2. If a window is conveniently available in the radiograph room, orient the cephalostat so that the patient will be looking out the window when a lateral film is taken. Otherwise, place a mirror of reasonably generous size (18 inches square or larger) on the wall of the radiograph room so that the patient will be looking into it when the film is taken.
3. Place a chain at the midsagittal plane of the cephalostat so that it hangs vertically at the front end of the radiographic field, in front of the patient's nose (Fig. 4-14).
4. Place the patient in the cephalostat with the ear rods out and check to be sure that the ears are level. Almost all patients have symmetrically positioned ears, but occasionally one does not. If the ears are symmetric, place the ear rods lightly into the ear canals, as would be done in standard cephalometric technique. If they are not, do not use the ear rods. Instead, position the patient behind the chain, so that the image of the face is bisected by the chain as the patient looks into the mirror. This will establish transverse position

without tilting the head in line with the malpositioned ear canals.
5. Establish the vertical orientation of the head by having the patient look at the horizon or into his or her own eyes in the mirror, tilting the head up and down until a relaxed natural position is achieved. When patients look at an object on the horizon or into their own eyes in a mirror, and are relaxed in doing so, they are automatically in their NHP. At that point, the patient is holding his or her eyes level, as determined physiologically. If the ear rods are in use, the nasal-bridge holder then can be locked into place so that the patient is held in the NHP in the cephalostat as the radiograph is taken.

The major objections to NHP are that it is less reproducible and more technique-sensitive than the standard anatomic positioning. This is undeniably true, but if the NHP is established carefully, it is acceptably reproducible. The operator must not accept the vertical position until the patient is relaxed and orienting the head to look into the mirror, not just compensating with eye movements for a strained head position. With good technique, the chance of an error severe enough to compromise diagnostic evaluation is much less than the chance of a diagnostically significant error using anatomic positioning.

The lateral head film should be taken with lips relaxed and the jaws in retruded contact position. Often patients must be coaxed into relaxing their lips, but rehearsal will produce a film that is superior for diagnostic and planning purposes. Mandibular deficient patients often habitually posture the jaw forward—at least 10% have 2 mm or more difference between CR and CO. If the patient has difficulty in maintaining the retruded contact position, the best plan is to make a wax bite with the jaws in the correct position for the radiograph, and send this to the radiology technician with the patient. Unless the patient is significantly overclosed, the bite wafer should be thin.

Temporomandibular Joint Radiographs

TM joint radiographs are not obtained routinely for patients with dentofacial deformities but instead are reserved for those whose TM joint symptoms require further evaluation. There are five major types of TM joint images, each with advantages and disadvantages: (1) transcranial radiographs, (2) tomographs (laminographs), (3) computed tomographic (CT) scans, (4) arthrographic evaluations, and (5) magnetic resonance images (MRI). Specific indications are discussed in Chapter 19; an overview is provided here.

Transcranial Radiographs

Although the simplest and least expensive way to obtain a view of the TM joint is a transcranial radiograph, the severe limitations of this method make it rarely useful for patients with dentofacial deformities. As discussed above, TM joint films are indicated only for patients who have signs or symptoms of internal joint problems, and in this circumstance, transcranial radiographs often are distorted and inadequate diagnostically. These films can give a reasonably clear view of the integrity of the bony surfaces of the joint, but only of the lateral third of the condyle (the medial pole routinely is obscured). The transcranial radiograph is an unreliable way to determine condylar position,[19] so these films cannot be used to evaluate whether the condyle is centered. Both false-negative and false-positive images can be a problem. The difficulty in both instances results from the number of superimposed structures, particularly if the orientation is not exactly correct or if patient anatomy is unusual.

Tomographs (Laminographs)

Tomographic images of the TM joint provide true lateral or PA images without the distortion or superimposition that is characteristic of transcranial views, and because lateral tomographic views can be readily obtained with a combination laminographic-cephalometric unit, some orthodontists have used radiographs of this type in recent years.[20] Unfortunately, the same feature that produces an obstructed image of the mandibular condyle and associated area of the temporal bone also is the greatest weakness of these films: the cut

through the condyle shows only a small portion of its total surface. Furthermore, because the image typically is obtained perpendicular to the midsagittal plane but the long axis of the condyle is inclined anteriorly and superiorly, the location of the tomographic cut is critical in determining exactly what will be visualized.

For ideal tomographic imaging, multiple views of the condyle at various depths are needed, but the radiation exposure necessary to do this becomes an important consideration, and only one or two views of each condyle typically are obtained. False-positive findings of pathologic changes affecting the joint are unlikely, but false negatives are quite possible. For example, a clear and normal appearance of the condyle near its medial pole does not mean that there are no degenerative areas or bone spurs centrally or at the lateral pole. Although some authors have stressed the diagnostic importance of the condyle being centered in the fossa in the lateral laminographic projection, this also can be affected by the depth of the cut, and the validity of reduced joint space as a diagnostic criterion for disk displacement or other pathology has been questioned.[21] In short, although laminographic films are preferable to transcranial radiographs, these also may not be diagnostic, particularly when internal derangements are suspected.

Computed Tomography

CT scans of the TM joint probably provide the clearest imaging of the hard tissues available at present (Fig. 4-15). The advantages are the multiple cuts available from a single scan and the soft-tissue imaging capability. The amount of radiation, though not negligible, is quite low for the multiple images of the joint that are obtained, and the joint can be visualized both laterally and anteroposteriorly during the same scan. The main disadvantage of CT scans is the extreme cost of the necessary equipment, which restricts it to hospitals, and the correspondingly high cost to the patient of a TM joint series (typically $300 to $500).

Although in theory CT scans also can provide useful information about the intracapsular disk and other soft tissues, direct visualization of the soft tissues on CT scans remains difficult, and interpretation of the soft-tissue image may not be accurate. Techniques to obtain direct visualization of the disk have improved rapidly, and a CT scan could be particularly advantageous if it could provide the same information that would be achieved from a combination of a conventional tomographic series and an arthrographic examination.[22] When a direct view of the soft tissue is needed, however, MR imaging may be the best method.

Arthrography

Visualization of the soft tissues of the TM joint, particularly the disk, can be greatly improved by injecting contrast material into the joint space before obtaining

Fig. 4-15. **A,** A close-up view of a sagittal CT scan of the right TM joint in the closed position in a patient with an anteriorly displaced disk. In this view, the displaced disk can be visualized at the inferior portion of the articular eminence, anterior to the condyle. The bone is seen as white, the disk as a darker mass. **B,** Direct sagittal CT scan of the same joint in the open position. Now the condyle has translated forward, and the disk is in its normal position over the condylar head. The arrows point to the anterior and posterior bands of the disk.

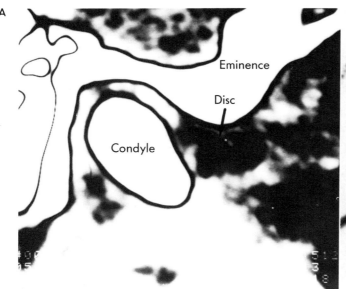

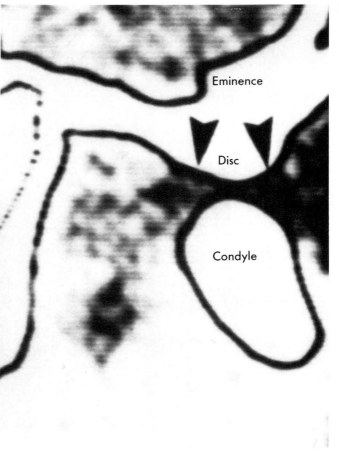

tomographic views (Fig. 4-16). Until the 1970s, the role of disk displacement in TM joint problems was not appreciated. With its recognition came an increased interest in arthrography as a way of demonstrating the correlation between disk movments and TM joint sounds and of documenting disk position.

Arthrography is a relatively safe but nonetheless invasive procedure. The joint space must be penetrated to inject the contrast material, and complications may result. Now that the results of arthrographic investigations have documented the relationship between disk movements and TM joint sounds,[23] the diagnosis of disk displacement often can be made on clinical grounds without the necessity for arthrography. Therefore at this point its use is limited to patients who are considered highly likely to need surgery for repositioning and/or repair of the disk, in whom there is some doubt on clinical grounds as to the condition of the disk.

Magnetic Resonance Imaging

It is possible to obtain surprisingly precise images of internal hard and soft tissues with the new and still rapidly developing method of magenetic resonance imaging. MRI is based on the relaxation time of protons

in body fluids that were temporarily brought to a higher energy state by the application of a strong external magnetic field. Because of differing fluid compositions and rate of fluid transfer within varying tissues, most soft-tissue and hard-tissue elements have a characteristic MRI "signature," which can be resolved into images via computer analysis. No ionizing radiation is required with MRI, and the image is displayed on a computer screen from data stored in computer memory. The images can be recalled at any time, reviewed and manipulated as desired, and returned to computer memory.

At this writing, MRI for the TM joint remains a promising development for the future rather than a currently valid clinical tool.[24] It seems highly likely, however, that MRI will prove useful for TM joint evaluation, just as it has for other tissues of the body. Like CT, MRI requires elaborate and costly equipment available only at major medical centers and therefore is expensive. The expense is magnified by the long exposure time (30 to 45 minutes) needed to obtain a TM joint image (i.e., only a few patients per day can be studied with a diagnostic tool that costs over $1 million at present).

An additional complication with MRI is that mag-

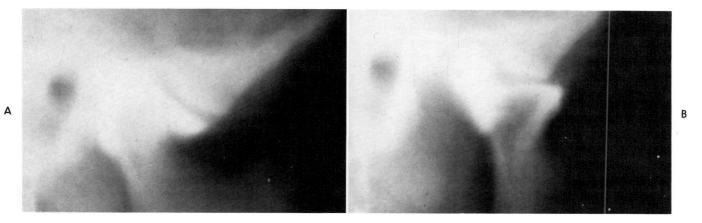

Fig. 4-16. **A,** Inferior joint–space arthrogram of right TM joint in the closed position. An accumulation of dye anterior to the condyle represents an anterior disk displacement, with some folding of the disk anteriorly. **B,** Arthrogram of the same patient in the open position, with minimal dye remaining anterior to the condyle. This demonstrates reduction of the disk to its proper location in the fully open position; that is, the patient has anterior disk displacement with reduction.

netically active metals must be excluded from the powerful magnetic field needed to generate the images. Although there are special techniques to minimize the difficulty and at least theoretically allow a satisfactory image, the presence of ferrous metals in the mouth, such as the stainless steel usually employed in orthodontic appliances, creates considerable difficulty. For this reason, MRIs of many patients with dentofacial deformities may be compromised by the orthodontic treatment that they are already undergoing. It seems likely that these limitations can and will be overcome in the future. If so, because the strong magnetic fields necessary for MRI seem to cause no tissue damage, MRI may well be the preferred technique for TM joint imaging in the future.

Application of these techniques in specific circumstances is illustrated in more detail in Chapter 19.

Dental Casts: Articulator Mounting?

Dental casts are an essential part of the diagnostic records. They should be obtained in the standard fashion for orthodontic records, with maximum reflection of the soft tissue so that the alveolar process is revealed as much as possible. The casts, like the photographs, are invaluable as a permanent record of the condition before treatment began. They also provide a better view of dental relationships than can be obtained on clinical examination and thereby serve to provide more details of what can be seen rather grossly on clinical examination. In this instance, they are rather like the cephalometric radiograph. Finally, the dental casts are essential in the treatment planning steps that call for trial repositioning of the teeth and jaws (model surgery), and they may need to be duplicated for this purpose (see Chapter 5).

It is fair to say that whether and when dental casts should be mounted on an articulator is the most controversial aspect of diagnosis and treatment planning at present. To some excellent clinicians, mounting the casts is important for almost every patient. Other clinicians of equally high repute rarely employ articulator mounting and discount the value of any additional information this procedure might provide. Is there a rational way to decide if and when the articulator is needed?

There are two reasons for mounting casts on an articulator. The first is to record and document any discrepancy between the jaw relations at the initial contact of the teeth, which is the centric relation (CR), and the relations at the patient's full or habitual occlusion, centric occlusion (CO). The second is to record the lateral and anterior excursive paths of the mandible, documenting these and making the tooth relationships during the excursions more accessible for study.

The second purpose is very important when reconstructive dentistry is planned because the contours of replacement or restored teeth must accommodate the path of movement. However, this is less important for diagnosis and treatment planning in patients who will have orthodontics and surgery because jaw function may change in adaptation to surgery. Therefore the question for diagnosis in potential orthognathic-surgery patients is whether enough additional information about the CR and CO positions will be obtained to justify the additional time and expense of articulator mounting.

There is no particular difficulty in establishing a patient's CO, but CR is more problematic and controversial. The definition of CR has changed considerably in recent years. Currently there are strong advocates of three quite different concepts. The first, which was generally accepted until the mid-1970s, is that CR is the most posterior and superior position of the mandibular condyles to which the mandible can be manipulated without undue strain. The second, which is the most widely accepted now but has not achieved a consensus, is that CR is the most superior position to which the patient can bring the mandible, using his or her own musculature.[25] Typically, this position is close to but somewhat forward from the manipulated position. The third, definitely a minority opinion but with many advocates, is that CR is the position to which the mandible is brought when external electrical stimulation of the musculature is employed to overcome sensory cues that might otherwise complicate the situation and lead to a strained position for the mandible.[26] The condylar position produced by electrical stimulation often is considerably downward and forward from that produced by either of the other two methods, adding to the controversy.

There is also a controversy about the significance of a discrepancy between CO and CR. At one time, it was thought that the CR and CO positions should be coincident, particularly after extensive restorative dentistry. However, it is now generally accepted that in normal individuals the habitual occlusion is 1 to 2 mm forward from the condylar position to which the individual can be manipulated or that he or she can achieve.[27,28]

This difference is almost always present in untreated natural dentitions. It is probably important for optimum jaw function and patient comfort. A lateral shift from initial contact to complete closure is not normal, nor is a large forward shift. Because CR/CO differences large enough to be possibly significant are found frequently, and because TM joint problems may arise in such individuals (even if not so consistently that one can confidently speak of cause and effect), it is important to document such discrepancies. Articulator-mounted casts are one way to do that.

Our suggestions for articulator mounting of dental casts for diagnosis in patients with dentofacial deformities are as follows:

1. In patients who have no TM joint signs or symptoms, as assessed by the clinical evaluation method described above, and in whom there is neither a lateral shift nor a major (greater than 2 mm) anterior shift, articulator-mounted casts are unnecessary for surgical-orthodontic diagnosis. If lateral or anterior shifts are present but there are no symptoms, they should be documented and taken into account in planning treatment.

2. In patients who do have TM joint problems, articulator-mounted casts are desirable. In these individuals, it is advantageous to employ a disclu-

sion splint for a few days before making the CR record to be as sure as possible that muscle spasm and splinting is not distorting the condylar position. The technique for obtaining the registration in this way is described in some detail in Chapter 19.

3. Articulator-mounted casts may be needed for treatment planning in some patients who do not need them for diagnosis. This is particularly true in planning surgical treatment to reposition the posterior maxilla. The use of mounted casts in model surgery is discussed in Chapter 5.

4. When articulator mounting of casts is desired, a semiadjustable articulator (e.g., Hanau or Whip Mix) almost always is satisfactory. The articulator should accept lateral and protrusive check bites and provide for adjustment of condylar guidance. The more elaborate articulators sometimes used in restorative dentistry, with features such as the timing of the Bennett shift, are unnecessary.

DATA FROM DIAGNOSTIC RECORDS
Cephalometric Analysis in Perspective

Information from the lateral and (if indicated) PA cephalometric films is a major part of the data base for surgical-orthodontic treatment. For most items in the data base, direct observation or an informal analysis suffices to provide the desired information, but cephalometric films usually are analyzed in a more formal way, now often employing a computer. Because of its importance, we discuss here cephalometric analysis in some detail and present an analytic approach that combines components of several previously published methods.

It should be kept in mind that there are two reasons for obtaining a lateral cephalometric film before orthodontic or surgical-orthodontic treatment. The first, which is the focus of the discussion that follows, is to provide detailed information about the relationships of the parts of the dentofacial complex. These relationships can be observed on direct visual examination—a cephalometric film is not required to note the presence of severe mandibular deficiency—but the extent of the deficiency can be evaluated much more precisely from a cephalometric film.

The second reason for obtaining this radiograph is that it provides baseline data against which the later treatment response can be measured. A skilled clinician often can observe dentofacial relationships accurately enough for diagnosis and treatment planning without resorting to cephalometric analyis at all, though there is no doubt that the diagnosis can be done more precisely and reliably if cephalometric information is available. However, clinical impressions of treatment response are notoriously unreliable, and it is the use of

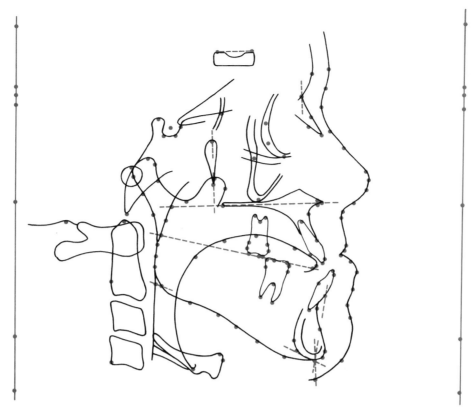

Fig. 4-17. The model used for digitization of cephalometric films for research at the University of North Carolina, which includes up to 156 points. The more points in a digital model, the greater the anatomic fidelity, but the greater the demands on the computer system and the more time it takes to enter the information. For diagnostic purposes, simpler models that employ 15 to 30 points are adequate. Treatment planning requires more points (see Chapter 5).

serial films to follow treatment response that is the compelling reason for using cephalometrics in routine orthodontic cases. The more complex the case, the greater the need for cephalometrics in diagnosis and treatment planning, and so it follows logically that there would be more need for cephalometrics in the severe cases that might require surgery. Even for these patients, however, evaluating treatment response is at least as important a reason for obtaining the cephalometric film.

Tracing versus Digitization

Preparing a tracing of a cephalometric film facilitates its uses for both the major purposes described above. For diagnosis, tracings allow easier visualization of the pattern of relationships and easier identification of landmarks used in measurements. For analysis of treatment changes, superimposition of tracings is the best way to observe exactly what happened.

With the widespread availability of office and home computers, it is a straightforward procedure to place cephalometric information in computer memory by digitizing the location of various landmarks and storing their coordinates in memory (Fig. 4-17). The computer equivalent of a tracing is produced by simply connecting the landmarks. The more points that are included in the digital model, the more the computer version will resemble an actual tracing.

The advantage of creating a digital model is twofold. First, once this has been done, an essentially unlimited number of calculations can be made quite rapidly, yielding any number of angular and linear measurements. Second, when a later cephalometric film becomes available for the same patient, after it has been digitized using the same model, superimpositions can be made within computer memory and plots produced to give the equivalent of superimposed tracings for visual analysis. Until recently, the creation of a computerized cephalometric data base of this type was limited primarily to research groups and universities, but cephalometric programs for office computers have rapidly changed this situation. It seems likely that cephalometric information will be stored and used, for both diagnosis and treatment planning as outlined below, more and more in digital form.

There is nothing conceptually different about measuring angular and linear relationships by hand or within a computer data base, nor is there any difference in planning treatment by moving templates within computer memory or on an overlay tracing. The advantage of the computer is convenience and speed, not different or better information. The clinician must remember that both the computed and manually generated measurements are not the desired product from cephalometric analysis, but an intermediate step toward generating it. The result of the analysis is the judged relationship of the component parts, not the measurement that was the basis for the conclusion.

Because the focus of cephalometric analysis must be on the observed relationships, the discussion below is not affected by whether the cephalometric films were digitized and placed into a computer data base or were traced and evaluated manually. The computer method offers potentially greater flexibility, speed, and convenience, but is not necessary for accurate diagnosis or adequate planning of treatment.

Template versus Measurement Analysis

If the goal of cephalometric analysis is to provide an accurate description of dentofacial relationships, one must specify exactly what relationships are of interest. This is done best by considering the head and face as composed of five major units: (1) the cranium and cranial base, (2) the nasomaxillary complex, (3) the mandible, (4) the maxillary dentition, and (5) the mandibular dentition (Fig. 4-18). The object of diagnosis is to detect and quantify disproportionate relationships among these units, and lateral cephalometric analysis offers a quantative and precise way of doing this in the anteroposterior and vertical planes of space. The result of the cephalometric analysis is a judgment as to the relationship of the parts, not the generation of a table of angular or linear measurements.

The detection of imbalances and disproportions in dentofacial relationships is based on comparing the data for the individual being analyzed with data for a normal or idealized reference. There are two ways to display the "normal" data. The first is in the form of tabulated measurements, with which measurements for the individual being analyzed can be compared. The second is to display the normal data in the form of a template, which is an average tracing for the reference group or perhaps a synthetic ideal.

Experienced clinicians often simply look at a cephalometric film and immediately recognize areas of disproportion. What they are doing, of course, is mentally placing a template of the appropriate relationships over the film in question, and then noting any discrepancies.

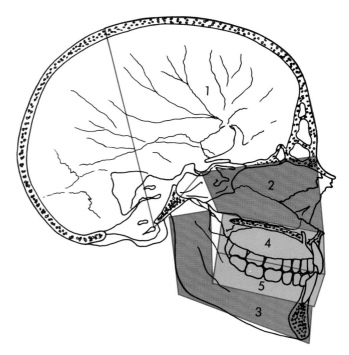

Fig. 4-18. The goal of lateral cephalometric analysis is to establish the anteroposterior and vertical relationships of the five major craniofacial units, as shown here. Many different methods for doing this have been proposed, none of which is satisfactory for all patients under all circumstances. For instance, in establishing how the maxilla relates to the cranium-cranial base, several methods could be used quite satisfactorily, and no single measurement is adequate for all patients. The goal is to establish the relationship, not to carry out some specific analytic procedure.

The accuracy of that approach is as good as the clinician's mental template. This presumably becomes better with time but can be affected by various experiences that were never analyzed systematically. When prepared templates such as those from the Bolton growth study[29] are the basis for comparision, or when tabulated measurements are compared, the quality of the information is determined by how well the individual fits the reference group. From this perspective, template analysis is more similar to analysis of tabulated measurements than might have been thought initially. The two methods are alternate ways of doing the same thing. They are discussed individually below.

Technique for Measurement Analysis
Anteroposterior Relationship of the Jaws to the Cranium

When cephalometric analysis was initially developed in the 1940s by Downs at Illinois,[30] the focus was largely on the relationship of the maxilla to the mandible, which was indirectly linked back to the cranium via the facial angle. This emphasis was in the Angle

TABLE 4-4 Comparative cephalometric values for three racial groups (in degrees)

Parameter	Caucasian	American black	Japanese
Frankfort-SN	6	6	—
SNA	82	85	81
SNB	80	79	77
ANB	2	6	4
Y axis	59	63	62
Facial plane	88	88	86
Mandibular plane (SNGoGn)	32	38	34
Occlusal plane to SN	14	—	20
1̅ to NA degrees	22	23	24
1̲ to NA mm	4	7	6
1̅ to NB degrees	25	34	31
1 to N̲B mm	4	10	8
1̲ to 1̅	131	114	120

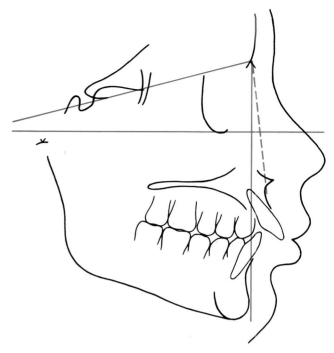

Fig. 4-19. Cephalometric tracing of a patient with maxillary protrusion in whom SNA and SNB angles could be misleading because of the inclination of the anterior cranial base relative to true horizontal. When the nasion perpendicular line is dropped across the face, the maxilla is well anterior to it and the mandible is just on it, indicating maxillary protrusion—but the SNA angle is normal and the SNB angle is low. Because the SN plane is inclined at 14 degrees to true horizontal, 8 degrees higher than normal, it is necessary to add 8 degrees to the SNA and SNB angles to obtain values that correctly reflect the skeletal relationships.

orthodontic tradition. Edward Angle, the founder of modern American orthodontics, had concluded that the position of the maxilla and maxillary dentition was all but invariant. This made the location of the mandible the key element in diagnosis. From this perspective, there was no reason to check the position of the maxilla.

However, experience with cephalometric radiographs soon made it clear that Angle had underestimated the amount of variation contributed by the maxilla. In 1952, Riedel[31] suggested using the sella-nasion line and its angular relationships to the anterior maxillary and mandibular landmarks (the SNA and SNB angles) to estimate the position of the maxilla and mandible to the cranium, and using the SNA-SNB difference (ANB) as an indicator of the relative anteroposterior position of the jaws. These measurements (normal values in Table 4-4) quickly became the cephalometric standard, and they still are widely used. The merits or demerits of ANB as an indicator of relative jaw position remains the subject of debate.[32]

The problem with using angular measurements to SN as an indicator of the anteroposterior position of the jaws is that this assumes a normal inclination of the anterior cranial base, which is not always the case. Because the inclination of the SN line to the true horizontal can vary considerably, an uncritical acceptance of SNA and SNB can lead to an error in determining which jaw is at fault in a discrepancy. For example, consider the patient shown in Fig. 4-19. For this individual, there is an obvious Class II malocclusion with relative protrusion of the maxillary anterior teeth. The SNA angle is 82 degrees, which is approximately nor-

mal, and the SNB angle is 74 degrees, 6 degrees less than normal. Therefore one might conclude that the problem is a mandibular deficiency.

However, the correct way to look at the same individual is provided by using a true horizontal orientation (the Frankfort plane or, even better, the true horizontal line from a NHP radiograph). If this is done, it can be seen that for this patient, the SN line is inclined upward at an angle of 14 degrees to true horizontal, versus a normal SN-Frankfort inclination of 6 degrees. If the SN line is corrected to its normal inclination to true horizontal, the effect is to add 6 degrees to the initial SNA and SNB angles. Now the corrected SNA is 88, well above normal, whereas the corrected SNB is 80, approximately the normal value. The problem is maxillary protrusion, not mandibular deficiency.

In modern cephalometrics, the SNA and SNB angles can be used only in this fashion, after correction for the inclination of the SN line to true horizontal. Otherwise, serious errors can result. The practical effect is to

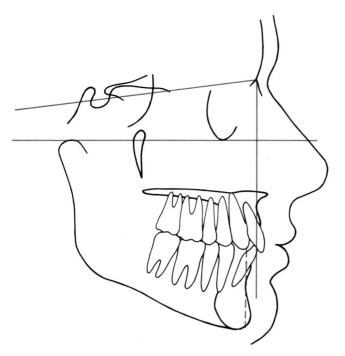

Fig. 4-20. A well-proportioned face, showing normal relationships of the anterior structures to the nasion perpendicular line. The normal A-B difference projected to the true horizontal is 4 mm. Point A usually is slightly (about 2 mm) ahead of the nasion perpendicular line, and point B about 2 mm behind it. When a true vertical line (which will be parallel to nasion perpendicular) is drawn through point B, the chin should be about 2 mm in front of it, and the tip of the lower incisor 2 to 4 mm in front of it. Small deviations from these ideal measurements are of no consequence.

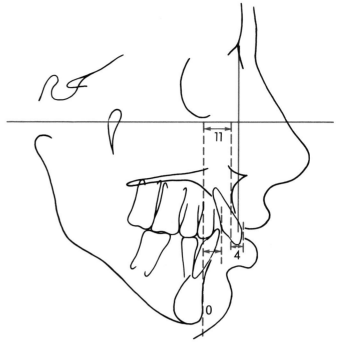

Fig. 4-21. A convex face with mandibular deficiency, although there is only moderate overjet. Point A is slightly behind the nasion perpendicular, but point B is over a centimeter behind it. The A-B difference projected to the true horizontal line is 11 mm as compared with the normal 4 mm. Note the protrusion of the lower incisors relative to a vertical line through point B and the lack of chin prominence (the incisor tip is 7 mm in front of the line, pogonion is 0 mm). The upper incisor is 4 mm anterior to the true vertical line through point A, which is normal.

relate the maxilla and mandible, not to the SN line, but to true horizontal.

If one accepts that the maxilla and mandible must be related to the cranium with the head oriented as it is in life, rather than arbitrarily tipped forward or backward according to the inclination of the anterior cranial base, there is an easier and more direct way to locate the jaws anteroposteriorly. This method, first published by McNamara,[33] relates the jaws to a true vertical line (perpendicular to true horizontal) dropped from nasion. (McNamara's published data are based on the Frankfort plane rather than on true horizontal, which was not available for his Michigan growth study reference sample. The origin of the Frankfort plane as an estimator for true horizontal has already been discussed above.)

For most normal Caucasian patients, the nasion perpendicular line passes slightly behind point A and 2 to 3 mm anteriorly to point B (Fig. 4-20). The normal A-B difference (i.e., distance between points A and B when both are projected to the true horizontal line) is approximately 4 mm. Therefore measurements to the

nasion perpendicular line can establish the anteroposterior relationships of the jaws to the cranium and to each other. An individual whose maxilla is slightly behind the line and whose mandible is well behind it can fairly be said to have mandibular deficiency with no component of maxillary protrusion (Fig. 4-21). An individual such as the one shown in Fig. 4-19, whose maxilla is 6 mm forward and whose mandible is 2 mm behind, should be diagnosed as having maxillary protrusion, not mandibular deficiency.

In some well-proportioned individuals with a posteriorly divergent profile (who often are of Scandinavian descent), the maxilla may be 3 to 5 mm behind the nasion perpendicular line and the mandible 7 to 10 mm behind it (Fig. 4-22). In individuals with anterior divergence, the maxilla may be 2 to 4 mm in front of the line and the mandible on or slightly ahead of it. As with clinical analysis of the profile, this facial divergence does not indicate jaw deformity. Blacks and Orientals normally have more prominence of the face relative to the cranium than do Caucasians, which is reflected in a tendency toward anterior divergence and

A

B

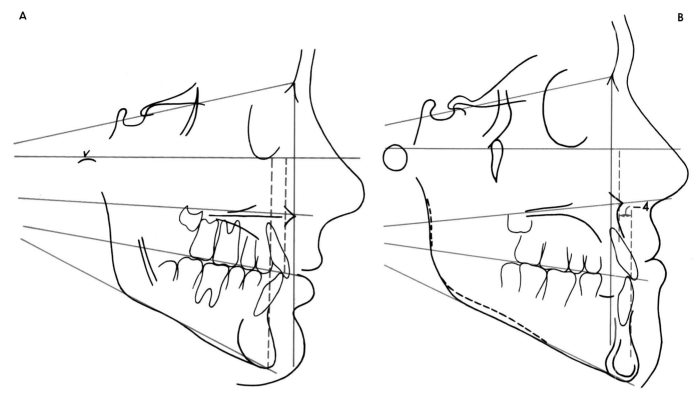

Fig. 4-22. **A,** A cephalometric tracing of an individual with a posteriorly divergent profile but excellent occlusion and facial esthetics. Point A is 4 mm behind the nasion perpendicular line, and point B is 10 mm behind it. The A-B difference is 6 mm. These numbers are quite different from the ideal, but there is no skeletal or dental problem. **B,** Tracing of an individual with an anteriorly divergent profile. Point A is 3 mm in front of the nasion perpendicular line, and point B is 7 mm in front. The A-B difference is -4 mm. Again, there is no problem.

somewhat different relationships of the jaws to the nasion perpendicular line. Similarly, northern Europeans have a tendency toward decreased facial prominence and posterior divergence that can affect the position of both jaws relative to the cranium. Only if the A-B difference is too large is there a problem.

To avoid the possibility of confusion because of facial divergence, first establish whether there is a jaw discrepancy. This is seen easily from the A-B difference in millimeters, as projected to the true horizontal line (Fig. 4-21). An A-B difference greater than 6 mm or less than -4 mm (B in front of A gives negative numbers) indicates a discrepancy. If there is a discrepancy, then decide which jaw is at fault by comparing their positions to the nasion perpendicular line.

A jaw discrepancy can result from a problem in the size of the jaw or from its position. Perhaps the most straightforward approach to evaluating the size of the jaws is Harvold's approach, which is incorporated into the McNamara analysis. Harvold[34] measured the distance from the posterior aspect of the condyle to the chin and to the anterior aspect of the maxilla, as shown in Fig. 4-23. The absolute distances are interest-

ing as a reflection of jaw size, but the difference in the mandibular and maxillary lengths is more significant in determining the extent of a jaw discrepancy. If the mandibular length is more than 30 mm or less than 15 mm greater than the maxillary length, the discrepancy may be too great for orthodontic correction. In using this approach, it must be kept in mind that the vertical separation of the jaws affects the measured distances.

Another way to evaluate size-versus-position relationships is given in the Wylie analysis of anteroposterior dysplasia,[35] first published in the 1940s and therefore one of the older cephalometric methods, but still valuable and less used than would be beneficial. Wylie projected maxillary and mandibular measurements to the Frankfort plane, which would be the true horizontal line in modern use, and subdivided the increments along the plane as shown in Fig. 4-24. It is possible for a mandible of normal size to be attached to the cranium anteriorly or posteriorly to its normal position, and this obviously would contribute to its relative prominence. Similarly, the maxilla could be projected more or less forward from its normal position. Disturbances in jaw position rather than in size can contrib-

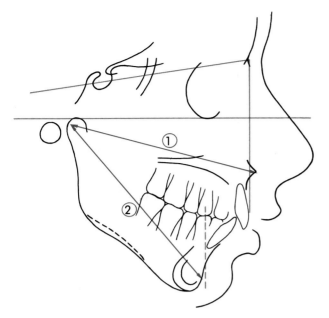

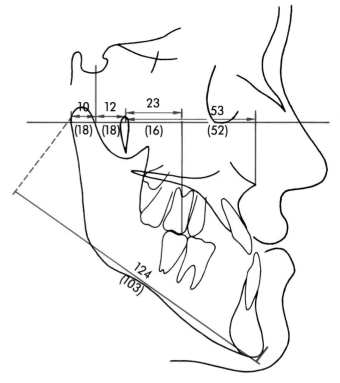

Fig. 4-23. The tracing of a patient with severe mandibular deficiency, showing the measurements for maxillary and mandibular unit length as advocated by Harvold and incorporated into the McNamara analysis. Maxillary length is measured *from* a point on the posterior contour of the temporal fossa behind the condyle *to* the point on the contour at anterior nasal spine where the bony tip is 2 mm thick. Mandibular length is from the same posterior condylar point to pogonion. For this patient, the maxillary length is 92 mm (normal for adult males is 114 mm) (see Table 4-6) and the mandibular length is 100 mm (normal is 127 mm). Both the maxilla and mandible therefore are quite small in size, the mandible more so in proportion than is the maxilla. The unit length difference of 8 mm (normal is 16 mm) is outside the range of possible orthodontic treatment. This information supplements what would be learned from using the nasion perpendicular, which suggests that the maxilla is slightly behind its normal position and the mandible far behind it. The A-B difference projected to true horizontal is 21 mm.

Fig. 4-24. Cephalometric analysis of a patient with a severe Class III malocclusion and maxillary deficiency, using the Wylie analysis of anteroposterior dysplasia. The patient's measurements are shown above the Frankfort (true horizontal) line, and the standards are below. Note that the sella-condyle distance is short, which projects the mandible excessively forward relative to the cranial base. The sella-PTM distance also is short, which means that the maxilla is not positioned forward as much as normal. The maxilla itself is of a normal size, but the mandible is large. The result is a severe jaw discrepancy resulting from a combination of a large mandible that also is positioned too far forward and a normally sized maxilla that is not positioned far enough forward. In this analytical method, if all the measurements are small or large respectively relative to the standards, there is no problem, but disproportions are significant. It provides a way to differentiate problems caused by the size of the jaws from problems caused by their anteroposterior position.

ute to jaw discrepancies, as Fig. 4-24 illustrates. This information is highly pertinent in establishing exactly what the problem is in some patients with severe problems.

Vertical Relationship of the Jaws to the Cranium

In the original forms of cephalometric analysis, vertical relationships did not receive nearly the attention as did anteroposterior relationships. Although this deficiency has been recognized in modern cephalometrics, there still is a tendency to place greater emphasis on the anteroposterior plane of space. More than anything else, this reflects the bias in classical orthodontics toward anteroposterior relationships that was exemplified in the Angle classification.

Vertical jaw discrepancies can be very difficult to correct with traditional orthodontic treatment, so the bias away from vertical evaluation also was reinforced in orthodontics by a tendency to avoid the untreatable. Vertical relationships can be changed as readily in surgical-orthodontic treatment as can anteroposterior ones, and vertical distortions must be recognized and quantified in the same way as are anteroposterior problems.

The first step in analyzing vertical relationships is to observe the orientation of the horizontal planes of the face: the cranial base (SN), Frankfort, palatal, occlusal, and mandibular planes (Fig. 4-25). In the late 1950s,

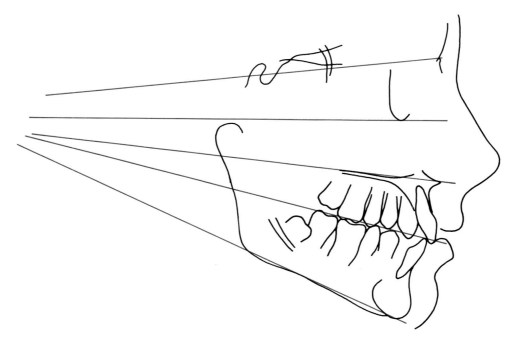

Fig. 4-25. In a well-proportioned face, the horizontal planes project posteriorly toward a common meeting point not far behind the back of the skull. The more parallel the planes (i.e., the further behind the skull they would meet), the greater the tendency toward anterior deep-bite malocclusion, thus the term skeletal deep bite for this condition. Conversely, the more rapidly the planes converge posteriorly (or diverge anteriorly, if you prefer to look at it that way), the greater the tendency toward anterior open bite, thus the term skeletal open bite.

Sassouni[36] contributed the idea that in a vertically well-proportioned face, the horizontal planes project toward an approximate common intersection located near the back of the skull. Sassouni pointed out that if these planes are nearly parallel, so that their point of convergence is well away from the face, anterior and posterior facial height will be nearly the same. This produces a predisposition toward deep bite anteriorly. Conversely, if the planes converge just behind the face, the patient is predisposed toward an anterior open bite because anterior facial dimensions will be considerably longer than posterior ones. In addition, if one part of the face is vertically disproportionate, the plane through it will not converge with the others.

Many patients with dentofacial deformities can be seen on inspection to have rotation of one or both jaws, as revealed by a palatal and/or mandibular plane that deviates from the intersection of the other planes (Fig. 4-26). Rotation of the mandible has been known for many years to contribute to dentofacial deformities. Only recently has it been appreciated that rotation of the maxilla also can be a major contributor. For instance, many patients with a long-face condition can be seen on inspection of the palatal plane to have a maxilla that is rotated down posteriorly and up anteriorly.

Downward rotation anteriorly is less common but can contribute to the short-face condition. Mandibular rotation may be partially or almost entirely secondary to maxillary rotation.

Inspection of the facial planes can immediately reveal deep or open-bite tendencies and whether jaw rotations are present, but it is only the first step in vertical analysis. It also is necessary to more precisely locate disproportions. For example, if the maxilla is rotated counterclockwise, is it because it is up anteriorly, down posteriorly, or some combination? This second step in vertical analysis requires the use of linear measurements (Fig. 4-27).

Measuring the contributions of the maxilla and mandible to total face height is an excellent way to establish whether anterior vertical disproportions are primarily in the maxilla or mandible. Note that these measurements are made along the true vertical line, not on any sort of angle (which of course would increase the distance if an anteroposterior deviation from normal jaw position was present).

Linear measurements from cranial-base reference points (sella and ethmoid points) can be useful in establishing the vertical position of the posterior maxilla (PNS) and mandible (Go). Measurements of this type

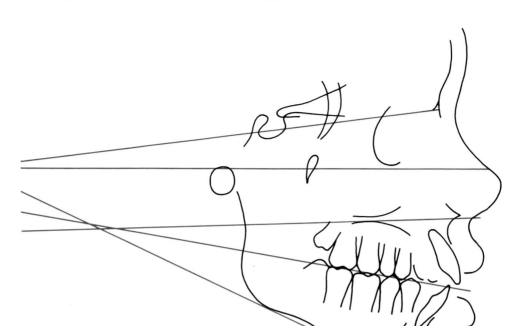

Fig. 4-26. Inspection of the horizontal planes quickly reveals vertical disproportions in the form of planes that do not project toward the common meeting point of well-proportioned faces. This patient has a maxilla that is rotated downward posteriorly and upward anteriorly, which predisposes toward anterior open bite and excessive face height (because the downward rotation of the maxilla posteriorly has caused the mandible also to rotate down and back).

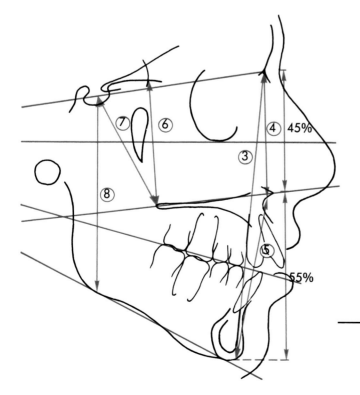

rarely have been included in published cephalometric analyses, despite their importance, and so tabulated data for standards are not widely available. The best source is the Michigan growth study,[37] which does include data for a number of millimeter measurments. A summary of pertinent Michigan linear measurement standards is included in Table 4-5. The measurements are illustrated in Figs. 4-27 and 4-28.

Interpretation of these measurements must be tempered by an appreciation for the proportionality of faces. Linear distances have some meaning in their own right, but they should be interpreted primarily in the context of proportional relationships within a particular individual. If the upper-face height is large, the lower-face height must also be large to provide reasonable balance, and one would expect both measurements to be larger in a tall individual than in a short one. Similarly, if anterior dimensions are large, one would expect posterior dimensions to be large also in a

Fig. 4-27. Linear measurements useful in establishing the source of vertical jaw disproportions. The measurements are keyed to Table 4-5, where normative values are given.

TABLE 4-5 Cephalometric linear measurements for adult caucasians (age 16) (see Figs. 4-27 and 4-28)

	Male	Female
1. Maxillary length (TM-ANS)*	114(4)	105(3)
2. Mandibular length (TM-Pg)*	127(5)	119(4)
3. Total face height (Na-Me)	137(8)	123(5)
4. Upper face height (Na-ANS)	60(4)	55(2)
5. Lower face height (ANS-Me)	80(6)	69(5)
6. Ethmoid point— PNS	55(4)	50(3)
7. Sella—PNS	56(4)	51(3)
8. Posterior face height (S-Go)	88(6)	79(4)
9. Palatal plane— menton	76(6)	67(4)
10. Palatal plane— upper molar	28(3)	25(2)
11. Palatal plane— upper incisor	33(3)	30(3)
12. PNS—ANS	62(4)	57(4)
13. Mandibular plane—lower incisor	49(3)	42(3)
14. Mandibular plane—lower molar	38(3)	33(3)
15. PTM vertical†	18(?)	18(?)

Standard deviation is in parenthesis.
Data, except as indicated, from Riolo ML, Moyers RE, McNamara JA, et al: An atlas of craniofacial growth, Ann Arbor, 1974, University of Michigan Center for Human Growth & Development.
*Data from Harvold EP: The activator in orthodontics, St. Louis, 1974, The CV Mosby Co.
†Data from Ricketts RM: Perspectives in the clinical application of cephalometrics, Angle Orthod 51:115-150, 1981.

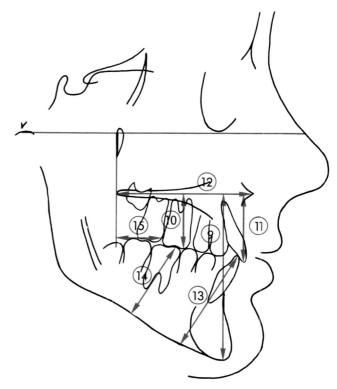

Fig. 4-28. Linear measurements to establish the anteroposterior and vertical position of the upper molar and the vertical position of the incisors and lower molars. Normative data are included in Table 4-5.

well-proportioned face. Given a reasonable amount of caution in this regard, however, the interpretation of the vertical measurements is quite straightforward. For example, if the upper jaw is rotated and the distance from nasion to ANS is normal (see Fig. 4-27), one could conclude that the maxillary rotation results from excessive vertical development posteriorly.

Relationship of the Maxillary Teeth to the Maxilla

Anteroposterior Relationships. From the beginning of use of cephalometric analysis, the amount of protrusion of the incisor teeth was recognized as important. Both angular and linear measurements for analyzing

this were suggested. In the early cephalometric analyses, angular measurements were preferred. Originally, the inclination of the upper incisor to the facial plane (N-Pg) was measured, but this related the maxillary incisor to the mandible more than to the maxilla. Measurement of the angle between the long axis of the upper incisor and the Frankfort plane, then later the SN plane, also was employed, but these measurements also did not really relate the upper incisor directly to the maxilla. The first cephalometric approach that specifically did so was the Steiner analysis,[38] which was introduced in the 1950s and still is widely employed. It was also the first to use linear as well as angular measurements. Steiner suggested that the upper incisor should be related to the NA line and that both its inclination to the line and the millimeter distance from the incisal edge to the line (Fig. 4-29) should be measured. The dual measurements indicate where the incisal edge is and whether the tooth was tipped or displaced bodily to that location—which is still what you need to know.

In contemporary use, we suggest that Steiner's NA line be replaced by the true vertical line through point A and that both the millimeter distance and angulation be measured to this line, in the same way that Steiner

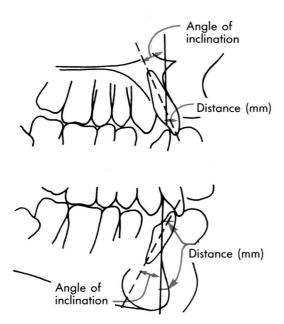

Fig. 4-29. The measurements used in the Steiner analysis to determine the position of the maxillary and mandibular incisors. Steiner used the NA and NB lines for the upper and lower incisors, respectively. This biases the measurements toward dental compensation for a skeletal discrepancy (i.e., the original Steiner method is increasingly unsatisfactory as the A-B difference increases). In modern analysis, we suggest that the true vertical line through points A and B be substituted for the NA and NB lines.

measured them. The true vertical line through point A often is the NA line in normal patients, but this is less likely in dentofacial deformity patients. Using the true vertical rather than the NA line is more accurate when the maxilla is displaced anteriorly or posteriorly.

It also is important in some patients to judge the anteroposterior position of the maxillary molar, especially when there is a question as to whether it has drifted mesially. A measurement from the center of the pterygomaxillary fissure to the mesiobuccal cusp of the upper first molar is included in Wylie's analysis of anteroposterior dysplasia (see Fig. 4-24). More recently, Ricketts[39] has suggested a measurement from the pterygoid vertical line along the distal margin of the fissure to the distal of the first molar (see Fig. 4-28), which amounts to the same thing. Both the Wylie and Ricketts measurements are satisfactory for establishing the anteroposterior position of the posterior maxillary teeth.

Vertical Position. Linear measurements from a superior reference plane to the maxillary incisor and molar are the best way to establish the vertical position of the teeth relative to the maxilla, and the palatal plane (ANS-PNS) is the preferred reference (see Fig. 4-28). Tabulated data for the distance from the molar and in-

cisor along a perpendicular plane to the palatal plane are available from the Michigan growth study (see Table 4-5).

Relationship of the Mandibular Teeth to the Mandible

Anteroposterior Relationship. In the early days of cephalometric analysis, there was a strong tendency to orient the mandibular teeth to the maxillomandibular position, rather than just to the mandible. For instance, the lower incisors often were evaluated by their relationship to the A-Pg line.[40] If a constant relationship to A-Pg is expected, the lower incisor would move backward or forward relative to the mandible, depending on the magnitude of the jaw discrepancy. The implication, of course, was that tooth position must accomodate the jaw relationship; that is, both growth modification and surgery were out of the question. Then the object of diagnosis would be to establish how much compensation for the jaw discrepancy was already present, which in treatment planning would determine how much more compensation should be created by orthodontic tooth movement.

The Steiner analysis, interestingly enough, provided a reasonably unbiased approach to measuring the position of the lower incisor to the mandible, despite the fact that Steiner then proceeded to discuss treatment planning from the perspective that jaw relationships could not be changed. Steiner measured the inclination and linear distance of the lower incisor to the NB line, analagous to the measurements for the upper incisor to NA (see Fig. 4-29). Soon thereafter, Holdaway suggested that the prominence of the bony chin to the NB line also should be considered, and this measurement was almost routinely incorporated into the Steiner analysis. These measurements remain useful today. Steiner suggested that in planning treatment, a compromise in incisor position in both arches would be determined by the magnitude of the jaw discrepancy, which is less relevant today, but he did analyze first and compromise second, instead of confusing the two steps.

In modern analysis, it is more logical to orient the lower incisor to the true vertical line, using the McNamara approach. The Steiner measurements to NB are not quite as reliable as those to NA in estimating the tooth-jaw relationship, simply because the NB line is more inclined. The large inclination of A-Pg and its underlying assumption make it still less valid.

The variations in the morphology of the mandible behind the dentition make it difficult to locate a posterior landmark, so the AP position of the mandibular molar is rarely evaluated from a cephalometric measurement. Arch length measured from the dental cast, coupled with analysis of incisor position, provides the same information.

Vertical Relationships. It is possible to measure the

vertical position of the mandibular incisor and first molar as a linear distance perpendicular to the mandibular plane (see Fig. 4-28), and tabulated data from the Michigan growth study provide a reference (Table 4-5). The inclination of the mandibular plane to the true horizontal gives these measurements a horizontal component, but they can help clarify some cases. A better measurement, particularly for the lower incisor, would be the distance from the lower border of the chin to the tip of the lower incisor along a true vertical line. Unfortunately, there are no standard reference data.

Racial Differences

When cephalometric measurements are used to establish relationships, the patient's numbers are compared with normal values. For some measurements, there are no significant differences between racial groups, but for many of the measurements outlined above, the Caucasian norms that usually are employed can be significantly different from the normal values of other population groups. The differences in cephalometric values can be grouped into three major areas: (1) the relationship of the jaws to the cranium and cranial base, (2) the prominence of the maxillary and mandibular teeth relative to the jaws, and (3) the vertical proportions of the face and jaws.

In general, Caucasian populations have less prominent faces than do the other racial groups, and so the normal values for the position of the maxilla and mandible relative to the cranium are higher for both blacks and Orientals than for whites. As Table 4-4 demonstrates, this means that normal values for SNA and SNB are lower for the white group. There also is a tendency for whites to have a less prominent mandible, which means that anterior divergence of the profile is more likely to be found in the other groups.

Blacks normally have more prominence of the dentition than do either whites or Orientals, and this difference can be seen well in the Steiner values for the relationship of the upper and lower incisors to the NA and NB lines. What would probably be considered excessive protrusion for most whites or Orientals is perfectly normal for blacks. The best judgment as to whether incisor prominence is excessive is not from cephalometric analysis of the tooth position relative to the jaws, but from analysis of the vertical and horizontal position of the lips. A diagnosis of excessive incisor protrusion should be made only if the lips are both horizontally protrusive and separated vertically.

The differences between the racial groups in vertical facial proportions are seen in two ways. First, the horizontal planes tend to converge more rapidly in blacks; that is, there is a tendency toward a skeletal open-bite relationship in this group as compared with a skeletal deep-bite tendency in whites. The epidemiologic data for open bite versus deep bite in whites and blacks reveal a striking difference. In the white population, only about 1% have an open bite greater than 2 mm, but this is found in nearly 10% of blacks. In contrast, less than 1% of blacks have an overbite greater than 6 mm, whereas 10% of whites have this problem. This undoubtedly reflects the underlying skeletal proportions. Orientals do not seem to be so strongly predisposed toward one kind of vertical problem.

Second, the vertical proportions of the anterior face height are somewhat different between the racial groups. In this regard, Orientals normally have a relatively short lower face as compared with whites, whereas blacks are at the other exteme, their lower faces normally being relatively long. These differences are neither good nor bad—all are compatible with good facial proportions. However, the racial differences must be kept in mind when reference values are employed. Tabulated reference data for most racial and national groups now are available, including English language sources of data for major groups.[41-43]

Template Analysis
Selection of a Template

A template is the visual equivalent of a table of standard values in measurement analysis. As with a set of numbers, the template has been prepared to represent the average of a group of reference individuals or perhaps a somewhat arbitrary ideal. It is more or less appropriate for any given patient, depending on how well that person is representative of the reference group.

For the Caucasian populations of North America and Europe, probably the best templates at present are those prepared from the Bolton growth study because of the extensive anatomic detail in the composite tracings and because of the well-characterized sample. The Bolton growth study was carried out in Cleveland in the 1940s and 1950s.[29] These templates also have the virtue of ready availability (from Kirtland Enterprises, 9058 Little Mountain Road, Kirtland Hills, OH 44060). Other templates are available from a smaller Alabama sample of roughly similar racial and ethnic background to the Bolton sample,[44] from the Michigan growth study[45] (but these are harder to use for diagnosis because of the lack of anatomic detail), from the Burlington growth study in Canada,[46] and perhaps from other American or European studies. At this writing, templates have not been prepared for other racial or ethnic groups, but this undoubtedly will occur in the future.

The following discussion, and the illustrations that accompany it, are based on use of the Bolton templates.

Template Analysis of Cranial-Jaw Relationships

The Bolton templates represent the data from a longitudinal growth study and therefore are a series of av-

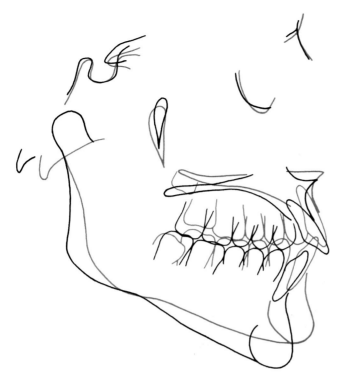

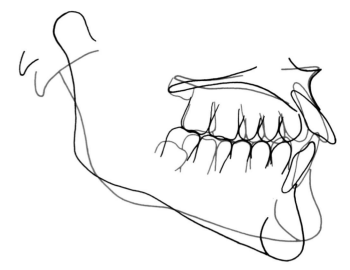

Fig. 4-30. A Bolton template *(red)* superimposed on the cranial base over the tracing of a 14-year-old boy with severe malocclusion *(black)*. In the Bolton series, templates are supplied for varying ages up to 18. To use the templates in diagnosis, the first step is to select the appropriate template, which is the one in which the SN distance approximately matches that of the patient (not necessarily the template for the patient's chronologic age). With the template superimposed on the SN line, the position of the jaws relative to the cranial base can be observed directly. For this patient, it is obvious that the maxilla is down and slightly back from the ideal position. The mandible is rotated significantly downward and backward, producing horizontal mandibular deficiency and excessive anterior face height.

Fig. 4-31. When the Bolton template is superimposed on the maxilla (on the palatal contour lingual to the upper incisors, along the palatal plane) of the patient in Fig. 4-30, two things can be observed: (1) the relationship of the mandible to the maxilla, and (2) the relationship of the maxillary teeth to the maxilla. This superimposition shows that relative to the maxilla, the mandible is still rotated down and back, but its posterior vertical dimensions are relatively short. The maxillary teeth are somewhat proclined but can be seen not to have erupted too much relative to the maxilla—their downward position relative to the cranial base entirely results from downward rotation of the palate.

erages for people from the ages of 3 to 16. The first step in using them for diagnosis is to select the template with the same S-N distance as that of the patient. If the patient's anterior cranial base length is greater than any of the templates, the largest one is used.

With the template superimposed on the SN line at N, the antero-posterior and vertical relationships of the maxilla and the mandible can then be observed directly (Fig. 4-30). For example, if the patient's maxilla is further down and back than the one on the template, the diagnostic conclusion is downward and backward displacement of the maxilla. If the mandible is rotated down and back, it will be obvious immediately as a difference between the patient and the template.

It may also be desirable to check the relationship of the maxilla to the mandible. For instance, the question might arise whether downward and backward rotation of the mandible is only secondary to downward dis-

placement of the maxilla, or whether the mandible has some distortion in its own right. This can be seen by superimposing the template on the maxilla and then examining the position of the mandible (Fig. 4-31). It could be done equally logically, actually, by superimposing on the mandible and observing the relative position of the maxilla, but the thought process is more direct the first way. Whichever the superimposition, the relative position of the other jaw is immediately apparent.

A patient who has an extremely severe deformity can be more difficult to evaluate with templates than is a more normal individual, simply because the template is so different. At first it can look as if everything is affected, which makes it hard to decide where the major contributors to the deformity are located. If this is the case, superimposing on the cranial base initially and carefully evaluating the maxilla, then superimposing on the maxilla while evaluating the mandible, can make things less complex. The mandible-cranium relationship is no less valid for having been obtained indirectly.

Template Analysis of Dental-Skeletal Relationships

For analysis of the position of the maxillary teeth relative to the maxilla, superimposing the template on the outline of the maxilla provides the necessary infor-

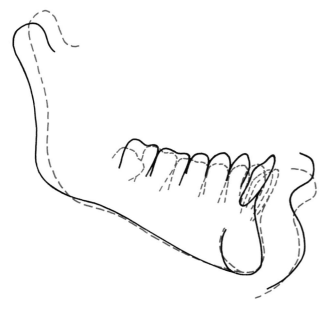

Fig. 4-32. Superimposition of the Bolton template on the mandible (on the inner part of the symphysis and along the mandibular plane) shows the vertical and horizontal relationship of the mandibular teeth to the mandible and the general mandibular morphology as compared with what is normal. Note that for this patient (the same as in Figs. 4-30 and 4-31) the incisors are supererupted and slightly lingually positioned, the mandibular body is slightly long, and the ramus is short.

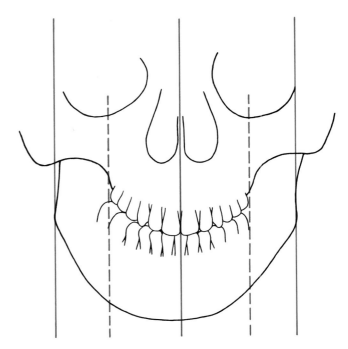

Fig. 4-33. For analysis of the PA cephalometric film, a tracing is made and vertical planes are used to illustrate transverse asymmetries. Drawing the midsagittal plane and planes through the angles of the mandible and the outer borders of the maxillary tuberosity, as shown here, often helps to establish where the asymmetry lies. The analytic technique is simply to draw vertical planes parallel to the midsagittal plane through any pair of landmarks that are suspected of being asymmetric. For this patient, the chin and dentition deviate to the right, but the mandibular angles are symmetric.

mation. Both the anteroposterior and vertical relationships of the teeth to the underlying bone can be visualized directly (see Fig. 4-31).

For analysis of the mandibular teeth in relation to the mandible, the template is superimposed on the inner surface of the symphysis and along the lower border of the mandible (Fig. 4-32). It would be better to use the shadow of the inferior alveolar neurovascular bundle rather than the lower border to align the template posteriorly, but unfortunately this information is not provided in the templates.

The information from a template analysis may appear to be less scientific than that from a table of measurements. In fact, the template is the visual analogue of a table and is just as valid. The question is not whether template analysis is useful—it is quite useful in the right situation—but whether the sample from which the template was derived is applicable to the patient under evaluation. The limitations of template analysis as compared with measurement analysis are based much more on the limited number of samples available in template form than on any inherent superiority of the measurement method. What the template does is place the emphasis on the analysis itself; that is, deciding what the distortions are, rather than on an intermediate measurement step that too often becomes an end in itself rather than just a means to the end.

Analysis of PA Cephalometric Films

The primary indication for obtaining a PA cephalometric film is the presence of facial asymmetry. Therefore the analysis of the film is oriented primarily toward quantifying and locating any asymmetry that may be present. As Fig. 4-33 shows, an excellent beginning in analysis is to draw vertical planes to visually illustrate transverse asymmetries. One way to clarify the source of asymmetry is to relate the midline landmarks (i.e., nose, chin, dental midlines) to the midsagittal plane. Vertical planes through the angles of the mandible and the outer borders of the zygomatic arch will highlight asymmetry in the position of these structures.

Vertical asymmetry can be observed readily by drawing the transverse planes at various vertical levels and observing their relative orientation (Fig. 4-34). This is analogous to the Sassouni approach for the lateral film, and the interpretation is equally straightforward. For instance, it can be seen whether the entire maxilla is tipped, or whether a canted occlusal plane results only from failure of maxillary teeth on one side to erupt as much as on the other.

It is possible to make linear measurements on the PA cephalometric film, but precise measurements of details

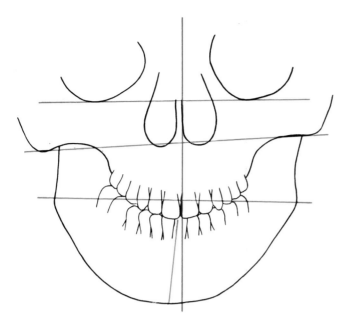

Fig. 4-34. On the PA tracing, horizontal planes connecting bilateral landmarks are useful to illustrate vertical asymmetry. As applied to this particular patient, this method shows the extent to which the maxilla is canted at the level of the zygomatic arches as compared with the cant of the occlusal plane and the mandibular angles.

are as likely to be misleading as helpful. Reference data are sparse, and there is a chance that the apparent distance will be affected by a tilt of the head in the head-holder, which is harder to control in PA than in lateral films. However, one point to keep in mind is the relationship between the width and height of a well-proportioned face. Bizygomatic width should be 85% to 90% of face height[13] (see Table 4-3), and these measurements can be checked readily on a PA film if they were not recorded directly from the patient.

Analysis of Hand-Wrist Radiographs

Hand-wrist radiographs are used to estimate a patient's skeletal age when there is reason to suspect delayed or, less frequently, accelerated maturation. The multiple bones of the hand and wrist present a constantly changing pattern of ossification events that provide a detailed chronology for this area and, by analogy, the rest of the skeleton. However, the analogy between hand-wrist development and jaw development is not perfect, and this limitation must be kept in mind. The appendicular skeleton follows Scammon's general body growth curve quite accurately, but the growth of the jaws is influenced by neural as well as by general body growth. Nonetheless, the correlation between hand-wrist development and jaw development is on the order of 0.8,[47] strong enough to make it helpful in analyzing some patients even if it is weak enough to leave some doubt about the true state of facial growth.

A major question for most orthodontic applications of hand-wrist films is whether the patient has reached the adolescent growth spurt and, if so, whether its peak has passed. This can also be important in the diagnostic evaluation of some surgical-orthodontic patients, particularly those with maxillary or mandibular deficiency for whom the earliest feasible surgery is projected. More commonly, however, the question for a patient with a dentofacial deformity is not where the patient is relative to the adolescent growth spurt, but whether he or she has reached adult status and therefore will have minimal further growth. The second question is harder to answer with hand-wrist films than is the first.

Although a number of methods for relating the stage of hand-wrist development to the adolescent growth spurt have been suggested, the most recent and probably the best is that proposed by Grave and Brown in Australia.[47] This is based on detailed examination of particular bones, primarily the hamate (Fig. 4-35). Other ossification events, especially the appearance of the ulnar sesamoid bone, have been proposed as markers for the adolescent growth spurt, but these are less reliable.

A more general approach to hand-wrist films, and the only one that is applicable to the timing of surgery in late adolescence, is the comparison of the pattern of ossification in the patient's radiograph with the series in a standard atlas such as that of Greulich and Pyle.[48] With reasonable accuracy, this can be used to obtain a skeletal age plus or minus 6 months. An apparently immature 14-year-old with a hand-wrist age of 11 years, 6 months, is indeed quite immature skeletally.

However, the accuracy declines toward the adult end of the scale, the very point where greatest accuracy is needed for timing of orthognathic surgery. Furthermore, there is reason to believe that patients with dentofacial deformities often have a pattern of growth that is systematically different from that of the normal children on whom the atlas is based. Those who develop mandibular prognathism, for instance, seem to have not only more mandibular growth than is normal, but also growth that continues for a longer period. Because of that, it is one thing to judge that a person with normal mandibular development who has reached the hand-wrist stage comparable with age 17 will have little or no further horizontal mandibular growth, and another to make a similar conclusion about a patient with prognathism. In the prognathic patient, the hand-wrist film can be misleading. We suggest that hand-wrist films be used with caution for establishing the onset of adult growth status.

The most accurate measure of growth of the jaws in patients with mandibular prognathism is obtained from superimposing tracings of lateral cephalometric films. In the 17- to 19-year-old patients who state that they have not increased in height within the past 12

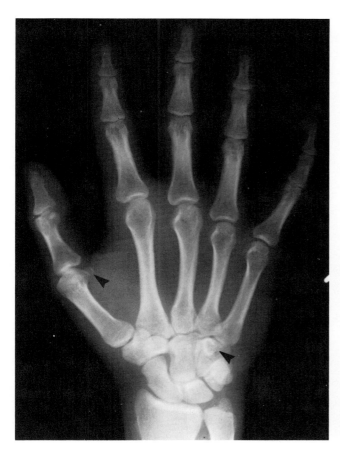

Fig. 4-35. Hand-wrist film of an immature-looking 16-year-old boy with mandibular deficiency. Ossification of the bones indicates that he is past the adolescent growth spurt, as indicated by the presence of the ulnar sesamoid bone *(arrow)* and ossification of the hook of the hamate *(arrow)*. The general appearance of the film is consistent with his chronologic age.

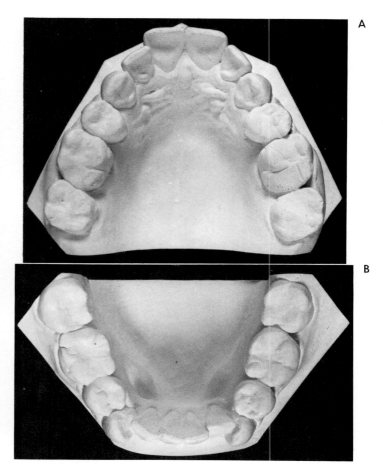

Fig. 4-36. The first step in classification with the Ackerman-Proffit system is to view the casts from the occlusal view. For this patient (case 1, Figs. 4-39 to 4-42), one can see that there is reasonable symmetry of both arches with severe crowding of the mandibular incisors, mild irregularity of the maxillary incisors, and a very tapered maxillary arch form.

months, successive 6-month tracings with no change in jaw growth provide good confirmation that growth of the jaws has declined to the very slow adult level.

CLASSIFICATION: DERIVING A PROBLEM LIST FROM THE DATA BASE

When all diagnostic records have been obtained and when the necessary preliminary analysis has been accomplished, the process of abstracting a problem list from the data can begin. A systematic approach should be used to ensure that this is both thorough and accurate. Systematic organization of the diagnostic data is, of course, the process of classification.

The first step in classification is to separate pathologic from developmental problems, placing problems resulting from disease or degenerative processes in a separate category. Periodontal disease, psychosocial disorders, degenerative changes in the TM joints—all are important, must be recognized, and will require consideration before treatment of the developmental

problems can start, but are not part of the surgical-orthodontic treatment plan itself.

The second step is to systematically examine the data base, including data from the interview, clinical evaluation, and diagnostic records. For this part of classification, we advocate the Ackerman-Proffit method.[49] In it, the five major characteristics of malocclusion are described in sequence, skeletal versus dental contributions to the deformity are specifically considered, and interactions among the various components are taken into account. To carry out the classification, the five major components of a malocclusion/dentofacial deformity are considered in order.

Alignment and Symmetry of the Dental Arches

The first step in the classification procedure is to examine the dental casts from the occlusal view. Any deviations from symmetry within the arches are noted, and if there is crowding and malalignment, its severity is judged (Fig. 4-36). If desired, the technique of space

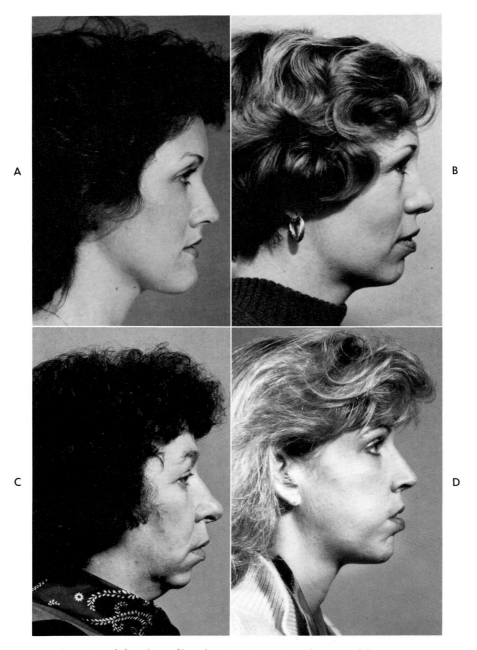

Fig. 4-37. A series of facial profiles showing increasing degrees of lip protrusion. **A,** A straight profile with flat, almost retrusive lips. **B,** Moderately full lips with a convex profile. **C,** Prominent but competent lips with a very convex profile. **D,** Prominent and incompetent lips. The patient in **C** has chin deficiency, not excessive protrusion of incisor teeth. Because of her lip competence, there would be little or no change in lip prominence if the incisors were retracted. In contrast, the patient in **D** has excessive incisor protrusion. It is important to keep in mind that lip protrusion and profile convexity are not the same thing.

analysis can be used to quantitate arch length discrepancy, but usually it is sufficient to grade the crowding as mild, moderate, or severe in each dental arch or area of the arch.

Effect of the Dentition on Facial Esthetics

The effect of the dentition on facial esthetics is evaluated primarily from the clinical examination data, with reference to the facial photographs and lateral cephalometric radiograph. The major focus is on the relative prominence of the lips and their degree of separation at rest, if protrusion is present (Fig. 4-37). Why should this receive such specific consideration? Simply because if there is not enough room for the teeth, there are only two possibilities. Either the teeth remain upright and well related to their supporting bone but are crowded into malaligned positions, or they align themselves anteriorly at the expense of the lips, in essence trading protrusion for crowding. The extent to which this has occurred, and therefore the true extent of crowding in the arches, can be evaluated only by looking critically at the facial profile.

Some individuals normally have more lip protrusion than others. This varies with racial and ethnic background. However, lip protrusion is excessive when the lips are both prominent and incompetent (separated excessively at rest). In other words, if the incisors are positioned forward and the lips are prominent but not separated at rest, there is not excessive protrusion (nor will retraction of the incisors for such a patient reduce the lip prominence). But if the lips are protrusive and separated at rest, excessive incisor protrusion exists and should be noted as a problem.

At this point in the classification, a dental or skeletal asymmetry that affects esthetics also would be noted, as would other special features of esthetics such as a soft-tissue deficit or excess in a specific area.

Transverse Dental and Skeletal Relationships

For the next step in the classification, the dental casts are placed in occlusion and the dental and skeletal relationships are evaluated in all three planes of space, beginning with the transverse. The essence of the analytic approach is to note initially any deviation from normal occlusal relationships and then determine whether that occlusal imbalance is caused by a displacement of the teeth relative to their supporting bone, a displacement of one or both jaws, or some combination of both.

For analysis of transverse relationships, the occluded dental casts are viewed from the front, and the focus is on the posterior crossbite and anterior midlines. How the dental midlines relate to the face is part of the clinical examination data. If a PA cephalometric radiograph was taken, this also is considered at this stage.

The most common crossbite is with the maxillary

TABLE 4-6 Arch width measurements (young adults)

Tooth	Maxillary (mm)		Mandibular (mm)	
	Male	Female	Male	Female
Canines	32*	31	25	23
First premolar	37	35	33	31
Second premolar	41	40	38	36
First molar	47	45	43	42
Second molar	52	49	49	47

*All distances are measured between the centroids of the teeth; standard deviation is approximately 2 mm for all measurements. Data from Moyers RE, van der Linden FPGM, Riolo ML: Standards of human occlusal development, Ann Arbor, 1976, University of Michigan.

teeth lingual rather than buccal to the mandibular teeth, which can be caused either by too wide a mandibular arch or too narrow a maxillary arch. If this point is in doubt, reference to a table of standard arch widths[50] (Table 4-6) can help.

One of the reasons that PA cephalometric radiographs are not needed routinely is that skeletal as well as dental dimensions can be seen on the casts, provided properly extended impressions were taken (Fig. 4-38). The mandibular molars normally are positioned somewhat lingual to the underlying body of the mandible, which is seen in the undercut areas below the molar teeth. The absence or diminution of these undercuts would suggest some narrowing of the mandible, whereas extreme undercuts would suggest either a widening of the mandible itself or, more likely, a narrowing of the dentition. Extreme undercuts in a patient with an intermolar distance that is much smaller than normal would be interpreted as dental displacement from a relatively normal mandibular base width.

Skeletal-width dimensions can be seen easily in the maxillary cast because the height of the palatal vault and its contours are clearly revealed. In a crossbite caused by a narrow maxillary arch (the vault is narrow and the maxillary alveolar processes tip outward), one would conclude that the crossbite is skeletal in origin rather than caused by displacement of the teeth. On the other hand, if the palatal vault is wide and the maxillary alveolar processes tip inward, the crossbite is dental rather than skeletal. The distinction is important, of course, because of its implication for the focus of treatment.

Dental versus skeletal midlines can be observed on the PA cephalogram, but in many ways this is judged better from clinical examination of the patient. The problem with judging dental midlines from the PA film

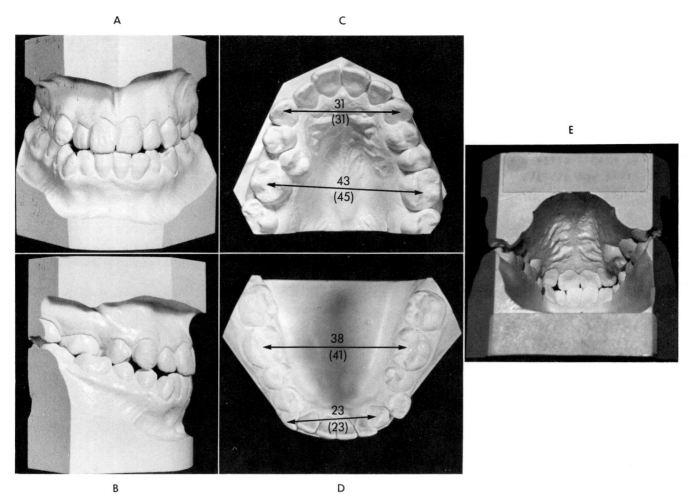

Fig. 4-38. Skeletal-width dimensions can be ascertained, at least to some extent, from observation of the dental casts. **A** and **B,** Casts in occlusion showing a unilateral posterior crossbite. **C,** The maxillary intermolar width is decreased (actual measurement above the line, norm for adult females in parentheses below it), while **D,** the mandibular intermolar width is normal. **E,** Observation of the mandibular cast from the rear shows the lower molars positioned slightly lingual to their supporting bone, which is the normal relationship. An increase in the relative undercut in the mandibular posterior *(arrow)* would indicate some narrowing of the dental arch relative to the bone; no undercut at all would indicate the arch was relatively wide. In contrast, it is obvious from inspection of the maxillary cast in this view and in **C** that the palatal vault is narrow and that the maxillary alveolar processes tilt outward. Therefore we can conclude that the crossbite is caused by the maxillary arch and that the problem is largely a skeletal one caused by a narrow palate. The displacement of the maxillary right second premolar just adds to the underlying problem.

is that a slight twisting of the patient's head can make an apparent difference of 1 to 2 mm in the cephalometric midline, which is enough sometimes to affect the determination of whether a midline discrepancy is caused by the upper or lower teeth. The clinical observation is likely to be more accurate. As with any other diagnostic point, if there is a disagreement between the clinical notes and the diagnostic records, the patient should be examined further to resolve the discrepancy.

Anteroposterior Relationships

With the dental casts in occlusion, the amount of overjet or reverse overjet is noted. Then cephalometric information is used to deduce the extent to which the problem is primarily dental (caused by displacement of the maxillary or mandibular incisors) or skeletal (caused by a displacement of one or both jaws). For example, consider the patient shown in case 1 below. There is a full-cusp Class II relationship of the posterior teeth, with 9 mm of overjet. The cephalometric analysis (see Fig. 4-42) shows that point A is almost exactly on the nasion perpendicular line, whereas point B is 14 mm is behind it instead of the expected 4 mm. The analysis also shows that the maxillary incisors are 5 mm in front of the true vertical line through point A, about where they should be, and that the mandibular incisors are 2 mm more prominent than pogonion and therefore also are close to a normal relationship to the mandible and chin. Therefore one would conclude that the excess overjet is entirely caused by a distal position of the mandible.

Vertical Relationships

With the casts in occlusion and referring to the lateral cephalometric radiograph, the analysis now is of open bite or deep bite. As always, the idea is to locate the precise anatomic cause of the problem.

For example, consider the patient shown in case 2 below. There is a 6 mm anterior open bite. Analysis of the cephalometric film (see Fig. 4-46) shows that the lower anterior face height is increased and that the mandible is rotated downward and backward. The in-

clination of the palatal plane shows that the maxilla is rotated downward posteriorly. The mandibular teeth are vertically well related to the mandible, but the maxillary teeth have supererupted anteriorly and posteriorly. Therefore the open bite results from the downward rotation of the maxilla posteriorly and excessive eruption of the maxillary posterior teeth, which has forced a downward rotation of the mandible and separated the anterior teeth. The upper incisors have compensated partially by supererupting. The patient's excessive overjet also results from the mandibular rotation, so one is led immediately toward an initial step in treatment planning, the realization that both the open bite and the overjet could be corrected by elevating the maxilla posteriorly.

ILLUSTRATIONS OF PROBLEM-ORIENTED DIAGNOSIS

The diagnostic process outlined above is illustrated in the following two cases. A diagnosis in the form of a completed problem list is established here for these two patients. The treatment plan for the same two patients will be developed in Chapter 5.

Case 1 (Figs. 4-39 to 4-42)

Interview. D.J., a 32-year-old elementary school teacher, sought consultation because of her concern about the protrusion of her upper incisors, crowding of her lower teeth, and contact of her lower incisors with the palate behind the upper incisors. She had had orthodontic treatment about 20 years previously, with the extraction of first premolars. She reported that her teeth had come together for a short time after treatment, then relapsed. She had not sought retreatment orthodontically because she thought it would fail again, and had only recently heard that surgical correction might be possible.

She was well adjusted emotionally and realistic in her expectations of improved function and esthetics. There was no significant medical or dental history.

Clinical examination

Facial proportions and esthetics. Fig. 4-39 shows the four standard facial photographs recommended for surgical-orthodontic patients as the best record of the patient's appearance during the clinical evaluation. The face was symmetric and slightly short vertically in the lower third. On profile examination, the lips were slightly everted, and mandibular deficiency was evident.

Health of the hard and soft tissues. Numerous restorations were present, but there was no active caries. Probing depths were normal. There was an area of gingival recession and minimal attached gingiva in the lower anterior area.

Jaw function and TM joints. Maximum opening was 45 mm with normal protrusive and lateral movements. There were no joint sounds or areas of pain on palpation.

Evaluation of diagnostic records: systematic description

Dental alignment and symmetry. (This would be observed from the occlusal view of the dental casts—see Fig. 4-36.) There was mild maxillary and very severe mandibular anterior crowding. The arches were symmetric.

Dental protrusion and facial esthetics. (This is taken from the records of the clinical examination, supplemented by viewing the facial photographs and cephalometric film and tracing—Figs. 4-39 and 4-42.) The profile was severely convex, resulting almost entirely from mandibular deficiency. The incisors were reasonably upright in both arches. There was an appearance of mild overclosure, resulting in slight eversion of the lips.

Continued.

Case 1—cont'd.

Transverse relationships. (This would be observed from the dental casts placed in occlusion and viewed from the front and further evaluated by comparing skeletal and dental widths as visible on the casts— see Fig. 4-36 for an example, using another case.) No crossbites were present.

Anteroposterior relationships. (These would be observed from the dental casts placed in occlusion and also on

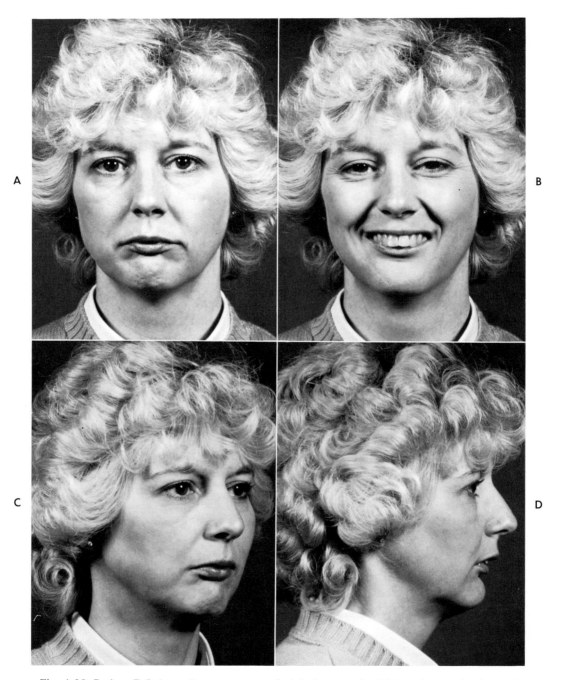

Fig. 4-39. Patient D.J. (case 1), pretreatment facial photographs. This is the standard set of four photographs that we recommend for potential surgical-orthodontic patients (unless there is significant facial asymmetry, in which case additional views are needed to document it).

Case 1—cont'd.

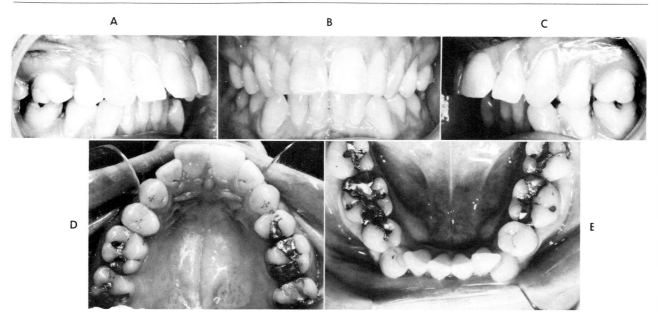

Fig. 4-40. Patient D.J., pretreatment intraoral photographs. We recommend this standard set of five views. The occlusal views must be taken using a mirror, and mirror views of the posterior occlusal relationships provide a better record if access is limited.

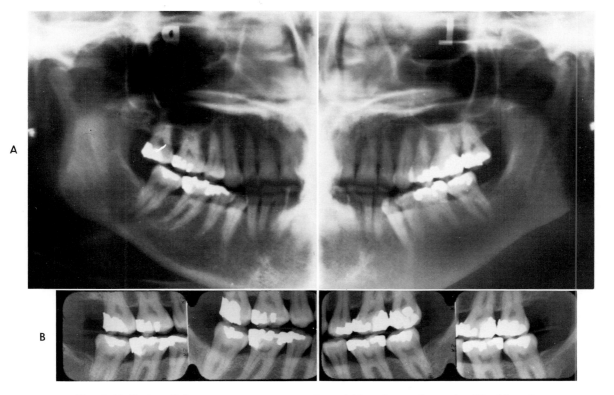

Fig. 4-41. Patient D.J., pretreatment panoramic and bite-wing radiographs. The bite-wings are required because of the previous caries experience, but a full intraoral series is not necessary in the absence of active periodontal disease at this time.

Continued.

Case 1—cont'd.

the lateral cephalometric film and tracing.) There was a full-cusp Class II relationship of molars and incisors, with 8 mm overjet. Cephalometrically, the maxilla was normal in size and position, and the mandible was small and deficient in projection (Fig. 4-42). The teeth of both jaws were well related to their supporting bone.

Vertical relationships. (These would be observed in the same way as anteroposterior relationships.) There was 6 mm overbite with palatal impingement. There was a mild tendency toward skeletal deep bite, with the excessive curve of Spee caused more by infraeruption of mandibular posterior teeth than by excessive eruption of the lower incisors. Anterior face height was slightly short.

Problem list. In the order in which they placed into the data base, D.J.'s problems were:

- Gingival recession and inadequate attached gingiva, mandibular anterior region
- Mild maxillary, severe mandibular anterior crowding
- Skeletal Class II mandibular deficiency
- Deep bite, skeletal and dental, mildly deficient anterior face height.

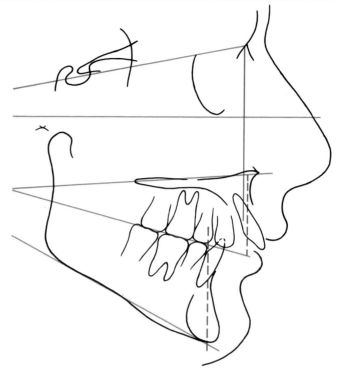

Fig. 4-42. Patient D.J., cephalometric tracing and analysis. The radiograph is taken in her NHP so that the true horizontal and vertical lines can be established. The pattern of dentofacial relationships can be observed in the anteroposterior and vertical relationships of the jaws to the horizontal and vertical reference planes. Cephalometric measurements: nasion perpendicular line to point A (N perp to A), 1 mm; N perp to pogonion *(Pg)*, 10 mm; AB difference projected to the true horizontal line, 15 mm; upper face height (nasion to a point opposite the anterior nasal spine, measured on the true vertical line) *(UFH)*, 51 mm; lower face height (ANS to a point opposite menton, measured on the true vertical line) *(LFH)*, 66 mm; max-mand length difference (Harvold), 25 mm; mandibular plane (GoGn to true horizontal), 30 degrees; maxillary incisor relationship to a true vertical line through point A (MxI to A vert), 5 mm (from incisal edge), 29 degrees (to long axis of tooth); mandibular incisor to true vertical line through point B (MnI to B vert), 4 mm, 28 degrees.

Case 2 (Figs. 4-43 to 4-46)

Interview. S.S., age 28 years, 3 months, sought treatment because of her concern that "my teeth protrude and don't meet in front." She had recently had her photograph appear in the local newspaper when she and her husband moved to a new community, and this (plus improved economic circumstances coincident with the move) was her reason for seeking treatment at this time. She seemed well adjusted and happily married. Her oldest child had a cleft palate that had been surgically repaired, and was doing well. There was no history of serious illness or current medications beyond occasional mild pain relievers.

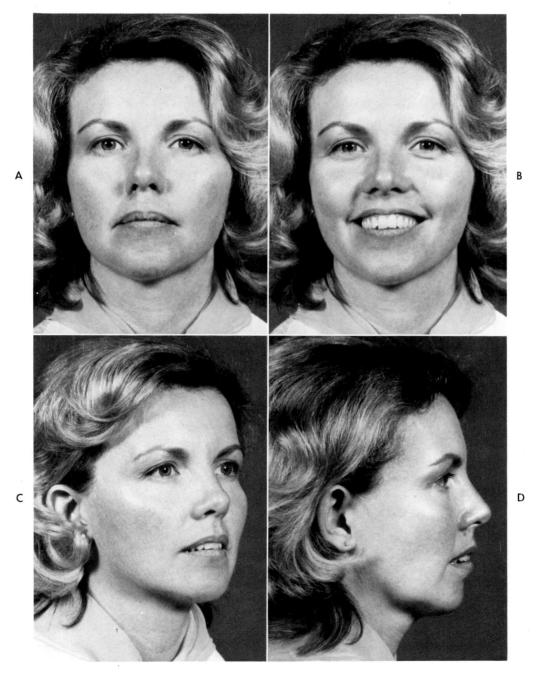

Fig. 4-43. Patient S.S. (case 2), pretreatment facial photographs.

Continued.

Case 2—cont'd.

Clinical examination

Facial proportions and esthetics. There was good facial symmetry, and the dental and skeletal midlines were correct. The lower face was slightly long, as shown by the increased distance from the base of the nose to the chin as compared with the height of the midface. Face height was slightly excessive relative to width. There was 6 mm of lip incompetence at rest. The profile was convex, with the deviation being caused primarily by backward deviation of the chin.

Health of hard and soft tissues. Several teeth had been restored previously, but there was no active caries. There was moderate recession of gingival tissues over the maxillary central incisors, with adequate attached gingiva there and elsewhere. Periodontal probing depths were normal in all areas.

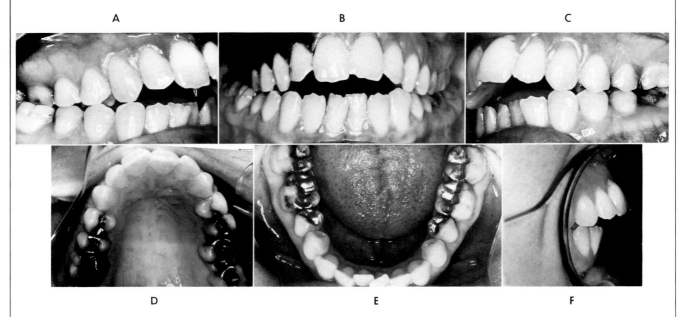

Fig. 4-44. Patient S.S., pretreatment intraoral photographs. The true lateral view *(F)* is an optional but often desirable addition to the photographic series.

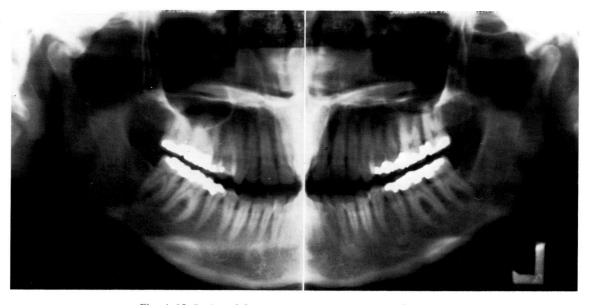

Fig. 4-45. Patient S.S., pretreatment panoramic radiograph.

Case 2—cont'd.

Jaw function and TM joints. There was no limitation of motion, no joint sound or report of joint pain, and no areas of soreness on palpation. Maximum opening was 50 mm, with free lateral and protrusive movements. There was no lateral shift on closure.

Evaluation of diagnostic records: systematic description

Dental alignment and symmetry. (This would be observed from the dental casts, examined from an occlusal view—see Fig. 4-44, *D* and *E* for the same information here.) The maxillary arch showed mild irregularity with good symmetry; the mandibular arch had 5 mm incisor crowding.

Dental protrusion and facial esthetics. (This would be observed clinically, with further reference to the cephalometric film and tracing.) The profile was convex, with mild protrusion of the lower lip and 5 mm of lip incompetence at rest.

Transverse relationships. There was a unilateral lingual crossbite on the right side resulting from a narrowing of the maxillary dental arch in that area. There was no mandibular shift, so the crossbite was truly unilateral.

Anteroposterior relationships. The dental casts showed a full Class II relationship of molars and canines, with 7 mm overjet. Cephalometric analysis showed that the maxilla was well related to the cranium and cranial base and that the mandible was distally positioned to the maxilla and to the cranium. The maxillary teeth were well related to the maxilla, and the mandibular teeth were mildly protrusive relative to the mandible.

Vertical relationships. There was a 4 mm anterior open bite, with no contact forward from the first molars. Cephalometric analysis showed the maxilla tipped down posteriorly. The mandible was rotated down and back, and anterior face height was excessive.

Problem list

The problem list, which is the initial diagnosis, is produced simply by listing the positive findings from the data base. S.S's problems are:

● Gingival recession, maxillary anterior region
● Moderate mandibular and mild maxillary incisor crowding
● Maxillary right lingual crossbite, dental; lingual displacement of maxillary teeth
● Skeletal Class II mandibular deficiency, 7 mm overjet
● Skeletal open bite, maxilla rotated down posteriorly

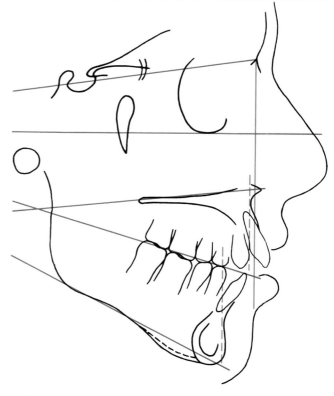

Fig. 4-46. Patient S.S., initial cephalometric tracing and analysis. Note the rotation of the palatal plane, lip separation at rest, and protrusion of the mandibular incisors relative to the mandible. In addition to relationships that can be observed directly, the following measurements are pertinent: N perp to A, 2 mm; N perp to Pg, 12 mm; AB difference, 9 mm; UFH, 56 mm; LFH, 74 mm; mand plane, 29 degrees; MxI to A vert, 7 mm, 23 degrees; MnI to B vert, 20 mm, 35 degrees; sella to PNS, 52 mm; ethmoid point to PNS, 53 mm; palatal plane to upper molar, 24 mm; palatal plane to upper incisor, 31 mm; mandibular plane to lower molar, 33 mm; mandibular plane to lower incisor, 38 mm; sella to gonion, 82 mm.

REFERENCES

1. Macgregor FC: Social and psychological implications of dentofacial disfigurement, Angle Orthod 40:231-233, 1970.
2. Behrents RG: A treatise on the continuum of growth in the aging craniofacial skeleton, Ann Arbor, 1985, University of Michigan Center for Human Growth and Development.
3. Gorlin RJ, Pindborg JJ, Cohen MM, Jr: Syndromes of head and neck, ed 3, New York, 1990, McGraw-Hill.
4. The selection of patients for x-ray examination: dental radiographic examination, HHS Pub FDA 88-8273, Rockville, Md., 1987, US Food and Drug Administration, Center for Devices and Radiologic Health.

5. Douglas CW, Gillings D, Sollecito W, et al: National trends, the prevalence and severity of the periodontal diseases, J Am Dent Assoc 107:403-412, 1983, and suppl.

6. Socransky SS, Haffajee AD, Goodson JM, et al: New concepts of destructive periodontal disease, J Clin Periodontol 11:21-32, 1984.

7. Lang NP, Joss A, Orsanic T: Bleeding on probing. A predictor for the progression of periodontal disease, J Clin Periodontol 13:590-596, 1986.

8. Rugh JD, Solberg WK: Oral health status in the United States: temporomandibular disorders, J Dent Educ 49:398-405, 1985.

9. Mohlin B, Thilander B: The importance of the relationship between malocclusion and mandibular dysfunction and some clinical applications in adults, Eur J Orthod 6:192-204, 1984.

10. Riolo ML, Brandt D, Ten Hoeve IR: Associations between occlusal characteristics and signs and symptoms of TMJ dysfunction in children and young adults, Am J Orthod 92:467-477, 1987.

11. Williamson EH, Evans DL, Barton WA, et al: The effect of bite plane use on terminal hinge axis location, Angle Orthod 47:25-33, 1977.

12. Farkas LG: Anthropometry of the head and face in medicine, New York, 1981, Elsevier Science Publishing Co, Inc.

13. Farkas LG, Munro JR: Anthropometric facial proportions in medicine, Springfield, Ill, 1987, Charles C Thomas, Publisher.

14. Hellman M: Variations in occlusion, Dent Cosmos 63:608-619, 1921.

15. Tyndall DA, Matteson SR, Soltmann RE, et al: Exposure reduction in cephalometric radiography: a comprehensive approach, Am J Orthod Dentofacial Orthop 93:400-412, 1988.

16. Tyndall DA, Matteson SR, Bechtold W, Proffit WR: Cephalometric dose reduction with prepatient rare earth filtration, J Clin Orthod 21:470-473, 1987.

17. Solow B, Tallgren A: Natural head position in standing subjects, Acta Odontol Scand 29:591-607, 1971.

18. Moorrees CFA, Kean MR: Natural head position: a basic consideration for analysis of cephalometric radiographs, Am J Phys Anthropol 16:213-234, 1958.

19. Aquilino SA, Matteson SR, Holland GA, et al: Evaluation of condylar position from temporomandibular joint radiographs, J Prosthet Dent 53:88-93, 1985.

20. Isberg A, Widmalm SE, Ivarsson R: Clinical, radiographic and electromyographic study of patients with internal derangement of the temporomandibular joint, Am J Orthod 88:453-460, 1985.

21. Heffez L, Jordan S, Rosenberg H, Miescke K: Accuracy of temporomandibular joint space measurements using corrected hypocloidal tomography, J Oral Maxillofac Surg 45:137-142, 1987.

22. Tucker MR, Guilford WB, Thomas PM: Versatility of CT scanning for evaluation of mandibular hypomobilities, J Oral Maxillofac Surg 14:89-92, 1986.

23. Laney TJ, Kaplan PA, Tu HK, Lydiatt DD: Normal and abnormal temporomandibular joints: quantitative evaluation of inferior joint space arthrography, Int J Oral Maxillofac Surg 16:305-311, 1987.

24. Katzberg RW, Schenck J, Roberts D, et al: Magnetic resonance imaging of the temporomandibular joint meniscus, Oral Surg Oral Med Oral Pathol 59:332-335, 1985.

25. Williamson EH, Steinke BM, Morse PK, et al: Centric relation: a comparison of muscle-determined position and operator guidance, Am J Orthod 77:133-145, 1980.

26. Jankelson B: Three dimensional orthodontic diagnosis and treatment. A neuromuscular approach, J Clin Orthod 18:627-636, 1984.

27. Okeson, JP: Fundamentals of occlusion and temporomandibular disorders, St. Louis, 1985, The CV Mosby Co.

28. Mohl ND: A textbook of occlusion, Chicago, 1988, Quintessence Publishing Co, Inc.

29. Broadbent BH, Sr, Broadbent BH, Jr, Golden WH: Bolton standards of dentofacial developmental growth, St. Louis, 1975, The CV Mosby Co.

30. Downs W: Variation in facial relationships: their significance in treatment and prognosis, Am J Orthod 34:812-840, 1948.

31. Riedel RA: The relation of maxillary structures to cranium in malocclusion and normal occlusion, Angle Orthod 22:142-145, 1952.

32. Jarvinen S: Floating norms for the ANB angle as guidance for clinical considerations, Am J Orthod 90:383-387, 1986.

33. McNamara JA, Jr: A method of cephalometric evaluation, Am J Orthod 86:449-468, 1984.

34. Harvold EP: The activator in orthodontics, St. Louis, 1974, The CV Mosby Co.

35. Wylie WL: The assessment of anteroposterior dysplasia, Angle Orthod 17:97-108, 1947.

36. Sassouni VA: A classification of skeletal facial types, Am J Orthod 55:109-123, 1969.

37. Riolo M, Moyers RE, McNamara JA, et al: An atlas of craniofacial growth, Ann Arbor, 1974, University of Michigan Center for Human Growth and Development.

38. Steiner CC: The use of cephalometrics as an aid to planning and assessing orthodontic treatment, Am J Orthod 46:721-735, 1960.

39. Ricketts RM: Perspectives in the clinical application of cephalometrics, Angle Orthod 51:115-150, 1981.

40. Williams R: The diagnostic line, Am J Orthod 55:458-476, 1969.

41. Drummond RA: A determination of cephalometric norms for the Negro race, Am J Orthod 54:670-682, 1968.

42. Cotton WH, Takano WS, Wong MW, Wylie WL: The Downs analysis applied to three other ethnic groups, Angle Orthod 21:213-220, 1951.

43. Engel GA, Spolter BM: Cephalometric and visual norms for Japanese population, Am J Orthod 80:48-60, 1981.

44. Jacobson A: The proportionate template as a diagnostic aid, Am J Orthod 75:156-172, 1979.

45. Ackerman RJ: The Michigan school study norms expressed in template form, Am J Orthod 75:282-290, 1979.

46. Popovich F, Thompson GW: Craniofacial templates for orthodontic case analysis, Am J Orthod 71:406-420, 1977.

47. Grave KC, Brown T: Skeletal ossification and the adolescent growth spurt, Am J Orthod 69:611-619, 1976.
48. Greulich WW, Pyle SI: Radiographic atlas of skeletal development of the hand and wrist, ed 2, Stanford, Cal, 1959, Stanford University Press.
49. Ackerman JL, Proffit WR: The characteristics of malocclusion: a modern approach to classification and diagnosis, Am J Orthod 56:443-454, 1969.
50. Moyers RE, van der Linden FPGM, Riolo ML, et al: Standards of human occlusal development, Ann Arbor, 1976, University of Michigan.

CHAPTER 5

Treatment Planning:
The Search for Wisdom

William R. Proffit

The goal of treatment planning is to develop the plan that will maximize benefit to the patient. It must, of course, be based on the diagnostic truth that has been established previously. If an important diagnostic point has been missed, the treatment plan is likely to be seriously flawed.

The following discussion of treatment planning is divided into four major sections: (1) surgical treatment possibilities, (2) the logical sequence in planning surgical-orthodontic treatment, (3) the treatment planning techniques of cephalometric prediction and cast prediction, and (4) illustrative cases. The objective is to provide pertinent background material about what can be done, and then to illustrate general principles and methods. More details about planning the interaction between surgeon and orthodontist are included in Chapter 6, and further information about specific types of cases is presented in the clinical chapters that follow.

SURGICAL TREATMENT POSSIBILITIES

It is not possible to begin planning surgical-orthodontic treatment without considering what the possibilities are for treatment. The envelope of discrepancy presented in Chapter 1 (see Fig. 1-2) illustrates the anteroposterior and vertical limitations of surgery accurately but too superficially for planning treatment and provides no information about the transverse plane of space.

Until the mid-1970s, there were major technical limitations on what could be done by orthognathic surgery. Earlier, the sagittal split and its modifications made most mandibular movements possible, and the LeFort I down-fracture technique provided essentially all movements of the maxilla and maxillary dentoalveolar units. Mandibular posterior dentoalveolar surgery was the last frontier. Until a way was developed to expose and protect the inferior alveolar neurovascular bundle and, if necessary, gently lift it out of the way, it was not technically possible to free the mandibular posterior teeth from the body of the mandible and reposition them. When this barrier was overcome, both posterior and total mandibular dentoalveolar osteotomies became possible, and it was at least technically possible to reposition both jaws, the chin, and dentoalveolar processes in all three planes of space.

It is one thing to move a jaw or dentoalveolar segment in the operating room, and something else to get it to heal correctly and remain stable in its new position. As techniques have improved, the limitations on orthognathic surgery have become more and more related to physiologic adaptation (jaw function and soft-tissue adaptability). Perhaps the best way to illustrate these limitations is to consider the possible movements of the jaws, chin, and dentoalveolar processes in all three planes of space. Let us look at what is now feasible, what is not, and why that is the case.

Changes in Width
Maxilla

Consider first the transverse plane of space for the maxilla (Fig. 5-1). Surgically, it is possible both to widen and to narrow the maxilla. Narrowing it is technically more difficult because it is necessary to remove bone to bring the two sides closer together, but this movement is entirely feasible. Although widening the maxilla leaves a space somewhere in the palate, healing usually is adequate without a bone graft. The major constraints on transverse change are the palatal soft tissues and, to a lesser extent, the soft tissues laterally and superiorly. At the extreme, the maxilla can be widened or narrowed perhaps 15 mm, but 10 mm of change is a more reasonable expectation.

Not only the amount of change that can be created at surgery, but also the stability of the repositioned segments must be considered. When the maxilla is widened surgically, there is a considerable relapse tendency that is expressed in two ways. First, the two halves of the maxilla tend to move back together postsurgically even if a bone graft fills the gap and the position of the teeth is maintained. This skeletal relapse is permitted by orthodontic tooth movement. Usually, the teeth move relative to stable bone, but in this instance the movement of the bone relative to the stabilized teeth allows the bone to slip back toward the midline. Second, there is a tendency toward dental relapse after the fixation is released. The combination of these two effects typically leads to approximately a 40% decrease in the intermolar width that was established at surgery.[1,2] This can be overcome, if at all, only by using extraordinary fixation methods. Although RIF may improve the relapse tendency, more data are needed to substantiate this clinical impression.

It is interesting to compare surgical expansion with what happens when the maxilla is widened, in a patient young enough to make this possible, by the orthodontic (dentofacial orthopedic) technique of maxillary expansion. If relatively heavy force is applied across the maxillary molars, the midpalatal suture widens and new bone fills in at that location. This effectively widens the palate and the dental arch. Following orthopedic expansion, the separated halves of the maxilla relapse back toward the midline even though the position of the teeth is maintained, as the bone moves relative to the teeth because of the orthodontic force created by stretched tissues in the palate.[3,4] When retention is released, the teeth also tend to relapse. There is approximately a 40% decrease in the intermolar width that was established immediately after the expansion. The relapse after orthopedic expansion, in other words, is remarkably similar to what happens after surgical expansion.

If the result of surgical or orthopedic expansion is

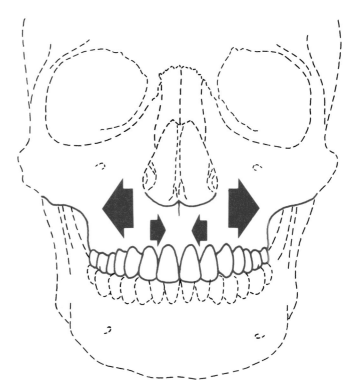

Fig. 5-1. Surgically, it is possible both to widen the maxilla and to narrow it. As the diagram suggests, widening is more easily accomplished. Technically, it is more difficult to remove bone to bring the segments together. Rarely is it necessary to place a graft when the segments have been separated to create expansion.

similar, which should be chosen? In the younger patients for whom it is feasible, maxillary orthopedics is an effective approach and should be used. The orthopedic technique is effective until the late teens. After that, it is increasingly difficult to separate the suture, and expansion occurs only by movement of the teeth. Therefore, in older patients, orthopedic expansion is not really an alternative. If the palate needs to be widened, surgery is the only possibility.

As patients get older, orthopedic expansion is limited by the increasing interdigitation of the maxillary sutures, not just in the palate, but also laterally. It seems reasonable that if the resistance of either the midpalatal or the lateral sutures could be reduced, as by an osteotomy in these areas, orthopedic force might still be able to widen the palate. In this method of surgically assisted orthopedic expansion, the orthodontist would place an expansion appliance immediately after an osteotomy, and orthopedic expansion would then occur.

The first attempts to do this employed a midpalatal incision to open up the interlocked suture. Although palatal expansion usually became possible, there was a considerable risk of wound dehiscence following sur-

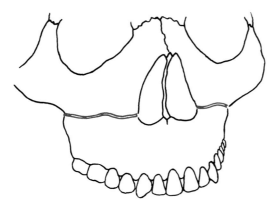

Fig. 5-2. The difficulty in orthopedically expanding the mid-palatal suture in older patients is caused by a combination of resistance from the suture itself and from other areas of the maxilla. Expansion across the midpalatal suture requires compensatory changes at the lateral and superior maxillary sutures also. As these sutures become increasingly interdigitated with age, palatal expansion is impeded. If an osteotomy is done bilaterally from the piriform rim of the nasal fossa to the pterygomaxillary fissure, as shown diagrammatically here, it nearly always is possible then to open the palatal suture with a jackscrew. This is a more practical approach to surgically assisted rapid maxillary expansion than is making a surgical cut in the palate. (Redrawn from Glassman AS, Nahigan SJ, Medway JM, et al: Conservative surgical orthodontic adult rapid palatal expansion: sixteen cases, Am J Orthod 86:207-213, 1984.)

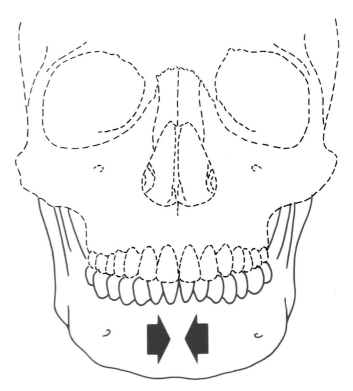

Fig. 5-3. Surgically, it is possible to narrow the width of the mandible anteriorly, but for all practical purposes it is impossible to widen it. The difficulty is a technical one: it is extremely difficult to obtain adequate soft-tissue coverage of the necessary bone graft.

gery because the soft tissue over the suture is quite thin and not well vascularized. As an alternative, an osteotomy in the lateral buttress of the maxilla was proposed to reduce the resistance from this area (Fig. 5-2). An osteotomy in the lateral maxilla, including separation at the pterygomaxillary region, did reduce resistance enough to allow the desired orthopedic expansion, and wound dehiscence was no longer a problem.[5] When surgically assisted expansion is indicated, this now is the preferred method.

The question remains whether surgically assisted expansion is better than surgery alone. Does it combine the benefits of surgery and orthopedics to produce a superior result? Or does it combine the costs and risks of both, without a compensatory increase in benefit? In our view, the latter view is more correct. There is no evidence that surgically assisted expansion is more stable than orthopedic or surgical expansion alone, and there is evidence that segmenting the maxilla during a LeFort I osteotomy so that it can be widened does not affect anteroposterior or vertical stability.[6] We suggest that orthopedic expansion be used when possible to widen the maxilla. If the patient is too old for orthopedics to succeed without surgical assistance, the better plan is to continue the surgery to the point that the bony segments and teeth can be placed in their desired

position, eliminating the need for the expansion device. When the patient also needs an osteotomy to reposition the maxillary segments vertically and/or anteroposteriorly, which usually is the case, surgical expansion is easily accomplished with little added morbidity. This topic is discussed in more detail in Chapter 8.

There is little or no alternative to surgery to narrow a maxilla that is too wide. If the orthodontist places a constricting force across the maxillary molars, the teeth will move toward the midline, but remodeling of the suture so that the maxilla itself becomes narrower does not occur. In very young patients, an appliance might succeed in reducing width by interfering with the normal widening, but growth in width of the maxilla occurs quite early. By the end of the adolescent growth spurt, surgery is the only possibility for significantly narrowing the maxilla.

Mandible

Changes in mandibular width are not as easy to make as are maxillary width changes. There are two major limitations: (1) the soft-tissue envelope, and (2) the TM joint. It is possible to narrow the mandible anteriorly and to widen or narrow the alveolar process somewhat posteriorly (Fig. 5-3). However, it is not

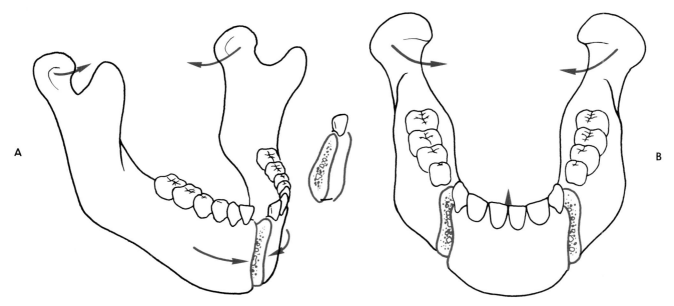

Fig. 5-4. **A,** An ostectomy in the mandibular symphysis, using either the space created by extraction of a mandibular incisor or an existing edentulous space, allows the mandible to be narrowed as the segments rotate slightly inward. **B,** A body ostectomy in the premolar region also leads to a narrowing of the mandible because when the canine is brought into contact with the second premolar, the condylar fragments must rotate inward to prevent an outward step in the dental arch. For most patients with mandibular prognathism, this is an undesirable side effect. Occasionally, when the mandible is too wide, it is an advantage. Excessive mandibular width may be an indication to select the body procedure over the more commonly used ramus osteotomy.

possible to significantly widen the mandible or the dental arch anteriorly.

Technically, it would not appear difficult to separate the mandible in the vicinity of the symphysis and insert a bone graft to widen it. The problem comes in obtaining soft tissue to cover the graft. In a patient with all the teeth present, it is difficult to the point of being almost impossible to stretch the gingiva and alveolar mucosa enough to significantly widen the mandibular intercanine distance. If there is an edentulous area, an infrequent clinical situation, the problem is not quite so intractable because soft tissue can be mobilized from adjacent areas for wound closure, allowing 3 to 4 mm of expansion.

The opposite movement, removing bone from the symphysis area so that the mandible can be narrowed, is quite feasible[7] (Fig. 5-4, *A*). Extraction of an incisor may be necessary to provide the necessary space, or the surgery can be used to reduce or eliminate an existing edentulous space. When the mandible is narrowed in this way, condylar width is maintained and the condyles rotate slightly on their vertical axis.

A body ostectomy at any point along the mandible makes it narrower because of the geometry of the bone (Fig. 5-4, *B*). The mandible tapers as it comes forward. If a segment of the body is removed in the premolar re-

gion, as sometimes is done to correct mandibular prognathism, the posterior segments will have to rotate inward to reestablish continuity of the dental arch when the anterior segment is set back. In most circumstances this would be a disadvantage, but the procedure is ideal when the mandible would otherwise be too wide.

Anteroposterior and Vertical Changes
Maxilla

The possible anteroposterior and vertical changes of the maxilla are illustrated diagrammatically in Fig. 5-5. Although movements in both direction are possible, they are not equally feasible.

Surgically, the entire maxilla can be moved forward and upward. The key to success is an osteotomy that frees it from its posterior and superior attachments. When this has been accomplished, the maxilla can be moved forward up to 10 mm with good stability and upward 10 to 15 mm with excellent stability. The surgery is technically exacting but not otherwise problematic.

The major limitation to moving the maxilla forward is the resistance of the soft tissue anterior to it, primarily the upper lip. The tighter the lip, the greater the difficulty in advancing the maxilla. This is particularly pertinent in a patient with a cleft lip and palate, who is

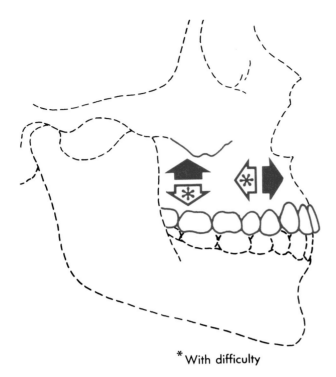

*With difficulty

Fig. 5-5. Surgically, it is quite feasible to move the entire maxilla upward or forward following a total maxillary osteotomy. It is difficult to move it backward because of the structures behind it, a technical difficulty that can be overcome by segmentation, and difficult to move it downward because of postsurgical instability.

likely to have maxillary deficiency and therefore may be a candidate for advancement. Although the maxilla can be advanced in these patients, the quality of the lip repair and the extent of scarring in the lip is an important consideration.

Another aspect of maxillary advancement is its potential effect on velopharyngeal closure during speech. Failure to achieve a seal between the soft palate and the posterior pharyngeal wall allows leakage of air through the nose and causes "cleft-palate speech." Although there was concern in the 1970s that maxillary advancement could cause cleft-palate speech in normal patients because the soft palate would be moved away from its area of contact, this has proved not to be a problem in patients with a normal velopharyngeal mechanism. On the other hand, patients with cleft palates who have a marginal seal before advancement are likely to have an air leak afterward. If that occurs, a second surgical procedure to establish a pharyngeal flap probably will be required (see Chapter 18 for additional details).

The potential problem patient is the one with an unrecognized submucous cleft before maxillary advancement. Taking a lateral cephalometric film while the patient is producing a vowel sound (Fig. 5-6) is one way

to quickly screen for normal function. If there is any remaining doubt, testing for the area of contact[8] can be done in the laboratories associated with many cleft-palate centers, and if it is minimal, the patient should be warned about the possibility of a disturbance of speech postsurgically. Only patients with cleft palates appear to be at risk of this complication.

When surgery to superiorly reposition the maxilla was first considered, there was great concern that neuromuscular adaptation would not occur. The question was whether the postural position of the mandible would change so that the mandible would rotate upward at rest as well as in function. If it did not, there would be no decrease in face height, just an increase in the freeway space between the teeth when the jaw is in its postural position. These fears were heightened by the common experience that, when dentures are being made, the mandibular postural position responds minimally if at all to changes in the height of the replacement teeth.

Fortunately, mandibular posture does adapt to surgical changes in the vertical position of the maxilla, and freeway space stays about the same after the maxilla is repositioned.[6] The key difference from the prosthodontic patient who does not respond is the presence of the natural teeth. We do not know exactly how the necessary signal to the central nervous system is generated (Fig. 5-7). It seems likely that pressure receptors in the periodontal ligament of the maxillary posterior teeth are important. Perhaps their output is integrated with muscle and TM joint proprioception to establish the postural position of the mandible. Whatever the precise mechanism, when the maxilla is moved up, the mandible rotates up along with it, and the surgical results are remarkably stable.

The entire maxillary dentition can be moved backward surgically, but posterior bony interferences limit this, and the maximum is only 3 to 5 mm. However, it is almost never really necessary to move the entire maxilla back. Instead the objective is to retract the protruding anterior portion, and this can be accomplished by sectioning the maxilla and removing bone across the palate. Then the anterior segment can be brought back posteriorly while the posterior segment(s) remain in position or move anteriorly (Fig. 5-8). The difficulty in moving the maxilla back is technical, in other words, and this can be overcome by performing a segmental osteotomy along with the LeFort I procedure. Some concern has been expressed that a multisegment osteotomy might be less stable than a one-piece osteotomy, but current research data indicate that stability is quite similar whether or not the maxilla is segmented[6] (see Chapter 8 for more details).

Orthodontic management interacts with surgical management in all types of surgical-orthodontic treatment, but particularly so when segmental maxillary sur-

Fig. 5-6. **A,** Cephalometric film during phonation of /oo/ in a child with a submucous cleft of the soft palate. Note the failure of the soft palate to contact the posterior pharyngeal wall. This causes leakage of air through the nose during some speech sounds, creating cleft-palate speech. **B,** Phonation cephalometric film in a noncleft adolescent with maxillary deficiency for whom maxillary advancement was planned. Note the normal area of contact of the soft palate with the pharyngeal wall. Advancement for this patient was done without any disturbance in speech, as can be expected when there is normal velopharyngeal function before surgery.

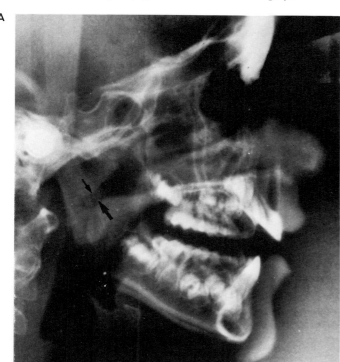

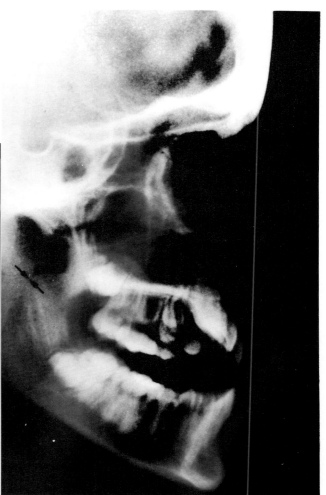

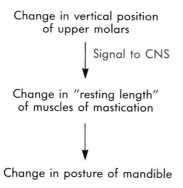

Fig. 5-7. Neurophysiologic adaptation when the maxilla is moved upward leads to a new postural position of the mandible, so freeway space before and after the surgery is changed only slightly if at all. The nature of the signal that causes this adaptation is unknown but presumably is based in some way on the pressure receptors in the periodontium of the upper posterior teeth.

gery is planned. A two-segment maxilla is used primarily to correct a transverse problem, so when this is planned, there is no reason for the orthodontist to expand the maxilla presurgically. Three maxillary segments are needed when the anterior and posterior segments must be moved differentially, either to retract the incisors or to deal with a vertical step in the dental arch. The osteotomy cuts to create the segments usually are made bilaterally through a premolar extraction site.

Should the premolars be extracted when presurgical orthodontic treatment is begun, or should the extractions be delayed until the time of the orthognathic surgery? For esthetic reasons, it might seem desirable to leave the premolars in place until the last possible moment. However, as a general rule, it is better to go ahead with the premolar extractions before presurgical orthodontics begin so that the extraction space can be partially used in correcting the axial inclination of the

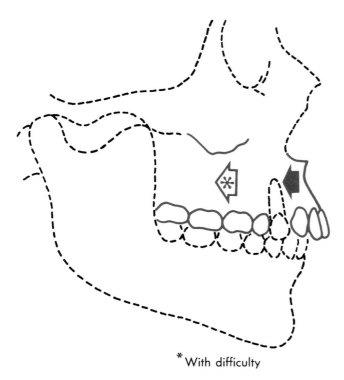

*With difficulty

Fig. 5-8. The difficulty of moving the maxilla back is overcome by segmenting it horizontally so that the protruding anterior segment can be retracted. Adding segmentation to a total maxillary osteotomy means that the posterior segments can be moved forward somewhat at the same time that the anterior segment(s) moves posteriorly, allowing precise control of the final position of the anterior segment.

incisors. As Fig. 5-9 shows, if the surgeon must rotate the anterior segment to position the incisors correctly, the canines will be lifted up off the occlusal plane and the roots will be separated at the extraction site. This can cause major problems and delays in the finishing orthodontics. In contrast, if the segments can be brought together without rotation, orthodontic finishing is facilitated. It is perfectly acceptable to close up to half the extraction space during the presurgical orthodontics—but the space cannot be totally closed without compromising the surgery.

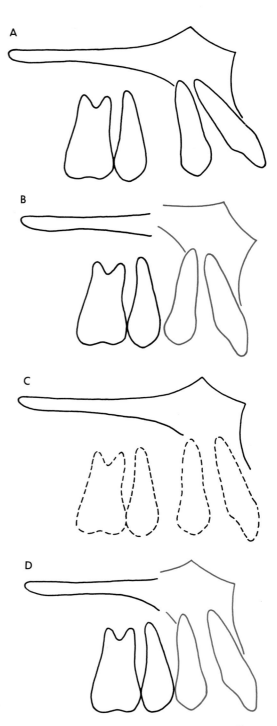

Fig. 5-9. When anterior and posterior segments will be created during a maxillary osteotomy, it usually is better to extract the premolars first so the protruding incisors can be tipped back to the proper inclination during the presurgical orthodontics. **A,** Tracing of a maxilla with protruding incisors. **B,** The effect of surgically retracting the anterior segment and rotating it at the time of surgery to obtain the correct inclination of the incisors. The canines are lifted up out of occlusion, and the canine and second premolar roots are separated. **C,** The tooth movement likely to occur if the incisors are tipped back presurgically, correcting their inclination. There also will be some forward movement of the posterior teeth, which does not matter in this context. **D,** Superimposition showing surgical closure of the remaining extraction space after the tooth movement in C. Now the teeth fit correctly without rotating the segments, and finishing orthodontics is minimized.

Moving the entire maxilla down is technically feasible, although an interpositional bone graft is required. No particular problem exists in obtaining satisfactory healing. The lack of soft tissue that is a problem in the mandibular symphysis does not apply in this region. This movement is difficult for a different reason—it is not stable postsurgically. When the maxilla is moved up, it does not tend to come back down, and indeed is remarkably stable in its superior position.[6] But when it is moved down, there is a strong tendency for it to move back up.[9]

The reason for this instability is not known with certainty. It seems likely, however, that it is related to the stretch of soft tissues that is created when the maxilla is moved downward. Even if neuromuscular adaptation occurs (as should be the case if the vertical position of the upper teeth is an important determinant), the skin, connective tissue, vessels, and nerves are stretched by increasing face height. This would create a gentle but constant force to move the maxilla back up, and the neuromuscular system would immediately adapt to readjust mandibular posture in concert with any relapse that occurred. Whether or not this hypothesis is correct, the fact remains that when the maxilla is moved down, there is a strong tendency for it to relapse upward postsurgically.

This instability does not mean that moving the maxilla down is impossible—it can be accomplished with extra attention to measures that enhance stability.[10,11] Technical modifications for this purpose include using additional fixation to stabilize both the maxilla and mandible against vertical changes and graft materials that increase mechanical stability. These methods are discussed in some detail in Chapters 7, 8, and 12 on surgical technique and clinical treatment. For treatment planning purposes, however, the difficulty with this movement should be kept in mind, and more stable alternatives should be selected when they are possible.

Mandible

The possibilities for surgically moving the mandible anteroposteriorly and vertically are shown in Fig. 5-10. As the diagram indicates, the mandible can be moved forward or back. The chin or inferior border can be moved up or down. The gonial angle area can be moved up, but moving it down is so difficult that, for all practical purposes, it is impossible.

The vertical position of the gonial angle rarely is an important problem for patients with dentofacial deformities. It therefore may be surprising that changes in this area are extremely important in planning mandibular surgery. The reason for mandibular surgery usually is to move the mandible forward or back, but changes in the vertical position of the chin and gonial angle occur along with the horizontal movement, and the vertical changes are the primary determinants of postsurgical stability.

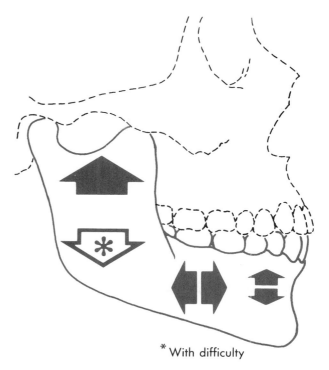

* With difficulty

Fig. 5-10. Surgically, the mandible can be moved forward or back, up or down anteriorly, but only upward in the gonial angle area. The difficulty with moving the gonial angles downward is not technical—it is straightforward to move the angles down at surgery. The problem is a strong relapse tendency when this is done. Moving the mandible forward or back nearly always causes vertical changes, and the pattern of vertical change is a major determinant of postsurgical stability.

When the mandible is moved forward or back, there are three possibilities for vertical reorientation (Fig. 5-11): (1) the mandibular plane can increase as the chin moves down and/or the gonial angle moves up, (2) it can remain approximately the same, as the mandible is repositioned along the existing mandibular plane, or (3) it can decrease as the chin moves up and the gonial angle moves down.

The rotation pattern has a major effect on postsurgical stability.[12] Mandibular surgery that rotates the mandible down anteriorly and up posteriorly (in a way that would correct a deep bite anteriorly in addition to making anteroposterior changes) has excellent stability. Surgical movements along the existing mandibular plane, particularly advancements, are not quite as stable but still are acceptable. Surgery that rotates the mandible up anteriorly and down posteriorly (so that an anterior open bite is corrected) is notoriously unstable and should be avoided whenever possible.

This variation in stability following mandibular surgery is related both to neuromuscular adaptation and to soft-tissue stretching. Note in Fig. 5-11 the effect of

A   B   C

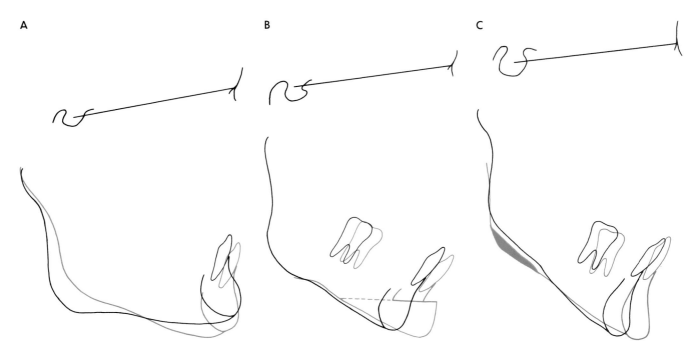

Fig. 5-11. There are three possibilities for rotating the mandible when it is advanced (or set back). **A,** Rotation so that the chin goes down and the gonial angles up (increasing the mandibular plane angle and correcting a deep bite anteriorly) produces the most stable movement. **B,** Advancing the mandible along the mandibular plane is less stable but satisfactory. An inferior border osteotomy, as used in this patient to achieve better chin-lip balance and advance the chin more than the incisor, has no effect on stability. **C,** Rotation so that the chin goes up and the gonial angles down (decreasing the mandibular plane angle) is highly likely to lead to relapse. This movement should be avoided when at all possible.

the various rotations on the soft tissues. When the chin moves down and the gonial angle moves up, the muscles attached to both areas are shortened and the soft tissues are relaxed. When these structures move in the opposite direction, the muscles and associated soft tissues are stretched.

In the case of downward movement of the maxilla, there was reason to believe that neuromuscular adaptation occurred, and yet instability still was experienced. When ramus surgery is used to rotate the mandible so that the muscles are stretched, neuromuscular adaptation does not occur, and problems caused by stretch of other soft tissues are magnified by muscle pull in a relapse direction. The direction of vertical movement of the gonial angle is particularly important. The effect of pull of the muscles at the chin is trivial when compared with the effects of the powerful mandibular elevator muscles that insert posteriorly. Failure of the elevator muscles to adapt to movement of the mandible creates almost irresistable relapse tendencies (Fig. 5-12).

If the hypothesis of soft-tissue stretch as a cause of instability is correct, we would expect better stability when the mandible is moved back than when it is advanced. Some tissue stretching must occur when the mandible is moved forward, but moving it back should

tend to relax soft tissues. This is in fact the case. All other things being equal, setting the mandible back is a more stable movement than is advancing it.[13] Even with a mandibular setback, however, it is possible to stretch tissues at the gonial angle. This occurs because if the mandible is rotated up in front to close an open bite, it tends to rotate around a fulcrum at the molar teeth, and this causes the gonial-angle area to move downward. Muscle pull and/or the elasticity of the other soft tissues will pull the gonial angle back up. The result is a postsurgical tendency toward open bite.

Unless there was an unfavorable rotation, the mandible tends to stay reasonably close to its postsurgical position when it is moved posteriorly.[13] More precisely, any relapse tendencies are related more to how successfully the condyle was maintained in the temporal fossa than to soft-tissue effects. When the mandible is advanced, however, even if the rotation was favorable, the inevitable stretch of soft tissues at the chin that accompanies forward movement creates a relapse tendency.[14,15] If the teeth are wired together, tooth relationships are maintained while healing occurs, but orthodontic tooth movement allows the jaw to slip posteriorly. The maxillary incisor teeth are retracted relative to the maxilla, the mandibular incisors tip for-

A

B

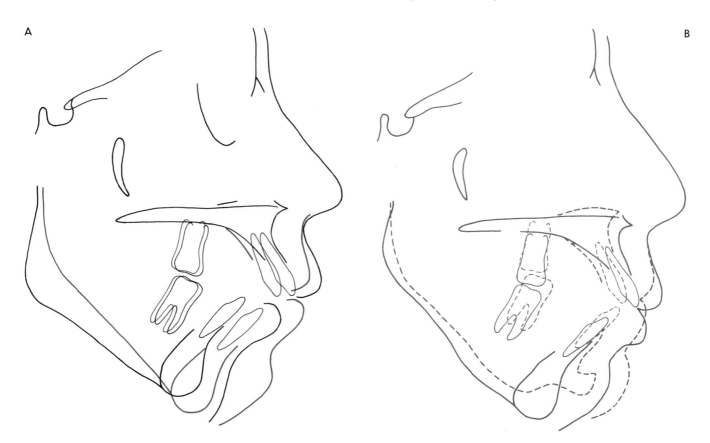

Fig. 5-12. Cephalometric superimposition showing the result of mandibular advancement in a patient who had "wrong-way" rotation. **A,** Superimposition of presurgery tracing *(in black)* with 3-month postsurgery tracing *(in red).* Three points are of interest: (1) the surgery succeeded in advancing the chin anteroposteriorly; that is, despite the relapse tendency, the chin is further anteriorly after the surgery than before, (2) rotating the chin up and the gonial angles down, so as to close the open bite, was unsuccessful—there has been significant relapse into open bite, and the ramus now is much shorter than before surgery, and (3) the pull of stretched soft tissues during fixation led to significant retraction of the upper incisors and proclination of the lower incisors, an effect analagous to the use of heavy Class II elastics. **B,** Superimposition showing subsequent orthognathic surgery for this patient, in which maxillary posterior and anterior segmental osteotomies, with extraction of maxillary first premolars, was used to correct the overjet and open bite. A genioplasty also was performed. This produced a stable result.

ward relative to the mandible, and the mandible moves back (Fig. 5-13). This change continues until bone continuity at the osteotomy site is reestablished, typically at about 6 weeks after surgery.[16] At that point, the bone can withstand the soft-tissue pressure, the relapse tendency disappears, and the mandible tends to move forward again in the patients in whom it slipped posteriorly.[15] With RIF, the mandible is more stable during the first 6 weeks after surgery, and there is no rebound after fixation release.[17] This pattern of postsurgical change is described in detail in Chapter 12.

Two important guidelines for treatment planning are evident from the preceeding discussion:

1. Whether the mandible is moved forward or back, lengthening the ramus by rotating the mandible down posteriorly should be avoided. The technique of cephalometric prediction, which is discussed in detail below, shows whether the ramus would be lengthened by mandibular surgery. RIF cannot be relied on to overcome the relapse tendencies created by wrong-way rotation.

2. If a necessary movement of the mandible would lengthen the ramus, this can be avoided by also planning surgery to elevate the posterior maxilla. For this reason, surgery on both jaws often is needed in patients with Class II or III open-bite problems.

A more general guideline for treatment of patients with short faces or long faces also can be derived from a consideration of vertical stability. All other things be-

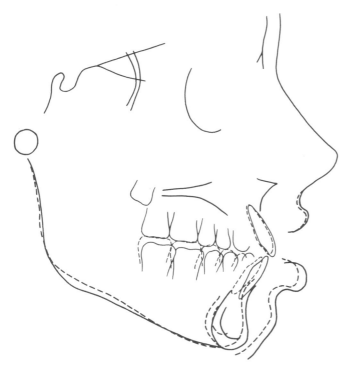

Fig. 5-13. Cephalometric superimposition showing typical changes during the first 6 weeks following mandibular advancement with wire fixation in a patient whose mandible came straight forward without unfavorable rotation or lengthening of the ramus. This change occurred during maxillomandibular fixation as a result of light continuous pressure from stretched soft tissues. The occlusal relationships were maintained, but the upper incisors tipped lingually and the lower incisors tipped labially, and the orthodontic tooth movement allowed the chin to slip back. See Chapter 12 for a more complete discussion of stability following mandibular advancement.

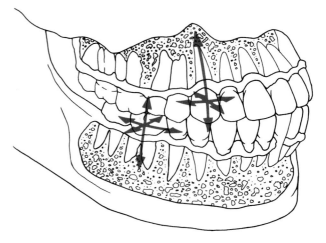

Fig. 5-14. Surgery to reposition dentoalveolar segments in all three planes of space now is possible. The key is maintaining an adequate blood supply to the bone and teeth through intact labial or lingual mucosa. In the mandibular posterior area, temporarily lifting the inferior alveolar neurovascular bundle out into the cheek allows cuts to be made safely beneath the teeth. Although the nerve supply to the involved teeth is interrupted, sensation usually returns and endodontic treatment almost never is required (see Table 5-1).

Dentoalveolar Surgery

Dentoalveolar segments now can be repositioned surgically in all three planes of space (Fig. 5-14), but there are limitations both on the distance that the segments can be moved and on the size of the segments themselves.

As a general rule, the distance that a dentoalveolar segment can be moved surgically is approximately the same as the distance those teeth could be moved orthodontically. If this seems surprising at first, consider that the ultimate limit on moving teeth is the amount of soft-tissue adaptation that will occur.[18] The teeth cannot be put in a position that the soft tissues will not accept—if they are, relapse is inevitable. Therefore the limits shown for tooth movement in the diagram of the envelope of discrepancy are applicable to surgery and to orthodontics (see Fig. 1-2).

If that is true, why would surgical movement of dentoalveolar segments ever be indicated? For at least two related reasons: anchorage and time. Orthodontic tooth movement requires care to prevent reaction forces from displacing dental units that should not be moved; that is, to keep from moving anchor teeth as well. Extraoral anchorage (headgear) may be required, which increases the demands on patient cooperation and makes treatment less pleasant. Surgically repositioning segments places essentially no demands on anchorage. Extensive orthodontic tooth movement also

ing equal, it is better to treat a short-face problem with mandibular rather than maxillary surgery. This would increase anterior face height by a stable movement, rotating the mandible down anteriorly, rather than by the unstable one of moving the maxilla down. But it is better to treat a long-face problem with maxillary surgery, moving the maxilla up and allowing the mandible to rotate upward and forward. This would decrease the mandibular plane angle without the instability associated with lengthening the ramus.

This general guideline is just that, not a rigid rule. Much of the discussion that follows in this chapter is aimed at determining how the total picture for a patient fits together. Other considerations may affect the final treatment plan. The guideline does suggest a way to maximize stability of the surgical result in patients with vertical discrepancy problems.

TABLE 5-1 Tooth relapse and vitality after segmental alveolar surgery

	Number of teeth	Not responding at 12 months	Requiring endodontics	Requiring extraction
Kohn and White[20]	189	28 (15%)	4 (2.1%)	1 (0.5%)
Pepersack[21]				
Maxillary	588	31 (5.3%)	1 (0.2%)	0
Mandibular except Kole	245	68 (28%)	3 (1.2%)	0
Kole procedure	178	84 (47%)	2 (1.1%)	5 (2.8%)

will require a considerable amount of time, whereas the same movement could be done more quickly surgically.

A rational guideline for dentoalveolar surgery would be that the more difficult and prolonged the equivalent orthodontic tooth movement would be, the more one would consider surgical repositioning of dentoalveolar segments. Because it is harder to intrude teeth orthodontically than to extrude them or move them anteroposteriorly, large intrusive movements are particularly favorable for dentoalveolar surgery.

An additional indication for surgically repositioning dentoalveolar segments is when teeth cannot be moved orthodontically. A small segment osteotomy is the only way to move an ankylosed tooth. Occasionally teeth that are not ankylosed will not respond to orthodontic force because some abnormality in the periodontal ligament causes the condition of primary failure of eruption,[19] or perhaps because of fibrotic gingiva that impedes movement. Larger segments sometimes can be repositioned surgically in these patients to solve occlusal problems that otherwise would be untreatable (see Chapter 10 for further information).

The size of surgical segments is an important consideration. The smaller the segment, the greater the chance of problems because of compromised blood supply. In theory, the surgeon could create segments as small as a single tooth, but in practice, segments that contain fewer than three teeth are increasingly hazardous. We suggest that the treatment plan should not call for more than four dentoalveolar segments within a single arch and that three-tooth segments should be the minimum if more than two segments are being created. In other words, it may be all right to reposition one two-tooth segment, but surgically creating six two-tooth segments in the same arch would not be wise.

Although the blood supply to the teeth is maintained after dentoalveolar surgery, the nerve supply is interrupted. The teeth routinely do not respond to an electrical pulp tester for a few months postsurgically. However, the nerve supply regenerates. After 6 months, nearly all the teeth in or adjacent to maxillary segments

and the majority of those in mandibular segments once again respond to stimulation (Table 5-1).[20] Of the minority that do not respond, only a few have necrotic pulps that require endodontic therapy.[21,22] General dentists who are not used to encountering vital but denervated teeth, which is the condition that exists following alveolar surgery, must be warned not to equate vitality with the response to pulp testers. Pulp vitality can be demonstrated by other means, as for instance by carefully measuring the temperature of the tooth, detecting the warmth associated with blood flow in the pulp.

On occasion, the technique of corticotomy, which is the surgical creation of multiple small partial segments, has been advocated as a way to speed up orthodontic tooth movement.[23] With this method, labial flaps are raised and interdental osteotomy cuts are made between each tooth, but the segments are not totally freed. Then orthodontic forces are applied. Unless the base of the segments fractured due to the orthodontic force, so that the entire segment could displace rapidly—which does not occur—faster tooth movement following the surgery presumably would result from some general stimulation of bone metabolism related to the healing process. The evidence that this happens is tenuous at best, and there is a risk of creating periodontal defects and/or gingival recession. Corticotomy, in other words, suffers from the same problem as does surgically assisted maxillary expansion: it combines the disadvantages, not the advantages, of surgery and orthodontics. If the small segments are totally freed so the surgeon can reposition the teeth instantly, it becomes a risky variant of the small-segment osteotomy approach, with too many segments.

Chin Surgery

The position of the chin can be changed in two ways: by adding some extraneous material to it (e.g., bone, cartilage, any of several alloplastic materials), or by using an inferior border osteotomy to free it so that it can be repositioned. The inferior border osteotomy always is preferred when this surgery is possible.

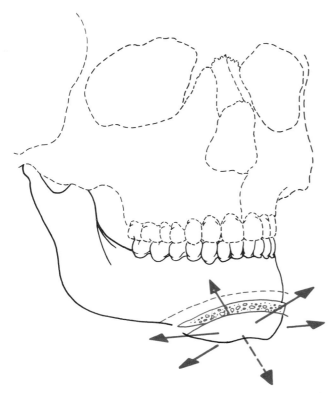

Fig. 5-15 Inferior border osteotomy allows the chin to be re-positioned in all three planes of space. If the osteotomy cut is angled upward anteriorly, moving the chin forward creates a horizontal augmentation simultaneously with a vertical reduction, which is a highly desirable combination for many long-face, chin-deficient patients. If further vertical reduction is needed, it is best to remove a wedge of bone above the chin rather than remove bone from the lower border. A graft can be placed in the rare instance that the chin needs to be moved down away from the teeth.

As Fig. 5-15 shows, the chin can be repositioned in all three planes of space with an inferior border osteotomy. An asymmetry can be corrected by sliding it sideways and/or repositioning it vertically, a deficiency by moving it forward or downward (which may require an interpositional graft), and an excess by moving it backward or upward (which is done best by removing a wedge of bone above the chin).

Laterally repositioning the chin to conceal mandibular asymmetry can be quite effective because the position of the chin is obvious at a glance, whereas a casual observer will not notice the location of the gonial angles (Fig. 5-16). As with most aspects of surgical treatment, judgment is required as to whether the best plan is to correct the problem, which in the case of a mandibular asymmetry might require bilateral ramus surgery, or merely conceal it, as could be done by an inferior border osteotomy. If the occlusion is satisfactory, the considerable esthetic benefit and much less complex

surgery make inferior border osteotomy an attractive alternative in many instances.

When the chin is moved forward by an inferior border osteotomy, it also goes up (Fig. 5-17). The extent of vertical shortening can be controlled to some extent by the angle of the osteotomy cut. Many patients with long faces have a combination of horizontal deficiency and vertical excess of the chin, so the combination of horizontal augmentation and vertical reduction is ideal for them. Conversely, when the chin slides posteriorly, it also moves down. A reduction inferior border osteotomy therefore is also to some extent a vertical augmentation, which may or may not be advantageous. Excessive lengthening during horizontal reduction can be prevented by removing a wedge of bone.

One of the advantages of genioplasty via inferior border osteotomy is that the ratio of soft-tissue to hard-tissue change is quite predictable.[24] When the chin is advanced, the soft tissue moves forward about 60% as much as does the hard tissue, with remarkably little individual variation. Reduction genioplasty is not as precise, but the anteroposterior soft-tissue reduction is about 50% of the hard-tissue change.[25] Vertically, the soft tissue moves approximately the same amount as does the hard tissue. It must be remembered, however, that the patient sees the chin from in front, and profile prediction is far from the whole story in evaluating the three-dimensional soft-tissue effect.

In situations of extreme deficiency, there may be no alternative to adding material to the chin. Autogenous bone grafts require an additional donor site. Results with autogenous and allogeneic bone grafts from the iliac crest or a rib have been unpredictable. Autogenous membrane bone from the cranium seems to retain its contour more predictably, but additional clinical experience with this approach is needed. In some cases, alloplastic materials are the only choice. They can be combined with other grafts. Hydroxylapatite grafts show promise; the rate of migration and secondary infection seems less than with alloplastic materials used previously. See Chapter 10 for additional details.

Implications of Incomplete Growth

The implication of incomplete growth for a patient who may need orthognathic surgery is straightforward: growth following the surgery is quite likely to cause relapse because the growth pattern that caused the problem in the first place will still be present. When the situation is not complicated by previous trauma or the presence of chronic disease, most orthognathic surgical procedures have remarkably little impact on the magnitude or direction of subsequent growth.

It would be advantageous if a ramus osteotomy to correct mandibular prognathism also eliminated the potential of the jaw to grow afterward. Unfortunately, the osteotomy does not do that, which means that unless

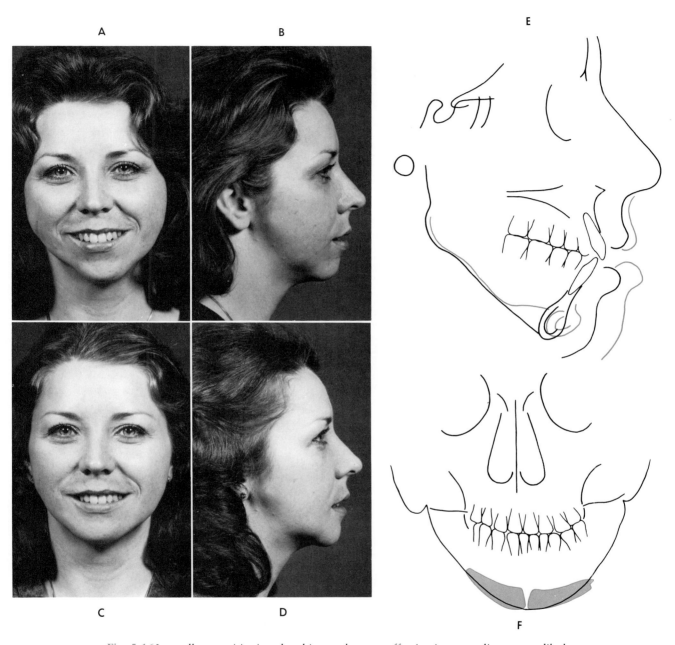

Fig. 5-16. Laterally repositioning the chin can be very effective in concealing a mandibular deficiency even though an asymmetry at the angles persists because most observers notice the chin and not the posterior areas. This woman was concerned about her deviated chin, but the dental occlusion was reasonably good following previous orthodontic treatment. **A** and **B,** Facial appearance before inferior border osteotomy to move the chin laterally and forward. **C** and **D,** Facial appearance after surgery. **E,** Lateral cephalometric tracing with surgical changes in red. Some postsurgical edema still is present. **F,** PA cephalometric tracing.

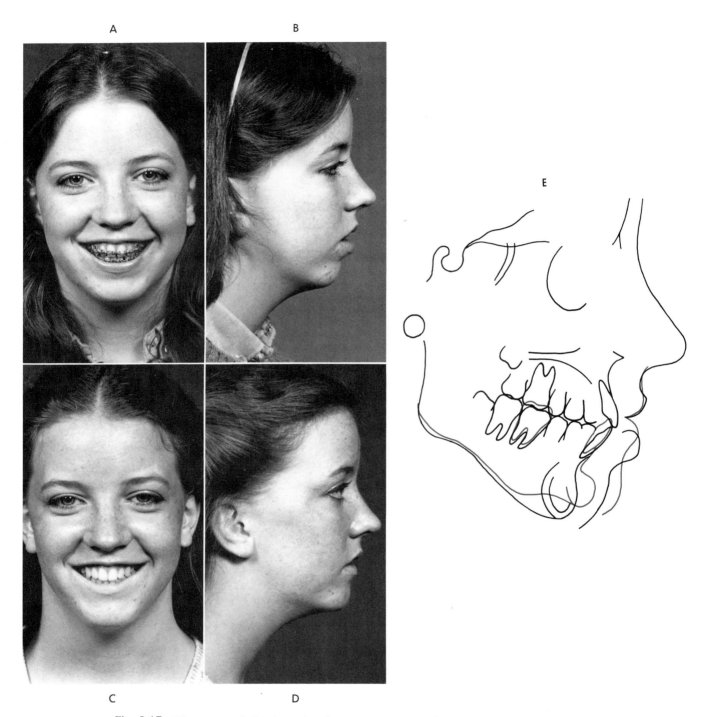

Fig. 5-17. When an angled inferior border osteotomy is used to move the chin forward, it also moves up, shortening face height. In a patient such as this girl with chin deficiency and excessive lip separation at rest, both changes can be important in improving facial esthetics. **A** and **B**, Facial appearance, age 15 years, 6months. **C** and **D**, Age 16 years, after inferior border osteotomy. **E**, Cephalometric tracing showing the change produced by the surgery.

A   B

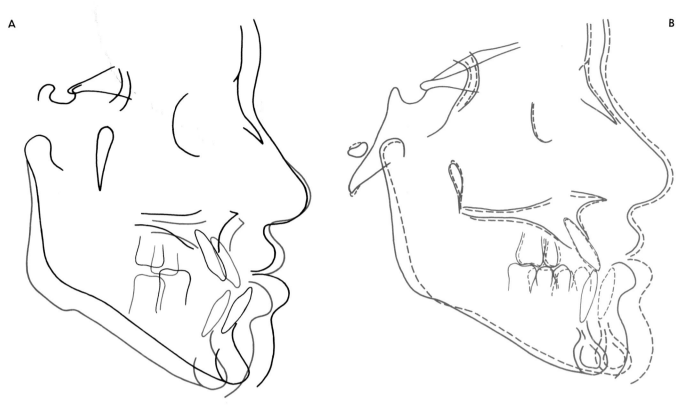

Fig. 5-18. If correction of mandibular prognathism is carried out before growth is completed, as it was because of the severity of the problem in this 15-year-old male, subsequent
growth may lead to relapse. **A,** Cephalometric superimpositions showing the changes made
at surgery, when the maxilla was advanced and the mandible was set back. **B,** Superimposition showing the change over the next 3 years, as rapid mandibular growth led to a partial
recurrence of the problem. Note that the maxillary advancement was stable, but the maxilla
showed very little subsequent growth. A second mandibular surgery, after growth has
stopped, will be needed.

growth of the mandible is complete or nearly so at the
time of surgery to shorten the mandible, subsequent
growth is almost certain to cause relapse. This does not
necessarily rule out correcting a severe Class III problem
before growth is completed. It may be necessary to do
this for psychologic reasons, but, if so, a second surgical
procedure later may be needed (Fig. 5-18). Similarly, it
would be convenient if early surgery to correct a vertically long maxilla also prevented later vertical growth.
Although surgery to correct long-face problems can be
done earlier than can that for mandibular prognathism
(see Chapter 2), there is a chance of relapse caused by
continued growth in this condition also.

On the other hand, if a jaw deformity is caused by a
deficiency in growth, early surgical intervention should
cause no problems because postsurgical growth would
be quite possible. But this situation is not so clear-cut.
Early surgery probably will not reduce the already deficient growth even further, but neither will it magically
change an aberrant growth pattern to a normal one, so
continued growth of the normal jaw could again leave

the deficient one behind. For example, the mandible
grows after preadolescent mandibular advancement,
but the growth direction nearly always is more vertical
and less horizontal than is normal, which can create a
relapse tendency if there is significant forward maxillary growth.[26-28] Even in deficiency situations, therefore, it is better to wait until after the adolescent
growth spurt. However, at that point the surgery can
be done sooner in deficiency than in excess growth
problems. This subject is discussed in some detail in
Chapter 6.

The possibilities for orthodontic and surgical treatment are a necessary background for treatment planning because there is nothing to be gained from attempting treatment that will be problematic at best and
a failure at worst. However, knowing what can and
cannot be done does not tell you what should be done.
In the following sections of this chapter, the focus is on
a treatment planning process designed to take all pertinent information into account in deciding what would
be best for any individual patient.

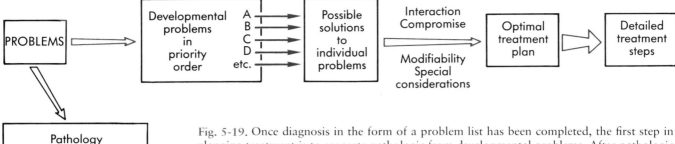

Fig. 5-19. Once diagnosis in the form of a problem list has been completed, the first step in planning treatment is to separate pathologic from developmental problems. After pathologic problems are brought under control, a series of logical steps is used to develop the plan for the developmental problems, beginning with ranking the developmental problems in priority order.

LOGICAL SEQUENCE OF TREATMENT PLANNING
Pathologic versus Developmental Problems

The first step in the logical sequence for planning treatment (Fig. 5-19) is the differentiation between pathologic and developmental problems. Although the focus of this chapter is on the treatment of the patient's developmental problems, any pathology must be explicitly recognized and treated first. A critical principle of treatment is that oral and systemic diseases must be brought under control before treatment of developmental problems begins.

For our purposes here, disease problems and their associated pathologies can be divided into three major groups: (1) chronic systemic disease states or metabolic derangements, of which arthritis and diabetes, respectively, are the best examples, (2) local conditions specifically affecting oral health, such as periodontal disease, and (3) psychologic or emotional problems, such as distorted perceptions of reality that lead to unrealistic expectations for treatment.

Chronic Systemic Diseases

Chronic Degenerative Problems: Arthritis. The inflammatory and destructive forms of arthritis (rheumatoid arthritis or one of the related types) can and often do involve the TM joint. If this happens in childhood, a facial deformity is almost certain to develop[29,30] (Fig.

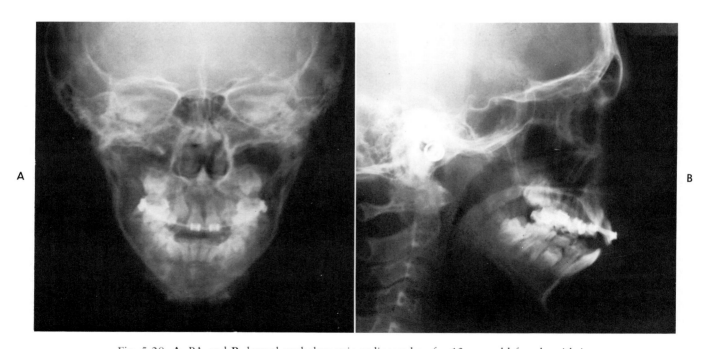

Fig. 5-20. **A,** PA and **B,** lateral cephalometric radiographs of a 12-year-old female with juvenile rheumatoid arthritis. Note the destruction of the condylar process and consequent downward and backward rotation of the mandible, creating excessive overjet and anterior open bite.

A

B

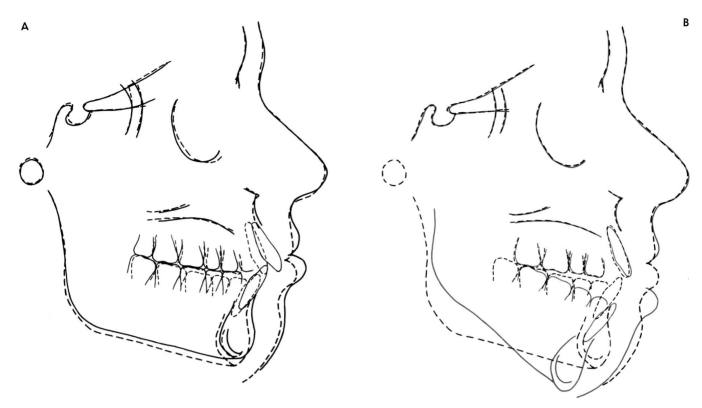

Fig. 5-21. Cephalometric superimposition showing the changes produced by progressive rheumatoid arthritis in a young woman. **A,** Changes during orthodontic treatment in the late teens (*black,* pretreament; *dashed black,* posttreatment). **B,** Posttreatment changes caused by the arthritic degeneration of the TM joint (*dashed black,* posttreatment; *red, 7 years later*). As the arthritis destroyed the condylar processes, the mandible rotated downward and backward, producing a severe anterior open bite and facial deformity. Although the primary problem is in the mandible, surgical corrrection in such patients requires elevating the posterior maxilla—mandibular surgery should be avoided. (Courtesy Dr. J.R. Greer.)

5-20), and a deformity may occur in older patients if arthritic degeneration is severe enough[31] (Fig. 5-21). In contrast, the osteoarthritis that often accompanies aging may lead to disturbances in TM joint function but almost never causes a dentofacial deformity.

Classic rheumatoid arthritis and its variants are autoimmune diseases. The destruction seems mediated by an attack from the immune system on body elements, particularly joint membranes, whose surface markers have become altered so that they are no longer recognized as self. Why this occurs, and why the disease affects some joints more than others, is simply unknown. The accompanying inflammatory process results in the formation of granulation tissue in the joint spaces and destruction of cartilaginous and bony components of the joint. In some patients, rapid and severe destruction occurs, though in episodic fashion, whereas in others the disease progresses very slowly or may disappear for years after an initial flare-up. As Fig. 5-21 illustrates, the entire condylar process of the mandible may be lost in severe cases.

An important principle in planning treatment for patients with inflammatory and destructive arthritis is that manipulation of the TM joint should be as limited as possible. In its simplest form, the principle is that any changes in an arthritic joint are likely to be for the worse, and treatment plans have to be developed with this in mind. In a child with juvenile rheumatoid arthritis, functional appliances to advance the mandible in the hope of stimulating better growth are not recommended because, in the arthritis patient, stimulating increased bone turnover in the joint area may cause a net loss of skeletal tissue rather than the desired net gain. For the same reason, surgical advancement of the deficient mandible should be avoided if possible because this inevitably results in some repositioning of the condyle in the fossa and a compensatory acceleration in remodeling. (See Chapter 9 for a description of the condylar rotation that usually accompanies ramus osteotomies.) A better surgical plan might be superior repositioning of the maxilla combined with an augmentation genioplasty.

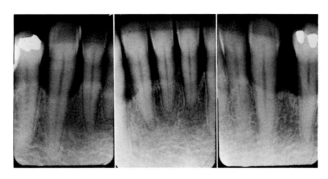

Fig. 5-22. Periapical radiographs showing the bone destruction that occurred in the lower arch during a period of uncontrolled diabetes in this woman in her early twenties. (Courtesy Dr. I. Aukhil.)

Diabetes and Other Metabolic Diseases. Diabetes is a deceptively simple metabolic problem. The defect, a relative lack of insulin, is well understood, but this affects glucose metabolism and thereby a major portion of the entire body's energy utilization mechanism. The widespread effects of this are still being discovered.[32] Problems may arise not only because of a lack of production of insulin by the endocrine cells of the pancreas, but also because insulin receptors on various target cells are blocked or inadequate, making control difficult even if exogenous insulin is supplied. The spectrum of diabetes runs from mild insulin lack or insulin resistance in many middle-aged or older individuals to severe problems in some children whose pancreatic islets have been destroyed at an early age by an apparent autoimmune process.

There are two major implications of diabetes in a potential surgical-orthodontic patient. First, healing is decreased when diabetes is not well controlled. This is an obvious contraindication to elective surgery, but it should be noted that the contraindication is for surgery in an uncontrolled or poorly controlled diabetic, not in a patient whose disease is well controlled. Second, rapid and severe periodontal bone loss can occur in uncontrolled diabetics.[33,34] (Fig. 5-22). Orthodontic appliances add to stress on the periodontium by making oral hygiene more difficult. Active orthodontic tooth movement complicates the situation even further. If diabetes is not under good control, presurgical and/or postsurgical orthodontic treatment could lead to unanticipated and possibly severe periodontal problems. For the orthodontic as well as the surgical phases of treatment, therefore, it is important to ascertain any diabetic tendencies during the diagnostic process and to scrupulously maintain control measures if treatment is undertaken.

Diabetes is the most important metabolic disease of patients with dentofacial deformities because of its frequency and potential severity, but it is by no means the

only one. Other possibly significant hormonal imbalances and metabolic problems are summarized in Table 5-2.

Chronic systemic disease by no means contraindicates surgical-orthodontic treatment for many patients, but clinical management of these individuals obviously requires close cooperation with their physicians. Systemic disease can affect both the orthodontic and surgical phases of treatment. It is important that all concerned understand the implications of any disease and that the patient be monitored carefully and frequently.

Suggestions for interaction with the physician in several specific disease states that may be encountered in orthodontic-surgical patients are discussed in Chapter 6.

Local Conditions

Local oral conditions must be considered carefully in planning treatment for surgical-orthodontic patients because of the importance of the patient's oral health care. These can be divided into two major categories: (1) problems caused by trauma and (2) the local disease states of caries and periodontal disease.

Trauma. A history of trauma to the teeth and jaws is important for two reasons. First, teeth that have been traumatized are more likely to undergo pulpal changes and root resorption than are other teeth.[35] The stress of orthodontic tooth movement may cause a pulpal situation that was borderline previously to degenerate irreversibly. Severe root resorption accompanying orthodontic tooth movement is much more likely in teeth that were traumatized previously, particularly if there is any sign of resorption before the orthodontic treatment begins. Patients must be warned about these possible complications. As with everything else, if you are told before it happens, it is an explanation. Afterward, it is just an excuse.

Second, a history of trauma is important in the evaluation of growth status. In an adult, the results of trauma are immediately apparent. In a child, the ultimate impact of trauma may be much greater than its apparent extent soon after the injury because of subsequent distortions of growth. This is particularly important because it is so easy to overlook fractures of the condylar process in children, who, for instance, may have suffered an injury of that type when a baseball also damaged the teeth. Chapter 2 includes a discussion of the potential impact of trauma and the role of surgery and orthodontics in managing subsequent problems.

Local Disease States. Orthodontic or surgical-orthodontic treatment is futile unless dental caries and periodontal breakdown can be controlled. Adult patients who are serious about surgical-orthodontic treatment usually are not difficult to motivate to take care of their mouth. On the other hand, the presence of orth-

TABLE 5-2 Medical problems significant for surgical-orthodontic treatment

Condition	Significance	Comments
Diabetes mellitus	Susceptible to periodontal breakdown during orthodontic treatment; decreased resistance to infection; poor wound healing	Maintenance of excellent control necessary
Hyperthyroidism	Increased metabolic rate, tendency to osteoporosis	Infection may create crisis; psychologic instability possible
Adrenal insufficiency	Decreased stress tolerance, delayed healing	Knowledge of steroid dosage important
Pregnancy	Major hormonal changes, increased susceptibility to periodontal breakdown	Defer surgical treatment; limited orthodontic treatment acceptable but careful periodontal monitoring required
Rheumatic heart disease, other heart disease	Susceptible to endocarditis	Antibiotic coverage required for invasive procedures; in orthodontics, for banding but not for bonding or routine adjustments
Bleeding disorders (e.g., hemophilia, von Willebrand's disease, thrombocytopenia)	Susceptible to bleeding	Replace missing clotting factors before surgery; in orthodontics, bonded attachments instead of bands, avoid aspirin and related drugs for pain control
Sickle cell anemia	Susceptible to sickle cell crisis, bone loss	Not good candidates for general anesthesia, therefore usually not considered for orthognathic surgery
Allergy-immune problems	Excessive reaction to drugs, other antigens	Rarely, nickel content in stainless steel orthodontic appliance causes problem
Rheumatoid arthritis	Episodic involvement of multiple joints, possible destruction of TM joint	Manipulation of TM joint tends to exacerbate problem; avoid functional appliances, Class II elastics, and mandibular advancement
Osteoarthritis	Progressive involvement of multiple joints, possibly including TM joint, with increasing age	Orthodontics or orthognathic surgery has little effect for better or worse on involved TM joints
Behavioral disorders	Depends on degree of control; patients often on potent medications	Drug effects may slow orthodontic tooth movement; bizarre reactions to surgery possible

In all instances, surgical-orthodontic treatment would be undertaken only after these and related conditions were under medical control.

odontic appliances adds another level of difficulty to maintaining oral hygiene. For some patients, a definite treatment plan for the developmental problems should be deferred until it is clear that the local condition can be maintained.

Not all dental treatment should be done before orthodontics and surgery. The general principle is that whatever endodontic, periodontic, and/or restorative procedures are necessary to bring oral health problems under control should be done before beginning orthodontic treatment (Fig. 5-23). This is exactly analogous to the guideline for systemic disease. Once control of local disease has been achieved, surgical-orthodontic treatment can begin, with some periodontic therapy and

definitive restorative procedures deferred until the occlusion has been established by orthodontics and surgery.

Measures to bring local disease under control and the sequence of restorative, periodontic, orthodontic, and surgical treatment are discussed in detail in Chapter 6.

Psychologic Problems

Managing patients with psychologic problems can be difficult, time consuming, and troublesome for all concerned. The greatest difficulty is likely to occur in a patient who was not diagnosed as having a psychologic problem until treatment was well advanced. For those who are identified as having psychosocial problems

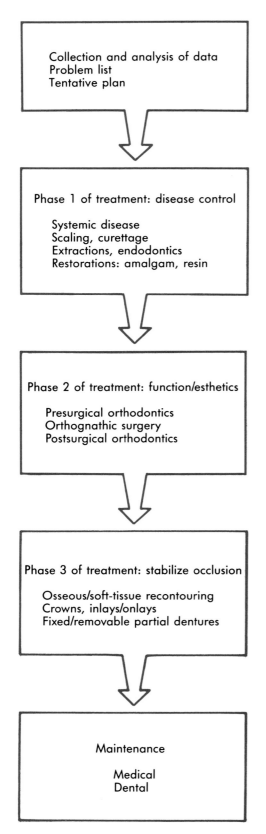

Collection and analysis of data
Problem list
Tentative plan

Phase 1 of treatment: disease control

Systemic disease
Scaling, curettage
Extractions, endodontics
Restorations: amalgam, resin

Phase 2 of treatment: function/esthetics

Presurgical orthodontics
Orthognathic surgery
Postsurgical orthodontics

Phase 3 of treatment: stabilize occlusion

Osseous/soft-tissue recontouring
Crowns, inlays/onlays
Fixed/removable partial dentures

Maintenance

Medical
Dental

Fig. 5-23. The sequence is important in planning restorative, periodontic, orthodontic, and surgical treatment for patients with complex problems involving all these specialties. The principle is that oral disease must be brought under control first. Then the final occlusion is established with appropriate surgical-orthodontic treatment, and finally the definitive periodontic and restorative procedures are carried out to complete the treatment.

during the diagnostic workup (see Chapters 3 and 4), we suggest considerable caution in proceeding with elective surgical treatment. It is difficult to refer a patient in midtreatment for psychologic counseling or psychiatric treatment, but if the patient's perception of reality is distorted enough, this may be necessary. Proceeding with treatment without adequate psychosocial evaluation is poor judgment indeed.

In borderline situations, as with a patient who might benefit from psychologic counseling but is not willing to accept it, sending the patient a detailed letter outlining the consultation and explicitly stating both the reality and what the patient apparently prefers to believe can help communication. The documentation in a letter may or may not prevent later conflict, but it can make problems easier to manage if they develop.

Prioritizing the Developmental Problem List

Once problems related to pathology have been dealt with, treatment planning for the developmental problems can begin (see Fig. 5-19). The first step is to place the patient's problems in priority order so that the most important problem is considered first.

The importance of this step cannot be overstated. The same problem list, prioritized differently, will produce a totally different treatment plan. There is no single correct treatment plan for a given set of problems, simply because the relative importance of the items on the list will vary in different circumstances. The object of treatment planning is to maximize benefit to the patient. That means treating the most important things first, and if it is not possible to correct everything, emphasizing treatment for high-priority rather than for low-priority items. The orthodontist and the surgeon must work together to produce the prioritized problem list and subsequently the treatment plan. If extensive restorative dentistry and periodontal treatment are anticipated, the dentists expected to provide this treatment should be involved. Multidisciplinary treatment is difficult, but a coordinated effort leads to the best result for the patient.

The patient's chief complaint must be considered carefully at the stage of prioritizing the problems. This does not mean that it automatically must receive the highest priority for treatment, as patients often do not understand their situation well enough to make an intelligent ranking. It does mean, however, that the chief complaint cannot be ignored. The clinicians' best judgment after carefully considering the patient's complaint must be used in deciding what is most important for a particular patient.

If the clinicians are not careful, a bias toward making some things more important than others can appear in the formulation of the problem list itself. As an example, consider what may happen when a patient with a prominent chin and an anterior crossbite visits an orthodontist or a surgeon. Whatever the patient's complaint, the orthodontist is quite likely to make a diagnosis of Class III malocclusion, which implicitly emphasizes the dental component of what probably is also a skeletal problem, whereas the surgeon probably will label the patient as having mandibular prognathism. The bias, of course, can extend to an almost automatic assumption that a particular type of treatment is needed. The orthodontist will tend to focus on correcting what he or she has already labeled as a dental problem, whereas the surgeon usually thinks first about changing the jaw relationship. Perhaps the clinicians cannot help being biased toward their own area of treatment, but they can at least recognize the potential bias. Good treatment planning requires considering the patient's complaint against the perspective of the clinician's views.

The patient must understand and agree with the final ranking, particularly if the chief complaint does not receive the highest priority for treatment. It is one thing to assume that the patient would agree with the doctor's ranking if he or she understood it, and something else to verify that assumption. The consultation at which the proposed treatment plan is presented to the patient should be structured in the form of first outlining the problems and then discussing their importance. This approach gives the patient an opportunity to agree or disagree with the proposed ranking. Informed consent, which is discussed in more detail in Chapter 6, begins at this level.

As an example of a relatively frequent clinical situation, consider the problems of the patient in case 2, whose diagnostic evaluation was illustrated in Chapter 4 and whose treatment planning is continued at the end of this chapter (see Figs. 4-43 to 4-46 and 5-39 to 5-42). The patient's chief complaint was that her upper front teeth protruded, and she sought orthodontic consultation about this problem. Although the patient did not recognize it explicitly, the diagnostic evaluation makes it plain that the maxillary incisor protrusion is as much vertical as it is horizontal; that is, the maxillary incisors not only protrude forward beyond the lip, they also hang down beneath it. It would be possible to correct the horizontal component of the protrusion by extracting two upper premolars and retracting the maxillary anterior teeth, correcting the overjet. Correcting the vertical component of the protrusion, however, would require surgical elevation of the maxilla.

The clinician may well think that the vertical problem should be the first priority, but the more complex treatment to correct that as well as the horizontal protrusion obviously should be undertaken only if the patient understands and agrees with that assessment. If both the doctor and the patient judge the vertical incisor protrusion as the priority problem, a plan to elevate these teeth (involving both orthodontics and surgery) will almost inevitably follow. On the other hand, if the horizontal protrusion is the priority item and the

vertical problem is given a lower priority or ignored, the treatment plan is likely to be just retraction of the incisors into the extraction space. But if the patient sees the vertical problem as a high priority, whether or not she can put this in words, and the clinician's plan does not address it, the treatment will be inadequate. The patient almost surely will be dissatisfied because she did not receive maximum benefit.

As a practical matter, prioritizing the problem list is usually neither difficult nor time consuming. The patient's chief complaint is balanced against the clinician's judgment of problem severity and importance, and a priority ranking emerges. At this stage, the goal is to set priorities as objectively as possible, avoiding the temptation to automatically arrange things in the direction of the clinician's favorite treatment plan.

Potential Solutions to Problems

The next step in treatment planning is to review the possible solutions to each individual problem, considering each problem as if it were the only problem the patient had, and beginning with the most important (see Fig. 5-19). This approach does two things: (1) it breaks down what initially can be an almost overwhelmingly complex problem list to manageable dimensions, and (2) it encourages the clinicians to think broadly about what could be done to correct the problems, rather than focusing immediately on their particular treatment approach.

Continuing with the example of the patient in case 2, if the patient's priority problem is vertical protrusion of the upper incisors, what are the possible solutions? Treatment would require upward movement of the incisors. This could be accomplished surgically by a total maxillary osteotomy or by an anterior maxillary segmental procedure, or orthodontically by intrusion of the incisors with segmental arch mechanics or perhaps by extra-oral force. Which would be best? That can be determined only by looking at the other items on the problem list and their possible solutions, and judging how the possible solutions to the first problem would fit with the solutions to the other problems. For instance, if the patient had a deep bite anteriorly, intruding the anterior teeth or repositioning the anterior segment may be satisfactory. Because this patient's bite is open anteriorly, it will be necessary to elevate the posterior maxilla also, to prevent anterior open bite.

Possible solutions to the second problem of maxillary incisor overjet are orthodontic or surgical retraction of the maxillary anterior segment following extraction of premolars; or forward positioning of the mandibular teeth by orthodontically displacing the mandibular teeth forward with orthodontic elastics, by surgically advancing the mandible, or by vertically elevating the maxilla, allowing the mandible to rotate upward and forward.

When the solutions to the second problem are compared with those for the first problem, it is clear that one of the solutions to the most important problem, a total maxillary osteotomy to elevate the maxilla, also is a solution to the second problem because it would allow the mandible to rotate upward and forward. The positive interaction does not necessarily make this the preferred solution because other factors have to be considered, as in the continued planning process for case 2. This does illustrate how the solution to one problem can affect another.

This is the stage of the treatment planning process when it is most helpful to predict the outcomes of various possible solutions to problems. Prediction is primarily based on cephalometric tracings and secondarily, but importantly, on dental casts. Methods for cephalometric and cast prediction are discussed later in this chapter, and their use is shown in the two cases.

Interaction, Compromise, Therapeutic Modifiability: The Introduction of Practical Considerations

An idealistic approach, though admirable, often can be criticized as not practical and therefore not really in the patient's best interest. Cost, risk, and other practical matters must be taken into account before a wise decision can be reached. It is not wise to exclude some possibilities too hastily as impractical, and the diagnostic and planning procedures to this point have focused on preventing that occurrence. But the practical matters must be included at the proper time, which is when the potential solutions are brought together into the final treatment plan. Three different aspects need to be considered: (1) *interaction* among the potential solutions, (2) the *compromise* necessary because not all problems can be solved, and (3) the *cost-risk/benefit* or therapeutic modifiability (see Fig. 5-19).

Interaction

The interaction among various treatment possibilities has been cited and partially illustrated above. When individual solutions to multiple problems are considered, one solution to the most important problem may also be a solution to the second or third problem. Conversely, at least one possible solution to the most important problem might result in the second or third problem becoming worse. All other things being equal, solutions that interact positively by solving multiple problems are preferred, whereas solutions that interact negatively should be avoided.

Consider, for instance, the patient whose dental occlusion and lateral cephalometric tracing are shown in Fig. 5-24. She has a Class III malocclusion with edge-to-edge incisors, moderate mandibular incisor crowding, and a protruding chin. One solution to the Class III relationship and anterior crossbite tendency would be to extract the first premolars in the lower arch and

retract the lower incisors, which also would solve the crowding problem—but as the tracing shows, this would make the protruding chin look even more prominent. This is negative interaction. It is also highly significant because the chin is the patient's chief complaint and should be considered her most important problem. Interactions, both positive and negative, usually are observed most readily from cephalometric predictions. As Fig. 5-24, *D* shows, another solution, which would be preferred for this patient, would be extraction in both arches to retract the upper incisors but resolve the lower crowding without further retraction, followed by a surgical setback of the mandible to correct the chin position.

As the effect on low-priority problems of various solutions to high-priority problems is observed and recognized, a pattern of broadly beneficial treatment steps usually will begin to take shape. These need to be tested against the additional practical considerations discussed below.

Compromise

The term *compromise* can have negative connotations in planning clinical treatment. The implication is that the doctors did not do their best or that the patient chose second-rate treatment. In the sense of maximizing benefit to the patient, compromise has a different meaning. Then it relates to the real possibility that it will not be possible to solve all of the patient's problems. When that is the case, the best plan focuses on the patient's more important problems at the expense of less important ones, compromising the less important problems in favor of the more important ones. It is wise, if you cannot treat everything, to treat the most important things. The relationship of this approach to prioritizing the problem list is obvious.

A common but not trivial orthodontic illustration relates to the decision to treat crowding and protrusion with or without the extraction of teeth. All other things being equal, extracting dental units and retracting incisors tends to improve the stability of dental alignment, but it may have a negative effect on facial esthetics and will reduce occlusal function. Conversely, arch expansion rather than extraction may enhance function, at the expense of stability and perhaps esthetics also. Knowing that, should one extract teeth? The obvious answer is that it depends on the relative importance of these three factors. Sometimes extraction of teeth is the preferred approach, sometimes nonextraction is better.

A surgical illustration along similar lines might relate to two-jaw versus one-jaw surgery. Repositioning one jaw often will correct a Class II or Class III dental relationship quite satisfactorily. If both jaws were moved surgically, facial esthetics might be better, but the surgical result might be less stable, and there are additional risks with the more extensive surgery. Which is

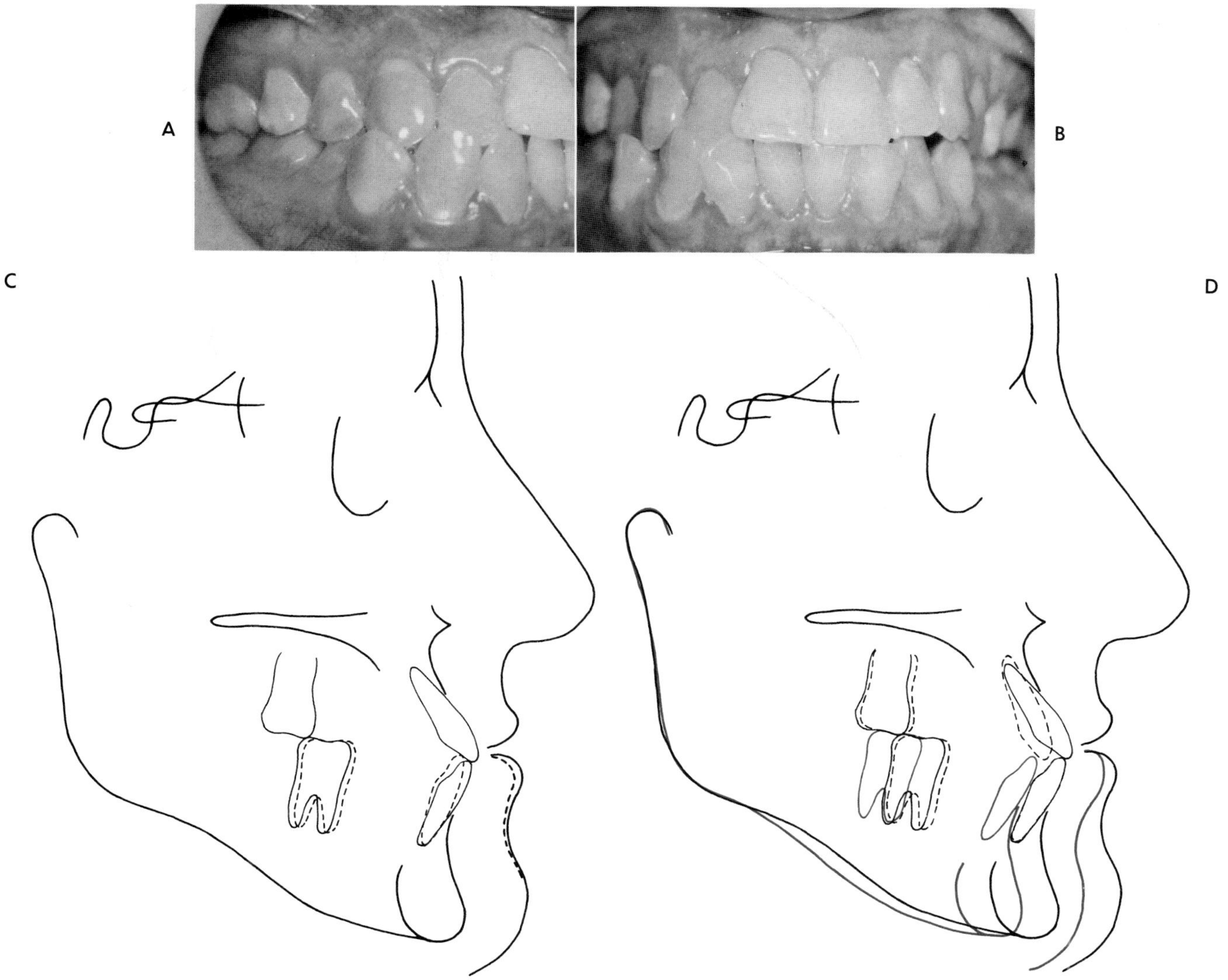

Fig. 5-24. **A** and **B,** Dental relationships and **C,** cephalometric tracing of a young woman with a Class III malocclusion, anterior crossbite tendency, and prominent chin (which is her chief complaint). The tracing makes it clear that her skeletal Class III relationship results primarily from excessive growth of the mandible, which has been partially compensated by protrusion of the maxillary incisors. If lower first premolars were extracted and the lower incisors were aligned and retracted, satisfactory alignment and incisor relationships could be achieved (as shown in the dashed line, a prediction of this treatment result). In a classic example of negative interaction among solutions to problems, this would make the apparent prominence of the chin worse, because the lower lip but not the chin would be retracted. **D,** Cephalometric prediction of the result of extracting maxillary and mandibular first premolars, creating reverse overjet by more retraction of the upper than the lower incisors *(dashed black),* and then setting the mandible back surgically *(red).* This avoids the negative interaction from orthodontic treatment alone and deals with the patient's chief complaint.

better? Again, it depends on the relative importance of esthetics, stability, and occlusal function.

Cost-Risk/Benefit

Benefit. Some treatment procedures have the potential to produce a great deal of benefit despite the fact that they are simple and all but risk-free. In the same patients, other complex, risky, and expensive procedures would produce only a small improvement at best. Obviously, the former would be preferred.

This type of thinking is instinctively adopted by both patients and doctors. Specifically considering cost and risk factors versus benefit is entirely appropriate, and the best decisions result from doing this explicitly. Cost in this context must be taken broadly, as more than just economic factors. Cost is not only finances, but also morbidity, pain, discomfort, etc. Risk is the chance of causing harm rather than benefit, creating a problem where none existed before. Calculation of benefit must relate to how well the treatment will solve the patient's problems and produce the desired result. This also is highly germane to the prioritization of the problem list. Whatever the treatment, if it will not solve the patient's most important problems, its benefit is limited, and this must be taken into account in evaluating the benefit part of the cost-risk ratio. Orthodontic treatment is more conservative than surgical treatment; that is, surgery has greater risk. On the other hand, if conservative orthodontic treatment would produce little or no benefit but surgical treatment great benefit, the risk/benefit ratio nevertheless would favor surgery (or, if the risks were judged unacceptable, no treatment at all).

Risks of Orthodontics. The risks of surgical-orthodontic treatment are a combination of the risks from orthodontics and surgery. The major risks associated with orthodontic treatment are damage to the enamel surface of the teeth from plaque buildup around orthodontic appliances and consequent decalcification, and root resorption during treatment. Periodontal breakdown during orthodontic therapy is less likely but not impossible.

Enamel decalcification is a risk only in patients with poor oral hygiene, and periodontal problems also are strongly associated with inadequate care of the mouth. Poor oral hygiene is more a problem with reluctant adolescent orthodontic patients than with adult surgical-orthodontic patients, whose high motivation usually leads to excellent hygiene during treatment. The risk of periodontal problems also increases in patients with uncontrolled systemic disease. With control of systemic and local factors, damage to teeth and gums is unlikely.

Root resorption is a different story. Recent data show that during orthodontic appliance therapy, a small amount of root resorption occurs on essentially every tooth incorporated into the appliance.[35,36] Tooth movement depends on remodeling of bone adjacent to the teeth in response to an altered environment created by gentle but prolonged pressure. At one time, it was believed that the cementum on the roots of teeth was so highly resistant to attack by resorptive cells that loss of root structures rarely occurred. It is clear now that all teeth undergo some remodeling of cementum as well as bone. Scalloped-out areas within the cementum are created as teeth move. These may extend into the dentin but rarely penetrate to any significant depth. Along the sides of the root, these deficits are then filled in by new cementum. Typically, when an orthodontic appliance is activated, force levels decline after a few days, and then there is a relative passive period until the next activation. Cemental repair seems to occur during this time.[37]

Resorption at the root apex is different only in one way: areas of cementum at the apex can be cut off as the edge of a crater extends around the curvature of the root tip. These isolated bits of cementum are not replaced when the residual crater on the root tip is filled in. This leads to a shortening of the roots that is roughly proportional to the duration of treatment: the longer the treatment, the greater the root shortening. An average tooth loses approximately 1 mm per year during typical treatment. This is clinically inapparent as well as insignificant, and changes can be detected only by careful studies using precisely oriented radiographs. For all practical purposes, therefore, this is of no consequence and creates no risk.

In a few patients, however, root resorption is much more accentuated (Fig. 5-25). A noticeable shortening of at least 1 root occurs in perhaps 10% of patients. Multiple teeth are affected in 2% to 5%, and half or more of the root is lost in a few extreme instances.[35,36] We still do not know why this happens. If orthodontic forces are heavy, the tendency toward root resorption appears to be accentuated. Significant loss of root structure as a consequence of heavy forces probably occurs primarily when the heavy force is also prolonged, so that the repair process is impeded. Although excessive orthodontic force is a potential contributing factor, most patients with severe resorption have not experienced this, nor do they have the other predisposing factors (e.g., hormonal imbalances, metabolic diseases) that have been suggested at various times.

Some individuals have spontaneous root resorption in the absence of orthodontic treatment. They are much more susceptible to excessive loss of root length during orthodontic treatment. Therefore, in patients who already have had some resorption before treatment, keeping the orthodontic treatment to the absolute minimum is prudent.

Surgical Risks. Broadly speaking, the sequelae and risks of surgical treatment can be divided into three major categories: predictable sequelae, unanticipated surgical complications, and catastrophic events.

The events surrounding hospitalization, anesthesia, surgery, and the immediate recovery period are largely predictable and can be explained to the patient before surgery. Some discomfort, surgically induced edema, temporary neurosensory deficit, and compromised nutrition routinely accompany surgery. Patients will accept these sequelae if discussed before the fact. In addition, patients may have surgical complications—for example, wound infection, wound dehiscence, or prolonged facial edema—which could not be anticipated.

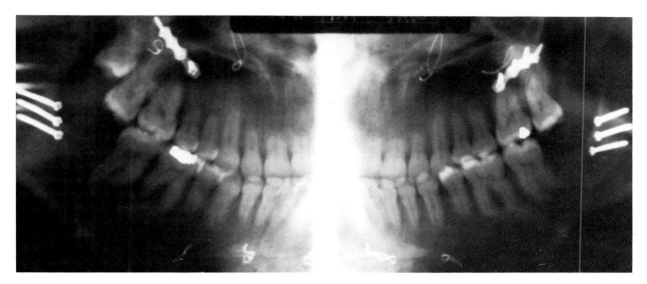

Fig. 5-25. During surgical-orthodontic treatment to correct a long-face/mandibular-deficiency problem, this patient had severe resorption of maxillary incisor roots and moderate root resorption elsewhere. Fortunately, generalized resorption of this extent occurs rarely. Because the reasons are unknown, it is all but impossible to predict.

With more or less inconvenience to the patient, these conditions can be resolved, sometimes requiring additional treatment. Catastrophic events—for example, nonunion of bony segments, loss of bone and teeth, or life-threatening anesthesia complications—occur very infrequently, but these must also be considered in the context of a decision for treatment. It can be argued that catastrophic events are a part of life. If so, perhaps important life decisions should not include such considerations because all of us are at risk for serious, unanticipated accidental injury and death at any time. Nevertheless, patients should be reminded that catastrophic events are possible though highly improbable. Most patients will understand and appreciate the context in which risks are presented and will not decide whether or not to have treatment based on the chance of a catastrophic event.

Intangible Costs. The costs of treatment include not only money, but also the intangibles (including the life adjustments) associated with wearing an orthodontic appliance and undergoing surgery. For orthodontic treatment, these nonmonetary costs include both the social impact of wearing an orthodontic appliance for a relatively prolonged period and the discomfort associated with treatment. For surgery, they include the anxiety, discomfort, and inconvenience associated with the hospital experience and the period of physical rehabilitation that inevitably follows surgery.

The Nonmonetary Costs of Orthodontic Treatment. Until relatively recently, it was quite rare to see an adult with braces on his or her teeth, and it was generally thought that adults could not tolerate orthodontics because of the social difficulties this would cause. However, adult orthodontics has become more and more accepted in recent years, despite the fact that most orthodontic appliances are obvious to any observer.

The amount of psychologic distress caused by wearing braces as an adult is very much a function of the patient's personality and attitudes.[38] The more confident an individual is, and the greater the benefit that he or she expects as a result of treatment, the more positive an attitude he or she will project. Because others react to what is expressed, this affects the social feedback they receive. When an adult wearing orthodontic appliances confidently and securely meets another person, conveying the attitude that "I'm OK, braces are no big deal," the response is minimal or positive, "Oh, she's got braces, no big deal." The same adult, obviously concerned and insecure, projecting the concern "What will he think about my braces" evokes "Hey, braces on her teeth! Poor lady!" and may suffer a social handicap because now she will be treated differently. Using an appliance that makes the patient feel more confident—which some people need more than others—can reduce this psychologic cost of orthodontics.

Patients with dentofacial deformities severe enough to require orthodontics and surgery usually are quite convinced of the benefit of treatment (at least those who seek treatment feel that way).[39] In addition, as was discussed in Chapter 3, these individuals tend to be more confident and positive than the average individual. As a result, the psychologic cost of visible appliances for these patients is minimal, and there is little or no need to make the appearance of the appliance a key factor in planning treatment. As a rule, the more severe the deformity, the less the concern about the esthetics of the appliance to treat it, and vice versa.

In some circumstances, appliance visibility is a benefit, not a cost. The best illustration is the teenager with mandibular prognathism who desperately wants treatment but whose surgery is being delayed until growth slows down. For that patient, having obvious braces on the teeth during the wait for surgery is a silent statement, "So I've got a big jaw. We're working on it, somebody cares!" To an extent, this kind of feeling probably contributes to the positive attitude that is so characteristic of surgical-orthodontic patients.

Considerable progress has been made recently in developing more esthetic fixed appliances, which can reduce the social cost of orthodontics. Selection of an appliance for patients with dentofacial deformities is discussed in some detail in Chapter 6. For most patients who need surgery, the esthetics of the appliance is not a major concern, but for a few it can be very important.

The Intangible Costs of Surgical Treatment. The intangible costs of surgical treatment involve anxiety over hospital admission and a surgical procedure, disability during the immediate recovery period, and the additional effort and adjustment in life-style required to return to full use of the jaws. Anxiety before surgery can be resolved by the surgeon, assisted by the orthodontist and all involved staff. A careful description of the steps leading to hospital admission and the events in the hospital and frank discussion about anesthesia, surgery, postsurgery morbidity, and the postsurgical recovery period can help the patient through this stage of treatment. Often, discussion with another patient who has had a similar surgery provides an important perspective, but some level of anxiety cannot be avoided and must be considered a cost of surgical treatment.

Following discharge from the hospital, most patients require 10 to 14 days before they can return to work. Early in this time, even the most simple tasks are tiring, and a short period of postsurgical depression is common. Encouragement from the surgeon and the patient's family and friends is most helpful in this period. RIF that allows early mobilization of the jaws shortens this period of disability, but some period of adjustment must take place.

Recovering full use of the jaws may take 6 months after surgery, until the finishing orthodontics has been completed or nearly so. Adapting to new speech and chewing patterns, adjustments in the use of facial muscles, recovery from neurosensory deficits, and accepting a different facial appearance require patience and added effort on the part of the patient. Usually, the benefits of treatment are obvious at this time, and they provide more than adequate motivation. But this final effort is also a cost of surgical treatment.

TABLE 5-3 Hospital charges for orthognathic surgery (1985)

Parameter	Mean	Range
Length of stay—days		
Sagittal split	3.2	2 to 4
LeFort I	3.7	2 to 5
Sagittal split/LeFort I	4.1	3 to 6
All	3.6	2 to 6
Total charges		
Sagittal split	$3086	$1997 to 4561
LeFort I	3538	2297 to 4046
Sagittal split/LeFort I	4778	3778 to 7325
All	3801	1997 to 7325

From Dolan P, White RP, Jr, Tulloch JFC: An analysis of hospital charges for orthognathic surgery, Int J Adult Orthod Orthogn Surg 1:9-14, 1987.

Economic Costs. In dollar terms, it is instructive to compare the cost of orthodontics in a patient who also will have surgery with the cost of orthodontic treatment alone. In most instances, surgical-orthodontic treatment has a smaller requirement for orthodontic tooth movement than does orthodontic treatment for the same problems, and the duration of treatment from braces on to braces off tends to be less. On the other hand, the orthodontic phase of surgical treatment often is more complex. In addition, there is an increased time commitment of the orthodontist immediately before surgery, when stabilizing arch wires and splints must be fabricated, and immediately after surgery, when the stabilization must be removed and working arch wires placed again. This more than balances out the shorter treatment duration, and the general guideline is that the fee for orthodontics combined with surgery is about the same or slightly more than the fee for treatment of a similar malocclusion by orthodontics alone.

The surgeon's fee for orthognathic surgery is similar to the orthodontist's professional fee except in the most complex surgical cases where surgery must be carried out in both jaws. Major medical insurance should include coverage for the surgeon's fee with the usual copayments applied. Dolan and colleagues recently reported on hospital charges for orthognathic surgery.[40] Mean hospital charges in fiscal year 1985 in this study were $3086 to $4778, with the range being $1997 to $7325 (Table 5-3). With the analysis of charges from this and similar studies, surgeons have altered practice patterns to keep hospital charges to a minimum. Major medical insurance should cover hospital charges as well.

CEPHALOMETRIC AND CAST PREDICTION AS A TREATMENT PLANNING TOOL

For most potential surgical-orthodontic patients, the practical considerations described above cannot be fully assessed without predicting the results of various treatment approaches. This is done by using cephalometric tracings and dental casts to simulate the effects of the orthodontic and surgical treatment. Cephalometric prediction allows direct evaluation of both dental and skeletal movements, whereas cast predictions show in more detail the dental relationships that indirectly reflect underlying skeletal changes.

Cephalometric Prediction

Cephalometric prediction can be done manually in two ways, by repositioning an overlay tracing or by moving templates. It also can be done by computer, using several different currently available software programs, alone or in combination with video images to obtain a picture of the probable result that is easier for patients to understand. The manual methods are described in some detail below, and then the computer methods are discussed.

Tracing Overlay Method

The tracing overlay approach is the simplest way to simulate the effects of mandibular surgery. The final prediction tracing is produced without any intermediate tracings. This method is limited to surgery that does not affect the vertical position of the maxilla (i.e., the mandible does not rotate around the condylar axis). The steps in preparing a prediction tracing in this way are illustrated (using case 2) in Fig. 5-26.

Several aspects of this method are worth additional comment:

1. It helps to have dental casts available when the cephalometric prediction is carried out. The critical step in the prediction is orienting the repositioned mandibular teeth to the maxillary teeth when the overlay tracing is moved to its new position. Observing the dental relationships when the casts are repositioned can make it easier to place the overlay tracing in the best position. It is important to trace the incisal and cusp outlines of all the teeth so the occlusal plane is visible. The dental casts also help in doing this task.

2. If major orthodontic tooth movement is anticipated before surgery, so that the orientation of the incisor teeth will change, it helps to have this simulated on dental casts in the form of an orthodontic diagnostic setup as discussed below before the cephalometric prediction. In patients with severely malaligned teeth, it is not possible to reposition the casts to simulate surgery until tooth interferences have been eliminated as they will be by presurgical orthodontics. It is possible to reorient cephalometric tracings even though some teeth overlap, but it is much easier to do this when you can refer to casts on which the teeth have been repositioned. The diagnostic setup also provides a guide to the amount that the mandibular incisors should be retracted or flared forward on the prediction tracing before movement of the overlay begins.

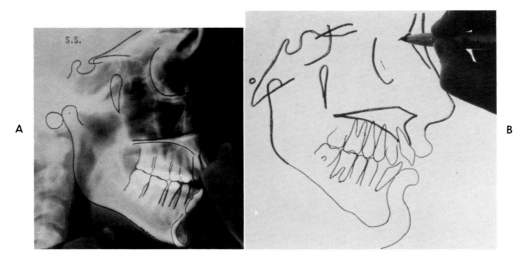

Fig. 5-26. Steps in cephalometric prediction using the overlay method (the patient is case 2). **A,** Trace the film, being sure to include all teeth (at least their occlusal surfaces). **B,** With a new sheet of tracing paper over the original tracing, trace the structures that will not be changed by the mandibular surgery: the cranial base, maxilla and maxillary teeth, mandibular ramus down to the angle, and soft-tissue profile down to the base of the nose. Do not trace the mandible or the soft tissue below the nose.   *Continued.*

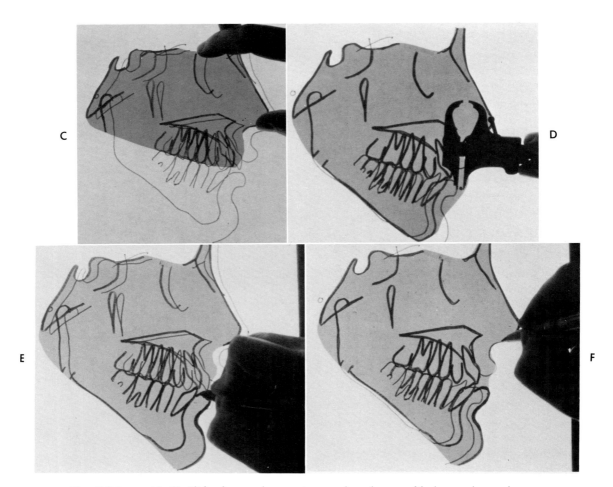

Fig. 5-26, cont'd. **C,** Slide the overlay tracing so that the mandibular teeth can be seen through it in their desired postsurgical position and trace the lower teeth and jaw. **D,** Superimpose the overlay tracing back on the cranial base and measure how far the lower incisor moved forward. The lower lip will go forward two-thirds as far. Make a mark that distance forward of the lip. **E,** Superimpose again on the mandible. Draw in the soft-tissue chin and complete the lower lip outline through the marked point. **F,** Superimpose again on the cranial base. Complete the soft-tissue profile, using Table 5-4 as a guide, keeping in mind that the upper lip probably will come back and down very slightly. This completes the prediction tracing. The actual prediction for mandibular advancement for this patient is shown in Fig. 5-40, *B.* Note the assumption in the procedure outlined above that presurgical orthodontics would not change the position of the incisors relative to the maxilla and mandible. In fact, for this patient, the lower incisor would either go slightly forward if the crowding were corrected without extraction, or would be retracted somewhat with premolar extraction. To take that into account, it is necessary to reposition the lower incisor before beginning the prediction sequence, as illustrated in Fig. 5-27.

3. Whatever the prediction method, producing the predicted soft-tissue outline is more of an art form than a scientific exercise. At best, the estimates for change in lip position shown in Table 5-4 are rough guidelines. It is important to remember that these estimates are based on changes in the position of the lips at rest. If the original cephalometric film was taken with the patient straining to bring the lips together, prediction of the postsurgical relaxed lip position is all but impossible.

Template Method

The use of templates for intermediate tracings between the original and final prediction tracing is mandatory when the maxilla will be repositioned vertically, very helpful when major movements of the teeth must be simulated or when the chin is repositioned, and

---

TABLE 5-4 Current concepts of facial growth

Treatment	Soft-tissue change	Notes
Anteroposterior movement of incisors: maxillary or mandibular, forward or back, surgical or orthodontic	60 to 70% of incisor movement	1, 2
Vertical movement of incisors	Minimal unless jaw rotates	3, 4, 5
Mandibular advancement	Soft tissue: chin 1:1 with bone, lower lip 60% to 70% with incisor	6
Maxillary advancement	Nose: slight elevation of tip Base of upper lip: 20% of point A Upper lip: 60% of incisor protraction, shortens 1 to 2 mm	7, 8
Mandibular setback	Chin: 1:1 Lip: 60%	5
Maxillary setback	Nose: no effect Base of upper lip: 20% of point A Upper lip: 60% of incisor Advancement lower lip: variable, may move back	3
Mandibular setback plus maxillary advancement	Changes similar to a combination of the two procedures separately	
Maxillary superior repositioning	Nose: usually no effect Upper lip: shortens 1 to 2 mm Lower lip: rotates 1:1 with mandible	7
Mandibular advancement plus maxillary superior repositioning	Chin: 1:1 Lower lip: 70% of incisor Upper lip: shortens 1 to 2 mm 80% of any incisor advancement Nose: slight elevation of tip	9

Mandibular inferior border repositioning	Soft tissue forward: 60% to 70% bone
	Chin: Up—1:1 with bone
	      Back—50% bone
	      Laterally—60% bone
	      Down—?	

1. Little difference with surgery or orthodontics.
2. If both upper and lower incisors are retracted (bimaxillary protrusion), lip movement stops when lips come into contact.
3. Lip shortens 1 to 2 mm with vestibular incision (more if surgical technique is poor).
4. Lip rotates with mandible 1:1.
5. If face height increases, lip may uncurl and lengthen.
6. If lip uncurls, it will go forward less.
7. Nose change is usually temporary.
8. Less soft-tissue change occurs after cleft-lip repair.
9. Data from Jensen AC, Sinclair PM, Wolford LM: Soft tissue changes associated with double jaw surgery, Am J Orthod Dentofac Orthop [in press].

quite possible when only the mandible is being moved. Templates, in other words, can be used for any type of prediction. The only reason for not employing this method generally is that it is more time-consuming to prepare a template than to proceed directly to a finished prediction tracing, as is done with the overlay method in uncomplicated mandibular surgery.

The steps in preparing and using templates for pre-

diction of maxillary surgery are described and illustrated in Fig. 5-27, using case 2.

Typically, templates are made for the entire maxilla if a one-piece or two-piece maxillary osteotomy is planned (the two-piece osteotomy is used to change width, which does not affect a lateral cephalometric prediction). If a three-piece maxillary osteotomy is planned, it is necessary to make an anterior and a pos-

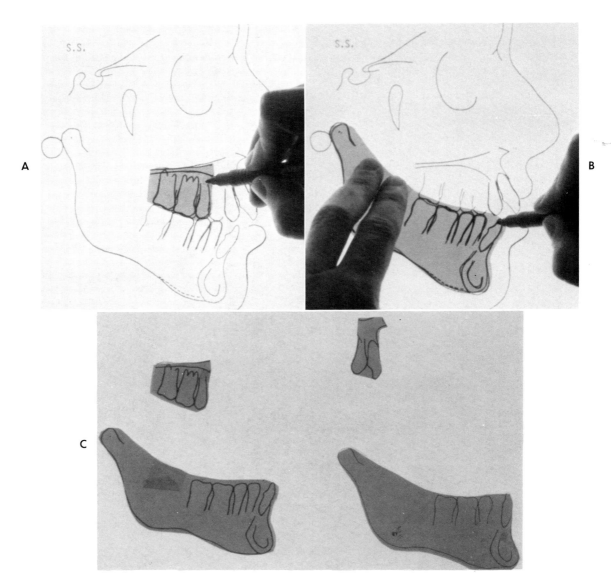

Fig. 5-27. The steps in cephalometric prediction, using templates to predict the effect of maxillary segmental surgery (the patient is case 2). **A,** Prepare the maxillary templates by tracing the posterior (second premolar/second molar) segment, as shown here, and similarly tracing the maxillary anterior (central incisor/canine) segment. **B,** Prepare two mandibular templates, one with the crowding resolved without extraction (the incisors therefore must be advanced slightly), as shown here, and one with extraction (the incisors retracted). **C,** The four templates ready for use.

terior maxillary template. Usually, first premolars are extracted, so the posterior template would show the palatal plane from the posterior nasal spine forward to the second premolar and also show three teeth, the first and second molars and the second premolar. The anterior segment includes the anterior nasal spine, the bony contour through point A, and the lingual contour of the alveolar process behind the incisors. If the arch is segmented at a different site, the templates must contain the appropriate teeth for the segment that will be created. In the mandibular arch, the template includes the mandibular teeth and the entire outline of the mandible, including as accurate a representation of the mandibular condyle as is possible.

In the prediction procedure, the mandible will be rotated around the condyle, hence the importance of locating this structure as accurately as possible. If the possibility of repositioning the chin via an inferior border osteotomy is to be explored, a template of this region is made by tracing the anterior and inferior outlines of the chin up to a mark that represents the putative osteotomy cut.

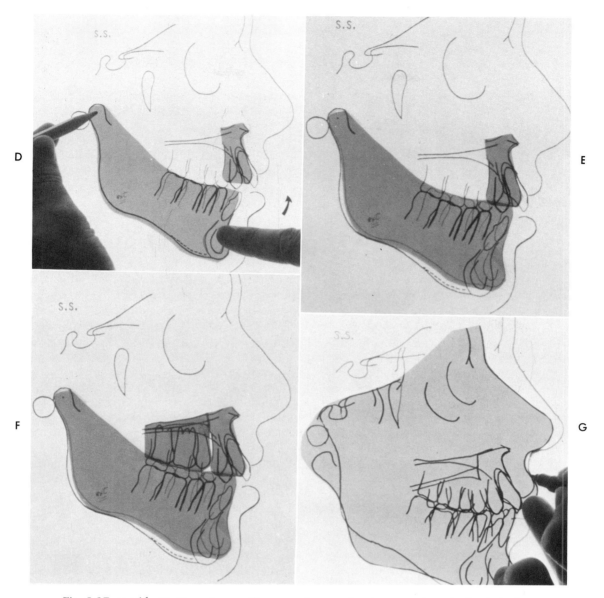

Fig. 5-27, cont'd. **D,** Place the maxillary anterior template in approximately the desired position, about 2 mm below the lip line and in approximately the original anteroposterior position. When the nonextraction template is rotated up to the anterior maxillary template, the relationship is not good. Either the maxillary anterior segment must be placed too far forward, or there is an anterior crossbite tendency. With the extraction template, the maxillary anterior segment can be retracted somewhat. **E,** When the extraction template is rotated up to the anterior maxillary template as shown here, the teeth fit nicely. It is clear that the prominence of the upper anterior teeth will be a function of how much the mandibular incisors are retracted and how far up the maxilla is moved. **F,** Position the maxillary posterior template. **G,** With a clean sheet of tracing paper over the original and the templates, complete the prediction tracing. Use the guidelines in Table 5-4 to complete the soft-tissue outline. Here, the upper lip is being drawn in, using a superimposition on the maxilla.

If preparatory orthodontics will alter the position of the teeth, particularly the incisors, this must be simulated when the templates are prepared. One of the questions that cephalometric prediction can help decide is the extent of preparatory orthodontic tooth movement that is needed, but it may be necessary to prepare more than one template to see this clearly, perhaps showing the position of the incisors with or without extraction, or with the lower arch leveled primarily by elongation of canines and premolars versus being leveled primarily by intrusion of incisors.

Variations in the amount of tooth movement can be produced by variations in orthodontic technique, and this must be kept in mind when the prediction is being prepared. The prediction procedure can give valuable information about the orthodontic mechanotherapy as well as the surgical treatment by establishing exactly where the teeth should be positioned.

Special considerations with the use of templates for cephalometric prediction include:

1. It is very helpful if the templates are a different color from the original tracing. If the original tracing was in black pencil, the templates might be traced in red or green.

2. Similarly, the completed prediction tracing is easier to interpret if different colors are used to indicate what structures were repositioned. The colors on the final tracing, however, should not be those of either the original tracing or the template. Different colors make it much easier to keep up with exactly where you are as the various tracing and template layers are manipulated.

3. When a mandibular template is prepared, the approximate center of the condyle on the original tracing should be marked, and this mark transferred to the template. The mandibular template can be rotated around this point.

A number of studies have been carried out in an attempt to discover the true center of mandibular rotation when the maxilla is repositioned vertically. Although the results are variable, the center of rotation usually appears to be posterior and inferior to the condyle in the mastoid region.[41,42] The calculation of the true center of the rotation is difficult. It requires locating the point of intersection of two nearly parallel lines that are projected from the presurgical and postsurgical positions of an anterior mandibular landmark, usually the lower incisor. A small error in tracing the anterior landmark becomes a large error in the presumed center.

Although one might conclude that using a center of rotation away from the condyle would improve the accuracy of prediction,[43] there are two problems with doing so. First, the apparent condylar displacement observed in the studies of center of rotation may not have been the desired result, but instead was the result of poor control of the condyle during surgery. In that case, building it into the planning would be unwise. Second, as a practical matter, the location of the center of rotation makes surprisingly little difference in the predicted location of the anterior mandible after autorotation. The best prediction seems to result from using the center of the condyle, and extreme precision in locating that point is unnecessary. Deliberately choosing an arbitrary center of rotation some distance from the condyle has as great a chance of increasing as of reducing prediction error.

Computer Prediction

The first step in using a computer program for cephalometric prediction is to enter a digital model of the patient's tracing into computer memory. The details of the digital model vary among the several currently available software programs, but all use a relatively limited number of coordinate points (x,y) to represent the tracing (Fig. 5-28). The more points in the digital model, the 5 greater the anatomic fidelity of that model. On the other hand, the more points that are digitized, the more time it takes to enter the tracing into the computer, and the more memory is required for processing. The programs available for use in orthodontic and surgical practices have improved rapidly and now are quite powerful and effective.

A digital model that is quite adequate for cephalometric analysis (i.e., it contains enough digitized landmarks to allow the calculation of an impressively large number of cephalometric angles or distances) may not be adequate for cephalometric prediction. For the prediction of segmental maxillary surgery, it is necessary to know the position not only of the crowns, but also of the roots adjacent to the osteotomy site (which is typically but not always the first premolar area; if so, the canine and second premolar outlines are needed). In addition, the incisal and cusp outlines of maxillary and mandibular teeth should be recorded so that the potential dental interferences can be observed. More generally, digitization of many points on the soft-tissue profile is necessary to obtain a smooth outline.

Once an adequate digital model has been created, most computer programs operate quite analogously to the template method illustrated above. The difference is that the program is used to develop the template, which can then be stored as a separate item and recalled as necessary. The cursor keys or a mouse can be used to move the electronic template to a new position, which is much easier in some programs than in others. Presurgical orthodontics must be simulated before the simulated surgical repositioning is done, exactly as it would be with manual templates.

For cephalometric prediction of mandibular surgery alone, the computer only repositions the mandibular template. For simulation of maxillary surgery with autorotation of the mandible, the sequence of moves is the same with the computer method as it is manually. The maxillary anterior template is moved to its new position and adjusted as desired; then the mandible is rotated and also repositioned anteroposteriorly if necessary. If the maxilla is segmented, the maxillary anterior template, the mandible, and then the maxillary posterior template are moved into position. If a genioplasty also is to be simulated, this is the final step in the prediction sequence.

The computer method has two major advantages. First, the software programs often include automatic

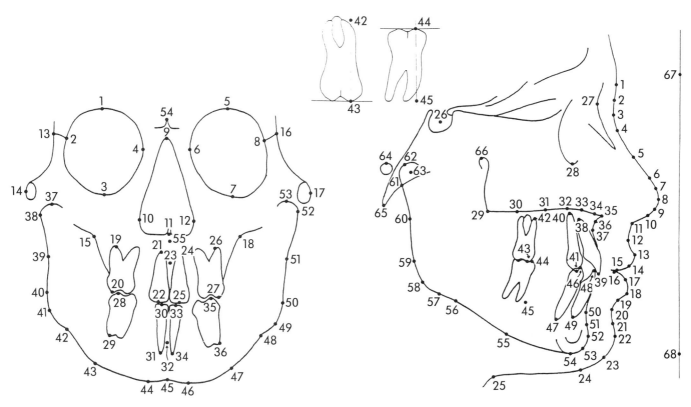

Fig. 5-28. The standard lateral and frontal digitization models used in a current cephalometric prediction program (Dentofacial Planner). This program allows up to 180 points in either model, and both can be customized for different approaches; that is, a more extensive model can be employed for patients requiring surgical treatment planning than is needed for routine orthodontic patients. (Courtesy Dr. R. Walker.)

adjustments in the soft-tissue profile, in essence incorporating the information given in Table 5-4. This can speed up the prediction process and make it more consistent. Second, with the digital model in computer memory, it is easy to produce several slightly different cephalometric predictions, so the impact of minor changes can be examined in more detail. The more predictions that are to be made, the more advantageous it is to have the cephalometric data in an appropriate digital model.

Another potentially significant advantage of the computer method is that it can help integrate information from the dental casts with the cephalometric information. It is a straightforward procedure to digitize the occlusal surface of the dental casts, thus placing the equivalent of an occlusogram in the computer memory. One way to accomplish this is to place the cast on a copying machine with the teeth down and make an image. The error in this transfer is amazingly small. The two-dimensional image than is digitized exactly as a cephalometric tracing would be, using an appropriate model. In the computer, moving the incisors or molars on the cast can then simultaneously produce the appropriate changes on the cephalometric tracing, and vice versa.

The disadvantages of the computer approach are the cost of the necessary hardware and software and the limitations of the existing programs. A modern orthodontic or surgical practice is quite likely to have a computer system for monitoring patient accounts and other business aspects. Although it is possible to run a cephalometric program on the same machine, which would reduce hardware costs to the digitizing pad and plotter (or laser printer), this often is not feasible. The cephalometric software requires a specific operating environment that may be incompatible with the business software. A remote terminal often is not satisfactory for cephalometric applications on a small computer system. Instead, the main computer must be used, which is awkward if it is out at the reception desk or in the business office. The new operating systems (e.g., OS/2 and Unix) that now are becoming available will help overcome these problems. At this writing, however, a dedicated and reasonably fast microcomputer is the preferred hardware for computer cephalometric prediction.

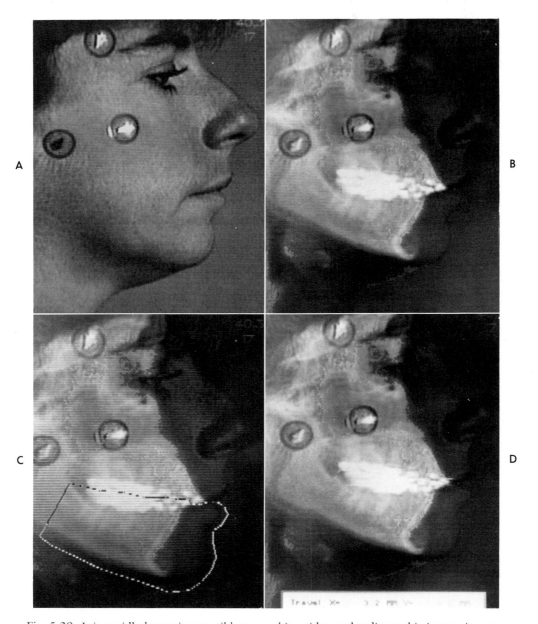

Fig. 5-29. It is rapidly becoming possible to combine video and radiographic images in computer memory and display, so both can be manipulated during prediction. **A,** Video image of a female with mandibular deficiency (the original is in color). The markers on the face are used to superimpose this image with the cephalometric film taken with the same markers in place. **B,** Superimposed video and radiographic images of this patient. **C,** Outline on computer screen of area to be repositioned (which is created with the computer mouse, allowing the operator to use a drawing motion). **D,** Prediction of mandibular advancement. The box on the lower portion of the screen gives the quantitative amount of advancement.

On the software side, present programs remain relatively costly and somewhat inflexible. Even with the best programs, automatic soft-tissue adjustments can be misleading if the clinician forgets that these are based on a series of highly arbitrary judgments incorporated into the program. It seems reasonable to assume that rapid progress in prediction software will continue so that the programs will become increasingly easier to use and less rigid in their internal structure.

Patients want to know what they would look like after surgery. It is possible to cut photographs and move the sections in a way that somewhat simulates surgery, but this allows no way to change soft-tissue contours as will occur after treatment, and the unavoidable gaps

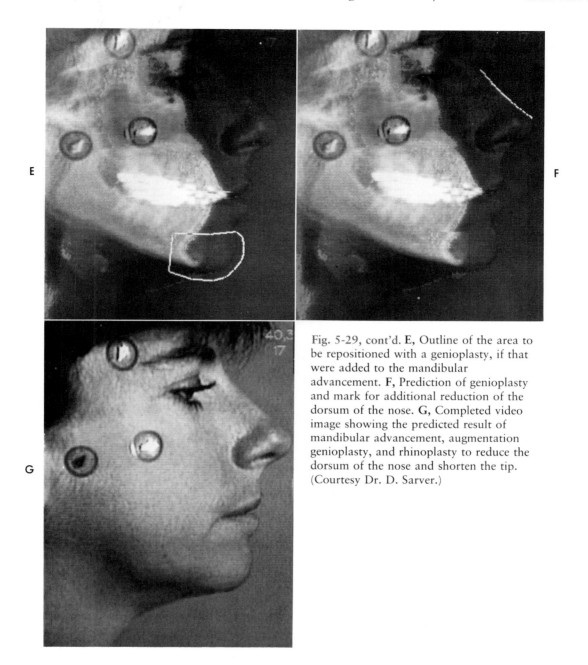

Fig. 5-29, cont'd. **E**, Outline of the area to be repositioned with a genioplasty, if that were added to the mandibular advancement. **F**, Prediction of genioplasty and mark for additional reduction of the dorsum of the nose. **G**, Completed video image showing the predicted result of mandibular advancement, augmentation genioplasty, and rhinoplasty to reduce the dorsum of the nose and shorten the tip. (Courtesy Dr. D. Sarver.)

in the cut-up photographs are a problem. Recently it has become possible to accurately superimpose radiographic images on a computer screen with video images and to automatically produce soft-tissue changes in the video image as the jaws and/or teeth are moved within the computer program (Fig. 5-29). The video image is much more realistic than is photographic simulation, and it is much easier for a patient to comprehend than just the soft-tissue profile on a cephalometric tracing. A danger might be that patients would be led to expect too much from predictions that were too realistic, but this does not seem to be borne out when these methods are used in practice.[44] It is quite possi-

ble, given the speed of recent technologic change, that in a few years the combination of video and radiographic images in a computer format will become the standard method of cephalometric prediction.

As with computer cephalometrics in general, it is important to keep in mind that computer prediction methods provide no information that could not be obtained by doing the prediction manually. The choice of a manual or computer approach is based largely on convenience and, to a lesser extent, speed and patient education versus cost. It is as fast or faster to do a single tracing by hand for a patient who will have mandibular surgery rather than to digitize the cephalomet-

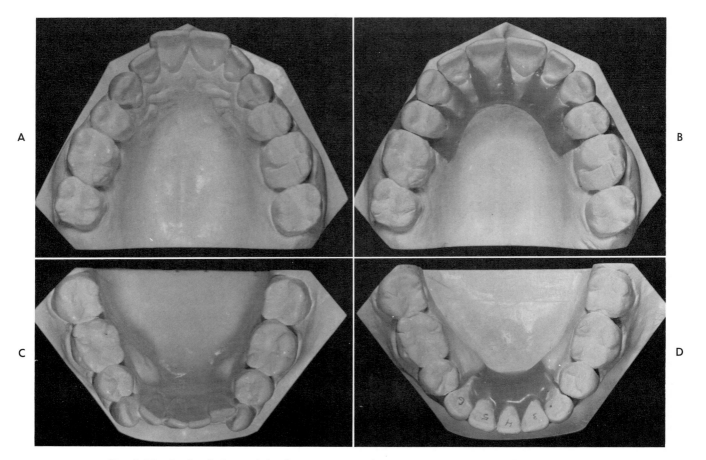

Fig. 5-30. Occlusal views of the diagnostic setup for patient D.J. (case 1). Before treatment, she had very severe mandibular incisor crowding but only mild maxillary incisor crowding. The setup is used to evaluate the result of extracting one mandibular central incisor (see Fig. 5-32).

ric film, create a mandibular template, and manipulate it at the keyboard. Speed becomes a significant advantage when multiple similar predictions are being made. Patient education may become a greater advantage as the computer methods improve. A software program also is no substitute for knowing what surgical movements are possible and practical in an individual case. Many things can be simulated, manually or on a computer, that cannot or should not be done. Good judgment and knowledge of possible options remain the basis for decision making, even though the computer may carry out the manipulations.

Cast Prediction (Model Surgery)
Diagnostic Setup

A diagnostic setup is employed to be sure that it will be possible to get the teeth to fit together if a given orthodontic treatment plan is employed. The usual reason for doing a setup, which is not required routinely, is to examine how the teeth would fit if a particular approach to a tooth-size discrepancy were used (Fig. 5-

30). For example, in a patient such as the one in case 1 below, who has a relative tooth-size excess in the mandibular anterior region, one possibility would be to extract one mandibular central incisor and close all space. Another possibility would be to align the upper and lower incisors and leave a 1 mm space mesial and distal to each maxillary lateral incisor so that these teeth could be built up with composite resin. Cephalometric prediction would reveal how prominent the teeth would be with each plan, but a cast prediction with the teeth repositioned would be necessary to evaluate the dental occlusion.

The first step in a diagnostic setup is to carefully remove the teeth from the dental cast in the region where significant tooth movement would occur, being careful not to change tooth dimensions. It is better not to remove all the teeth. In the example of an anterior tooth-size discrepancy, leaving the molars in their original position would make it easier to keep track of the overall occlusion without affecting the outcome of the anterior teeth. Even if the arches are quite crowded and ir-

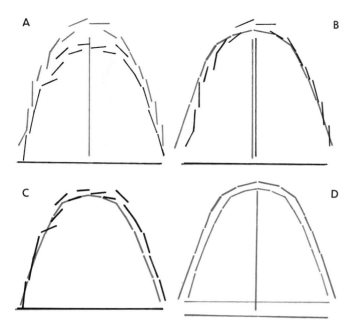

Fig. 5-31. Occlusogram tracings showing the repositioning of teeth necessary for treatment of a patient with mandibular deficiency and severe crowing. The position of each tooth is shown as a line segment (a drawing of this type can be made from a Xerox copy of the dental cast). **A,** Original malocclusion: the maxillary arch is black and mandibular arch is gray. **B,** Changes in the maxillary arch: pretreatment is in black and posttreatment is in red. **C,** Changes in the mandibular arch: pretreatment is in black and posttreatment is in red. **D,** Posttreatment occlusion: the maxillary arch is red and the mandibular arch is pink. Note that premolar extraction was carried out in the mandibular but not the maxillary arch, and then the mandible was advanced. This method allows detailed planning of the orthodontic tooth movement necessary for successful treatment and also allows a precise evaluation of the posttreatment occlusion that could be produced.

regular, so that all teeth must be moved, it usually is preferable to leave the terminal molar on the original cast as a landmark from which movement of other teeth can be measured.

The teeth are then reset in wax so that their alignment and interdigitation can be observed. A relatively soft wax, one that allows the teeth to be moved with finger pressure but is firm enough so that they will remain where they are put, is ideal. The harder waxes used in prosthodontics make the setup unnecessarily time consuming. The object is to experiment with various arrangements of the teeth to find the one that would fit best. Only if a permanent record is required is there any reason to add harder wax or plaster.

A "paper setup" sometimes can provide valuable information without the laboratory time and expense of the actual diagnostic setup described above. The occlusogram provides a two-dimensional representation of the planned posttreatment dental arch form and alignment[45] (Fig. 5-31). Dental casts can be digitized in the same way that cephalometric tracings are digitized, and as this computer method becomes more widely available, occlusograms or their equivalent are likely to be used routinely. The two-dimensional view of tooth position and arch form can illustrate visually the amount of retraction of incisors or change in the position of individual teeth that would occur under various circumstances. This makes the three-dimensional setup necessary only in the most extreme cases, primarily those which have complicated tooth-size problems.

Model Surgery

Model surgery is the dental cast version of cephalometric prediction of surgical results. How complicated it is to do this with dental casts depends both on the type of surgery and on the amount of tooth movement that will occur later.

In its simplest form, model surgery requires nothing more than articulating the pretreatment casts by hand in a possible postsurgical position. Mandibular advancement can be simulated, for instance, by sliding the lower cast forward relative to the upper cast (Fig. 5-32). It is easier to study the possible tooth relationships if the casts are mounted temporarily on an arbitrary articulator so that they are held in the desired position. The better the occlusion without any tooth movement, the easier it is to articulate the casts by hand, and vice versa.

When the teeth are highly irregular or when the maxillary and mandibular arch forms are incompatible, model surgery is impossible without simulating the presurgical orthodontic treatment. In this case, a diagnostic setup is done first, then the setup models are moved as they might be at surgery, as shown in Fig. 5-32.

For the model surgery that is done immediately before surgery, it is important in many cases to use a facebow transfer to mount the casts on a semiadjustable articulator so that the condyle-tooth relationships are recorded (Fig. 5-33). It rarely is necessary to do this at the initial treatment planning stage. Doing the cephalometric prediction and articulating the casts by hand to check for arch compatibility nearly always is sufficient. The technique for model surgery on articulated casts is shown in detail in Chapter 6.

The application of these treatment planning methods is illustrated in the case presentations below. Further examples of specific problems are provided in the clinical chapters in Section IV (Chapters 12-19).

ILLUSTRATIVE CASES

The treatment planning process is illustrated on pp. 181-189 for the same two patients for whom problem lists were derived in Chapter 4.

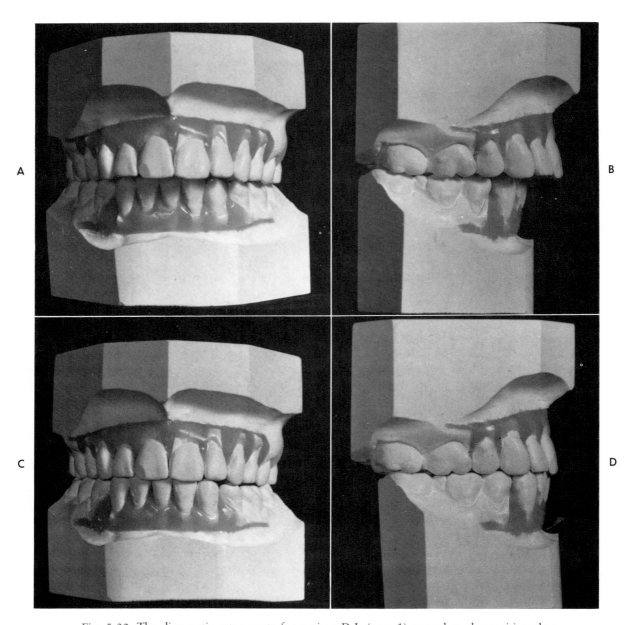

Fig. 5-32. The diagnostic setup casts for patient D.J. (case 1) moved to the position they would be in after mandibular advancement. This is the simplest form of model surgery. When model surgery is done before beginning treatment, which may be necessary for some patients as it was for this one, a diagnostic setup must be used if there will be significant orthodontic tooth movement. Most model surgery is done on the immediate presurgery models, when the tooth movement has been completed.

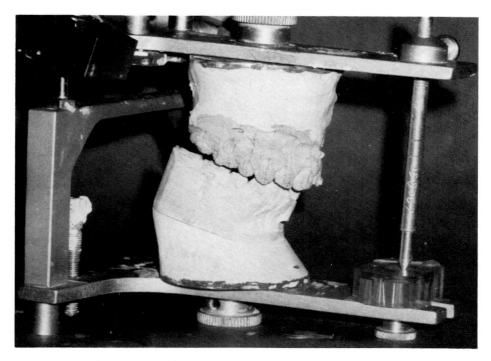

Fig. 5-33. Casts for a patient who will have superior repositioning of the maxilla and mandibular advancement, mounted on a semiadjustable articulator in preparation for model surgery. When maxillary surgery is planned, an articulator mounting with the aid of a facebow is needed for maximum accuracy. This is necessary at the final surgical planning stage, immediately before surgery, but rarely is it needed during the initial treatment planning. The technique for model surgery on mounted casts is shown in Chapter 6.

Case 1 (Figs. 4-39 to 4-42, 5-34 to 5-38)

The diagnostic evaluation for D.J. was presented in Chapter 4. See Figs. 4-39 to 4-42 for the initial diagnostic records.

The problem list was as follows:
- Gingival recession and minimal attached tissue, mandibular anterior region
- Severe mandibular, mild maxillary incisor crowding
- Mandibular deficiency, 8 mm overjet (relapse after previous orthodontic treatment)
- Deep bite, skeletal and dental, with palatal impingement

Taking the steps in treatment planning in order:

1. *Separation of developmental from nondevelopmental problems.* The irritation of palatal tissues behind the upper incisors and the tendency to gingival recession apparent in the lower incisor region were felt to require periodontal treatment before the surgical orthodontic treatment could begin. Because of her desire to have surgery during the Christmas holidays 9 months later and because the lower incisors were so irregular, it was decided to do preliminary periodontal scaling, then begin alignment of the lower incisors before placing the necessary gingival graft (see below).

2. *Prioritization of problem list.* Her chief complaint was the protrusion of her upper teeth, but she also referred to the irritation caused by the overbite and to the lower incisor crowding. The priority problem clearly seemed to be the mandibular deficiency, with the overbite and incisor crowding both secondary but important. The prioritized list was:
   (1) Mandibular deficiency, excessive overjet
   (2) Deep bite, skeletal/dental
   (3) Mandibular incisor crowding

3. *Possible solutions to individual problems.* Considering the mandibular deficiency and excessive overjet first, the possible solutions were:
   (1) Camouflage via retraction of maxillary teeth and proclination of mandibular teeth (but this was done once previously and failed—there is no reason to think that retreatment would produce a stable result)
   (2) Mandibular advancement (possibly satisfactory: need to review prediction)

Continued.

A cephalometric prediction of mandibular advancement (Fig. 5-34) shows that the pattern of rotation is favorable and the esthetic result should be satisfactory. (See Fig. 5-26 for an illustration of the steps in making this prediction).

Consider the possibilities for the second problem, the deep bite:

(1) Mandibular advancement with rotation down anteriorly (prediction looks satisfactory but may need slight depression of lower incisors in advance to prevent excessive face height after treatment)

(2) Other possibilities: ? none available

Consider the possibilities for the third problem, the incisor crowding:

(1) Arch expansion (possibly satisfactory for the upper arch but unlikely to be stable in the lower arch)

(2) Extraction (first premolars already removed: what?)

Although it is possible to close the space orthodontically after both first and second premolars have been extracted, it is better to avoid this if possible. With the severity of the lower incisor crowding, extraction of one lower incisor was considered a possibility, especially because there was a mild tooth-size excess (from Bolton analysis) in the mandibular anterior region. A diagnostic setup (Figs. 5-30 and 5-32) was done to verify that satisfactory occlusion could be achieved with only three lower incisors. Cephalometrically, the other incisors would have to be advanced slightly if only one were extracted, and a new prediction was made with this position, which would slightly decrease the amount of mandibular advancement that would occur

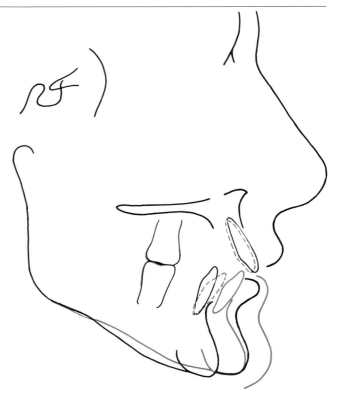

Fig. 5-34. Cephalometric prediction, D.J. (See Fig. 5-26 for the steps in the prediction procedure). This prediction simulates the effect of mandibular advancement following alignment of the lower incisors with extraction of one incisor *(dashed line),* which still requires slight advancement of the other incisors. The mandibular rotation is satisfactory because ramus height is unchanged.

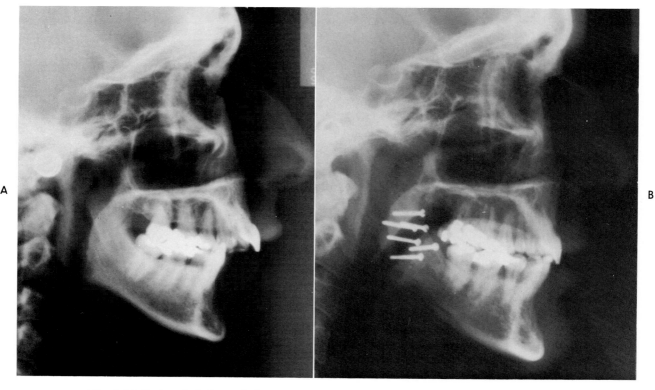

Fig. 5-35. Patient D.J. **A,** Cephalometric radiograph before treatment. **B,** Cephalometric radiograph following treatment including mandibular advancement.

at surgery. Both the occlusion and the cephalometric result looked satisfactory.

4. *Integration of treatment possibilities into a final plan.* Based on the interaction of the possible solutions and incorporating the necessary periodontal treatment, the final plan was:
   (1) Periodontal disease control
   (2) Extraction of the mandibular right central incisor
   (3) Preliminary alignment of the lower incisors
   (4) Free gingival graft to the lower incisor area
   (5) Completion of presurgical orthodontics, with closure of the extraction space
   (6) Bilateral sagittal-split osteotomy for mandibular advancement and downward rotation anteriorly, with RIF (lag screws)
   (7) Finishing orthodontics
   (8) Orthodontic retention, prolonged in the lower anterior region.

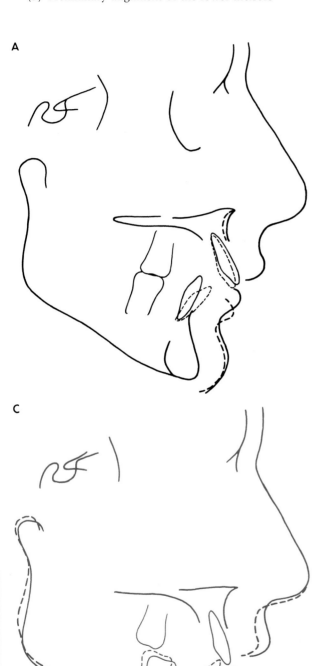

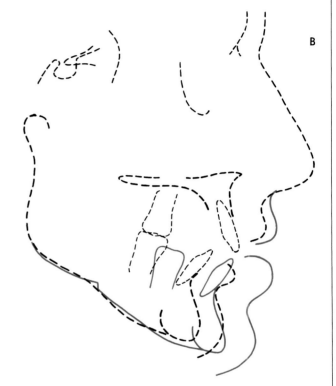

Fig. 5-36. Patient D.J. **A,** Cephalometric superimposition pretreatment to presurgery *(dashed line).* **B,** Superimposition presurgery to immediately postsurgery *(solid line).* **C,** Superimposition postsurgery to end of treatment *(dashed line).* After the screws used for rigid fixation were in place, the maxillomandibular fixation was released and the interocclusal splint was wired to the maxillary arch so she could function into it. The splint was present when the postsurgical cephalometric film (Fig 5-35, *B*) was taken. Its presence then, and removal later, can be seen in the vertical changes in mandibular position from postsurgery to the end of treatment.

Continued.

Case 1—cont'd.

The sequence of treatment was as follows:

Time	Stage of treatment
Feb.	Present treatment plan
Mar.	Preliminary periodontics completed, start orthodontic alignment
April	Gingival grafts placed

Dec.	Mandibular advancement
Feb.	Resume orthodontic treatment
June	Deband, orthodontic retainers

The results of this treatment are shown in Figs. 5-35 to 5-38.

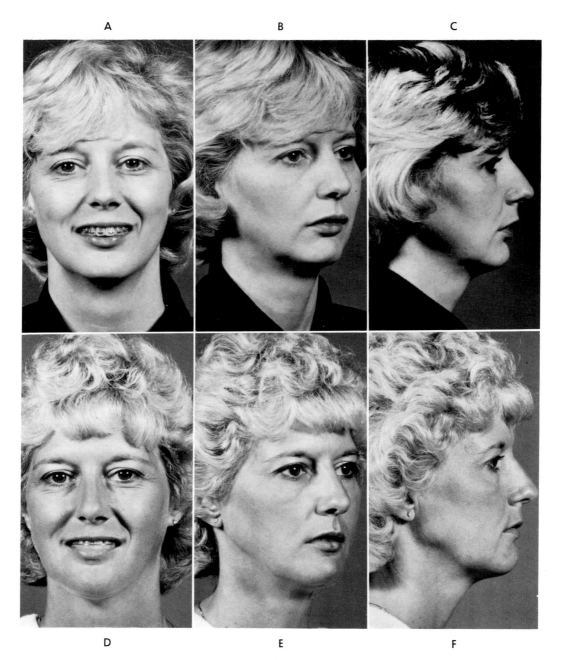

Fig. 5-37. Facial photographs, D.J. **A** through **C**, Immediately before surgery. **D** through **F**, 6 months later, when orthodontic appliances were removed.

Case 1—cont'd.

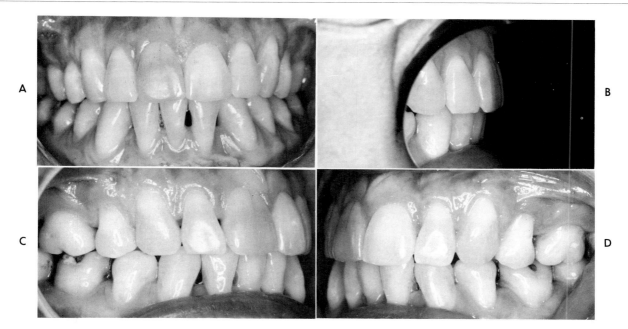

Fig. 5-38. Intraoral photographs, D.J., at the completion of orthodontic treatment.

Case 2 (Figs. 4-43 to 4-46, 5-39 to 5-42)

The diagnostic evaluation for S.S. is reviewed in detail in Chapter 4. See Figs. 4-43 to 4-46 for the initial diagnostic records.

The problem list was as follows:
- Gingival recession, maxillary incisors
- Moderate mandibular incisor crowding and protrusion; mild maxillary incisor crowding and protrusion
- Unilateral lingual crossbite, maxillary right
- Skeletal Class II malocclusion, mandibular deficiency, 7 mm overjet
- Skeletal open bite, lip incompetence, excessive anterior face height, maxilla rotated down posteriorly, mandible rotated down and back

Taking the steps in treatment planning in order:

1. *Separation of developmental from nondevelopmental problems.* The mild gingival recession around S.S.'s maxillary central incisors was reviewed with a periodontist. Because there was good attached gingiva and because further recession was considered unlikely even with surgical-orthodontic treatment, no treatment was recommended.

2. *Placing the developmental problems in priority order.* The chief complaint was "My teeth protrude and do not meet in front," thus the patient was emphasizing the prominence of the upper incisors and also recognizing the open bite. Which is more important, the horizontal mandibular deficiency and excessive overjet, or the skeletal open bite that causes the lip incompetence and contributes to the mandibular deficiency? Reasonable clinicians might argue about vertical versus horizontal jaw discrepancy, but clearly these skeletal problems are more important than the crossbite (which is causing no functional problems) or the incisor irregularity.

We suggest that for S.S., and for many patients who complain about the prominence of the maxillary incisors, the vertical exposure of these teeth is as important as the horizontal exposure and overjet. The complaint that "my upper front teeth stick out" should not be interpreted as referring entirely to the horizontal plane. This is what patients say when they dislike the vertical exposure of the teeth, as well as being a complaint about overjet. In addition, in S.S.'s case, the mandibular deficiency and excessive overjet are caused to a large extent by downward and backward rotation of the mandible secondary to the vertical maxillary position. Therefore the priority problem is the skeletal open bite and downward maxillary rotation. The Class

Continued.

II/excessive overjet component of the chief complaint should receive second priority.

The functional importance of a unilateral posterior crossbite in the absence of a mandibular shift and any TM joint problems is debatable. In planning treatment, deciding which problem is the first priority is more important than differentiating between the lesser problems. In our view, the crossbite and the incisor crowding are of approximately equal importance, with the incisor crowding slightly more significant because of the component of mandibular incisor protrusion that accompanies it. Therefore the prioritized problem list for S.S. is:

(1) Skeletal open bite, lip incompetence, excessive anterior face height, maxilla rotated downward posteriorly

(2) Skeletal Class II malocclusion, mandibular deficiency (mandible rotated down and back)

(3) Moderate mandibular incisor crowding and protrusion, mild maxillary incisor crowding

(4) Unilateral lingual crossbite, right side.

3. *Possible solutions to individual problems.* Consider first the possibilities for the most important problem. These are:

(1) Camouflage: move the teeth to close the anterior open bite

(2) Surgical correction (at her age, growth modification cannot be considered a possibility)

   (a) Mandibular advancement

   (b) Maxillary intrusion

   (c) Other?

At this stage, cephalometric prediction becomes important because it lets the clinician see the probable result of a given treatment option. For S.S., both the sliding overlay and the template methods illustrated in Figs. 5-26 and 5-27 respectively were employed.

Fig. 5-39, *A* (prepared using a maxillary anterior template) shows the predicted result of orthodontic treatment alone. With the extraction of upper first premolars, it would be possible to retract the upper incisors and close the open bite by elongating them and also elongating the lower incisors. In the absence of growth, the vertical dimension would change little if any, so the change from treatment can be simulated easily by repositioning templates of the teeth. It is apparent that this would make the upper teeth even more prominent vertically, so facial esthetics probably would be worse. In addition, closing an open bite in this way in an adult often produces an unstable result, so relapse into open bite and overjet would be likely. From inspection of the probable result, if not from previous knowledge, this approach can be rejected.

Fig. 5-39, *B* shows the result of a ramus osteotomy to advance the mandible (the prediction procedure is shown in Fig. 5-26). Notice that to close the open bite, it is necessary to rotate the mandible up anteriorly. It rotates around a fulcrum in the molar region, so the gonial angles are forced downward. This is the pattern of rotational advancement that is notorious for relapse. The prediction tracing clearly shows that lengthening of the ramus, though not an objective of the treatment, will occur if the mandible is advanced in this pa-

tient. Mandibular advancement, therefore, should be avoided.

In doing a prediction of maxillary surgery to elevate it and allow the mandible to rotate upward and forward, it is necessary to consider the position of the mandibular incisors at the conclusion of preparatory orthodontics. If the lower arch is treated without extraction, the incisors will be slightly advanced; if extractions are employed, the incisors can be aligned and also slightly retracted if desired.

Note in Fig. 5-39, *C* that when the lower arch is treated without extraction, the upper teeth must be moved considerably forward when they are elevated surgically. When the lower incisors are retracted, as they could be with premolar extraction and good anchorage control (Fig. 5-39, *D*), the upper incisor prominence can be reduced. Lower arch extraction therefore is required.

Based on these predictions, it is clear that the best solution to the problem of open bite and vertical prominence of the upper teeth would be surgery to elevate the maxilla.

Now consider the possible solutions to the second problem of mandibular deficiency, excess overjet and Class II malocclusion, and examine them in comparison with the solutions to the most important problem:

(1) Camouflage by upper incisor retraction (rejected: poor esthetics, probably unstable)

(2) Mandibular advancement (rejected, rotation wrong way)

(3) Maxillary intrusion (satisfactory: the forward rotation would bring the mandible far enough forward without ramus surgery)

Now consider the third problem, the incisor crowding, especially in the mandibular arch. The possible solutions are:

(1) Arch expansion (rejected for lower arch; ? upper)

(2) Premolar extraction (necessary in lower arch)

The final problem, the maxillary unilateral crossbite, could be corrected by:

(1) Reciprocal tooth movement via cross-elastics (but this would elongate the posterior segments that need intrusion)

(2) Orthopedic maxillary expansion (but this would produce bilateral movement where unilateral is needed and might need surgical assistance in any case in a patient of this age)

(3) Posterior maxillary segmental surgery (satisfactory in a patient who needs total maxillary osteotomy anyway—this would require extraction of first premolars for access)

4. *Integration of the individual possibilities into a final plan.*

When the possible solutions to the individual problems are reviewed, it is apparent that all the problems can be solved and that segmental maxillary surgery with premolar extraction is required. Therefore the final plan is:

(1) Extraction of maxillary and mandibular first premolars

(2) Preparatory orthodontic treatment to align the teeth, close the mandibular extraction space with

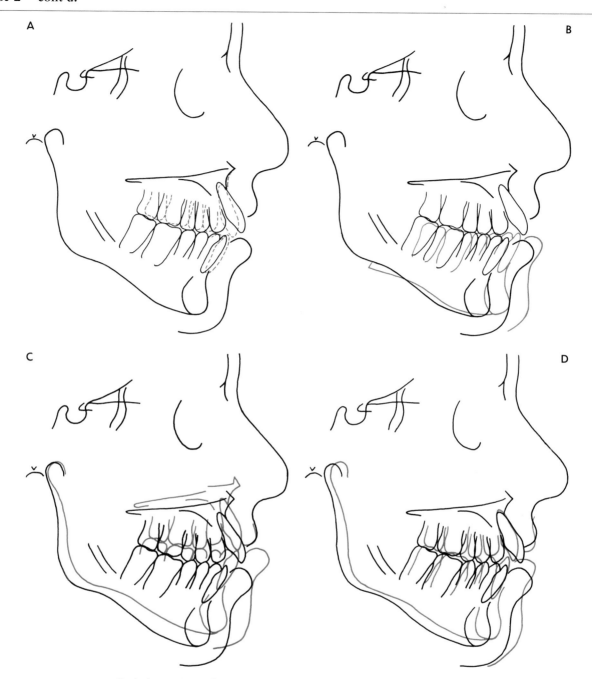

Fig. 5-39. Cephalometric predictions, patient S.S. (All were made using templates as demonstrated in Fig. 5-27.) **A,** Prediction of orthodontic treatment alone, using extraction of upper premolars to retract the upper incisors. This perhaps could bring the teeth together but would make the prominence of the upper incisors worse by elongating them relative to the lip. Closing an anterior open bite in this way rarely gives a stable result, so relapse also would be a problem. **B,** Prediction of mandibular advancement alone. Note the wrong-way rotation of the mandible and lengthening of the ramus. This treatment would almost surely lead to relapse and postsurgical problems. **C,** Prediction of superior repositioning of the maxilla with nonextraction treatment in the lower arch (which would bring the incisors forward). Note that when the mandible rotates upward and forward, there are incisor interferences unless the maxillary anterior segment is advanced to an undesirable extent. **D,** Prediction of superior repositioning of the maxilla with premolar extraction in the mandibular arch and slight retraction of the lower incisors. With the lower incisors retracted, the anterior maxilla can move up without being advanced—thus extraction in the lower arch would be the preferred plan.

Case 2—cont'd.

A   B   C

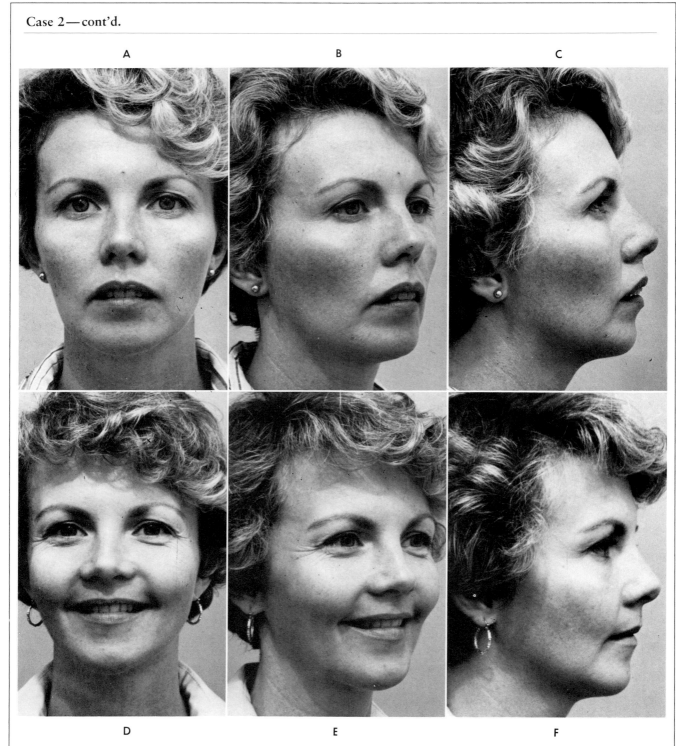

D   E   F

Fig. 5-40. Facial photographs, S.S. **A** through **C**, Immediately before surgery. **D** through **F**, 1 year later, when orthodontic appliances were removed.

39. Kiyak HA, McNeill RW, West RA, et al: Personality characteristics as predictors of sequelae of surgical and conventional orthodontics, Am J Orthod 89:383-392, 1986.

40. Dolan P, White RP, Jr, Tulloch JFC: An analysis of hospital charges for orthognathic surgery, Int J Adult Orthod Orthognath Surg 1:9-14, 1987.

41. Brewka RE: Pantographic evaluation of cephalometric hinge axis, Am J Orthod 79:1-19, 1981.

42. Sperry TP, Steinburg MJ, Gans BJ: Mandibular movement during autorotation as a result of maxillary impaction surgery, Am J Orthod 81:116-123, 1982.

43. Rekow ED, Worms FW, Erdman AG, et al: Treatment-induced errors in occlusion following orthognathic surgery, Am J Orthod 88:425-432, 1985.

44. Sarver DM, Johnston MW, Matukas VJ: Video imagining in planning and counseling in orthognathic surgery, J Oral Maxillofac Surg 46:939-945, 1988.

45. Marcotte MR: The use of the occlusogram in planning orthodontic treatment, Am J Orthod 69:655-667, 1976.

CHAPTER 6

Combined Surgical-Orthodontic Treatment: Who Does What, When?

William R. Proffit
Raymond P. White, Jr.

The previous chapters in this section have focused on diagnosis and the formulation of a plan to maximize benefit to the patient. In this chapter the emphasis is on the general sequence of treatment from initial disease control through postsurgical orthodontics and retention and on the interaction between orthodontist, surgeon, and other practitioners. Although some details of treatment differ depending on the patient's specific problems, the flow of treatment described in this chapter is basically the same for all surgical-orthodontic patients.

PRESENTING TREATMENT POSSIBILITIES TO THE PATIENT: INFORMED CONSENT

Having a patient's consent based on adequate information is a prerequisite to elective treatment. The patient must have information about the risks and costs as well as the benefits of the proposed treatment. If the doctors do not provide information about problems that might arise during the course of treatment, the patient can bring successful legal action for damages, as a number of well-publicized malpractice suits have demonstrated in recent years. Informed consent is first of all an ethical requirement, but it is also a well-established legal one.

Although there is a legal and ethical necessity to obtain the patient's informed consent, there are no strict guidelines on exactly how this should be done. Most practitioners now use a prepared form that they discuss with the patient before both sign the document. The signed form indicates that the content of the form was discussed, but the fact that the patient signed the form does not prove informed consent. Patients may assert at a later time that they did not understand the content of the discussions. Nor does the absence of a form indicate that the patient's consent was uninformed. A standard outline or a signed note in the chart can be used to document the consultation and the provision of adequate information.

We suggest that informed consent be obtained during the consultation to explain the treatment plan by discussing, in the following sequence: (1) the patient's problems, (2) the proposed treatment for those problems, and then (3) explicitly and in order, the benefits (functional and esthetic), risks (physical and psychologic—e.g., change in appearance), and costs (financial

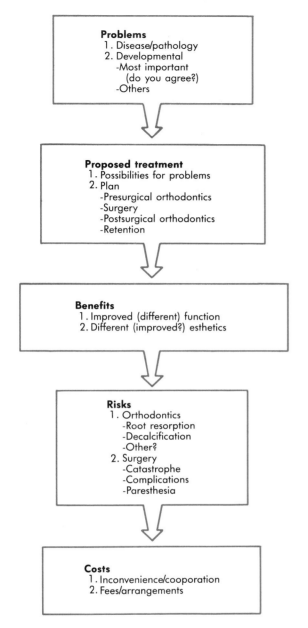

Problems
1. Disease/pathology
2. Developmental
   -Most important
    (do you agree?)
   -Others

Proposed treatment
1. Possibilities for problems
2. Plan
   -Presurgical orthodontics
   -Surgery
   -Postsurgical orthodontics
   -Retention

Benefits
1. Improved (different) function
2. Different (improved?) esthetics

Risks
1. Orthodontics
   -Root resorption
   -Decalcification
   -Other?
2. Surgery
   -Catastrophe
   -Complications
   -Paresthesia

Costs
1. Inconvenience/cooporation
2. Fees/arrangements

Fig. 6-1. The flow chart for consultation that ends with informed consent.

and intangible) of the treatment. The consequences of no treatment must be addressed, providing as much information as is known.

A consultation structured in this way (Fig. 6-1) is highly compatible with the diagnostic and treatment planning approach that we have outlined in the previous chapters. The advantage of discussing the patient's problems first, then the proposed treatment and the benefits to be obtained from that treatment, is that this provides ample opportunity to be certain that the patient and the doctor are in agreement as to the objec-

tive of the treatment. Risks and costs are also important, but informed consent is incomplete if the prioritization of the patient's problems and the benefits to be obtained from treatment have not been presented clearly.

At this stage, a generous amount of time with the patient must be available for discussion. More problems arise from misunderstandings by the patient and family about the patient's problems and expectations of treatment than from failure of patients to clearly understand risks. If possible, both the surgeon and the orthodontist should participate in the same presentation of the treatment plan, although separate consultations are adequate if the doctors communicate well enough with each other so as to not confuse the patient. Some surgeons and orthodontists now use audiovisual presentations (video tape or interactive videodisc—see Chapter 3 for more information) to explain the procedures and sequence of treatment. These can be quite helpful, as long as the patient's problems are adequately presented and time is allowed for discussion.

Patients should be encouraged to bring a list of questions to the consultation, take notes, and call later with lingering questions. It also is a good idea for them to bring a spouse, parent, other family member, or close friend to the consultation. This individual has the patient's best interests in mind and often asks important questions that the patient has forgotten. Following the appointment, this third party may help the patient organize his or her thoughts during the process of making a decision about treatment. Opinions vary as to whether a patient should be encouraged to delay a decision about treatment until after the initial presentation of the plan. Patients should always be given adequate time for their decision. If this means a second appointment, the delay can be accommodated if the patient has made a better decision.

Following the initial orthodontic phase of treatment, the surgeon will discuss again with the patient the surgical procedure, course of events in the hospital, and immediate postsurgery period. Any deviations from the initial plan must be thoroughly explained. Often both the hospital and the surgeon have written consent forms for surgery which must be signed and witnessed at this time.

CONTROL OF PATHOLOGIC PROBLEMS

In Chapter 5 we emphasized the necessity to control systemic or local disease before beginning treatment for developmental problems and discussed the implications of various pathologic conditions for treatment planning. In the following discussion, the emphasis is on the interaction among the various practitioners and the sequence of treatment, to be certain that disease control is established and maintained.

Systemic Disease

Chronic systemic disease requires continuing medical care, and surgical-orthodontic treatment for patients with such problems must be coordinated with the patient's physicians. The major interaction centers around the severity and control of the chronic disease and medication the patient may be taking. Restrictions on diet and physical activity also can be important.

To achieve the best health status, the patient and physician may need to work together to make adjustments in the medical regimen. For example, a patient with hypertension might have both diet and drug regimen altered, or an insulin-dependent diabetic counseled to improve compliance with therapy.

Pregnancy also must be ruled out before surgery because a general anesthetic may have deleterious effects on the developing fetus. If the patient becomes pregnant after orthodontics has begun, plans should be altered so that surgery occurs 4 to 6 months following delivery. This allows the patient to recover physiologically, including building up an adequate red blood cell volume, and to make plans for the care of the new baby during the surgery and postsurgical recovery.

The possibility of drug interactions during surgery is obvious and is discussed in Chapter 7. Orthodontic treatment also can be affected by certain drugs. Because prostaglandins serve as a stimulus for the bone remodeling that makes orthodontic tooth movement possible, it may be difficult to move teeth in patients who are taking prostaglandin inhibitors. These fall into two classes: (1) corticosteroids and nonsteroidal antiinflammatory agents that interfere with prostaglandin synthesis, and (2) other agents that have mixed agonistic and antagonistic effects on various prostaglandins.

In the body, prostaglandins are formed from arachidonic acid, which in turn is derived from phospholipids. Corticosteroids reduce prostaglandin synthesis by inhibiting the formation of arachidonic acid, whereas indomethacin, aspirin, and related nonsteroidal drugs tend to block the conversion of arachidonic acid to prostaglandins. Definitely in experimental animals,[1] and almost certainly in human patients as well, these drugs slow the rate of orthodontic tooth movement. Steroidal and nonsteroidal antiinflammatory agents are encountered most often in patients with chronic arthritis, but are used frequently in other diseases as well. Most of the common pain relievers are prostaglandin inhibitors to some degree, including aspirin and most of the newer nonsteroidal agents. Because a drug's effectiveness for arthritis does not seem to be directly proportional to its inhibition of prostaglandin synthesis, it may be possible to substitute another medication if difficulty in moving teeth is encountered. Indomethacin has 8 to 10 times the antiprostaglandin effect of aspirin, for example, making chronic aspirin dosage much more compatible with orthodontic treatment.

Tricyclic antidepressants (e.g., doxepin, amitriptyline, imipramine), antiarrhythmic agents (e.g., procaine), antimalarial drugs (e.g., quinine, quinidine, chloroquine), and methyl xanthines have some agonistic and more potent antagonistic effects on prostaglandins.[2-4] All of these may be encountered in adults who are candidates for surgical-orthodontic treatment. Although there are no definite reports, it is possible that unusual responses to orthodontic forces would be encountered in patients taking any of these medications.

Other drugs also have the potential to affect orthodontic treatment. The gingival overgrowth commonly seen during therapy with diphenylhydantoin (Dilantin) and related drugs for control of seizures often is exacerbated in the presence of orthodontic appliances.[5] This delays tooth movement and can create both esthetic and periodontal health problems. Interestingly, seizure disorders are less of a contraindication for orthognathic surgery now than they were a few years ago because the problems that might arise if a seizure occurred while a patient was in maxillomandibular fixation are avoided with rigid internal fixation.

Dryness of the mouth, a common side effect of many drugs used for chronic disease states, can complicate orthodontic treatment. Orthodontic appliances at best are somewhat annoying to patients. If there is inadequate saliva, the potential for irritation of the lips, cheeks, and tongue increases. If the side effect of the medication (i.e., dry mouth) cannot be reduced, additional attention to smoothing the appliance to minimize projections into the mouth, use of additional protective materials such as wax over brackets, and greater emphasis on oral hygiene all may be necessary.

The most important thing to remember in treating patients who have chronic systemic disease is the necessity for excellent communication with the physician, so that the physician understands the long-term orthodontic as well as the short-term surgical implications of treatment and so that the orthodontist and surgeon are well aware of the patient's systemic condition, the progression and prognosis of the disease, and how it is being treated.

Dental Disease

As with systemic disease, oral health problems must be brought under control before surgical-orthodontic treatment begins, and that requires coordinated treatment with other dental practitioners. Three specific circumstances relative to dental disease are worth additional comment.

Caries Control

Controlling active caries usually requires only the establishment of proper oral hygiene, which is necessary also for periodontal health and is the key to maintenance of oral health during other treatment.

Especially if caries has been a problem recently, it is wise to prescribe a fluoride rinse to prevent further de-

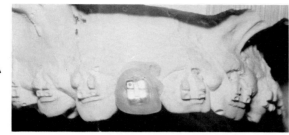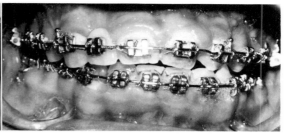

A

B

Fig. 6-2. During orthodontic treatment, the best way to handle a missing anterior tooth that must be replaced for esthetics is to prepare a plastic pontic that can be tied to the orthodontic arch wire. **A,** Preparation of the pontic on a cast. After it is properly contoured, an orthodontic attachment is bonded to it. **B,** The pontic in the mouth. A rectangular arch wire or a loop or spur in a round wire is needed to prevent rotation of the pontic from rotating on the wire.

calcification of teeth during orthodontic treatment. There now are good studies to show that decalcification can be reduced by a combination of good toothbrushing and either a stannous or sodium fluoride (NaF) rinse.[6] We recommend that a 0.05% NaF rinse be used routinely during orthodontic treatment and particularly that its use be maintained during any period of intermaxillary fixation accompanying surgery.

Should surgical-orthodontic patients who have had trouble maintaining good hygiene be encouraged to use a powered toothbrush? The original reciprocal action electric toothbrushes did not prove effective, but two newer rotary designs seem to have some advantages for patients who have difficulty in proper cleaning—which includes many patients who are wearing orthodontic appliances.[7,8] Brushes of this type, used in conjunction with a fluoride rinse program, can help in controlling decalcification around brackets and bands. They are not needed by the majority of patients.

Temporary Restorations

Carious teeth must be restored before orthodontic treatment begins, but definitive restorations should not be placed until the final dental occlusion has been established; that is, until completion of the surgical and orthodontic phases of treatment. Caries control calls for temporary restorations that are compatible with the relatively prolonged orthodontic and surgical treatment. Amalgam or composite resin materials are satisfactory. Temporary cement restorations (zinc phosphate and similar materials) may not last through the orthodontic treatment, and cast inlays, onlays, or crowns should be deferred until the final occlusion has been established.

Missing Teeth

In a patient who already has fixed bridges anchored by crowns to abutment teeth, it may be necessary to start by sectioning the bridge and removing pontics if abutment teeth are to be repositioned in the orthodon-

tic phase of treatment. Whether to preserve or sacrifice a bridge, of course, is a function of its possible utility afterward. Given the cost of fixed prostheses, it is worthwhile to save a bridge if possible. In addition, patients often object to being without a replacement tooth because of esthetics. It is poor judgment, however, to go to such lengths to preserve an existing bridge if the benefits of surgery and orthodontics are compromised. Decisions about resin-bonded bridges are less difficult because they are neither as permanent nor as costly as bridges anchored by crowns on abutment teeth.

During orthodontic treatment, the esthetic objection of a space previously filled by a bridge pontic can be overcome by placing an orthodontic bracket on a replacement tooth contoured to fit the space and simply tying this to the orthodontic arch wire (Fig. 6-2). When extremely flexible initial round wires are employed, stabilizing the replacement tooth may be difficult, but even with a round wire, it is possible to use a small loop, soldered spur, or modified ligature tie to hold the temporary pontic in position. The patient must realize that the pontic is strictly for appearance, not for function. As soon as enough initial alignment has been achieved to allow the use of a rectangular wire—which can be quite early with the use of rectangular Nitinol or a braided rectangular wire—most of the difficulty with a pontic of this type disappears. Tying a pontic to an arch wire is preferred to the alternative of a "flipper" type removable appliance.

Crowns on abutment teeth, or full crowns in general, can create a problem in the placement of an orthodontic appliance. If enough roughness of the surface of a metal crown could be created, it might be possible to bond to it, but usually this is not feasible, so a tooth with a full metal crown must be banded. Unless it is possible to span the orthodontic appliance across a posterior bridge with metal crowns to a more posterior single tooth, there may be no alternative to removing the bridge pontic so that orthodontic control of that

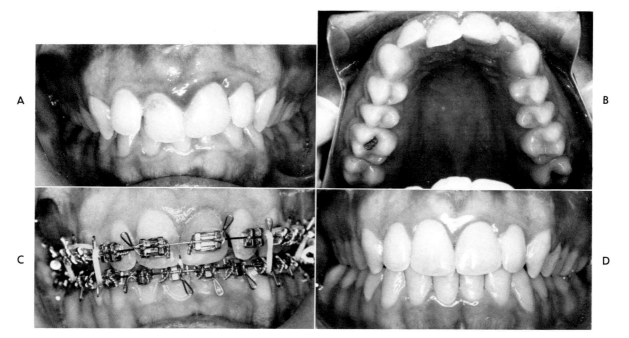

Fig. 6-3. **A,** The poor crown on the left central incisor and the resulting gingival inflammation contributed to this patient's esthetic problems. **B,** The excessive thickness of the original crown also was a problem: it would not have been possible to align the incisors when the excess overjet was corrected. **C,** Before surgical-orthodontic treatment began, the crown was replaced with a plastic temporary crown with acceptable margins. It functioned satisfactorily throughout treatment, as here during the postsurgical finishing. **D,** After the orthodontic appliances had been removed, a permanent replacement crown was made.

area can be obtained. It is possible to bond orthodontic attachments to porcelain surfaces, using a silane coupling agent before placement of the bonding adhesive.[9] If the porcelain surface is slightly roughened before the attempt to bond to it, a more reliable bond can be achieved, but of course the surface will have been permanently scratched.

As a general rule, it is better to maintain an exisiting crown, even though it will have to be replaced later, than to remove it and place a plastic temporary one. Sometimes there is no alternative because poor crown margins or an exaggerated contour make orthodontic repositioning impossible. For example, a thick anterior crown can make correcting excessive overjet impossible. No problem exists in bonding an orthodontic attachment to a plastic replacement crown, and a well-made plastic temporary crown usually will serve satisfactorily during surgical-orthodontic treatment (Fig. 6-3).

Periodontal Disease

The guideline for periodontal treatment is the same as for caries control: everything necessary to bring the patient's condition under control must be done before beginning surgical-orthodontic treatment, but some de-

finitive periodontal procedures, primarily osseous recontouring, may be better deferred until the final occlusion has been established.

In a patient with active periodontal disease, initial scaling, curettage, flap procedures to allow removal of calculus and granulation tissue, and anything else necessary to bring periodontal disease to the point that the patient can be maintained during orthodontic treatment should be done before an orthodontic appliance is placed. A patient who has had difficulty in maintaining proper oral hygiene must demonstrate the ability to do so. In patients who have previously neglected their mouth but now say they will do whatever it takes to maintain a damaged dentition, their willingness to improve oral hygiene foreshadows their willingness to cooperate with the other phases of treatment. Elaborate orthodontics has no place in the treatment plan for an individual who cannot or will not maintain the dentition over a long period.

For some patients with an extremely compromised periodontal situation, however, orthognathic surgery to reposition the jaws may be the key to successful removable prosthodontics to replace most or all of the teeth. The fact that a tooth will have to be removed eventually does not automatically mean that it should

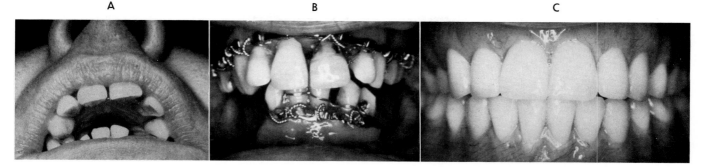

Fig. 6-4. In a patient with teeth that are hopelessly involved periodontally, orthognathic surgery may be indicated to create a situation that can be managed prosthodontically. In that circumstance, the teeth should be maintained if at all possible until after the surgery. **A,** Extreme overjet before treatment. Severe periodontal disease requires extraction of almost all remaining teeth. **B,** Occlusal relationships 10 weeks after surgery. **C,** Upper and lower dentures in place after surgery.

be removed before orthognathic surgery. Sometimes a tooth that is hopelessly involved periodontally can be useful one last time as a temporary abutment during surgical stabilization (Fig. 6-4). Periodontally mobile teeth tied together with orthodontic arch wires or arch bars give better control of jaw position at surgery than the alternative, a treatment partial denture. In such a patient, orthodontics may be rather limited, but even then, some preliminary or finishing orthodontics may help in the final positioning of any teeth that can be maintained. This topic is explored in more detail in Chapter 17.

Periodontal Control Measures

Although most patients who need surgical-orthodontic treatment do not have severe periodontal problems, the fact is that 12% to 15% of a typical adult population do have some areas of severe periodontal breakdown,[10] and there is no reason to think that this is significantly different for those with dentofacial deformities. In potential surgical-orthodontic patients, periodontal control measures are directed toward three main areas: (1) arresting the progression of periodontal attachment and bone loss, (2) improving hygiene and home care so that the results of the periodontal therapy can be maintained, and (3) preventing the loss of gingival attachment in areas that could be stressed to this level by orthodontic and/or surgical treatment.

The presence of periodontal pockets seems to be critical to the progression of bone loss because this is related to the different (anaerobic) bacterial flora in those areas. There is increasing evidence that specific microorganisms are involved in periodontal breakdown and that the causative organisms are much more prevalent in deep pockets,[11] a subject that continues to receive great attention in the literature. The primary goal of treatment, therefore, is control of the subgingival bacteria through control of subgingival plaque.

In broad terms, there are three ways to do this: (1) promote repair of the pockets by some sort of regeneration of the lost bone, (2) eliminate the pockets surgically, or (3) reduce pocket depth by conservative treatment measures and teach the patient how to maintain a less pathogenic environment in the pockets. Regeneration of a new connective-tissue interface between bone and tooth would be the ideal treatment but remains a distant goal, despite continuing progress in this direction. Surgical treatment, the mainstay of periodontics 20 years ago, has proved less successful in the long term than was expected initially, and it now is clear that even after surgery, long-term maintenance still is the key variable in determining success.[12] Gingivectomy and osseous recontouring therefore are used less now in patients with moderate pocket depths. At present, the most effective approach and the one most applicable to the majority of surgical-orthodontic patients is maintenance therapy. The critical pocket depth appears to be 5 to 6 mm. Patients can successfully maintain pockets of that magnitude, but greater depths are not manageable and must be reduced to at least that level.[11]

Maintenance Procedures

Maintenance of pockets in the 3 to 6 mm range is based on some combination of professional cleaning at 8- to 12-week intervals and the use of topical chemical agents such as chlorhexidine. The rationale for professional cleaning is that there is a relationship between the supragingival and subgingival plaque and that, following scaling and cleaning the teeth, it takes some weeks for bacterial recolonization to occur in the pockets. Although systemic antibacterial agents such as metronidazole and tetracycline can be used during periods of acute periodontal breakdown, these have no place in

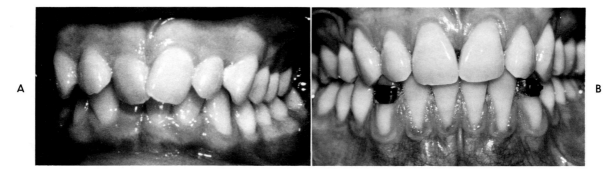

Fig. 6-5. Gingival recession problems in a short-face, deep-bite patient treated by orthodontic expansion of the dental arches. **A,** Pretreatment intraoral views. **B,** Posttreatment, 2 years later. The gingival recession in the lower incisor region is related at least partially to the stress created by the expansion. It is better to prevent problems of this type by periodontal treatment to augment the gingival attachment than to try to correct the recession later.

long-term maintenance therapy.[13] Topical chemical inhibition, however, is proving quite successful as a maintenance procedure.

Fluoride preparations can be used for this purpose, but by far the most effective agent for topical inhibition of oral bacteria is chlorhexidine, which also is both low in cost and quite safe. Its greatest disadvantage is that it stains the teeth to the point that periodic professional cleaning is required—not a serious problem, of course, in a surgical-orthodontic patient who would require regular maintenance visits anyway. Although chlorhexidine is more effective if injected directly into the pockets rather than used just as a rinse, because it penetrates better into the depths that way,[14] this is not yet a practical approach. Using it with a water-jet irrigating device requires very large quantities of the material, and patients may do more harm than good attempting to inject it themselves with a blunt syringe. The best method appears to be regular rinses after brushing and flossing the teeth.

For surgical-orthodontic patients, the key to maintenance of the 4 to 6 mm pockets that may remain after active periodontal disease is brought under control is regular periodontal recall for cleaning and scaling. This should be done at 2- to 3-month intervals. In patients with the most severe problems, the recall schedule may need to be supplemented with chlorhexidine rinses or perhaps another topical approach.

Mucogingival Considerations

A special periodontal consideration for surgical-orthodontic patients is the quantity and quality of attached gingiva (see Chapter 4, Fig. 4-4). Gingival grafts may be needed before surgical-orthodontic treatment to provide an adequate attachment.

The gingival attachment is stressed by orthodontic procedures that expand the dental arch labially or buccally (Fig. 6-5) and by surgical incisions in the vestibule

for orthognathic procedures. The usual reason for arch expansion is mild to moderate crowding, but additional space in the dental arch also is needed to level an excessive curve of Spee. Expansion typically moves incisors labially and/or premolars laterally. The gingival attachment is particularly at risk when incisors are advanced in a patient whose attachment is initially minimal. A good example is the patient with mandibular prognathism whose lower incisors have tipped lingually as the problem developed (Fig. 6-6). Moving these incisors labially without first being sure there is adequate attached gingiva is inviting a periodontal problem characterized by gingival clefting and loss of bony support to the teeth.

Incisions in the maxillary vestibule are a feature of maxillary surgery. When the amount of facial attached gingiva is marginal in the maxillary anterior and premolar regions, and particularly when gingival recession already is present, a free gingival graft to the area to improve tissue quanitity and quality must be considered before orthodontic treatment.

In the mandibular arch, a vestibular incision is required for inferior border or subapical osteotomy. Patients with a chin deficiency tend to have labially positioned lower incisors as part of the usual dental compensation for skeletal deformity, and these incisors often have a reduced facial gingival attachment. Because of this, chin-deficient patients who require a lengthening of the inferior border of the mandible are quite likely to need gingival grafts before their orthodontic and surgical treatment (see case 1, Chapter 5, Figs. 5-30 to 5-37).

Planning a gingival graft as a preventive procedure is a much better approach than going ahead with orthodontics or orthognathic surgery and then having to deal with the consequences of rapid and severe gingival recession. Although the majority of patients with dentofacial deformities do not need gingival grafts, in our

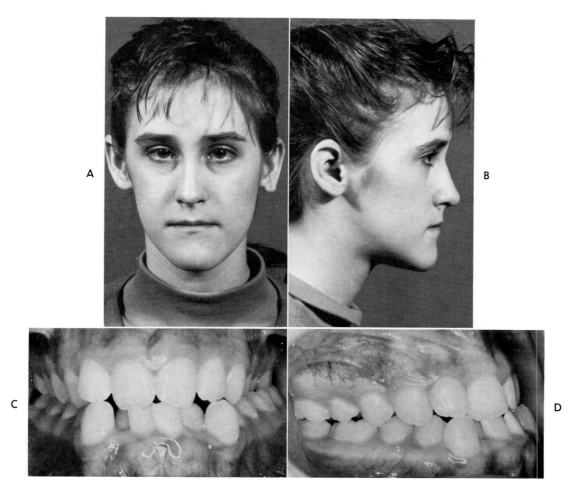

Fig. 6-6. In this 16-year-old girl with skeletal Class III malocclusion caused by a combination of maxillary deficiency and excessive mandibular growth, the lower incisors have tipped lingually during development. **A** and **B,** Facial appearance. **C** and **D,** Intraoral views. In removing the dental compensation in preparation for orthognathic surgery, it is desirable to advance the lower incisors and correct the crowding without extraction—but if this is done, the gingival attachment will be stressed severely. Gingival grafts before treatment probably will be required.

experience, facial gingival grafts are needed in up to 25% of patients who will have a mandibular inferior-border osteotomy and in 5% to 10% of those who will have a LeFort I downfracture procedure.

Sequence of Treatment

Several specific questions about the sequencing of periodontic with orthodontic and surgical treatment can arise:

If a gingival graft is needed in an area, but a tooth must be extracted in that area for orthodontic reasons, should the extraction or the graft be done first? This question arises most frequently in a patient who has minimal attached gingiva in the lower incisor area and who also has so much crowding of the lower incisor teeth that extraction of one lower incisor is part of the

orthodontic treatment plan (see case 1, Chapter 5). As a general rule, a better graft will result if the alveolar bone in the area has not been disturbed by a recent extraction and if the periodontist does not have to contend with an orthodontic appliance, so doing the graft first usually is preferred. On the other hand, if the teeth are extremely crowded and irregular, and particularly if there is a labial defect where the extraction will be done, it may be better to extract the tooth and proceed with orthodontics to obtain at least preliminary alignment of the teeth before placing the graft. Once gingival recession has begun, the graft placement may not restore gingival attachment or supporting bone, so any delay should be minimal.

For the periodontist, performing a free gingival graft for a patient who is wearing orthodontic appliances

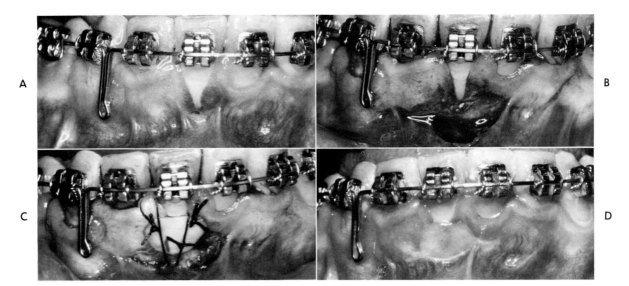

Fig. 6-7. **A,** Gingival recession beginning to appear in a patient whose orthodontic preparation for surgery is nearly complete. **B,** Preparation of a bed for a free gingival graft. **C,** The graft (from the palate) sutured into position. **D,** Healing 2 weeks later. Although it is technically more difficult to place a graft with the orthodontic appliance in place, periodontal treatment should not be delayed in a situation such as this one. (Courtesy Dr. John Moriarty.)

has pluses and minuses (Fig. 6-7). With the appliance in place, it is technically more difficult to position the graft. The orthodontist will need to remove an arch wire containing any loops near the graft site and should not use brackets with integral hooks that project gingivally. On the other hand, an orthodontic appliance does provide an excellent way to hold periodontal dressings in place, and the improved protection in some cases facilitates healing. The quality of the graft result should not be compromised by the presence of the appliance. Whether a graft is placed initially or after preliminary tooth alignment, its presence causes no difficulty in carrying out orthodontic tooth movement.

In a patient with a severely compromised periodontal situation, what schedule of periodontal maintenance is required? Periodontal maintenance obviously must be varied to meet the individual's needs, but it is likely that scaling, curettage, and related treatment will be required more frequently during surgical-orthodontic treatment. The orthodontist must see to it that the patient receives the necessary attention and that periodontal control is maintained. In the most severe cases, orthodontic and periodontic appointments may be on the same schedule (i.e., approximately once per month). More frequent visits to the periodontist may be needed while active disease is being treated, but it would be poor judgment to attempt surgical-orthodontic treatment on a patient who had to be seen by the periodontist more than once a month in order to main-

tain control of disease. Orthodontic treatment in the presence of active periodontal disease should be avoided.

What are the implications for orthodontic treatment of reduced bone support around the teeth? The implication is simple—the greater the amount of periodontal breakdown and bone loss that has already occurred, the more careful the orthodontist must be to keep forces light. Pressure within the periodontal ligament space, not the force that is applied to the crown of the tooth, is the key factor in determining the physiologic response. If the periodontal ligament area has been reduced by 50% because of periodontal disease, the orthodontist's typical force against the crown of a tooth would produce twice as much pressure in the remaining periodontal ligament area (Fig. 6-8). Because the center of resistance would be located further down the root, moment-to-force ratios also have to be adjusted when bone loss has occurred. Careful control of orthodontic force levels is an absolute necessity for periodontally involved patients.

In addition, though it seems not to have been documented in the literature, our experience suggests that root resorption may be more likely in orthodontic patients who have had previous periodontal bone loss than in those with a normal periodontium. Whether this is caused by an increased susceptibility to root resorption because of the periodontal disease, or by the tendency for routine orthodontic forces to create greater pressure in the periodontal ligament, or per-

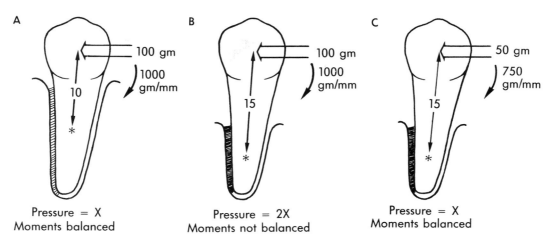

Fig. 6-8. **A,** For optimal bodily movement of a premolar whose center of resistance is 10 mm apical to the bracket, a 100 gm force and a 1000 gm-mm moment is needed. **B,** The same force system is entirely inappropriate for an identical premolar whose bone support has been reduced by periodontal disease so that the periodontal-ligament area is half as large and the center of resistance is 15 mm apical to the bracket. For such a tooth, the 100 gm force would produce twice the optimal pressure in the PDL and the moment would not be large enough to prevent tipping. **C,** The correct force system for the periodontally involved tooth would be a 50 gm force and a 15 × 50 = 750 gm-mm moment. Orthodontic movement of periodontally involved teeth can be done only with careful attention to forces (lower than normal) and moments (larger than normal).

haps is just another spurious clinical observation, remains unknown at this time. Patients who have had periodontal breakdown, however, should receive a special warning about the possibility of root resorption during surgical-orthodontic treatment.

What periodontal treatment should be left until surgery and orthodontics have been completed? The general rule is that if osseous recontouring is planned as part of the periodontal treatment, it should be deferred until the postsurgical orthodontic treatment is completed. Again, the reason is straightforward: the bone remodeling that accompanies orthodontic tooth move-

ment often reduces the amount of surgical bone recontouring that would be required. In some cases, orthodontic treatment can eliminate the need for this aspect of periodontal surgery. Defects along the mesial of tipped molar teeth are particularly likely to improve as the teeth are uprighted, turning what otherwise would have been an area needing osseous recontouring into one that does not (Fig. 6-9).

As with all good rules, this one has exceptions. Some patients have scalloped-out areas in the alveolar process that simply must be smoothed to bring the overall periodontal situation under control, and in that cir-

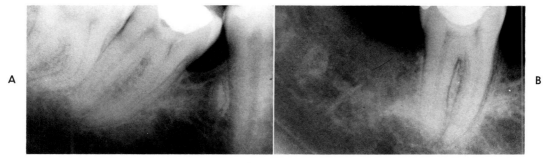

Fig. 6-9. **A,** Before treatment, probing indicates a 4 mm pocket on the mesial of the tipped second molar in this 20-year-old patient. **B,** After extraction of the third molar and uprighting of the second molar, the pocket has been eliminated. The bone on the mesial of the molar went with it as it was uprighted. Because of changes of this type in bone contour, periodontal surgery to recontour the alveolar bone usually should be deferred until after orthodontic tooth movement is completed.

cumstance, there is no alternative to doing the osseous contouring before orthodontics. Where natural remodeling can be induced by orthodontics, however, it is preferable to surgical recontouring because the amount of bone loss is likely to be less.

Impacted or Unerupted Teeth

Impacted or unerupted teeth are significant for surgical-orthodontic patients to the extent that their presence could complicate or compromise the surgery. Although orthognathic surgery is not indicated except in rare instances until after the adolescent growth spurt (see Chapter 2), another reason for delaying it is that the osteotomy cuts could encounter many normal unerupted teeth in a younger child.

A LeFort I osteotomy poses a threat to maxillary canines until eruption of these teeth is almost complete. In a postadolescent patient with maxillary deficiency, this can delay surgery for which the patient is otherwise ready. Occasionally, the teeth must be uncovered so that an orthodontic bracket or other attachment can be bonded (a ligature around the tooth is a much less desirable alternative).[15] Then the tooth is brought into position during the presurgical orthodontics.

In an adult patient, the decision to remove or leave an impacted maxillary canine should be made in the context of the best total patient care (which usually but not always indicates removal). Removing the tooth before LeFort I osteotomy is necessary only if the position of the tooth compromises orthodontic preparation of the patient. If the tooth is encountered after downfracture of the maxilla, it can be removed if easily accessible. If not, its presence should not impair healing.

Impacted maxillary third molars do not complicate a LeFort I osteotomy, and removal of these teeth is not necessary before surgery. Often the teeth are easily removed after the downfracture. If not, they can be removed selectively at a later time. Impacted or unerupted mandibular third molars in patients who will have a ramus or posterior subapical osteotomy are more problematic. Unless these teeth are well positioned and almost in occlusion, so that they would be of some value for function postsurgically, it is better to remove them. The question is whether to do this before the osteotomy or at the same time.

For a sagittal-split osteotomy, it usually is better to remove mandibular third molars 6 months or more before the orthognathic surgery, so that the area is well healed by that time. In some cases, removing the teeth at surgery causes no problems, but the situation is unpredictable. Three complications are possible if these teeth are removed during the osteotomy or left in place at that time: (1) the presence of the tooth or the defect left by its removal may influence the bone at the osteotomy site, increasing the chances of a "bad split," (2) if

the tooth is removed in the operating room after the osteotomy, the chance of infection in the area may be increased, and (3) the third molar may make the use of rigid internal fixation more difficult or impossible. The space occupied by an impacted third molar weakens the lingual plate, making it prone to fracture. After osteotomy and tooth removal, the third molar socket often leaves a space where bone screws might be placed for rigid fixation.

For a transoral vertical ramus osteotomy and other ramus procedures, similar considerations also dictate removing unerupted third molars before orthognathic surgery. The teeth are less likely to be encountered than during a sagittal-split osteotomy, which may make retaining them a more viable option, but there still is the possibility of a complication because of the third molar. For a posterior subapical osteotomy, it is necessary to remove the third molars, which can be done at that time if the teeth are in a reasonable position.

When the sequence of treatment is planned, the orthodontist and surgeon should consider impacted teeth carefully. Removing these teeth at the beginning of treatment, before the presurgical orthodontics begins, usually is the best plan. Often this can be done when other teeth are extracted for orthodontic purposes. Even if it adds another surgical procedure to an already long treatment sequence, this is preferable to a complication during osteotomy.

PRESURGICAL ORTHODONTICS

The goals of presurgical orthodontics are to align the teeth, establish the desired anteroposterior and vertical position of the incisors, and achieve arch compatibility. However, it is important to keep in mind that it is neither necessary nor desirable to set things up so perfectly that no postsurgical orthodontics will be required.

The general guideline for contemporary treatment is that every patient will need a relatively constant period of postsurgical orthodontic treatment to bring teeth into their final positions. The period of presurgical orthodontics, in which the tooth movement necessary to get the patient ready for surgery is carried out, is much more variable. This pattern of treatment offers the greatest possible efficiency. If the patient is not properly prepared, surgery cannot be carried out effectively, the quality of the result is diminished, and the postsurgical orthodontic treatment time is increased. On the other hand, beyond a certain point of preparation for surgery, the orthodontist is merely wasting time. Beyond this optimal point, approximately the same amount of postsurgical orthodontics will be required no matter how precisely the teeth are positioned. Extending the presurgical orthodontics simply increases the total treatment time without appreciably benefiting the patient.

The steps in presurgical and postsurgical orthodontics, with an indication of some procedures that can be done either before or after surgery, are summarized in Table 6-1. Specific points relative to presurgical treatment are described below.

Selection of the Appliance

Two major fixed orthodontic-appliance systems are in use at present: (1) the edgewise appliance, with its myriad of variations, and (2) the Begg appliance. The two differ significantly in the method by which an arch wire is attached to the bracket on a tooth and in how precisely the wire fits. In the edgewise appliance, a round or rectangular wire is tied into a bracket slot. A small round wire fits loosely, a full-dimension rectangular wire quite tightly. As a result, the appliance is well adapted both for tooth movement and for stabilization of teeth. In the Begg appliance, the attachment is significantly different. The arch wire is held in a vertically oriented slot by a pin that allows the tooth to slide or tip freely on the wire. The result is maximum ability for the teeth to move relative to the arch wire, but little or no capacity for stabilization.

The orthodontic appliance for surgical-orthodontic patients is used not only to move teeth but also to stabilize them against the stresses encountered at surgery and during maxillomandibular fixation. The difficulty of doing this with the Begg appliance is a strong argument against its use for surgical patients. It is not impossible to do good surgical-orthodontic treatment using the Begg appliance, but it is significantly more difficult and problematic. We recommend that a modern preadjusted edgewise appliance be used for surgery patients. Other characteristics of an acceptable appliance for surgery patients are discussed below.

Esthetic Appliances?

Presumably, the less visible the orthodontic appliance, the less impact it should have on social adjustment. Removable appliances can be totally invisible if they are removed on socially sensitive occasions, but this is not compatible with surgical treatment. The only way to keep a fixed appliance from being seen is to put it on the inside rather than the outside of the teeth. Lingual fixed appliances have been under intense development in the last decade and are becoming better adapted to routine orthodontic treatment in adults.[16,17]

A lingual appliance is ill-suited for surgical-orthodontics, however, for several reasons. First, it is almost impossible to use the appliance to stabilize the jaws at the time of surgery. If a lingual appliance is being used, it will be necessary to place a labial appliance as well, at least temporarily, for use in the operating

TABLE 6-1 Presurgical versus postsurgical orthodontics

Procedure	Comment
Necessary before surgery	
Alignment	Primarily by tipping: flexible round wire (16 mil austenitic NiTi best)
Intrusion (leveling)	Segmented arch technique required; stabilizing lingual arches needed; Burstone depressing arch (17×25 TMA or steel) suggested
Arch compatibility	Be careful regarding: Second molars' vertical position (don't elongate upper second molars!) Canine widths
Before and/or after surgery	
Posterior crossbite correction	No orthodontic expansion before surgery in a patient who will have surgical expansion
	Okay to leave up to half-cusp crossbite for correction after surgery
Extrusion (leveling)	Easier and more efficient after surgery; partial leveling with continuous arch wires can be done before surgery
Necessary after surgery	
Extrusion (settling, leveling)	Should complete in 4 to 6 months
Root paralleling at osteotomy sites	
Detailed tooth positioning	

room and in the immediate postsurgical rehabilitation period. Postoperatively, patients often have limitations on opening, particularly in the first few months when the postsurgical orthodontics must be done. This greatly complicates the already difficult process of using a lingual appliance. Whatever the orthodontist's feelings about fixed lingual appliances for other adult treatment, by themselves they are a poor choice for surgery patients.

Fixed labial appliances cannot be made invisible, but they can be made less visible. Excellent progress has

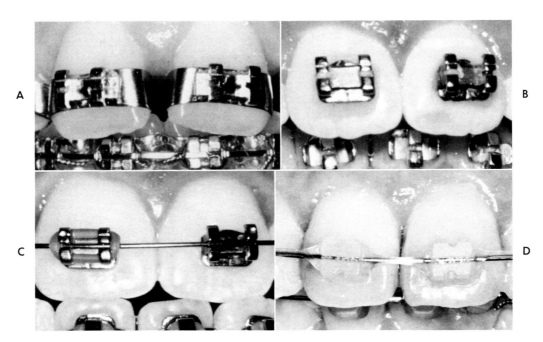

Fig. 6-10. A progression of increasingly esthetic but still mechanically effective edgewise brackets. **A,** Twin bracket on an anterior band (1975). **B,** Bonded twin bracket (1981). **C,** Bonded mini-twin bracket (1985). **D,** Bonded ceramic bracket (1988).

been made in this direction in two ways: (1) by eliminating metal anterior bands and reducing the size of metal attachments, and (2) by replacing metal with clear or tooth-colored attachments (Fig. 6-10).

When it became possible in the 1970s to replace anterior bands with bonded brackets, the visibility of the labial appliance was considerably reduced and esthetics consequently improved. Enhanced esthetics has been a factor in the increasing acceptance of adult orthodontics. In the 1980s, even better esthetics was the primary reason for a trend toward further reducing the size of bondable anterior brackets, accomplished primarily by reducing the mesiodistal width. Unfortunately, in some cases this reduction was carried to an extreme. It is a mistake to use metal brackets that have been made so small in search of esthetics that their mechanical qualities are compromised (see Fig. 6-13, *D*).

Mesiodistal width is needed in a bracket for two purposes: to allow control of rotations and to provide the means for mesiodistal root movement. Of the two, rotation control is usually the more important for posterior teeth, whereas root position is particularly important for obtaining maximum esthetics with upper incisors. Although rotation control can be accomplished with mesial and distal wings or extensions from a narrow bracket, the extensions must contact the arch wire. In some recent brackets, the extensions were made so small in an attempt to be inconspicuous that adequate rotation control was lost because the arch wire could lie above or below the rotation-controlling

portion of the bracket. Such a bracket makes it very difficult, for instance, to close a maxillary midline diastema without also rotating the centrals in a decidedly unesthetic way. These brackets also can cause problems during postsurgical finishing, when small but precise root movements are needed.

Clear or tooth-colored plastic brackets have been available since the 1970s. These are not well suited for complex adult orthodontic treatment or for surgical orthodontics for two reasons: (1) the plastic brackets themselves tend to fail, typically by breakage within the bracket itself, and (2) the bracket slot is not rigid enough to provide good torque control. The latter problem can be mitigated but not totally overcome by using a plastic bracket with a metal slot; the former has proved intractable. In addition, plastic brackets are much more esthetic when first placed than later because the brackets tend to discolor with time. For these reasons, plastic brackets are not recommended for surgical-orthodontic patients.

The recent introduction of ceramic brackets promises to overcome many of the limitations of tooth-colored plastic brackets. The ceramic brackets are strong enough to reduce the chance of failure in use. The bracket itself is rigid enough to give good torque control, and color stability is not a difficulty. Despite its great strength, however, the ceramic material is brittle, and the brackets are susceptible to fracture.[18] They require greater care to avoid impacts that may cause fracture (which often occur in the operating room) but can be adequate for surgical-orthodontic treatment.

In terms of stability of the appliance, metal brackets still are more reliable than ceramic ones. For surgical-orthodontic treatment, we recommend routine use of stainless steel twin brackets that are half the width of the tooth, or metal single brackets with wings rather than extensions of the base (Lewis or Lang brackets). When an esthetic labial bracket is needed for maxillary anterior teeth to improve the social acceptability of an appliance, ceramic brackets that are approximately half the width of the tooth are the best choice.

18-Slot or 22-Slot Appliance

The rigidity of a 17×25 steel arch wire in an 18-slot appliance is entirely adequate for surgical stabilization. (Arch wire and bracket slot sizes here and elsewhere in the text are given in mils; i.e., 17 mils = .017 inch.) A 21×25 beta-titanium (TMA) or steel wire is satisfactory in a 22-slot appliance. Often it is easier to finish a case with the 18-slot appliance because the smaller slot size makes precisely fitting steel wires more flexible. The 22-slot appliance can be advantageous, however, when segmented arch mechanics are needed for complex movements, particularly in patients with severe periodontal breakdown. In that circumstance, the greater ability to stabilize small units of the arch with a segment of 21×25 wire is helpful in controlling anchorange and obtaining precisely determined forces. With that exception, either an 18-slot or a 22-slot appliance is satisfactory for nearly all patients.

Bands versus Bonds

Directly bonded attachments for anterior teeth have become the routine in orthodontic practice in recent years, and patients with a fully bonded fixed appliance are seen frequently. Experience has shown that bonded appliances are entirely compatible with surgical orthodontics. The stress on bonded brackets at surgery may lead to an occasional failure, but the same is true with bands, the primary difference being that a loose bracket is immediately apparent, whereas a loose band may not be. Bonding posterior teeth is more difficult because higher tissue attachments and moisture control problems are found and stresses are greater. Although a fully bonded appliance can be satisfactory for surgical patients, we recommend bonded attachments for anterior teeth and bands for posterior ones. Usually the transition is at the first premolar so that it is bonded whereas the second premolar is banded, but occasionally both premolars are bonded, with bands only on the molars.

The presence of periodontal problems is a contraindication to the posterior bands that are recommended otherwise. It is harder for patients to clean around bands than bonded attachments, and the difference could be significant in a periodontally compromised patient. A fully bonded appliance is preferred in that circumstance, despite the greater chance of appliance problems.

Modifications in the Appliance

In the 60 years since Edward Angle introduced it, the edgewise appliance has undergone constant adaptation and modification. Not all of the bewildering variety of edgewise brackets and tubes now available are equally adaptable to surgical orthodontics. We recommend that the appliance used for surgical-orthodontic treatment have the following features:

1. Angulation, torque, and in-out compensation built into the brackets. Although the original edgewise appliance is perfectly satisfactory for surgical orthodontics, the advantages of the contemporary prescription appliance are at least as great for surgical as for nonsurgical patients. The same prescription can be used in the appliance for both types of patients, but there are some precautions for the surgical patients.

   As a general rule, extreme prescriptions should be avoided. Particularly, the "extraction series" brackets that have high root paralleling angulation should be avoided on maxillary canines and premolars in patients who will have a maxillary segmental osteotomy. In many instances, it is desirable to partially close the extraction space during the presurgical orthodontics, using some of the space to align the incisors and tip them lingually so as to gain the proper inclination. The roots must not be brought together before surgery when an interdental osteotomy is planned, and it is relatively easy to have greater root than crown proximity after partial space closure with the severely angulated brackets (Fig. 6-11). If roots converge too closely, the interdental osteotomy is impossible. On the other hand, there is no reason to exaggerate the separation of the roots, as would happen if the right and left canine and premolar brackets were deliberately reversed during presurgical treatment. That is likely to result in an unnecessary degree of postsurgical root paralleling, even after the brackets have been changed. The best approach is simply to use standard canine and premolar brackets with a regular prescription.

   The same principle applies more generally to brackets and tubes for other teeth. The objective of presurgical orthodontics is to arrange things first to facilitate the surgery, and then the finishing orthodontics. Exaggerated tooth positions are not desirable for either procedure. The prescription appliances, in short, are likely to be maximally effective for surgical patients if a regular prescription is used.

2. Bands or bonded attachments for all teeth, including second molars. Lower second molars should be

A   B

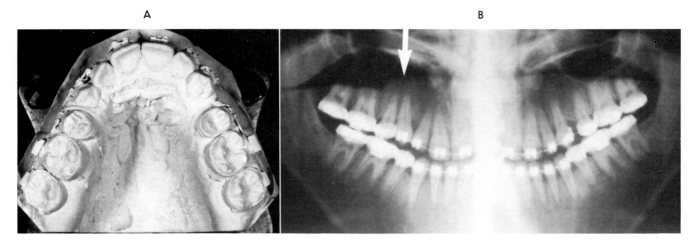

Fig. 6-11. Problems caused by bracket angulation in a patient being prepared for maxillary segmental surgery. The plan was to partially but not completely close the upper first premolar extraction spaces, leaving room for the surgical cuts. **A,** Presurgical dental cast, showing that the extraction spaces have not been totally closed. **B,** Presurgical panoramic radiograph. On the right side *(arrow)*, because of excessive angulation in the bracket prescription combined with incorrect placement, there is not enough room for the surgical cuts, and further orthodontic preparation to separate the roots is required.

banded routinely before surgery. Upper second molars usually need to be included in the appliance during finishing but often can be left unbanded until after surgery. If they are banded earlier, they should be kept vertically depressed with a step in the arch wire (Fig. 6-12) to prevent occlusal interferences as jaws are repositioned at surgery.

3. Auxiliary tubes and lingual attachments on upper and lower first molars. The lower molar should have a convertible bracket slot for the main arch wire and an 18×25 auxiliary tube. The upper molar needs a convertible bracket slot, a headgear tube

of 45 or 51 mil diameter, and an 18×25 auxiliary tube. The molar bands also require a lingual attachment (cleat, hook, or button) so that elastics from the lingual surface can be employed if necessary. A major reason for banding rather than bonding molars is to supply this lingual attachment without having to bond twice to the same tooth and without risking that an isolated lingual attachment would become detached and then swallowed or aspirated.

4. Adequate mesiodistal width of brackets to provide good rotation control. This can be achieved by using either medium-width twin brackets (brackets

A   B   C

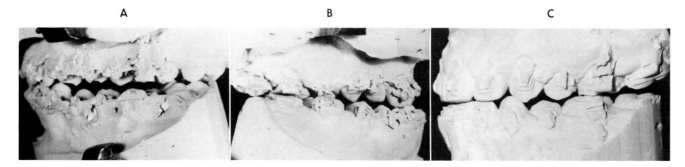

Fig. 6-12. **A,** Interference at model surgery created by a mandibular second molar that is above the occlusal plane of the other teeth. **B,** Interference created by a banded maxillary second molar that has been brought down to the level of the first molar (the reverse overjet cannot be corrected without encountering the elongated second molar). **C,** Model surgery casts for a patient whose upper second molars have been kept depressed by a bend in the arch wire so that interference is avoided when the casts are repositioned at model surgery. These teeth can be elongated into occlusion readily after the surgery, but removing interferences can be a major last-minute problem.

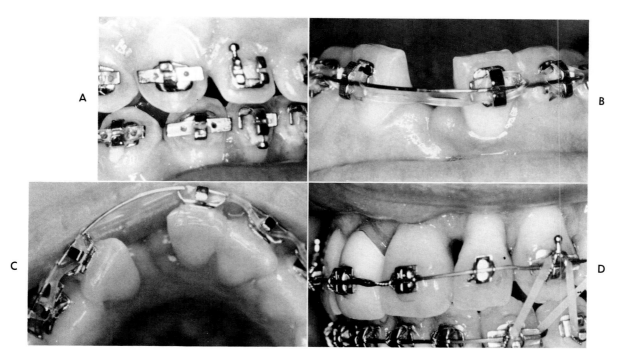

Fig. 6-13. Edgewise bracket possibilities for anterior teeth. **A,** Lang brackets for maxillary and mandibular canines; twin and Lewis brackets with integral hooks for maxillary and mandibular lateral incisors, respectively. **B** and **C,** Lewis bracket for mandibular lateral incisor. These winged brackets provide satisfactory rotation control with maximal inter-bracket span. **D,** Mini-brackets for the maxillary central and lateral incisors. With such small brackets, esthetics are improved at the cost of rotation control—these brackets are not recommended for surgical patients. Note the integral hook on the canine bracket, however, which can be quite helpful in surgical treatment.

half the width of the tooth, as provided in most contemporary twin-bracket–appliance setups) or single brackets with wings large enough to provide good rotational control (Fig. 6-13). Smaller brackets may be more esthetic, but the greater difficulty of controlling rotations makes them a poor choice for treatment as complex as often is needed in conjunction with surgery.

5. Integral hooks. Now that most brackets are cast rather than milled, it is not particularly difficult to include a hook built into the bracket itself, and brackets of this type do offer advantages for surgical orthodontics (Figs. 6-13, *A* and *D* and 6-14). A built-in hook definitely should be part of the standard assembly for molar teeth, and such hooks are quite helpful for surgical stabilization and postsurgical finishing. Hooks on other brackets can be useful for the intra-arch elastics needed in postsurgical orthodontics. Using them for maxillomandibular fixation at surgery, however, can pose some problems. If an auxiliary stabilizing arch wire is used at surgery, as in a multiple-segment maxillary osteotomy, the hooks built into the brackets are not long enough. As a consequence, maxillomandibular fixa-

tion is difficult in a situation where ease of application is most needed. Some surgeons feel that bonded brackets are more likely to be displaced in the operating room if fixation is applied to ingegral hooks rather than to lugs on a stabilizing arch wire. A major problem with integral hooks is that they extend gingivally in a way that complicates keeping the mouth clean. Small hooks are better, and excellent patient cooperation in maintaining oral hygiene is necessary if these are employed. The high level of motivation of surgical patients makes them good candidates for such brackets.

In contrast, several features of brackets are essentially irrelevant for surgical cases. These include the depth of the slot, the precise location on the tooth where the attachment is placed (but the orthodontist needs to be consistent with appliance placement), and whether the bracket is steel or ceramic. Plastic brackets should be avoided.

Alignment: The First Step in Treatment

In the traditional description of the stages of orthodontic treatment, alignment and leveling usually are joined in the first stage. It is quite common to begin

A   B   C

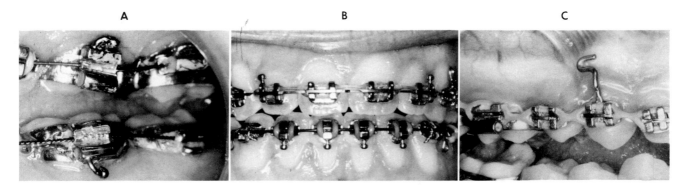

Fig. 6-14. **A**, Integral hooks on first and second molar attachments. Note the auxiliary tubes, on the first molars, which are essential for the segmented arch mechanotherapy that surgical-orthodontic patients often require. **B**, Integral hooks of the optimal small size incorporated into mandibular incisor and maxillary lateral incisor brackets. **C**, Large integral hook ("power-arm") on a maxillary canine. Large hooks are not recommended for surgical-orthodontic patients because of their potential to cause gingival problems. Small integral hooks (see Fig. 6-13) are adequate for interarch stabilization during surgery if multiple dentoalveolar segments are not created as part of the surgical procedure.

correcting vertical discrepancies at the same time as alignment, and we do not wish to imply that this is undesirable in any way. For discussion here, however, alignment and leveling are separated to clarify the presentation. A more integrated approach will be presented in the later clinical chapters.

From the orthodontist's perspective, alignment is not different for patients who will have surgery. The guiding principle is a simple one: preliminary alignment should be achieved by tipping the crowns of the teeth toward their proper position in the arch. Bodily movement is not only unnecessary, it is positively undesirable. The reason is that the tooth buds nearly always were reasonably well aligned. Malalignment developed as the erupting teeth were displaced from their normal path of eruption because of lack of space. As a result, the crowns of the teeth will be more out of line than will be the roots, and proper alignment can be achieved best by tipping the crowns into position.

With the edgewise appliance, it follows logically that the initial alignment arch wire should have several characteristics. It should be: (1) round rather than rectangular, to minimize inadvertent root movement, (2) undersized relative to the bracket slot, so that teeth can tip mesiodistally as well as labiolingually, and (3) highly resilient, so that light forces are created even if the wire is bent several millimeters to reach a malaligned tooth. The more resilient the wire, the fewer the number of adjustments that will be needed to complete the alignment.

Great progress has been made recently in developing arch wires with these characteristics. Austenitic nickel-titanium (NiTi) arch wires, introduced in the late 1980s, have the remarkable property of superelasticity and are almost ideal for initial alignment. Like most

metals, NiTi undergoes phase transformations with temperature change, and the ability of NiTi alloys to "remember" their shape in one phase when transformed to another has been used in many applications outside dentistry. The original NiTi alloys were developed by the Naval Ordinance Laboratory as spacecraft antennae, and the phase transition induced by the cold of outer space was exploited in designing an antenna that would unfold in space after being tightly compressed for launch. Despite intriguing demonstrations of phase changes induced in orthodontic arch wires by immersing them in a hot liquid, there have been no practical uses of temperature-induced phase changes in orthodontic treatment. The martensitic NiTi orthodontic wires that have been available since the mid-1970s are useful because of the elastic properties of that phase of the material.

However, phase changes are utilized in the new austenitic arch wires. Unlike the original martensitic orthodontic wires, austenitic NiTi has the amazing property whereby a partial phase change can be induced by internal stress.[19,20] The result is that when an austenitic NiTi arch wire is stressed, as would occur when it is tied into the brackets on malaligned teeth, some martensite forms within the basically austenitic material. In essence, this allows the elasticity of the martensite to be added to that of the austenite, thus the term *superelasticity*. The result is an amazingly flat load-deflection curve, so the wire can be displaced a considerable distance without developing excessive force (Fig. 6-15). Furthermore, although the unloading curve lies some distance below the loading curve (i.e., the wire produces even lighter forces than might first be thought from standard experiments), nearly 100% springback is achieved after very large deflections. The difference

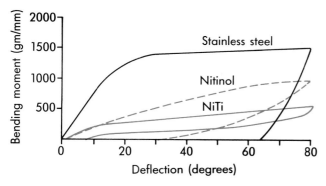

Fig. 6-15. Load deflection curves for equivalent-size stainless steel *(black)*, martensitic nickel-titanium (Nitinol, *dashed red*), and austenitic nickel-titanium (Ni-Ti, *red*). Both types of NiTi have significantly better elastic properties than does stainless steel, but the austenitic NiTi is better than the original martensitic form of this material. It has two advantages: its load-deflection curve is flatter, and its recovery is more complete. (Redrawn from Burstone CJ, Qin B, Morton JY: Chinese NiTi wire—a new orthodontic alloy, Am J Orthod 87:445-452, 1985.)

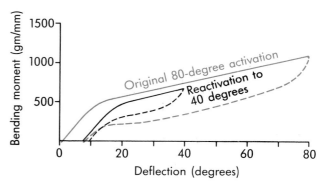

Fig. 6-16. Force-deflection curves for austenitic NiTi, showing how the wire can be reactivated merely by releasing and then retying it. This almost magical property results from the superelasticity created by stress-induced phase changes within the material. (Redrawn from Burstone CJ, Qin B, Morton JY: Chinese NiTi wire—a new orthodontic alloy, Am J Orthod 87:445-452, 1985.)

between the loading and unloading curves produces a second amazing effect: if desired, an austenitic NiTi arch wire can be reactivated (i.e., manipulated to increase the force on a tooth after it has been partially moved into position) simply by releasing the ligature tying it to the tooth, allowing it to spring back to its original shape, and then retying it (Fig. 6-16).

These advantages of austenitic NiTi make it particularly valuable for patients with severe malalignment (Fig. 6-17). Although the material is relatively costly as compared with steel wires, its greater efficiency makes it well worth the cost when significant tooth movement is required. Single-strand steel wires are too stiff for preliminary alignment unless loops are bent in them at points where large deflections are needed. Loops make steel wires extremely efficient, so this is still an excellent way to achieve alignment, especially when one

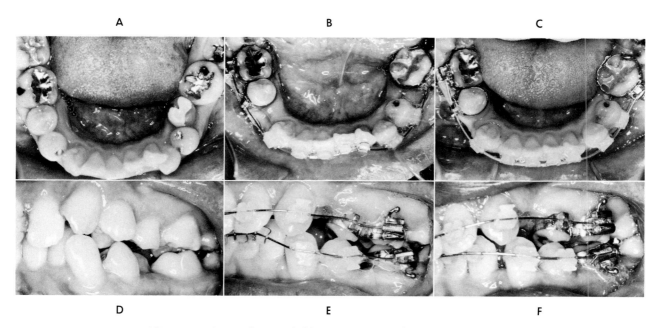

Fig. 6-17. Alignment of severely crowded lower incisors with austenitic NiTi in a mandibular-deficient patient before surgery. **A-C,** Occlusal and **D-F,** lateral views before treatment, 2 months after beginning treatment, and 4 months after beginning treatment.

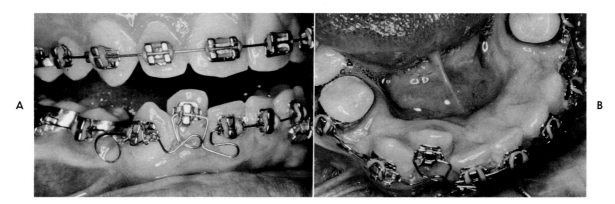

Fig. 6-18. When one tooth is severely out of line and the others are reasonably well aligned, loops in a 14-mil steel wire are preferred over a continuous NiTi wire because the former is less likely to distort arch form. **A,** Labial view. **B,** Occlusal view of alignment loops in a patient who has one lower lateral incisor crowded lingually. The rolled loop in the extraction site is being used to tip the canine distally, creating space for alignment of the lateral incisor.

tooth is far out of line while the others are in good position (Fig. 6-18). As a rule, however, it is not time-efficient to bend a large number of alignment loops.

A more practical alternative is multistrand steel wires. These can be quite effective with the 22-slot appliance when there is only moderate irregularity. They are less efficient in the 18-slot appliance because the total bulk of the multistrand wires tends to fill the smaller bracket slot more than is compatible with free sliding.

Rectangular NiTi or multistrand steel arch wires that would be flexible enough for initial alignment can be obtained. Superficially, it is attractive to think that a rectangular wire would be better from the beginning because it would provide better control of root position. When the teeth are malaligned, this almost never is the case. The risk that a root apex inadvertently will be moved to an undesired position already has been mentioned. This would require active torque or root paralleling to correct later. Even if displacement of the roots did not occur, a rectangular alignment arch wire would produce unnecessary back-and-forth movement of the root apices as the teeth moved into position, slowing the process and perhaps increasing the possibility of root resorption. It is said that any good rule has exceptions, and certainly there are exceptions to this one—for instance, torque to the upper central incisors in a patient with Class II, division 2 malocclusion may be needed from the beginning—but in general rectangular initial arch wires should be avoided.

The characteristics of initial alignment wires are summarized in Table 6-2.

Vertical Position of the Teeth: Level the Arch

In nonsurgical orthodontic treatment, leveling the dental arches to remove the excessive or reverse curve of Spee that characterizes most malocclusions is a standard procedure. In patients who will have surgery, it often is advantageous to use the surgery rather than just tooth movement to make vertical changes. If so, the orthodontist should not, indeed must not, automatically level the arches during the presurgical treatment. A better result may be achieved by completing the leveling postsurgically.

The steps in developing an appropriate treatment

TABLE 6-2 Initial alignment arch wires

Wire (dimension in mils)	Comments
16 NiTi (austenite/super-elastic)	Outstanding load-deflection characteristics; best all-around
16 NiTi (martensite)	The original material; all but obsolete for initial alignment but still valuable as an intermediate wire
17.5 twist steel	Good properties at low cost
19.5 coaxial steel	Properties similar to 17.5 twist steel but higher cost
14 steel with loops	Excellent properties but requires time for fabrication

NOTE: The preferred wire size for a standard fixed appliance setup is indicated. Smaller interbracket spans (wide brackets) or longer spans (missing teeth, very large teeth with narrow brackets) may require a compensatory decrease or increase respectively in wire size. All these wires can be used in the 22-slot edgewise appliance; all but 19.5 coaxial steel are useful in the 18-slot appliance.

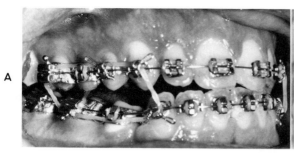
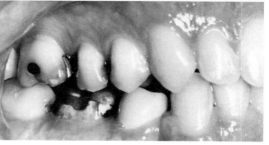

Fig. 6-19. Postsurgical leveling by extrusion. **A,** Working arch wires (16 steel) in place immediately after the surgical stabilizing wires were removed. In this patient with mandibular deficiency and a deep bite, lower first premolars were extracted during the presurgical orthodontics, but the arch deliberately was not leveled. Posterior box elastics (⅜-inch light) are worn full time at this stage, and a cross-elastic to the molars is added if needed, as it was here. **B,** Leveling and postsurgical orthodontics completed 4 months later.

plan for patients with vertical facial disproportions and open bite-overbite problems were discussed in some detail in Chapter 5. The orthodontist must remember that when the mandible is moved forward or back surgically, the vertical position of the lower incisors will determine face height. In short-face patients, where an increase in face height is desired, the lower incisors should not be depressed before surgery. Instead, leveling the arch should be done by extruding canines and premolars, and this usually can be accomplished better after surgery (Fig. 6-19). In a patient with normal or excessive face height, however, leveling the arch by intruding the incisors should be done before surgery. The

goal is to establish, before surgery, the desired postsurgical vertical position of the incisors.

Although there is less variation in the way the orthodontist would manage the upper arch, the same guideline does dictate leveling or lack of it in that location also. For example, a long-face patient with an anterior open bite who will have segmental surgery in the maxilla should not have the upper arch leveled before that surgery. Differential vertical movement of the segments can correct most of the discrepancies, and the object would be to level only within the segments (Fig. 6-20).

For the orthodontist, the difference between leveling

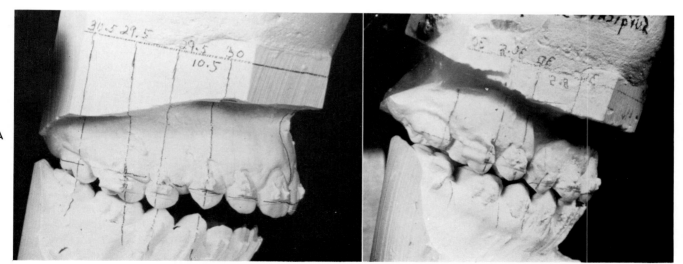

Fig. 6-20. A patient with a vertical discrepancy within the maxillary arch who is being prepared for a three-segment maxillary osteotomy should have leveling only within each segment. It is neither necessary nor desirable to level the entire arch. **A,** Casts mounted on an articulator for model surgery after completion of presurgical orthodontics. Note that the extraction space was partially closed as the correct inclination of the upper incisors was established, but the arch has not been leveled. **B,** Model surgery completed. The leveling is accomplished surgically rather than orthodontically.

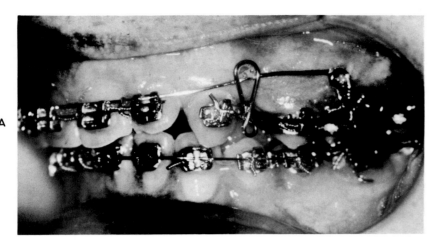
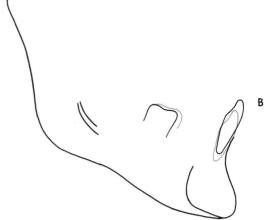

Fig. 6-21. **A,** Burstone intrusion arch to intrude the maxillary incisor segment. The buccal segments are stabilized with a full-dimension rectangular steel segment and also with a lingual arch. The four incisors are controlled with a flexible rectangular segmental wire. The depressing arch (for this patient, 17 × 25 steel with a helical loop; 17 × 25 TMA without the loop is an alternative) fits into the auxiliary tube on the first molars and is tied beneath the anterior segmental wire. Note that the depressing arch is tied distal to the centrals rather than in the midline—the location of the ties is determined by how much tipping of the teeth is desired. **B,** In a patient for whom a similar intrusion arch was used to depress the lower incisors before mandibular advancement, cephalometric superimposition on the mandible shows the excellent ratio between intrusion of the incisors and elongation of the molars obtained in this patient.

by extrusion and leveling by intrusion of incisors is largely a difference between continuous and segmented arch wires. With continuous arch wires, leveling occurs almost entirely by extrusion. A small amount of intrusion of incisors may occur, but the majority of the leveling will occur by elongating the other teeth. Significant depression of incisors is likely to occur only in patients with a short face and powerful masticatory muscles, whose heavy biting force tends to inhibit posterior extrusion. These are the very patients, of course, in whom elongating the infraerupted canines and premolars often is most desired. It is much easier to level the lower arch, especially in these patients, when the teeth to be elongated have been taken out of occlusion by repositioning the jaw at surgery.

Orthodontic intrusion is difficult primarily because light and precisely controlled forces are necessary. Successful intrusion requires a vertically directed force of 10 to 20 gm per tooth, depending on the size of the root (10 to 15 gm for lower incisors, 15 to 20 gm for upper incisors). If heavier forces are applied, intrusion is inhibited and the reaction forces then cause extrusion of the putative anchor teeth. This is the reason that continuous arch wires level largely by extrusion. Over the short interbracket distance between adjacent teeth, even a resilient multistrand or NiTi wire produces forces of 40 to 50 gm or more, too much for intrusion but excellent for extrusion.

The key to intrusion is keeping forces light by in-

creasing the distance between attachments. To intrude incisors, the orthodontist must use an appliance setup in which the arch wire bypasses the canines and premolars, spanning from the molars forward to the incisors (Fig. 6-21). One way to do this is not to place an attachment on the teeth to be bypassed. The other, which is preferable in surgical patients, is to use segments of arch wire to avoid undesirably rigid connections during intrusion. Rigid connections will be needed later, of course, and the appliance must provide that capability when it is required.

Two basically similar but subtly different mechanisms are the primary means of producing intrusion: (1) the utility arch, which is tied into the brackets on the incisor teeth,[21] and (2) the Burstone intrusion arch, which is tied beneath the brackets[22] (Fig. 6-21). Both are attached posteriorly to an auxiliary tube on the first molar. The use of this tube in intrusion is a major reason for having it as a standard part of the orthodontic appliance.

Although both mechanisms are quite effective, the Burstone design is more versatile because the force direction relative to the center of resistance can be varied. As Fig. 6-22 shows, when an intrusion force is applied to the brackets on the central incisor, the teeth tend to tip labially as they intrude because the line of force is anterior to the center of resistance. The utility arch produces just this effect because it is tied into the brackets. An exactly equivalent effect is achieved when

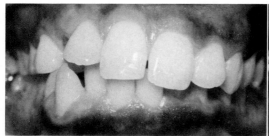

Fig. 6-22. Diagrammatic representation of an intrusion arch. The necessary light force is created by the long span from the molars forward to the incisor region. If the intrusion arch is tied in the midline, or if the utility arch design is used so that the intrusion arch fits into the brackets on the anterior teeth, the line of force is anterior to the center of resistance of the anterior teeth *(line 1)* and the teeth tend to tip labially. If the intrusion arch is tied more distally, as between the lateral and canine on each side *(line 2)*, the line of force is closer to the center of resistance and the tendency to tip is less. If the intrusion arch is tied still more posteriorly *(line 3)*, the teeth may actually tip lingually instead of labially because the line of force is now behind the center of resistance.

the Burstone depressing arch is tied in the midline. The labial tipping can be overcome by lightly cinching back on the utility arch, at the cost of some strain on posterior anchorage. It also is possible to tie the Burstone arch more posteriorly, changing the relationship of the line of force to the center of resistance of the anterior segment so that the teeth do not tip as they intrude, without straining the anchorage. Furthermore, if the teeth within the anterior segment are not vertically aligned, the Burstone design makes it easy to vary the number of teeth to which the intrusion arch is tied. If a vertical asymmetry exists, the auxiliary intrusion arch can be tied on only one side and will then produce an asymmetric intrusion (Fig. 6-23).

Whatever the intrusion mechanism, adequate posterior anchorage is important. Successful intrusion of maxillary incisors requires a buccal stabilizing segment in the molar and premolar brackets; that is, a rectangular steel full-dimension wire. In addition, a transpalatal

lingual arch is needed if more than a minimal amount of intrusion is required. Similar stabilizing segments are required in the mandibular arch, and a stabilizing lingual arch is highly desirable.

Anteroposterior Incisor Position

Just as the position of the incisors vertically will determine postsurgical face height because the surgeon must bring the teeth together at the time of the operation, so the anteroposterior position of the incisors will affect how much the jaws can be moved anteroposteriorly at surgery.

One of the major goals of presurgical orthodontics is to reduce or eliminate dental compensation that would limit surgical correction. As a result, the teeth often are moved during surgical preparation opposite to what would have been needed for nonsurgical treatment. In patients with Class II malocclusion, upper incisors usually are left in their original position or advanced, but lower incisors are retracted. This increases the overjet and thereby increases the distance that the mandible can be advanced surgically and produces better chin-lip balance. In Class III problems, the lower incisors are advanced but the upper incisors retracted, increasing the reverse overjet and the amount of change that can be produced surgically. The effect on treatment planning was discussed in some detail in Chapter 5 but bears repeating here: if extraction of premolars is employed, the approach for surgical orthodontics is often just the opposite of what would have been done with orthodontic treatment alone.

One difference between patients with Class III and Class II problems is that there is an alternative to retracting the protruding lower incisors in the Class II group. Protrusion of the lower incisors is relative to their supporting bone; that is, to the chin. The options therefore are to retract the incisors or to advance the chin via an inferior border osteotomy. In the upper arch, if the incisors protrude, there is little alternative to retracting them—nasal surgery rarely is a feasible substitute. The subtleties of planning treatment that involves removal of dental compensation are explored more fully in the chapters on specific types of problems.

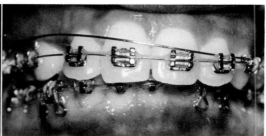

Fig. 6-23. If the anterior segment is vertically asymmetric, as in this patient, an auxiliary depressing arch can be tied only on the side where greater intrusion is needed.

Except that the goal of the treatment often is not to reduce but to increase the overjet or reverse overjet before surgery, the orthodontic mechanotherapy needed to establish presurgical incisor position is no different from what is done in routine treatment. The amount of incisor retraction is a function of the anchorage available, which the orthodontist must control. Either sliding or loop mechanics can be used to vary the anteroposterior position of the incisors, depending on the needs of the patient and the orthodontic appliance that has been selected.

Inevitably, a slight rebound follows orthodontic tooth movement, and this is accentuated by forces against the teeth when patients are in maxillomandibular fixation following surgery. For this reason, modest overtreatment of incisor position is desirable. As a general rule, in preparation for mandibular advancement, retract the lower incisors a millimeter or so further than their desired final position because these teeth will tend to tip forward later. In the same patient, it is better to have the upper incisors slightly prominent—they will tend to tip lingually following the advancement. The reverse is true in preparing for correction of mandibular prognathism: the lower incisors should be slightly prominent, and the upper incisors slightly over-retracted. If a little bit is good, however, a whole lot is not necessarily better. Overtreatment of this type should be minimal.

From a practical perspective, maximum anchorage often is needed in the arch where incisors are to be retracted. Reinforcement of anchorage with lingual arches and/or extraoral force, and the appropriate use of Class III elastics in Class II problems or Class II elastics in Class III problems, can help in achieving the necessary incisor movement. Extraoral force for anchorage control in presurgical treatment rarely is necessary because the teeth in one arch are being retracted while the other arch needs proclination. Interarch elastics usually provide this force very effectively if their vertical side effects can be kept under control. And if the jaws are being repositioned vertically anyway, the extrusive effect of elastics is not a major problem because the surgery can correct it.

Arch Compatibility

The final step in presurgical orthodontics is achieving reasonable arch compatibility so the teeth will fit together satisfactorily after surgery. Similar maxillary and mandibular arch forms and compatible arch widths must be established.

Often the arch form must be changed, particularly in the maxilla. In many patients with mandibular deficiency and excessive overjet, the maxillary arch is narrow and V-shaped, constricted across the canines and premolars. The same individuals usually have a more ovoid mandibular arch. The reverse pattern of a ta-

pered mandibular and a more rounded maxillary arch may occur in Class III patients with negative overjet, though less severely. During the presurgical orthodontics, it is necessary to expand the constricted areas in the more tapered arch, and to do this, relatively heavy rectangular arch wires are required.

If arch wires with coordinated arch forms are used during the progression toward the full-dimension rectangular wires used for stabilization at surgery (see Table 6-3), arch compatibility is produced almost automatically—but keep in mind that changes in arch form occur slowly and that the larger wires must be in place for more than a few weeks to accomplish this change. When major changes are needed, exaggerating the arch form in intermediate wires can help. If the teeth are merely tipped buccally, the lingual cusps will be elongated and interferences may result, so rectangular arch wires and torque control are necessary. Occasionally, a heavy labial auxiliary placed in the headgear tubes can help to accentuate the effect of the lighter base arch wire.

Dental expansion of constricted areas within an arch is easier to acccomplish than expansion across the molars. Torquing the molars out is difficult, but interferences from lingual cusps are likely to be a problem if torque is inadequate. In surgical-orthodontic patients, skeletal expansion at surgery is an option. As a general rule, orthodontic expansion should be limited to 2 to 3 mm per side (4 to 5 mm total); that is, not more than a half-cusp crossbite. If this is not adequate, segmental surgery will be needed.

On the other hand, when orthodontic expansion would be sufficient, it does not have to be done before surgery, and often it is easier to do this postsurgically. Before surgery, the existing occlusion often opposes the expansion; afterward, there are no interferences. When splints are used as outlined below, perfect transverse compatibility of the arches is not necessary at surgery. The guideline is that not more than a half-cusp crossbite should be left for postsurgical corrrection.

Up to that amount of transverse change can be produced relatively easily and predictably. More than that amount is likely to be a problem. Judging arch compatibility clinically can be difficult. When mandibular advancement is planned, patients can hold their mandible forward so the orthodontist can judge the transverse relationships, but usually only the anterior teeth come into contact, and molar widths have to be estimated. In patients who will have maxillary surgery or mandibular setback, the only way to check compatibility is to take study casts. Doing this toward the end of the presurgical orthodontics, before sending the patient for the final presurgical records, can prevent surprises at that late stage (see below).

At the conclusion of presurgical orthodontics, when the goals outlined here have been met, the patient

TABLE 6-3 Typical arch wire sequences before surgery (wire sizes in mils)	
18 slot	**22 slot**
1. 16 NiTi (austenitic) or 14 steel loops (asymmetric crowding)	17.5 twist steel or 16 NiTi (austenitic) (severe crowding)
2. 16 steel	16 steel 18 steel
3. 17 × 25 TMA	21 × 25 TMA
4. 17 × 25 steel	21 × 25 steel

should be in full-dimension rectangular steel arch wires. These arch wires, which produce the final presurgical alignment and establish arch compatibility, also will be used for stabilization at surgery. Typical arch wire sequences during presurgical orthodontics are outlined in Table 6-3.

FINAL SURGICAL PLANNING AND PREPARATION
Presurgery Records

When the orthodontist feels that the presurgical orthodontics are complete, the next step is to obtain the records necessary for the final surgical planning. At a minimum, these include panoramic and lateral cephalometric radiographs, dental casts, and facial and intraoral photographs. If there is significant asymmetry, a PA cephalometric film will be needed. The panoramic film is used to verify that root positions will not interfere with any planned osteotomy cuts and to check for any pathologic changes that might have developed. This film is supplemented with periapical radiographs to view interdental osteotomy sites. The cephalometric film is necessary so that the cephalometric predictions can be repeated in preparation for model surgery, and the dental casts are required for use in the model surgery itself. If a total or posterior maxillary osteotomy is planned, or if the mandibular dental arch will be segmented or interrupted as with a subapical or body osteotomy, a facebow transfer for articulator mounting of the casts is necessary (see further discussion below).

An ideal time to obtain the final presurgical records is approximately 2 weeks before the tentative surgery date, after the final rectangular orthodontic arch wires have been in place long enough to be passive (ideally, 3 weeks or more). At that point, the arch wires are removed temporarily to have lugs added for interarch stabilization (which is necessary unless integral hooks are used throughout the appliance). The impressions then can be taken with the arch wires out, providing

better casts for the model surgery and splints. The other records can be obtained at the same appointment.

Cephalometric Predictions and Model Surgery

The final surgical planning must include both cephalometric prediction and model surgery, in that order. The surgeon has the major responsibility for carrying out these steps. The cephalometric predictions are done in precisely the same fashion described in Chapter 5, using the manual or computer method most appropriate for the particular situation. Cephalometric prediction must be done before the model surgery because information from it is needed to position the casts.

A key question for model surgery is whether and when it is necessary to use a facebow transfer to mount the casts on a semiadjustable articulator so that the condyle-tooth relationships are recorded. The answer is that this depends on the type of surgery. If the condyles will be separated from the dentition by the mandibular surgery, there is no advantage in maintaining this relationship while doing the model surgery. For this reason, an arbitrary articulator is quite satisfactory for dental-cast simulation of mandibular ramus surgery. But if the condyle-dentition relationship will be preserved at surgery and the mandible will rotate to a new position, which occurs primarily when the posterior or total maxilla is repositioned, it is important for this rotation to be simulated as accurately as possible. Then the casts should be mounted on a semiadjustable articulator. Remember that in two-jaw surgery, the mandibular position with the condyles intact is the guide for repositioning the maxilla before mandibular surgery is completed.

In model surgery to simulate mandibular rotation after repositioning of the maxilla, the first step is to measure from the cephalometric prediction tracings the anteroposterior and vertical movement of the maxillary central incisor and first molar so that the same movements can be made on the mounted casts. A facebow transfer is used to mount the casts on the articulator; the maxillary teeth are cut off the cast, in one piece if a one-piece maxillary osteotomy is planned, or in the planned segments if segmental osteotomies are included; and the model surgery is carried out as shown in Fig. 6-24. The measurements and tooth relationships on the mounted casts and the prediction tracing should be the same. If they are, it is good assurance that the surgery actually will turn out as predicted. If they are not, an error has been made in either the cephalometric prediction or the cast simulation, and both should be checked to find and eliminate it.

The model surgery serves two purposes: (1) to verify that the planned movements are possible, and (2) to relate the casts in the position where the occlusal wafer splints for surgery will be made. Once both the surgeon

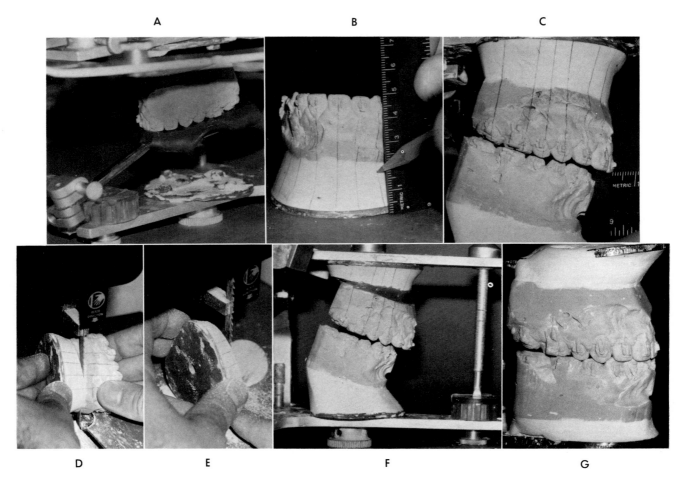

Fig. 6-24. The steps in model surgery for a patient who will have a total maxillary osteotomy and a mandibular advancement. **A,** The casts are mounted on a semiadjustable articulator, using a facebow transfer. **B,** Reference lines are drawn on the mounted casts, and the distance from the mounting rim to each cusp is recorded. **C,** The distance from the articulator pin to the incisal edge of the maxillary central incisor also is measured and recorded so that the magnitude of all movements can be evaluated precisely. **D,** The upper cast is cut away from the mounting ring, using a saw. **E,** An additional wedge of mounting material is cut away, giving room to reposition the upper cast vertically. **F,** The upper cast is remounted in the desired position, with the measurements checked against the cephalometric prediction for this patient. This is the projected result of the first stage of the surgery, and an intermediate splint is made to this mounting (after the upper cast is stabilized with plaster in its final position). **G,** The casts are mounted as they will be after the second stage of the surgery, the mandibular advancement. The second splint is made to this mounting. Note the position of the upper second molars, which were deliberately kept depressed during the orthodontic preparation so there would be no problems with second-molar interferences at this stage.

and orthodontist are satisfied with the position of the teeth, the dental casts must be held firmly together while the splint is made so that this relationship can be duplicated precisely in the operating room. This means that the casts, which were held with wax during the model surgery so that changes could be made, must be stabilized with plaster or stone before the splints are made.

If both jaws are to be repositioned (see Fig. 6-24), the maxillary cast is moved first and fixed on the articulator. This position generates the first occlusal wafer splint for surgery (or the first stage of a two-stage splint). Then the mandibular cast is repositioned to oppose the maxillary cast. It is easier to use a second identical set of casts, mounted in a hinge-type articulator, for this second stage. If either the mandibular or maxillary cast has been segmented, the second-stage cast is made from the first cast (rather than from the original impression). The final occlusal wafer splint (or the second stage of a combined splint) is constructed

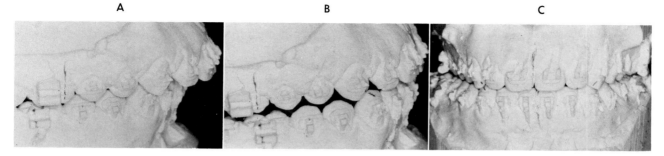

Fig. 6-25. At model surgery in a girl scheduled for mandibular advancement, interference because the maxillary canines are slightly narrow causes too much opening of the bite anteriorly. **A,** Presurgical occlusion. **B,** Model surgery, lateral view. **C,** Model surgery, frontal view. The alternatives are to delay surgery while the canines are stepped out, remove the interferences with grinding, or accept the position shown and manage the occlusion postsurgically. The third alternative was possible in this case because of the relatively minor problem, but with major interferences, delaying the surgery for a few weeks while the teeth are repositioned slightly often is the best solution.

using the casts positioned as they will be at the completion of surgery. The details of splint construction are illustrated in Chapters 7 and 11.

Prediction tracing and model surgery must be done very carefully. The best orthodontics and the most skillful surgery can be negated by poor presurgical planning. Both the orthodontist and the surgeon should be satisfied with positions of the teeth and jaws at this stage as predicted by tracings and model surgery.

Common Problems at this Stage

Although it is unlikely that problems requiring further orthodontics will be uncovered at model surgery, one of the reasons for doing model surgery is to discover precisely that sort of problem. If dental interferences would prevent putting the jaws or jaw segments in the right place, there is no alternative to correcting them orthodontically before proceeding with surgery. In our experience, there is approximately 1 chance in 20 that preliminary model surgery will show a need for additional orthodontic treatment.

By far the most common problem encountered at the stage of model surgery is interferences on second molar teeth (see Fig. 6-12). Interestingly enough, these problems usually relate to a *lack* of bands on the lower second molars or to the *presence* of bands on upper second molars. The orthodontist should band lower second molars early in treatment and align them with the first molars if they are elongated, as they usually are in mandibular deficiency. On the other hand, upper second molars usually are above the occlusal plane. Elongating them is a mistake, but this will happen if these teeth are banded and a straight arch wire is placed. The upper second molars should remain ramped upward to prevent interferences at surgery; they easily can be settled into position postsurgically.

Elongated second molars can be a serious problem, not just a trivial one. If these teeth force the mandible down posteriorly, the mandibular ramus may be elongated at surgery, a major source of instability. Sometimes the molar interference can be eliminated by reducing cusp heights with a dental stone in a handpiece. If severe grinding would be required, it is far better for the orthodontist to temporarily go back to a lighter arch wire and step the molars to their proper position.

A second relatively frequent problem at model surgery is incompatible canine widths. The orthodontist can observe whether canine widths are compatible by having the patient posture the jaw forward before surgery, so this rarely is a problem in Class II patients, but it does occur (Fig. 6-25). (The molars usually do not touch when the mandible is postured forward. It is not possible to observe the type of second-molar interferences alluded to above, hence their occasional discovery only at model surgery.) Class III patients, who cannot simulate the postsurgical position, are most likely to have unsuspected canine interferences at model surgery. The typical problem is a maxillary intercanine width that is slightly narrow relative to the mandibular width, so that the casts cannot be positioned without creating an anterior open bite. In that circumstance, there may be no good alternative to expanding the upper canines a bit more before surgery.

A third potential problem at model sugery is lack of space for interdental osteotomy cuts (see Fig. 6-11). The surgeon needs 4 to 5 mm of separation of roots to cut between them without undue risk of problems. Problems with root proximity usually result from improper orthodontic bracket placement that caused root movement that was not detected clinically. In this circumstance also, no choice exists but to go back to orthodontics to open the necessary space.

Whenever problems are discovered at model surgery,

the temptation is to try to work around them, either by reshaping teeth or changing the jaw position at surgery. Rescheduling the surgery to make some orthodontic change is at best a nuisance and at worst a public relations problem because the patient is annoyed. On the other hand, the surgeon, the orthodontist, and the patient need to remember that total treatment time, not the precise date of the surgery, is the important variable. Getting things set up properly often means accepting a few more weeks of presurgical orthodontics to avoid what could be months of additional finishing orthodontics and a compromised result.

Stabilizing Arch Wires and Splints

As a practical matter, passive stabilizing arch wires are in place at the time the model surgery is done (and will have to be removed and adjusted if any further changes turn out to be needed) (see Table 6-3). It is logical to discuss them and the surgical splints at the same time because both contribute significantly to stabilization following surgery. Although it is not strictly necessary to have an orthodontic arch wire in place at the time of surgery, this provides so much better control than the alternatives that it is preferred when possible.

The stabilizing arch wire should have the following characteristics.

1. Full-dimension rectangular wire; that is, at least 21×25 in a 22-slot appliance and 17×25 in an 18-slot appliance. The effectiveness of stabilization is to a large extent determined by how tightly the wire fits within the bracket, and round wires or smaller rectangular wires do not provide the same degree of stabilization. No problems usually occur in fitting a 17×25 steel wire into an 18-slot appliance, but many orthodontists, recognizing the extreme stiffness of 21×25 steel, are reluctant to use so heavy an arch wire. A 19×25 wire is better than nothing, but does not give the control of 21×25 wire. One way to deal with the excessive stiffness of 21×25 steel is to substitute 21×25 TMA, either as the surgical stabilizing wire or as an intermediate before placing 21×25 steel, which then will fit passively enough to be accepted by the patient with reasonable comfort.
2. Attachments for maxillomandibular fixation. Even if maxillomandibular fixation will be used only briefly or not at all following surgery, it is necessary for the surgeon to tie the teeth together into the splint during the final stages of the operation, and hooks must be provided for this purpose. These are even more critical for RIF (see Chapter 7). With modern appliances, integral hooks incorporated into the brackets often are employed, and these are quite helpful during the postsurgical orthodontics. For maxillomandibular fixation at surgery, however, attachments on the arch wire are preferred,

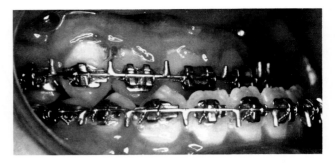

Fig. 6-26. Stabilizing arch wires with soldered brass hooks, in place just before surgery.

particularly when multiple dentoalveolar segments will be created at surgery.

Modified ligature hooks on the brackets (Kobayashi hooks) are quite satisfactory for attaching orthodontic elastics and are excellent during presurgical and postsurgical orthodontics, but they are prone to distort at critical times during the surgery itself. The ease with which they can be placed does not make up for potential problems in the operating room.

Soldered brass spurs are the preferred attachments to the arch wire itself (Fig. 6-26). These are placed in each interproximal area where there is no integral hook, except that in the lower arch there is no need to place a hook between the central and lateral incisors. An alternative is commercially prepared slide-on hooks that can be welded or soldered into position. The slide-on hooks are satisfactory only if they are firmly attached; they must not be left to slip around on the arch wire.

Crimp-on hooks, which can be placed over the stabilizing arch wire without removing it, are a tempting but dangerous option. Two big problems exist with these hooks. First, crimping alone may not hold the hook tightly enough in position, so that it slips in the operating room at a critical time when segments are being manipulated into place. Second and even worse, the act of crimping the hook over the arch wire has the potential to distort the wire, and if the hook is placed without removing the arch wire from the mouth, the distortion probably will not be noted. The result is likely to be a cascade of problems, starting with a splint that does not fit properly in the operating room.

The stabilizing wire must fit passively to be effective. If it creates any tooth movement after the model-surgery/splint-construction impressions have been made, the splint will not fit. The one circumstance in which it is better judgment to take the patient to surgery with no wire at all is when the surgery must be done and a well-fitting rectangular wire is not available (lost, destroyed, or just never made for whatever reason). A new rectangular wire inevitably will not be completely passive, and no wire at all is better than one that creates tooth movement just before surgery. In that case,

A   B   C

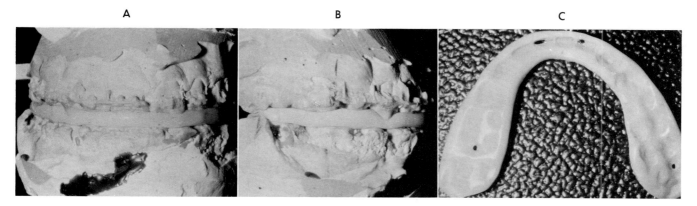

Fig. 6-27. **A-C,** Frontal, lateral, and occlusal views of the splint for a patient with a deep-bite, mandibular-deficiency problem whose lower arch will be leveled postsurgically. In this case, the splint is the thinnest possible: the teeth cut through it both anteriorly and posteriorly. The thickness of the splint in the middle part of the arch is adequate for strength. If the arches are level, approximately 2 mm separation of the teeth is correct.

the orthodontic attachments on the teeth and the splint can give adequate if inferior stabilization. If multiple dental segments are planned at surgery, consideration must be given to delaying surgery until a new passive arch wire is in place and model surgery can be repeated.

An occlusal wafer splint is used in the operating room to help in positioning the teeth and add to stabilization. The splint is made on the dental casts that show the result from the model surgery—the second reason for doing the model surgery is to enable construction of the splint, as has been discussed. Remember that the casts must be stabilized after the model surgery so that they cannot shift while the splint is being made.

Although it is not strictly necessary to have one, splints have such significant advantages that we recommend using them routinely. With a splint, the teeth can be put in any desired position, and there is no judgment in the operating room as to exactly how the teeth are supposed to fit. Without one, the teeth must be put in a position where there is some reasonably stable occlusion, and the surgeon may have to choose among several options for positioning the jaws without being able to assess midlines and posterior symmetry.

All other things being equal, the splint should be thin, producing the least amount of separation of the teeth that is compatible with the other objectives of the surgery. The reason is simple: the thicker the splint, the greater the possibility of error as the mandible rotates into occlusion when the splint is removed. The splint for a patient with a deep bite and a lower arch that will be leveled postsurgically can have the teeth cut all the way through it at the terminal molars and at one or two points anteriorly (Fig. 6-27). This is feasible because the splint will be thick enough along the rest of

the occlusal table to give it adequate strength. For other patients whose arches have been leveled before surgery, the thinnest practical splint has 1 to 2 mm of material between the teeth, the minimum necessary to keep the splint from breaking easily while it is being used. A wire in the edge of the splint can be added to provide greater strength if the splint is quite thin.

A uniformly thick splint rarely is a good idea, but occasionally it is desirable to make the splint thicker in one area than in another. For instance, if the patient has a vertical asymmetry that will be corrected by mandibular surgery only, the splint will have to be made thicker on the previously short side so that there will be a space into which those teeth can be extruded postsurgically (see Chapter 2, Fig. 2-3). With mandibular advancement or setback, some feel it is desirable to make the splint slightly thicker posteriorly than anteriorly so as to leave some room for upward displacement of the condyle when function begins. If this is done at all, it should be only in patients who will have wire osteosynthesis and maxillomandibular fixation, and then we recommend that the posterior separation be only slightly greater (2 mm or less) than is the anterior. If rigid internal fixation is used, there should be no additional separation of the posterior teeth. Too much posterior interocclusal space can become a problem during the orthodontic finishing if the surgeon correctly seats the condyle during the operation and no superior condylar movement follows.

The patient should wear the splint until he or she returns to the orthodontist for the postsurgical orthodontics. Removing it too soon can cause major problems in finishing the orthodontic treatment (see discussion below). With RIF, the patient may be allowed to resume jaw function well before the final phase of orthodontics starts, but the splint should be tied to the maxillary (usually) or mandibular arch so that the patient continues to function into it, guided by elastics. Modifications of the splint for use in function are discussed in Chapter 7. Special splint modifications also are discussed in later chapters.

SURGICAL AND POSTOPERATIVE CARE

The patient's care during surgery and the immediate postsurgical period is covered in detail in Chapter 7. The following discussion of the hospital experience, the early healing phases, and the period of rehabilitation focuses on the interaction among the orthodontist, surgeon, and patient at those times.

The surgeon must explain to the patient the events surrounding surgery and the weeks immediately following. At the time of initial case presentation, these topics can be covered in a general way, with only the steps in the planned surgery, usual sequelae, and complications explained in detail. Immediately before surgery, these topics are reviewed again with more detail on the hospital stay and the subsequent period. Often during the period of presurgical orthodontics, the orthodontist is asked questions regarding surgery and the hospital. Some questions are easily answered, but the orthodontist should defer complex questions to the surgeon. Having the patient make a list is a good way to ensure that legitimate questions are not ignored or forgotten.

Some orthognathic surgery procedures (e.g., mandibular inferior border osteotomy), do not require an overnight stay if a responsible adult is available to help the patient in the immediate postsurgical period. If any question exists about the postoperative care, the patient should remain in the hospital overnight after surgery. Additionally, more patients are now being admitted to the hospital on the day of surgery in preference to spending the night before in the hospital.

This choice is the patient's if no medical reason exists to dictate otherwise. Most of the presurgical evaluation, including ancillary laboratory tests, autologous blood donation, history and physical exam, and anesthesiology consultation, can be accomplished as an outpatient on the days preceding surgery. In some cases, third-party insurance carriers dictate that the patient be admitted on the day of surgery, and a maximum length of stay also is prescribed. Typically, orthognathic-surgery patients are hospitalized 2 to 3 days for one-jaw surgery and 3 to 4 days for two-jaw procedures, with a range for both of 2 to 6 days.[23]

Following discharge from the hospital, most patients return to at least limited activity within 2 weeks following surgery, and some are back to work at 1 week. Most facial edema is gone in 2 to 3 weeks, and the the final edema resolves as the patient returns to full jaw function, which occurs more quickly with the early jaw function allowed with rigid fixation. The jaws may not be healed enough for mastication until 6 to 8 weeks after surgery, and full bony remodeling takes 6 months or longer. Specific recommendations about rehabilitation and information regarding postsurgery sequelae are found in the chapters on surgical principles and techniques (Chapters 7 through 11).

POSTSURGICAL ORTHODONTICS

Postsurgical orthodontics can begin when the surgeon thinks the healing has reached the point of satisfactory clinical stability. With wire osteosynthesis and maxillomandibular fixation, clinical healing to this level requires 6 to 8 weeks after mandibular osteotomy, perhaps a bit less with maxillary osteotomy. With RIF, healing probably does not occur more quickly, but the bony segments are more stable from the beginning, allowing the patient limited early function. Finishing orthodontics may be possible at 4 or even 3 weeks after surgery, rather than beginning at 6 to 8 weeks. This remains a matter of the surgeon's judgment, pending more information on healing and rehabilitation with rigid fixation.

If there is doubt about the healing, it is better to err on the side of caution and delay. In the context of a total treatment time of 15 to 21 months, which is typical for surgical-orthodontic patients, 1 or 2 weeks for additional healing after surgery is trivial, particularly if problems might arise because of premature orthodontic forces that ultimately could delay completion.

The first step in postsurgical orthodontics is to remove the splint and the stabilizing arch wires (Fig. 6-28). These should be removed at the same time, by the orthodontist, who can immediately make any necessary repairs to the orthodontic appliance (it is not unusual to have a loose band or bracket at this stage) and then place the working orthodontic arch wires that are needed.

This sequence is important. Remember that the purpose of the stabilizing arch wires is to prevent the movement of teeth. The combination of the heavy arch wires and interocclusal splint gives the maximum resistance to tooth movement while at the same time providing the patient a solid occlusion with multiple contacts. So long as the splint is in place, the patient has maximum intercuspation at the position established at surgery, which should be centric relation or very close to it. When the splint is removed but the stabilizing arch wires remain, the teeth are held rigidly, often in a position where only two or three teeth contact when the mandibular condyles are seated. Then the patient unconsciously searches for a new habitual occlusal position that gives greater intercuspation.

In short, the price of removing the splint without taking out the stabilizing arch wires can be a centric relation-centric occlusion discrepancy that complicates the postsurgical orthodontics. The surgeon has just

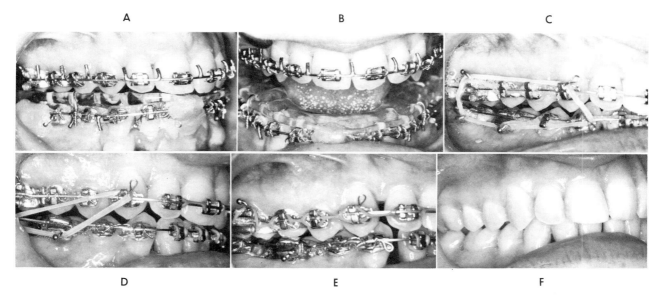

Fig. 6-28. The sequence of postsurgical orthodontics in a typical deep-bite, mandibular-advancement patient. **A** and **B,** Patient functioning into the splint (here tied to the lower arch) at the time of return to the orthodontist 5 weeks after surgery. **C,** Same appointment, working arch wires (16 steel) and posterior box elastics in place. The elastics are worn full time including eating. **D,** Four weeks later, with the light wires replaced by rectangular ones and a Class II component to the elastics. **E,** Four weeks later. **F,** Appliances removed, 2 months later.

gone to great lengths to prevent that by working to seat the condyles at surgery. Allowing a shift to develop by removing the splint too soon or by failing to remove the stabilizing wires when it is time to remove the splint is counterproductive.

The first postsurgical orthodontic appointment is necessarily a long one. The splint must be removed, arch wires changed, and repairs made to appliances if necessary. For this reason, the surgeon cannot simply decide that the patient is ready and unexpectedly send him or her back to the orthodontist, at least not if the necessary work is to be done that day. There are two satisfactory ways to coordinate the return to the orthodontist. The best is for the surgeon to provide at least a few days' notice so the orthodontist can set up the long appointment. Failing that, the patient should arrive to see the orthodontist with the splint still in place. The orthodontist then has the option to go ahead with all the appliance changes if there is time, or to reschedule the patient a few days later if there is not. A problem arises only if the surgeon has removed the splint. In that case, there is no option but to go ahead with the arch wire changes, or take a chance on centric relation-centric occlusion problems.

Once the splint and stabilizing wires have been removed, the orthodontist needs to place working arch wires and begin the process of settling the teeth into full occlusion. Typical working wires are 16 steel, which are flexible enough to produce the necessary

elongation of some teeth (see Fig. 6-28). When torque control of maxillary anterior teeth is particularly needed, it may be better to use a flexible rectangular arch wire—braided multistrand steel or NiTi are good choices. If movement of teeth in only the lower arch is desired, the stabilizing arch wire can be retained in the upper arch and a flexible wire placed only in the lower.

The final step at the first postsurgical appointment is placing the patient on light vertical elastics to the posterior segments and also to the anterior segment if there is any open-bite tendency. Modified ligature ties (Kobayashi hooks) are an excellent way to provide attachments for these elastics. Patients find it easier to place one large elastic than two or three small ones, so usually it is better to use a ⅜-inch box elastic (Fig. 6-29). Initially, these elastics should be worn even when eating, if the patient will accept that—most will, with no problem—and at all other times without exception.

The elastics serve two purposes. First, they help bring the teeth into a solid occlusion, reinforcing the settling produced by the arch wires. Equally important, they override the patient's proprioceptive drive toward positioning the mandible in maximum intercuspation. As long as the elastics are being worn, there will not be a tendency to shift into a relationship that is different from the centric relation.

It may be desirable to run the posterior box elastics in a Class II or Class III direction, rather than straight vertically, if the postsurgical occlusion is slightly off in

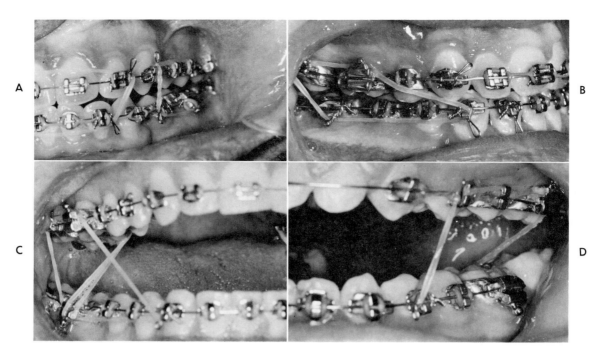

Fig. 6-29. Elastic use in postsurgical orthodontics. **A,** Typical use of anterior and posterior box elastics at the first postsurgical orthodontic appointment. The posterior elastics are worn full time, the anterior elastics only at night in most cases. **B,** Posterior box elastics in a Class III pattern, settling molars into occlusion. **C,** Posterior cross-elastic added to the box elastics to correct a mild postsurgical crossbite. **D,** An alternative when crossbite is present is to attach one corner of the box elastic lingually.

one direction or the other (see Fig. 6-29). It may also be desirable to begin correcting a posterior crossbite tendency. A separate cross-elastic is one possibility, and hooking one corner of the posterior box on the lingual rather than the buccal is another.

By the second postsurgical appointment, considerable settling typically has occurred and maximum intercuspation already is at the desired jaw position (see Fig. 6-28). It is no longer necessary to wear the box elastics as consistently. They can be omitted while eating in nearly every case, and if the occlusion has settled well, can be worn only at night. At this point, small vertical-step bends in the working arch wires may be needed to allow some teeth to come into occlusion.

By the third appointment, the teeth usually have settled into occlusion. For some patients, the postsurgical orthodontics is essentially completed at this point. Most will require at least one more set of minor adjustments in the arch wires, but will not need to go back to heavier rectangular arch wires. If there is enough of an anteroposterior discrepancy that heavier Class II or III elastics will be needed, it usually is good judgment to place rectangular arch wires before increasing the elastic force. By this time, the finishing problems for a surgery patient are not different from what is encountered in routine orthodontic treatment, and the use of elas-

tics and arch wires is the same as it would be in any patient.

An important special point during orthodontic finishing is the management of patients who have had transverse expansion of the maxilla at surgery. The maxillary expansion is unstable for approximately 6 months. If the stabilizing arch wires are replaced with light round working arch wires after a few weeks, as is necessary for settling the patient into good occlusion, there is nothing to prevent transverse relapse, and this can happen distressingly quickly. Transverse control can be maintained by using a heavy labial auxiliary wire (36 mil or heavier), which is placed in the headgear tubes on the molar bands (Fig. 6-30). Because it does not contact the other teeth, such an auxiliary arch does not interfere with vertical settling. It should be maintained until arch wires stiff enough to maintain control of arch form are placed or until the patient is ready for retainers.

As with any orthodontic patient who has worn interarch elastics, it is a good idea to observe the patient without elastics for 4 to 6 weeks after the final occlusion apparently has been achieved before removing the appliances, to ensure that there are no unsuspected relapse tendencies or shifts in occlusion. In a typical uncomplicated case, the patient is ready for appliance re-

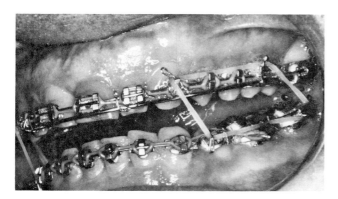

Fig. 6-30. If the maxillary arch has been expanded surgically, as in this patient who had a two-segment maxillary osteotomy in addition to mandibular advancement, it is important to maintain the width during the finishing orthodontics. The light orthodontic arch wires used for finishing are not stiff enough for this requirement. The problem can be overcome by maintaining a heavy labial wire (typically 36 mil) in the headgear tubes while light working arch wires and vertical elastics are used to settle the teeth into occlusion and complete the leveling of the lower arch.

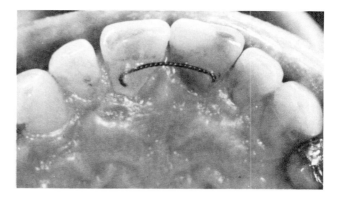

Fig. 6-31. If a maxillary midline diastema has been closed during surgical-orthodontic treatment, and particularly if a two-segment maxillary osteotomy has been used to widen the maxilla in such a patient, permanent retention is needed to keep the space closed. A bonded but slightly flexible wire, used here in the same patient shown in Fig. 6-30, is the preferred method.

moval and retainers 4 months after returning for postsurgical orthodontic treatment. The minimum is 3 months. If postsurgical orthodontics take longer than 6 months, either complications have arisen at some point or the patient was not sufficiently prepared before the surgery.

Although there is nothing wrong with using a positioner in a surgical patient as the final finishing step, this rarely is necessary if the procedure outlined above has been followed because the elastics and flexible arch wires bring the teeth into tight occlusion. Compared with routine patients, postsurgical patients may have increased difficulty in adapting to a positioner for two reasons: (1) some areas of paresthesia may still be present in the gingiva and/or lips a few months postsurgically, at the time a positioner would be used, and (2) biting force is variably affected by surgery.[24] If bite force decreases, as sometimes occurs, the positioner would be less effective. As a general rule, using elastics for final settling of the occlusion, perhaps with the posterior segments of the wires removed for a few days, and then going directly to a retainer is better for surgery patients.

RETENTION

Except for particular care to prevent transverse relapse in patients who had surgical maxillary expansion, there is nothing special about retention in surgical patients. As with everyone who has had fixed-appliance therapy, retainers should be worn full time except during eating for 3 to 4 months after the appliances are removed. It takes that long for reorganization of the pe-

riodontal ligament to be completed. Unless there is severe periodontal breakdown, in which case a full-time splint is preferred, it is counterproductive to have a patient wear a retainer while eating because periodontal ligament (PDL) reorganization is impeded by having teeth splinted together. The splinting produced by an orthodontic appliance is part of the reason for the PDL changes that persist after active tooth movement is completed. The teeth need to move independently of each other in function to develop the optimal ligament-bone interface.

After 3 to 4 months, the amount of time the retainers are worn can be reduced, and if the teeth are stable, retention can be discontinued a few months thereafter. If they are not stable, part-time retention may be needed indefinitely. In that case, it may be wise to consider a fixed rather than a removable retainer. A fixed retainer is often the only way to keep a maxillary midline diastema closed, and a bonded wire can maintain many other dental corrections that are almost impossible to keep from partial relapse with removable retainers (Fig. 6-31).

The broad outline of treatment provided in this chapter is meant to outline principles that can be applied to all types of dentofacial deformity treatment. More details of specific approaches to various types of problems are provided in the clinical chapters that follow.

REFERENCES

1. Chumbley AB, Tuncay OC: The effect of indomethacin (an aspirin like drug) on the rate of orthodontic tooth movement, Am J Orthod 89:312-314, 1986.

2. Horrobin DF, Manku MS: Roles of prostaglandins suggested by the prostaglandin agonist/antagonist actions of local anaesthetic, anti-arrhymthic, anti-malarial, tricyclic anti-depressant and methyl xanthine compounds. Effects on membrances and on nucleic acid function, Med Hypotheses 3:71-86, 1977.

3. Manku MS, Horrobin DF: Chloroquine, quinine, procaine, quinidine, tricyclic antidepressants, and methylxanthines as prostaglandin agonists and antagonists, Lancet 2:1115-1117, 1976.

4. Hwang EC, van Woert MH: Role of prostaglandins in the antimyoclonic action of clonazepam, Eur J Pharmacol 71:161-164, 1981.

5. Modeer T, Dahllof G: Development of phenytoin-induced gingival overgrowth in non-institutionalized epileptic children subjected to different plaque control programs, Acta Odontol Scand 45:81-85, 1987.

6. Strateman MW, Shannon IL: Control of decalcification in orthodontic patients by daily self-administered application of a water-free 0.4 per cent stannous fluoride, Am J Orthod 66:273-279, 1974.

7. Glavind L, Zeuner E: The effectiveness of a rotary electric toothbrush on oral cleanliness in adults, J Clin Periodontol 13:135-138, 1986.

8. van Venrooy JR, Phillips C, Christensen J, Mayhew M: Plaque removal with a new powered toothbrush for orthodontic patients in fixed appliances, Compendium Contin Educ Dent Suppl 6:S142-S146, 1985.

9. Smith GA, McInnes-Ledoux P, Ledoux WR, et al: Orthodontic bonding to procelain—bond strength and refinishing, Am J Orthod Dentofacial Orthop 94:245-252, 1988.

10. Douglass CW, Gillings D, Sollecito W, Gammon M: The 1960 to 1962 and the most recent national health surveys are compared in an indepth analysis to determine trends of periodontal diseases in the United States, J Am Dent Assoc 107:403-412, 1983.

11. Lindhe, J: Textbook of clinical periodontology, Copenhagen, 1983, Munksgaard, International Booksellers & Publishers, Ltd.

12. Becker W, Becker BE, Berg LE: Periodontal treatment without maintenance, J Periodontol 55:505-509, 1984.

13. Walsh MM, Buchanan SA, Hoover CI, et al: Clinical and microbiologic effects of single-dose metronidazole or scaling and root planing in treatment of adult periodontitis, J Clin Periodontol 13:151-17, 1986.

14. Eakle WS, Ford C, Boyd RL: Depth of penetration in periodontal pockets with oral irrigation, J Clin Periodontol 13:39-44, 1986.

15. McDonald F, Yap WL: The surgical exposure and application of direct traction of unerupted teeth, Am J Orthod 89:331-340, 1986.

16. Gorman JC: Treatment of adults with lingual orthodontic appliance, Dent Clin North Am 32:589-620, 1988.

17. Sinclair PM, Cannito MF, Goates LJ, et al: Patient responses to lingual appliances, J Clin Orthod 20:396-404, 1986.

18. Scott GE, Jr: Fracture toughness and surface cracks. The key to understanding ceramic brackets, Angle Orthod 58:5-8, 1988.

19. Burstone CJ, Qin B, Morton JY: Chinese NiTi wire—a new orthodontic alloy, Am J Orthod 87:445-452, 1985.

20. Miura F, Moga M, Ohura Y, et al: The super-elastic Japanese NiTi alloy wire for use in orthodontics, Am J Orthod Dentofacial Orthop 94:89-96, 1988.

21. Ricketts RM, Bench RW, Hilgers JJ: Mandibular utility arch. The basic arch in the light progressive technique, Proc Found Orthod Res pp. 130-125, 1972.

22. Burstone CR: Deep overbite correction by intrusion, Am J Orthod 72:1-22, 1977.

23. Dolan P, White RP, Jr, Tulloch JFC: An analysis of hospital charges for orthognathic surgery, Int J Adult Orthod Orthognath Surg 2:9-14, 1987.

24. Proffit WR, Turvey TA, Fields HW, Phillips C: The effect of orthognathic surgery on occlusal force, J Oral Maxillofac Surg [in press].

SURGICAL TREATMENT

Surgical procedures for repositioning the mandible and maxilla were described early in this century and have been performed with increasing frequency since 1950. Improved methods in anesthesia, pre- and postoperative surgical care, surgical instrumentation, and surgical technique have led to the routine and successful use of surgical procedures for correcting discrepancies in the size and position of the jaws. For two decades before 1965, surgeons had managed deformities of the mandible largely through extraoral incisions. The work of Kole, Walker and Murphey, and Mohnac coupled with the special impetus given to the field by Obwegeser's seminars in the United States in 1965 and his publications in the English language heightened the interest in intraoral orthognathic surgical procedures.[1-4] The work of these pioneers coupled with the work of Bell in the early 1970s developed important surgical principles for intraoral surgery which are the basis for the array of surgical procedures in common use today.[5]

The first chapter in this section presents accepted surgical principles for managing orthognathic surgery patients. The discussion is particularly informative for orthodontists and other nonsurgeons who may not be familiar with the complexity of the surgical procedures and the principles that undergird the successful management of patients during the surgical phase of treatment. The remaining chapters in Section III detail the surgical technique for the procedures commonly performed today.

CHAPTER 7

Principles of Surgical Management for Dentofacial Deformity

Myron R. Tucker
Raymond P. White, Jr.

Presurgical patient management
    Psychologic preparation for surgery
    Anesthesia considerations
    Autologous blood and blood products
Patient management at surgery
    Preservation of blood supply
    Protection of teeth, bone, and neurovascular structures
    Wound management
    Use of bone grafts
    The immediate postsurgical period
    Nutrition
Stabilization after osteotomy
    Planning for jaw repositioning
    Traditional fixation and stabilization
    Rigid internal fixation techniques
        Rigid fixation techniques for maxillary osteotomy
        Screw fixation techniques for mandibular osteotomy
        Bone plate techniques for fixation of mandibular osteotomy
    Advantages and disadvantages of rigid internal fixation
        Advantages
        Disadvantages
Postsurgical management
    Occlusion and rehabilitation of the jaws

Successful surgical procedures depend on a strict adherence to surgical principles. In orthognathic surgery as in other surgery, management of the patient before, during, and after the surgical procedure is as important as the details of the surgical technique. Important aspects of patient management include psychologic preparation of the patient; preservation of blood supply to the mobilized teeth and jaw segments; proper wound management; protection of teeth, bone, and neurovascular structures; fixation methods for bony segments; proper occlusion control; and rehabilitation to full jaw function. The use of appropriate anesthesia, blood products, and bone grafts also is an important adjunct to surgery. Good pre- and postoperative nutrition promotes good healing and a quick return to function following surgery. All of these topics are covered in this chapter.

PRESURGICAL PATIENT MANAGEMENT
Psychologic Preparation for Surgery

The first step in psychologic preparation of the patient for surgery is taken when the treatment plan is presented. At that time, the surgeon discusses the surgical procedures in general terms with the patient and family members. The probable location of incisions, identity of the surgical procedures (e.g., LeFort osteotomy), surgical sequelae and common complications, period of hospitalization and recovery, and expectations for rehabilitation before returning to the orthodontist should be covered in this discussion. Specific details of the surgery may be omitted (e.g., linear distances the jaws are moved) because such details can be better explained after presurgical orthodontic preparation is completed. All questions should be answered directly. During the presurgical orthodontics, the surgeon can encourage further dialogue and be available to discuss items of specific concern to the patient. The orthodontist often is queried by the patient regarding surgery. Obviously, general questions can be answered, but the orthodontist must defer to the surgeon for answers to specific questions.

In spite of every effort by the surgeon and orthodontist to get the patient's perspective before a plan of treatment is developed, occasionally the orthodontist and surgeon realize during the presurgery treatment that the patient's expectations differ from the plan. Once identified, the issues must be addressed directly and the patient's wishes accommodated if at all possible. Even when no discrepancy exists between the patient's expectations and the plan, a continuing dialogue during the presurgery orthodontic phase also can help prepare the patient for surgery.

In the weeks immediately before surgery, the surgeon must discuss with the patient and involved family the details of the hospitalization and the surgical procedures that are planned. If at all possible, this discussion should be held prior to the day before surgery. On the day before surgery, the patient must sign the surgical consent form. Obviously, this is the final opportunity to discuss details of the surgery and the hospitalization. At this point, the surgeon can discuss items important immediately after surgery (e.g., diet, level of physical activity immediately after recovery from anesthesia and surgery). These subjects are discussed in more detail following surgery, but the initial discussions do help the patient to adjust to the abrupt shifts in life-style that occur in the 4 to 6 weeks following hospitalization. After surgery most patients can expect to return to limited activity in the first 2 weeks and some are back to work or school within the first 10 days. Facial edema is disturbing to many patients. Most of the facial edema resolves in the first 3 weeks after surgery with the residual edema disappearing as the patient returns to full jaw function. Residual edema may resolve within the first month after surgery if rigid internal fixation (RIF) allows the patient some jaw function. With 6 to 8 weeks of maxillomandibular fixation, residual edema may remain for several months.

Audiovisual aids can be utilized to help the surgeons and the orthodontist prepare the patient for the phases of treatment. But remember these aids are not a substitute for the dialogue between the patient and the surgeon and orthodontist.

Almost all patients have a period of depression following surgery, beginning as early as the second postsurgery day and usually lasting only a few days. Anesthesia, medications taken following surgery (e.g., steroids, analgesics), abrupt changes in activity level and eating habits, and the major changes in jaw function and appearance all contribute. Patients should be warned that this is likely to occur. Most patients will recover from this depression when they discover that they can resume their normal level of activity. In un-

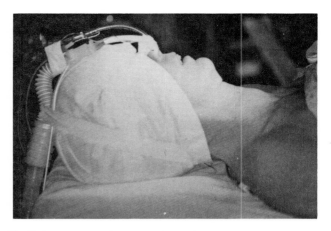

Fig. 7-1. Patient under general anesthesia before orthognathic surgery. Special modifications of the nasoendotracheal tube, conducting tubing, esophageal stethoscope, and CO_2 monitoring transducer provide the anesthesiologist with good control of the airway, but access for the surgeons is not hampered.

usual cases, patients may need referral for special counseling.

Major changes in jaw function and esthetics can accompany orthognathic surgery. Proper psychologic preparation takes time, good rapport, and communication with the patient. If patients feel well informed, their recovery and adjustment following surgery are facilitated (see Chapter 3 for a more thorough discussion).

Anesthesia Considerations

Advances in anesthesiology including patient monitoring have contributed as much to the effectiveness of orthognathic surgery today as refinements in surgical technique. Specific adaptations, including special nasoendotracheal tubes, CO_2 monitoring, and mechanical ventilation, allow the anesthesiologist to control the airway even though the surgeon is moving the patient's head during the procedure and the airway is in the midst of the surgical field (Fig. 7-1). The endotracheal tube is left in place following surgery until the patient is fully awake and has intact protective reflexes to control the airway and maintain adequate ventilation.

Noninvasive monitoring devices assist the anesthesiologist in assessing the cardiovascular and respiratory systems. Continuous electrocardiographic (ECG) recording, monitoring of heart-breath sounds with an esophageal stethoscope, repetitive measurements of blood pressure, and pulse oximetry to measure hemoglobin oxygen saturation are used routinely (Fig. 7-2). When the surgical procedure is predicted to last longer than 4 hours, an indwelling urinary catheter allows monitoring of urinary output. Occasionally an arterial line is placed (e.g., in the radial artery) for intermittent

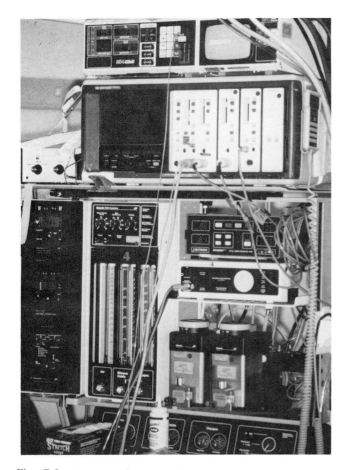

Fig. 7-2. Automated monitoring devices, including blood pressure recording, ECG, pulse oximetry, and end-tidal CO_2 monitor, assist the anesthesiologist in monitoring the cardiovascular and pulmonary systems.

sampling of arterial blood for measurement of blood gases, pO_2, pCO_2, and pH.

When multiple surgical procedures are performed or with LeFort I osteotomy, blood loss can be excessive because of the vascularity of the region. Deliberate hypotensive anesthesia techniques which reduce the blood pressure while maintaining adequate tissue perfusion, including kidney function, minimize blood loss and improve vision in the surgical field. The reader is referred to an excellent review of this subject by Anderson.[6]

Following surgery, monitoring of the patient continues in the postanesthesia care unit. Specially trained nurses and technicians aid the surgeon and anesthesiologist in managing the patient in this critical period until the patient can manage his or her own airway. Usually within a few hours, the patient can return to a surgical floor. Occasionally additional monitoring is required in a surgical intensive care unit. Repeated inservice training for all members of the surgical and anesthesia teams is another important component of the care of orthognathic surgery patients. It is the sur-

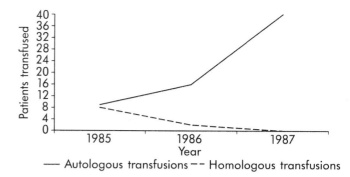

Fig. 7-3. Patients transfused at UNC with autologous and homologous blood. An autologous donor program can eliminate the use of homologous blood and the risks of transfusion. (Modified from Hegtvedt AK, Collins ML, White RP, Jr, Turvey TA: Minimizing the risk of transfusion in orthognathic surgery: use of predeposited autologous blood, Int J Adult Orthod Orthognath Surg 2:185-192, 1987.)

geon's responsibility to see that the team is informed, but the orthodontist may be called to assist in this education process.

Autologous Blood and Blood Products

Patients having orthognathic surgery may lose sufficient blood to require transfusion of blood products. Hegtvedt and others[7] have reported on the use of both autologous and homologous blood in 278 orthognathic surgery patients. Forty-one of 155 patients having surgery in the maxilla received one or more units of packed red cells. None of the 123 patients having mandibular surgery alone was transfused. Serious potential health hazards exist for patients receiving homologous blood, which can be prevented if autologous blood is substituted. Based on these data, we recommend that all patients having orthognathic surgery be offered the option of predepositing one unit of blood (Fig. 7-3). Any patient having LeFort I surgery, alone or in combination with other procedures, is strongly encouraged to predeposit at least one autologous unit during the 3 weeks before surgery.

PATIENT MANAGEMENT AT SURGERY
Preservation of Blood Supply

Surgical experience with patients suffering maxillofacial trauma demonstrated that multiple jaw segments would heal if soft tissue pedicles remained attached to the mobilized segments. Bell's pioneering work in experimental animals provided a biologic basis for these clinical impressions.[8-11] Maxillary and mandibular surgical procedures were carried out in experimental animals through intraoral incisions, and blood flow to soft tissue, bone, and teeth was studied with perfusion techniques. When an adequate soft tissue pedicle remained attached, collateral circulation maintained open vascu-

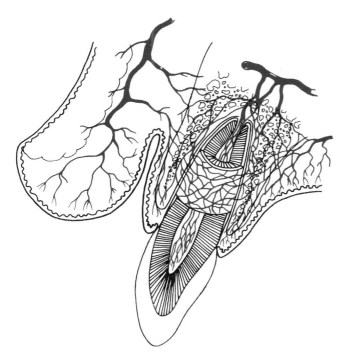

Fig. 7-4. Blood supply to bone, periodontal ligament, and dental pulp from soft-tissue pedicles.

lar channels to the mobilized bony segments, soft tissue, and teeth (periodontal ligament and dental pulp). Only a transient ischemia occurred at the osteotomy sites.

Subsequent studies attempting to quantitate blood flow have demonstrated that separating the jaws into multiple small dentoalveolar segments lessens the blood supply to the mobilized segments. As a general rule, it is unwise to create more than four dentoalveolar segments within a single arch or to have only a single tooth in a segment. In addition, it is clear now that penetrating vessels from the mandibular elevator muscles are important in the blood supply to the mandibular ramus, and surgical techniques for ramus osteotomies have been modified in recent years to minimize the amount of muscle stripping (see Chapter 9). The general principle remains that bone and soft tissue will heal appropriately if a sufficient soft tissue pedicle is left attached to mobilized bone at the time of osteotomy (Fig. 7-4).

Protection of Teeth, Bone, and Neurovascular Structures

Surgical procedures on the mandible are designed to protect neurovascular structures, particularly the facial nerve with extraoral approaches, and the sensory supply to the patient's lower lip. In some surgical procedures, the surgeon must work quite close to the inferior alveolar neurovascular bundle, for example, in the sag-

ittal split osteotomy or subapical osteotomy. In these osteotomies very careful attention must be paid to preserving this structure. As maxillary procedures evolved, equal attention was given to preservation of the infraorbital nerves to retain sensory supply to the upper lip.

Teeth in mobilized dental segments seem at risk for losing their vascular supply. Bell has demonstrated that keeping osteotomy cuts 3 to 5 mm away from root apices will preserve vascular supply to the dental pulps.[8-11] It has also been shown that damage to the apices of teeth during osteotomies may heal with adequate revascularization of the dental pulp.[12] Clinical studies have demonstrated that teeth do retain their blood supply and their sensory response although the teeth adjacent to osteotomy sites are at greatest risk.[13,14]

At surgery, careful attention must be paid to protecting alveolar bone between the teeth and surrounding tooth apices. Adequate periodontal ligament function can be maintained, and bony healing without ankylosis of teeth will follow interdental osteotomy, only if the periodontal ligament space is not violated by an osteotomy cut. The presurgical orthodontic preparation should leave 3 to 4 mm of bone between teeth where an interdental osteotomy is planned. Adequate separation of teeth at the root apices, not just at the alveolar crest, is required.

It also is important to position alveolar segments so that the height of the alveolar bone contour is consistent from one segment to another. Moriarty has shown that this is necessary to minimize postsurgical peridontal pocketing (Fig. 7-5).[15] If this guideline is not followed, pocketing with bone loss is almost inevitable.

Wound Management

Incisions through the skin of the face are necessary in special circumstances for surgical access to the facial bones, particularly in the submandibular approach to the ramus, preauricular approaches to the TM joint, and coronal flaps for exposure of the upper face. Extraoral approaches are clean surgical procedures and general surgical principles should be followed. These include appropriate preparation of the surgical site before surgery, sharp incisions through skin with careful dissection of underlying tissue planes, sharp incisions through periosteum as the mandible and other bones are approached, and careful wound closure following osteotomy eliminating dead space in the wound. Both skin and intraoral incisions may be needed for some surgical procedures. In these instances, special care must be taken to prevent unnecessary contamination of the wounds with oral fluids.

The majority of orthognathic surgical procedures for the mandible and maxilla are carried out with intraoral incisions through mucosa. Adequate lighting is necessary, and this makes fiber optic illuminated retractors

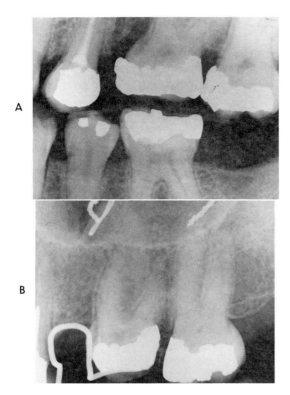

Fig. 7-5. Teeth and alveolar bone must be aligned at surgery to prevent bony periodontal defects. **A,** Bony periosteal defect between premolar and molar following maxillary posterior subapical dentoalveolar osteotomy. **B,** Periodontal defect corrected by removing bone from distal of premolar. Bony margin outlined by gutta percha.

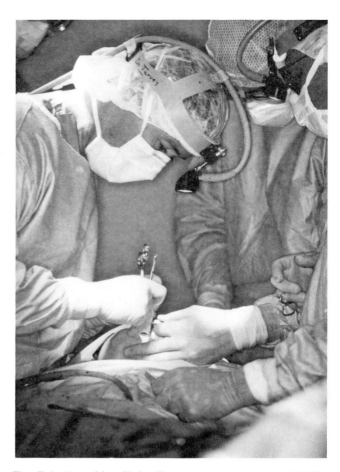

Fig. 7-6. Use of headlight illumination to improve visibility during surgical procedure.

or surgical headlights almost mandatory for intraoral surgery (Fig. 7-6). Even with ideal exposure and lighting, the surgical site is often clearly visible only to the operating surgeon, with limited access for assistants.

Intraoral surgical wounds are considered clean contaminated. Immediately before surgery, the incision sites require preparatory cleansing and disinfection. Even though all of the resident microbial flora cannot be eliminated, the numbers of oral microorganisms and the chance of a subsequent infection can be reduced. Before a mucosal incision is created, the surgical site is infiltrated with a vasoconstrictor, usually a local anesthetic containing epinephine, to help control bleeding. Standard surgical blades are used for most mucosal incisions, but a thermal knife such as a Shaw scalpel offers the advantage of an adequate mucosal incision with better control of bleeding from the wound edges (Fig. 7-7).[16] Depending on the surgical site, muscle tissue may be separated with blunt or sharp dissection under direct visualization, followed by sharp dissection through periosteum down to the bone where osteotomy cuts are planned.

Gentle retraction of soft tissues with instruments de-

signed specially for intraoral surgical approaches minimizes trauma to soft tissues and to the patient's lips during surgery. Lubrication of the lips with petrolatum or steroid cream also protects mucosa and skin from abrasion from the surgeon's gloves and instruments. Copious saline irrigation is needed to minimize thermal damage to bone when osteotomy cuts are carried out

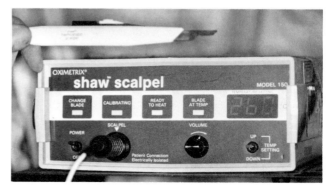

Fig. 7-7. Shaw thermal knife and control box.

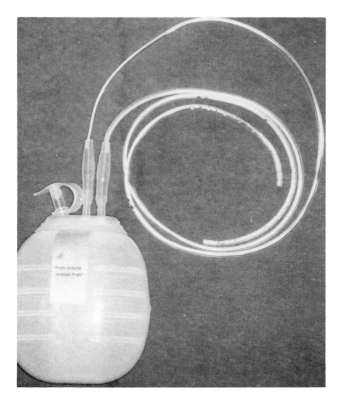

Fig. 7-8. Suction device and small drainage tubing to be placed in an intraoral wound.

with surgical burs and reciprocating or oscillating saws.

Following appropriate placement and fixation of bony segments in their planned new positions, bleeding is controlled and incisions are closed in layers with resorbable sutures, eliminating dead space as much as is possible. Occasionally, soft rubber drains or suction drains are needed to prevent excessive accumulation of blood in dead space in the wound (Fig. 7-8). These drains are generally removed within 48 hours of surgery to prevent wound contamination. Mucosal edges of surgical wounds are usually closed with running sutures of 3-0 or 4-0 diameter. Resorbable sutures do not require removal, an advantage in the immediate post-surgery period when access to the surgical sites may be difficult. Chromic gut sutures are satisfactory, but polyglycolic or polygalactic sutures of a similar diameter, which are retained in the wound about twice as long as surgical chromic gut, may be used to advantage when wound dehiscence may be a problem (e.g., following inferior border osteotomy for lengthening the mandible or LeFort I osteotomy for increasing vertical face height). A suture of greater diameter and strength may be selected for special applications (e.g., nasal alar base cinch suture).

High-dose corticosteroids help minimize surgical edema. If these are administered for only 24 to 36 hours, the hypothalamic-pituitary-adrenal mechanism for responding to stress is minimally altered. Ideally, administration of steriods should begin 8 to 12 hours before surgery, but giving the first dose after the intravenous (iv) line is started is generally acceptable. When the iv line is discontinued, an intramuscular slow-release dose completes steroid treatment. Prophylactic antibiotics aid in controlling wound contamination and postoperative infection in clean contaminated wounds. Antibiotics are administered to the patient intravenously during surgery and in the immediate postoperative period and are followed by oral dosage forms when the iv is discontinued. A suggested dosage schedule is shown in Table 7-1.

Wound dressings of gauze and elastic bandage usually are needed to support wounds for the immediate postsurgery period (1 to 5 days). Dressings are particularly important for wounds at high risk for dehiscence (e.g., the surgical approach inside the lower lip for access to the anterior, inferior aspect of the mandible).

TABLE 7-1 Perioperative corticosteroids and antibiotics

Stage of treatment	Corticosteroids	Antibiotics
Presurgery	Decadron 8 mg po hs	When iv started
At surgery	Solumedrol 125 mg iv	Penicillin G 1 M units iv
		or
		Kefzol 1.0 gm iv
Postsurgery	Solumedrol 125 mg iv q 4h × 24h then Depomedrol 80 mg im	Penicillin G 1 M units iv q 4h × 24h then 500 mg po q 6h × 1-5d or Kefzol 1.0 gm iv q 8h × 24h then 500 mg po q 8h × 1-5d

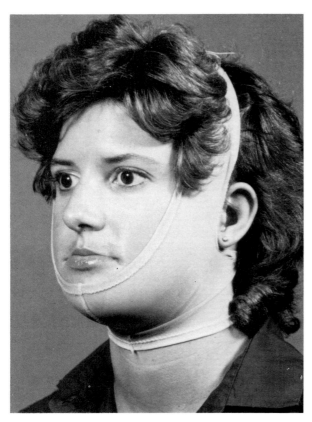

Fig. 7-9. Specially designed head dressing of elastic bandage and velcro. (Polli Chin-Neck Support, Caromed International, Inc., 308-D West Millbrook Road, Raleigh, NC 27609.)

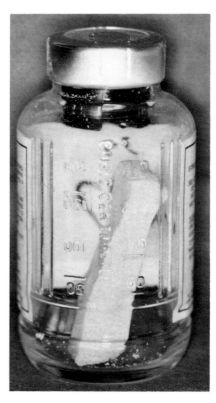

Fig. 7-10. Freeze-dried allogeneic bone in container for preservation until rehydration.

Specially designed head dressings of elastic bandage and velcro are the best choice for this area (Fig. 7-9). Because they are easily removed, cleaned of debris, and reapplied, patients accept wearing these dressings more readily.

Use of Bone Grafts

Both autogenous and allogeneic bone are used in orthognathic surgery to help stabilize bony segments at osteotomy sites and enhance bony healing. It is important to keep in mind that whatever the bone graft material, it serves only as a scaffold. The patient's own bone must replace the graft as healing progresses.

Because it is resorbed and replaced reasonably quickly (i.e., within 6 months) but more slowly than autogenous bone, freeze-dried allogeneic bone serves well for stabilization of osteotomy sites. It is particularly indicated for areas where there is a gap between bone segments following osteotomy and soft tissue forces may cause the segments to shift, as when the maxilla is repositioned inferiorly with LeFort I osteotomy.

Freeze-dried allogeneic bone can be purchased in sterile containers from certified tissue banks. A regu-

larly updated list of sources is available from the American Association of Tissue Banks (1350 Beverly Road, Suite 220A, McLean, VA 22101). This material is rehydrated with sterile saline in the operating room at the time of surgery (Fig. 7-10). Because this bone is harvested under sterile operating room conditions and precautions are taken to test the donors, the risk of transmitting infectious disease is almost nonexistent. Bone from the iliac crest is most suitable for orthognathic surgery. Autogenous bone grafts can be substituted for allogeneic bank bone if it is not available, but an additional surgical procedure is required to harvest the bone.

When rapid healing is a necessity, as in a repeat orthognathic procedure, cortical and particulate autogenous bone is preferred. Although knowledge of the details of bone biology following grafting is still evolving, healing with autogenous bone grafts is more predictable in these special situations. Small amounts of cortical autogenous bone can be obtained from osteotomy sites or from accessible adjacent areas, but particulate cellular bone from orthognathic surgery sites is extremely limited. When a large quantity of particulate cellular bone is required, extraoral donor sites such as the iliac crest or the parietal bone are necessary.

Some surgeons recommend implant materials (e.g.,

hydroxylapatite blocks) to stabilize osteotomy sites.[17] These materials are not replaced by bone and may give stability over a longer time period than bone. But wound dehiscence seems to occur more often over the implant materials and the lack of bone at the implant site in the long term can pose a problem in bony healing.

When augmentation of facial contour is the goal of surgery, autogenous bone may be preferred over bank bone because the contour after healing is more predictable. Many surgeons feel that autogenous bone from alternative donor sites behaves differently in the healing process. Grafts taken from membranous bone (e.g., parietal bone) seem to heal and retain their shape more predictably than allogeneic bone or autogenous bone from endochondral harvest sites.[18] Other surgeons would choose freeze-dried cartilage or specially contoured alloplastic implant materials to augment facial contour because no change in shape follows placement. Specific examples of the use of these materials will be discussed further in the clinical chapters that follow.

The Immediate Postsurgical Period

When the patient is released from the postanesthesia care unit and returns to the surgical floor, fluid intake and output are monitored carefully. Often with maxillary surgery, a nasogastric tube is left in place and attached to low suction for the first 12 to 24 hours to prevent nausea from blood and secretions accumulating in the stomach. Patients are strongly urged to take fluids by mouth almost immediately even though edema and numbness of the lips make this difficult. Once fluid intake is deemed adequate by the surgeon, the iv line is discontinued.

Patients having orthognathic surgery usually do not have prolonged severe pain. In the immediate postoperative period, parenterally administered opioids such as demerol may be necessary for adequate analgesia. Mild analgesics (e.g., acetaminophen with codeine) generally control pain after the first postsurgery day. Antibiotics can be continued by mouth once the iv line is discontinued and the final steroid dose is administered (see Table 7-1).

With LeFort I surgery, some slight oozing of blood is typical for 24 to 48 hours following surgery. This fluid accumulates in the maxillary or paranasal sinuses and causes a "stuffiness" and drainage from the nares or into the pharynx for 10 to 14 days. Although it is annoying, patients will accept this sequelae if the cause is explained to them. Nasal and sinus congestion can be controlled with a nasal spray (e.g., 0.1% xylometazoline) and oral decongestant combinations (e.g., brompheniramine, phenylephrine, phenylpropanolamine), making patients more comfortable.

Early ambulation is encouraged immediately after surgery. Movement minimizes the chance of pulmonary atelectasis. Patients seem to regain their appetite and energy more quickly if they resume daily activities as quickly as possible.

Some orthognathic surgery procedures (e.g., mandibular inferior border osteotomy) do not require an overnight hospital stay if a responsible adult is available to assist the patient at home. It is not unusual for patients having one-jaw surgery to go home on the day following surgery having spent only one night in the hospital, but a 1- to 3-day stay following surgery is the norm. Dolan and others studied details of the hospital stay in orthognathic surgery patients.[19] Patients were hospitalized 2 to 3 days for one-jaw surgery and 3 to 4 days for two-jaw surgery with a range of 2 to 6 days. In this study, all patients spent the night before surgery in the hospital, a practice now discouraged by many insurance carriers.

Postsurgery radiographs (e.g., panoramic, lateral cephalogram, PA cephalogram) are taken the day following surgery or as soon thereafter as practical. Close attention is paid to the position of jaw segments and the condyles. Management of specific complications is discussed fully in the following chapters on surgical technique.

Once patients are discharged from the hospital, they return to the surgeon for follow-up visits during the first week. Typically, additional visits are scheduled biweekly until the patient is ready to return to the orthodontist. During the first week the focus of the surgeon's attention is on wound healing, nutrition, and the specific complaints unique to each patient. Once the jaws are mobilized, full rehabilitation to function is the goal and focus of treatment. Rehabilitation is discussed more fully later in this chapter.

Nutrition

Good nutrition is mandatory in the postsurgery period to reverse the catabolic metabolism surrounding surgery and promote good healing. In reaction to the stress of surgery, the patient's nutritional requirements go up—at the very time that impaired function of the jaws makes nutritional intake difficult, particularly if the patient's teeth are held tightly in maxillomandibular fixation for 6 to 8 weeks.

In the immediate postsurgery period, fluid intake is the most important consideration. At a minimum, patients should be encouraged to consume more than 3000 cc of fluid each day, with the goal increased in hot weather. Additionally, each patient should be given a goal for caloric and protein intake. Reasonable goals for a patient are 2500 to 3000 calories and 1.0 to 1.5 g protein/kg body weight/day. Patients should be encouraged to plan five to six meals each day to meet nutritional goals. The goal may be difficult to meet at first, but supplementation with a nutritionally complete liquid such as Ensure (Ross Laboratories, Division of Abbott Laboratories, Columbus, OH 43216) will help.

Body weight is a good guide to adequate fluid and nutrition intake. If patients consume a nutritionally balanced diet after surgery, they can maintain body weight, a clinical sign that anabolic metabolism is achieved.[20] Patients can benefit from dietary consultation, and both the patient and the individual responsible for meals in the week after surgery should participate in the consultation. Excellent recipe books prepared especially for jaw surgery are available (e.g., *Drink to Your Health* by DL Wolford, published by Arlington Century Printing, Arlington, TX 760l3), and patients appreciate the surgeon's providing them this information.

STABILIZATION AFTER OSTEOTOMY

Satisfactory healing of a bone after it has been sectioned or split, whether by trauma or osteotomy, requires a period of immobilization. The specific need is to minimize the movement of one bony segment relative to the other; otherwise, a fibrous rather than a bony union is likely to result. In management of dentofacial trauma and orthognathic surgery, immobilization has been obtained through a combination of wire sutures to stabilize the fragments and maxillomandibular fixation. Recently, it has become possible to use a combination of bone screws and small bone plates to obtain rigid internal fixation (RIF), so that the position of the segments is maintained even if jaw movements continue. In the following section, we review the traditional approach and describe the newer rigid fixation methods in detail.

Planning for Jaw Repositioning

Whatever the method of fixation, the first surgical principle is to position the bone fragments correctly, so that they heal in the correct position. In orthognathic surgery, prediction tracings and model surgery are used to plan exactly where the jaws are to be positioned, and it is essential to transfer this plan as precisely as possible to the operating room. The two keys to doing this are establishing measurements that can be used during the surgery and fabricating an occlusal splint or splints to control the relationship of the teeth. From the prediction tracings, planned movements of the jaws are carried out on mounted dental casts. If the dental casts can be positioned as the tracings predict (model surgery), then millimeter measurements of the movements are recorded for use in surgery. An occlusal acrylic wafer splint is constructed to fit the position of the teeth at completion of model surgery. In general, at surgery the millimeter measurements guide the vertical and anteroposterior positions of the jaws and the occlusal splint controls the transverse and anteroposterior positions. Both millimeter measurements and the splint are relied on at surgery to position the jaws.

The use of an occlusal splint makes it possible to put the teeth in any planned position at surgery, regardless of whether the teeth interdigitate without the splint. In fact, the most desirable position for postsurgical orthodontic finishing often is not the one in which the occlusion would be most stable in the setup of articulated presurgical models. This is the reason that the splint is so desirable for most patients who receive coordinated surgical and orthodontic treatment. In addition, an appropriate splint makes the surgeon's job easier in the operating room by establishing a clearly visualized goal. In two-jaw surgery, an intermediate splint can be used to help establish the intermediate jaw position at the end of the first phase of the surgery. Finally, the splint assists in occlusal rehabilitation of the patient.

The splint is made on the casts as they have been related by model surgery. After these have been checked by the surgeon and the orthodontist (it is important for the orthodontist to agree with the proposed postsurgical occlusion), the first step in splint construction is to stabilize the casts with plaster or stone so they cannot shift as the splint is being fabricated. Then the articulator is opened to allow for enough thickness of splint material so that it does not break while in use. Thick splints potentially can introduce errors if the articulator mounting is not perfectly accurate. Splints should be designed with only enough thickness and bulk to prevent breakage in the operating room and in the weeks following surgery. The steps in fabrication of a typical splint are shown in Fig. 7-11. See Chapter 6 for additional discussion of splint design.

Traditional Fixation and Stabilization

The traditional fixation methods are based on a combination of transosseous wire fixation, skeletal wire fixation, and maxillomandibular immobilization for 6 to 8 weeks. The combination allows for good bony healing of maxillary and mandibular segments following orthognathic surgery. Special care always is given to positioning bone and tooth segments exactly as dictated by presurgical planning, and an occlusal wafer splint is a key to accomplishing this. Stainless steel wire (24- to 26-gauge) placed across osteotomy sites in combination with maxillomandibular fixation provide good stability to bony segments. With two-jaw surgery, skeletal suspension wires must be added from sites with dense cortical bone such as the piriform nasal rim, and circummandibular wires usually are needed to provide further support for the mandible (Fig. 7-12). Placement of these skeletal wires is discussed further in Chapter 11.

For mandibular ramus surgery, 5 to 7 weeks of maxillomandibular fixation is necessary before healing is adequate to allow mobilization of the jaws and the return of the jaws to function (see Chapter 9). With LeFort I osteotomy alone, healing may be more rapid and some surgeons suggest mobilization of the jaws as early as the third postsurgery week. This subject is discussed in more detail in Chapter 8.

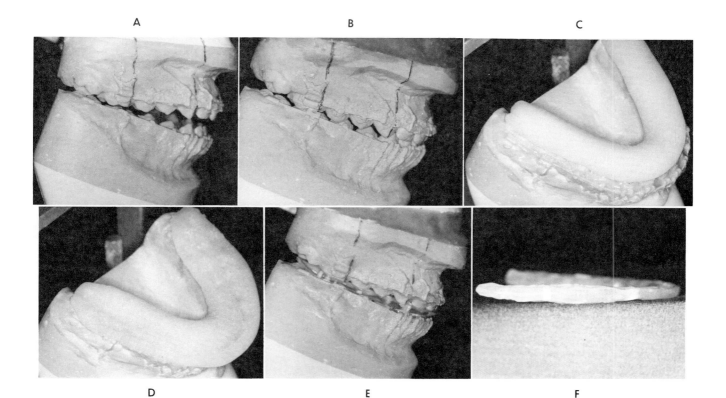

Fig. 7-11. Steps in occlusal splint construction, using the casts as related by the model surgery (in this case, a segment maxillary osteotomy is planned). **A,** Presurgical models. **B,** Occlusion following model surgery. **C,** To fabricate the splint, lay a roll of uncured acrylic on the occlusal surface. The casts are closed into it. The casts must be firmly secured to the articulator—if the casts shift, the splint will dictate the wrong position at surgery. **D,** The untrimmed splint with occlusal indentations. After the acrylic has cured, trim away excessive bulk labially and lingually. **E,** Trim the occlusal surfaces so that only shallow occlusal indentations remain. Place bur holes along the labial and buccal surface for attaching the splint to the arch wires. **F,** Completed splint.

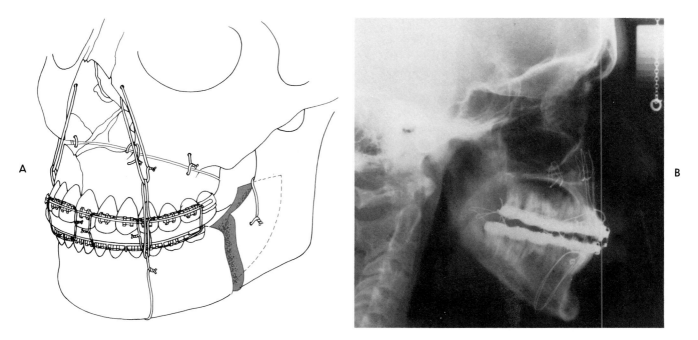

Fig. 7-12. Skeletal suspension wiring. **A,** Diagram. **B,** Postsurgery radiograph showing maxillary and mandibular skeletal suspension wires joined by intermediate connecting wire.

Rigid Internal Fixation Techniques

The use of small bone plates and screws for direct fixation of bony segments at the time of surgery is a recent development in the surgical correction of dentofacial deformities. The technique is termed *rigid internal fixation.* By directly and rigidly fixing bony segments together, the period of maxillomandibular fixation and jaw immobilization can be greatly reduced or even eliminated after the surgery is completed. Rigid fixation techniques are discussed in general terms in the following pages. Specific applications are covered in the chapters on surgical techniques and in the clinical chapters.

The application of RIF techniques requires great attention to detail by the orthodontist and surgeon in the planning stages. Presurgical orthodontic preparation of the orthognathic surgery patient is essentially the same whether conventional wire osteosynthesis and maxillomandibular fixation or RIF is anticipated. Because conditions at the time of surgery may prevent the use of RIF, patients should be prepared, both psychologically and in terms of the orthodontic appliance setup, for a full period of maxillomandibular fixation. The planned use of RIF should not become an excuse to minimize the orthodontic preparation of the patient. The extra manipulation required for application of RIF demands a precise, secure occlusion, made possible by presurgical orthodontic preparation which includes rectangular arch wires and vertical lugs for secure intraoperative maxillomandibular fixation (see Fig. 6-26). At surgery, the surgeon must position bony segments exactly as planned since RIF will not allow modification during the postsurgery healing period.

Rigid Fixation Techniques for Maxillary Osteotomy

Two basic types of rigid fixation exist for maxillary osteotomies, pin systems and the use of small bone plates. A variety of techniques for application of small bone plates to maxillary osteotomies have been described.[21-24] When application of plates for maxillary osteotomies is planned, minor modifications in osteotomy design may be desirable,[22] to allow placement of plates in areas of maximum bone thickness without jeopardizing adjacent anatomical structures such as teeth or the infraorbital nerve. Locating the osteotomy cuts at a higher level or using a step osteotomy often facilitates putting the plates in sturdier bone (Fig. 7-13).

For application of bone plates after completion of the osteotomy the maxilla is placed against the mandible with firm maxillomandibular fixation and with the maxillomandibular complex rotated to the proper position. At this point, the maxilla and mandible must be correctly positioned as determined by preoperative cephalometric prediction and model surgery, the

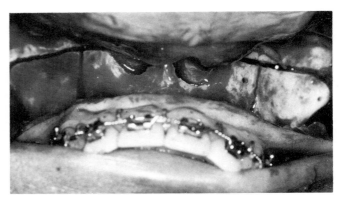

Fig. 7-13. Maxillary osteotomy modified to allow sufficient bone beneath the cuts for placement of plates.

condyles must be properly located in the fossa, and the mandible must be securely held against the maxilla. When there is no doubt that the maxilla is in the right place, the bony segments can be wired in position temporarily (usually preferred) or held in place by hand. Then bone plates are contoured to adapt passively to areas of maximum bony thickness along the lateral walls of the maxilla, usually in the piriform rim or zygomatic buttress area. After the plates are properly adapted, holes are drilled and screws placed to secure the plates to the maxilla. Plates of multiple configurations allow placement in different locations and patterns (Fig. 7-14), and a variety of plate sizes and shapes are particularly helpful in stabilizing segmental maxillary osteotomies. Each segment may be stabilized with an individual plate or segments can be tied together with a plate. After all plates are in place and before wounds are closed, maxillomandibular fixation must be released and the occlusion checked. Failure to complete this important step may lead to a late discovery of malpositioned bony segments which could have been corrected. Reoperation to correct the bony segment malposition and the associated malocclusion may be the only recourse.

Pin systems have been used successfully for stabilization of maxillary osteotomies.[25-27] Although this is a rigid fixation technique, it is not a rigid internal technique in that a portion of the stabilization device is exposed intraorally and future removal of the pins is mandatory. The pin system is adapted to the maxilla after repositioning bony segments into their desired position. The system then is secured with screws to the lateral maxillary walls and fixed to orthodontic appliances or the interocclusal splint (Fig. 7-15). This allows the surgeon to adjust the position of the maxilla postsurgically, which usually is done by bending segments of the wire with three-prong orthodontic pliers. Although the ability to adjust this fixation device can be helpful, precise adjustments are difficult and it is better to do everything possible to position the segments ex-

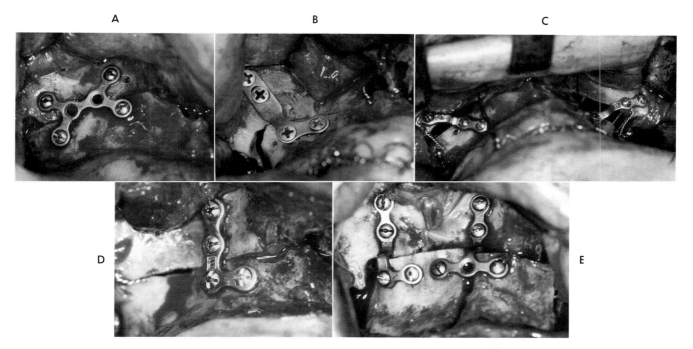

Fig. 7-14. Plate configurations and positions to stabilize maxillary osteotomies. **A** and **B,** Maxillary advancement. **C,** Maxillary setback. **D,** Maxilla superiorly positioned. **E,** Multisegment maxilla.

actly at surgery, rather than depending on adjusting them later.

Screw Fixation Techniques for Mandibular Osteotomy

The use of RIF for bilateral sagittal ramus osteotomies was first described by Spiessl in 1974.[28] Two basic techniques are used today for screw fixation of sag-

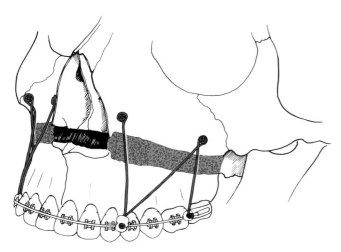

Fig. 7-15. Adjustable pin fixation system for stabilization of maxillary osteotomies. (Adapted from Bays RA: Rigid stabilization system for maxillary osteotomies, J Oral Maxillofac Surg 43:60-63, 1985.)

ittal osteotomies, the lag screw and the position or bicortical screw techniques.

The lag screw technique involves placing a screw so that its threads bind only in the medial bony cortex, and the screw rotates freely without binding in the lateral bony segment. This allows compression of the lateral bony segment between the head of the screw and the medial cortex of the mandible. The lag technique is accomplished in one of two ways. In the first approach, the same size hole is drilled in both segments and a true lag screw, one with only threads on the tip, is employed. This produces free rotation of the head in the lateral bony segment and compression as the screw is tightened (Fig. 7-16). An alternative technique involves using a fully threaded screw and enlarging the hole through the lateral bony segment so the screw threads will bind only in the medial segment (Fig. 7-17).[28]

A position screw or bicortical screw technique incorporates a fully threaded screw which binds in both the lateral and medial cortices.[23] As the screw is tightened, no compression is possible, because with the screw threads' engaging both segments, the distance between them is maintained (Fig. 7-18). Compression of the fragments with a lag screw is thought to facilitate healing, but as discussed more completely in Chapter 9, some benefit may be gained from a position screw in preventing displacement of the condyles as the screw is tightened (Fig. 7-19).

Both of these screw techniques can be accomplished

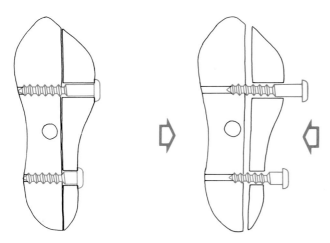

Fig. 7-16. Coronal section of mandible showing lag screw technique. True lag screw inserted with inner portion engaging medial cortex and nonthreaded outer portion rotating freely in lateral segment. When screw is tightened, lateral cortex is compressed against medial aspect of the mandible.

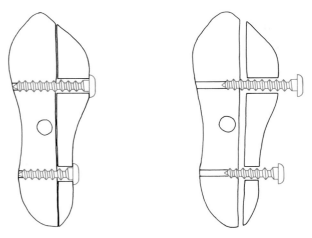

Fig. 7-17. Fully threaded screw used in a lag screw technique (outer cortex is enlarged to a size slightly greater than the outer diameter of the screw).

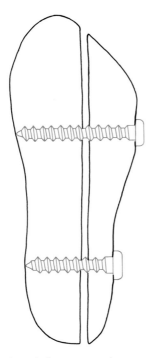

Fig. 7-18. Fully threaded screw used as a positioning or bicortical screw. Both the lateral and medial cortices are engaged, fixing the bone segments, but the interbone gap is maintained.

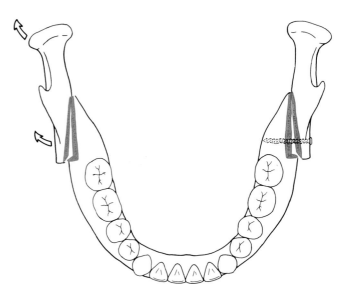

Fig. 7-19. Diagram of sagittal osteotomy with flaring of the condyle-ramus segment as a result of bone contact with mandibular advancement. Placing a position screw in the anterior portion of the osteotomy will maintain the position of the segments and prevent the screw from compressing the bone anteriorly at the screw, which would result in lateral displacement of the condyle.

through a transoral or percutaneous approach. When stretching the lips, osteotomy design, and the desired location of the screws all allow adequate access through the surgical incision, the transoral approach is preferred (Fig. 7-20). When intraoral access is limited or when a more perpendicular orientation of the screws to bone is desirable, a percutaneous approach is the option of choice. Access is gained by placing a small stab incision in the skin beneath the angle of the jaw, then inserting a trocar, allowing for instrumentation through its cannula (Fig. 7-21).

Screws can be placed in a linear or triangular pattern (Fig. 7-22), depending on the configuration of the bone. Three screws are generally used for stablization of each osteotomy site. A variety of screw designs are

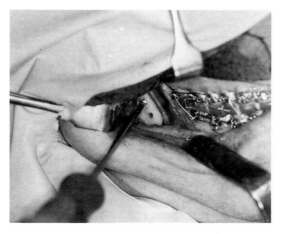

Fig. 7-20. Access for placement of screws in a sagittal osteotomy using the transoral technique.

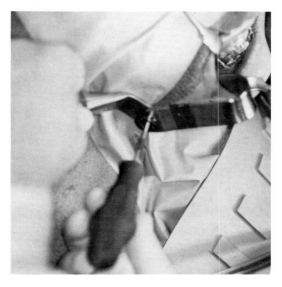

Fig. 7-21. Use of a percutaneous trocar for placement of screws in a sagittal osteotomy.

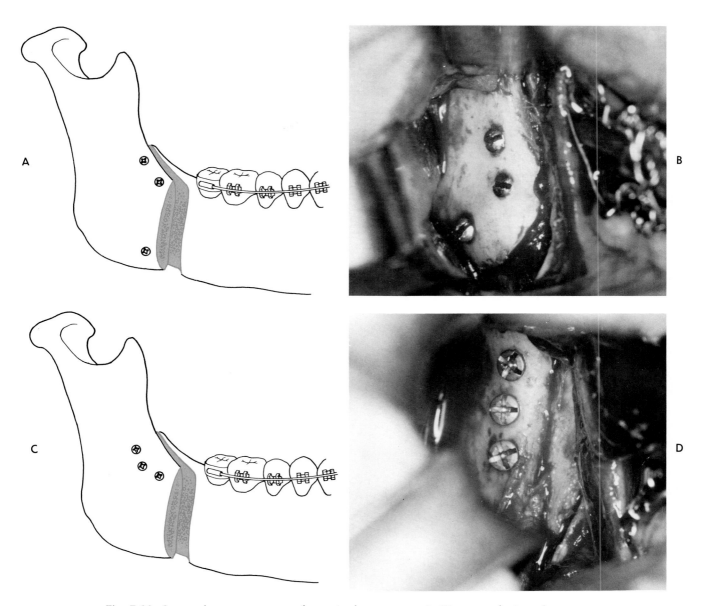

Fig. 7-22. Screw placement patterns for sagittal osteotomy. A, Diagram of triangular pattern. B, Clinical photograph of triangular pattern. C, Diagram of linear pattern at superior border. D, Clinical photograph of three screws in a linear pattern.

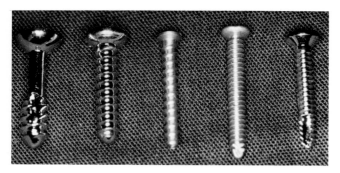

Fig. 7-23. Variety of screws used for fixation of sagittal osteotomies. From left to right: Osteo 3.5-mm lag screw, Synthes 2.7-mm screw, Wurzburg 2.0-mm screw, Synthes 2.0-mm screw, and Osteo self-threading 2.0-mm screw.

available. Screw sizes from 2.0 mm to 3.5 mm in diameter have been used successfully for fixation of sagittal osteotomies (Fig. 7-23). The smaller screw size and an intraoral approach for screw placement are preferred if this is technically feasible. At present, there are no data to indicate better stability with larger screws or a percutaneous approach.

Bone Plate Techniques for Fixation of Mandibular Osteotomy

When repositioning of bony segments results in bony overlap, as in a sagittal osteotomy, screw fixation techniques alone are adequate. If overlap of bony segments does not occur, bone plate techniques frequently can be adapted for mandibular stabilization. Application of plates is possible in a variety of ramus, subapical, body, and inferior border osteotomies (Fig. 7-24). As with all bone plate techniques, passive contouring of the plates to the repositioned bony segments is mandatory. Reconstruction of mandibular abnormalities with grafts (e.g., stabilization of a costocondral graft for reconstruction of a mandibular ramus-condyle area) is facilitated with bone plates (Fig. 7-25).[29]

Advantages and Disadvantages of Rigid Internal Fixation
Advantages

The ability to rigidly fix and stabilize bony segments has a number of advantages for the patient, orthodontist, and surgeon:

1. Improved comfort and convenience. The most obvious result of reducing or eliminating maxillomandibular fixation is improved postoperative airway control, nutrition, speech, and hygiene, all of which are facilitated by the patient's ability to open the mouth in the immediate postsurgical pe-

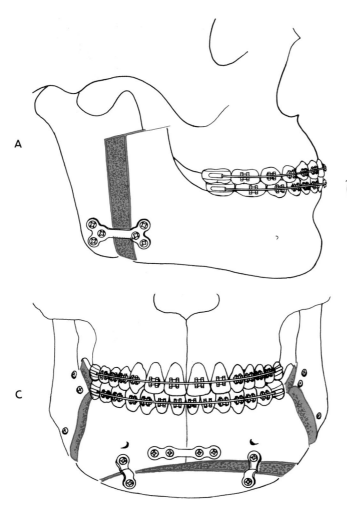

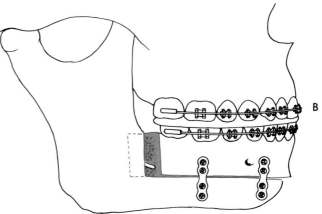

Fig. 7-24. Bone plate techniques for stabilization of mandibular osteotomies. **A,** Inverted L osteotomy. **B,** Total subapical osteotomy. **C,** Bilateral sagittal-split osteotomy and anterior mandibular midline osteotomy combined with a mandibular inferior border osteotomy.

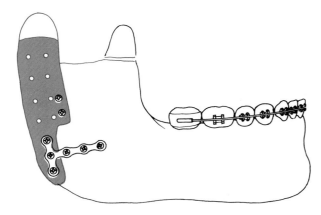

Fig. 7-25. Stabilization of a costochondal graft using small bone plate fixation.

riod. Reducing fixation time also significantly improves the patient's psychologic reaction to the orthognathic surgical experience. The length of maxillomandibular fixation may vary from no postoperative fixation at all (i.e., immediate intraoperative removal of wires at completion of surgery) to 2 to 3 weeks of maxillomandibular fixation. The length of time patients' teeth are wired depends on the type of procedure performed, the method of osseous fixation, and the surgeon's clinical judgment.

2. Increased safety in the immediate postoperative period. Without maxillomandibular fixation, postoperative management of the patient's airway is easier and safer. In rare cases when excessive hemorrhage or vomiting occurs, the easy access to the mouth and pharynx for suctioning of the airway is of significant benefit.

3. More rapid bony healing. The histologic pattern and mechanical properties of bone healing under the influence of compression (i.e., when lag screws or compression plates are used) are somewhat different from bone healing with conventional wire osteosynthesis techniques.[30] Healing during wire osteosynthesis is the result of a secondary bone healing process in which the first step is the formation of a callus. This then is followed by generation of new osteoblastic activity, deposition of bone, and eventual remodeling. Under the influence of compression, bone appears to heal primarily, without an obvious endosteal or periosteal callus. In an experimental model, osteotomies stabilized with rigid techniques demonstrated the histologic difference mentioned above as well as improved mechanical properties. At 6 weeks postoperatively, the strength of rigidly fixed osteotomies was approximately twice that of similar osteotomies treated with conventional wire osteosynthesis.[31,32]

4. Evaluation of postoperative occlusion in the operating room. Bony segments which inadvertently may have been poorly positioned at the time of surgery can be detected and corrected, since the occlusion can be checked easily after maxillomandibular fixation is released, before the wound is closed.

5. The ability to stabilize bony segments which would otherwise be difficult to control. In cases where bony contact is insufficient for direct wiring of osteotomy segments, plates, screws, or a combination can be used to adequately stabilize bony segments.[33] This is especially helpful when complications resulting from unanticipated fractures during maxillary or mandibular osteotomies arise (Fig. 7-26).[34,35]

6. Improved control of bony segments. Counterclockwise rotation of the proximal segment in mandibular osteotomies has been noted with several transosseous wiring techniques.[36] Although this may still occur, the problem appears to be decreased with rigid fixation techniques.[37,38]

7. Increased stability. Initially it was hoped that RIF techniques would eliminate relapse following surgery to correct skeletal abnormalities. Most studies indicate that immediate postoperative stability may be improved with the use of RIF. However, it appears that with certain bony movements some relapse occurs even after RIF.

Improved postoperative stability following mandibular setback with RIF compared with wire fixation was reported by Paulus and Steinhauser.[39] Van Sickles and others reported an apparent increase in stability using RIF techniques for sagittal osteotomies to advance the mandible.[37,40] While showing some improvement in stability with RIF, they also demonstrated skeletal relapse with both techniques, with the greatest change correlated with the amount of mandibular advancement. A recent study reporting 1-year follow-up data suggests that following mandibular advancement, RIF cases are more stable than those with traditional fixation during the first 6 weeks postsurgically (i.e., while the conventional cases are in maxillomandibular fixation). But in this study, the differences between the two groups all but disappeared at 1 year. In a significant number of patients with conventional maxillomandibular fixation, the mandible slipped back during fixation but came forward again at 1 year, while the RIF patients showed less of either type of movement.[41]

In addition to improved skeletal stability, a decrease in postsurgical dental change has been demonstrated with screw fixation techniques for mandibular advancement. Thomas and others[38] demonstrated that less maxillary incisor retroclination

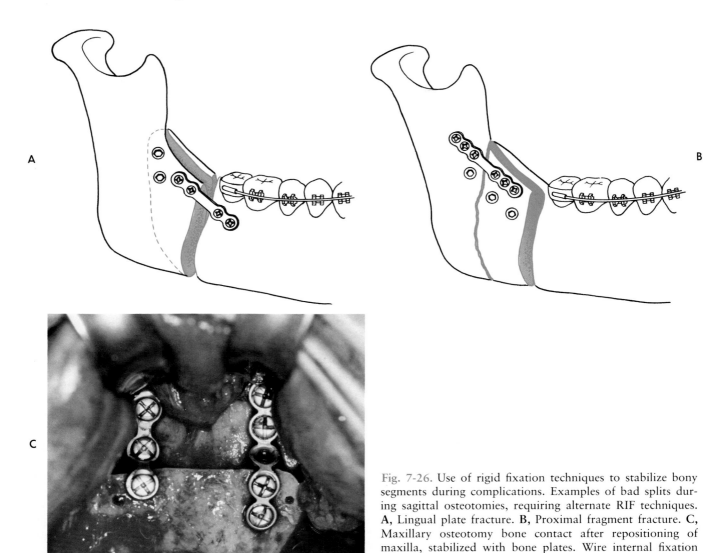

Fig. 7-26. Use of rigid fixation techniques to stabilize bony segments during complications. Examples of bad splits during sagittal osteotomies, requiring alternate RIF techniques. **A,** Lingual plate fracture. **B,** Proximal fragment fracture. **C,** Maxillary osteotomy bone contact after repositioning of maxilla, stabilized with bone plates. Wire internal fixation would not be adequate because of telescoping of bone at osteotomy sites.

and lower incisor proclination occurred during the first 6 weeks postsurgically in patients undergoing sagittal osteotomy mandibular advancements when RIF and no maxillomandibular fixation were used, compared to those patients treated with wire osteosynthesis and 6 weeks of maxillomandibular fixation. During maxillomandibular fixation after mandibular advancement, the light but steady pull of the stretched soft tissues is transmitted to the teeth and results in tooth movement remarkably similar to that produced by Class II elastics. It seems reasonable that with no maxillomandibular fixation, this would no longer occur.

Few studies exist in the literature that adequately document long-term stability of maxillary osteotomies with RIF. A slight decrease in postoperative movement has been described by Larson and others[42] and Harsha and Terry[21] in patients undergoing maxillary osteotomies with bone plates. Bays demonstrated increased stability of maxillary osteotomies when an adjustable pin fixation system was used.[25]

8. Greater staging flexibility. Since the mandible can be adequately stabilized with screw or plating techniques, it is possible to mobilize the lower jaw first in two-jaw cases, followed by positioning of the maxilla against the mandible, which has been moved to the desired new postsurgical position.[43] This sequence may be an advantage in multisegmented maxillas or when the anticipated bone contact in the maxilla is minimal. Additional detail on this technique is provided in Chapter 11.

9. Faster reduction of postoperative edema. Although assessment of postsurgical swelling is largely sub-

jective, rapid animation of facial muscles made possible by early jaw mobility appears to result in faster resolution of facial edema.

10. Rehabilitation of muscles and the TM joint. Immediate jaw function after surgery with gradual progression to normal ranges of jaw motion seems to allow for a quicker and more complete return to normal jaw function. Rehabilitation is discussed further, later in this chapter.

Disadvantages

Despite the number of positive aspects of RIF, several potential disadvantages exist with these techniques.

1. Technical difficulties. Plates must be contoured so they adapt passively to all areas of bone contact. If not, bony segments will be displaced by RIF. Screws improperly positioned across mandibular osteotomy sites can displace the mandibular condyles during the final tightening. If plating or screw techniques result in a malposition of bony segments postsurgically, adjustment of these segments and the associated occlusal disharmony may be difficult if not impossible without reoperation. In contrast to wire osteosynthesis, once bony segments are held in position with bone plates and screws, little movement can be expected and there is no prospect of the spontaneous improvement that often occurred with traditional fixation.

2. Increased costs. Plates and screws are expensive, in part because they are made from high-grade metal (usually titanium alloys), but largely because of the costly technology necessary to produce miniaturized plates and screws. Special instruments customized for use in the jaws also are needed to use RIF. The costs must be passed on to the patient.

3. Increased risk of infection. Although many surgeons consider that the placement of a foreign object leads to an increased risk of infection, little documentation from elective osteotomies of the facial region exists to support this notion.[22,44] There is little postsurgical infection in orthognathic surgery, with or without the use of RIF. Buckley and others[45] found only a 2% postsurgery infection rate following maxillary surgery, similiar for both RIF and wire fixation. Infection following mandibular osteotomy was 9% for RIF, compared with 3% for wire fixation, but all of the infections were readily managed with local measures and antibiotics.

4. Possible need for plate removal. Removal of plates and screws postoperatively is rare, 7% following mandibular osteotomy and 2% after maxillary surgery.[45] Reasons for removal include the bothersome presence of a plate or screw that can be palpated through the skin or mucosa, persistent wound infection, and the presence of a metal sensitivity. Metals currently used for rigid fixation appliances include stainless steel, vitalium, and titanium, all of which are biocompatible. Although stainless steel appears to have a slightly higher incidence of corrosion and postoperative tissue reaction, this problem is minimal in the maxillofacial region. Microcorrosion and tissue reaction are essentially nonexistent. Since plates and screws become nonfunctional after bone healing has occurred, minimal plate movement also is not a problem, if it occurs.

5. Neurosensory disturbances. Trauma to nerves within or close to the surgical field is possible from compression within bony segments or direct trauma from placement of the screw or plate. This is particularly true in the case of the inferior alveolar nerve in mandibular surgery. Paulus and Steinhauser reported a slight increase in postoperative neurosensory disturbances in transoral vertical osteotomies and sagittal osteotomy setbacks when screw fixation was compared to wire osteosynthesis.[39] Nishioka and others[46] also reported a greater incidence of neurosensory deficit in patients undergoing rigid fixation for sagittal osteotomies.

6. Tooth devitalization. Trauma to adjacent teeth with resulting devitalization is possible from bone plate and screw placement in both maxillary and mandibular surgery. There are currently no reports in the literature to document the incidence of such problems. A review of 150 patients treated with RIF at the University of North Carolina revealed 4 teeth devitalized following surgery,[45] which is a higher incidence than has been reported in previous accounts of traditional fixation. However, the damage may have occurred during the bony cuts for segmental osteotomies rather than from the rigid fixation techniques.

7. Postoperative TM joint symptoms. Torquing, distraction, or rotation of the condylar segments due to screw or plating techniques may result in postoperative TM joint symptoms. These problems can be prevented. This subject is discussed more completely in Chapter 9 on mandibular ramus surgery and in subsequent clinical chapters.

POSTSURGICAL PATIENT MANAGEMENT
Occlusion and Rehabilitation of the Jaws

Return of the jaws to full function is an important goal which has received more attention since the advent of RIF. It is not surprising that patients may have difficulty finding a new occlusal position after surgery because of the changed skeletal and dental segments; altered proprioception in the dental, skeletal, and muscular apparatus; and tissue edema. Postsurgically, patients find it easier to function into the new occlusal position when guided into a proper occlusal splint with light training elastics.

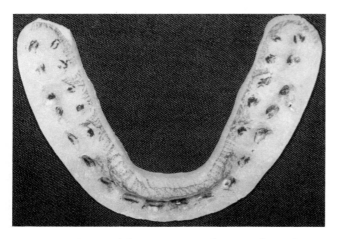

Fig. 7-27. Splint modification. Areas of potential interference are lightly marked for removal (lingual-distal aspects of indentations); cusp tips and incisal edge indentations (heavily marked) are to remain.

We strongly suggest that even if the patient's maxillomandibular fixation is released before he or she leaves the operating room because of successful RIF, the occlusal splint remain in place until the orthodontic stabilizing arch wires are removed (see Chapter 6 for more details on sequencing the surgical and orthodontic treatment). This does require some modification of the splint from the type that was used routinely with traditional fixation. Three steps are important: (1) reduction of the depth of the occlusal index of the splint, to remove potential interferences on the distal and lingual aspects of posterior teeth as well as the lingual aspect of incisor teeth—the patient must be able to go into lateral excursions as well as bite up and down (Fig. 7-27); (2) provision of adequate splint thickness

so that it does not break in function—although thin splints are the ideal, in instances where patients are to function into the splint just after surgery, the splint must be at least 2 mm thick and reinforced with wire if at all possible; and (3) provision for removal of the splint for cleaning (except in segmented cases)—this can be accomplished most easily by adding ball clasps to the splint, so that the patient can take the splint out, clean it, and put it back (Fig. 7-28).

Although patients are cautioned to remain on a soft diet for 6 to 8 weeks following surgery, progressive jaw rehabilitation with increasing range of motion should begin as soon as maxillomandibular fixation is released. The importance of physical therapy in the form of prescribed jaw exercises, for postoperative rehabilitation of muscle and joint function in the orthognathic surgical patient, is now generally accepted.[47]

The elimination of maxillomandibular fixation and the use of RIF techniques may shorten the time necessary for return to normal jaw function, a concept supported by clinical as well as animal studies.[48,49] Van Sickles and others suggest that an acceptable schedule for vertical opening after rigid fixation is 20 mm at 2 weeks, 30 mm at 4 weeks, and 40 mm or greater at 8 weeks postoperatively. Other parameters such as lateral function and protrusion must also be considered.[24]

The progression of postoperative rehabilitation depends on several factors, including type of surgery, stability of segments at time of surgery, age, and patient motivation. In general, mandibular surgical procedures alone or in combination with maxillary surgery result in more limited function and patients require more attention in rehabilitation than those with isolated maxillary procedures. Patients who have had procedures resulting in good bone contact and stabilization of segments can increase their range of motion more quickly

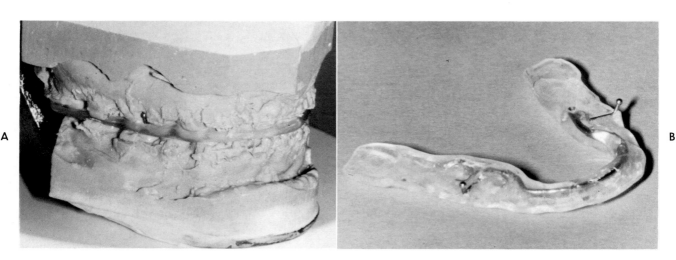

Fig. 7-28. **A** and **B,** A splint with ball clasps for a patient with RIF who will function into the splint for several weeks before the stabilizing arch wires are removed and the finishing orthodontics resume.

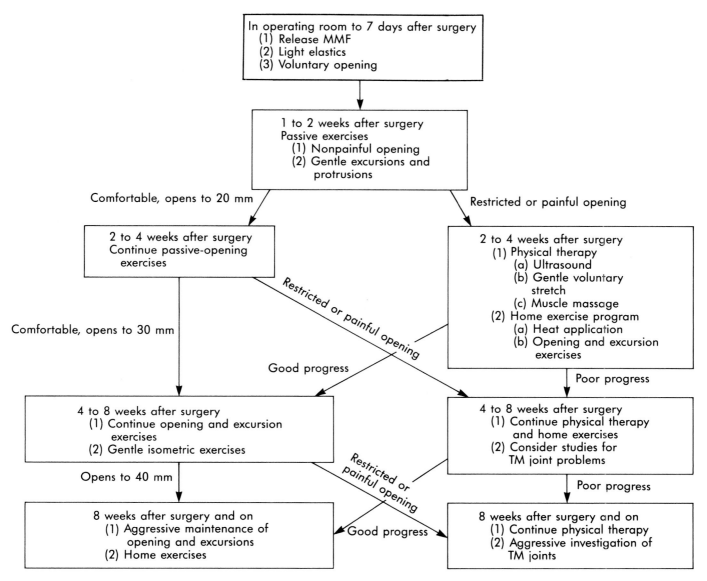

Fig. 7-29. Flow chart for jaw rehabilitation.

in the immediate postoperative period. Even when rapid and aggressive rehabilitation of jaw function is possible, it must be remembered that complete bony healing takes place over several months and excessive force used to assist jaw function may cause movement at the osteotomy sites in the first 2 months after surgery.

A typical sequence of rehabilitation exercises is summarized in Fig. 7-29. The sequence begins with passive jaw motion primarily in the vertical direction. Over the first 2 weeks after release of maxillomandibular fixation, lateral excursions and light active stretching are added. Some patients do have difficulty increasing their range of motion, and professionally administered physical therapy is helpful. Techniques such as ultrasound, spray and stretch, muscle massage, and range of mo-

tion exercises can be instituted early in the postoperative rehabilitation schedule for those who are adapting slowly, but these must be supervised by an experienced therapist.

To maintain the desired postoperative occlusion, light elastics are employed to guide the patient into the proper position in the occlusal splint (Fig. 7-30). These should be worn full-time initially. Some patients have no difficulty functioning into their new occlusion. Others require close observation and assistance with the direction of their guiding elastics. Once the patient can function into the splint easily, the guiding elastics can be reduced and then eliminated. At first, he or she may leave the elastics off 2 to 3 hours each day, usually around mealtimes. This may be in the second postsurgery week with RIF. Subsequently, the patient can

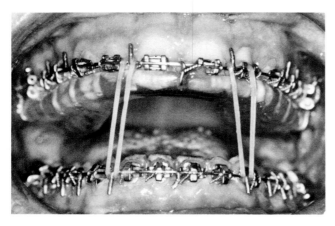

Fig. 7-30. Use of light guiding elastics in combination with interocclusal splint for control of postoperative occlusion.

eliminate the elastics during the day. If at any point the patient cannot find his or her established occlusion in the splint, elastics should be reapplied full-time and an immediate appointment sought with the surgeon to assess the problem.

With wire osteosynthesis and maxillomandibular fixation, it still is a good idea to have the patient function into the splint for at least a few weeks when jaw function resumes. This is particularly true after mandibular advancement, which seems to require the greatest adaptation. Two weeks of function into the splint, following 6 weeks of maxillomandibular fixation, is not an inordinate delay in resuming the orthodontic treatment and may save considerable time in the long run. On this schedule, the earliest the patient would return to the orthodontist is 8 weeks postsurgically.

With RIF, the return to the orthodontist can be sooner, depending on the surgeon's assessment of healing. Experience with this aspect of treatment is being gained rapidly, but as yet there are no definite guidelines to suggest how much advantage there is in resuming the orthodontic treatment more quickly: there may not be any. We suggest that the patient should retain the surgical stabilizing arch wires and function into the splint for at least 3 weeks following surgery, and 4 to 5 weeks may be more prudent. At that time, the splint is removed when the surgical arch wires are replaced with light flexible wires and light elastics once again are worn full-time. See Chapter 6 for further details of the surgeon-orthodontist interaction at this point of transition.

REFERENCES

1. Kole H: Surgical operations on the alveolar ridge to correct occlusal abnormalities, Oral Surg Oral Med Oral Pathol 12:277-288, 1959.

2. Murphey PJ, Walker RV: Correction of maxillary protrusion by ostectomy and orthodontic therapy, J Oral Surg 21:275-290, 1963.
3. Mohnac AM: Maxillary osteotomy in the management of occlusal deformities, J Oral Surg 24:305-317, 1966.
4. Trauner R, Obwegeser M: The surgical correction of mandibular prognathism and retrognathia with consideration of genioplasty, Oral Surg Oral Med Oral Pathol, 10:677-689, 787-792, 1957.
5. Bell WH: LeFort I osteotomy for correction of maxillary deformities, J Oral Surg 33:412-426, 1975.
6. Anderson JA: Deliberate hypotensive anesthesia for orthognathic surgery: controlled pharmacological manipulation of cardiovascular physiology, Int J Adult Orthod Orthognath Surg 1:133-159, 1986.
7. Hegtvedt AK, Collins ML, White RP, Jr, Turvey TA: Minimizing the risk of transfusion in orthognathic surgery: use of predeposited autologous blood, Int J Adult Orthod Orthognath Surg 2:185-192, 1987.
8. Bell WH: Revascularization and bone healing after anterior maxillary osteotomy: a study using rhesus monkeys, J Oral Surg 27:249-255, 1969.
9. Bell WH, Levy BM: Revascularization and bone healing after posterior maxillary osteotomy, J Oral Surg 29:313-320, 1971.
10. Bell WH: Biologic basis for maxillary osteotomies, Am J Phys Anthropol 38:279-289, 1973.
11. Bell WH, Fonseca RJ, Kennedy JW, Levy BM: Bone healing and revascularization after total maxillary osteotomy, J Oral Surg 33:253-260, 1975.
12. Hitchcock R, Ellis E III, Cox CF: Intentional vital root transection: a 52-week histopathologic study in Macaca mulatta, Oral Surg Oral Med Oral Pathol 60:2-14, 1985.
13. Kohn MW, White RP Jr: Evaluation of sensation after segmental alveolar osteotomy in 22 patients, J Am Dent Assoc 89:154-156, 1974.
14. Pepersack WJ: Tooh vitality after alveolar segmental osteotomy, J Maxillofac Surg 1:85-91, 1973.
15. Moriarty J: Personal communication.
16. Gallo WJ, Moss M, Gaul JV: The Shaw scalpel: thermal control of surgical bleeding, Int J Oral Maxillofac Surg 15:588-591, 1986.
17. Holmes RE, Woldrop RW, Wolford LM: Hydroxylapatite as a bone graft substitute in orthognathic surgery. Histologic and histomorphometric findings, J Oral Maxillofacial Surg 46:661-671, 1988.
18. Harsha BC, Turvey TA, Powers SK: Use of autogenous cranial bone grafts in maxillofacial surgery: a preliminary report, J Oral Maxillofac Surg 44:11-15, 1986.
19. Dolan P, White RP, Jr, Tulloch JFC: An analysis of hospital charges for orthognathic surgery, Int J Adult Orthod Orthognath Surg 2:9-14, 1987.
20. Kendell BD, Fonseca RJ, Lee M: Postoperative nutritional supplementation for the orthognathic surgery patient, J Oral Maxillofac Surg 40:205-213, 1982.
21. Harsha BC, Terry BC: Stabilization of LeFort I osteotomies using small bone plates, Int J Adult Orthod Orthognath Surg 1:69-77, 1986.

22. Van Sickles JE, Jeter TD, Aragon SB: Rigid fixation of maxillary osteotomies: a preliminary report and technique article, Oral Surg Oral Med Oral Pathol 60:262-265, 1985.
23. Schilli W, Niederdellmann H, Harle F, Goos U: Stable osteosynthesis and treatment of dentofacial deformity. In Bell WH, editor: Surgical correction of dentofacial deformities, vol 3, Philadelphia, 1984, WB Saunders Co.
24. Van Sickles JE, Jeter TS: Rigid osseous fixation of osteotomies. In Bell WH, editor: Surgical correction of dentofacial deformities, vol 3, Philadelphia, 1984, WB Saunders Co.
25. Bays RA: Maxillary osteotomies using the rigid adjustable pin (RAP) system: a review of 31 clinical cases, Int J Adult Orthod Orthognath Surg 1:275-297, 1986.
26. Bays RA: Rigid stabilization system for maxillary osteotomies, J Oral Maxillofac Surg 43:60-63, 1985.
27. Bennet MA, Wolford LM: The maxillary step osteotomy and Steinman pin stabilization, J Oral Maxillofac Surg 3:307-311, 1985.
28. Spiessl B: Mediane Ostektomie zur Verkleinerung des Unterkieferbogens bei Dysgnathie, Fortschr Kiefer Gesichtschir 18:163, 1974.
29. Terry BC: Personal communication, 1987.
30. Perren SM: Physical and biological aspects of fracture healing with special reference to internal fixation, Clin Orthop Related Res 138:175-195, 1979.
31. Reitzik M: Cortex to cortex healing after mandibular osteotomy, J Oral Maxillofac Surg 41:658-663, 1983.
32. Reitzik M, Schoorl W: Bone repair in the mandible. A histologic and biometric comparison between rigid and semirigid fixation, J Oral Maxillofac Surg 41:215-218, 1983.
33. Frost DE, Koutnik AW: Alternative stabilization of the maxilla during simultaneous jaw mobilization procedures, Oral Surg Oral Med Oral Pathol 56:125-127, 1983.
34. Tucker MR, Ochs, MW: Use of rigid internal fixation for management of intraoperative complications of mandibular sagittal split osteotomy, Int J Adult Orthognath Surg 2:71-80, 1988.
35. Van Sickles JE, Jeter TS, Theriot BA: Management of an unfavorable lingual fracture during a sagittal split osteotomy, J Oral Maxillofac Surg 43:807-809, 1985.
36. Singer RS, Bays RA: A comparison between superior and inferior border wiring techniques and sagittal split ramus osteotomy, J Oral Maxillofac Surg 43:444, 1985.
37. Van Sickles JE, Larsen AJ, Thrash WJ: Relapse after rigid fixation of mandibular advancement, J Oral Maxillofac Surg 44:698-702, 1986.
38. Thomas PM, Tucker MR, Prewitt JR, Proffit WR: Early skeletal and dental changes following mandibular advancement and rigid internal fixation, Int J Adult Orthod Orthognath Surg 3:171-178, 1986.
39. Paulus GW, Steinhauser EW: A comparative study of wire osteotsynthesis versus bone screws in the treatment of mandibular prognathism, Oral Surg Oral Med Oral Pathol 54:2-6, 1982.
40. Van Sickles JE, Flanary CM: Stability associated with mandibular advancement treated by rigid osseous fixation, J Oral Maxillofac Surg 43:338, 1985.
41. Watzke I, Turvey TA, Phillips C, Proffit WR: Stability of mandibular advancement by sagittal osteotomy with screw and wire fixation: a comparative study, J Oral Maxillofac Surg 48:108-121, 1990.
42. Larson AJ, Van Sickles JE, Thrash WJ: Postsurgical maxillary movement: a comparison study of rigid and nonrigid fixation, Am J Orthod [in press].
43. Buckley MJ, Tucker MR, Fredette SA: An alternative approach for staging simultaneous maxillary and mandibular osteotomies, Int J Adult Orthod Orthognath Surg 2:75-78, 1987.
44. Rosen HM: Mini-plate fixation of LeFort I osteotomies, Plast Reconstr Surg 78:748-754, 1986.
45. Buckley MJ, Dolan PJ, Tucker MR, White RP: Complications associated with rigid internal fixation used for orthognathic surgery, Int J Adult Orthod Orthognath Surg 4:69-75, 1989.
46. Nishioka GM, Zysset MK, Van Sickles JE: Neurosensory disturbance with rigid fixation of the bilateral sagittal split osteotomy, J Oral Maxillofac Surg 45:20-26, 1987.
47. Bell WH, Gonyea W, Finn RA, et al: Muscular rehabilitation after orthognathic surgery, Oral Surg Oral Med Oral Pathol 56:229-235, 1983.
48. Ellis E: Mobility of the mandible following advancement and maxillomandibular or rigid internal fixation. An experimental investigation in Macaca mulatta, J Oral Maxillofac Surg 46:228-123, 1988.
49. Timmis DP, Aragon SB, Van Sickles JE: Masticatory dysfunction with rigid and nonrigid osteosynthesis of sagittal split osteotomies, Oral Surg Oral Med Oral Pathol 62:119-123, 1986.

CHAPTER 8

Maxillary Surgery

Timothy A. Turvey
Raymond P. White, Jr.

HISTORICAL DEVELOPMENT

The downfracture osteotomy technique for maxillary surgery originated with Cheever, who in 1864 reported an osteotomy technique to resect a nasopharyngeal mass in two patients.[1] Although employed to gain access to the nasopharynx for tumor resection and not to correct a deformity, the surgical procedure was truly a remarkable feat, especially considering the state of surgery and anesthesia at the time. An entire century passed until the LeFort I osteotomy of the maxilla with downfracture became popular in the United States to correct dentofacial deformities.[2,3]

In 1921, a German surgeon, Herman Wassmund, reported his initial attempt to correct a dentofacial deformity by maxillary osteotomy, 70 years after Simon Hullihen introduced the mandibular subapical osteotomy.[4-6] Wassmund did not mobilize the maxilla after osteotomy; he employed orthopedic traction during the postsurgical period to position the maxilla. In 1934, Auxhausen, a student of Wassmund's, related his expe-

rience with mobilization of the maxilla for correction of open-bite deformity.[7] It was not until 1952 that an American surgeon, Converse, reported on maxillary osteotomy.[8]

Although early reports of the stability following correction of open-bite deformity by maxillary surgery were not good, Stoker and Epker indicated encouraging results.[8-10] Their success, along with the favorable experiences of others with LeFort I downfracture (e.g., Wilmar, Obwegeser, Bell), led American surgeons to adopt total maxillary osteotomy procedures.[3,11,12]

The option of LeFort I osteotomy provides surgeons the techniques to correct skeletal jaw deformity where it exists. Before 1965 dentofacial deformity was treated by mandibular surgery alone, although the skeletal problem presented by the patient may be partly or almost entirely in the maxilla. The final result often was not satisfactory. LeFort I osteotomy with maxillary downfracture allows the surgeon to move the maxilla in all three planes of space. Dentofacial deformity involving the maxilla can be satisfactorily corrected by maxillary surgery, alone or in combination with mandibular surgery.[13] Results are predictably good and most maxillary and mandibular skeletal corrections are stable.

The refined surgical techniques for maxillary and mandibular surgery have benefited patients and the specialty of oral and maxillofacial surgery. Fifteen years ago, only a few residency training programs included the teaching of maxillary surgical techniques. Today, every oral and maxillofacial surgery residency program in the United States has incorporated the teaching of maxillary surgery into their curriculum, and accreditation standards demand that residents obtain sufficient experience with both maxillary and mandibular surgery. Through continuing education efforts, surgeons who did not benefit from maxillary surgery experience in their residency have learned the procedures and incorporated them into practice.

VASCULAR CONSIDERATIONS

The major concerns of surgeons who first performed maxillary surgery to correct dentofacial deformities were intraoperative bleeding, and revascularization and healing of the maxilla. A better understanding of the vascular perfusion of the maxilla and the anatomy of the maxillary artery and its terminal branches has helped refine surgical techniques to minimize the risks of hemorrhage and maximize the potential for healing. Turvey and Fonseca reported on the anatomy of the maxillary artery and its relevance to maxillary surgery. Their study of cadaver specimens suggested that the LeFort I level osteotomy could be conducted safely, providing the surgeon paid strict attention to the anatomy in the posterior maxilla.[14] Although dynamic blood flow studies by Nelson and others indicated significant reduction in blood flow immediately following osteotomy, perfusion gradually increased during the postsurgical phase.[15] The revascularization studies of Bell indicated that the maxilla could be sectioned and mobilized after downfracture and could be expected to heal as long as large soft-tissue pedicles remained attached to the mobilized segments.[16] If basic surgical principles are followed meticulously, the problems of necrosis of bone and teeth and nonunion of mobilized jaw segments are rare following LeFort I osteotomy.

LE FORT I OSTEOTOMY: SURGICAL TECHNIQUE

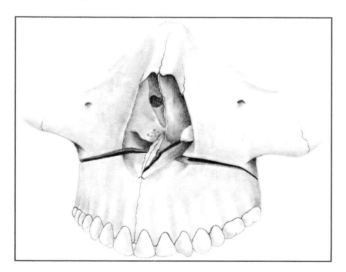

Tissue Dissection

At the outset of the procedure, a dilute solution of epinephrine (usually 2% lidocaine with 1:100,000 epinephrine) is infiltrated into the mucobuccal tissues along the entire facial surface of the maxilla to minimize bleeding from soft tissue following the incision. Palatal soft tissues form an important vascular pedicle to the maxilla and should not be injected with vasoconstrictor. By combining tissue infiltration with a vasoconstrictor, elevation of the head of the operating table approximately 15 degrees, and modified hypotensive anesthesia to control the systolic blood pressure (about 90 mm Hg), total blood loss can be reduced significantly during surgery.[17] Patients having maxillary surgery are encouraged to predeposit autologous blood. This subject is discussed more thoroughly in Chapter 7.

The incision is made from the zygomatic maxillary buttress region above the first molar, to the midline of the maxilla above the central incisors. After the incision, a broad pedicle of buccal tissue above the teeth (generally wider posteriorly) remains to perfuse the maxilla. With this incision, it is best to err by having too broad a soft-tissue pedicle rather than one that is too narrow (Fig. 8-1). A scalpel or a calibrated thermal knife for this incision yields predictable results with good healing (see Chapter 7). The use of electrocautery for the incision is discouraged since it may adversely affect wound healing by promoting excessive scar formation beneath the upper lip and nasal alar base.

Once the incision is carried through mucosa, muscle, and periosteum, the lateral wall of the maxilla is exposed superiorly with a periosteal elevator from the zygomatic maxillary buttress to the anterior nasal spine. The infraorbital neurovascular bundle is identified and carefully protected when exposing the zygomatic maxillary buttress. No dissection of tissue is done inferior to the incision. Remember this soft-tissue pedicle will perfuse the maxilla when it is repositioned. The dissection continues posteriorly toward the maxillary tuberosity and pterygoid plate with the direction of dissection angled inferiorly behind the zygomatic maxillary buttress on the posterior maxilla. The dissection posterior to the zygomatic maxillary buttress is tunneled to preserve a broad based intact mucosal pedicle. It is critical to perform this dissection subperiosteally and un-

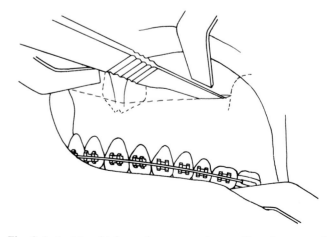

Fig. 8-1. Incision high on the zygomatic-maxillary buttress of the anterior maxilla across the midline to end on the opposite buttress.

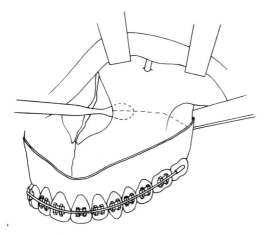

Fig. 8-2. Incision open: infraorbital nerve exposed, retractor at pterygomaxillary junction, and nasal aperture with anterior nasal spine exposed. Dashed line indicates planned osteotomy.

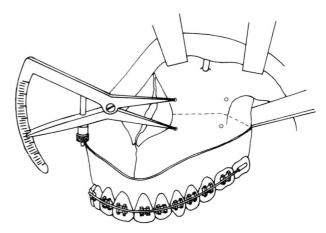

Fig. 8-3. Calipers mark vertical reference points: bur holes in bone at maxillary buttress and piriform nasal aperture. Dashed line indicates planned osteotomy.

der direct vision. Preventing superior dissection at the junction of the maxilla and pterygoid plates minimizes the risk of excessive hemorrhage or nerve injury. Occasionally, the buccal fat pad will be exposed, obscuring the surgical field. A moistened gauze can be placed over the fat pad to contain it and both can be retracted laterally to improve access and visibility.

Next, the nasal aperture is exposed with careful dissection along the piriform rim and lateral nasal wall under the inferior turbinate (Fig. 8-2). Similarly, mucosa and periosteum from the floor of the nose are elevated as far as the nasal crest of the maxilla in the midline. The septopremaxillary ligament and transverse nasalis muscle are transected to expose the anterior nasal spine. Careful reflection and dissection of nasal mucosa with as few perforations as possible minimize blood loss and postoperative discomfort. Once the soft-tissue dissection is completed unilaterally, reference landmarks are established before osteotomy.

Osteotomy

Vertical reference landmarks are placed at the piriform region and the zygomatic maxillary buttress (Fig. 8-3). Vertical reference marks are critical since vertical orientation is lost when osteotomy is complete and the maxilla is mobilized. Horizontal references are not necessary since the teeth and occlusal splint guide the correction in the sagittal plane. The landmarks are placed in bone with a bur, 10 to 15 mm apart, depending on the amount of vertical repositioning planned.[5] If the maxilla is to be superiorly repositioned and segments of bone removed, the reference holes must be farther apart than if the maxilla is inferiorly repositioned.

The osteotomy of the lateral maxilla begins posteriorly at the zygomatic maxillary buttress, just above the

inferior vertical reference mark, usually about 35 mm above the maxillary occlusal plane. With a reciprocating saw or surgical bur, the osteotomy advances through the thicker bone at the buttress and the thin bone of the lateral maxillary wall to the piriform rim where the bone thickens again. A portion of the lateral nasal wall also is sectioned with the saw as the piriform rim is approached. A periosteal elevator inserted subperiosteally into the piriform aperture approximately 2 cm protects the nasal mucosa as the piriform rim and lateral nasal wall are sectioned (Fig. 8-4). If the maxilla is to be repositioned superiorly, the amount of bone to be removed from the piriform rim region is measured, scored on the maxilla with a periosteal elevator, and removed with a saw or bur (Fig. 8-5). Because of the anatomy of the lateral maxillary wall and the propensity for the maxilla to telescope at the zygomatic maxillary buttress region and the posterior max-

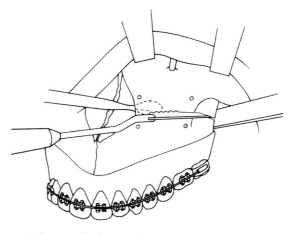

Fig. 8-4. Periosteal elevator in nasal aperture; reciprocating saw performing osteotomy along lateral wall.

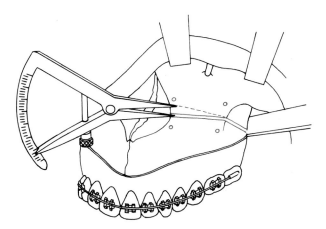

Fig. 8-5. Caliper measuring amount of bone to be removed at piriform region after initial osteotomy.

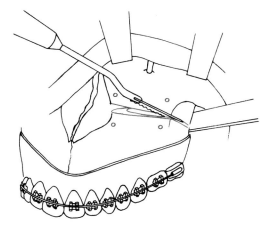

Fig. 8-7. Reciprocating saw completing osteotomy from maxillary buttress to posterior maxilla, heading inferiorly under the flap.

illary wall, less bone than the desired superior maxillary movement is removed posterior to the piriform rim (Fig. 8-6).

Before sectioning the posterior lateral wall of the maxilla, a toe out retractor is placed subperiosteally at the junction of the maxilla and pterygoid plate. Under direct vision, the osteotomy is directed inferior and posterior, from the zygomatic maxillary buttress to the junction of the maxilla and pterygoid plate to minimize the risk of damaging the maxillary artery or any of its

terminal branches (Fig. 8-7). The osteotomy only need be 5 mm superior to the second molar (which is approximately 25 mm long) to minimize the risk of devitalizing this tooth. If impacted third molars are present, their position should not alter the osteotomy design. Third molars may be removed after maxillary down-fracture if they interfere with repositioning the maxilla. After the reciprocating saw sections the posterior lateral maxillary wall, its direction is reversed so that the blade placed into the maxillary sinus cuts laterally

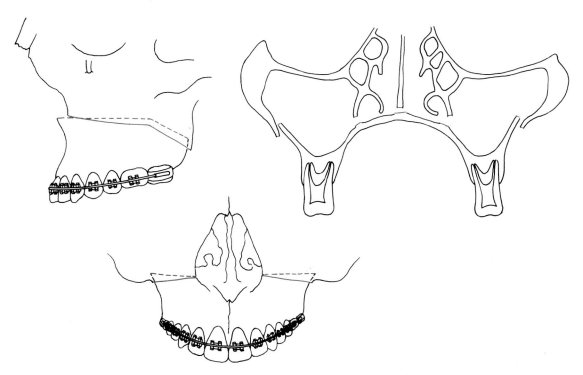

Fig. 8-6. Maxilla repositioned superiorly; telescoping of bony segments at maxillary buttress.

Fig. 8-8. Reciprocating saw reversed so cutting is from inside the maxillary sinus to outside at posterior maxilla.

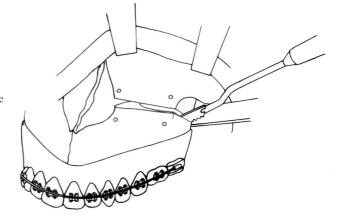

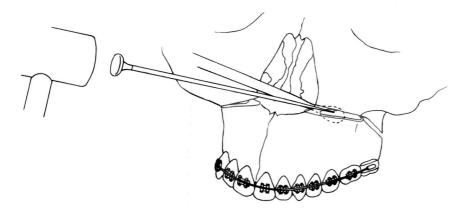

Fig. 8-9. Spatula osteotome sectioning the lateral nasal wall with elevator protecting the nasal mucosa.

from the sinus to the outside. This maneuver permits easy sectioning of the posterior wall of the maxilla (Fig. 8-8). When bone cuts are complete, the wound is packed with a moistened gauze and the same steps are repeated in an identical fashion on the opposite side.

Attention is then directed to the nasal cavity. A periosteal elevator protects the nasal mucosa while the lateral nasal wall is sectioned with a spatula osteotome directed posterior and inferior, along the lateral nasal wall toward the perpendicular plate of the palatine bone (Fig. 8-9). The lateral nasal wall is thin and offers little resistance to sectioning until the palatine bone is reached. Resistance to the advancing osteotome as well as an audible change in sound when malleting the osteotome indicate that the palatine bone has been encountered. Partial section of the perpendicular part of the palatine bone is sufficient. If the osteotome is malleted too far posteriorly, injury to the descending palatine vessels may result in hemorrhage, which is difficult to control until the maxilla is mobilized. After the opposite lateral nasal wall is sectioned similarly, attention is directed to the nasal septum. With care to reflect nasal mucosa intact, a septal osteotome is malleted posteriorly, freeing the cartilaginous septum and sectioning the bony septum at the nasal floor (Fig. 8-10).

Once the septum and lateral nasal walls are free, the maxilla must be released from the pterygoid plates. The packs previously placed at the lateral maxilla are removed and a retractor is placed subperiosteally at the junction of the maxilla and pterygoid plate. Under direct vision, a curved osteotome is positioned and directed medial and inferior, at the lowest part of the junction between the maxilla and the pterygoid plate. For orientation prior to malleting, an index finger

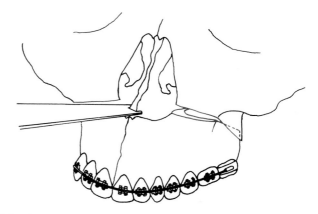

Fig. 8-10. Nasal septal osteotome freeing cartilaginous and bony septum.

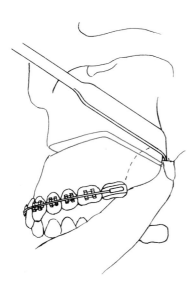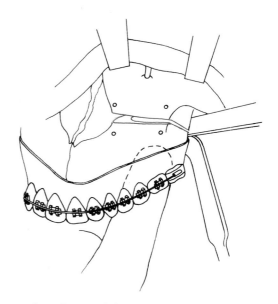

Fig. 8-11. Separation of maxilla at pterygoid plates with malleting of the osteotome. Finger tip should feel lower edges of osteotome.

placed on the palate at the hamular notch region should feel the tip of the osteotome. The osteotome is malleted to achieve bony separation (Fig. 8-11). Moist packs are placed in the wound, and the procedure is repeated on the opposite side. The maxilla is ready for downfracture.

By utilizing finger pressure on the anterior aspect, the maxilla is forced down. Simultaneously, the remaining attached nasal soft tissues are elevated care-fully from the nasal floor (Fig. 8-12). With a rongeur any remaining vomer and the nasal crest of the maxilla are removed, particularly if superior repositioning of the maxilla is planned (Fig. 8-13). The anterior nasal spine may require reduction if the maxilla must be moved forward or in a superior direction, but it is not intentionally removed otherwise. Similarly, the lateral nasal walls are reduced with a rongeur to permit visualization of the perpendicular portion of the palatine bone and to facilitate any superior movement. Then maxillary distraction and mobilization devices are placed bilaterally on the buccal side at the posterior aspect of the maxilla, and under direct vision the maxilla

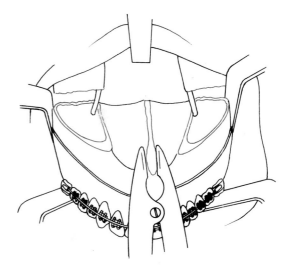

Fig. 8-12. Maxilla forced down with hand pressure; nasal mucosa elevated to expose nasal floor.

Fig. 8-13. Rongeur to reduce septal crest of the maxilla and lateral nasal wall.

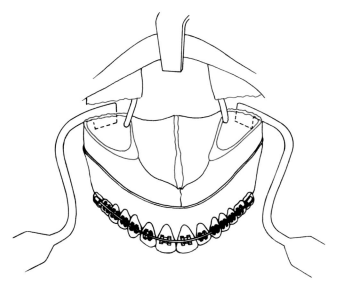

Fig. 8-14. Mobilizers pulling maxilla forward, fracturing remaining bony attachments.

is brought forward, fracturing any remaining posterior bony attachments (Fig. 8-14).

The descending palatine neurovascular bundle commonly is visualized posterior and medial to the maxillary sinuses. Bone should be removed carefully from the posterior maxilla and from around the descending palatine vessels with a rongeur, osteotome, or bur. If possible, these vessels should be preserved to enhance blood supply to the maxilla through the soft-tissue pedicle on the palate (Fig. 8-15). If the descending palatine vessels are violated, bleeding can be controlled by vascular clamps or packing. When bone is removed from the pterygoid plate, bleeding may be encountered

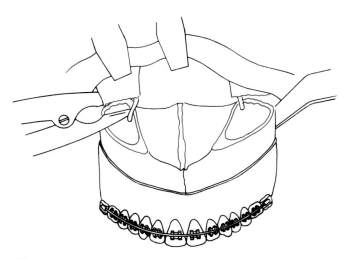

Fig. 8-15. Removal of bony interferences from posterior maxilla with ronguer: descending palatine vessels should be kept intact.

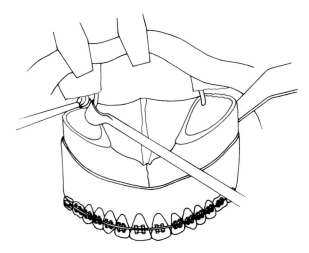

Fig. 8-16. Removal of bone from pterygoid plate with bur. Instrument protecting descending palatine vessels.

from the pterygoid muscles. This bleeding can be controlled by injecting a dilute epinephrine solution (usually 2% lidocaine with 1:100,000 epinephrine) into the soft tissue and gauze packing. If superior or posterior repositioning is planned, it is critical to remove a sufficient quantity of bone at the posterior and medial maxilla (Fig. 8-16). Bony interference is common in this area, preventing planned repositioning of the maxilla. When insufficient bone is removed, faulty positioning of the maxilla and the mandible may result. The mandible and its condyles are easily displaced inferiorly from the fossa by this bony interference as the mandibular-maxillary complex is repositioned (Fig. 8-17).

The sequence of performing these osteotomies (lateral maxillary walls, nasal septum, lateral nasal walls, pterygomaxillary junction) should permit easy and quick mobilization of the maxilla if excessive hemorrhage is encountered during the procedure. Previous studies with cadaver specimens have demonstrated that LeFort I osteotomy can be performed without an excessive risk to the maxillary arteries.[14] The vessels at greatest risk for hemorrhage are the descending palatine artery and vein.

After maxillary mobilization and bony reduction and insertion of the occlusal wafer splint, the maxilla and mandible are held together by utilizing 25-gauge wire for maxillomandibular fixation. The mandible with the maxilla secured to it is then rotated closed superiorly. The surgeon must look for deviations or bony interferences, palpating for premature bony contact which may distort the position of the maxilla (see Fig. 8-17). When the mandible is rotated closed, it should be held at the inferior border, just anterior to the angles bilaterally, and guided so that the condyles remain seated. If deviations or premature bone contacts are detected, sufficient bone must be removed from the maxilla to

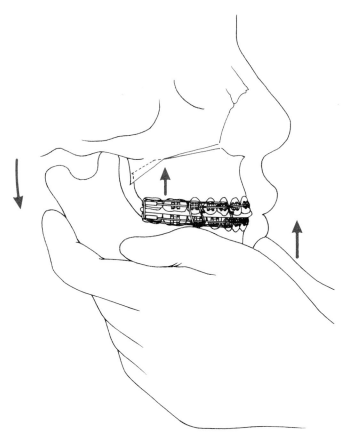

Fig. 8-17. When the maxilla and mandible are wired together in maxillomandibular fixation, if there is a bony obstruction at the posterior maxilla, the mandibular condyle will be displaced.

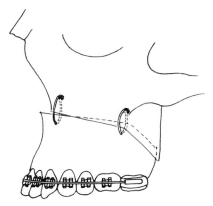

Fig. 8-18. Maxilla repositioned vertically. Butt joints at piriform rim and telescoping at maxillary buttress and tuberosity.

allow the maxillomandibular complex to be repositioned passively.

The distance between the vertical reference holes is measured to be certain that the expected amount of repositioning has occurred. By incremental removal of bone, good bone contact can be obtained anteriorly at the piriform region even with telescoping of the maxillary walls posteriorly (Fig. 8-18). Large defects in the maxillary walls may result from overzealous removal of the bone from the lateral maxilla and zygomatic maxillary buttress region. This is to be prevented if possible.

Attention is then directed to the nasal septum area. If the maxilla is repositioned superiorly, bone from the nasal crest of the maxilla and bone and cartilage from the nasal septum should be resected, sufficient to allow the maxilla to be elevated. This reduction will assist in maintaining the nasal septum in the midline without buckling. If septal spurs are present on the inferior part of the septum, they also can be removed. Extensive submucosal dissection of the septum is not suggested since unnecessary bleeding may occur. The nose cannot

be packed to control bleeding when maxillomandibular fixation is placed. Additional room for the nasal septum can be gained by removing bone from the septal crest of the maxilla with a bur.[18] If more than 5 mm of superior maxillary movement is planned, an osteotomy freeing the nasal floor from the remaining maxilla is suggested. With a bur, a U-shaped section of bone is mobilized but left attached to palatal mucosa. As the maxilla moves up this bony segment is displaced inferiorly.

If the inferior turbinates are interfering with repositioning the maxilla, they may be trimmed with a Mayo scissors following exposure through the nasal mucosa (Fig. 8-19). Incisions and any gross tears in the nasal mucosa should be repaired with 4.0 chromic gut suture to minimize nasal bleeding in the immediate postsurgery period.[18]

Maxillary Segmentation. If the maxilla must be segmented to facilitate expansion or contraction, leveling of the occlusal plane, or space closure, further osteotomy is done after the maxilla has been mobilized. Paramidline sagittal osteotomy is planned when transverse expansion or contraction with minimal alteration in the occlusal plane is needed. With the maxilla downfractured, bilateral paramidline osteotomies through the nasal floor are followed by a planned midline interdental osteotomy (Figs. 8-20 to 8-22). Bilateral osteotomy minimizes the bony defect in the palate following expansion and disperses the resulting soft-tissue tension across the entire palate rather than concentrating it to a single area adjacent to only one osteotomy site. Additionally, the soft tissues under the lateral nasal floor are thicker and less likely to rupture than the midline soft tissues.[19]

To level the occlusal plane and close interdental spaces, several dentoalveolar segments must be created. Osteotomy cuts between indicated teeth are added to the paramidline sagittal osteotomies. Leveling, when

Fig. 8-19. Turbinate resection after incision in nasal mucosa.

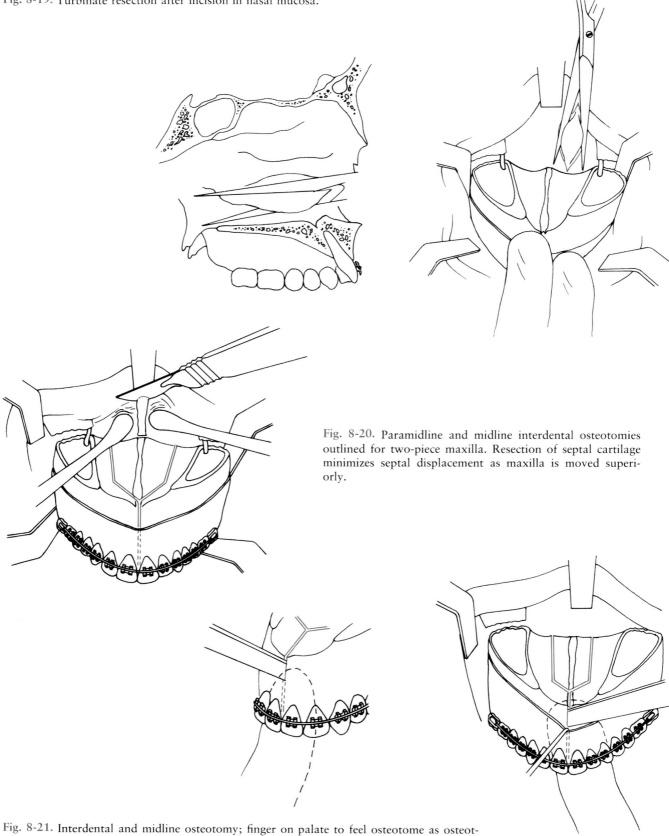

Fig. 8-20. Paramidline and midline interdental osteotomies outlined for two-piece maxilla. Resection of septal cartilage minimizes septal displacement as maxilla is moved superiorly.

Fig. 8-21. Interdental and midline osteotomy; finger on palate to feel osteotome as osteotomy is complete.

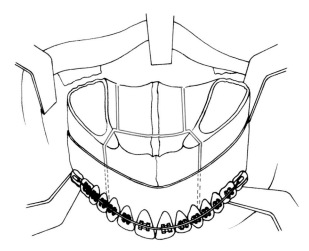

Fig. 8-22. Paramidline and interdental osteotomies outlined for three-piece maxilla.

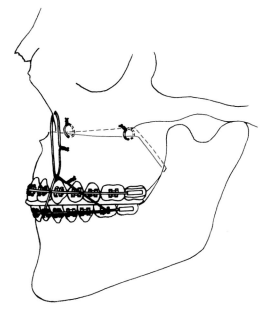

Fig. 8-23. Four osseous wires are usually sufficient to immobilize the maxilla. One piriform suspension wire with an intermediate wire directed to the mandibular arch will control the mandibular movement, which could displace the maxilla.

needed, almost always is required bilaterally. Simple space closure may be necessary unilaterally or bilaterally and the osteotomy must be designed accordingly.

An important part of segmenting the maxilla is to be certain that there is sufficient room between the roots of teeth at the proposed osteotomy site. The orthodontist must keep tooth roots parallel or even divergent at planned interdental osteotomy sites. Previous studies of the effect of interdental osteotomies on periodontal tissues indicate that leaving at least 3 mm of bone between the roots of adjacent teeth allows osteotomy without excessive risk to the teeth and supporting tissues[20] (see Chapter 7 for further discussion).

After very careful exposure of interdental bone at osteotomy sites with minimal reflection of mucoperiosteum, a small fissure bur (e.g., 701) is used to score the lateral cortical bone. With a spatula osteotome, the interdental osteotomy is completed. A finger is placed on the palatal tissues to palpate the tip of the osteotome as it passes through the palatal bone (see Fig. 8-21). The segments are mobilized with finger pressure or the bone spreader. If interdental bone is to be removed, particular care must be taken not to remove the bone over the roots of the adjacent teeth, especially at the alveolar crest. Tissue pedicles to dentoalveolar segments must remain intact. Creating more than four maxillary dentoalveolar segments is inadvisable.

Following osteotomy to segment the maxilla, the occlusal wafer splint is used to configure the maxillary dental arch holding the segments into a preplanned position. The palatal soft-tissue pedicle is checked to make certain that folds in the palatal mucosa, which could reduce blood supply, are eliminated. Often freeing mucosa with a Freer elevator at osteotomy sites reduces tissue folding. With the maxillary segments held into the splint with finger pressure, maxillomandibular

fixation is secured with 25-gauge wires. Additional stability for the segmented maxilla is obtained from a prefabricated auxiliary stabilizing wire (36 or 40 mil) fixed into headgear tubes on molar bands and secured to the segmented orthodontic arch wires. The mandible with the maxilla secured to it is rotated closed superiorly. As with an unsegmented maxilla, the surgeon must look for bony interferences as the maxilla is repositioned. Interferences must be removed to allow passive positioning of the maxilla into its planned new position.

Stabilization and Fixation

Stabilization of the maxilla following superior repositioning usually is accomplished with transosseous 26-gauge wire sutures. Before transosseous fixation wires are placed, the nasal floor, exposed maxillary sinuses, and posterior maxillary areas should be flushed copiously with saline to remove accumulated blood clots. Any points of bleeding must be controlled, usually with electrocautery. Wire sutures are placed through holes in the thick areas of the piriform region and the zygomatic maxillary buttress which retain the wire well. In addition, a unilateral skeletal suspension wire (24-gauge) placed in the piriform region is also inserted, brought into the maxillary mucobuccal fold, and a loop left exposed above the wire twist. Subsequently, the suspension wire loop is connected to the mandibular arch wire, minimizing the effect of mandibular movement on the position of the maxilla (Fig. 8-23).

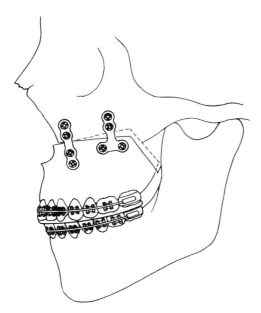

Fig. 8-24. Two plates on each side, one at the piriform region and one at the maxillary buttress, are adequate to secure the maxilla in position.

Bone plates are an alternate means of internal osseous fixation. Usually small semirigid bone plates are placed in the maxilla after the osteotomy sites are fixed with transosseous wire sutures. The plates must be bent to conform as closely as possible to the walls of the maxilla. When improperly contoured plates are secured with screws, they may displace the maxilla and produce an unanticipated occlusion. If possible the plates should be secured with two screws on either side of the osteotomy site. Fixation can be adequate with only one screw holding the plate to the repositioned maxillary segment, but two are preferred. When the maxilla has not been segmented, one plate on each side will fix the maxilla securely if good bone contact exists bilaterally. With multiple maxillary segments, a plate to fix each bony segment may be necessary. Four plates (two bilaterally) in the piriform rim and zygomatic maxillary buttress areas will hold the maxilla firmly (Fig. 8-24).

When rigid fixation with bone plates is completed, maxillomandibular fixation should always be removed and the occlusion into the acrylic splint checked. With pressure on the inferior border of the mandible bilaterally, just anterior to the angles, the mandible should be rotated until the teeth firmly occlude into the splint. If deviation of the mandible occurs or an open bite exists, the position of the maxilla must be checked carefully. If the maxilla is not in the correct position (as is indicated by the occluding mandible), the screws holding the plates must be removed on one or both sides of the osteotomy, maxillomandibular fixation reestablished,

and the maxillomandibular complex rotated into position. Often a bony interference is found posteriorly and medially. The interference should be removed and the jaws rotated closed again until the surgeon is convinced that the maxilla is in the correct position. Rigid fixation is reapplied with new screw holes, maxillomandibular fixation released, and the occlusion checked again. This sequence is repeated until the occlusion is adequate to allow the patient to function into the splint. The occlusal splint may be at fault but the surgeon must not assume that an unanticipated occlusion at this point in the procedure is the result of a poor splint. Usually the problem is with the position of the maxilla.

The occlusal wafer splint must be modified when early jaw function is anticipated, removing all interferences from the surface occluding with the mandibular teeth. Occlusal splints and their modifications are discussed in Chapters 6, 7, and 11.

Bone Grafts for Stabilization. When the maxilla is advanced or positioned inferiorly more than a few millimeters so that the piriform rim and zygomatic buttress are not in contact, or when there are significant defects in the lateral maxillary walls at the completion of surgery, bone grafts should be placed to bridge the defects and stabilize the new position of the maxilla. Bone grafting will promote more rapid healing of bone at the osteotomy sites and may improve the stability of the result.

The walls of much of the maxilla are thin and osseous union is often incomplete following osteotomy and repositioning. But the bone at the piriform rim and zygomatic buttress is relatively thick. When these areas are in contact after maxillary repositioning, bone heals well with osseous union. Bone over the premolars may heal with fibrous tissue leaving bony defects. Usually these defects do not affect maxillary stability or the health of the maxillary sinus.

Defects at the piriform rim and the zygomatic buttress need bone grafts for stabilization. The grafts should be mechanically locked between bone segments or should be supported with wire or screw fixation. The grafts are most easily held in place with 26-gauge transosseous wire sutures. The bone graft is shaped to fit the defect and sandwiched between the wires before they are secured (Fig. 8-25). Bone plates alone across a maxillary defect usually are not enough to promote good bony healing. When bone plates are used, they are adapted over the grafts at the piriform rims and zygomatic buttress sites. After the maxilla has been stabilized in its new position and the occusion checked, additional bone can be placed over defects in the remaining lateral maxillary walls. Grafts should not be placed unsupported in defects where they may be dislodged into the maxillary sinus. Bone grafts which dislodge into the sinus will eventually sequestrate, but displaced

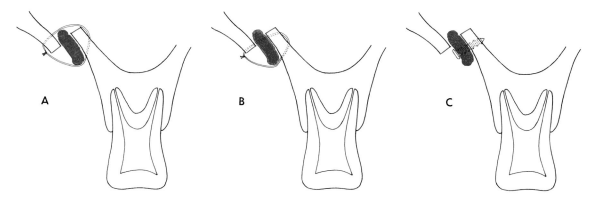

Fig. 8-25. **A** and **B**, Bone grafts at osteotomy sites supported by wire sutures or **C**, by a bone screw.

grafts do little to enhance the healing of maxillary wall defects. Additionally when sequestration occurs, patients will complain of nasal discharge and a foul odor. If this does not resolve within 10 to 14 days, the graft may have to be removed from the maxillary sinus. If a graft at the piriform rim or zygomatic buttress is displaced, maxillary instability and an unintended occlusion may result.

There is little question that autogenous bone grafts revascularize more rapidly than allogeneic bone grafts or alloplasts and ensure the best chance of osseous union. The ileum and cranium are common autogenous bone donor sites. The mandible provides another good donor source and should not be overlooked. Corticocancellous grafts are readily obtained from the body or symphysis regions, especially when vertical reduction of the mandibular inferior border is performed.

Allogeneic bone grafts (bank bone) have also been utilized to obliterate maxillary osteotomy defects with success. The increased availability of this material from commercial sources and the advantage of not having an added donor site make its use attractive for maxillary osteotomy. Vascularization of the allogeneic bone graft and healing are delayed when compared with that of autogenous bone grafts, but final results are similar to those observed with autogenous graft material. The infection rate after surgery, which one might expect to be higher with allogeneic bone grafts, is comparable with autogenous donor bone and bank bone.

The alloplastic material hydroxylapatite has also been used in maxillary osteotomy defects.[21] Although clinical reports suggest favorable results, all experimental studies do not support its use as an interpositional graft material. The hydroxylapatite will stabilize the defects at osteotomy sites (e.g., piriform rim, zygomatic buttress, palate), but the material is not replaced by bone. With a significant bony defect, the alloplastic material may actually prevent bony healing. Tissue dehiscence also seems to be higher over the alloplastic material.[21] With good local wound care, the surgical

sites will close after dehiscence, but stability at the osteotomy site may be compromised if the material is lost. Additional discussion on the use of bone grafts is found in Chapter 7.

Wound Closure

Lip Considerations. Initial studies assessing lip length following maxillary surgery suggested that the lip shortened, especially when the maxilla was superiorly or anteriorly repositioned.[22] Some authors indicated that lip shortening occurred because of the residual scar in the mucobuccal fold and recommended suture techniques which minimized excessive scarring. Others claimed that failure to suture the transected muscles of facial expression resulted in not only a shorter lip but also a wider nasal alar base.[23] Recently, Cosby and Wolford suggested that the nasal flare resulted from alteration of the bony architecture supporting the alar base when the maxilla is moved, and their data justified adding an alar base cinch suture when closing the wound.[24]

In our experience, soft-tissue response following repositioning of the maxilla, especially lip posture, is variable. The United States does not have a homogeneous population. Those who have thicker lips and greater dependency on tooth position for lip support will experience a different soft-tissue to hard-tissue change than those with short, thin lips whose lip posture is more dependent on the nasal tip and columella for support.

A recent study conducted in our laboratory on the effect of wound closure on lip length and nasal alar base changes endorses the use of muscle resuturing, especially the transverse nasalis muscle, and V-Y closure of the mucosa to maintain lip length.[25] When this technique was compared with simple mucosal closure, the vermilion height was better maintained as was the alar width. The muscle suturing technique employs the use of musculoperiosteal 3.0 chromic gut sutures (two on each side) placed diagonally so when they are tight-

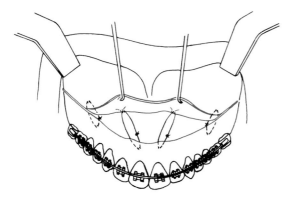

Fig. 8-26. Four musculoperiosteal sutures aid in restoring upper lip form and controlling the width of the alar bases.

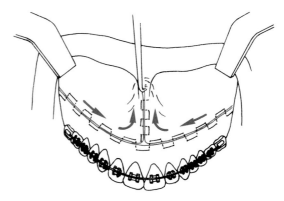

Fig. 8-27. The V-Y mucosal closure maintains the amount of vermilion lip at the midline at the expense of the lateral lip surface. Additionally, the prominence of the philtral columns is supported.

ened, they pull the lip medially (Fig. 8-26). The posterior suture begins at the first molar region in the superior part of the wound where the needle is passed through the periosteum and the muscle syncitium. When the suture is placed in the inferior wound edge, it should be inserted farther medially, at the premolar or canine region, passing through the muscular and periosteal layers. At this region, the muscular layer may not be well defined but the suture should help anchor the superior aspect of the wound forward. The next suture should be started farther anteriorly at the canine region passing initially through the superior edge of the transverse nasalis muscle, identified distinctly as muscle just under the alar base. The needle is then placed through the inferior wound edge after identifying the muscle just lateral to the anterior nasal spine. When securing this suture, an assistant should support the skin over the alar rim pushing in a medial direction as the suture is tightened and tied. If the tissue in the inferior wound edge will not support the suture, placing it in a bur hole through the base of the anterior nasal spine will secure it to a firm base. Identical sutures should be placed on the opposite side.

The V-Y mucosal closure with 4.0 chromic gut suture begins posteriorly with the vector of closure pulling the superior mucosal edge anteriorly. A skin hook placed in the midline of the superior wound edge allows an assistant to apply traction during the closure. As the closure proceeds to the midline, the superior edge of the wound on one side should be anchored above the midline before beginning closure of the opposite side. The resulting excess tissue is closed in a straight line (Fig. 8-27). Sutures through the mucosa should be placed close to the wound edge in a running horizontal mattress fashion to minimize the resultant scar. This wound closure pattern transfers mucosa from the posterior aspect of the wound anteriorly to minimize retraction of the vermilion surface and to provide support for the philtrum of the lip.

The single V-Y suture as described has been effective but lip bulk in the midline is developed at the expense of the loss of vermilion surface from the lateral lip areas. To minimize this problem for patients with very thin lips, a double V-Y mucosal closure has been employed (Fig. 8-28).[26] The suture is placed similarly to the single V-Y suture but leaves an arm extension just lateral to the height of the cupids bow bilaterally. Although this pattern of closure advances mucosa from the posterior aspect of the wound, it distributes it more evenly across the entire lip, minimizing vermilion surface deficiency laterally. The bulk of the advancement is not concentrated in the midline. The indications and effectiveness of the double V-Y closure have not been studied thoroughly, but it may be useful in special circumstances where lip bulk is very limited.

When no bone plate fixation is used, a unilateral skeletal suspension wire should be attached to the mandible following wound closure (see Fig. 8-23). One suspension wire minimizes mandibular movement and limits traction on the maxilla from the mandible. If RIF

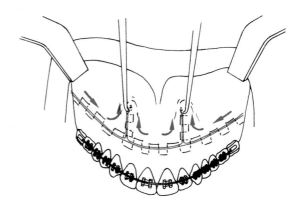

Fig. 8-28. A double V-Y closure disperses the advanced mucosa over a greater part of the lip surface rather than concentrating it in the midline.

has adequately stabilized the maxilla, the surgeon has the option of limiting mandibular movement with elastics or maxillomandibular fixation wires. Limiting jaw motion for at least 72 hours aids soft-tissue wound healing. When surgery has taken place in both jaws, additional skeletal fixation is required to stabilize bone at osteotomy sites. This subject is covered more thoroughly in Chapter 11. In short, without RIF in both maxilla and mandible, bilateral skeletal suspension wires are necessary.

At the completion of surgery a nasogastric tube is placed and secured, usually while the patient is still anesthetized. This tube is connected to low intermittent suction and left in place as long as it is productive, usually 10 to 15 hours following the surgery. Even with the best surgical technique, mucosal edges continue to ooze immediately after surgery and bleeding may continue from the nasal mucosa or sinuses. The nasogastric tube prevents blood (50 to 200 cc) from collecting in the gastrointestinal tract, helping to minimize nausea in the immediate postsurgery period. If only maxillary surgery is done, wound dressings may not be needed. With surgery in the mandible also, elastic bandages, form fitted and secured with velcro, are useful to help support the wounds and lower lip.

Postsurgery Sequelae

Patients can have considerable facial edema after Le-Fort I osteotomy. Often the edema does not correlate with the degree of difficulty of the procedure. The surgical edema usually peaks on the second or third postsurgery day and much of it resolves within 2 weeks. A change in position of bone and teeth is obvious to careful observers immediately after surgery. But soft tissues of the face, including the lips, take 6 to 12 months to adapt to new positions, a time frame much greater than might be expected by the patient and their family.

Every effort must be made to keep the nasal airway clear immediately following surgery. Crusting from dried blood and secretions should be removed with a moist cotton applicator tip and suction. Nasal decongestants (e.g., systemic phenylpropanolamine combinations) and topical medications (e.g., xylometazoline nasal spray) can be helpful. On rare occasions a nasopharyngeal airway is needed. In this circumstance, the nursing staff must clean the nasopharyneal airway frequently (every hour at least) or it will become an airway hazard.

Almost all patients have an altered sensation in the upper lip and paranasal areas just following surgery. Return of sensation may be rapid, occurring in a few weeks, or may continue to return over 12 to 18 months. Clinically, return of sensation is readily assessed with a cotton applicator tip with the end twisted into the shape of fine brush. If the patient can discern brush stroke direction, 85% or more of sensation has

returned. Intraoral tissues including teeth supplied by the infraorbital and superior alveolar nerves may also exhibit decreased sensory response immediately after surgery. This sensation should also return in 12 to 18 months, but the healing response is quite variable. As is the case with edema after surgery, return of sensation does not correlate with the degree of difficulty of the osteotomy procedure.

With wire fixation at osteotomy sites, maxillomandibular fixation supplemented with a single skeletal suspension wire attached to the mandible is required. Following one piece LeFort I osteotomy, the jaws can be mobilized early, 1 to 3 weeks. Guiding elastics are utilized at this time and continued as long as necessary until the patient functions easily into the occlusal splint, the new jaw position. With a multiple segment osteotomy, the period of maxillomandibular fixation may be longer, 5 to 8 weeks. In either case when fixation is released, the maxilla can feel "springy" as displacing pressure is applied. With another 2 to 3 weeks of healing and with some function, the maxilla will feel firm, resisting displacement. Appropriate physical therapy to assist the patient to regain a full range of jaw mobility is discussed in Chapter 7.

If RIF with small bone plates has been applied, patients may be held tightly in maxillomandibular fixation for a short time, 2 to 7 days, to allow early, undisturbed soft-tissue wound healing or they may be allowed to function immediately. In both instances guiding elastics are applied after release of maxillomandibular fixation to help the patient function into the occlusal splint, which dictates the new occlusal relationship. Active physical therapy may be delayed for a month to allow for initial bony healing. Additional information on the postsurgery period is available in Chapters 6 and 7.

Complications

Unanticipated bleeding in the first 12 hours following surgery is an uncommon event. When bleeding occurs, every attempt must be made to identify its point of origin. In most instances, the bleeding will originate from the nose, around the base of the septum or the posterior lateral wall. Simple pressure across the alar base, pinching the nostrils, can stem bleeding from the anterior septum. Bleeding posteriorly may require packing, but initially a topical vasoconstrictor spray (e.g., phenylephrine 0.5%) or topical solution (e.g., phenylephrine 0.5% or cocaine 4%) applied on a cotton applicator stick may be tried. Good light and suction with direct vision are most helpful. Reassuring the patient and having him or her lie quietly assists in controlling bleeding. If such measures fail, the surgeon must be prepared to release maxillomandibular fixation so that the patient can be reintubated and the osteotomy site explored under general anesthesia to identify the bleeding point.

Excessive trauma during surgery to separate the posterior maxilla from the pterygoid plates can result in pterygoid plate fracture and even trauma to the base of the skull. Late vascular complications that may follow are discussed by Lanigan.[27] Careful positioning of the pterygoid osteotome and judicious malleting can minimize the possibility of these complications. Some surgeons advocate hand malleting of the pterygoid osteotome to better control force. Fortunately, late vascular complications are quite rare.

When the maxilla is raised superiorly, the septum may be displaced or buckled if adjustments are not made in the septum itself or the nasal floor. When a septal deviation not present before surgery is recognized after surgery, it should be corrected. Often the septum can be repositioned on the first or second postsurgery day with a bayonet forceps under topical anesthesia (e.g., cocaine 4%). If this is not possible, reoperation may be required.

Every patient should have radiographs (panoramic, lateral and PA cephalometric) taken within 1 to 2 days after surgery to assess the position of maxillary segments and the mandibular condyles. If bony segments or the mandibular condyles are displaced from the planned positions, reoperation may be required to align segments satisfactorily.

MAXILLARY SINUS CONSIDERATIONS

The condition of the maxillary sinus is a legitimate concern with maxillary surgery. Young and Epker, and Nustad and others in retrospective studies, concluded that the incidence of sinus disease following maxillary orthognathic surgery was no greater than that in the general population.[28,29] Our experience with maxillary sinusitis following maxillary surgery is similar.

In the southeastern part of the United States, the incidence of sinusitis in the general population is greater than in other regions of the world and, therefore, patients have sinus disease both before and after surgery. We recommend routinely removing diseased sinus membranes at the time of maxillary surgery and sectioning the lateral nasal wall if extensive sinus membrane pathology is present to allow for improved sinus drainage following surgery (Fig. 8-29).

Wire sutures or small bone plates used to immobilize the maxilla at surgery may contribute to the increase in sinus symptoms following surgery. Removal of these foreign bodies may be helpful if symptoms persist for more than a few weeks. Obviously, if sinus disease occurs, it should be treated appropriately.

NASAL AIRWAY CONSIDERATIONS

A possible complication of superior repositioning of the maxilla would be an adverse effect on nasal breathing because space within the nasal cavity is decreased when the palate is moved up. However, studies

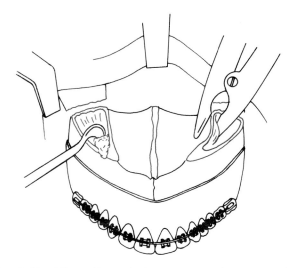

Fig. 8-29. When diseased sinus mucosa is present, it is stripped and removed and a large nasal antrostomy is placed through the lateral nasal wall to allow for drainage.

of nasal airway resistance[30,31] and the percentage of nasal versus oral breathing[32] indicate that this almost never occurs. Instead, nasal resistance usually decreases and air flow through the nose is facilitated. The explanation for this apparently paradoxical effect is the effect on the shape of the nostril, which is the liminal valve of the nasorespiratory system. When the maxilla is moved superiorly, the alar base widens. This opens the nostril, decreasing the resistance to air flow through the nose even though the volume of the nasal cavity may decrease (Fig. 8-30). For most patients, the percentage of nasal breathing actually increases following superior repositioning or advancement of the maxilla. Such effects can be expected as long as the nasal septum is repositioned in its presurgical position (see nasal considerations, discussed previously).

Excessive flaring of the alar base is unesthetic, and this now is controlled by resuturing the transverse nasalis muscle or placing an alar base cinch suture. Our airway data suggest that these procedures may have some limited effect on airway exchange. In those patients who have had resuturing of the transverse nasalis

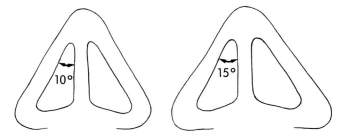

Fig. 8-30. When the maxilla is advanced or superiorly repositioned, the alar bases gain more support and therefore dilate. This opens the liminal valve and enhances nasal breathing.

muscle following LeFort I osteotomy, the nasal airway resistance decreased and the percentage of nasal breathing improved, but not as much as that of those patients whose alar bases were allowed to flare uncontrollably. But there is no evidence that controlling the width of the alar base causes any difficulty with nasal breathing. The decision to employ either of these suture techniques should be made with primary emphasis on esthetics, not on nasal breathing.

The following chapters discuss mandibular ramus surgery, segmental jaw surgery, and the special steps required when surgery is done in both the maxilla and mandible. Applications of maxillary surgery to clinical conditions will be more thoroughly discussed in the clinical chapters in Section IV.

REFERENCES

1. Moloney F, Worthington P: The origin of the LeFort I maxillary osteotomy. Cheever's operation, J Oral Surg 39:731-734, 1981.
2. Epker BN, Wolford LM: Middle third facial osteotomies: their use in the correction of acquired and developmental deformities and cranio-facial deformities, J Oral Surg 33:491-514, 1975.
3. Bell WH: LeFort I osteotomy for correction of maxillary deformities, J Oral Surg 33:412-426, 1975.
4. Wassmund M: Frakturen und Luxationen des Gesichtsschadels, Berlin, 1927.
5. Wassmund J: Lehrbuch der praktischen chirurgie de Mundes und der Kiefer, vol 1, Leipzig, 1935, Meusser.
6. Hullihen SP: Case of elongation of the under jaw and distortion of the face and neck, caused by a burn, successfully treated, Am J Dent Sci 9:157, 1849.
7. Auxhausen G: Zur Behandlung veralteter disloziert geheitter Oberkieferbruche, Dtsch Zahn Mund Kieferheilk 1:334-339, 1934.
8. Converse JM, Shapiro HH: Treatment of developmental malformations of the jaws, Plast Reconstr Surg 10:316-353, 1952.
9. Schuchardt K: Experiences with the surgical treatment of deformities of the jaws: prognathia, micrognathia, and open bite. In Wallace AG, editor: Second Congress of International Society of Plastic Surgeons, London, 1959, E & S Livingstone.
10. Stoker NG, Epker BN: The posterior maxillary osteotomy: a retrospective study of treatment results, Int J Oral Surg 3:153-157, 1974.
11. Willmar K: On LeFort I osteotomy, Scand J Plast Reconstr Surg Suppl 12, 1974.
12. Obwegeser H: Surgical correction of small or retro-displaced maxillae, Plast Reconstr Surg 44:351-365, 1969.
13. Turvey TA: Simultaneous mobilization of the maxilla and mandible: surgical technique and results, J Oral Maxillofac Surg 40:96-99, 1981.
14. Turvey TA, Fonseca RJ: The anatomy of the internal maxillary artery in the pterygopalatine fossa: its relationship to maxillary surgery, J Oral Surg 38:92-95, 1980.
15. Nelson RL, Path MG, Ogle RG, et al: Quantitation of blood flow after LeFort I osteotomy, J Oral Surg 35:10-16, 1977.
16. Bell WH, Fonseca RJ, Kennedy JW, Levy BJ: Bone healing and revascularization after total maxillary osteotomy, J Oral Surg 33:253-260, 1975.
17. Anderson JA: Deliberate hypotensive anesthesia for orthognathic surgery: controlled pharmacologic manipulation of cardiovascular physiology, Int J Adult Orthod Orthognath Surg 1:133-159, 1986.
18. Turvey TA: The management of the nasal apparatus during maxillary surgery, J Oral Maxillofac Surg 38:331-335, 1980.
19. Turvey TA: Maxillary expansion: a surgical technique based on surgical-orthodontic treatment objectives and anatomic considerations, J Maxillofac Surg 13:51-58, 1985.
20. Dorfman H, Turvey TA: Alterations in osseous crestal height following interdental osteotomies, Oral Surg 48:120-125, 1979.
21. Holmes RE, Wardrop RW, Wolford LM: Hydroxylapatite as a bone graft substitute in orthognathic surgery: histologic and histometric findings, J Oral Maxillofac Surg 46:661-671, 1988.
22. Schendel SA, Eisenfeld JH, Bell WH, Epker BN: Superior repositioning of the maxilla: stability and soft tissue osseous relations, Am J Orthod 70:663-674, 1976.
23. Schendel SA, Williamson LW: Muscle reorientation following superior repositioning of the maxilla, J Oral Maxillofac Surg 41:235-240, 1983.
24. Guymon M, Crosby DR, Wolford LM: The alar base cinch suture to control nasal width in maxillary osteotomies, Int J Adult Orthod Orthognath Surg 3:89-95, 1988.
25. Phillips C, Devereux JP, Tulloch JFC, Tucker MR: Full face soft-tissue response to surgical maxillary intrusion, Int J Adult Orthod Orthognath Surg 1:299-304, 1986.
26. Hackney FL, Nishioka GJ, Van Sickels JE: Frontal soft tissue morphology with double V-Y closure following LeFort I osteotomy, J Oral Maxillofac Surg 46:850-855, 1988.
27. Lanigan DT: Injuries to the internal carotid artery following orthognathic surgery, Int J Adult Orthod Orthognath Surg 3:215-220, 1988.
28. Young RA, Epker BN: The anterior maxillary osteotomy: a retrospective evaluation of sinus health, patient acceptance, and relapse, J Oral Surg 30:69-72, 1972.
29. Nustad RA, Fonseca RJ, Zeitler D: Evaluation of maxillary sinus disease in maxillary orthognathic surgery patients, Int J Adult Orthod Orthognath Surg 1:195-202, 1986.
30. Walker D, Turvey TA, Warren D: Alterations in nasal respiration and nasal airway size following superior repositioning of the maxilla, J Oral Maxillofac Surg 46:276-281, 1988.
31. Turvey TA, Hall DJ, Warren DW: Alterations in nasal airway resistance following superior repositioning of the maxilla, Am J Orthod 85:109-114, 1984.
32. Lints RM: The effect of orthognathic surgery on nasal breathing, master's thesis, 1989, University of Michigan.

CHAPTER 9

Mandibular Ramus Surgery

Bill C. Terry
Raymond P. White, Jr.

HISTORICAL DEVELOPMENT

Surgical procedures to correct mandibular skeletal deformity were described early in this century, but osteotomy to correct mandibular prognathism was not performed routinely until the 1950s.[1,2] Probably because of ease of access and the prevalence of missing mandibular teeth, body ostectomy became the first popular surgical procedure for shortening the mandible.[3-5] This procedure is performed intraorally today in special circumstances and will be discussed in Chapter 10. Following Caldwell and Letterman's paper in 1954 on vertical subcondylar osteotomy, extraoral approaches to the ramus of the mandible, which had the advantage of minimizing trauma to the inferior alveolar neurovascular bundle, replaced body ostectomy for correcting mandibular skeletal excess.[6-9] This procedure has great versatility and is still used today, particularly where extreme prognathism or asymmetry requires correction.

Extraoral surgery for lengthening the skeletal mandible also had its early proponents.[10,11] But surgical procedures to lengthen the mandible did not become common until after intraoral orthognathic surgery was popularized by European surgeons, particulaly Trauner and Obwegeser.[12,13] The bilateral sagittal split osteotomy of the ramus of the mandible was a lengthy procedure when first performed by American surgeons in the 1960s. Modifications in osteotomy design, the evolution of special instrumentation, and the versatility of the procedure allowing for corrections in three planes of space make the sagittal split osteotomy the mandibular procedure most often performed today.[14,15] The osteotomy can be accomplished quickly, usually in less than 2 hours. With the advent of RIF, patients have maxillomandibular fixation for a minimum time once they leave the operating room.

As intraoral orthognathic surgery became more common, an intraoral approach to vertical subcondylar osteotomy was described.[16] Subsequent modifications in design of the surgery and the availability of special instruments allow correction of mandibular excess with a length of surgery similar to that of the sagittal split osteotomy.[17-19] To date, rigid fixation techniques for this procedure are difficult. Until this technical problem is solved and the controversy over the best technical management of the proximal condylar segment is settled, it is unlikely that the transoral vertical subcondylar osteotomy will be adopted more widely.

Extraoral approaches for lengthening the mandible, usually a modification of a "C-type" osteotomy, have their application and can be quite effective in special circumstances.[20,21] Procedures performed today incorporate elements of the sagittal split and the use of RIF with both small bone plates and lag or positional screws.

Sagittal Split Osteotomy: Surgical Technique

In the following sections, the major surgical procedures in use today to lengthen or shorten the skeletal mandible and their sequelae and complications are described. The application of the surgical procedures to solve clinical problems is discussed in Section IV.

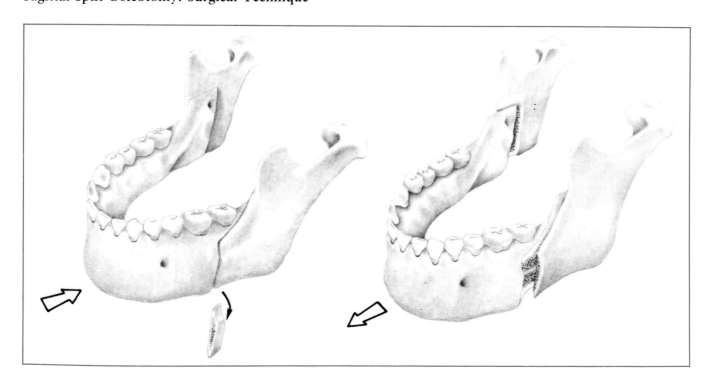

Sagittal split osteotomy of the mandibular ramus was originally described to American surgeons by Obwegeser when he toured the United States for a series of seminars in 1965. Since then, osteotomy design and surgical technique have been modified and newer methods for reduction, stabilization, and fixation of the segments have been adopted, but the basic surgical concepts and advantages of the procedure remain the same: (1) great flexibility in repositioning the distal tooth-bearing segment, (2) broad bony overlap of the segments after repositioning the jaws, and (3) minimal alterations in the position of the muscles of mastication and the TM joint. As the procedure has evolved, surgeons have focused on obtaining a more consistent bony split, providing greater protection for the neurovascular bundle, fixating the proximal segment to minimize unfavorable condylar position and enhancing bone healing. The addition of RIF to stabilize bony segments has great benefits for the patient as the period of maxillomandibular fixation is minimized. But rigid fixation techniques are exacting and require great attention to detail by the surgeon. RIF as applied to mandibular surgery will be discussed more thoroughly later in this chapter.

Soft-Tissue Dissection

An incision is made over the anterior aspect of the ramus of the mandible beginning at about midramus and continuing down onto the external oblique ridge and then curving into the facial vestibule, ending at approximately the first molar region (Fig. 9-1). Retracting the soft tissues laterally over the anterior ramus before the incision prevents initial exposure of the buccal fat. There may be an advantage to sharply incising only the mucosa at first. After extending sharp dissection down and through periosteum over the body of the mandible, the thicker tissue over the ramus, including buccinator muscle, is dissected with curved scissors down to periosteum. Then incision through the periosteum to bone is completed.

Periosteal dissection is begun laterally, reflecting the thinner tissue over the body of the mandible, extending to the inferior border just below the second molar and posteriorly over the anterior aspect of the ramus, free-

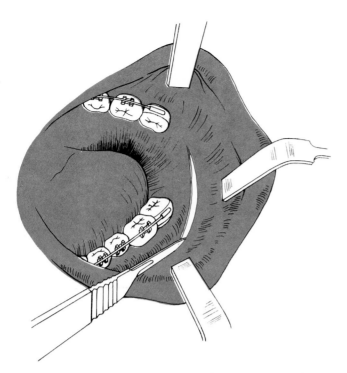

Fig. 9-1. Sagittal split osteotomy. Soft-tissue incision for access to the medial ramus and lateral posterior body of the mandible.

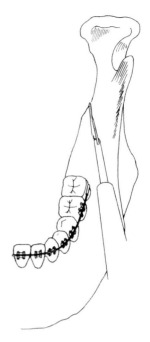

Fig. 9-2. Horizontal osteotomy with the reciprocating saw, through the medial cortical bone of the ramus.

ing the temporalis muscle attachment to a point about level with the greatest concavity. Dissection of the masseter and reflection of periosteum over the lateral ramus are minimal, sufficient only to provide access and vision. When rigid fixation devices are planned, more exposure of the lateral aspect of the mandible may be required. The dissection on the medial side of the ramus is carried beneath periosteum above the lingula and mandibular foramen almost to the posterior border of the mandible.

The lingula usually lies on a horizontal level with the greatest concavity in the anterior aspect of the mandibular ramus. This medial dissection must be above the mandibular foramen to allow for medial retraction without tension of the neurovascular bundle. Identification of the sigmoid notch with an instrument also can help the surgeon stay oriented anatomically. The medial dissection is started with a smaller periosteal elevator such as a flexible Freer. Once the initial periosteum has been lifted, a larger elevator can be used to tunnel posteriorly. Care must be taken to elevate the periosteum; penetrating it increases not only hemorrhage but also the possibility of damage to the neurovascular bundle. Finally, a large, broad elevator with a smooth end (e.g., a Seldin) is inserted for medial retraction.

When a circumramus-body wire is planned for stabilizing and fixing the segments, the mucoperiosteum is lifted with a Freer elevator on the medial side of the distal mandible just behind the third molar region and extended to the inferior border, taking care not to damage the lingual nerve.

Osteotomy

The basic osteotomy pattern includes cuts through the mandibular cortical bone first on the medial side above the lingula, down the anterior ramus onto the superior aspect of the body of the mandible, and then curving inferiorly through the lateral cortical plate, including the inferior border (Figs. 9-2 through 9-4). These cuts may be made with a rotary instrument or with the reciprocating saw and should extend only through the cortex and slightly into medullary bone. Before making the medial bony cut, the bone on the medial anterior ramus and temporal crest can be reduced with a rotary instrument. This step is indicated when there is a prominent bony shelf extending so far medially that it is difficult to obtain visibility for the medial cortical cut. The horizontal osteotomy in the ramus should extend posteriorly a half to two-thirds the anteroposterior dimension of the ramus. The vertical component of the osteotomy in the body of the mandible should include the inferior border.

The position of the inferior alveolar neurovascular bundle just under the lateral cortical plate of the body of the mandible dictates that the vertical osteotomy be just through the cortical plate. The bone over the neurovascular bundle is greatest over the area of the sec-

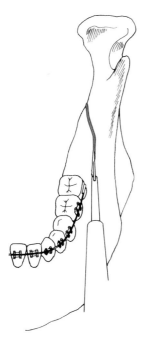

Fig. 9-3. Osteotomy extended into medullary bone of the anterior ramus and superior surface of the body of the mandible.

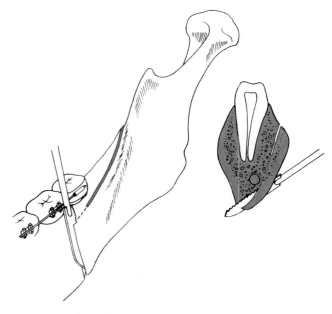

Fig. 9-4. Making the vertical cut tangential to the surface of the bone improves visibility and access for positioning the osteotome to split the mandible.

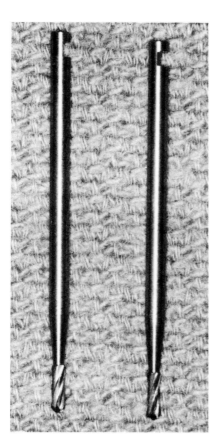

Fig. 9-5. Steiger-type burs, side cutting, and rounded cutting end, will cut bone with minimal damage to soft tissue.

ond molar and the vertical cut should be made here unless special circumstances dictate otherwise.[22] If a rotary instrument is selected for osteotomy, a Steiger-type bur is a good choice. The bur is rounded on the end but capable of both side and end cutting, designed to protect soft tissue but remain an efficient cutting instrument (Fig. 9-5). If the vertical osteotomy can be tangential rather than at right angles to the surface of the bone, there is better visibility through the osteotomy into the medullary bed (see Fig. 9-4). This access will enhance placement of the osteotome during the later stages of the procedure. A short body retractor with a cup that fits under the inferior border of the mandible gives good visualization and tissue retraction to prevent laceration of facial vessels or damage to the mandibular branch of the seventh nerve during the vertical bone cut.

Following the completion of the osteotomy pattern through cortical bone, a thin spatula osteotome malleted into the osteotomy sites better defines the cuts, beginning in the medial cut, working down the ramus, continuing on to the body and into the vertical cut (Fig. 9-6). Care is taken to keep the spatula osteotome directed just beneath the cortical plate to prevent damage to the neurovascular bundle. Next, the larger, bibeveled osteotomes are used to pry the fragments apart gently and carefully using only the cortical bone anterior to the vertical cut as a fulcrum (Fig. 9-7). Moderate pressure should separate the bone.

As the mandible splits, care is taken to visualize the course of the neurovascular bundle, making certain

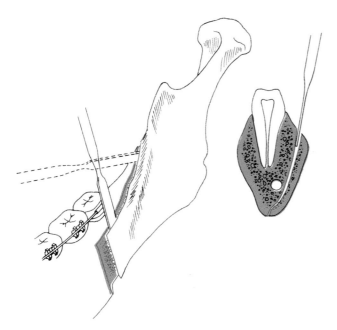

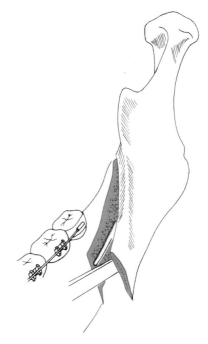

Fig. 9-6. **A,** Bony cuts completed. Initial separation with thin spatula osteotomes. **B,** Coronal section of mandible in second molar area; relationship of lateral cortical cut to neurovascular canal. Notice that the inferior border of the mandible is left with the proximal condylar segment.

Fig. 9-7. Bibeveled osteotome to pry mandibular segments apart. Only bone anterior to the vertical cut should be used as a fulcrum.

that portions of it are not contained in the proximal condylar segment. If the bundle is found to be attached to the proximal segment in some areas, the covering bone should be removed and the nerve freed with an instrument such as a #2 Molt curette. Once the neurovascular bundle is free from the proximal segment, osteotomes can be used more vigorously in a wedging fashion until the split of the ramus is completed.

The osteotomy is repeated on the opposite side of the patient's mandible. At this point, the distal mandible is repositioned. The teeth are secured into maxillomandibular fixation with 25-gauge wire and the aid of an occlusal wafer splint. The distal tooth-bearing segment should move easily to the new position. If not, the completeness of the separation at the osteotomy should be reassessed. Occasionally, the mandible will "green stick" fracture and bone must be separated at the inferior border near the angle.

If the mandible is advanced, the medial pterygoid muscle should be released at the inferior aspect of the distal segment with a periosteal elevator or a specially designed J stripper. If the mandible is set back, release of the medial pterygoid muscle and the masseter muscle at the inferior border may be necessary to prevent displacement of the condylar segment posteriorly. With a mandibular setback, bone must be trimmed from the anterior aspect of the proximal condylar segment, enough to allow the segment to rest passively against the tooth-bearing segment with the condyle in proper position.

Stabilization and Fixation

Following basic principles, bony parts must be reduced in the desired position, stabilized, and then fixed in that same position. To establish the condylar position, the proximal fragment is gently positioned and stabilized. A ramus pusher holds the proximal segment in position in the illustration (Fig. 9-8). A periosteal elevator or a wire director also can be used to position

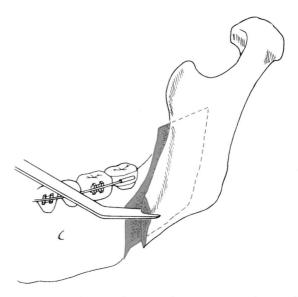

Fig. 9-8. Manipulation of proximal segment into place with a ramus pusher.

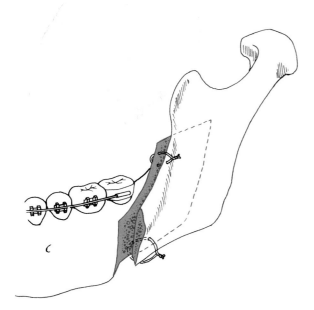

Fig. 9-9. Wire fixation at superior and inferior borders following movement of the distal tooth-bearing segment into its new position. Usually a wire at the superior or the inferior border is sufficient for stabilization.

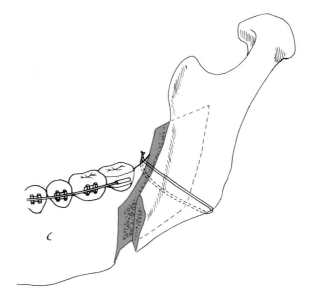

Fig. 9-10. Circumramus-body wire for fixation.

the segment, which includes the condyle. Four methods of interosseous fixation will be discussed: upper border wiring, lower border wiring, circumramus-body wiring, and RIF with lag screws, position screws, or small bone plates.

An upper border wire is placed by drilling a hole through the cortex of the proximal segment as well as through the cortex of the distal tooth-bearing segment. The hole in the distal tooth-bearing segment should be higher than the hole in the proximal condylar segment so that when the wire has been placed and tightened, it will tend to seat the proximal segment and condyle more superiorly. Some surgeons prefer adding a second hole in the distal segment, threading the wire suture back through this hole before tightening. Firm maxillomandibular fixation with the teeth in the planned occlusion must be established before upper border wire is tightened. This type of wiring with all its modifications only fixes the bone at the superior border and allows flaring at the lower border area (Fig. 9-9).

A lower border wire can be placed only if the split has left sufficient bone at the inferior border of the distal segment. Often the split occurs just below the neurovascular canal and no bone remains at the inferior aspect of the distal segment to retain a wire suture. When sufficient bone permits, the proximal segment is held in the desired position against the distal segment, a hole is drilled through the inferior border of both bony cortices, and a wire is placed and tightened. The lower border wire affords stability and fixation only in that area and can be technically difficult to place.

A circumramus-body wire more completely conforms to principles of stabilization and fixation. When such a wire is used as illustrated, both segments are approximated with tension over a broad area (Fig. 9-10). This wire is more easily placed before wiring the jaws into maxillomandibular fixation; then the wires are tightened after the patient's teeth are fixed together. A special wire-passing instrument (Walter Lorenz Surgical Instruments, Inc., 9850 Interstate Center Drive, Jacksonville, FL 32218) aids in placing the 24-gauge wire. The wire is threaded through the instrument with the end turned back on itself forming a loop. The instrument is directed to the inferior border beneath the periosteum on the medial aspect of the mandible behind the third molar area, through the periosteum in that area. The loop of wire is visualized below the inferior border between the segments. The loop of wire is picked up with a long, curved hemostat, pulled into the osteotomy site and around the lateral surface of the proximal segment. Then the wire-passing instrument is removed and both ends of the circumramus-body wire are tagged. The same procedure is completed on the opposite side following the split. At this point the planned maxillomandibular fixation is established. The proximal segment is firmly but not forcibly held against the distal segment, and the wire is tightened. An instrument (e.g., ramus pusher) placed on the face of the vertical cut on the proximal segment allows positioning of this segment with the condyle seating in an acceptable position.

Screw fixation can be accomplished either transorally or extraorally. When there is limited access intraorally or when there has been an unusual split, it is advisable to use the extraoral route. Screws may be

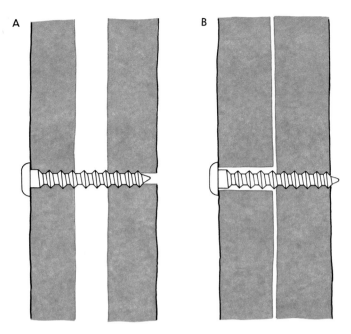

Fig. 9-11. **A,** Position screw. The screws threads maintain separation of bony segments. **B,** Lag screw. The screw head compresses the condylar segment against the bone of the tooth-bearing segment.

placed as position screws or as lag screws (Fig. 9-11). When there is good bony contact between segments with the condyle in the proper position, lag screws are ideal. Lag screws of any of the commonly available sizes—2 mm, 2.7 mm, 3.5 mm—will provide compression and fixation (see Chapter 7).

Concern has been expressed that compression of the bony segments can damage the neurovascular bundle and cause serious neurosensory disturbances. Theoretically, this is possible; practically, enough irregularities exist in the reapproximated bony surfaces that the two parts cannot be so tightly squeezed together as to cause such injury even with the most effective lag screws. But the bony surfaces along the course of the neurovascular bundle should be inspected for any sharp spicules that might project into the neurovascular canal and damage the nerve and vessels. Any projecting bone should be recontoured.

To place lag screws of 2.0 mm diameter, a 1.9 mm wire-passing bur (Stryker Lord, Kalamazoo, MI, 49001) is used to make an initial hole in the proximal condylar segment after the segment is positioned carefully against the distal segment with the condyle in position. Then the #61 bur is replaced in the handpiece with a 1.5 mm bur (Stryker Lord). Without turning the bur, the bone in the distal segment should be probed. Once cortical bone is felt, a pilot hole in the distal segment is made with the #59 bur. All bur holes must be made under copious saline irrigation. The sequence of using the #61 bur followed by the #59 bur

allows the surgeon to change direction slightly, drilling the pilot hole with the #59 bur to take advantage of the best available cortical bone. Screws are placed in each hole and tightened sequentially.

Position screws can provide adequate fixation. The proximal and distal bony segments must be kept aligned and held together as the screw engages both segments of cortical bone. If this is not possible, the segments will be displaced as the screw enters the distal segment. In addition, fixation may not be adequate if the screw does not engage sufficient bone in the distal segment to stabilize and fix the bone at the osteotomy site. To place 2.0-mm diameter screws as position screws, a #59 wire-passing bur is used to place the pilot hole through both the proximal and distal segments. The surgeon must take extra care to see that the segments remain aligned and do not move until the screw engages both segments. If the segments slip, it is difficult to engage the underlying distal segment and at least some distraction of segments occurs.

After placing lag screws or position screws, the osteotomy site should be carefully inspected. If the segments come apart after gentle prying in the osteotomy site with a periosteal elevator, some other method of fixation must be attempted.

Circumstances exist in which both lag screws and position screws are used at the same osteotomy site. When lag screws are used, they must only be placed where there is bone contact with the proximal condylar segment in the proper position. When bony contact between the two segments is minimal, as in some asymmetric movements, a position screw placed initially may protect against condylar displacement. As an alternative, an intervening bone graft (a piece of autogenous bone removed from the ramus or body of the mandible or a piece of allogeneic bone) can be placed as a shim so the condylar segment is not displaced at the screw is tightened, or the proximal or distal segments recountoured so that bone is in contact. Lag screws then can be inserted to achieve fixation (see Chapter 7 for further discussion).

Usually three screws are placed at each osteotomy site in a pattern that best stabilizes the proximal to the distal segment (Fig. 9-12). If bone available at the site for screw placement is minimal, two fixation screws may be adequate, but the surgeon must carefully assess stability before wound closure, prying in the osteotomy site with a periosteal elevator and looking for mobility of the segments. Greater care in this circumstance is required if the patient is allowed early jaw function. If screw fixation is not adequate, the elevator muscles of the mandible will displace the proximal condylar segment.

In most circumstances, retraction of tissue provides adequate access for placement of screws intraorally. When an extraoral approach is selected, access to the

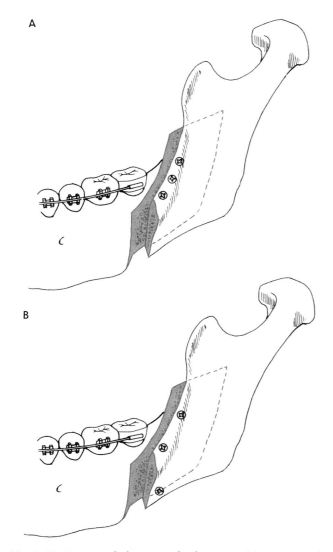

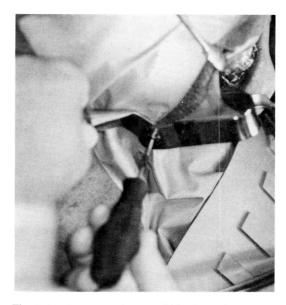

Fig. 9-13. Access to the mandible through a trocar.

Fig. 9-12. Pattern of placement for lag or position screws. **A,** Three screws can be placed at the superior border, or when bone contact is limited there, **B,** a third screw may be placed below, avoiding the neurovascular canal.

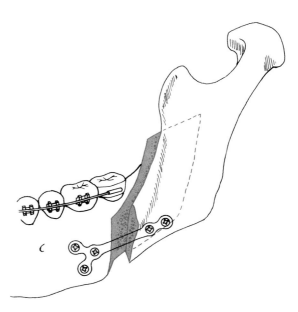

Fig. 9-14. Bone plate fixation across the osteotomy site.

osteotomy site for screw placement can be gained through a small stab incision just above the inferior border of the mandible (Fig. 9-13). Following tissue infiltration with a local anesthetic and dilute vasoconstrictor (usually 2% lidocaine with 1:100,000 epinephrine), a 3- to 5-mm incision is made only through the skin. A pointed trocar is introduced through the lumen of the drill guide and bluntly dissected through the underlying muscle and periosteum (see Fig. 9-13). Once the end of the drill guide is exposed intraorally, a self-retaining retractor that holds the cheek tissues on the inner side away from the end of the drill guide is placed, allowing excellent visualization. All necessary screw holes on a side can be drilled and screws placed

through one skin penetration. After removal of the drill guide, one or two vertical mattress skin sutures or steristrips are adequate to close the stab wound. The incision heals with minimal scar.

Small bone plates can fix the proximal and distal segments (Fig. 9-14). For maximum stability, the plate should be placed near the inferior border of the mandible bridging the osteotomy site and secured with at least two screws on either side of the osteotomy. Bicortical screws provide the most stability, but it may not be possible to place these without damage to the teeth. In most cases, screws placed only through the lateral

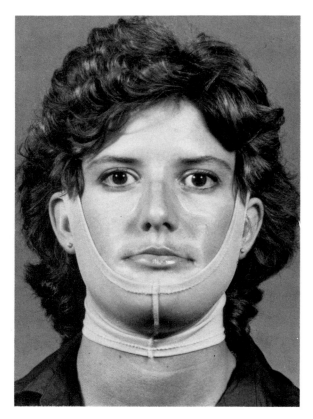

Fig. 9-15. Elastic bandage, form fitted and attached with velcro to support the wound.

cortical plate provide adequate stability. The plate must be adapted exactly to the bone contour to prevent condylar displacement when the screws are tightened. If one plate does not fix the mandible rigidly enough to allow function, a second plate can added to provide additional stability.

After the segments have been stabilized and fixed, the wounds are irrigated and inspected for continued hemorrhage. Bleeding from obvious vessels in the wound edges is controlled with cautery. If for any reason slight hemorrhage from muscle or medullary bone continues, an active suction drain is indicated, placed on the lateral surface of the mandible and brought out through a stab incision just in front of the closed intraoral incision. The drain is generally left in place for 12 to 24 hours or until it is not productive.

Wounds are closed with 3.0 chromic gut sutures in a horizontal mattress fashion. Restrictive external pressure dressings are not used following the sagittal split procedures primarily because swelling, if it does occur, should be allowed to expand laterally and not medially to compromise the airway. Elastic bandages, form fitted and attached with velcro, are useful to support the wounds (Fig. 9-15). Patients are encouraged to wear these dressings for 72 hours following surgery. Addi-

tional discussion of surgical principles is found in Chapter 7.

The total period of maxillomandibular fixation varies according to the needs of the patient, the fixation methods at the osteotomy site, and the time required for clinical bony healing. It usually is 4 to 6 weeks if wire osteosynthesis only has been used for stabilization and fixation of the segments. Following release of maxillomandibular fixation, the osteotomy sites should be assessed for adequate healing. The jaw should feel quite firm on manipulation. If clinical healing is judged adequate, the patient should wear guiding elastics bilaterally until he or she can function without deviation into the occlusal wafer splint, the established occlusion.

When rigid fixation methods are used, the surgeon must release the maxillomandibular fixation at surgery and determine that the mandible will rotate into its planned position with minimal force and without evidence of condylar distraction or translation. When an occlusal wafer splint is used, it must be cleared of all occlusal interferences to allow cuspal interdigitation. (See Chapter 7 for a discussion of occlusal splints and their modifications.) To rotate the mandible into the splint without distracting the condyle, pressure should be applied only beneath the angles, carefully noting initial occlusal contact. If there is evidence of mandibular shift to achieve maximum occlusion, the rigid fixation devices must be removed, maxillomandibular fixation established, and the proximal condylar fragment repositioned. Once again rigid fixation is applied. Adjustments must continue to be made until the mandible can be rotated into the planned position repeatedly with a minimum of effort and without shifting.

When RIF is used to fix the segments, patients may be maintained in maxillomandibular fixation for a short period of time or allowed to function immediately. In either event, guiding elastics are used to direct the mandible into its new functional relationship. The elastics may be angled as required to guide the mandible. Patients who have undergone mandibular advancement may function at first in a more protrusive position. The reason for this is not clearly understood, but it may be related to edema in the TM joint and slight alteration of muscle positions or to a habit of posturing the mandible forward. Guiding elastics are utilized as long as necessary until the patient functions easily into the new position.

Postsurgery Sequelae

Most patients experience considerable facial edema following sagittal split osteotomy. Often the edema does not correlate with the duration or the degree of difficulty of the procedure. Much of the edema resolves within 2 weeks following surgery, with the area near the angle of the mandible the last to resolve. Changes in the position of the jaws and teeth achieved at surgery are obvious to careful observers. Soft tissues of the face including the lips may take months to adapt to new positions, a time frame much greater than might be expected by patients and their families. Casual observers may see no changes at all in facial appearance even though major movement of the teeth and the bony skeleton has occurred.[23]

Almost all patients have diminished sensation in the lower lip over the distribution of the mental nerve just after surgery. Return of sensation may be rapid, may occur over a few weeks, or may occur gradually over 12 to 18 months. Clinically, return of sensation is readily assessed with a cotton applicator tip with the end twisted into the shape of a fine brush. If the patient can discern brush stroke direction on the skin of the lower lip, 85% or more of the sensory perception has returned. Intraoral tissues including teeth that are supplied by the inferior alveolar and buccal branches of cranial nerve V may also exhibit decreased sensory response immediately following surgery. If recovery of sensory function is assessed critically after a year, more than two-thirds of the patients will demonstrate deficits. Perhaps more important, patients do adjust to the sensory deficit and have a positive opinion about their overall results of treatment.[24]

Other important considerations following surgery, including oral hygiene, diet, and physical therapy needed to return to full jaw function, are discussed in Chapter 7.

Complications

The most often encountered complications in the sagittal split osteotomy are unanticipated bony splits at the osteotomy site, laceration of the neurovascular bundle, and malpositioning of the proximal segment, including the condyle. Significant bleeding is a rare complication and usually involves the inferior alveolar or facial vessels. These complications will be addressed separately.

Unanticipated bony splits occurred with about the same frequency as neurovascular bundle transections, 3.1% and 3.5%, respectively, in a series of 256 patients reported by Turvey.[25] During the separation of the mandible with osteotomes, a poor split may occur on the distal tooth-bearing segment or the proximal condylar segment but usually not both. In the distal segment, the lingual cortical bone extending posteriorly may split just as it joins the intact mandible usually just behind the last molar tooth. Most often this fracture occurs as a third molar is being removed during the osteotomy. If practical, impacted or nonfunctional third molars should be removed as a separate procedure more than 6 months in advance of the planned osteotomy. If the schedule will not allow this, extreme care must be taken in removing the third molar at osteotomy to prevent a fracture of the lingual segment. If the

lingual plate fracture occurs, lingual soft-tissue dissection in the area should be kept to a minimum so that the bone retains a good blood supply. If sufficient bone exists, a wire suture may be placed, tying the fractured segment to the remaining mandible. Rigid fixation is much more complicated with a lingual plate fracture and inadequate rigid fixation at the osteotomy site may commit the patient to 6 to 8 weeks of maxillomandibular fixation.

Unintended splits of the proximal segment may occur before or after the mandible has been separated. Access to the bone on the lateral mandible is usually good and the poor split may be prevented if the surgeon sees it developing. Perhaps the greatest cause of a poor split is improper wedging with osteotomes, using bone within the split as the fulcrum. Only bone on the facial surface anterior to the vertical osteotomy can safely serve as a fulcrum to separate the mandible (see Fig. 9-7). Once a poor split of facial bone occurs, the surgeon must determine whether the proximal condylar segment is separated from the distal tooth-bearing segment. If the mandible is still intact, usually bone at the inferior border below the neurovascular bundle must be cut. Access can be difficult, but with great care the mandible can be separated with reciprocating saws, a bur, or an osteotome. After the distal segment of the mandible is repositioned and teeth held together in maxillomandibular fixation, bony segments at the osteotomy site can be tied together with wire sutures, taking care to minimize soft-tissue dissection from the segments and making certain the condyle is in its proper position. Sometimes a bone graft from the opposite osteotomy site can help stabilize the site of the bad split. Rigid fixation techniques for repairing poor bony splits have been reviewed by Tucker and Ochs.[26] With position and lag screws, and small bone plates, the osteotomy site can usually be stabilized following a poor bony split. In this circumstance, the fixation must be carefully evaluated before allowing mandibular function. Usually, extraoral access for screw placement is required, as described previously in this chapter.

If the mandibular neurovascular bundle is lacerated, extreme care should be taken in completing the procedure to maintain continuity of the neurovascular bundle. After repositioning the mandible, the damaged neurovascular bundle should be gently manipulated into position. Adequate healing with return of sensory function usually follows. If the neurovascular bundle is completely transected, an attempt should be made to reapproximate the ends by using fine sutures (6.0 nylon) in the perineurium. A microanastomosis under an operating microscope or magnification provides the ideal repair, but this may not be practical in all circumstances. Patients with repositioned and repaired transected neurovascular bundles recover sensation, though the healing period is prolonged.

Malposition of the proximal condylar segment occurs occasionally after the repositioning of the distal mandible, even in the hands of the most accomplished surgeons. In most patients, the proximal segment is easily positioned with an instrument applying gentle pressure, and it is obvious to the surgeon that the condylar position is correct. Even in the best clinical circumstances, however, the proximal segment can be displaced subsequently as fixation at the osteotomy site is applied. Wire sutures improperly placed will distract the condyle. However, during the weeks of maxillomandibular fixation, the wire suture will allow masticatory muscles to reposition the condyle when displacement of only a few millimeters exists. With rigid fixation improperly placed, no adjustment by muscles is possible. As was advocated earlier in this chapter, it is important to check carefully the occlusion and position of the condyles before wound closure after rigid fixation is applied. During placement of rigid fixation, considerable force can be exerted with the screw driver, which can displace bone segments and stretch wires holding the jaws in maxillomandibular fixation. With careful attention, this problem can be prevented.

Occasionally, it is not possible to tell at surgery what is the proper position of the condyle. In fact, in some patients, especially those who postured their jaw forward for years to chew food and compensate for a mandibular deficiency, it is not possible to find a repeatable condylar position before surgery. Several intraoral fixation devices to be applied before the osteotomy have been suggested. The difficulty with this solution is finding the proper condylar position even before the special device is applied.

A radiograph, usually a panoramic film, should always be taken on the first or second postsurgery day to assess the position of the osteotomy segments, including the condyle. If the segments are distracted from the planned position by more than a few millimeters, the patient should be returned to surgery and the problem corrected. Even the most careful surgeons find distracted segments that were not apparent at surgery. Immediate correction of the problem once identified is always the best course of action.

Excessive bleeding during surgery and the need for blood transfusions are rare during sagittal split osteotomy. Bleeding may occur from the inferior alveolar neurovascular bundle and sometimes from the medullary bed of bone or muscle, but this bleeding can be controlled by local measures. As has been mentioned, the facial vessels can be lacerated beneath the mandible. Bleeding is easily stopped with pressure on the skin over the area, but brisk bleeding follows when hand pressure is released. If at all possible, these vessels should be clamped and tied. This may require a skin incision for access. Packing the intraoral wound to apply pressure may be an alternative. The packing can be slowly removed over the first 3 postsurgery days in a setting where bleeding can be managed if it occurs.

Less common is hemorrhage from the retromandibular vein, which lies immediately adjacent to the posterior ramus border. Injury to this vessel can occur during the final phase of the splitting procedure by penetration with the osteotome. Tamponade with a gauze sponge and/or placement of a hemostatic material such as microfibrillar collagen hemostat (Avitene) or an absorbable gelatin sponge (Gel Foam) is usually sufficient to control bleeding. Hemoclips also may be directly applied to the injured vessel. Rarely it is necessary to appproach his vessel extraorally for hemorrhage control.

Transoral Vertical Ramus Osteotomy: Surgical Technique

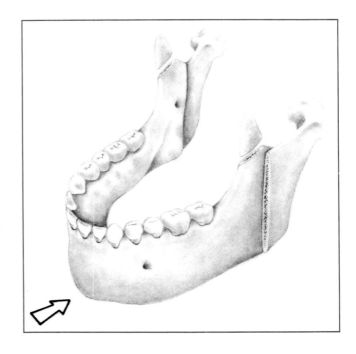

Vertical osteotomy of the ramus of the mandible accomplished via a transoral approach has proved to be an effective surgical procedure for correction of mandibular prognathism. The procedure is useful alone or in combination with a sagittal split osteotomy on the opposite side for mandibular repositioning to correct asymmetry. The intraoral approach has the same advantages of the vertical ramus osteotomy accomplished extraorally, without the disadvantages of facial scarring and jeopardy to the marginal mandibular branch of the facial nerve. An additional advantage is the reduced operating time as compared with that of the extraoral procedure. Disadvantages include difficulty in visualization and access to the ascending ramus. The surgery has been made easier with the development of special instrumentation, including retractors and saws. Studies have shown that the procedure accomplished intraorally or extraorally for mandibular prognathism has a high degree of stability and minimal chance of permanent injury to the mandibular neurovascular bundle.

Modifications of the procedure originally described by Winstanley continue to be adopted.[16,17] However, the basic osteotomy remains the same. The bone is divided from the sigmoid notch to the inferior aspect of the angle or posterior ramus of the mandible, staying behind the entrance of the mandibular neurovascular bundle at the lingula. With the condylar segment displaced laterally, posterior repositioning of the mandible following the osteotomy allows varying degrees of bony overlap and contact. One modification described by Wilbanks[27] included a more sagittal design of the osteotomy, which afforded a broader bony contact. While broad bone contact of the segments is desirable, bony healing follows even when there has only been minimal contact of the overlapping segments.[7] RIF techniques have thus far been difficult to apply to the transoral vertical ramus osteotomy because of difficult access and potential damage to the neurovascular bundle. Sophisticated instrumentation for RIF has been reported by Steinhauser[28] and Kraut.[29] An additional problem with RIF as well as with other stabilization procedures is potential condylar displacement. These technical problems probably will be solved, allowing RIF to be used routinely for fixing the segments and a reduced period of maxillomandibular fixation or even immediate function.

Soft-Tissue Dissection

The initial incision exposing the anterior ramus and posterior body of the mandible is as described for the sagittal split procedure. Then periosteum is reflected from the lateral aspect of the ramus of the mandible from the sigmoid notch to the inferior border, extending back to the posterior border. A pterygoid-masseteric sling J stripper is used to free the periosteum from the inferior border. This not only provides greater access and vision but also relaxes the soft-tissue envelope so that there is less danger of iatrogenic injury to the marginal mandibular branch of the seventh nerve, the facial artery and vein, or the retromandibular vein. When a circumramus wire or suture is planned to stabilize the proximal fragment against the lateral ramus, the periosteum is reflected on the medial aspect of the mandible to the posterior border above the neurovascular bundle. The width of this reflection need be no more than a few millimeters to allow introduction of an instrument to carry the suture or wire on the medial aspect of the mandible to the posterior border. All periosteal reflections should be completed before commencing the bony cuts.

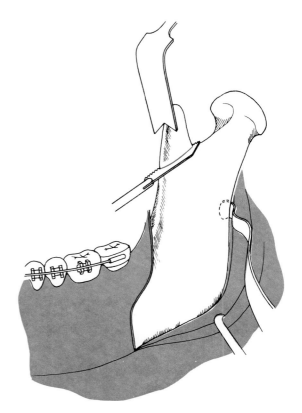

Fig. 9-16. Transoral vertical ramus osteotomy; with a reciprocating saw the coronoid process is released and allowed to retract.

Osteotomy

After the soft tissue is reflected, the lateral surface of the mandible is examined for access and visibility. An estimate of the corresponding position on the lateral surface, of the medial entrance of the neurovascular bundle into the mandible must be made, generally indicated by a slight bony elevation midramus. If visibility and access are compromised or if there is to be more than a few millimeters of mandibular repositioning, the coronoid process should be released. With a small reciprocating saw, a cut to release the coronoid is made from the sigmoid notch at the base of the coronoid process extending through the anterior ramus (Fig. 9-16). Bone is relatively thin in this area and the osteotomy is accomplished easily. After this cut has been completed, the coronoid fragment with attached temporalis muscle is allowed to retract.

A retractor such as the Merrill-Levassuer or others similar to the one originally described by Moose that cups around the posterior border of the mandible can be used to retract the soft tissues laterally.[30] The Merrill-Lavassuer retractor has a lateral step which is approximately 5 mm from the end fitting around the posterior border. This provides an excellent marker for directing the line of the osteotomy, which extends from

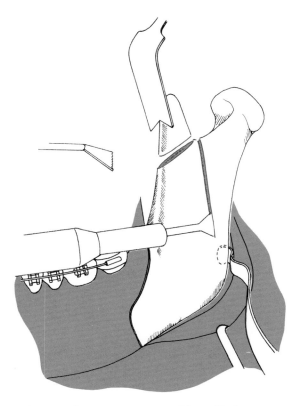

Fig. 9-17. Ramus osteotomy with oscillating saw.

an area in front of the condyle to a point at or near the angle of the mandible. A fan-shaped oscillating saw is recommended for sectioning the ramus. This saw, which projects at about a 30-degree angle to the shaft, is preferable to a saw at a 90-degree angle (Fig. 9-17). The rounded corners of the saw blade reduce chattering, do not bind easily, and allow a smooth, controlled cut. The osteotomy cut begins at the superior aspect of the ramus where visibility is usually excellent, particularly after releasing the coronoid process. The cut is carried through the mandible, continuing down to a point at or near the angle. The design of the saw blade and the rapid short oscillating motion limit soft-tissue injury on the medial aspect. The surgeon should verify the direction of the osteotomy before completion, as it is easy to become disoriented and make the cut too close to the posterior border or too far anteriorly. If the osteotomy is directed too far posteriorly, a subcondylar-type osteotomy can occur. Although there may be less bony contact of the overlapping segments, this should not present insurmountable problems. If the osteotomy is directed too far anteriorly, increased danger of injury to the inferior neurovascular neurovascular bundle exists. Care should be taken also to see that the mandible is transected throughout the entire osteotomy line.

Some surgeons prefer a reciprocating saw for the osteotomy. A number of reciprocating saw blade designs

exist, and the resulting oblique bone cut allows for greater bony contact of the overlapped segments. The design of the osteotomy cut does not affect the healing response. The choice of osteotomy design is the preference of the individual surgeon.

When the osteotomy has been completed, the proximal condylar fragment may tend to displace medially. If this happens, the surgeon can distract the mandible anteriorly, allowing an instrument (e.g., a periosteal elevator) to be placed in the osteotomy site so that the proximal fragment can then be positioned laterally. Often it is necessary to strip some of the remaining periosteal and muscle attachments from the inferior medial aspect of the proximal condylar fragment as well as along the posterior border to allow the fragment to remain in a lateral position. At this time, a suture or wire to stabilize the proximal fragment against the distal segment is placed by using the special wire-passing instrument as described in the sagittal split procedure.[28] The wire or suture is passed beneath the periosteum on the medial aspect of the mandible, picked up at the posterior aspect of the ramus, and carried around and lateral to the proximal segment. The wire or suture is tagged, the wound packed, and the same procedure repeated on the opposite side. Placement of the wire or suture prior to maxillomandibular fixation is preferred because of ease of access.

Stabilization and Fixation

Following sectioning of the rami bilaterally, the mandible is repositioned and secured with maxillomandibular fixation. Next, the osteotomy sites are examined and the position of the overlapping proximal segments verified. When there has been a preexisting asymmetry, an exaggerated flare of the proximal condylar segment may exist with the inferior aspect of that segment extending laterally. This flaring can be reduced by removing bone from the lateral side of the distal segment. If the inferior aspect of the condylar fragment is still prominent, the inferior portion can be removed. The bone segments should be in contact, but an exact cortex to cortex fit is not necessary. Bone remodels during healing and no residual deformity results.

After determining that the proximal condylar fragments are not distracted, a decision must be made as to stabilizing the proximal fragment against the residual ramus. Some surgeons prefer no stabilization, allowing the muscles to maintain the position of the condylar fragment against the distal ramus. Others prefer a suture or wire to hold the condyle segment against the ramus. No clinical data exist to support either approach. If a circumramus wire or suture is used, it is important to determine the anteroposterior relationship of the condylar fragment to the underlying ramus. If the posterior border of the condylar fragment in its reduced

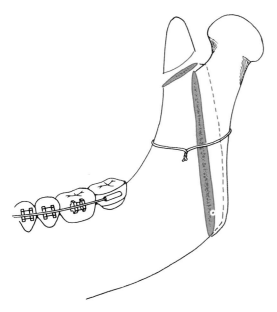

Fig. 9-18. Circumramus wire in place following maxillomandibular fixation.

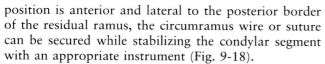

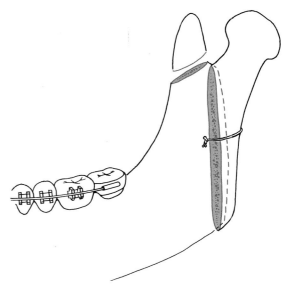

Fig. 9-19. Wire suture stabilizing condylar segment when mandibular movement is only a few millimeters.

position is anterior and lateral to the posterior border of the residual ramus, the circumramus wire or suture can be secured while stabilizing the condylar segment with an appropriate instrument (Fig. 9-18).

If the mandible was set back only a few millimeters and the posterior border of the condylar segment lies posterior to the distal segment, use of circumramus fixation is not recommended. If a circumramus suture or wire is tightened in this situation, it will displace the proximal condylar fragment forward. When only a minimal mandibular setback is planned, the proximal condylar fragment can be stabilized by a suture placed in a hole made with a wire-passing bur, which penetrates the distal segment just anterior to the repositioned proximal condylar fragment. This wire or suture, brought around the posterior border of the condylar fragment and secured, assures that the condylar segment and distal segment cannot be displaced anteriorly (Fig. 9-19).

Securing the proximal fragment with some type of wire or suture does prevent it from rotating forward or displacing medially, especially in the event of a postsurgical problem during the immediate recovery period when maxillomandibular fixation must be released and the mandible distracted. With no fixation of the segments and release of maxillomandibular fixation, there is great likelihood that the proximal condylar fragments would displace medially and prevent reestablishment of the desired mandibular position. In this case, reoperation would be required.

Although RIF is not commonly used to fix the proximal and the distal ramus fragments, lag screws, posi-

tion screws, or small bone plates can be placed.[28-29] We predict that RIF will eventually be adopted for routine use in this procedure.

Wound closure, use of drains, and application of dressings are similar to those discussed with the sagittal split procedure. As with any surgical procedure to reposition the mandible, radiographs (usually a panoramic and a lateral cephalometric film) are taken on the first or second postsurgery day to assess the position of the condyles and relationship of the bony segments. In the event there has been major anterior and/ or inferior displacement of the condyle (more than a few millimeters), it is advisable to attempt immediate repositioning. However, some slight anterior and inferior distraction of the condyle is common. Condylar position will adjust during healing and no further intervention is required.

Patients undergoing this procedure with only wire or no fixation at osteotomy sites usually are left in maxillomandibular fixation for a period of 4 to 6 weeks. When maxillomandibular fixation is released and the patient allowed to function, guiding elastics are used until the mandible functions without deviation into the occlusal splint and there are no shifts from the planned occlusion. The patient should be examined at frequent intervals, at least every 5 to 7 days, to be certain the occlusion remains as established. Instability at the osteotomy site can cause shifts in occlusion which can be corrected with elastic traction if the problem is recognized immediately. Most patients can tell when they are not occluding correctly and will return for adjustment if cautioned to do so. When it is determined that the osteotomy site is clinically stable, the occlusal wafer splint is removed and finishing orthodontics begun.

A vertical ramus osteotomy should not be selected if the prognathism includes an anterior open bite necessitating a counterclockwise mandibular rotation. In addition, difficulties may exist with the transoral approach when 15 mm or more of posterior repositioning is necessary or when there is a significant asymmetry. In such situations, an extraoral vertical osteotomy is preferred. The extraoral approach provides greater flexibility in managing any unusual problems encountered and excellent access can be obtained for RIF methods.

Complications

Complications encountered with transoral vertical ramus osteotomy include excessive bleeding, damage to the inferior alveolar neurovascular bundle, unanticipated bony splits, and distraction of the proximal condylar segment. As with any surgery, complications of hemorrhage can occur, usually from the masseteric and inferior alveolar vessels or the retromandibular vein. Bleeding is controlled with direct pressure from gauze sponges and application of hemostatic agents and hemoclips. Injury to the maxillary artery as it crosses medially at about the level of the condylar neck is very uncommon. Except for an anomalous course of that vessel, injury should not occur if the surgery is performed as outlined. If the maxillary artery should be lacerated or severed, hemorrhage would be profuse but could be controlled by packing and direct pressure. Only in unusual circumstances would ligation of the external carotid artery on the affected side be required.

Severance of the inferior alveolar neurovascular bundle is a rare but more significant complication. If this does happen, reanastomosis with microsurgical techniques is almost impossible because of difficulty with access and visibility. With careful design of the osteotomy, this complication should not occur.

Unanticipated bony splits may occur when the osteotomy is not carried completely through the ramus in all areas. With patience and careful examination of the osteotomy site, residual areas of bony bridging can be identified. Care must be taken in completing the osteotomy. When there are residual bony connections, it is easy to fracture off the facial cortex or even fracture the lower part of the proximal condylar fragment, resulting in a free bony segment. The oscillating saw should always be moving when it is placed into a bony cut. It should never be used as a wedge to separate the segments when it is thought that the osteotomy has been nearly completed. Wedging or binding of the saw blade can result in its separating from the shaft, and if the blade has been fully extended through the ramus when this happens, recovery may be difficult.

Distraction of the proximal condylar segment may

occur soon after surgery, several weeks after surgery, or even after the patient begins jaw function. Presumably, the combination of heavy muscular forces and instability at the osteotomy site aggravated by minimal bony contact contribute to the problem. Clinically open bite or an asymmetry may follow. When recognized after beginning jaw function, this complication can be corrected if treated aggressively with elastic traction. Reoperation may be required to reposition the condylar segment.

Extraoral Vertical Ramus Osteotomy: Surgical Technique

Vertical ramus osteotomy accomplished extraorally was one of the most common procedures used for mandibular repositioning.[6-11] Without RIF, a period of maxillomandibular fixation from 4 to 6 weeks was required for bony healing. Scars from skin incisions and possible damage to the marginal mandibular branch of the seventh nerve are disadvantages of the procedure. With careful surgical technique, these disadvantages are minimized. Although the procedure was designed primarily for the correction of prognathism, modifications in the osteotomy design and the use of RIF have made it possible for this approach to be used for mandibular advancement, particularly for management of extreme mandibular sagittal deficiency.[21] The major modification employed today includes only a partial vertical ramus osteotomy with a sagittal split of the remaining portion of the ramus and body of the mandible added to the procedure. This surgical combination is discussed in the next session of this chapter.

Soft-Tissue Dissection

A 2.5-cm skin incision is made approximately 1.5 cm below the angle and posterior body of the mandible. When possible, this incision is placed in an existing skin line. The incision is carried down to the platysma muscle, which is divided. A major structure beneath the platysma is the marginal mandibular branch of the seventh nerve, which runs parallel with the lower border of the mandible, sometimes above but usually just below the inferior border crossing superficial to the facial vessels as the nerve courses superiorly. Although the incision and dissection plane is usually inferior to the mandibular branch of the seventh nerve and avoids it, every attempt should be made to identify and preserve this structure. A nerve stimulator may help locate the mandibular branch (VII). The facial artery and vein may or may not require ligation for surgical access.

After definite identification and protection of the marginal mandibular branch (VII), the dissection is carried down to the mandible and the periosteum is incised over the angle, posterior border, and inferior border. The insertion of the masseter muscle is released and the periosteal reflection carried superiorly, exposing the lateral ramus up to the level of the sigmoid notch. A channel retractor with the cupped end placed in the sigmoid notch is helpful in retracting the tissues over the lateral ramus.

No consensus exists over the need to detach the coronoid process. In all but very small movements, we recommend freeing the coronoid process to eliminate the tethering effect of the temporalis muscle. The coronoid process can be scored with a rotary instrument at its base and then fractured with an osteotome, allowing it to retract with the temporalis muscle. The temporalis muscle reattaches in this area during healing, often with radiographic evidence of a new coronoid process.

Osteotomy

Good visibility of the lateral ramus is imperative. A bulge of bone on the lateral surface opposite the lingula identifies the mandibular foramen, the beginning course of the neurovascular bundle in the mandible. The osteotomy is performed with a reciprocating saw along a line approximately 5 mm in front of the posterior border and behind the neurovascular bundle entrance, extending from the sigmoid notch to a point at or near the angle of the mandible. After the osteotomy has been completed and the condylar ramus segment displaced laterally, the attachments of the medial pterygoid muscle and periosteum are stripped from the posterior border sufficiently to allow this proximal segment to overlap the distal ramus freely without interposed soft tissues. The wound is packed and the same procedure repeated on the opposite side. After completing both osteotomies, the mouth is entered, the distal segment repositioned, and the teeth placed in maxillomandibular fixation. Then the extraoral wounds are inspected with careful attention to the position of bone segments and the degree of bony overlap.

Management of the proximal fragment varies greatly among surgeons. Some prefer to use no internal fixation, allowing the condylar segment to lie free in its overlapped position. However, if asymmetry has been corrected and lateral displacement of the condylar segments exists, the bone over the distal ramus segment should be relieved, allowing the proximal fragment to assume a more normal vertical position, maximizing bony contact of the segments. If the inferior aspect of the proximal fragment is prominent laterally, it can be recontoured. Some surgeons prefer to decorticate the lateral aspect of the distal ramus and the medial bone of the proximal fragment to allow broader bone contact and a more normal position of the condyle. Boyne has demonstrated in animal experiments that there is no difference in the healing rate of cortex to cortex compared with decorticated to decorticated bone in the vertical ramus osteotomy procedure.[7] Van Zile suggested removing a section of the distal ramus after the

mandible has been repositioned in its planned maxillomandibular relationship to allow the proximal condylar segment to resume as normal a relationship as possible.[31] This works well except in situations where the osteotomy and movement have been such that removal of this bone would jeopardize the inferior alveolar neurovascular bundle. The modification offers the best position of the condyle in the glenoid fossa.

Stabilization and Fixation

Surgeons who advocate fixation of the proximal condylar fragment in mandibular setback have used direct wiring and, more recently, screws or small bone plates for RIF. With the Van Zile modification, two small bone plates bridging the proximal and distal segments give excellent stability. With RIF techniques, the period of maxillomandibular fixation is greatly reduced or eliminated. With wire or no direct fixation, a period of 4 to 6 weeks of maxillomandibular fixation is required. When a patient is allowed to function, elastics guide the mandible into the planned new occlusion.

Wound Closure

Following completion of the bony surgery, care is taken to carefully close the tissues in layers. If the skin surface is reapproximated with a continuous subcuticular suture, additional skin sutures may not be required. If skin sutures are used, they should be of a monofilament type of 6-0 or smaller. A gauze dressing lubricated with petrolatum or an antibiotic ointment covers the incision and steristrips reduce tension across the incision. A pressure dressing incorporating gauze fluffs over the incision area is worn for the first 24 to 48 hours. Active drains are required rarely in this procedure. If drains are placed, the end of the drain is brought through the skin from a separate stab incision below the incision line. Sutures in the skin are removed in 3 to 5 days and the wound is supported with steristrips for an additional week.

Complications

Because of excellent access and good visibility from proper soft-tissue retraction, surgical complications should be minimal. Occasionally, hemorrhage results from injury to the masseteric artery as it courses laterally through the sigmoid notch. The possibility of injury to the retromandibular vein exists. Bleeding from these vessels or other structures can be controlled as previously discussed.

After surgery, there may be a transitory decrease in function of the marginal mandibular branch (VII). If this is due to retraction of the nerve during surgery, full function should return. If the nerve is inadvertently sectioned and this is recognized at surgery, a microsurgical repair should be attempted.

In rare instances, an unfavorable scar may occur. If

possible, an extraoral approach for correction of mandibular deformities should not be used in individuals who may form keloids. Care should also be taken in siting the primary incision. A vertical skin incision crossing existing skin and tension lines will result in a poor scar and require subsequent revision.

Combined Vertical Ramus and Sagittal Osteotomies: Surgical Technique

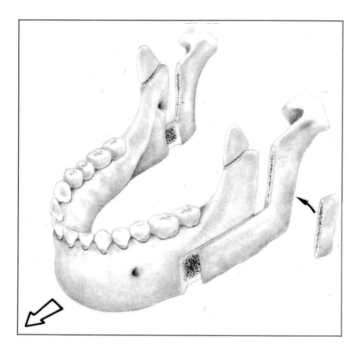

When there is need for mandibular advancement greater than 10 to 15 mm, an extraoral procedure combining components of the vertical ramus and sagittal osteotomy has proved very effective.[21] This procedure also may be considered when there has been previous ramus surgery or when there are other factors (e.g., an unusual asymmetry) that may complicate the surgery through a transoral-only approach. More flexibility in surgical options is available with this combined procedure. But the combined procedure carries the disadvantages associated with the sagittal split as well as the extraoral vertical ramus osteotomy. These have been discussed previously.

Soft-Tissue Dissection

The incision for exposure of the lateral ramus and the posterior body of the mandible is as previously described. To accommodate a major advancement, the skin incision and dissection must be extended to expose the body of the mandible as far forward as the mental foramen. Ligation of the facial artery and vein is required. Precautions are taken to preserve the marginal mandibular branch (VII).

Osteotomy

At the outset, the coronoid process is separated, allowing it to retract with the temporalis muscle. Then an osteotomy is carried through the ramus from the sigmoid notch about 5 mm in front of the posterior border to a point just below a line that would identify the ramus body juncture. Beginning at the termination of this ramus osteotomy, a cut through the lateral cortex only is made, extending anteriorly in the body of the mandible on a line just below the root apices of the teeth. Depending on the amount of advancement, this cortical cut can extend up to the mental foramen or until the mandible curves at the parasymphysis. The cut through the lateral cortex then curves downward to the inferior border. Then the inferior border is sectioned back to a point in the inferior border directly below the vertical bone cut in the ramus. The periosteum is reflected on the medial surface of the ramus and the cortical cut is continued superiorly through the medial cortical bone, connecting with the previously made through-and-through vertical ramus cut (Fig. 9-20). The osteotomies are examined to make certain that the vertical portion in the ramus is completely through the mandible and that the lateral and medial cortical cuts in the body have extended into medullary bone.

With a thin spatula osteotome, working from the inferior border, the cortical plates are separated and finally pried apart with broader osteotomes. Care is taken to not injure the inferior alveolar neurovascular bundle. Neurovascular bundle injury should be minimal with this approach if care is taken with the cortical osteotomies. When the bony separations have been completed, the proximal segment will contain the condyle, a portion of the posterior ramus, and the anterior projection of the lateral cortical plate of the body of the mandible. This same procedure is then repeated on the opposite side.

Stabilization and Fixation

After completion of the osteotomies, the mandible is advanced and placed into maxillomandibular fixation as planned with the aid of an occlusal splint. Wide overlap of the proximal and distal segments in the mandibular body region should allow direct wire osteosynthesis or RIF using lag screws (Fig. 9-21). At least three lag screws should be placed on each side. The bony gap in the ramus area should approximate the amount of mandibular advancement, and the gap can be grafted with either autogenous or allogeneic bank bone.

Allogeneic bone has been found to be very acceptable as a graft material, especially in this situation, where there is an excellent coverage by the pterygomasseteric muscle sling providing a rich blood supply. If the advancement was extreme to the extent that

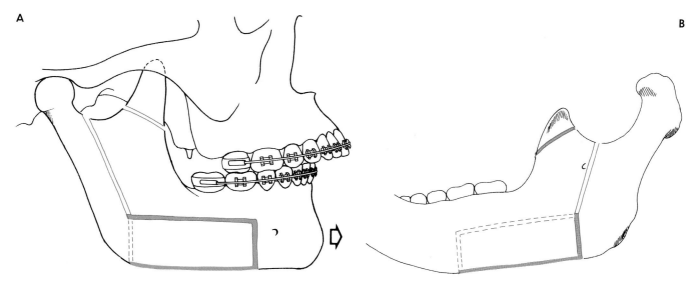

Fig. 9-20. Osteotomy cuts for combined vertical ramus and sagittal osteotomy. **A,** Lateral and **B,** medial view of the mandible.

there is minimal overlap or no overlap of the bony segments, bone plates can be placed to provide RIF and bridge this gap. Grafts also can be placed in any bone-deficient areas in the body region. Following completion of fixation, the wound is closed in layers and dressed as has been described. If rigid fixation is satisfactory, the period of maxillomandibular fixation may be reduced or eliminated entirely. If wire osteosynthesis only is used, maxillomandibular fixation will be required for at least 4 to 6 weeks. The use of guiding

elastics with jaw function is imperative as the jaws are mobilized, as discussed previously.

Complications

The combined procedure incorporates the risks associated with both the transoral sagittal split osteotomy and the extraoral vertical ramus osteotomy. However, because of the excellent access and visibility, there is less danger of injuring the inferior alveolar neurovascular bundle than with the transoral sagittal split proce-

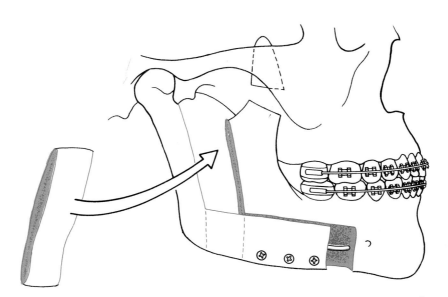

Fig. 9-21. Mandibular segments secured with lag screws following mandibular advancement.

dure. In the unlikely event of an injury, excellent access exists for a microsurgical repair.

Another potential complication is an unanticipated bony split, producing a fracture of the anterior projection of the lateral cortical plate anterior to the ramus segment. If this occurs, the segments can be stabilized with bone plates. As previously stated, this open approach to the ramus and body of the mandible allows complete versatility and flexibility in managing any unusual situations or complications that might present, with much better access than through the transoral route.

The following chapter will discuss segmental mandibular and maxillary procedures. Applications of mandibular surgery to clinical conditions will be more thoroughly discussed in the clinical chapters in Section IV.

REFERENCES

1. Blair VP: Operations on jaw bones and face: study of aetiology and pathological anatomy of developmental malrelations of maxilla and mandible to each other and to facial outline and of operative treatment when beyond the scope of the orthodontist, Gynecol Obstet 4:67-78, 1907.
2. Blair VP: Underdeveloped jaw with limited excursion, JAMA 17:178-183, 1909.
3. New GB, Erich JB: The surgical correction of mandibular prognathism, Am J Surg 53:2-12, 1941.
4. Dingman RO: Surgical correction of mandibular prognathism, an improved method, Am J Orthod Oral Surg 30:683-692, 1944.
5. Burch RJ, Bowden GW, Woodward HW: Intraoral one-stage ostectomy for correction of mandibular prognathism: report of case, J Oral Surg 19:72-76, 1961.
6. Caldwell JB, Letterman GS: Vertical osteotomy in the mandibular rami for correction of prognathism, J Oral Surg 12:185-202, 1954.
7. Boyne PJ: Osseous healing after oblique osteotomy of the mandibular ramus, J Oral Surg 24:125-133, 1966.
8. Hinds EC, Girotti WJ: Vertical subcondylar osteotomy: a reappraisal, Oral Surg 24:164-168, 1967.
9. Smith AE, Robinson M: Surgical correction of mandibular prognathism by sub-sigmoid notch ostectomy with sliding condylotomy: a new technique, J Am Dent Assoc 49:46-62, 1954.
10. Robinson M: Micrognathism corrected by vertical osteotomy of ascending ramus and iliac bone graft: a new technique, Oral Surg 10:1125-1130, 1957.
11. Robinson M, Lytle JJ: Micrognathism corrected by vertical osteotomies of the rami without bone grafts, Oral Surg 15:641-645, 1962.
12. Trauner R, Obwegeser H: The surgical correction of mandibular prognathism and retrognathia with consideration of genioplasty, Oral Surg 10:787-792, 1957.
13. Dal Pont G: Retromolar osteotomy for the correction of prognathism, J Oral Surg 19:42-47, 1961.
14. Hunsuck EE: A modified intra-oral sagittal splitting technic for correction of mandibular prognathism, J Oral Surg 26:249-252, 1968.
15. Epker BN: Modifications in the sagittal osteotomy of the mandible, J Oral Surg 35:157-159, 1977.
16. Winstanly RP: Subcondylar osteotomy of the mandible and the intraoral approach, Br J Oral Surg 6:134-136, 1968.
17. Herbert JM, Kent JN, Hinds ED: Correction of prognathism by an intraoral vertical subcondylar osteotomy, J Oral Surg 28:651-653, 1970.
18. Hall HD, Chase DC, Payor LG: Evaluation and refinement of the intraoral vertical subcondylar osteotomy, J Oral Surg 33:333-341, 1975.
19. Hall HD, McKenna SJ: Further refinement and evaluation of intraoral vertical ramus osteotomy, Oral Maxillofac Surg 45:684-688, 1987.
20. Caldwell JB, Hayward JR, Lister RL: Correction of mandibular retrognathia by vertical L-osteotomy: a new technique, J Oral Surg 26:259-264, 1968.
21. Hayes P: Correction of retrognathia by modified "C" osteotomy of the ramus and sagittal osteotomy of the mandibular body, J Oral Surg 31:682-686, 1973.
22. Rajchel J, Ellis E, Fonseca RJ: The anatomical location of the mandibular canal: its relationship to the sagittal ramus osteotomy, Int J Adult Orthod Orthognath Surg 1:37-47, 1986.
23. Dunlevy HA, White RP, Proffit WR, Turvey TA: Professional and lay judgment of facial esthetic changes following orthognathic surgery, Int J Adult Orthod Orthognath Surg 2:151-158, 1987.
24. Zaytoun HS, Jr, Phillips C, Terry BC: Long-term neurosensory deficits following transoral vertical ramus and sagittal split osteotomies for mandibular prognathism, J Oral Maxillofac Surg 44:193-196, 1986.
25. Turvey TA: Intraoperative complications of sagittal osteotomy of the mandibular ramus: incidence and management, J Oral Maxillofac Surg 43:504-509, 1985.
26. Tucker MR, Ochs MW: Use of rigid internal fixation for management of intraoperative complications of mandibular sagittal split osteotomy, Int J Adult Orthod Orthognath Surg 2:71-80, 1988.
27. Wilbanks JL: Correction of mandibular prognathism by double-oblique intraoral osteotomy: a new technique, Oral Surg 31:321-327, 1971.
28. Steinhauser EW: Bone screws and plates in orthognathic surgery, Int J Oral Surgery 11:209-216, 1982.
29. Kraut RA: Stabilization of the intraoral vertical osteotomy using small bone plates, J Oral Maxillofac Surg 46:908-910, 1988.
30. Moose SM: Surgical correction of mandibular prognathism by intra-oral sub-condylar osteotomy, Br J Oral Surg 1:172-176, 1964.
31. Van Zile WN: Triangular ostectomy of the vertical rami: another technique for correcting mandibular prognathism, J Oral Surg 21:3-10, 1963.

CHAPTER 10

Segmental Jaw Surgery

Raymond P. White, Jr.
Bill C. Terry

HISTORICAL DEVELOPMENT

Although segmental jaw surgery has been performed for most of this century, surgical procedures to correct the position of the jaws did not become common until after World War II. Performed in the tooth-bearing area of the lower jaw, body ostectomy was the first popular surgical procedure to shorten the skeletal mandible.[1-4] This procedure has only special applications today and will be described in this chapter. Mandibular anterior, posterior, and total subapical dentoalveolar osteotomy were performed in the United States after Kole's publication in English in 1959.[5] Improvements in instrumentation have allowed surgeons to make the required precise bony cuts, minimizing damage to teeth, periodontal structures, and the inferior alveolar neurovascular bundle. The subapical procedures described in this chapter have limited, but very useful indications. Their clinical application will be discussed more fully in the clinical chapters in Section IV.

Osteotomy of the inferior border of the mandible to shorten or lengthen the jaw also has been performed frequently in the United States since the publications by Kole, and Trauner and Obwegeser.[5,6] Inferior border osteotomy may be performed alone or in combination with other orthognathic surgery procedures. Bone grafts (autogenous or allogeneic bone) and alloplastic graft materials may be incorporated with this surgery to modify the shape of the jaw. Inferior border osteotomy with its common modifications in technique are described in this chapter. Applications of mandibular inferior border osteotomy are discussed in almost every chapter in Section IV.

Segmental surgery in the maxilla was described in the European literature over 50 years ago.[7] Kole's publication and the work of Murphey and Walker, and Mohnac led to anterior maxillary subapical osteotomy's being performed frequently in the decade of the 1960s.[5,8,9] The procedure improved occlusion and function, but esthetics were compromised because the anterior teeth were retracted too much. When the maxilla is segmented after a LeFort I osteotomy, the surgeon can partially close the premolar extraction space by bringing the posterior segment forward. By the 1980s, this greater flexibility of Lefort I osteotomy had relegated anterior maxillary supapical osteotomy to use only in special circumstances. Surgical procedures for anterior maxillary subapical osteotomy, modified from those originally reported by Wassmund and Wunderer, are described in this chapter.[10,11]

Isolated posterior maxillary subapical osteotomy also has its special indications.[12,13] The procedure is used most often today to reposition maxillary posterior dentoalveolar segments before prosthodontics or to correct isolated unilateral posterior crossbite. Descriptions of these surgical procedures are included in this chapter. The clinical applications of maxillary anterior and posterior subapical osteotomy are discussed in Section IV.

SURGICAL TECHNIQUES: MAXILLA
Anterior Subapical Osteotomy

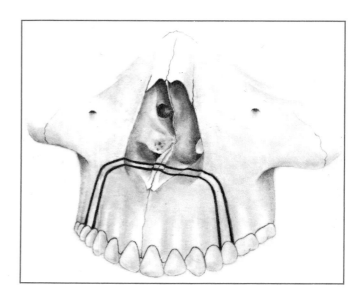

Anterior maxillary subapical osteotomy is a reliable surgical technique useful today in special clinical situations. Bell provided an excellent review for the interested reader.[14] Most often the anterior maxillary procedure is performed with mandibular anterior subapical osteotomy in conjunction with orthodontics to correct bimaxillary protrusion. The procedure also can be used to advantage in the patient with a partially edentulous maxilla to correct maxillary protrusion before the construction of removable partial dentures. After osteotomy or ostectomy, the anterior maxillary dentoalveolar segment is most easily moved in a posterior or inferior direction, which also allows a tipping movement of the bone and teeth. With difficulty, the segment can be moved in a superior direction. Anterior movement of the dentoalveolar segment is almost impossible because stabilization and fixation of the segment even with bone grafting are difficult, and soft-tissue pedicles are often insufficient to cover the surgical defects. Posterior and/or inferior movement of the anterior maxillary dentoalveolar segment can be accomplished by using modifications of the Wassmund or Wunderer surgical techniques.[12,13] The Wassmund technique maintains a more extensive soft-tissue pedicle with its accompanying vascular supply. The Wunderer technique is less difficult technically when the transverse palatal bony cut must be made posterior to the premolar region. Both techniques as modified from Wassmund and Wunderer are described in this section.

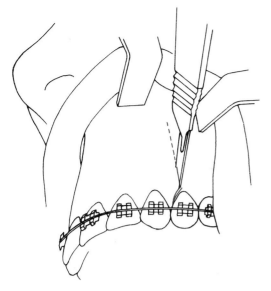

Fig. 10-1. Vertical mucoperiosteal incision to expose alveolar bone above the canine root.

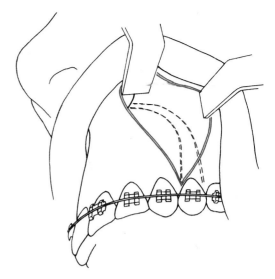

Fig. 10-2. Mucosa reflected to expose lateral aspect of the piriform aperture.

Soft-Tissue Dissection and Osteotomy/Ostectomy

Wassmund technique. The Wassmund technique maintains both facial and palatal soft-tissue pedicles to provide vascular supply to the mobilized dentoalveolar segment. After infiltrating the mucosa with vasoconstrictor (usually 2% lidocaine with 1:100,000 epinephrine) above the canines and premolars bilaterally, a vertical mucosal incison is made between the canine and premolar from the gingival margin superiorly to the level of the anterior nasal floor, superior to the root apex of the maxillary canine (Fig. 10-1). No vasoconstrictor should be injected into the palatal tissue. Bleeding is usually minimal from the palate since the palatal vessels are preserved in the dissection. Attention is directed to the facial aspect of the anterior maxilla. Keeping the gingival papilla distal to the canine attached to bone, mucoperiosteum is reflected superiorly until the apical third of the maxillary canine is reached. At that point, the anterior superior margin of the mucoperiosteal incision is reflected, tunneling forward subperiosteally until the nasal piriform aperture is exposed (Fig. 10-2). If possible the mucoperiosteum just inside the nasal aperture should be released with a flexible Freer elevator. If planned the first premolar should be removed, preventing root fracture if possible, so the alveolar bone remains intact. If no tooth removal is planned, presurgical orthodontic tooth movement should provide 3 to 5 mm of space for vertical bony cuts between retained teeth and for removal of palatal bone. Adequate bone between the roots is demonstrated easily in periapical radiographs taken just before surgery. Before removing alveolar bone, the pala-

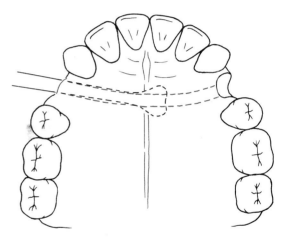

Fig. 10-3. Palatal mucosa reflected to just past the midline after removal of premolar teeth.

tal mucosa is reflected to just past the midline (Fig. 10-3). As palatal mucosa is detached, special care should be taken where the palatal aspect of the alveolus and the horizontal palatal bone meet, so the anterior palatine vessels are not injured. On occasion these vessels are partially enclosed in bone and must be dissected free before the palatal mucosa can be mobilized.

The surgeon has the option of performing the osteotomy/ostectomy with a bur or combinations of reciprocating and oscillating saws. Bony cuts between the teeth should be carefully done, leaving 1 to 2 mm of bone over adjacent teeth and removing no more than the planned amount of alveolar bone necessary to reposition the anterior dentoalveolar segment. Once bone in the area of the alveolus has been removed, the

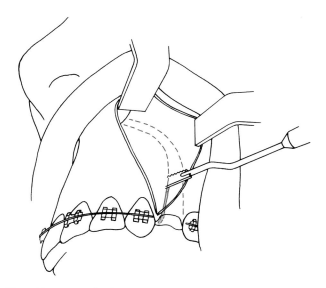

Fig. 10-4. Facial alveolar bone removal, including bone above the canine to the piriform rim.

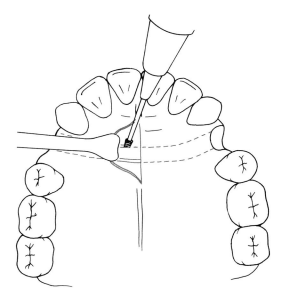

Fig. 10-6. Midline mucoperiosteal incision on the palate for access to bone at the midpalate.

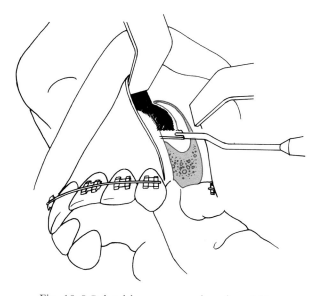

Fig. 10-5. Palatal bone removed to the midline.

bone cut is extended above the teeth, forward to the lateral aspect of the nasal aperture staying at least 4 mm above root apices (Fig. 10-4). If more than 1 to 2 mm of superior movement is planned, a measured amount of bone must be removed from the piriform rim area. Next, attention is directed to removing palatal bone from the alveolus to the midline. Although bone removal directly across the palate in a transverse direction suffices, surgical access is often easier if the cuts are directed posteriorly about 45 degrees from the midsagittal plane (Fig. 10-5). No more than the measured amount of bone required for repositioning the anterior dentoalveolar segment should be removed.

The palatal bony cuts can be made with a Steiger bur, a reciprocating saw, or an osteotome. Bone can be thick at the midline. If any difficulty is encountered in removing bone at the midline of the palate, a small anteroposterior midpalatal incision can be made for access (Fig. 10-6). The palatal vascular pedicles are not compromised by this additional incision.

A similar osteotomy/ostectomy is accomplished on the opposite side. Following the bony cuts, the anterior dentoalveolar segment occasionally can be disarticulated from the nasal septum with hand pressure. Usually, a small vertical mucoperiosteal incision is required over the anterior nasal spine. After careful reflection of the mucoperiosteum from the anterior nasal spine and the inferior aspect of the cartilaginous nasal septum with a flexible Freer elevator, a nasal septal osteotome is malleted above the nasal spine to free the anterior dentoalveolar segment from the nasal septum.

If required, the anterior dentoalveolar segment can be split in the midline into two pieces. After carefully tunneling in the midline beneath the mucoperiosteum to the crest of the alveolar bone between the maxillary incisor teeth, a fine bony cut is made through the facial plate of bone only with a 701 fissure bur (Fig. 10-7). A fine spatula osteotome malleted in the midline through the alveolar bone to the palate produces two anterior dentoalveolar segments (Fig. 10-8). The anterior segments should be mobile and easily repositioned into the occlusal splint. Bony interferences may prevent this. Often they occur near the midline on the palate. Interfering bone can be removed judiciously with a bur. Once the segments are positioned manually into the occlusal splint, the palatal soft-tissue pedicle should be

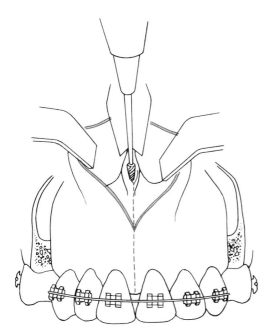

Fig. 10-7. Anterior midline mucoperiosteal incision for access for a bur cut through the facial cortical bone.

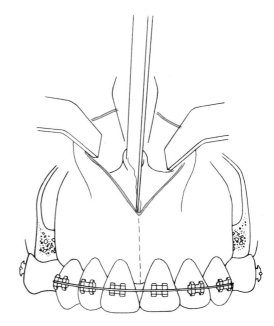

Fig. 10-8. Anterior dentoalveolar segment split in the midline with an osteotome.

inspected to make certain that it is not folded on itself, compromising blood supply. The facial soft-tissue pedicle should still be attached to the anterior dentoalveolar segment.

Wunderer Technique. Facial soft-tissue incisions for access to the lateral maxilla and the piriform nasal aperture are similar to those of the Wassmund technique. Following exposure of facial bone, palatal mucosa is reflected only from the alveolar bone. If planned, the posterior tooth in the osteotomy site should be removed. If not, presurgical orthodontics must have prepared space adequately between teeth. A minimum of 3 to 5 mm of bone must be available for osteotomy/ostectomy in the dentoalveolar aspect of the maxilla. The measured amount of alveolar bone is removed with either a bur or a combination of reciprocating and oscillating saws. The osteotomy is extended anteriorly to the nasal aperture. Special care must be taken to keep bony cuts more than 4 mm above the apices of all teeth to be included in the mobilized dentoalveolar segment (Fig. 10-9). With osteotomy posterior to the first premolar the maxillary sinus is exposed. Exposure alone should pose no problem as long as meticulous wound closure is accomplished at the completion of the procedure.

A similar procedure is repeated in the lateral maxilla on the opposite side. Attention then is directed to the palate. After propping the patient's mouth open wide for access, a mucoperiosteal incision is made transversely across the palate just anterior to the planned osteotomy/ostectomy site (Fig. 10-10). Bleeding from

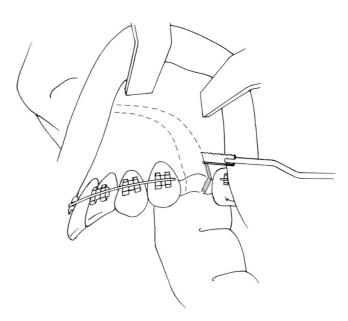

Fig. 10-9. Bone removed from the alveolus at the second premolar site and from the lateral maxilla above the apices of the teeth to the piriform aperture.

palatal vessels should be controlled with pressure or hemostats and cautery. If necessary, vasoconstrictor can be injected directly into the tissue at the point of transection of the palatal vessels to control bleeding. The palatal mucosa posterior to the incision is raised with a periosteal elevator, taking care to preserve palatal vessels. Occasionally this can be difficult because

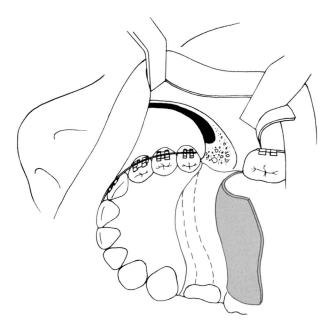

Fig. 10-10. Palatal incision and mucoperiosteal reflection for access for palatal bony cuts.

other. Access to the palatal bone is excellent at this juncture and allows for bony cuts as far posterior as the second molar. Palatal bone should be removed carefully with as little trauma to the nasal mucosa as possible. Bone is thicker in the midline, where the nasal crest of the maxilla intersects with the nasal septum. Usually a greater thickness of bone must be removed at this point to complete the osteotomy/ostectomy. Once all bony cuts are complete, the anterior maxillary dentoalveolar segment can be mobilized manually, carefully separating the nasal septum from the segment through the palatal osteotomy site (Fig. 10-11).

If necessary, the segment can be divided in the midline. This may be required for transverse expansion to widen the distance between the canines. When expansion is planned, a full palatal mucoperiosteal flap is reflected from the gingival margin of the anterior teeth to as far posterior as necessary for access to the transverse palatal bony cut. The palatal midline cut is made with a small fissure or Stieger bur, using a thin spatula osteotome to complete the separation. Care must be taken to maintain the soft-tissue pedicle to the facial aspect of the mobilized segment since this provides the only blood supply. For this reason the facial portion of the described osteotomy is always completed first and adequacy of the perfusion of the soft-tissue pedicle confirmed before proceeding to the palatal osteotomy. If the soft-tissue perfusion is questionable, palatal cuts must be made as a second stage procedure. Sectioning the segment in the midline also can be more difficult

the palatal vessels can lie in a groove in the bony palate separated from the thick keratinized tissue over them. Just enough palatal mucosa posterior to the incision should be elevated to allow the planned osteotomy/ostectomy. With the Wunderer technique, a premolar might be removed on one side and a molar on the

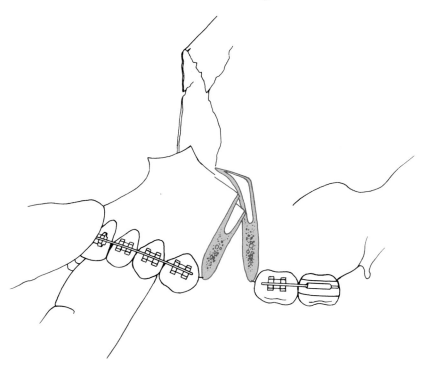

Fig. 10-11. The anterior dentoalveolar segment is carefully mobilized to preserve the attachment of the facial vascular pedicle.

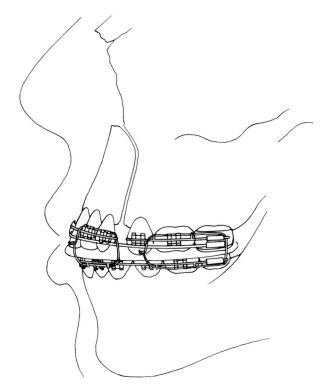

Fig. 10-12. Anterior maxillary segment repositioned in the occlusal splint, stabilized with an auxiliary orthodontic arch wire and maxillomandibular fixation.

technically than with the Wassmund technique because the segment is mobile.

Once mobilized the anterior maxillary dentoalveolar segment is manually positioned into the prepared occlusal splint. Interfering bone is removed judiciously with surgical burs. The palatal soft tissue anterior to the transverse palatal incision and the facial soft tissue should remain attached to bone to provide adequate vascular perfusion to the mobilized segments.

Stabilization and Fixation Methods

After the anterior dentoalveolar segments have been positioned and wired into the occlusal splint, the surgeon may choose to place the patient in maxillomandibular fixation. A previously prepared orthodontic auxiliary arch wire is inserted into buccal headgear tubes on molar teeth and ligated to place. Then the repositioned dentoalveolar segment held in the occlusal splint is ligated to the auxiliary arch wire (Fig. 10-12). At this point, the mandibular teeth should occlude appropriately into the underside of the occlusal splint.

Wound closure is less difficult if the patient is not in maxillomandibular fixation. Palatal incisions are closed first with interrupted simple or vertical mattress sutures. Continuous sutures may be used to close the vertical incisions on the facial aspect of the maxilla, but continuous sutures on the palate should be avoided if

there is any chance of compromising blood supply to the palatal vascular pedicle. If a full palatal flap has been reflected in the Wunderer technique to allow transverse expansion, the flap is reapproximated with interdental sutures. A petrolatum gauze pack may aid in maintaining the palatal flap against underlying bone and preventing hematoma formation. The pack can be held in place with light wire or nonresorbable suture material extending across the palate and anchored or tied around the adjacent teeth. The pack should be retained for 5 to 7 days then removed. Usually the maxilla has been repositioned posteriorly, and the excess tissue remaining allows wound closure. In most instances, no additional maxillomandibular fixation is required. But some surgeons choose to replace the maxillomandibular fixation, leaving it for a few days during the initial stages of soft-tissue healing.

Postsurgery Sequelae

Anterior maxillary subapical osteotomy rarely produces significant postsurgery pain. However, facial edema can be excessive and abrasion of the mucosa of the lips from retraction at surgery is common. Protecting soft tissues with specially designed retractors and moistening the lips with petrolatum or steroid cream can minimize soft-tissue trauma, but the amount of postsurgery edema may not be correlated with the trauma of the surgical procedure. Edema usually subsides rapidly, with most of it usually gone within 2 weeks. A minimum amount of residual edema may remain for up to 6 months as the lips learn to function with the dentoalveolar segments in a new position.

Sensory supply to the anterior teeth and mucosa may be altered for 6 months to a year. Remember that vascular supply to the bone, periodontal ligament, and teeth is maintained, and teeth may have an adequate vascular supply while responding negatively to electrical or cold stimuli. See Chapter 7 for further discussion.

When jaw function is resumed, patients are encouraged to restrict themselves to a soft, nonchew diet for a minimum of 4 weeks. Between 4 and 6 weeks, the anterior dentoalveolar segment should be clinically firm and bony healing should be adequate to allow the patient to increase the consistency of the diet, beginning function on the repositioned segment. The instructions of the surgeon must be followed closely since bony healing in some patients may be more rapid than others. Usually by 8 weeks the patient can return to the orthodontist for removal of the splint and the auxiliary arch wire and the initiation of postsurgical orthodontics.

Complications

Complications with anterior maxillary subapical osteotomy are rare. When they do occur, persistent periodontal defects in osteotomy sites between teeth and loss of blood supply to teeth adjacent to osteotomy cuts are reported most frequently. Every attempt must be made to leave adequate bone over teeth adjacent to bony cuts, preserving the periodontal ligament. When dentoalveolar segments are repositioned, alveolar bone between teeth must be aligned at the same vertical level (see Fig. 7-5). If a significant bony periodontal defect does occur, often it can be treated without loss of the involved teeth. Loss of vascular supply to the pulp of teeth adjacent to osteotomy sites does occur. The teeth may change color, abscess formation and drainage near the teeth may follow, or radiographic changes (e.g., periapical bone loss) may be the only presenting symp-

toms. Usually such teeth can be treated with traditional endodontic methods without loss of the affected teeth. Loss of blood supply to both teeth and alveolar bone in mobilized segments is a very rare complication. In these circumstances, teeth and segments of bone may be lost. When wound dehiscence occurs at osteotomy sites and the surgeon suspects a compromised vascular supply, usually heralded by a change in tone and color of the mucosa, every effort must be made to keep these sites clean and debrided. The process requires that patients be seen frequently over a period of several months. Usually bone and most of the involved teeth can be retained if wound care is meticulous. When bone and teeth are lost, the defect can be restored with prosthetic replacements.

Posterior Subapical Osteotomy

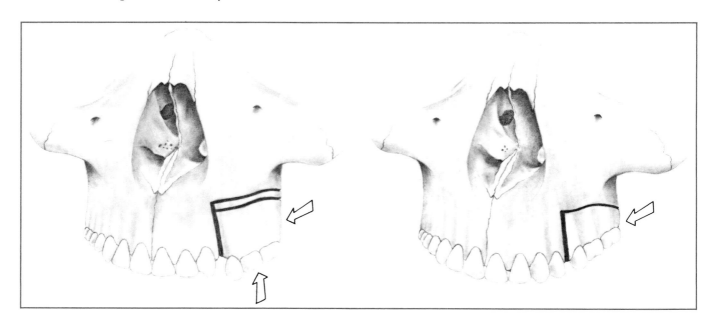

Posterior maxillary subapical osteotomy is utilized most often for correction of isolated unilateral posterior crossbite or for excessive eruption of posterior maxillary teeth as a result of missing mandibular posterior teeth.[12,13] Today LeFort I osteotomy is the preferred surgical procedure to correct true maxillary vertical excess. Posterior subapical osteotomy is a reliable surgical procedure which produces excellent results. The procedure may be performed under local anesthesia and conscious sedation without the patient's remaining in the hospital overnight as an alternative to surgery under general anesthesia. Usually the procedure is performed in conjunction with orthodontics to align teeth, provide space for interdental bone cuts, and aid in stabilizing bony segments at completion of osteotomy. Prosthodontic procedures must be coordinated to facilitate replacement of teeth in the maxilla

or in the opposing mandibular arch. Before surgery, periapical dental radiographs must demonstrate adequate bone, 3 to 5 mm, between teeth for planned osteotomy/ostectomy cuts.

Soft-Tissue Dissection

Following infiltration of a vasoconstrictor (usually 2% lidocaine with 1:100,000 epinephrine) at the height of the maxillary vestibule, a mucoperiosteal incision is made from the maxillary canine posterior beneath the zygomatic maxillary buttress to the tuberosity (Fig. 10-13). No vasoconstrictor is injected on the palate. With a periosteal elevator, mucoperiosteum is reflected superiorly, leaving the mucoperiosteum beneath the incision attached to bone. When tooth removal is planned anteriorly or posteriorly, the teeth are carefully removed at this time to keep alveolar bone in-

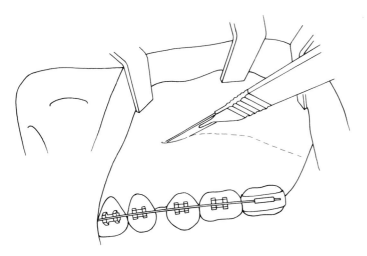

Fig. 10-13. Horizontal mucoperiosteal incision to expose bone above the maxillary posterior teeth.

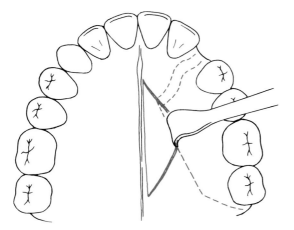

Fig. 10-14. Palatal incision if necessary to complete palatal bone cuts.

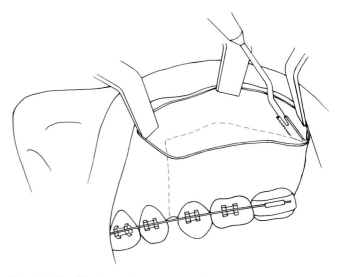

Fig. 10-15. Horizontal osteotomy above the segment to be mobilized.

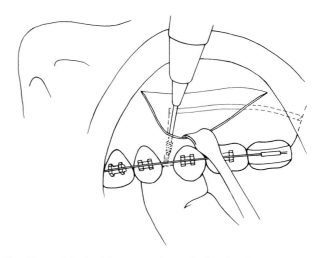

Fig. 10-16. Vertical bone cut through the alveolus anterior to the segment to be mobilized.

tact. With a flexible Freer periosteal elevator carefully reflecting mucoperiosteum inferiorly, bone in the area of the planned vertical cuts is exposed. Usually a palatal incision is not required. But when the posterior dentoalveolar segment must be moved medially more than a few millimeters, or it appears unlikely that the mobilized segment will telescope medially into position, palatal bone may need to be removed through a supplementary palatal incision made medial to the planned palatal cut usually extending from the canine posteriorly to the first molar (Fig. 10-14). With a periosteal elevator, the palatal mucosa is reflected, taking care to preserve the palatal vessels. Reflecting this palatal mucoperiosteal flap provides access to the bone removed with most difficulty from the lateral approach, the junction of the bony cuts in the palate with the anterior vertical cuts in the dentoalveolar segment.

Osteotomy/Ostectomy

After adequate exposure, horizontal osteotomy above the dentoalveolar segment to be mobilized is made through the thin lateral maxillary wall into the maxillary sinus with a bur or reciprocating saw (Fig. 10-15). If necessary, a measured amount of bone is removed to allow superior repositioning. Since the segment will usually telescope into the sinus, less bone removal is required than the distance the segment is to be moved superiorly. Attention is then directed to the planned vertical bony cuts. With a 701 fissure bur, bony cuts extend medially almost through the alveolar process (Fig. 10-16). Then with a thin spatula osteotome malleted into these cuts, the osteotomy is extended through to the palate, taking care to minimize

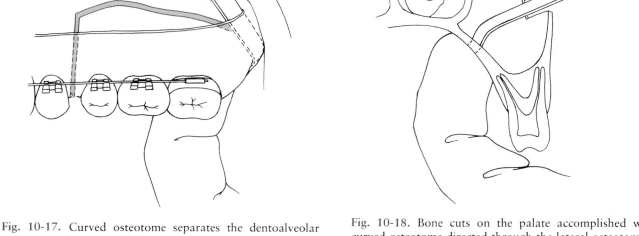

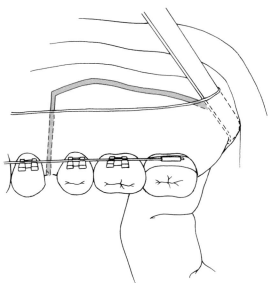

Fig. 10-17. Curved osteotome separates the dentoalveolar segment at the pterygoid plates.

Fig. 10-18. Bone cuts on the palate accomplished with a curved osteotome directed through the lateral osteotomy.

trauma to the palatal mucosa. When sufficient bone exists posterior to the terminal molar, vertical bone cuts may be made in this area. As an alternative, a curved osteotome may separate the maxillary tuberosity from the pterygoid plates (Fig. 10-17). Next, attention is di-

rected to the palatal bony cuts. In most circumstances, palatal bone can be cut with a curved osteotome directed through the lateral horizontal bony cut and the maxillary sinus (Fig. 10-18). By malleting the curved osteotome along the superior aspect of the palatal bone

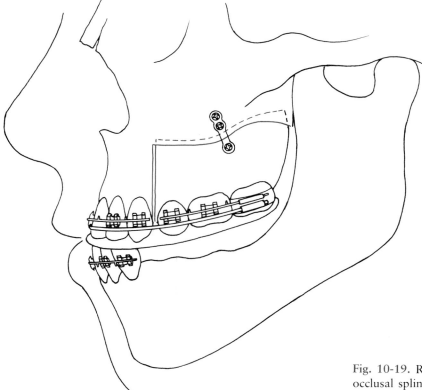

Fig. 10-19. Repositioned posterior maxillary segment in the occlusal splint, stabilized with an auxiliary orthodontic arch wire and a small bone plate.

from posterior to anterior, bony cuts are connected. If access through a palatal incision is required, bone cuts are completed on the palate with a bur or osteotome.

After appropriate bone removal, the posterior dentoalveolar segment is manually positioned into the prepared occlusal splint. Adequate vascular supply is maintained to the mobilized segment from both facial and palatal soft-tissue pedicles.

Stabilization and Fixation Methods

When sufficient numbers of teeth remain in the maxillary dental arch, the occusal splint is ligated to the teeth. It may be necessary to apply maxillomandibular fixation to stabilize the posterior maxillary segment. Usually an auxiliary orthodontic stabilizing arch wire can be inserted into buccal headgear tubes to stabilize the posterior dentoalveolar segment. Rigid fixation with bone plates or a vertical wire strut adds stability (Fig. 10-19). When the patient has multiple missing teeth or when lateral expansion of more than 5 to 7 mm of the maxillary segment has occurred, transpalatal orthodontic stabilization should be considered. By combining modifications in the occlusal splint, orthodontic arch wire stabilization, and rigid fixation, posterior dentoalveolar segments can be kept immobile until adequate clinical healing has taken place. In most circumstances maxillomandibular fixation is not required for more than a few days for isolated posterior subapical osteotomy. Following stabilization and fixation of the segment, soft-tissue incisions are closed with 4.0 chromic gut sutures. Wound closure is easier before establishing maxillomandibular fixation. Except when the posterior dentoalveolar segment is expanded laterally, adequate palatal mucosa exists for good wound closure. When lateral expansion does not leave enough palatal tissue for closure, additional mucoperiosteal incisions on the contralateral palate may be required to mobilize palatal tissue so that mucosa can be closed over the palatal osteotomy site. Care must be taken with wound closure to not compromise the vascular supply of the palatal tissue pedicle.

Postsurgery Sequelae

Significant postsurgery pain is unusual with posterior maxillary subapical osteotomy. However, facial edema on the operated side can be substantial and the lips can be abraded from retractors utilized for surgical access. Facial edema usually resolves quickly, most of the edema being gone in 2 weeks with the residual resolving over several months. Patients are restricted to a soft nonchew diet for a minimum of 4 weeks. If adequate clinical healing has taken place, the surgeon will allow the patient to increase dietary consistency over the next few weeks. Usually the patients return to the orthodontist for finishing orthodontic therapy at about 2 months. When fixed or removable prosthetic appliances are planned, they are completed following a period of orthodontic retention, within 6 to 12 months following surgery.

Complications

The most common complications are significant periodontal defects at vertical osteotomy sites and loss of vascular supply to teeth in the mobilized dentoalveolar segments. As has been discussed with anterior maxillary subapical surgery, these complications usually can be treated without loss of teeth or significant amounts of alveolar bone. Loss of blood supply to both bone and teeth is a rare complication. When this occurs, wound dehiscence or changes in tone and color of the mucosa herald the process. Every effort must be made to keep these sites clean and debrided. The healing process with a compromised blood supply can be protracted, requiring multiple patient visits, but usually loss of bone and teeth can be kept to a minimum.

SURGICAL TECHNIQUES: MANDIBLE
Inferior Alveolar Neurovascular Bundle Decompression

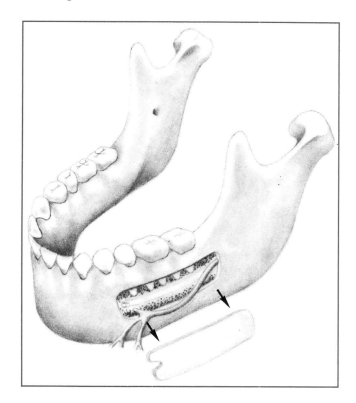

When an osteotomy, segmental or subapical, involves the body of the mandible, inferior alveolar neuvascular bundle decompression is necessary to minimize damage to this structure and the resultant neurosensory disturbances. In a few patients the mandibular neurovascular canal is positioned well below the apices of the molar and premolar teeth, sufficient to allow a subapical osteotomy without endangering the neurovascular bundle or compromising tooth vitality.[15,16] As a general rule, at least 4 mm of bone should be present between the osteotomy and the root apices to prevent damage to the roots. In most patients insufficient bone exists between the neurovascular canal and the root apices to allow a bone cut without creating additional space by surgical neurovascular bundle displacement.

In early experiences with body ostectomy the neurovascular bundle was sectioned; immediate anesthesia followed in the mental nerve distribution. Some patients had complete return of sensation with that approach.[17] However, neurosensory return when the bundle is sectioned is unlikely, and the nerve should be protected if possible. When subapical or body osteotomy/ostectomy at or behind the mental foramen is planned, decompression of the neurovascular bundle is accomplished first before the osteotomy/ostectomy procedure.

A method for exposing and decompressing the neurovascular bundle in its course through the mandibular body will be described. This approach has resulted in minimal long-term neurosensory disturbances and is recommended when segmental mandibular subapical surgery is performed in the posterior mandible or when a body osteotomy/ostectomy is performed at or proximal to the mental foramen.[18-22]

Soft-Tissue Dissection

After infiltrating the mucosa with vasoconstrictor (usually 2% lidocaine with 1:100,000 epinephrine), the soft-tissue incision in the mucosa begins at a point just superior and lateral to the ramus body juncture (Fig. 10-20). When both sides of the mandible are to be operated, the incision is carried well out into the unattached mucosa around the entire mandible to the contralateral ramus body junction. On approaching the region of the mental foramen, the incision should curve up and more medial to minimize the danger of injuring the mental neurovascular bundle. After the incision, the submucosal tissues are divided down to periosteum by using curved scissors. Care is taken in the dissection at the mental foramen to stay above the emerging nerve fibers while dissecting down to the superior aspect of the foramen. Once the bone is reached, the periosteum is incised and a mucoperiosteal flap developed inferiorly from the posterior mandible around to the contralateral side. Next the main trunk of the mental neurovascular bundle is exposed and mobilized with a series of incisions which run parallel to the course of individual nerve bundles. By dissecting with a scissors beneath the main nerve trunk and then spreading along the parallel incisions, the nerve trunk and its branches can be freed sufficiently to allow its retraction (Fig. 10-21).

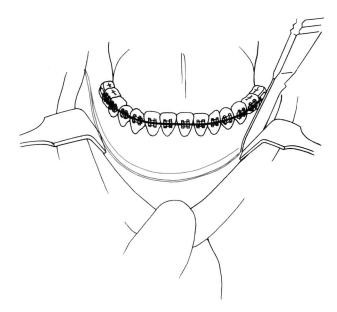

Fig. 10-20. Mucoperiosteal incision for total mandibular alveolar osteotomy, including inferior alveolar neurovascular bundle decompression.

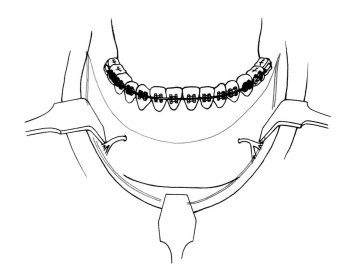

Fig. 10-21. Soft-tissue dissection complete.

Osteotomy/Ostectomy

The next step involves bony cuts to decorticate the lateral mandible to expose the mandibular canal and neurovascular bundle. The mandibular canal should be exposed proximally to just behind any planned vertical osteotomy. In the total subapical procedure this exposure must be carried proximal to the terminal molar teeth. In patients with second molars present, the exposure ends proximally where the neurovascular bundle turns medially and superiorly on its course through the ramus to the mandibular foramen at the lingula. Using a small Stieger or 701 fissure bur, bone cuts are out-

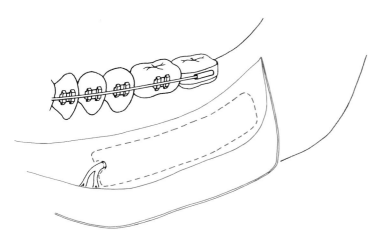

Fig. 10-22. Initial bony cortical cuts for neurovascular bundle exposure.

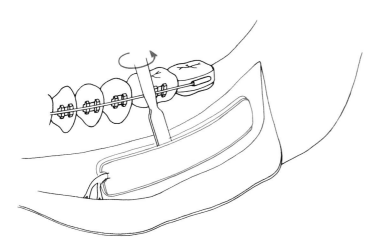

Fig. 10-23. Bony cuts complete. The lateral cortical bone is freed.

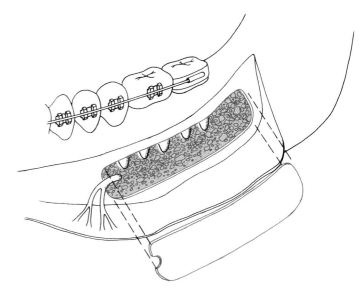

Fig. 10-24. Bony cortical plate removed to expose the neurovascular bundle.

neurovascular bundle is clearly visualized, a decision can be made as to whether or not there is sufficient room between the neurovascular bundle and the root apices to allow a subapical osteotomy.

Retraction of the Neurovascular Bundle

In most cases, it is necessary to lift the neurovascular bundle from the canal to safely carry out the subapical procedure. For a body ostectomy procedure with a vertical bone cut proximal to the mental foramen, the neurovascular bundle must be retracted. When the decision has been made to remove the neurovascular bundle the anterior continuation (incisive branch) of the neurovascular bundle must be severed, accomplished easily with a #11 blade.

Next the neurovascular bundle is lifted carefully from the canal using a #2 molt curette to a point just proximal to the extent of the planned osteotomy/ostectomy. During this freeing (decompression) procedure, the surgeon must be patient (Fig. 10-25). The small neurovascular bundle connections to the root apices must be severed. Magnification loops are recommended for optimum visualization. Some may prefer to use an operating microscope although we have not found this necessary. Once the bundle is lifted from the canal, retracted, covered, and protected with a moist gauze, the neurovascular bundle is decompressed on the contralateral side. The cortical plates of bone are preserved for later use before wound closure. Care must be exercised by both the surgeon and assistants not to injure the exposed neurovascular bundles while they are positioned laterally during the osteotomy/ostectomy procedure.

lined from the mental foramen proximally to the ramus body juncture (Fig. 10-22). The plate of bone to be removed over the neurovascular bundle should be 5 to 7 mm in width, extending only through the lateral cortical plate into the medullary bed. At the mental foramen area, the cut extends anterior to the foramen with both ends ending in the foramen proper. The cuts on the proximal end are connected in a gentle curve (Fig. 10-23). After completion of the cortical bone cuts, a wide osteotome is inserted at the middle of the superior bony cut. With a wedging action the cortical plate usually detaches from the mandible in a single piece. The notch cut into the mental foramen allows the cortical plate to be freed from around the mental nerve trunk (Fig. 10-24). Cancellous bone can now be scooped away from the neurovascular bundle with a #2 Molt curette or similar instrument. Once the course of the

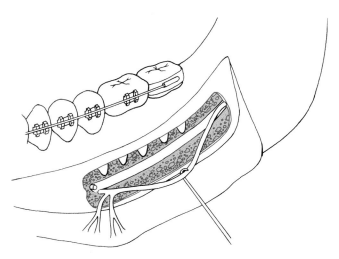

Fig. 10-25. Neurovascular bundle can be retracted after cutting the incisal branch.

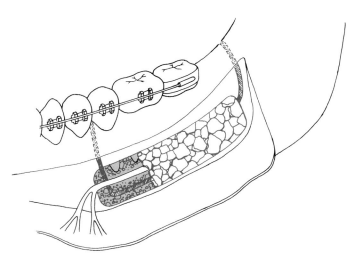

Fig. 10-26. Neurovascular bundle replaced and covered with bone graft at completion of procedure.

Repositioning of the Neurovascular Bundle

After completion of the planned bony surgery, the neurovascular bundles are replaced in the mandibular bodies. If space exists between the dentoalveolar and inferior mandibular segments (e.g., in a subapical procedure) a bone graft (autogenous or allogeneic bone) is placed on the medial aspect to fill the gap and help support the dentoalveolar segment in its new position. Then the neurovascular bundle is repositioned and covered with a graft of particulate bone. The facial bone removed initially to expose the neurovascular bundle can be cut into small particles with a rongeur or bone mill and used as a portion of this graft. This bone also can be cut into vertical struts and wedged between the segments laterally to help stabilize the repositioned segment (Fig. 10-26; also see Fig. 10-45).

Postsurgery Sequelae and Complications

Decompression of neurovascular bundles in this manner has resulted in minimal neurosensory disturbances in our series.[19] All patients are warned that they will have loss of sensation immediately following this procedure. After 6 months the patient can anticipate good recovery and return to normal neurosensory function. Devitalization of teeth has not been a problem in our experience, although some teeth never regain a normal sensory response. However, the potential for permanent nerve injury as well as need for endodontic treatment for devitalized teeth always exists. In this procedure, there is always the danger of neurovascular bundle disruption during its decompression. Microanastomosis of the disrupted nerve bundle is recommended in such circumstances. At a minimum the severed ends of the neurovascular bundle should be approximated in the mandibular canal before wound closure.

Body Ostectomy

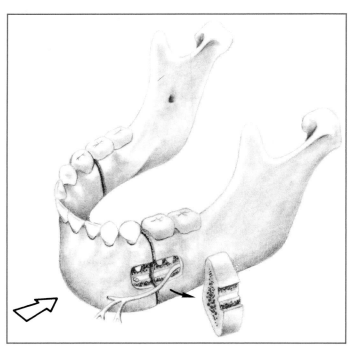

Body ostectomy was one of the first procedures performed in orthognathic surgery, usually to shorten the mandible.[1-4] As other more effective surgical procedures were developed, including subapical and mandibular ramus osteotomy, use of the body ostectomy became less common. The procedure has special indications today (e.g., with a ramus procedure to narrow the mandibular dental arch by removing a segment in the anterior mandible or to reposition malaligned molar and premolar segments). Occasional patients have a mandibular deformity which is primarily an elongation

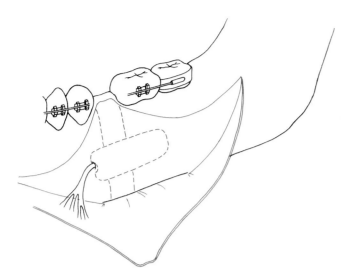

Fig. 10-27. Mucoperiosteal "finger flap" and outline of bone cuts for body osteotomy.

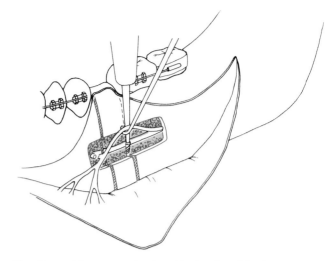

Fig. 10-28. Neurovascular bundle freed and body osteotomy being completed.

of the body of the mandible. Such patients benefit both esthetically and occlusally by shortening only that dimension. A predictable method for minimizing damage to the neurovascular bundle and the option of RIF for immediate repair of the continuity defect have encouraged surgeons to reconsider the option of the body procedure. When shortening the mandible with the body procedure, space must be available for the ostectomy and the planned amount of posterior repositioning of the anterior segment. Space must be created by removing a tooth or by preparing an adequate space with presurgical orthodontics. Lack of available space for bone removal remains the major reason why surgeons would choose another procedure to shorten the mandible.

Soft-Tissue Dissection

As has been discussed, body ostectomy usually requires decompression of the mandibular neurovascular bundle. The incision as described for exposure of the lateral mandible in the neurovascular decompression procedure is performed first. The incision for a body procedure alone usually ends anterior to the mental foramen in the region of the first premolar or canine teeth. If a tooth is removed to gain space for an ostectomy the incision can be modified to include a "finger flap" at the crest of the alveolus (Fig. 10-27). The facial mucoperiosteal flap is reflected to expose the inferior border of the mandible. Lingual mucoperiosteum is reflected at the site of the planned ostectomy to the inferior border. The sharp curved end of the flexible Freer periosteal elevator is very useful in following the lingual contour of the mandible, especially as it turns more laterally beneath the mylohyoid crest. Care should be taken not to tear the lingual mucoperiosteum so the mouth floor structures are protected.

Ostectomy

After removal of the neurovascular bundle from its canal proximal to the planned ostectomy site and elevation of the mucoperiosteum on the lingual side of the mandible, protecting it with a periosteal elevator, a planned amount of bone is removed with a Stieger bur or a reciprocating or oscillating saw sufficient to allow the correction (Fig. 10-28). Usually bilateral body ostectomies are required; the contralateral side is managed in a similar fashion. To improve bone contact following repositioning of the segments, the bony cuts may be configured in a step design. Following completion of the ostectomy and bone removal maxillomandibular fixation is established.

Stabilization and Fixation Methods

A heavy stabilizing arch wire secured in tubes on molar bands is placed to enhance fixation of the dental components after the planned occlusion has been established with the occlusal splint. Usually it is easier to place the auxiliary arch wire just before maxillomandibular wires are placed. Then the osteotomy sites are inspected. When the anterior segment has been repositioned posteriorly, a lateral step exists since the repositioned anterior segment is more narrow transversely across the canines than the mandibular posterior segments. It is possible to narrow the posterior transverse dimension, rotating both posterior segments around the condylar vertical axis. This movement requires very careful planning before surgery when the procedure is simulated on dental casts. The position of the vertical condylar axis must be estimated from submental vertex radiographs. The condylar post in a semiadjustable articulator may not represent the actual position of the vertical condylar axis.

RIF is the method of choice for fixing and stabilizing the bony segments in a body procedure. Small semi-

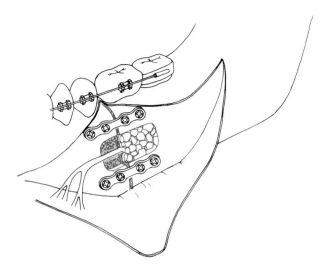

Fig. 10-29. Anterior mandibular segment repositioned and rigidly fixed with small bone plates.

rigid bone plates can be contoured to both the proximal and the distal segments. The semirigid bone plate must be long enough for placement of at least two screws on either side of the ostectomy site, and three screws are preferable. Two plates, one near the inferior border and the second just below the root apices, may be required if the patient is to function soon after surgery. Bicortical screws to secure the plates are preferred, but monocortical screws can be used in the superior plate to prevent damaging roots of teeth in the vicinity. Principles of bone plate adaptation and screw placement must be followed (Fig. 10-29). In some patients the segments are difficult to keep aligned while plates are contoured and placed. In such circumstances placing a 26-gauge wire suture at the inferior border through the lateral cortical plates will approximate the bone segments and stabilize the ostectomy site. The wire suture can be removed once the bone plates are in place. After RIF has been applied and before repositioning of the mandibular neurovascular bundle, maxillomandibular fixation must be released and the planned mandibular position and occlusion verified. If condylar distraction or other discrepancies are evident, RIF must be removed and segment(s) repositioned as required. Rigid fixation is replaced once the segments are properly positioned and the occlusion checked again. If minimal bony contact exists in the osteotomy site, autogenous or allogeneic bone grafts should be placed to fill the defects. Often sufficient bone can be obtained from the mandible adjacent to ostectomy sites. With a body procedure the neurovascular bundle usually is decompressed only a few millimeters along its course. Placing a graft over the exposed bundle is not mandatory in such circumstances. Incisions are closed with a running horizontal or interlocking mattress suture. When a tooth has been removed to gain

space for bone removal, special care must be taken to close the wound primarily at the superior aspect of the alveolus. The "finger flap" incision design facilitates wound closure in such circumstances.

Postsurgery Sequelae

As with other orthognathic surgical procedures, patients can have considerable facial edema following surgery, but severe pain is rare. The bulk of the edema subsides in 2 weeks. The lips and surrounding tissue adapt to the new jaw position over several months. All patients have immediate neurosensory alteration associated with the neurovascular bundle manipulations. Long-term neurosensory disturbance (greater than 6 months) is unusual but may occur if the neurovascular bundle is torn at surgery. Teeth adjacent to ostectomy sites and those in the repositioned anterior mandible usually maintain their blood supply, but sensory supply to the teeth, periodontal ligament, and surrounding mucosa may be altered for 6 months to a year.

When RIF is applied, the patient may be allowed to function immediately after surgery with guiding elastics. A liquid or soft diet is mandatory for at least 6 weeks before resuming normal mastication. If the RIF is not adequate for jaw function, the patient is placed in firm maxillomandibular fixation with 26-gauge wire loops for a period of 4 to 6 weeks. Whenever fixation is released rehabilitation of the jaws to full function is an important goal which must not be neglected (see Chapter 7).

Complications

A major complication peculiar to the mandibular body procedure is delayed bony healing or nonunion of the bony segments. Often the mandibular segments must be repositioned so only minimal bony contact exists at ostectomy sites. If this can be anticipated in advance, the design of the ostectomy cuts can be altered to facilitate bony contact after segments have been repositioned. Poor bone contact following ostectomy cannot always be anticipated even with the best planning. If poor bone contact exists before wound closure, bone grafts should be packed into the defects at the surgical site. Bone usually can be obtained from sites adjacent to the ostectomy, but autogenous bone from the cranium or iliac crest may be required. Allogeneic bone is not as useful in such circumstances when rapid bony healing is the goal.

RIF, effectively applied across the ostectomy sites, reduces the risk of protracted healing. If any question exists about the stabilization/fixation at the ostectomy site the patient must be checked at regular intervals to assess bony healing. Healing is slower in the body ostectomy as compared to a ramus osteotomy, a feature of the procedure easily forgotten when the surgeon performs the procedure infrequently. If nonunion follows ostectomy it may not be evident for 10 to 12 weeks.

When nonunion occurs the surgical site must be reoperated and grafted with autogenous bone.

Midline Osteotomy

In some patients, the mandible must be narrowed transversely when the deformity is primarily in the mandible, and maxillary surgery to accommodate mandibular width is not indicated. A midline osteotomy/ostectomy may be performed alone or in conjunction with bilateral procedures in the ramus or an inferior border osteotomy. Although the procedure is most commonly used to narrow the mandible, horizontal or transverse expansion of a few millimeters also may be attained, but mandibular expansion is difficult. If a midline osteotomy is contemplated for narrowing the mandible a space must be created orthodontically or, more commonly, an incisor tooth is removed to make space at the time of surgery. The available space must be sufficient for the desired movement. If multiple mandibular procedures are planned the midline osteotomy should be performed last, to allow greater stability of the mandible during other procedures (e.g., the sagittal split procedure involves more wedging and torsional forces to complete the osteotomy, an even more difficult task when the anterior mandible is in several pieces).

Soft-Tissue Dissection

After infiltrating the mucosa on the anterior mandible with a vasoconstrictor (usually 2% lidocaine with 1:100,000 epinephrine), a full mucoperiosteal flap is reflected from the necks of the teeth into the facial vestibule, exposing at least two teeth on either side of the planned osteotomy (Fig. 10-30). If the midline osteotomy/ostectomy is combined with an inferior border osteotomy, the incision for that procedure may be utilized for access to the midline of the alveolus. The mucoperiosteal reflection on the facial surface of the man-

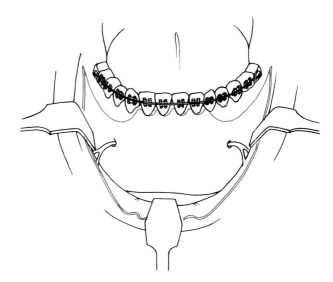

Fig. 10-30. Mucoperiosteal incision and dissection for mandibular midline osteotomy.

dible is carried to the inferior border. Next the lingual mucosa adjacent to the midline osteotomy site is reflected from the necks of the teeth, as described for the body osteotomy procedure, and the lingual tissues protected with a periosteal elevator down to the attachment of the genioglossus muscles.

Osteotomy/Ostectomy

After removal of a tooth if necessary, the mandible is divided with either a bur or a reciprocating or oscillating saw. A planned segment of bone is removed if the mandible is to be narrowed. If the mandible is to be widened, a step osteotomy design is utilized with the vertical portion through the alveolar bone, a horizontal limb to either the right or left side and continuing vertically through the inferior border (Fig. 10-31, *A* and

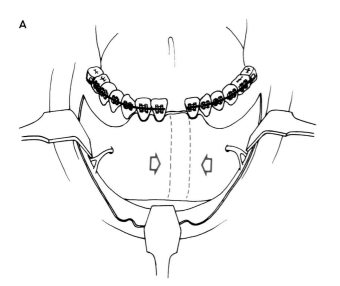
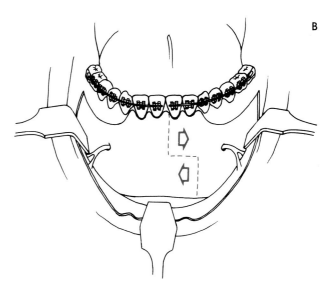

Fig. 10-31. Outline of bone cuts: **A,** to allow narrowing, and **B,** to allow expansion.

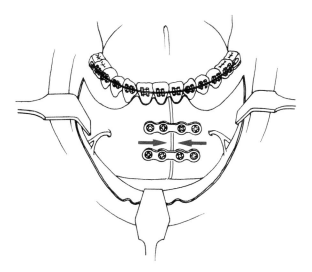

Fig. 10-32. Stabilization of midline osteotomy with small bone plates after narrowing.

B). This design provides good stability as the osteotomy allows the segments to slide along the horizontal component maintaining bone contact and eliminating a vertical continuity defect.

Stabilization and Fixation Methods

After all osteotomies are completed, the teeth are placed into the planned occlusal relationship with the aid of the occlusal splint and held securely with maxillomandibular wires. Additional stabilization can be gained from placement of a preformed auxiliary arch wire secured to tubes on molar bands. When both ramus and midline osteotomies are combined, the midline osteotomy site is stabilized first, then the ramus osteotomies. This sequence should reduce the tendency for buccal-lingual tipping of the tooth segments, which will occur when maxillomandibular fixation is applied. Semirigid bone plates and screws secure the midline osteotomy with plates long enough for at least two screws on either side of the osteotomy site (Fig. 10-32). A plate at the inferior border across the midline osteotomy is placed first. A second plate just below the root apices of the teeth may be added. If the mandible has been expanded, autogenous or allogeneic bone should be placed in the vertical defects of the osteotomy site. With RIF, maxillomandibular fixation is released after all segments have been stabilized and mandibular position and occlusion are verified. To begin wound closure, interdental sutures are placed to adapt the facial mucoperiosteal flap to the remaining teeth. The rest of the incisions are closed with interrupted mattress sutures.

Postsurgery Sequelae

Edema following midline osteotomy alone may not be as great as with body or ramus surgery. Additional support to the soft-tissue wounds can be gained from using a elastic velcro head dressing (see Chapter 7). Loss of sensory supply to teeth and soft tissue at the osteotomy site should be less than with a body osteotomy.

When RIF is adequate, the patient may function into the occlusal splint after surgery aided by guiding elastics. Patients must be restricted to a liquid or soft diet. If wire fixation alone is used across the osteotomy sites, the patient must remain in maxillomandibular fixation for 4 to 6 weeks.

Complications

Complications with midline osteotomy should be minimal since the osteotomy does not involve the mandibular neurovascular bundle except for the incisal branches. RIF decreases the chance of delayed healing or nonunion across the osteotomy sites.

Inferior Border Osteotomy

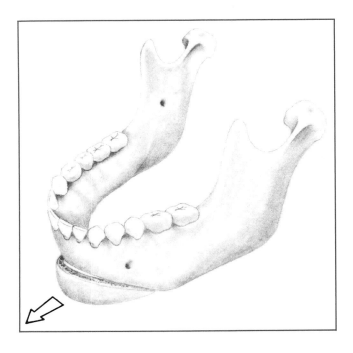

Inferior border osteotomy can be utilized for correction of abnormality in the anterior as well as the body of the mandible.[5,6] In the anterior mandible, the inferior border osteotomy can alter form in the vertical, transverse, or anteroposterior dimensions. The anteroinferior border osteotomy, also referred to as a *genioplasty,* may be carried out alone or in conjunction with other mandibular or maxillary procedures. The inferior border osteotomy in the body portion of the mandible is most commonly utilized to shorten the vertical dimension of one side (e.g., to correct conditions such as hemimandibular hyperplasia). Decompression and repositioning of the mandibular neurovascular bundle

A
B

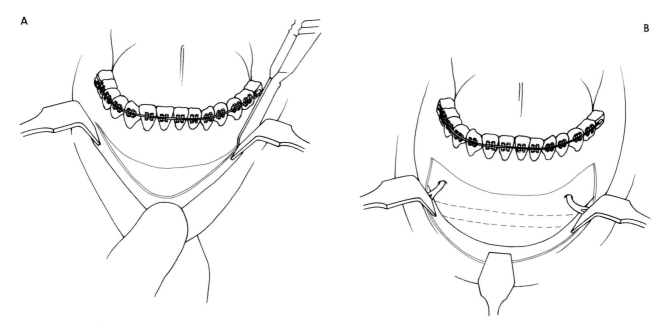

Fig. 10-33. Inferior border osteotomy. **A,** Mucosal incision. **B,** Dissection exposing anterior mandible with outline of bone cuts.

usually are not necessary except when a major vertical reduction of the mandibular body is planned.

Soft-Tissue Dissection

All bony movements following inferior border osteotomy in the anterior mandible are possible through a common incision and flap design. After infiltration of the mucosa with a vasoconstrictor (usually 2% lidocaine with 1:100,000 epinephrine) the incision begins well out into the facial mucosa, actually in the lower lip, from an area just anterior to the mental foramen of one side to the same point on the opposite side. After the initial incision through mucosa, dissection is carried through the submucosal tissues and muscle down to periosteum with scissors. The periosteum is sharply incised and periosteum is reflected from the anterior mandible to the inferior border. During this dissection care is taken to identify and protect the mental foramen and the emerging mental nerve bundles. Since the inferior border osteotomy usually extends posterior to the mental foramen, the mucoperiosteum at the inferior border must be freed at least to the anterior third of the body of the mandible (Fig. 10-33, *A* and *B*).

Osteotomy/Ostectomy

For *vertical reduction* of the anterior mandible, a horizontal osteotomy is first carried out just above the inferior border (Fig. 10-33, *B*). At its posterior limit the osteotomy should taper into the body rather than creating a vertical step, to preclude a defect after healing that could be noticeable in the overlying soft tissue. After the inferior border has been freed, it remains pedicled to the digastric muscle insertions and sometimes a portion of the geniohyoid muscle. For a vertical reduction, a measured amount of bone is removed from the anterior mandible with a second horizontal bone cut and the inferior border is repositioned superiorly. This approach is preferred to simple trimming of the inferior border because preserving the inferior border itself in a vertical reduction will produce the best soft-tissue adaptation and form (Fig. 10-34, *A* and *B*).

Along with the vertical reduction, the inferior border also can be repositioned anteriorly or posteriorly. The amount of repositioning is planned before surgery to meet the needs of the individual patient. Occasionally when the inferior border is repositioned posteriorly and superiorly, the facial surface of the mandible no longer has any contour. A facial-lingual concavity in the anterior mandible must be developed above the inferior border to give it form for the best lip function and esthetics. The concavity is carefully sculptured in bone with a bur.

Advancement of the inferior border of the mandible can be accomplished with an osteotomy. Once the bony segment is freed it is repositioned forward to the planned new position. Usually bone remains in contact, the facial plate of the mandible above in contact with the lingual plate of the inferior border segment. If additional bone contour is desired after advancing the inferior border, an onlay bone graft of autogenous or allogeneic bone is placed over the step area. If required, the inferior border can be advanced even farther than the width of the inferior border segment, leaving a gap be-

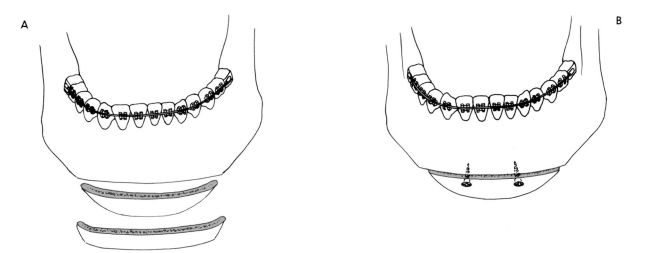

Fig. 10-34. **A,** For vertical reduction a measured amount of bone is removed. **B,** Inferior border repositioned and fixed with position screws.

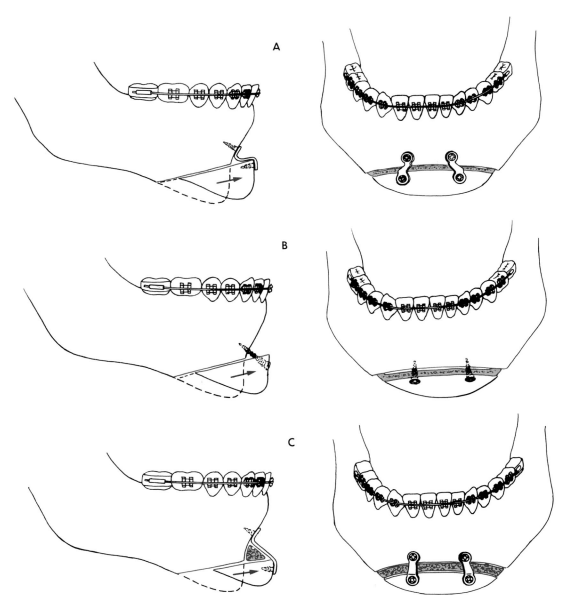

Fig. 10-35. **A,** Inferior border advancement stabilized with small bone plates. **B,** Position screw stabilization. **C,** Bone graft augmentation following rigid fixation and extreme advancement.

tween the lingual surface of the advanced segment and the facial surface of the intact mandible. When such an extensive advancement is made, the defect is filled with autogenous or allogeneic bone after the segments are stabilized and fixed (Fig. 10-35, *A* through *C*). To correct extreme retroposition of the anteroinferior border of the mandible, it is possible to make multiple bony slices, advancing and fixing each segment stepwise. With the availability of rigid fixation techniques using semirigid bone plates, such a tedious procedure is not necessary as the inferior border can be advanced and stabilized and the intervening gap filled with a bone graft.

Transverse width reduction of the anterior mandible in conjunction with an inferior border osteotomy usually involves removing a piece of bone at the midline of the inferior border segment to allow constriction in that area (Fig. 10-36, *A* and *B*).

A less common need for correction is *widening* the anteroinferior mandible in a transverse direction usually in conjunction with mandibular advancement. In this circumstance the freed inferior border segment is divided in the midline and then fixed to the mandible to acquire the increased transverse width. An extensive midline gap results between the segments. The defect is grafted with autogenous or allogeneic bone sup-

plemented with onlay grafts laterally if needed (Fig. 10-37).

Reduction of the inferior border of the mandible in the *AP plane of space* only can be accomplished by inferior border osteotomy and repositioning of the segment in a posterior direction. Though the osteotomy is not difficult, the soft tissue rarely follows the bone in a posterior direction in contrast to almost all other movements where soft-tissue adaptation is good. Because the soft-tissue results are not predictable, osteotomy to shorten the inferior border of the mandible in the AP direction is performed only occasionally (Fig. 10-38, *A* and *B*).

The reader is referred to the figures describing osteotomy cuts for anteroinferior border osteotomy, which include all of the possibilities discussed. With RIF the segments can now be repositioned as required and bone grafts placed in voids between the repositioned segment and the remaining mandible. Onlay grafts can be added to provide additional facial contour.

Correction of anterior mandibular inferior border *asymmetry* presents more complex problems. Following release of the inferior border of the mandible after osteotomy, the segment can be shifted to the right or

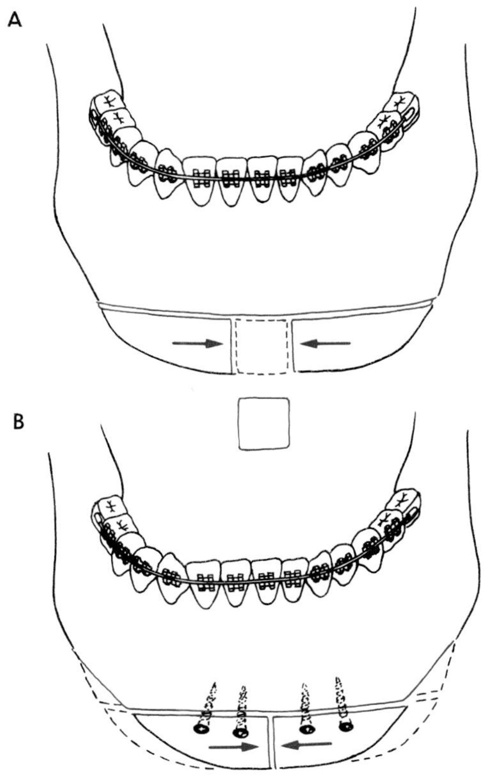

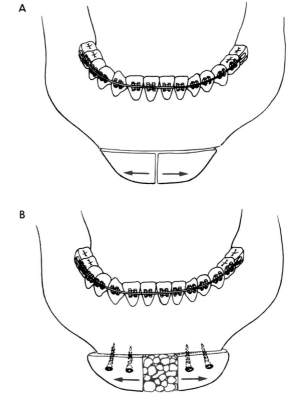

Fig. 10-36. **A,** Bone removed for transverse width reduction. **B,** Segments repositioned and rigidly fixed with position screws.

Fig. 10-37. **A,** Osteotomy for transverse expansion. **B,** Segments stabilized with position screws; bone graft placed in midline defect.

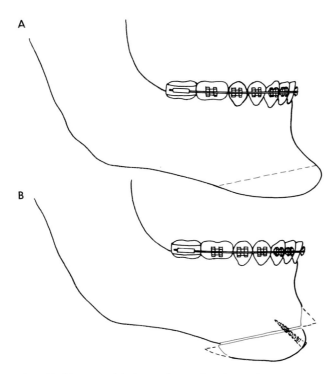

Fig. 10-38. Mandibular inferior border reduction in AP plane. **A,** Outline of bone cuts. **B,** Repositioned bony segment stabilized with position screws.

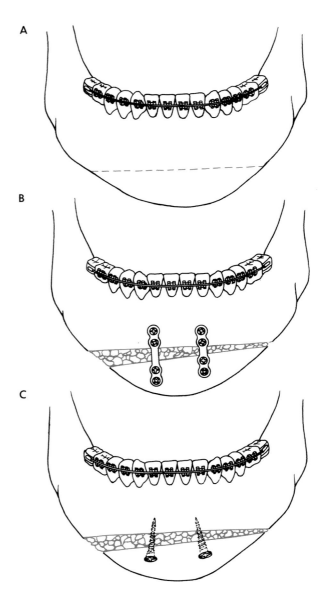

Fig. 10-39. A, Outline of bone cuts for correction of antero-inferior border asymmetry. **B,** Segment repositioned and rigidly fixed with small bone plates; bone graft interposed. **C,** Lag or position screw fixation of inferior segment; bone graft interposed.

left side, shortened or lengthened asymmetrically. In addition it can be advanced or retruded. Correction is often necessary in these situations in the vertical, transverse, and AP planes. The freed inferior border segment can be shifted to allow correction in all of these dimensions and then held exactly in the new position with RIF (Fig. 10-39, *A* through *C*). Defects then can be grafted as required. Before the use of RIF all bone cuts had to be coordinated to allow segment repositioning with maximum bone contact or interposing grafts had to be carefully sculptured to fit exactly the predetermined defects which corresponded to the amount of movement. Now the segment(s) can be positioned as desired, rigidly fixed, and bone grafts placed between the repositioned segment and intact mandible.

Vertical reduction at the inferior border of *the body* of the mandible, usually unilaterally (e.g., to correct hemimandibular hyperplasia) is more predictably done alone as a second surgery after mandibular repositioning. It is extremely difficult to plan the exact amount of bone removal at the inferior border until the mandible has been repositioned in the primary procedure and the soft tissues adapt to the new bone position, usually a minimum of 6 months.

Unilateral inferior border osteotomy in the body of the mandible is indicated to correct the deformity that often develops in a patient with hemimandibular hyperplasia. The first step is to remove the neurovascular

bundle from its bony canal before bone removal since the neurovascular bundle often has been displaced on the deformed side to near the inferior border. [23] Following the mucoperiosteal flap reflection, the inferior border is identified from the angle region to the symphysis; the periosteum underneath the inferior border is relieved with a J stripper. The neurovascular bundle is removed as previously described. Using a small reciprocating saw the inferior border is sectioned from the angle to the symphysis. The segment of bone is removed and the remaining bone is contoured with rotary instruments as necessary. Vertical reduction at the

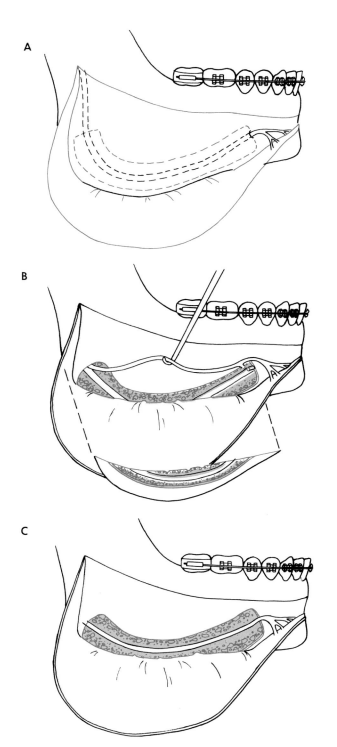

Fig. 10-40. **A,** Mucoperiosteal flap retracted for vertical reduction osteotomy of mandibular body inferior border with outline of bony cuts for neurovascular bundle exposure. **B,** Bone removal and contouring at inferior border. **C,** Neurovascular bundle repositioned.

inferior border of the body of the mandible is the exception to the rule of preserving and repositioning the inferior border (Fig. 10-40, *A* through *C*). If bilateral inferior border osteotomy is planned (e.g., reduction of one side and augmentation of the opposite side) the bone removed from the first side can be used to augment the opposite side. Since the osteotomy will usually involve the mandibular canal, the neurovascular bundle which has been retracted is replaced beneath the mandibular body before closure of the incision. Soft tissue adapts closely to the contour of the inferior aspect of the mandible after 6 months of healing.

Stabilization and Fixation Methods

Traditionally, figure-of-eight wire sutures, 25- or 26-gauge, have been used for fixation if bone remains in contact after the inferior border segment has been repositioned. Wire sutures placed through cortical plates in the midline and laterally provide firm fixation. Position screws or Kirschner wires through cortical plates of bone also provide excellent fixation. Position screws and wire sutures can be used together. Lag screws can be placed, but segments may be displaced as the screws are tightened. When a significant defect exists after repositioning of the segments, fixation is best managed with semirigid bone plates. The plate is adapted with one arm against the intact mandible above a second arm spanning the gap and the third over the facial aspect to allow one or two screws in both the repositioned segment and the intact mandible above. In some instances a single plate will suffice for fixation although two plates placed on the lateral aspects of the osteotomy are recommended to provide more rigidity. See Figs. 10-34 through 10-39 for examples of RIF for inferior border osteotomy.

Following completion of the osteotomy and fixation, the incision is closed in layers with deep sutures approximating the severed muscles and the mucosa is closed with a running horizontal mattress suture. An external pressure dressing is almost mandatory to provide wound support. The elastic-velcro dressing is ideal. Absolute hemostasis greatly reduces the danger of hematoma formation and subsequent wound breakdown. The external pressure dressing is maintained in place for a minimum of 5 days.

Postsurgery Sequelae

Soft-tissue edema can take several weeks to resolve after inferior border osteotomy. Often the lips also are repositioned with the procedure and they may take 3 to 6 months to adapt to function in a new position. Patients should be advised of this time sequence. Occasionally active lip exercises are prescribed to improve lip tone when it does not improve with usual daily activity. Since surgery usually exposes the mental nerve, patients have a sensory deficit in their lower lip following surgery. Sensation generally returns in 3 to 6 months, more rapidly than with sagittal split osteotomy. If ramus surgery which exposes the neurovascular bundle is performed with inferior border osteotomy, return of sensation may exceed 6 months.

Complications

Provided care is taken with the initial soft-tissue dissection and subsequent bony cuts, minimal complications accompany this procedure. Because dead space almost always is created after segments are repositioned, wound dehiscence is more likely with this procedure than with other orthognathic surgery procedures. If dehiscence occurs, meticulous wound care with frequent irrigations to prevent accumulation of food debris allows wound closure by secondary intention. Occasionally orthodontic tooth movement and the incision for inferior border osteotomy lead to a loss of keratinized tissue and periodontal defects over mandibular anterior teeth. The problem should be evaluated by a periodontist as soon as it is recognized. In most cases the situation can be corrected with a periodontal surgical procedure.

Rigid fixation techniques have lessened the possibility of shifting of repositioned inferior border segments following surgery, not an uncommon complication formerly, especially when the lingual cortical plate of an advanced segment was wired to the facial cortical plate of the intact mandible. Wire sutures alone did not prevent muscle tension from tipping the advanced segment inferiorly, reducing the amount of projection and causing vertical lengthening. When fixation is found to be inadequate, reoperation may be necessary to correct the problem.

Anterior Subapical Osteotomy

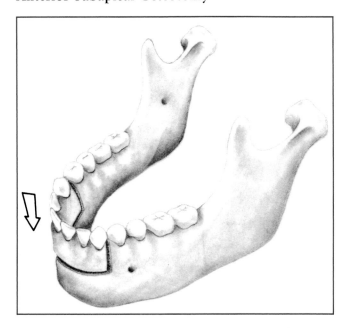

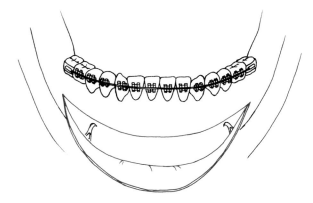

Fig. 10-41. Mucosal incision and dissection exposing anterior mandible without tooth removal.

Anterior subapical osteotomy in the mandible commonly has been used to close anterior open bite, to depress an elevated anterior dentoalveolar segment, or to retrude or advance a dentoalveolar segment.[5,6] The procedure often is combined with anterior maxillary subapical osteotomy for correction of bimaxillary protrusion. If the segment to be repositioned involves the premolar teeth, the mandibular neurovascular bundle is decompressed to a point proximal to the planned vertical component of the osteotomy. When the segment is to be repositioned posteriorly, a tooth usually is removed for space or space is created during the presurgical orthodontics.

Soft-Tissue Dissection

Two basic designs for incisions and mucosal flaps are used for access. Before the incision the facial mucosa is infiltrated with a vasoconstrictor (usually 2% lidocaine with 1:100,000 epinephrine). When it is not necessary to remove a tooth (space was created orthodontically), a vestibular incision is made, beginning in the first or second molar area and carried around to the opposite side. The incision is similar to the incision used for decompression of the neurovascular bundle, described previously. The facial mucoperiosteum over the osteotomy site in the alveolus can be lifted to the crest of the alveolus, allowing access for reflection of the mucoperiosteum and placement of an instrument for protection of lingual tissue. The dentoalveolar segment can be repositioned in a posterior, superior, or inferior direction with this surgical incision (Fig. 10-41). If a tooth must be removed for space to carry out the osteotomy or if the dentoalveolar segment is to be advanced, then a mucoperiosteal flap which includes a "finger flap" to the gingival margins must be utilized. The vestibular incision begins in the first or second molar region, extends up to the gingival margin at least one tooth away from the planned osteotomy site, con-

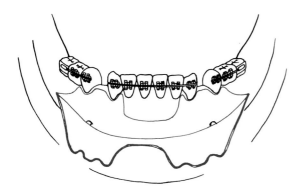

Fig. 10-42. Mucosal incision and dissection when a tooth is to be removed or the dentoalveolar segment advanced.

tinues around the gingival margins of the teeth, then extends into the vestibule to reproduce the same incision design on the opposite side. Mucoperiosteal flap reflections and the lingual subperiosteal dissection to protect the lingual mouth floor structures are carried out as previously described (Fig. 10-42).

If the vertical line of the osteotomy is anterior to the mental foramen, the neurovascular bundle need not be removed from the mandibular canal. If the vertical component of the osteotomy is proximal to the mental foramen and there is insufficient distance between the root apices and the neurovascular bundle for the bony cut, the bundle is removed from its canal and protected as has been described. The mucoperiosteal flap usually is reflected to the inferior border of the mandible to provide best visualization and access.

Osteotomy/Ostectomy

Using a bur or a reciprocating saw, a vertical osteotomy is carried through the alveolus bilaterally. A horizontal osteotomy 4 mm below the root apices connects the vertical osteotomy sites. A small oscillating saw can be used for this procedure, but a reciprocating saw with a blade long enough to cut through the entire width of the mandible is preferred. Once the dentoalveolar segment has been freed, it remains pedicled to the lingual mucosa and a portion of the genioglossus and geniohyoid musculature. The dentoalveolar segment then can be lowered by removing a measured amount of bone from the base of the mandible, retruded by removing the bone in the vertical component of the osteotomy, or elevated, leaving a defect beneath the segment. If the segment is to be advanced, the lingual mucoperiosteal reflection must be extended posteriorly through the molar area to allow the soft tissues to stretch with the repositioned segment. Occasionally an additional vertical release incision in the mucosa behind the second molar is needed.

Stabilization and Fixation Methods

After the segment is repositioned, maxillomandibular fixation is established in the planned occlusion with the aid of an occlusal wafer splint. A stabilizing arch wire is added, secured in tubes on molar bands. Osteotomy sites are inspected to confirm that segments are in the planned position. Segments may be secured with transosseous wires or stabilized by RIF utilizing semirigid bone plates and/or lag or position screws (Fig. 10-43, *A* through *D*). If the dentoalveolar segment has been repositioned superiorly to correct an anterior open bite, an autogenous or allogeneic bone graft is wedged between the repositioned segment and intact mandible. If the dentoalveolar segment has been advanced, bone is grafted into the vertical alveolar defects. As has been discussed for inferior border osteotomy, rigid fixation is an asset when bone grafts are planned because the stability of the segments is assured before bone grafts are placed. When RIF is used, maxillomandibular fixation is released and the stability and position of the segment are confirmed.

If a vestibular incision alone was used for access, closure is accomplished with a running horizontal mattress suture in the mucosa after reapproximating muscle layers. If any doubt exists as to the integrity of wound closure, a second running over and over suture is placed. Wound closure may be a problem when the dentoalveolar segment is repositioned in a superior and/or forward direction. In such cases a nonresorbable monofilament suture is used for the primary wound closure, followed by an oversew with a resorbable 4-0 chronic suture. If the incision and flap design include vertical incisions to gingival margins, closure over the edentulous portion of the alveolus is accomplished first with careful readaptation of the gingival papillae with sutures running from the facial to the lingual aspect. The remainder of the wound is closed as described previously. An external pressure dressing (e.g., elastic velcro type) is placed to support the wound and covering soft tissues for a minimum of 5 days.

Postsurgery Sequelae

Edema can be minimal with anterior mandibular subapical osteotomy, usually less than with inferior border osteotomy. The patient will have a sensory deficit in the gingiva, lower lip mucosa, and anterior teeth. The sensory deficit in the lower lip is proportional to the amount of manipulation of the mental nerve required by the procedure. Because the incisive nerve branches are severed, sensory deficit in the teeth and gingiva may take 6 to 12 months to recover. Teeth in the repositioned dentoalveolar segment usually retain their vitality. Teeth adjacent to vertical osteotomy cuts are at greatest risk for damage.

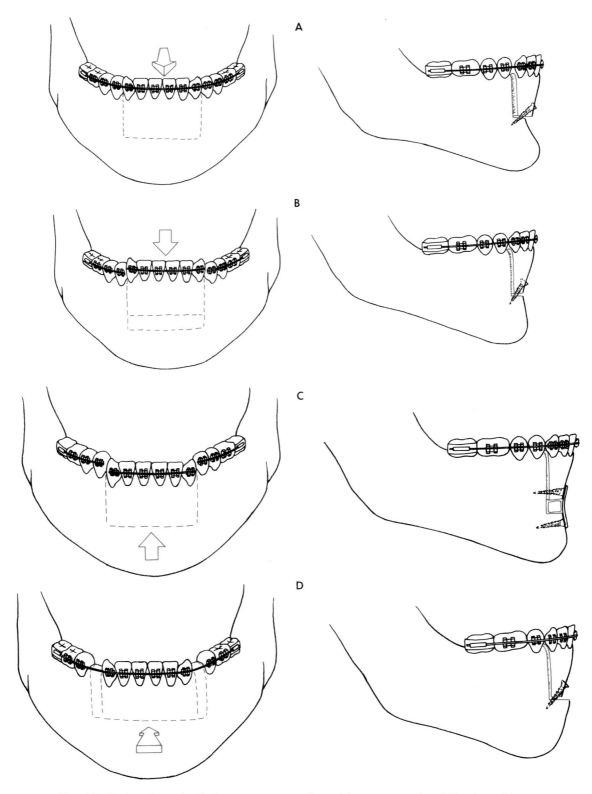

Fig. 10-43. Anterior subapical osteotomy—outline of bone cuts and stabilization of bony segments. **A,** Segment positioned anteriorly. **B,** Segment positioned inferiorly. **C,** Segment positioned superiorly. **D,** Segment positioned posteriorly.

When RIF is used the patient may resume jaw function immediately following surgery but should be cautioned to remain on a soft diet for 4 weeks. If transosseous wires are combined with a well adapted auxiliary orthodontic arch wire, the stability of the segment may be sufficient to allow some immediate function with restrictions to a liquid or soft diet. If the segment is not stable, a minimum of 4 weeks of maxillomandibular fixation is necessary before jaw function can begin.

Complications

With meticulous soft-tissue dissection, controlled osteotomy cuts, and careful management of the mobilized dentoalveolar segment, complications with the procedure are few. As with any segmental osteotomy, maintaining a vascular pedicle for perfusion is mandatory. Ordinarily this is not a problem with the anterior mandibular subapical procedure since the vascular pedicle contains the attachments of the genioglossus and geniohyoid musculature. Neurosensory deficits may be prolonged if trauma to the mental nerves was extensive. Good planning and execution of osteotomy cuts and protection of these neural structures during surgery should minimize the neurosensory problems.

Total Subapical Osteotomy

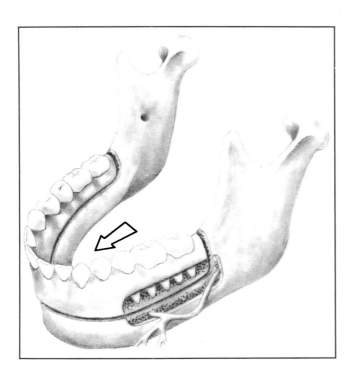

Total subapical osteotomy involving the total mandibular alveolus allows correction of mandibular dentoalveolar abnormalities in a manner similar to correction of maxillary problems via the LeFort I osteotomy. The major technical problems with the subapical os-

teotomy in the posterior mandible are management of the neurovascular bundle and potential for prolonged neurosensory disturbances.[15-22,24] When the neurovascular bundle is decompressed and retracted, as has been described earlier in the chapter, these hazards are greatly reduced or eliminated. The total mandibular subapical osteotomy can be used to shift the entire dentoalveolar segment anteriorly or posteriorly or to elevate it. If necessary the alveolus can be separated into several segments to accommodate a new occlusal relationship. The total subapical procedure is indicated when the deformity is confined to the dentoalveolar aspect of the mandible rather than involving the entire mandible, for example, a patient with a Class II type malocclusion and deep bite, but a satisfactory chin position (vertical as well as horizontal) and an overall length of the body of the mandible compatible with maxillary length. Anterior open bite from the terminal molars forward with an appropriate mandibular skeletal length can be corrected well with the total subapical procedure. Adequate bone must exist beneath the posterior alveolus to perform the procedure. For best results at least 10 mm of bone should be present between the inferior border of the mandible and the apices of posterior teeth.

Soft-Tissue Dissection

The first step in the total subapical osteotomy in the mandible is to expose the neurovascular bundle, as discussed previously in this chapter. If there is insufficient room between the neurovascular bundle and the root apices for the planned osteotomy (i.e., <4 mm), then the neurovascular bundle is removed from the canal to a point proximal to the planned vertical component of the osteotomy in the alveolus. Usually removal of the neurovascular bundle from the canal is necessary to provide room for the osteotomy and to assure preservation of the neurovascular bundle. Following retraction of the mandibular neurovascular bundle, the lingual mucoperiosteum is reflected from the medial surface of the mandible over the site of the planned vertical component of the osteotomy through the alveolus.

Osteotomy/Ostectomy

In a total subapical procedure the osteotomy is begun in a sagittal direction behind the most posterior tooth, using a small reciprocating saw or a micro-oscillating saw after protecting the lingual tissues and other mouth floor structures with an instrument beneath the periosteum. This tangential osteotomy cut extends from the alveolar crest posterior into the residual mandibular canal. By directing this cut tangentially, the lingual aspect of the osteotomy is well behind the terminal molar and the facial portion is just anterior to the exposed neurovascular bundle remaining in the residual canal. The mandibular canal is used as a reference

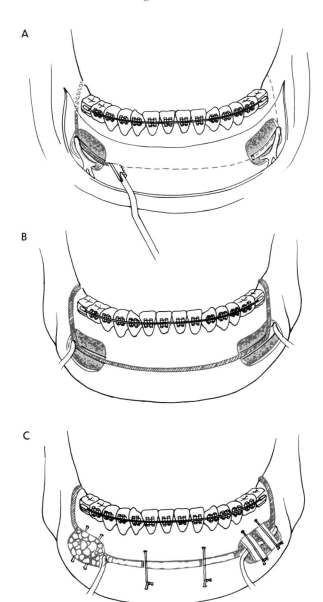

Fig. 10-44. **A,** Osteotomy with reciprocating saw after neurovascular bundle decompression. **B,** Repositioned dentoalveolar segment. **C,** Wire fixation and bone grafts; left side stabilizing bone struts and right side particulate bone graft overpacking.

for the subapical cut made with a reciprocating saw and carried beneath the posterior teeth and at the same level through the symphysis. A similar osteotomy is repeated on the opposite side (Fig. 10-44, *A*). At this point the dentoalveolar segment should be free. If the segment is not free, residual bone may be bridging in the proximal areas of the vertical cut through the superior portion of the alveolus or in the symphysis region where the bone is the thickest. Usually gentle prying in the osteotomy cut with an osteotome will reveal whether the bony connections require additional use of

the saw or whether the bone can be freed with osteotomes or fractured by wedging. If the alveolus is to be segmented, additional vertical bone cuts are made in the spaces created during presurgical orthodontics or by tooth removal.

Stabilization and Fixation Methods

Once the dentoalveolar segment has been freed, occlusion is established with maxillomandibular fixation aided by an occlusal wafer splint. The usual repositioning of the freed segment will be superiorly and anteriorly. If the segment is to be repositioned in a posterior direction or depressed, then bone must be removed. The remaining intact mandible is inspected, and the areas of bone contact with the mobilized and repositioned dentoalveolar segment are noted. Care must be taken to prevent condylar distraction as segments are repositioned. Formerly stabilization was achieved by direct transosseous wires extending through the facial plate of the dentoalveolar and inferior mandibular segments with intervening struts of cortical bone bridged between them. Stabilization with wires was a final step after the neurovascular bundles had been replaced into the body of the mandible. Particulate autogenous or allogeneic bone was placed to cover any residual lingual defects before repositioning of the neurovascular bundle. Patients were kept in maxillomandibular fixation for 4 to 6 weeks. This method is illustrated in associated figures (Fig. 10-44, *B* and *C*).

Today RIF is used for stabilizing the repositioned segments. Usually one or two semirigid bone plates are placed in the body regions and one or two bone plates or lag screws in the symphysis. Defects on the lingual side of the mandible are grafted and the neurovascular bundle is repositioned before the bone plates are secured. Bicortical screws secure the plates in the inferior border area, and monocortical screws are placed in the dentoalveolar portion of the repositioned segments. If possible, interdental spaces or edentulous areas should be chosen for placement of screws to prevent damage to tooth roots. After rigid fixation has been applied, additional bone is placed in residual defects on the lateral surface of the mandible (Fig. 10-45). Following placement of RIF, maxillomandibular fixation is released and the planned occlusion and mandibular position verified. If there is a discrepancy in the occlusion, then the rigid fixation must be removed, adjustments made, fixation reapplied, and the occlusion checked again. Facial muscles in the anterior mandible are reapproximated with 3-0 or 4-0 chromic gut suture. Mucosal wound closure is accomplished with a running horizontal mattress suture carried to the midline with a similar suture repeated on the opposite side. Following placement of the horizontal mattress suture, the wound is carefully inspected for any open areas. If several areas of the wound are open, an oversew resorbable su-

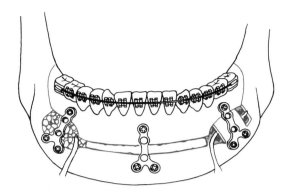

Fig. 10-45. Total subapical osteotomy; dentoalveolar segment stabilized with small bone plates to cover the neurovascular bundle after it is repositioned.

ture is placed over the entire wound. If one or two areas are open, interrupted sutures are placed to provide tight closure. An external pressure dressing, an elastic-velcro type, is placed and maintained for a minimum of 5 days.

Postsurgery Sequelae

Edema can be considerable following total subapical osteotomy, but the bulk of the edema should resolve in 2 weeks. Often lip position is altered and lip posture may continue to change for 3 to 6 months as the lips adapt to a new jaw position. Neurosensory change always is present following total subapical osteotomy. Recovery may take 6 to 12 months. Recovery of sensation usually is more rapid and complete than with sagittal split osteotomy. If RIF has been used to secure dentoalveolar segments, the patient is allowed to function into the occlusal splint with guiding elastics. The patient must stay on a liquid or soft diet for 4 to 6 weeks.

Stability following total subapical osteotomy has been excellent in the series of patients from our institution. Though not used frequently, the procedure has allowed correction of some dentoalveolar deformities which could not be corrected otherwise.

Complications

Complications are few with total subapical osteotomy. Disruption of the neurovascular bundle and long-term sensory disturbances are always possible. Preliminary data from our institution indicate that this risk is greater with sagittal split osteotomy.[19] Maintaining a vascularized pedicle to mobilized dentoalveolar segments is paramount. In this procedure, the attached lingual mucosa and musculature, which usually includes the mylohyoid as well as the genioglossus and a portion of the geniohyoid anteriorly, provide good perfusion of the denotalveolar segments.

Posteror Subapical Osteotomy

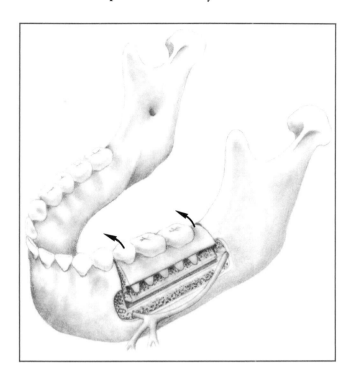

Subapical osteotomy in the posterior portion of the mandible is performed to shift the dentoalveolar segment(s) in multiple directions: medial or lateral, superior or inferior, anterior or posterior, or a combination of movements. Most often the procedure is performed to correct a problem that exists only on one side of the mandible. Once the vertical osteotomy sites are identified in the planning stages, the presurgical orthodontic preparation must include flaring of the roots of the teeth adjacent to the vertical osteotomy sites if an edentulous space does not exist, or the plan must include tooth removal.

Soft-Tissue Dissection

Before making the incision, the mucosa is infiltrated with a vasoconstrictor (usually 2% lidocaine with 1:100,000 epinephrine). To gain access for the osteotomy, the neurovascular bundle is managed as described earlier in this chapter. However, the incision-and-flap design is slightly different in that the incision extends to the gingival crest with a "finger flap" at least one tooth behind and in front of the planned vertical bony cuts through the alveolar segment (Fig. 10-46). Removal of the neurovascular bundle from its bony canal usually is required if insufficient space for osteotomy cuts (i.e., <4 mm) exists below root apices.

Osteotomy/Ostectomy

After the neurovascular bundle is retracted laterally, the lingual tissues opposite the terminal molar tooth

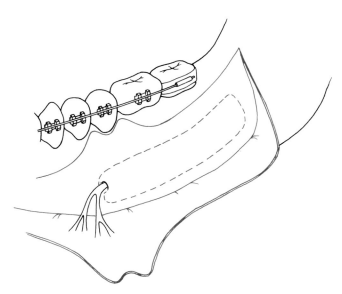

Fig. 10-46. Posterior subapical osteotomy; mucoperiosteal flap retracted and cortical bone cuts outlined for neurovascular bundle exposure.

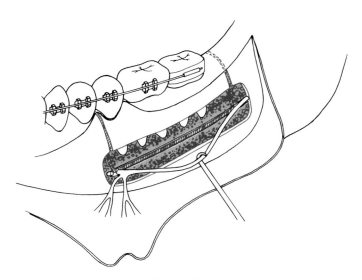

Fig. 10-47. Neurovascular bundle retracted, osteotomy completed.

are reflected from the medial side of the mandible and protected with an instrument during the vertical sectioning of the alveolus with the saw or rotary instrument, as previously described for total subapical osteotomy. The bony cut then continues horizontally through the residual canal (or between the neurovascular bundle or the root apices if there is sufficient room) to a point opposite the verical anterior component of the osteotomy. Once again the mucosa is reflected from the lingual side of the mandible opposite the anterior vertical osteotomy site and protected with an instrument while that bony cut through the alveolus is completed (Fig. 10-47). After the segment has been freed, it is repositioned as planned. If inferior movements must

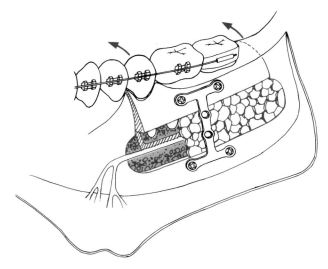

Fig. 10-48. Posterior dentoalveolar segment repositioned, neurovascular bundle replaced, interposed bone graft and stabilization with small bone plate.

be made, interfering bone is removed from the inferior aspect of the mandible. With anterior or posterior movement of the dentoalveolar segment, interdental bone in the alveolus must be carefully removed.

Stabilization and Fixation Methods

With the segment carefully positioned into the occlusal splint, maxillomandibular fixation is applied. A preformed auxiliary arch wire secured to tubes on molar bands may be added to improve stability if more than one dentoalveolar segment exists. Special care is taken to see that the segment(s) are exactly positioned into the occlusal splint. Bone grafts are placed in any defects remaining on the lingual aspect of the mandible before replacement of the neurovascular bundle. Grafts of particulate bone usually available from the removed cortical plate are placed over the neurovascular bundle occluding the bony defect. Additional autogenous bone or allogeneic bone also may be added. Fixation is achieved with either wire osteosynthesis or, preferably, with semirigid bone plates. A double T-plate, which allows two screws in the inferior border and two in the repositioned dentoalveolar segment, provides excellent stabilization (Fig. 10-48). A lingual acrylic splint which was made on dental casts following model surgery can be used for additional stabilization, but usually this is not required. The incisions are closed as described previously.

Postsurgery Sequelae

Edema ordinarily is minimal with an isolated posterior subapical osteotomy, but if access is difficult the lips may be abraded more than with other procedures. Edema should resolve rapidly, the bulk of it in 10 days following surgery. With adequate rigid fixation or special splint modifications, the patient may function just after surgery. If maxillomandibular fixation must be maintained, 4 weeks usually is sufficient to allow early bony healing. The patient should not begin mastication earlier than 4 weeks after surgery.

Complications

The isolated posterior subapical osteotomy can be a complex surgical procedure. With small dentoalveolar segments, maintaining the soft-tissue pedicle and the blood supply to the segment may be difficult. The dentoalveolar segment is pedicled from the lingual mucosa and a portion of the mylohyoid muscle. Great care must be taken in manipulating the segment so that these tissue attachments are not disrupted.

Since the blood supply may be easier to interrupt in an isolated posterior subapical osteotomy, a greater chance of segment devitalization exists. In our series loss of the segment has not occurred. Teeth may not respond to stimulation for 6 to 12 months following surgery. Teeth adjacent to vertical osteotomy cuts are at greatest risk of injury. Great care must be taken in planning for the repositioning of the dentoalveolar segments to prevent periodontal defects at the vertical osteotomy sites. Both the occlusal surfaces of the teeth and the height of the alveolar bone must be aligned to minimize periodontal defects.

Other postsurgical complications of this procedure are related to the neurovascular bundle decompression. With isolated posterior subapical osteotomy, surgical access can be more difficult than with a total subapical procedure. In our series the patients have had good sensory return 6 months following surgery, and sensory disturbances following the procedure are less than with sagittal split osteotomy.

AUGMENTATION WITH IMPLANTS

Bony defects or deficiencies in the maxilla or mandible may occur as part of a congenital or developmental problem or result from loss of bone substance due to trauma or as a complication of surgery. Bony defects are often expressed in the facial contours. An associated malocclusion may or may not be present.

In the maxilla contour deficiencies are seen commonly in the paranasal, infraorbital, and (malar) zygomatic (cheek bone) prominence areas. Onlay augmentation in these anatomic regions can significantly enhance soft-tissue contours and improve facial balance and function. When the maxilla is being repositioned via a LeFort I osteotomy, bony contour deficiencies may not be corrected entirely, and additional onlay augmentation is required for an optimum esthetic result. Onlay augmentation may preclude more extensive LeFort surgery.

Mandibular contour defects and deficiencies commonly involve the inferior border from the angle

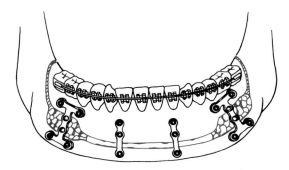

Fig. 10-49. After a total subapical osteotomy, insufficient bone exists (<10 mm) to allow an inferior border osteotomy for advancement without possible complications of mandibular fracture.

through the symphysis. Ramus involvement may occur (e.g., in hemifacial microsomia). In such circumstances a related soft-tissue deficiency often exists and correction may require more than bony augmentation. Defects sometimes follow mandibular orthognathic surgical procedures (e.g., in the posteroinferior border following a sagittal split osteotomy for advancement). If the split in the body region includes a good portion of the lingual plate in the proximal ramus segment, there may be inadequate soft-tissue support after the distal tooth-bearing segment is advanced, causing a notching deformity in the soft tissue overlying the area just anterior to the angle of the mandible. If a significant defect is recognized at surgery, immediate placement of a graft in the defect(s) can correct the problem. Secondary correction also is possible. Superior rotation of the proximal condylar segment with loss of prominence of the angle of the mandible is a complication of sagittal split osteotomy resulting from inadequate fixation at the osteotomy site. Obviously the malposition of the proximal segment should be corrected at surgery if recognized. But most often the rotation occurs in the first few weeks after surgery and subsequent surgery must correct the problem.

A similar complication can result in the inferior border of the mandible following an advancement. If the proximal portion of the osteotomy is not gently tapered into the body, as has been discussed earlier in this chapter, a notch is created, which may be reflected in the overlying tissue, especially in thin individuals. Carefully executed bony cuts to prevent this complication or immediate grafting at surgery is preferable to secondary correction. In selected patients in whom an inferior border osteotomy is not practical, an onlay augmentation may be considered to lengthen the mandible (e.g., when advancement is required along with a mandibular subapical procedure, there may be insufficient bone to maintain an intact mandible). Rather than causing a fracture or mandibular continuity defect, onlay augmentation should be considered (Fig. 10-49). The following discussion addresses the com-

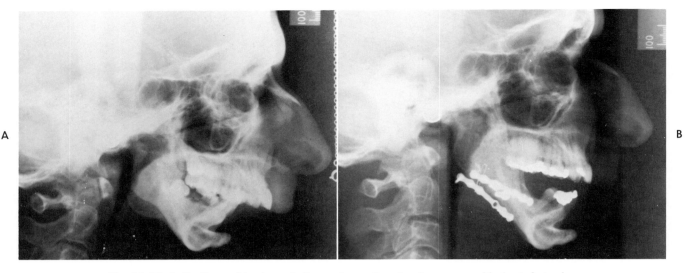

Fig. 10-50. **A,** Radiographic view of allogeneic cartilage implant to mandibular inferior border for camouflage correction of extreme mandibular AP deficiency, 35 years after placement. Note radiographic density suggesting calcification. **B,** Postmandibular advancement, extraoral sagittal ramus osteotomy (see Chapter 9 for details of the surgical technique).

mon problems identified in the maxilla and mandible; the same surgical principles apply to augmentation in other areas of the face.

Augmentation Materials

Materials used for contour augmentations include autogenous bone and cartilage, allogeneic bone and cartilage, and alloplasts. Alloplastic materials include Silastic, Proplast, and hydroxylapatite.[25] All implant materials have their limitations. Bone, autogenous and allogeneic, undergoes differing rates and degrees of resorption with unpredictable effects on contours of the covering soft tissues. Alloplasts may cause underlying bone resorption and migrate from the site of implantation. Usually alloplastic implants must be removed if they become infected. Autogenous or allogeneic cartilage appears to be most resistant to resorption, migration, and infection.[26,27] Cartilage appears to calcify over a long period of time without substantial change in shape (Fig. 10-50). Recent evidence indicates that calvarial bone may be more resistant to resorption than nonmembranous bone (e.g., iliac crest donor site).[28]

Paranasal Augmentation

Paranasal augmentation improves the soft-tissue support in the lateral and inferior aspects of the alar bases. Allogeneic cartilage is an excellent material for this use. A secondary donor site surgery is not required, the cartilage is resistant to resorption, and the material can be carved and shaped to the desired contour and heals firmly against underlying bone. Infection has not been as much of a problem with the cartilage as compared

to alloplasts. As the overlying tissues in this area are thin, almost a 1:1 ratio of implant size to soft-tissue change can be attained. Although clinical examination, photographs, facial moulages, and soft-tissue prediction tracings may help in determining the desired shape of the implant, the surgeon must use experience and clinical judgment in contouring the implant at surgery; the complexity of the decision can be compounded by the fact that LeFort I osteotomy is accomplished at the same time.

When a graft can be carved and shaped as a one-piece implant and placed in a carefully prepared subperiosteal pocket, it can be positioned and maintained only with the sutures used to close the vestibular incision. However, additional stabilization usually is necessary to lessen the chance of implant migration or displacement, which can occur with activity of facial muscles, edema, and/or a clot forming between the implant and bone. Displacement may not only affect the soft-tissue contour; an undesired asymmetry may result. One-piece implants can be stabilized easily with wire fixation or by placement of one or two small lag screws (Fig. 10-51).

When particulate implant material (e.g., autologous or allogeneic bone or hydroxylapatite) is used, a limited vestibular incision is made and the subperiosteal pocket carefully prepared only to the limits of the planned augmentation to contain the material within periosteum and prevent migration.[29] This approach allows limited augmentation especially in the areas lateral to the piriform rims and is not practical when LeFort I osteotomy is carried out at the same time. With a LeFort I osteotomy the contours in the lateral nasal

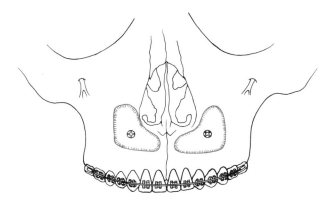

Fig. 10-51. Paranasal augmentations with carved autogenous or allogeneic bone, allogeneic cartilage, or alloplastic material; grafts fixed to underlying bone with lag screws.

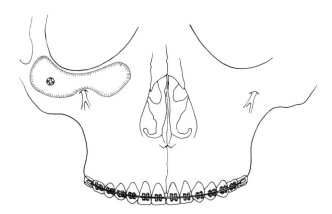

Fig. 10-52. Infraorbital-malar prominence augmented with carved autogenous or allogeneic bone, allogeneic cartilage, or alloplastic material; grafts secured with lag screws.

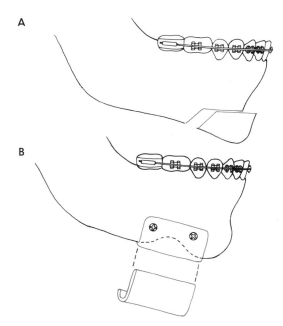

Fig. 10-53. **A,** Inferior border defect resulting from advancement of the mandibular inferior border where a step was created by the osteotomy design. **B,** Defect eliminated with autogenous bone, allogeneic cartilage, or an alloplast secured with lag screws.

areas are increased when the maxilla is advanced. Implants may be added for additional soft-tissue support.

Infraorbital Malar Augmentation

Properly contoured one-piece implant grafts are preferred for augmentation of the infraorbital malar region because the dissection needed to contain particulate material is not practical. A vestibular incision of sufficient length allows exposure of the infraorbital rim from the lateral nasal region to the malar eminence. The infraorbital nerve is carefully freed from overlying soft tissue for a short distance at its emergence from the foramen. The implant must be notched so that it fits around the infraorbital nerve without impingement. Once in place the implant can be secured with lag screws (Fig. 10-52). Wire fixation through the infraorbital rims also can be used, but wire placement can be difficult and requires more extensive soft-tissue dissection. Infraorbital zygomatic areas may be augmented along with a LeFort I osteotomy. Careful planning and

good clinical judgment at the time of surgery allow proper implant contour and placement. Use of particulate material is limited because containment of the material in the desired location is difficult.

Anteroinferior Mandibular Border Augmentation

Mandibular anteroinferior border defects are approached through a vestibular incision of sufficient length to allow access and clear visualization of the inferior border, taking care to protect the neurovascular bundle. The periosteum and other tissues attached to the inferior border in the area of the defect are dissected free. A J stripper or similar instrument is very useful in detaching tissue beneath the inferior border. Particulate material, autologous or allogeneic bone, alloplast (hyroxylapatite or Proplast) can be used for small defects. Containment of particulate material remains a problem. Properly contoured one-piece grafts provide more predictable results. When such implants are shaped to fit the defect at the inferior border, they become mechanically locked in place. If additional stabilization is required, lag screws can be placed through a percutaneous stab incision to secure the graft to the mandible. Access to the inferior border makes wire fixation difficult (Fig. 10-53, *A* and *B*).

Posteroinferior Mandibular Border Augmentation

Correction of a defect in the posterior mandible following a sagittal split osteotomy for advancement is

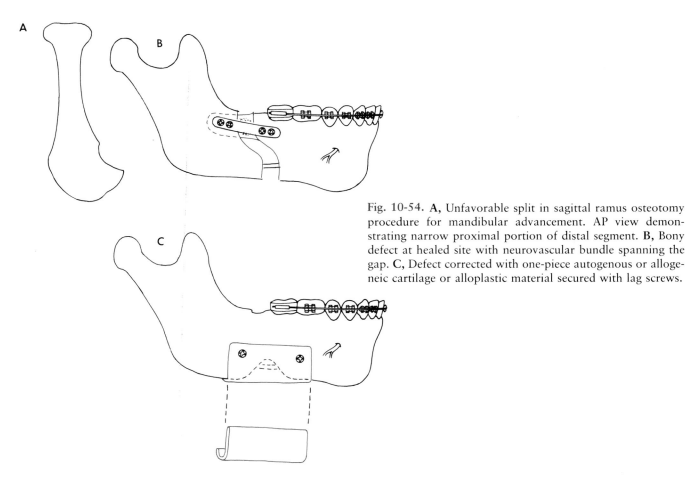

Fig. 10-54. **A,** Unfavorable split in sagittal ramus osteotomy procedure for mandibular advancement. AP view demonstrating narrow proximal portion of distal segment. **B,** Bony defect at healed site with neurovascular bundle spanning the gap. **C,** Defect corrected with one-piece autogenous or allogeneic cartilage or alloplastic material secured with lag screws.

usually managed through an incision in the scar from the previous surgery. Care must be taken in dissecting the tissues from the mandible and freeing the inferior border as the neurovascular bundle which crosses the defect may be attached to the covering tissues and is easily disrupted. Particulate graft material may be placed on the lateral surface of the mandible, but a properly contoured graft that bridges the defect and covers the inferior border for a short distance on either side provides the most predictable soft-tissue support (Fig. 10-54, *A* through *C*). Percutaneous placement of lag screws can fix the graft to the mandible if the graft is not mechanically locked in the defect.

The prominence of the angle of the mandible can be lost because of inadequate fixation and rotation of the proximal condylar segment following the sagittal split procedure. This is corrected most predictably with a cartilage graft. Some correction of a small, misshapen ramus can be gained with cartilage also. Because of muscle tension in this area, bone grafts tend to resorb and alloplastic material may cause underlying bone resorption. Particulate grafts are difficult to contain in the form required to provide the needed soft-tissue support. Following a soft-tissue incision as for a sagittal split procedure with more vestibular extension anteri-

orly for access, the subperiosteal dissection is carried to the inferior border. The soft tissue (masseter-medial pterygoid muscle sling) must be stripped completely free to allow the graft to fit around the inferior border. The graft is fitted to fill any obvious defect and provide the desired soft-tissue support. The muscular sling migrates superiorly after dissection in the area, and a loss of facial contour at the angle of the mandible follows. Bony resorption in the ramus also may occur. Overcontouring of the graft in this area is desirable. It is much easier to reduce the implant at a subsequent time than to add implant material. This implant is best stabilized with lag screws placed through a percutaneous approach (Fig. 10-55, *A* and *B*). Wire fixation is difficult at this site.

Anterolateral Mandibular Augmentation

Augmentation of the anterolateral surface of the mandible in the body or the chin region using bone grafts or alloplastic materials is possible though not indicated often. These areas are approached by the same incision and flap design as discussed for inferior border osteotomy procedures (see the discussion of inferior border osteotomy earlier in this chapter). Lateral placement of grafts will provide transverse augmentation of

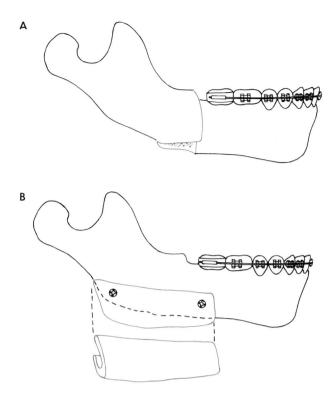

Fig. 10-55. **A,** Loss of mandibular angle prominence caused by superior rotation of proximal condylar segment following a sagittal ramus osteotomy. **B,** Defect corrected with implant of autogenous or allogeneic bone, allogeneic cartilage, or alloplastic material secured with lag screws.

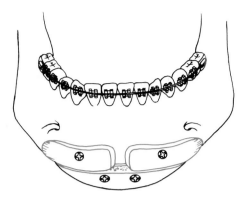

Fig. 10-56. Lateral onlay augmentation in conjunction with mandibular inferior border osteotomy. Graft secured with lag screws.

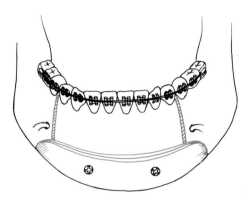

Fig. 10-57. Mandibular inferior border augmentation with laminated allogeneic cartilage slices secured to underlying bone with lag screws.

a narrow chin-parasymphysis area. Grafts used to onlay each side can be secured easily with bone screws usually placed via the transoral route (Fig. 10-56).

Chin Augmentation

Chin augmentation with an onlay graft is possible, but an inferior border osteotomy for mandibular advancement is preferred because it gives more predictable results. However, when chin augmentation is required along with a mandibular subapical osteotomy to preserve the continuity of the inferior mandible, augmentation with a graft is indicated, using any of the available materials. Allogeneic cartilage is easily contoured, can be laminated to provide the desired thickness, exhibits minimal resorption, unites with adjacent bone, and undergoes calcification with time (Fig. 10-57).[20] Autogenous and allogeneic bone grafts exhibit greater resorption when compared to cartilage but are satisfactory when combined with inferior border osteotomy. Alloplasts (Silastic, Proplast, or hydroxylapatite) can be satisfactorily placed but present an increased risk of infection and can cause underlying bone resorption. Shaped and fitted hydroxylapatite grafts may prove more satisfactory than other alloplasts.[24]

Infection following placement of alloplastic materials almost always dictates removal.

Hydroxylapatite plaster of Paris (HA-PP) implants may prove to be the alloplast of choice. As recently described for alveolar ridge augmentation, the HA-PP implant can be preformed and sterilized for implantation or can be custom formed at surgery from sterile materials. A major advantage of the HA-PP is that as the plaster is resorbed, HA particles become surrounded by fibrous connective tissue and the particles adjacent to bone become firmly fixed. The desired implant form is maintained and removal usually is not required if it becomes infected.[29]

Postsurgery Sequelae

Edema can be considerable following implant placement because dissection is extensive, particularly if surgical sites are entered for a second time. Most of the edema resolves within the first month after surgery, but residual edema may be present until the jaws and soft tissue return to full function, 6 months or longer. Patients seeking augmentation of contour defects are looking for immediate results and must be cautioned that soft-tissue contours may continue to change over many months.

Neurosensory deficits almost always follow implant placement if sensory nerves (e.g., infraorbital) are exposed in the dissection. Usually sensation returns in 6 months if the nerves were not disrupted. Long term sensory loss is possible and occurs in a small number of cases, but much less often than with sagittal split osteotomy.

Complications

Dehiscence of the incision is always possible following implant augmentation. Eliminating dead space with meticulous wound closure and proper placement of support dressings (e.g., elastic-velcro type) can minimize wound dehiscence. If dehiscence occurs with alloplasts, correcting the problem is difficult and loss of the implant may occur if the wound does not close by secondary intention. Once open the wound must be treated frequently with copious irrigation to keep it free of debris until wound closure follows.

Wound infection following implant placement can have more serious consequences. Infection following alloplast placement almost always means the implant must be removed. Copious irrigation of the wound may be tried for 7 to 10 days. If no progress toward resolution of the infection is seen, removal of the implant is the best course to take. Following healing, augmentation of the defect can be repeated. If the alloplastic implant has been in position for 8 to 12 weeks or longer, the soft-tissue contours may be maintained after implant removal and additional augmentation may not be necessary.

With careful planning and proper fixation of the implant at surgery, shifting or migration of the implant should be a rare complication. Particulate implants are difficult to contain as has been discussed, but they are not placed when proper soft-tissue dissection is not possible. Rigid fixation techniques (e.g., lag screws) can be used to great advantage to fix implants in place, usually with less technical difficulty than wire fixation.

At times, judging the correct contour of implants is difficult and the correction leads to soft tissue being overcontoured. At least 6 months of healing should be allowed following implant placement before additional surgery is considered. Edema often resolves slowly, and final tissue contour and form are not attained until the jaws and soft tissue return to full function. In most instances the implant can be recontoured with secondary surgery if that is required.

Long-term neurosensory disturbances are rare following implant placement if major sensory nerves (i.e., inferior alveolar, mental, lingual, infraorbital) are carefully preserved during dissection.

REFERENCES

1. Blair VP: Operations on jaw bones and face: study of aetiology and pathological anatomy of developmental malrelations of maxilla and mandible to each other and to facial outline and of operative treatment when beyond the scope of the orthodontist, Gynecol Obstet 4:67-78, 1907.
2. New GB, Erich JB: The surgical correction of mandibular prognathism, Am J Surg 53:2-12, 1941.
3. Dingman RO: Surgical correction of mandibular prognathism, an improved method, Am J Orthod Oral Surg 30:683-692, 1944.
4. Burch RJ, Bowden GW, Woodward HW: Intraoral one-stage ostectomy for correction of mandibular prognathism: report of case, J Oral Surg 19:72-76, 1961.
5. Kole H: Surgical operations on the alveolar ridge to correct occlusal abnormalities, Oral Surg 12:277-288, 1959.
6. Trauner R, Obwegeser M: The surgical correction of mandibular prognathism and retrognathia with consideration of genioplasty, Oral Surg Oral Med Oral Pathol 10:677-689, 787-792, 1957.
7. Cohn-Stock G: Die chirurgische Immediatre-gulierung der Kiefer, speziell die chirvrgische Behandlung der Prognathie, Vjschr Zahnheilk Berlin 37:320, 1921.
8. Murphey PJ, Walker RV: Correction of maxillary protrusion by ostectomy and orthodontic therapy, J Oral Surg 21:275-290, 1963.
9. Mohnac AM: Maxillary osteotomy in the management of occlusal deformities, J Oral Surg 24:305-317, 1966.
10. Wassmund J: Lehrbuch der praktischen chirurgie des Mundes und der Kiefer, vol 1, Leipzig, 1935, Meusser.
11. Wunderer S: Erfahrungen mit der operativen Behandlung hochgradiger Prognathien, Dtsch Zahn-Mund-Kiefer-heilk 39:451, 1963.
12. West RA, Epker BN: Posterior maxillary surgery: its place in the treatment of dentofacial deformities, J Oral Surg 30:562-575, 1972.
13. Bell WH, Turvey TA: Surgical correction of posterior crossbite, J Oral Surg 32:811-822, 1974.
14. Bell WH: Correction of maxillary excess by anterior maxillary osteotomy, Oral Surg Oral Med Oral Pathol 43:323-332, 1977.
15. MacIntosh RB: Total mandibular osteotomy—encouraging experiences with an infrequently indicated procedure, J Maxillofac Surg 2:210-218, 1974.
16. Booth DF, Dietz V, Gianelly AA: Correction of Class II malocclusion by combined sagittal ramus and subapical body osteotomy, J Oral Surg 34:630-634, 1976.
17. Kemper JW: Surgical correction of mandibular prognathism, J Oral Surg 5:29-32, 1947.
18. Fitzpatrick B: Total osteotomy of the mandibular alveolus in reconstruction of the occlusion, Oral Surg Oral Med Oral Pathol 44:336-346, 1977.
19. Terry BC, Gregg JM, Small EW: Neurosensory studies of trigeminal dysesthesia following accidental and iatrogenic injury. Abstract presented at the 4th Congress European Association for Maxillo-Facial Surgery, Venice, Italy, June, 1978.

20. Bell WH, Proffit WR, White RP: Surgical correction of dentofacial deformities, vol 1, Philadelphia, 1980, W.B. Saunders Co.
21. Piecuch JF, Tideman H: Correction of deep bite by total mandibular alveolar osteotomy: report of case, J Oral Surg 39:601-606, 1981.
22. Frost DE, Fonseca RJ, Koutnik AW: Total subapical osteotomy—a modification of the surgical technique, Int J Adult Orthod Orthognath Surg 2:119-128, 1986.
23. Obwegeser HL, Makek MS: Hemimandibular hyperplasia-hemimandibular elongation, J Maxillofac Surg 4:183-208, 1986.
24. Buckley MJ, Turvey TA: Total mandibular subapical osteotomy: a report on long-term stability and surgical technique, Int J Adult Orthod Orthognath Surg 3:121-130, 1987.
25. Moening JE, Wolford LM: Chin augmentation with various alloplastic materials: a comparative study, Int J Adult Orthod Orthognath Surg 4:175-187, 1989.
26. Dingman RO: Osteotomy for the correction of mandibular malrelation of developmental origin, J Oral Surg 2:239-259, 1944.
27. Sailer HF: Transplantation of lyophilized cartilage in maxillofacial surgery—experimental foundations and clinical success, Basel, Switzerland, 1983, S. Karger AG, Medical and Scientific Publishers.
28. Zins JE, Whitaker LA: Membranous vs endochondral bone: implications for craniofacial reconstruction, Plast Reconstr Surg 72:778-784, 1983.
29. Terry BC, Baker RD, Tucker MR, Hanker JS: Alveolar ridge augmentation with composite implants of hydroxylapatite and plaster for correction of bony defects, deficiencies and related contour abnormalities, Materials Res Soc Symp Proc 110:187-198, 1989.

CHAPTER 11

Combining Surgical Procedures in the Mandible and Maxilla

Raymond P. White, Jr.
Myron R. Tucker

HISTORICAL DEVELOPMENT

As intraoral surgical techniques were adopted by American surgeons in the 1960s, they began to work more closely with orthodontists to diagnose and treat problems in patients with dentofacial deformity. By the mid-1970s intraoral surgical procedures could correct skeletal problems in both the mandible and the maxilla. For the first time, the orthodontist and the surgeon could plan to treat dentofacial deformity where the problem existed. A maxillary skeletal deformity could be corrected by surgically aligning the maxilla, a mandibular deformity by surgery in the mandible. Initially surgical corrections of problems in both the maxilla and the mandible were performed as separate or staged procedures because of the complexity of presurgical planning, technical difficulty of the procedures, and time required to complete each procedure.[1] Then subapical orthognathic surgery in both jaws or mandibular ramus and maxillary subapical surgery were performed under the same anesthetic.[2-4]

As American surgeons became more adept at intraoral surgery and surgical instrumentation improved, LeFort I osteotomy and surgery in the ramus of the mandible were done in combination.[5-7] The need for very careful planning before surgery and the proper sequencing of two jaw procedures in the operating room became apparent. A series of papers by Turvey, Epker, LaBanc, Fish, and Hall summarized the experience of the 1970s and set the stage for frequent use of combined maxillary and mandibular orthognathic surgery procedures as we know them today.[8-11] This chapter focuses on the special planning required for two-jaw surgery and assumes the reader is familiar with the diagnostic and planning sequences suggested in Chapters 4 to 7, and the surgical procedures detailed in Chapters 8 to 10. Appropriate methods for stabilization and fixation, postsurgery sequelae, and complications of two-jaw surgery are discussed. Clinical applications of two-jaw surgery and a discussion of the decision to perform surgery in one or both jaws appear in almost every chapter in Section IV.

PLANNING FOR TWO-JAW SURGERY

The diagnostic process for a patient with dentofacial deformity may produce a problem list indicating a skeletal deformity in both the mandible and the maxilla. To correct the problems that exist in both jaws, the treatment plan may involve simultaneous two-jaw surgery. The decision to perform two-jaw surgery was discussed in the chapters in Section II. This section details the planning steps once the decision has been made. As has been discussed in detail in Chapter 5, the surgeon or the orthodontist must produce cephalometric prediction tracings as an initial step in planning treatment.

Once the presurgical orthodontics is complete, the surgeon must repeat the prediction tracings (Fig. 11-1).

Cephalometric Prediction

A maxillary template that includes the anterior nasal spine, palate and nasal floor, posterior nasal spine, and maxillary teeth is drawn. Anticipated orthodontic corrections of maxillary teeth must be incorporated into the maxillary template in the initial planning stages. Just before surgery, the orthodontic tooth movement is represented in the presurgical lateral cephalometric radiograph. The first step in producing the prediction tracing is to properly position the maxillary template, and the maxillary anterior teeth vertically and horizontally, to support the patient's upper lip. The proper angulation of the maxillary incisors must also be considered in this step. As a general guideline, point A should be ±2 mm from nasion perpendicular and the facial surface of the crown of the maxillary incisors should be approximately 4 mm anterior to a line drawn per-

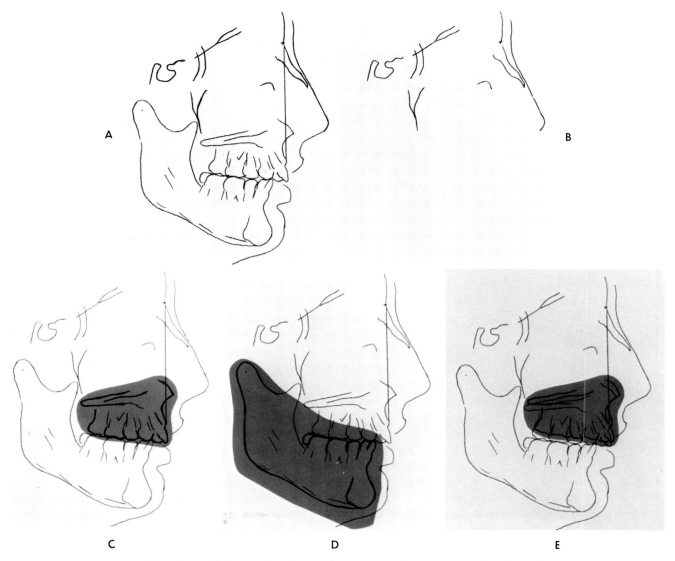

Fig. 11-1. Steps in prediction tracing for two-jaw surgery. **A,** Prepare a tracing from the presurgical lateral cephalometric radiograph. **B,** With a new sheet of tracing paper over the original tracing, trace the structures that will not be changed at surgery. **C** and **D,** Prepare maxillary and mandibular templates. Trace the occlusal surfaces of the teeth in both templates; the nasal floor, palate, and anterior and posterior nasal spines in the maxillary; and the ramus with the condyle, inferior border, and chin in the mandibular templates. **E,** Position the maxillary template over the first tracing to simulate proper support of the upper lip and esthetic exposure of the incisor teeth. *Continued.*

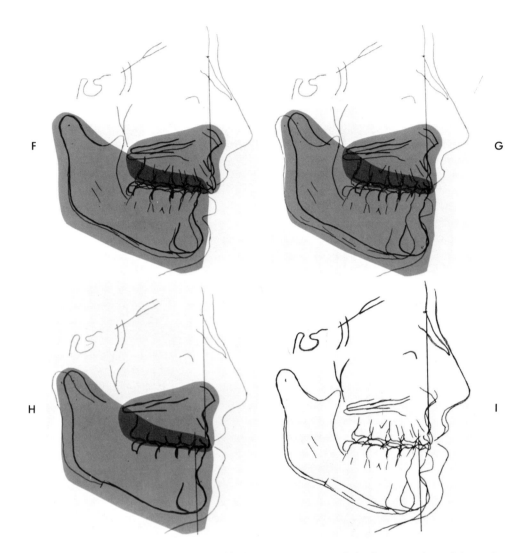

Fig. 11-1, cont'd. **F,** Rotate the mandibular template around the horizontal condylar axis. Note that the lower teeth are in a Class II occlusion with more overjet than is acceptable. Mandibular autorotation will not suffice and two-jaw surgery is indicated. **G,** Position the mandibular template to maximally occlude the teeth in a Class I occlusal relationship as indicated by the dental casts. **H,** Overlay the tracing as prepared in **B.** Trace the structures from the maxillary and mandibular templates. Add tracings of the lips and the soft tissue over the chin. Good balance exists between the mandibular incisors and pogonion. No inferior border osteotomy is needed. **I,** Superimpose the prediction tracing over the first tracing. Measure the change in position of the maxillary molars and anterior teeth. These measurements will dictate the movements of the casts in the model surgery (see Fig. 11-2). Remember that predictions based on a lateral cephalometric film only include AP and vertical movements. The transverse plane of space can be better assessed from the clinical exam, dental casts, and a PA cephalometric film. More detail on correcting transverse changes is available in Chapter 15.

pendicular through point A. A third to a half of the crown of the maxillary incisor should be exposed beneath the upper lip in its repose or rest position. Some judgment is required here. If the patient has a very active upper lip in facial animation, less of the incisor might be exposed with the lip at rest. However, not showing any incisor beneath the upper lip at rest is not esthetic. If the decision is difficult, more of the maxillary incisor should be exposed beneath the upper lip at rest than less. Once the maxillary template is in position, the mandibular template should be developed (with orthodontic correction simulated if in the initial planning stages) and positioned so that the maxillary and mandibular occlusal planes are aligned.

Autorotation of the mandible rather than mandibular ramus surgery is always a possibility with skeletal deformity in both jaws. The mandibular template should be rotated around the horizontal condylar axis to simulate such a movement. If the mandibular template can be rotated to an appropriate position, maxillary surgery only might be performed and mandibular surgery avoided. The maxillary template could be repositioned slightly in the anteroposterior plane to accommodate the rotated mandibular template. But remember that the position of the maxilla and support for the upper lip are primary, and surgery in two jaws is pre ferred to a compromise in the position of the maxilla. Discussion of the decision between surgery in one or two jaws is included in the clinical chapters in Section IV.

If two-jaw surgery is required, repositioning the mandibular template simulates mandibular surgery. Once the maxillary and mandibular templates are positioned appropriately, the need for mandibular inferior border surgery is assessed. If necessary, a template repositioning the mandibular inferior border is produced. As a general guide, the mandibular incisor tip should be about the same distance ahead of a vertical line through point B as pogonion. Variations in the morphology of the soft tissue of the chin may influence the decision as to the final position of pogonion. If the patient has considerable soft tissue over pogonion, the mandibular inferior border need not be advanced as much as in a patient with minimal soft tissue to achieve

the same result. Obviously, the clinical judgment of the surgeon and orthodontist and the patient's wishes take precedence over guidelines derived from cephalometric measurements. As a last step, the facial soft tissues are added to produce the final prediction tracing.

A computer software program also may be used to produce the final cephalometric prediction tracing. Remember that the sequence of jaw movement is the same with the computer method as is done manually. The prediction simulating the repositioning of the maxilla at surgery remains the most important step. Once the position of the maxilla is determined, the mandibular prediction is completed.

Cast Prediction

Cast prediction or model surgery is the next step in the planning sequence (Fig. 11-2). When both jaws are to be repositioned, the maxillary dental cast is mounted on a semiadjustable articulator with the aid of a facebow transfer from the patient. In the early planning stages, a mounting with a facebow is not mandatory. Just before surgery, the facebow mounting is required to allow the surgeon to make the most accurate measurements during model surgery to be used subsequently to reposition the jaws in the operating room. Next the mandibular dental cast is mounted with the aid of a bite registration taken with the patient's jaws in the retruded contact position or centric relation. With some patients this position can be difficult to establish. Patients with jaw deformity often posture their mandible forward to enable them to produce maximum dental interdigitation. Over a period of

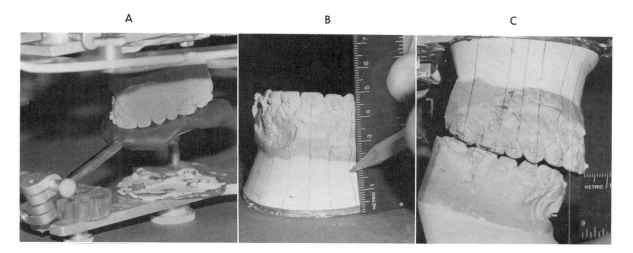

Fig. 11-2. The steps in model surgery for a patient who will have a total maxillary osteotomy and a mandibular advancement. **A,** The maxillary cast is mounted on a semiadjustable articulator, using a facebow transfer. **B,** Reference lines are drawn on the maxillary cast, and the distance from the mounting rim to each cusp is recorded. **C,** The distance from the articulator pin to the incisal edge of the maxillary central incisor also is measured and recorded. With the measurements, the magnitude of all maxillary movements can be evaluated precisely.   *Continued.*

D   E   F   G

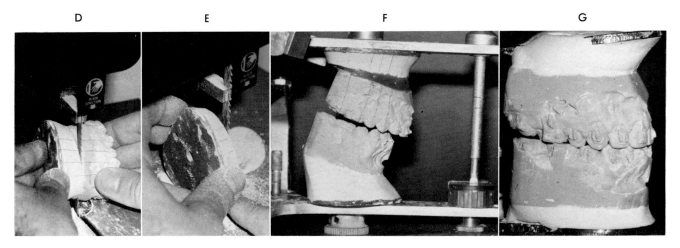

Fig. 11-2, cont'd. **D,** The maxillary cast is cut away from the mounting ring. **E,** An additional wedge of mounting material is cut away, giving room to reposition the maxillary cast vertically. **F,** The maxillary cast is remounted in the desired position, with the measurements checked against the cephalometric prediction for this patient. This is the projected result of the first stage of the surgery, and an intermediate splint is made to this mounting (after the upper cast is stabilized with plaster in its final position). **G,** The casts are mounted as they will be after the second stage of the surgery, the mandibular advancement. The second splint is made to this mounting. Note the position of the upper second molars, which were deliberately kept depressed during the orthodontic preparation so there would be no problems with second molar interferences at this stage.

years the patient may accommodate to this forward position of the jaws. The surgeon and the orthodontist may encounter difficulty repositioning the mandible posteriorly to find the appropriate retruded contact position. At times both the surgeon and the orthodontist accept a position that most closely approximates retruded contact position of the patient. This subject is discussed more thoroughly in Chapters 12, 13, and 14.

Model simulation of anticipated surgical movement is performed next. Before moving or sectioning of the mounted casts, several vertical reference lines and two horizontal reference lines should be drawn on the maxillary cast a measured distance apart. The distance between the facial surface of the maxillary incisors and the articulator pin is recorded. With these reference points the surgeon will be able to determine precisely the movement of the jaw segments after model surgery. The individual dental casts must be repositioned, duplicating the same movements of the jaws as depicted on the final prediction tracing. The sequence of movements is the same. The maxillary cast is repositioned first according to the measurements from the prediction tracing. Once the maxillary cast is fixed in the new position on the articulator, the mandibular cast is repositioned to oppose it in the planned occlusal relationship. The casts are then stabilized in the articulator with plaster.

In initial planning stages where significant tooth movement is planned before surgery, individual teeth should be positioned in the respective dental casts to simulate anticipated tooth movement (see Chapter 5, Fig. 5-32). But in planning just before surgery, the positions of individual teeth as depicted in the casts must be acceptable to both the surgeon and the orthodontist. If not, surgery must be postponed for further orthodontic preparation. Postponing surgery is often a better decision for the patient if the alternative is a protracted period of orthodontic finishing, that is, more than 6 months of orthodontics once the patient returns to the orthodontist following surgery. Additional discussion of this topic is found in Chapter 6.

The measured movement of the dental casts as repositioned in the articulator should be very close to the measurements obtained from the prediction tracing. A difference of a few millimeters is not critical in the early planning stages before orthodontic treatment. Just before surgery when the steps in prediction tracing and model surgery are repeated, there is no room for error. If any discrepancy exists between the prediction tracing and model surgery, the planning steps must be repeated until the reason for the error is detected. Errors undetected in planning usually cannot be corrected in the operating room and will be reflected in the positions of the jaws and teeth after surgery.

As has been mentioned, cephalometric prediction tracings and model surgery are performed during the planning stages for a patient before any treatment is begun. The same steps are repeated after the presurgical orthodontics and just before surgery to simulate jaw movements. But the presurgical model surgery has a second purpose, generating the occlusal wafer splints for use at surgery. When both jaws to are to be repositioned, the first stage or the intermediate occlusal wafer splint is generated after the maxillary cast is repositioned on the articulator (see Fig. 11-2). Then the mandibular cast is repositioned to oppose the maxillary cast simulating the final position of the jaws at surgery. This final position generates the final occlusal wafer splint for use at surgery and during the period of jaw rehabilitation following surgery. It is easier to use a second identical set of casts mounted in a hinge-type articulator for the final splint because the occlusal surfaces of the casts can be damaged in construction of the intermediate splint.

If the maxilla is to be repositioned in one piece at surgery, two separate splints (an intermediate splint and a final splint) to reposition first the maxilla and then the mandible are constructed. If the maxilla must be segmented at surgery, a combined, or two-stage, splint can be constructed. This technique involves construction of the final splint first (on a hinge articulator) followed by fabrication of the combined splint (Fig. 11-3).[12] This approach has the advantages of leaving the final occlusal wafer splint attached to the maxilla at surgery once the maxillary segments have been repositioned and stabilized.

The decision by the surgeon and the orthodontist to recommend two-jaw surgery to the patient requires clinical judgment. Just because two-jaw surgery will correct the patient's problem, it does not follow *a pri-* *ori* that two-jaw surgery should be done. All other alternatives should be considered. Simultaneous surgery in both jaws can be performed safely and practically. But additional surgical risks and greater potential for complications exist. The patient should realize significant benefit from two-jaw surgery over alternative plans for treatment involving only surgery in one jaw. Specific clinical indications for two-jaw surgery are discussed more thoroughly in most chapters in Section IV.

SEQUENCE OF JAW SURGERY

LeFort I osteotomy and bilateral sagittal split osteotomy are the most frequent operations performed in combination. With LeFort I osteotomy, the surgeon can move the maxilla in all three planes of space. Moving the maxilla in a posterior and superior direction is technically difficult but not impossible. The bilateral sagittal split osteotomy in the ramus of the mandible allows for alteration in mandibular length, vertical correction, and transverse movements for asymmetry correction. The sequence of jaw surgery for this combination evolved in the mid-1970s.[6-8] The soft-tissue incisions and the initial bony cuts are completed bilaterally for mandibular sagittal split osteotomy, delaying the separation of the tooth-bearing segment of the jaws from the proximal condylar segment. The wounds are packed with moist gauze and the LeFort I osteotomy completed. With an intermediate occlusal splint (or the combined two-stage splint) in place and the jaws held together in maxillomandibular fixation, the maxilla is repositioned and stabilized, usually with wire sutures in the piriform rim and zygomatic maxillary buttress

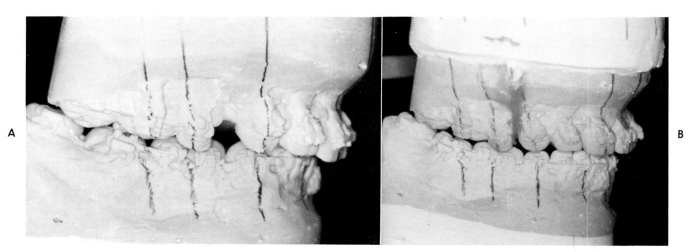

Fig. 11-3. The steps in construction of a combined two-stage splint for a patient who will have two-jaw surgery; a three-segment LeFort I osteotomy and a mandibular bilateral sagittal split osteotomy. **A,** The casts are mounted on a semiadjustable articulator with a face-bow transfer and reference lines are drawn on the casts. **B,** After cutting the upper cast from the mounting ring, the maxillary segments are repositioned as planned in occlusion with the lower cast and held with wax. Measurements are taken from the reference lines and checked against the cephalometric prediction tracing for this patient. *Continued.*

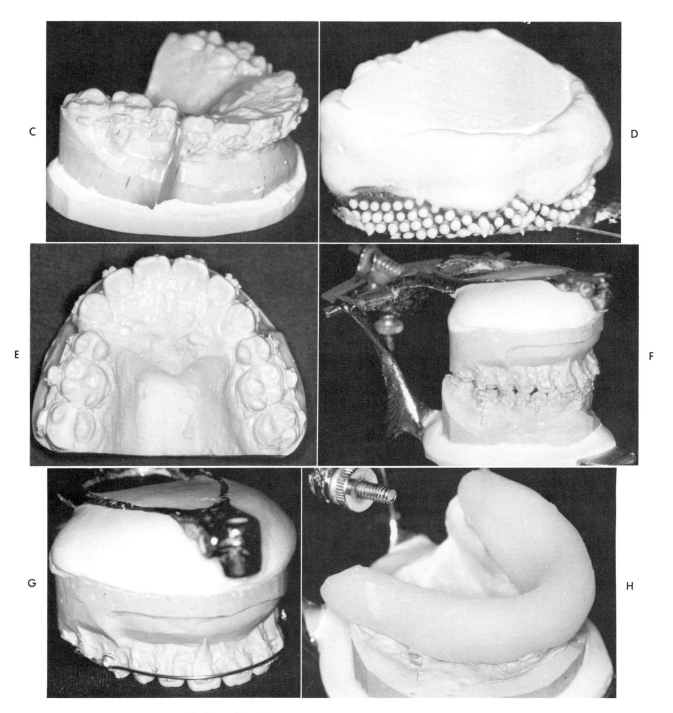

Fig. 11-3, cont'd. **C, D,** and **E,** The repositioned and segmented upper cast is reproduced by making an alginate impression and pouring new casts in dental stone, one for the final splint and one for the first-stage splint. **F,** To check position of the teeth and jaws and to construct the final splint for use at surgery, both upper and lower casts are mounted in a hinge-type articulator in the final position of the jaws at surgery. Space is left for the splint to intervene between teeth. Remember to keep the space between the casts at a minimum so the splint will be thin. **G,** The 40-mil maxillary auxiliary arch wire is constructed to lie passively against the facial surfaces of the teeth occlusal to the brackets. The wire will be secured in the headgear tubes in molar bands at surgery. The wire is constructed at this stage because the teeth are often damaged in the final steps of splint construction. **H** and **I,** After applying separating medium to the teeth, a roll of quick curing acrylic is adapted to the occlusal surface of one cast and the opposing cast is positioned into the soft acrylic by closing the articulator. Porosity in the splint can be minimized by allowing it to cure in a pressure cooker.

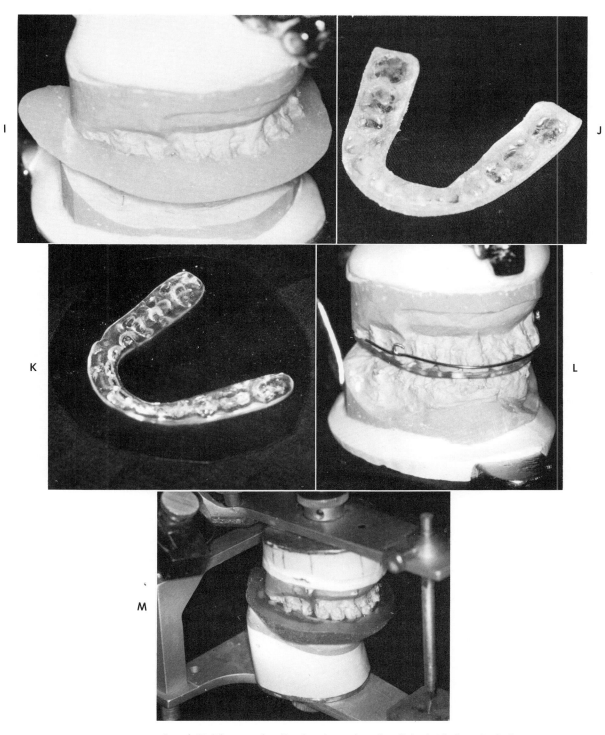

Fig. 11-3, cont'd. **J** and **K**, The cured splint is trimmed and polished. If plans include RIF and early function of the jaws, the undersurface of the final splint must be relieved so only indentions for mandibular cusp tips remain. Holes in the periphery of the splint are added at this point to enable the surgeon to tie the splint to the maxillary arch wire at surgery. Since the maxilla will be segmented, two holes adjacent to each maxillary segment are needed. Often the splint is not removed for 3 to 4 months following surgery, until healing is adequate to stabilize the multiple maxillary segments without the splint in place. **L**, The finished final splint with upper and lower casts occluded. **M**, The two-stage splint is constructed with the cast of the segmented maxilla repositioned in the semiadjustable articulator. The first stage of the combined splint is made with the final splint fixed to the segmented upper cast. If the first-stage splint can be made of a colored acrylic, this helps the surgeon see the interdigitations of the teeth and the two-stage splint in the operating room. *Continued.*

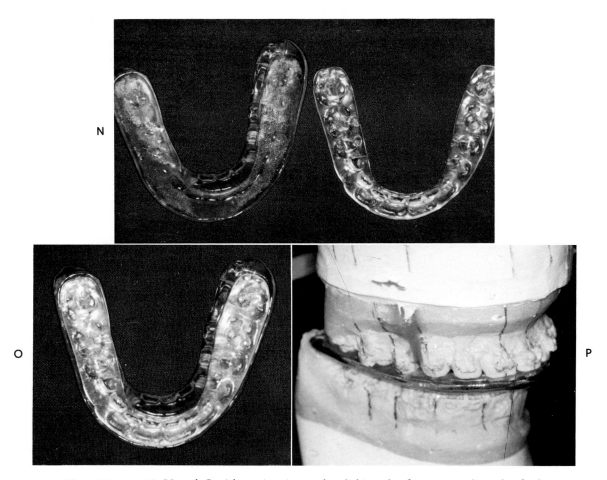

Fig. 11-3, cont'd. **N** and **O**, After trimming and polishing the first-stage splint, the final splint should interdigitate easily into the upper surface of the first-stage splint. **P**, Both splints together, the combined splint, with upper and lower casts occluded. This corresponds to the jaw position following LeFort I osteotomy, before completion of the sagittal split osteotomy. (**A** through **P** courtesy of Dr. Mark Ochs.)

areas. Fixation of the maxilla is completed with either skeletal stabilizing wires or semirigid bone plates (Fig. 11-4).

At this point, the maxillomandibular fixation is released. Sagittal split osteotomies are completed bilaterally in the mandible with osteotomes. The distal tooth-bearing segment of the mandible is repositioned using the final occlusal splint as a guide. With the patient's teeth again held firmly together in maxillomandibular fixation, the mandibular osteotomy sites are stabilized and fixed with either wire sutures, position or lag screws, or semirigid bone plates. See Chapters 8 and 9 for further details about the surgical technique and Chapter 7 for additional details about fixation and stabilization of the osteotomy sites and the return of the jaws to function in the postsurgery period.

Buckley and colleagues have suggested another sequence for two-jaw surgery.[13] The advent of RIF would allow the mandibular bilateral sagittal split osteotomies to be completed before LeFort I osteotomy. RIF with position or lag screws provides an intact, stable repositioned mandible. The intermediate splint in this instance uses the intact maxilla as the guide. With the mandible held in the new position with screws or bone plates, the final occlusal splint properly repositions the maxilla after LeFort I osteotomy. This alternative to staging in two-jaw surgery minimizes the chance of displacement of maxillary segments once they have been repositioned. Because LeFort I osteotomy is the last procedure performed, the chance of displacing maxillary segments while doing other procedures is minimized. This approach can be used to advantage when difficulty in stabilizing the maxilla after LeFort I osteotomy is anticipated, for example, in repeat LeFort I osteotomy when the maxilla must be moved forward and inferiorly with defects stabilized by bone grafts or alloplastic materials, or when a multisegment maxilla may not be stable enough to support

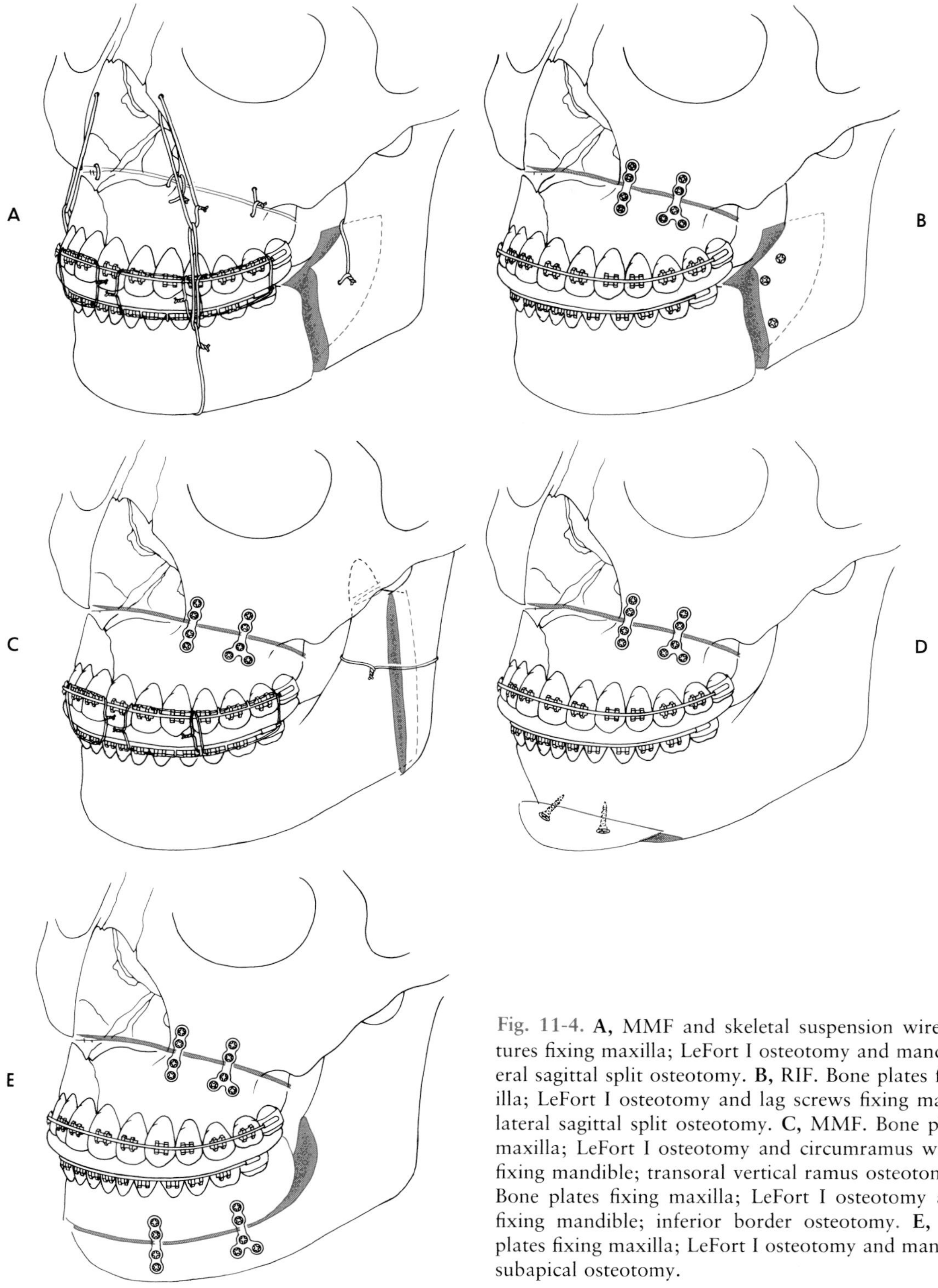

Fig. 11-4. **A,** MMF and skeletal suspension wires, wire sutures fixing maxilla; LeFort I osteotomy and mandible; bilateral sagittal split osteotomy. **B,** RIF. Bone plates fixing maxilla; LeFort I osteotomy and lag screws fixing mandible; bilateral sagittal split osteotomy. **C,** MMF. Bone plates fixing maxilla; LeFort I osteotomy and circumramus wire fixation fixing mandible; transoral vertical ramus osteotomy. **D,** RIF. Bone plates fixing maxilla; LeFort I osteotomy and screws fixing mandible; inferior border osteotomy. **E,** RIF. Bone plates fixing maxilla; LeFort I osteotomy and mandible; total subapical osteotomy.

the mandible while fixation across the mandibular osteotomy sites is applied.

LeFort I osteotomy and mandibular inferior border osteotomy are also combined frequently (see Fig. 11-4). Usually LeFort I osteotomy is performed first. After

fixation and stabilization of the maxilla, the inferior border osteotomy is the second surgical procedure. With this combination of procedures, the mandible autorotates around the horizontal condylar axis to occlude with the repositioned maxilla. The mandibular occlusion serves as a reference to help reposition the maxilla. The sequence of procedures can be reversed if the surgeon utilizes RIF (position screws or semirigid bone plates) to fix bony segments after inferior border osteotomy. If difficulty in stabilizing the maxilla is anticipated (e.g., in repeat LeFort I osteotomy, LeFort I osteotomy positioned inferiorly), the mandibular inferior border osteotomy should be performed first.

Transoral vertical ramus osteotomy also may be performed with LeFort I osteotomy (see Fig. 11-4). First maxillary surgery is completed. After stabilization and fixation of the maxillary segments, the mandibular ramus osteotomy is performed. As has been mentioned in Chapter 9, RIF remains a problem with transoral vertical ramus osteotomy. Once technical problems associated with RIF are solved, alternative approaches to staging these two procedures may be possible.

Two-jaw surgery may involve any combination of surgical procedures in the mandible and the maxilla. Often mandibular and maxillary subapical osteotomies are performed together, the sequence being dictated by the final positions of the teeth. For example, if anterior maxillary and mandibular subapical osteotomies are planned to correct a bimaxillary protrusion, moving the mandibular segment first is often less difficult because the repositioned mandibular segment allows the maxillary segment to be repositioned more easily at surgery.

STABILIZATION AND FIXATION METHODS
Traditional Fixation Methods

Stabilization and fixation across osteotomy sites are even more important in two-jaw surgery than with osteotomy in one jaw. If LeFort I osteotomy is completed first, the maxilla must be repositioned and stabilized before the osteotomy can be completed in the mandible. With traditional fixation methods, 26-gauge wire sutures are placed across maxillary osteotomy sites in areas of dense bone, usually the piriform nasal rim and the zygomatic-maxillary buttress. The maxilla should feel firm clinically at this point; otherwise, proceeding with the completion of the osteotomy in the mandible is hazardous and may lead to an instability in both jaws, compromising holding the postoperative position of the jaws during healing. If use of RIF is not contemplated, 24-gauge skeletal suspension wires must be added, particularly if there is any question about the adequacy of dense cortical bone in the maxilla to hold the wire sutures across osteotomy sites (see Fig. 11-4). The skeletal fixation wires should have as vertical a pull as possible. A wire can be placed bilaterally in the infraorbital rim or the nasal piriform rim above the osteotomy site. This wire can be attached initially to the maxillary arch wire or maxillary splint.

After completion of the mandibular osteotomy, suspension wires are connected to circum-mandibular wires.[8] Before the mandible is placed into MMF with the aid of the occlusal wafer splint, bilateral circummandibular wires, 24-gauge, should be placed with the aid of a mandibular awl. This step is most easily accomplished by passing the awl through the skin beneath the mandible into the floor of the mouth, picking up the circum-mandibular wire, bringing the wire just beneath the inferior border of the mandible without removing the awl and passing it into the facial vestibule, and passing the wire through the mucosa, facial to the premolar teeth. Once the wire is removed from the tip of the awl, the awl may be withdrawn though the skin. After grasping both ends of the wire with wire drivers, the wire should be pulled against the inferior border of the mandible in a sawing motion to make sure that soft tissue is not trapped between the wire and the lower border of the mandible. Wire on the tongue side of the mandible should be passed inferior to the contact of the premolar teeth but above the arch wire bilaterally. The mandibular suspension wires can then be twisted, leaving a loop just facial to the premolar teeth.

At this point, the tooth-bearing segment of the mandible is repositioned and held in place with with 24- or 25-gauge maxillomandibular wires with the occlusal wafer splint intervening. The proximal condylar segments of the mandible now can be appropriately positioned and 24- to 26-gauge stainless steel wire sutures tightened, twisted, and cut. As a final step before wound closure, a 26-gauge intermediate wire is placed to connect the circum-mandibular and the piriform rim skeletal suspension wires bilaterally. The stability of the fixation should again be inspected to make certain that the jaws are adequately immobilized. As the final step, soft tissues at surgical sites are closed in the mandible and the maxilla.

If mandibular subapical osteotomy is performed with LeFort I osteotomy, skeletal supension wires in addition to MMF are usually required for adequate stability and immobilization of the jaws. If segments of mandibular or maxillary teeth are not included in the osteotomy, stable vertical occlusal stops remain and skeletal suspension wires may not be necessary. Such combinations include anterior mandibular subapical osteotomy and anterior maxillary subapical osteotomy, and maxillary posterior subapical osteotomy and mandibular ramus osteotomy. Skeletal suspension wires are uncomfortable to the patient during the entire time they are in place, but adequate fixation and stabilization are mandatory for satisfactory healing of the jaws and must take precedence over patient comfort.

With traditional fixation methods for two-jaw surgery, 5 to 7 weeks of MMF is necessary before healing is adequate to allow mobilization of the jaws and return of jaws to function. Once MMF is released, the intermediate wire connecting the skeletal suspension wires is also removed. Healing across the osteotomy sites of the individual jaws should be clinically firm. Usually the patients are allowed to function into the occlusal splint aided by light elastics attached to lugs on the surgical arch wires. Skeletal suspension wires can also be connected with elastics. Some surgeons feel that elastics connecting the suspension wires minimize traction across the maxillary osteotomy site. But any movement of maxillary or mandibular skeletal suspension wires is painful to the patient. The potential advantage of connecting the suspension wires with elastics must be weighed against the discomfort such elastics produce. Once clinical healing is adequate, patients may increase the consistency of their diet and regain jaw function. See Chapters 7 to 10 for details regarding bony healing and return of the jaws to function. When the determination has been made that the jaws are healing adequately and the patient begins to regain some jaw function, usually 2 weeks following release of MMF, the skeletal suspension wires may be removed. Prophylactic antibiotics, usually penicillin G or a first-generation cephalosporin, are taken just before skeletal suspension wire removal and for one or two doses following.

Rigid Internal Fixation

The greater short-term stability provided by RIF can be particularly advantageous for two-jaw surgery. Most surgeons use the same sequence of surgical steps in two-jaw surgery, making the mandibular cuts without splitting the mandible as the first step, followed by completion of LeFort I osteotomy. Following repositioning of the maxilla, semirigid bone plates must stabilize the maxilla well before proceeding to complete the mandibular osteotomy. A minimum of one bone plate on either side of the maxilla usually is required for adequate stabilization and fixation. With multiple maxillary segments at least one bone plate must stabilize each segment. Once the maxilla appears clinically firm, the mandibular osteotomy may be completed and the tooth-bearing segment of the mandible placed in MMF with the intervening occlusal wafer splint. After the mandibular osteotomy sites have been adequately stabilized and fixed with position or lag screws, MMF must be released and the occlusion checked. Any deviation in the occlusion must be corrected before the completion of surgery even if it means removing the rigid fixation devices to correct the jaw position. See Chapters 8, 9, and 10 for details of applying RIF. If the occlusion is adequate, the surgical incisions may be closed. In most circumstances, skeletal suspension wires are not required with RIF. Some surgeons do advocate placing skeletal suspension wires, connecting them for 2 to 3 weeks, and not allowing the patient any jaw movement, all to improve stability at osteotomy sites. Long-term stability with skeletal suspension

wires added has not yet been shown to be superior to conventional RIF techniques.

In some instances, particularly with LeFort I osteotomy in one piece, bone contact at osteotomy sites is excellent after repositioning the maxilla. Wire sutures across osteotomy sites in areas of dense cortical bone may be adequate by themselves for maxillary stabilization in two-jaw surgery. Lag or position screws stabilize the mandible following osteotomy. The decision to not use semirigid bone plates in the maxilla is a clinical judgment, one that can only be made at the time of surgery. Preliminary data do suggest that RIF in the maxilla and mandible provides more short-term stability.

With RIF in both jaws, the period of MMF can be greatly reduced or eliminated. Most surgeons remove firm MMF within the first week after surgery and allow the patient some jaw function using light elastics to guide the patient into the planned new occlusion. Patients should regain jaw function with RIF in about the same timeframe as with one-jaw surgery, usually 4 to 6 weeks after MMF release. See Chapter 7 for details regarding return of the jaws to function.

POSTSURGERY SEQUELAE

Two-jaw surgery carries the sequelae of each of the individual surgical procedures performed and the additional risks of an increased operating time. For example, with LeFort I osteotomy nasal stuffiness is common for up to 2 weeks until blood is cleared from the maxillary and other paranasal sinuses. These symptoms are the same when LeFort I osteotomy is combined with mandibular surgery. Edema is greater than with surgery in a single jaw, but two-thirds of the edema should resolve within 2 weeks of surgery. Increased operating time, 4 to 6 hours, and multiple surgical procedures increase blood loss.[10] Predonation of autologous blood is recommended in two-jaw surgery. Hegtvedt and colleagues documented that 33 of 96 patients with two-jaw surgery were transfused with their autologous blood.[14] In that study, increased operating time with two-jaw surgery correlated with increased blood loss. Ten of eleven patients whose operating time exceeded 6 hours were transfused with their autologous blood.

Hospital length of stay is increased with two-jaw surgery with patients remaining in the hospital an additional day beyond that required for surgery in a single jaw. Dolan and colleagues also documented increased total hospital charges for two-jaw surgery.[15] Once the initial stages of healing in the first 2 weeks following surgery have passed, two-jaw surgery should pose no more problems than surgery in a single jaw.

COMPLICATIONS

Surgery in two jaws carries all of the complications associated with each of the surgical procedures performed. The most significant additional complication results from the problems in planning for two-jaw surgery. Prediction tracings and model surgery must be carried out very carefully. Any discrepancies in measurements and positions of the teeth and jaws should be discovered before the occlusal wafer splints are made and the surgery is begun. Two-jaw surgery is predicated on the patient's having a repeatable centric jaw relation or retruded contact position. Such a position may be quite difficult to establish in a patient who has had a habit of posturing the mandible forward for years. On rare occasions, the discrepancy in jaw position is not discovered until the patient is under general anesthetic after two-jaw surgery has been completed. Fortunately in these cases, the discrepancy is generally only 1 to 2 mm and postsurgery jaw function and esthetics are not compromised. If a more severe discrepancy exists, reoperation may be necessary.

Successful completion of two-jaw surgery is predicated on the surgeon being able to adequately stabilize and fix one jaw, for example, LeFort I osteotomy with bone plates, before the osteotomy in the second jaw is completed. If adequate stabilization and fixation are not possible for any reason, the osteotomy in the second jaw should be delayed. If this is not done, gross discrepancies may exist between the planned positions of both jaws and the positions produced during surgery. This circumstance requires at least one additional surgery to correct the problem.

In summary, two-jaw surgery can be safely and predictably carried out with excellent results. Both the surgeon and orthodontist must carefully assess the benefits gained from surgery in both jaws and discuss the situation openly with the patient. Additional discussion of the indications for two-jaw surgery is found in each of the clinical chapters in Section IV.

REFERENCES

1. Gross BD, James AB: The surgical sequence of combined total maxillary and mandibular osteotomies, J Oral Surg 36:513-522, 1978.

2. Mohnac AM: Maxillary osteotomy in the management of occlusal deformities, J Oral Surg 24:305-317, 1965.

3. Bell WH, Condit CL: Surgical-orthodontic correction of adult bimaxillary protrusion, J Oral Surg 28:578-590, 1970.

4. Kent JN, Hinds EC: Management of dental facial deformities by anterior alveolar surgery, J Oral Surg 29:13-26, 1971.

5. Connole PW, Small EW: Combined maxillary and mandibular osteotomies: discussion of three cases, J Oral Surg 29:572-578, 1971.

6. Epker BN, Wolford LM: Middle third face osteotomies: their use in the correction of acquired and developmental dentofacial and craniofacial deformities, J Oral Surg 33:491-514, 1975.

7. Oatis GW, Van Belois MJ, Sugg WE, Jr: Combined surgical procedures to correct facial deformities, J Am Dent Assoc 97:58-65, 1978.

8. Turvey TA: Simultaneous mobilization of the maxilla and mandible: surgical technique and results, J Oral Maxillofac Surg 40:96-99, 1981.

9. Epker BN, Turvey T, Fish LC: Indications for simultaneous mobilization of the maxilla and mandible for the correction of dentofacial deformities, Oral Surg 54:369-381, 1982.

10. Turvey T, Hall DJ, Fish LW, Epker BN: Surgical-orthodontic treatment planning for simultaneous mobilization of the maxilla and mandible in the correction of dentofacial deformities, Oral Surg 54:491-498, 1982.

11. LaBanc JP, Turvey T, Epker BN: Results following simultaneous mobilization of the maxilla and mandible for the correction of dentofacial deformities: analysis of 100 consecutive patients, Oral Surg 54:607-612, 1982.

12. Ripley JF, Steed Dl, Flanary CM: A composite surgical splint for dual arch orthognathic surgery, J Oral Maxillofac Surg 40:687-688, 1982.

13. Buckley MJ, Tucker MR, Fredette SA: An alternative approach for staging simultaneous maxillary and mandibular osteotomies, Int J Adult Orthod Orthognath Surg 2:75-78, 1987.

14. Hegtvedt AK, Collins ML, White RP, Jr, Turvey TA: Minimizing the risk of transfusion in orthognathic surgery: use of predeposited autologous blood, Int J Adult Orthod Orthognath Surg 2:185-192, 1987.

15. Dolan P, White RP, Jr, Tulloch JFC: An analysis of hospital charges for orthognathic surgery, Int J Adult Orthod Orthognath Surg 2:9-14, 1987.

CLINICAL TREATMENT

In order to discuss the treatment of specific types of cases, it is necessary to group them in some way, despite the fact that each patient has an individual set of problems that requires a unique response. Our approach to this dilemma has been to discuss in detail the clinical treatment procedures for the major problem of the three largest groups of surgical-orthodontic patients: those with (1) mandibular deficiency and short or normal face height; (2) excessive face height, whatever their vertical proportions; and (3) Class III problems due to mandibular excess and/or maxillary deficiency. These chapters then are followed by separate discussions of other treatment needs that may be encountered in patients whose major problem was discussed previously or in patients with this problem alone: asymmetries, transverse and open-bite problems, problems secondary to cleft lip-palate, and dentofacial deformities in patients with major prosthetic needs and or TM joint problems.

We hope that for the majority of surgical-orthodontic patients, almost all the relevant information about treatment will be found in a single chapter. We recognize that for a significant minority, more than one chapter must be consulted because multiple problems are involved. Our intent is to be as thorough as possible in discussing treatment methods, while minimizing redundancy by grouping similiar conditions together.

In each of the clinical chapters that follow, we have included detailed case reports to further illustrate specific types of problems and the methods used to solve them.

CHAPTER 12

Mandibular Deficiency in Patients with Short or Normal Face Height

William R. Proffit
Raymond P. White, Jr.

NEED AND DEMAND

Of all the problems that require surgical-orthodontic treatment, mandibular deficiency in individuals who do not have excessive face height is the most common. The limited epidemiologic data available at present, and the extrapolations from it discussed in Chapter 1, suggest that there are approximately 1.2 million Americans (about 0.5% of the population) who have a dent-ofacial deformity that would warrant surgical-orthodontic correction. Of these, approximately 650,000 have mandibular deficiency, either alone or combined with maxillary excess (see Chapter 1, Table 1-2). A significant minority of this mandibular-deficient group, approximately 25%, have excessive face height. Their horizontal mandibular deficiency is at least in part due to downward and backward rotation of the mandible because of excessive vertical development of the maxilla. If we exclude this group, we deduce that there are approximately 500,000 people in the U.S. population with mandibular deficiency and normal or short anterior face height. They represent, therefore, about 40% of the total pool of potential surgical-orthodontic patients.

Another way to estimate the relative importance of this group of mandibular-deficient patients is to look at their prevalence in the population who seek treatment.[1] At their initial evaluation, 573 of a group of 1102 patients (52%) evaluated through the Dentofacial Program at the UNC were judged clinically to have mandibular deficiency, and 28% had 7 mm or more overjet. Of the mandibular-deficient patients, a third were judged to have excessive anterior face height, and the remaining two-thirds had normal or decreased face height. Essentially similar results were obtained from later cephalometric analysis.

From these data, it appears that the number of individuals with mandibular deficiency and normal/short face height who seek and receive surgical-orthodontic treatment is about 35% of the total surgical-orthodontic patient pool, a bit lower than their representation in the population of potential patients. Why that occurs is not known. Perhaps it is related to the lesser esthetic

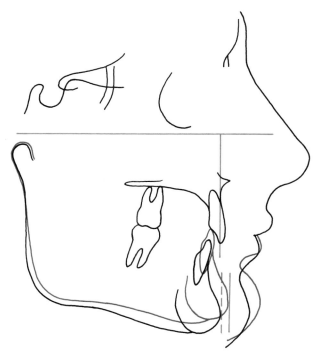

Fig. 12-1. Because of the geometry of the mandible, when normal or deficient face height is reduced even more by rotating the mandible upward and forward, the lower incisors move up more but forward less than the chin. In this tracing (*black*, original position; *red*, rotated up and forward), note that, with the face oriented to the true horizontal line, as the mandible rotated up and forward, the chin came forward 4 mm while the incisors advanced only 2 mm. A somewhat similar rotation occurs during the development of a short-face problem, contributing to the projection of the chin relative to the dentition that is characteristic of these patients.

impact of this condition as compared with mandibular prognathism, asymmetry, or the long-face pattern of deformity. Even so, this is the largest single group of surgical-orthodontic patients.

DIAGNOSTIC CHARACTERISTICS

In evaluating patients with normal or short anterior face height combined with mandibular deficiency, the strong interaction between the vertical and AP position of both the lower incisors and the chin must be kept in mind. When the mandible moves up, the chin moves forward an approximately equal amount, and when the mandible goes down, the chin goes back. The effect on the mandibular dentition is similar, but the geometry of the jaw, particularly when face height is short, produces a somewhat different effect: as the jaw rotates up or down, the motion of the incisors is more vertical than anteroposterior (Fig. 12-1). Mandibular-deficient patients with short anterior face height have experienced a relative upward and forward rotation of the jaw during growth. Developmentally, that is how

their problem arose. The result, therefore, is likely to be a relatively strong chin, especially in comparison to the lower lip, despite the mandibular deficiency.

On clinical examination, these patients are characterized by:

- Class II molar and canine relationship
- Anterior deep bite
- Increased overjet (but maxillary incisor malalignment often makes the overjet less than might be expected, given the skeletal discrepancy)
- Excessive curve of Spee in the mandibular arch, but a reduced or negative curve of Spee in the maxillary arch
- A tendency toward incisor crowding, often more severe in the upper than in the lower arch

Facially, the patient often has a surprisingly well-developed chin button, with an appearance of deficiency at the lower lip more than at the chin. Face height tends to be short, and the shorter it is, the greater the tendency for a curl of the lower lip that accentuates the labiomental fold (Fig. 12-2). The mandibular plane angle tends to be low, the gonial angle relatively square, and the elevator muscles of the mandible well developed.

The anterior deep bite, which is present whether face height is short or normal, has the potential to cause two different functional problems: (1) irritation of the gingival tissues behind the maxillary incisors (if the upper incisors are tipped lingually in the Class II, division 2 pattern, there may also be gingival irritation on the labial of the lower incisors); and (2) a tendency toward clicking within the TM joint, probably related to excessive distal positioning of the condyles on full closure.

The prevalence and importance of this second problem are unknown and highly debated. Some investigators have reported a modest but statistically significant correlation between excessive anterior deep bite and the presence of TM joint signs such as clicking, whereas others report that neither signs nor symptoms are increased in Class II deep-bite patients.[2-5] There seems to be no evidence that the sign of clicking is likely to extend into symptoms such as pain, crepitus, and limited motion unless the patient engages in clenching and grinding that overstresses the musculature. The deep bite, in short, may predispose to TM joint problems but is unlikely to be their sole cause. The tissue irritation, in contrast, is directly related to the trauma from teeth impacting against vulnerable soft tissues, and this can be blamed largely on the occlusal relationship.

Etiologically, the presence of a strong hereditary component is apparent both from an examination of the families of individuals with the problem, who tend to have somewhat similar facial features, and from an evaluation of the prevalence of the condition in various racial and ethnic groups. Mandibular deficiency with

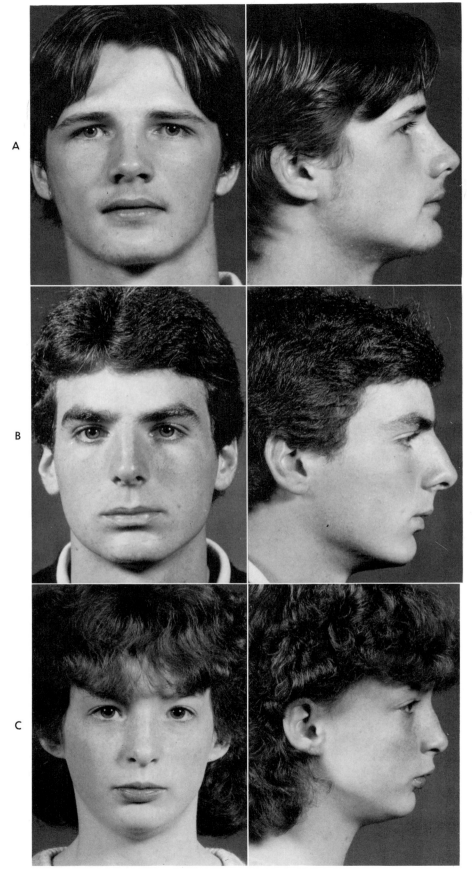

Fig. 12-2. This series of faces illustrates the effect of increasingly severe mandibular deficiency and decreased face height, from the moderate deviation in **A** to the severe problem in **D**. Note the increasing depth of the labiomental fold (curl to the lower lip) as face height decreases.

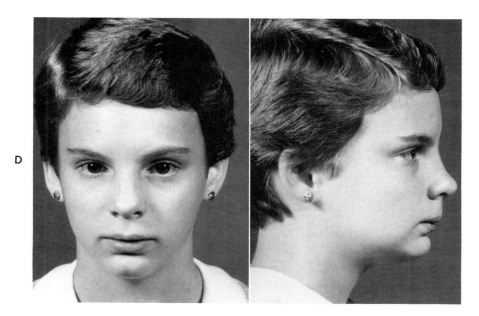

D

Fig. 12-2, cont'd. For legend, see opposite page.

short facial height is almost exclusively a Caucasian problem, occurring only rarely in blacks and Orientals, and it appears to be much more prevalent in some Caucasian groups (English, German) than in others (Scandinavian). To some extent, this can be explained by craniofacial proportions. All other things being equal, the "saddle angle," which reflects the flexure of the anterior lobes of the brain and the cranial base, will affect anterior face height (Fig. 12-3). This angle is slightly greater in Caucasians[6] who therefore would have some predisposition toward short-face, deep-bite problems. What is not explained, of course, is why a few develop a severe problem while the great majority with the same saddle angle do not.

It is very difficult to identify environmental contributions to this condition. Trauma that caused poor mandibular growth is highly unlikely. The normal/short face, mandibular-deficient patients are characterized by short anterior face height but a relatively long ramus, whereas patients who have suffered trauma to the mandible tend to have the opposite, a decrease in ramus height and a downward-backward rotation of the mandible. Habits of various types, respiratory difficulties, and interferences with tooth eruption also are not usual contributors to the development of the condition. When the mandible is deficient and anterior face height is short, the lower lip tends to interfere with the upper incisors. If the lip stays behind the incisors, they tip forward, creating a Class II, division 1 malocclusion and a tendency toward incisor spacing. If the lip stays in front of the incisors, they tip lingually, creating a Class II, division 2 pattern with crowding. Biting force has been reported to be higher than normal in patients

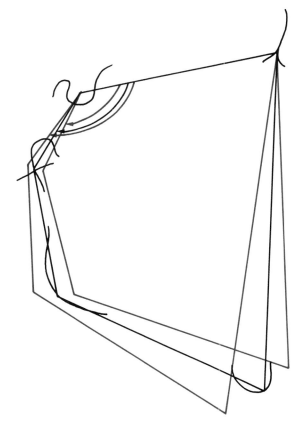

Fig. 12-3. This diagram illustrates the marked effect on face height of modest changes in the saddle angle, N-S-Ar (articulare). The black lines are traced from an individual with normal facial proportions. The red outlines show the effect on face height and chin prominence of increasing or decreasing the saddle angle by 5 degrees, keeping other angles and distances the same.

with short facial dimensions (see Chapter 2), and cephalometrically it often appears that posterior teeth have erupted less than the normal amount. Although it is tempting to think that this is cause and effect, there is no evidence to indicate this is the case. It is entirely possible that the relative lack of dental eruption and the change in biting force both are related to a third, as yet unknown, characteristic of these patients.

One possible factor in the development of the condition is that the mandible could become "trapped" by an impinging overbite. At least in theory, this could prevent the normal downward and forward displacement of the mandible that seems to be necessary for normal growth. Occasionally, when orthodontic treatment for a deep-bite Class II patient is begun by tipping the upper incisors forward and applying mechanotherapy to reduce the overbite, a considerable spurt of mandibular growth in a favorable direction occurs immediately, which gives some credence to an interference with growth from the occlusion as an etiologic factor. That does not explain, of course, how the overbite came into existence to start with, nor does it account for the majority of patients who do not show this type of growth when the overbite is corrected. Although we can conclude that a combination of hereditary tendencies and environmental influences seems to be involved in the etiology of these problems, that statement is not particularly satisfying given our lack of knowledge about details of the contributions on either side.

On cephalometric evaluation, the distinguishing characteristic for any group of mandibular-deficient patients is an increased A-B difference as projected to the true horizontal line. (This is much more reliable for evaluating jaw relationships than projecting the difference to the occlusal plane, as in the Wits analysis.) As that distance increases, it becomes more and more difficult to obtain proper jaw function or esthetics. The maximum A-B difference that is compatible with reasonable occlusion and esthetics is about 8 mm, which means that larger differences must be reduced at least to this level either by growth modification or surgery.

The relationship of the incisors to their supporting bone and the vertical relationship of the jaws and teeth also are important. Excessive overbite in these patients is more likely to be due to infraeruption of the posterior teeth than to supereruption of incisors, but this varies among individual patients and must be checked

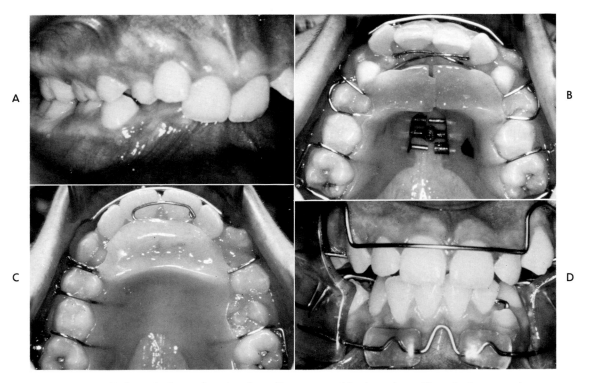

Fig. 12-4. Before placing a functional appliance, repositioning of maxillary incisors can be accomplished with a removable appliance. **A,** The incisor position in this Class II division 2 malocclusion makes a construction bite for a functional appliance impossible. **B,** A removable appliance with a jackscrew for lateral expansion and springs to tip the incisors forward is being used to prepare for later functional treatment. **C,** A second removable with a biteplate is being used to gain further bite opening. **D,** Frankel appliance in place with the mandible advanced. (**A-D,** courtesy Harry Orton, Kingston, England).

carefully. Decreased eruption of molars often accompanies a skeletal deep-bite pattern.

The cephalometric approach recommended for diagnostic evaluation is shown in detail in Chapter 4 and further illustrated in the case reports at the end of that chapter.

TREATMENT PLANNING
Preadolescents with Growth Potential

In a preadolescent child with severe mandibular deficiency, growth modification treatment certainly should be attempted. In a child with mandibular deficiency and an anterior deep bite, the key to treatment is eliminating the incisor interferences by opening the bite anteriorly and restraining forward maxillary growth while offering every encouragement for the mandible to grow downward and forward.

Three steps in treatment usually are required:

1. Align the upper incisors. Irregular and/or lingually tipped upper incisors can interfere with forward movement of the mandible, so this step is particularly needed in children with a Class II, division 2 problem. The necessary tooth movement can be accomplished with either fixed or removable appliances. All that is required in most instances is labial tipping of the incisors, perhaps coupled with some transverse expansion of the maxillary posterior segments. This can be accomplished with a removable appliance (Fig. 12-4), which may be advantageous for some patients. The ease with which brackets can be bonded to anterior teeth, however, also makes it entirely practical to place a fixed appliance to align the incisors and prepare the patient for a second stage of treatment with a removable functional appliance, even though this means that the fixed appliance is placed and then removed in a few months (Figs. 12-5 and 12-6). Because the fixed appliance is so much more effective in moving teeth than is a removable appliance, this usually is the preferred approach.

2. Modify jaw growth. The objective is to produce relative forward growth of the mandible by impeding growth of the upper jaw and facilitating growth of the lower. This also can be accomplished with either a fixed or removable (functional) appliance (Figs. 12-7 to 12-9). The typical fixed appliance consists of molar bands and bonded incisor attachments, with extraoral force to the upper arch. Functional appliances have in common a construction bite that positions the mandible forward. Although the theory of functional appliances (that they stimulate mandibular growth) is quite different from the theory of headgear (which is meant to impede maxillary growth), research has shown that the outcome of treatment with the two approaches seems to be remarkably similar.[7,8] Because of this, the choice of method can be based as much on practice efficiency and patient management as on any inherent difference in the two methods.

3. Allow posterior but not anterior teeth to erupt. Differential eruption of the posterior teeth, in concert with growth of the mandible, is the method for correcting the overbite (see Fig. 12-9). To the extent possible, eruption of the lower molars should be fa-

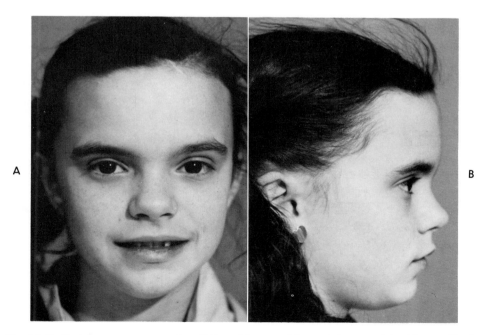

Fig. 12-5. Facial appearance, patient P.R., a 10-year-old preadolescent girl with mandibular deficiency, short face height, and Class II division 2 malocclusion.

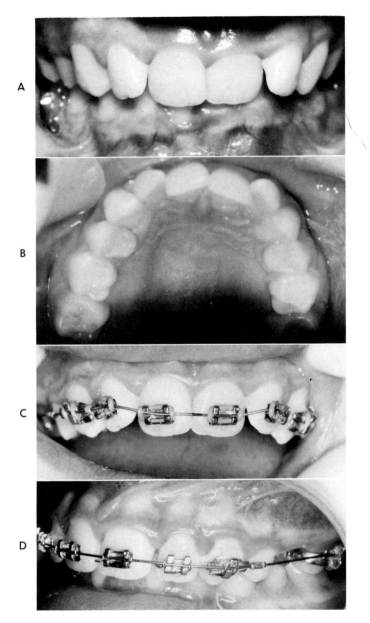

Fig. 12-6. Patient P.R. **A** and **B,** The lingual position of the maxillary incisors made it impossible to posture the mandible forward as required for the fabrication of a functional appliance. **C,** Bands were placed on first molars, bonded brackets were placed on incisors and canines, and a 16 NiTi wire was placed to align the incisors. **D,** Two months later, alignment was completed. The incisors had been tipped labially, creating the desired overjet.

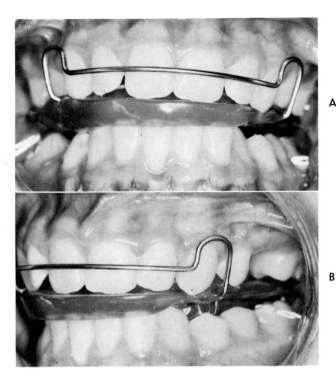

Fig. 12-7. P.R., activator appliance in place. Note the capping of the lower incisors to minimize their displacement labially and the shelf posteriorly that leaves the lower teeth free to erupt while impeding maxillary posterior eruption.

vored over eruption of the upper because an increase in the occlusal plane makes it easier to correct the Class II molar relationship. Differential eruption of the lower molar is easier with functional appliances. In a short-face, deep-bite patient, one would think first about using a cervical (low pull) headgear, which would tend to elongate the upper molar in addition to tipping it posteriorly and restraining maxillary growth. This tends to produce more eruption of the upper than of the lower molar, just the reverse of what is desired. In contrast, it is straightforward to design a functional appliance so that eruption of the lower but not the upper molars is facilitated.

The more severe the problem, the less the chance that growth modification treatment will be successful. On the other hand, at present there is no way to know how an individual patient will respond, and there are instances in which the amount of favorable growth seems almost miraculous. In severe problems, it is important to warn the parents that surgical treatment ultimately may be required, but it is wise to begin treatment of the type outlined here to take advantage of any possible favorable growth.

There is also a clear guideline for what should not be done in the treatment of a preadolescent patient of this type: removal of permanent teeth should be avoided except in the most extreme crowding situations. If a patient responds favorably to the growth modification treatment outlined above, labial and lateral expansion of the arches often makes it possible to incorporate all the teeth without extraction. If the response is unfavor-

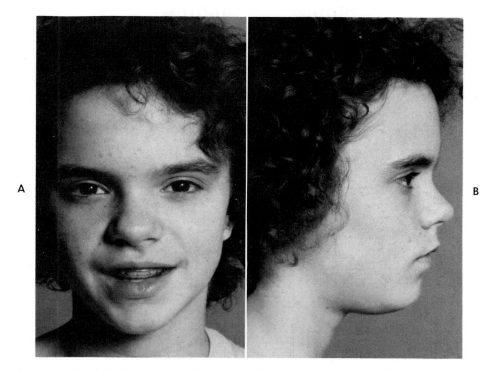

Fig. 12-8. P.R., facial appearance after 1 year of activator treatment. At this point, the Class II occlusal relationship was nearly corrected. A second stage of fixed-appliance orthodontic treatment was planned when the remaining permanent teeth erupted.

able, a choice between treatment with extraction for camouflage and surgery will be necessary. It is better to have all options open when this decision is made—which means that the decision should wait until growth potential decreases and the remaining permanent teeth erupt, during or following the adolescent growth spurt.

Adolescents with Questionable Growth Potential

Following the adolescent growth spurt, growth potential declines precipitously, and with it the chance of successful growth modification also drops. It can be very difficult to ascertain a patient's growth status, however, particularly in boys. In girls, the onset of menstruation is an obvious biologic marker that the peak of the adolescent growth spurt has passed. In boys, there is no such marker, and it must be kept in mind that boys often show considerable growth even into the late teens. Some girls also mature quite late, and the later the maturation, the broader and slower the adolescent growth spurt—which means that a girl who begins menstruation late nevertheless may have some growth left. Patients with questionable growth potential become a diagnostic dilemma.

The best approach to a patient of this type is to discuss the severity of the problems with the patient and parents, being sure they understand that surgery may be necessary, and then attempt nonextraction treat-

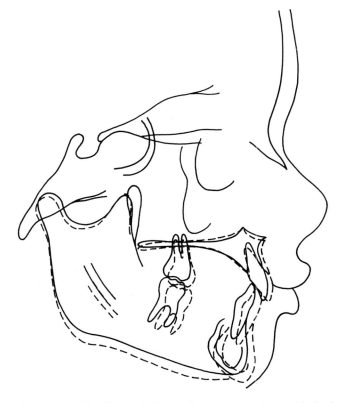

Fig. 12-9. P.R. The cephalometric superimposition *(dashed black)* illustrates the response to growth modification treatment.

ment with growth modification (Figs. 12-10 to 12-12). Six to 12 months' experience with that treatment approach will make it clear how much change it is likely to produce, and the best decision as to the next stage of treatment—camouflage with extractions or surgery to advance the mandible—is based on knowledge about the growth response (Figs. 12-13 to 12-15). As with the preadolescent patient, it is a mistake to proceed too quickly to premolar extractions and institute a plan that is based on camouflage. Treatment of that type will result in displacement of the teeth relative to their own jaw, retracting the upper incisors and proclining the lowers, in a way that can make ultimate surgical correction all but impossible. Before a camouflage treatment plan is undertaken, in other words, one

needs to be all but positive that it will succeed (see Chapter 1, Case 1).

When it is apparent that surgery to advance the mandible is necessary, we recommend (except in the unusual circumstances discussed in Chapters 2 and 16) that it be delayed until the adolescent growth spurt has been completed. That certainly does not mean that orthognathic surgery must be delayed until the late teens. If conservative therapy is instituted in an adolescent patient and there is little or no response within 6 to 12 months, the lack of response is evidence that the growth spurt is over. At that point, there is essentially no chance of enough future growth to correct the problem or to cause relapse after surgical correction, and proceeding with mandibular advancement, even at age 13 or 14, is perfectly satisfactory.

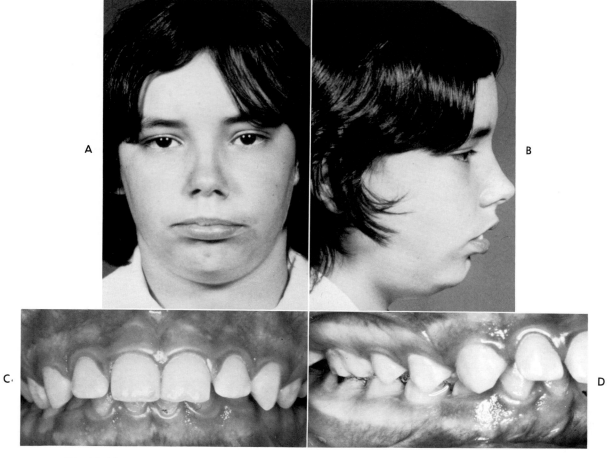

Fig. 12-10. Patient M.R. sought treatment initially at age 13 years, 10 months. His problems at that time were characterized as severe mandibular deficiency, maxillary dental protrusion with flared and spaced upper incisors, and deep bite anteriorly. **A** and **B**, Facial appearance initially. **C** and **D**, Initial occlusal relationships. Because he had not yet undergone puberty, there was at least a small possibility of favorable growth, and it was decided to attempt growth modification while avoiding extractions or tooth movements associated with orthodontic camouflage that would make later surgical correction more difficult if growth modification was unsuccessful.

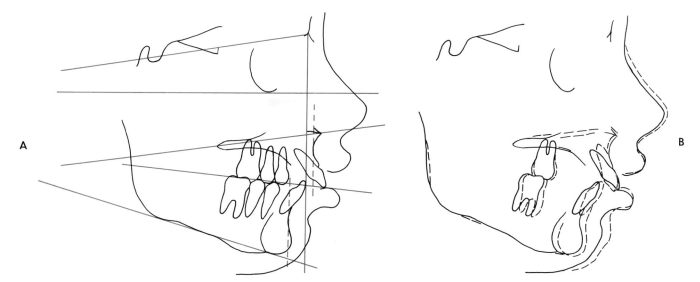

Fig. 12-11. M.R. **A,** Initial cephalometric tracing. Note the mandibular deficiency and the tipped palatal plane. Cephalometric measurements: nasion perpendicular line (N perp) to A, 3 mm; N perp to Pg, −7 mm; AB difference to true horizontal, 12 mm; upper face height (UFH), 54 mm; lower face height (LFH), 65 mm; mand plane (GoGn to true horizontal), 17 degrees; max incisor (MxI) to true vertical through point A (A vert), 7 mm, 37 degrees; mand incisor to true vertical through point B (B vert), 8 mm, 35 degrees. **B,** Superimposition ages 13 years, 10 months to 14 years, 10 months *(dashed black)*, the period of attempted growth modification. Note that favorable mandibular growth was obtained, which, however, was insufficient to correct the mandibular deficiency.

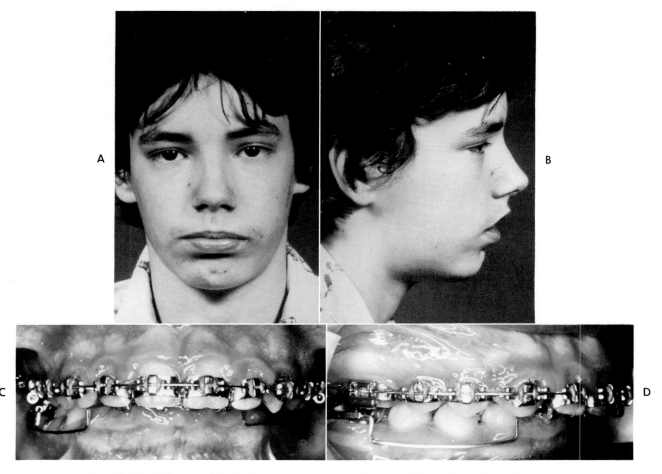

Fig. 12-12. M.R. **A** and **B,** Facial appearance age 14 years, 10 months, after orthodontic treatment with headgear and a partial fixed appliance (mandibular utility arch). **C** and **D,** Occlusal relationships. At this point, sexual maturation had occurred and the peak of the adolescent growth spurt had passed. Although the facial growth that occurred during the previous year was expressed in a favorable direction, there was now no doubt that surgical treatment was needed.

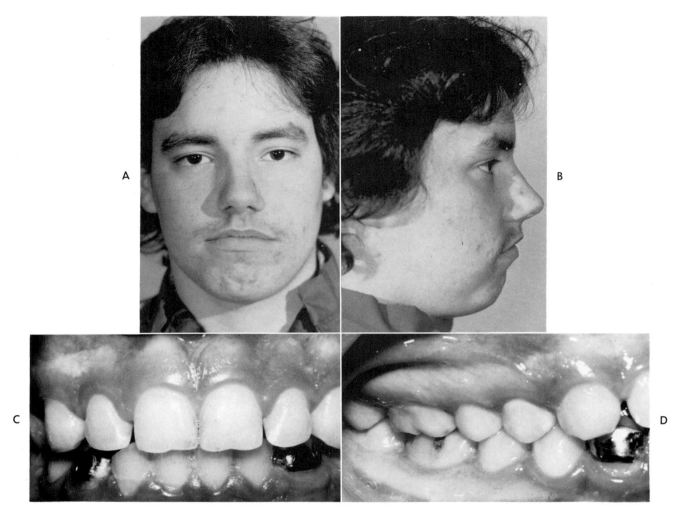

Fig. 12-13. M.R. **A** and **B,** Facial appearance at age 15 years, 6 months, after surgical mandibular advancement and completion of orthodontics. **C** and **D,** Occlusal relationships. In retrospect, chin augmentation could have further improved facial balance.

Adults with Little or No Growth Potential

Although the recent work of Behrents has shown that slow growth of the jaws does continue into adult life,[9] for all practical purposes growth modification ceases to be a possibility after adolescence. The key question for an older patient with mandibular deficiency and anterior deep bite therefore becomes whether the excessive overbite can be corrected orthodontically without the chin rotating backward too much—which is an esthetic judgment.

When no improvement in jaw relationship is possible, the orthodontist has two ways to correct excessive overjet, and three possibilities for correcting overbite. Overjet can be reduced by any combination of retraction of upper incisors and proclination of lower incisors. The limits for orthodontic tooth movement apply: it is unrealistic to expect that the upper incisors can be retracted more than 6 mm (less if they were upright

rather than flared to begin with), and lower incisors usually cannot be moved labially more than 2 mm without great risk of posttreatment instability. Overbite can be corrected by some combination of intrusion of upper or lower incisors and downward rotation of the mandible (i.e., an increase in lower face height and mandibular plane angle). The limits on these movements are even more stringent. It is extremely difficult to achieve more than 4 mm total bite opening by intrusion or to produce more than 2 mm downward rotation of the mandible in a patient who does not have a long-face tendency. Thus an adult who has more than 6 mm overbite or 8 mm overjet could be considered a candidate for surgery solely on the basis of dental relationships, without even considering facial esthetics. Esthetic limitations include vertical and AP tooth-lip relationships in addition to the effect of mandibular rotation on chin prominence.

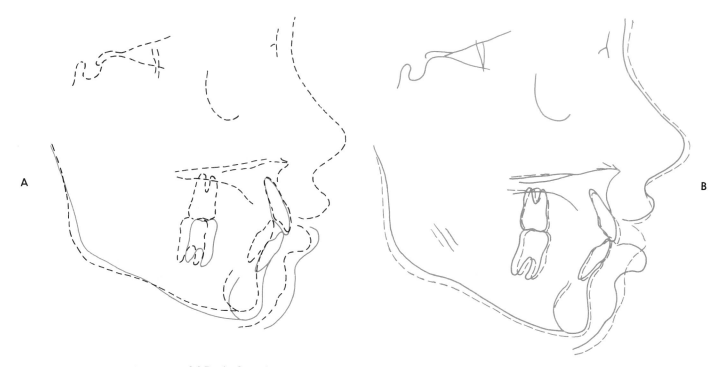

Fig. 12-14. M.R. **A,** Superimposition ages 14 years, 10 months, (presurgery) to 15 years, 6 months (completion of treatment) *(solid red).* **B,** Superimposition ages 15 years, 6 months to 20 years, 1 month (5-year recall) *(dashed red).*

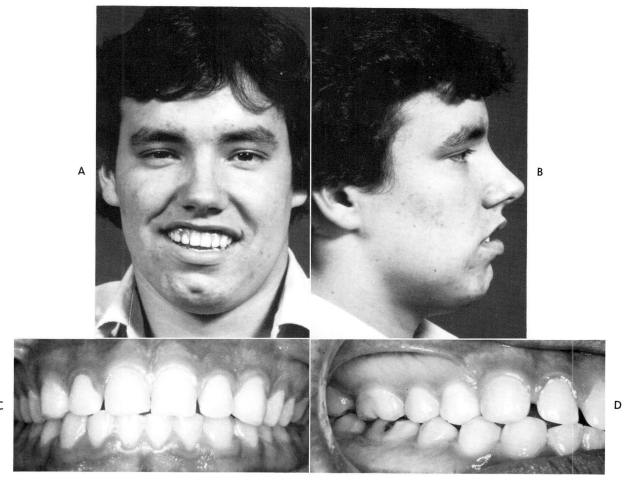

Fig. 12-15. M.R. **A** and **B,** Facial appearance age 20 years, 1 month, at 5-year recall. **C** and **D,** Occlusal relationships. Facial proportions and occlusal relationships were nicely stable.

In adults, it is important to decide in the beginning whether the treatment approach will be orthodontic or orthodontic-surgical. The reason is simple: from the beginning, the treatment will be quite different with the two approaches. Will extractions be necessary? Probably yes with orthodontics alone, particularly in the upper arch but perhaps not in the lower; often not with surgical-orthodontic treatment, perhaps in the lower arch but almost never in the upper. How should the overbite be corrected and the lower arch leveled? By intrusion of incisors, with orthodontics; by extrusion of premolars in the majority of cases, with surgical-orthodontic treatment. Will gingival grafts be needed before treatment begins? Perhaps, particularly when surgery is planned. In the younger patients discussed above, there is a positive benefit in beginning conservatively, trying orthodontic treatment and evaluating the result before proceeding to surgery. There is nothing to be gained, and potentially quite a bit to lose, in trying the same thing in adults.

Cephalometric prediction of the results of alternative treatment plans is the rational way to decide between them. Fortunately, it is much easier to predict outcomes when growth is not a variable. Accurate predic-

tions (see Chapter 5) can provide the information that the doctor and the patient need to make a decision.

PLANNING SURGICAL-ORTHODONTIC TREATMENT

In the conceptual framework of the treatment planning approach described in Chapters 5 and 7, we are now at the stage at which tentative solutions to the individual problems have been proposed, and these solutions are being integrated into a final treatment plan. For this group of patients, a surgical approach to the mandibular deficiency that is the most important problem has been chosen, and so the general plan for the surgery must be formulated before the details of the orthodontics can be established.

Surgical Approach

When a mandibular deficiency problem has no vertical component (i.e., when face height is essentially normal), analysis of the AP jaw and tooth relationships is straightforward. As facial dimensions become shorter (or longer), increasing care must be taken with the cephalometric analysis to avoid a misleading impression of the AP situation. Particularly in patients with

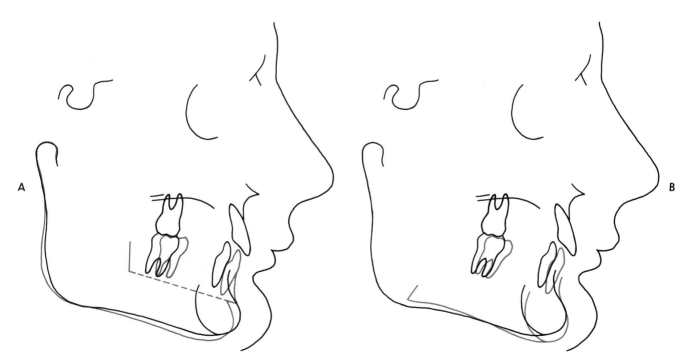

Fig. 12-16. When face height must be increased in treatment of a mandibular-deficient, short-face problem, a ramus osteotomy is likely to be more stable than a subapical osteotomy. When the mandibular plane angle is increased with a subapical osteotomy, the entire mandible is forced downward and backward, lengthening the muscles of the pterygomandibular sling as shown in **A** (surgical prediction, *red*). In contrast (**B**), with a ramus osteotomy the chin can move down but the gonial angle area up, relaxing the muscles in both areas.

very short face height, upward and forward rotation of the chin may partially or even totally conceal their mandibular deficiency (see Fig. 12-2). These patients may need to have their chin moved straight down. Even so, advancement of the mandible is needed. Otherwise, the chin would inevitably go backward as it moved downward because the mandible would rotate on an arc.

It is much more difficult to permanently increase anterior face height by rotating the mandible at the condyles than it is to rotate it within the body-ramus region via a ramus osteotomy. The first approach requires a lengthening of the elevator muscles, whereas the latter allows the muscles to shorten as the chin goes down but the gonial angles go up. In theory, the orthodontist should be able to produce a downward rotation of the mandible by elongating the posterior teeth, as with Class II elastics. The surgeon theoretically should be able to produce the same rotation with a mandibular subapical osteotomy that elongates the mandibular posterior teeth (Fig. 12-16). In fact, this sort of rotation of the mandible is much easier to produce in the long-face patients, in whom one does not wish it to happen, than in the short-face patients for whom it might be desirable. It is hard for the orthodontist to produce more than a modest amount of permanent rotation of the mandible in a short-face adult because of the difficulty in extruding posterior teeth in these patients. There may be more rotation during treatment, but often half or more of this is lost when active treatment ends and the extruded posterior teeth settle under the influence of biting forces. The result is a tendency for overbite to return.

Relapse of overbite correction following a mandibular subapical advancement also is likely to occur, for the same reason. One reason for considering a mandibular subapical advancement rather than a ramus osteotomy is the tendency for these patients to have a prominent chin relative to their dentition. The result is that often the dentition needs to come forward while the chin needs merely to move downward. If face height is only slightly short and overbite is not a major problem, the subapical osteotomy may be an ideal solution, but if significant vertical change is needed, a ramus osteotomy is preferred.

It is possible to advance the dentition more than the chin with a ramus osteotomy, and in fact this tends to occur almost automatically when a deep bite is corrected during the surgery. As the mandible is rotated to bring the incisors down while molar contact is maintained, the mandibular plane angle increases and the lower incisor is thrown forward relative to the chin. This is exactly what the patient needs for better chin-lip balance (see Chapter 1, Case 3, and Case 1 below). If the chin projection is still too great, a reduction genioplasty at the same time as the ramus osteotomy may

be indicated (Fig. 12-17). A lower border osteotomy to set the chin back requires a cut at an angle along the lower border, and when the chin goes back it also goes down, further increasing face height while reducing the horizontal prominence.

This reasoning is the basis for the usual surgical approach to these patients: after appropriate orthodontic preparation, the surgery will be a ramus osteotomy—almost always a sagittal-split, for reasons discussed in more detail below—to advance the mandible and rotate it downward anteriorly. For a few patients, a lower border osteotomy is needed at the same time to reduce chin prominence. Occasionally, when face height is essentially normal, a subapical advancement is indicated. Almost never in this type of patient is it desirable to move the maxilla downward. More specifically, the posterior maxilla should not be elongated in a way that stretches the pterygomandibular sling if this can be avoided. Rotating the maxilla so that the incisors are brought downward but the molars are not, can be used to solve an esthetic problem of infraerupted incisors without creating instability.

Another way to describe the skeletal deep-bite pattern is to note that posterior face height is relatively long as compared with anterior face height. In a few patients with mandibular deficiency and a short face anteriorly, the ramus is unusually long and the maxilla may actually be rotated down posteriorly. In these patients, two-jaw surgery to rotate the maxilla upward is needed, in addition to mandibular advancement with rotation that brings the chin downward and the gonial angle upward.[10]

Orthodontic Approach

The orthodontic approach is shaped by the need to properly position the maxillary and mandibular incisors presurgically, in both the AP and vertical planes of space. The surgeon will bring the incisors into occlusion, which means that their position determines the jaw position at surgery. Where the orthodontist puts the incisors will determine not only how much the mandible will be advanced, but also what will be the postsurgical face height.

In patients with deep overbite, there is nearly always an excessive curve of Spee in the lower arch, and occasionally a reverse curve in the upper arch as well. It is necessary to level this to obtain good occlusion. There are only two ways to do that: (1) intrude the incisors, or (2) elongate the posterior teeth, particularly the premolars. An important part of planning the orthodontic approach is deciding which method for leveling is to be employed. As a general rule, the shorter the face height, the greater the likelihood that leveling by extrusion is needed. Because most of these mandibular-deficient patients do need additional face height, most should be leveled by extrusion.

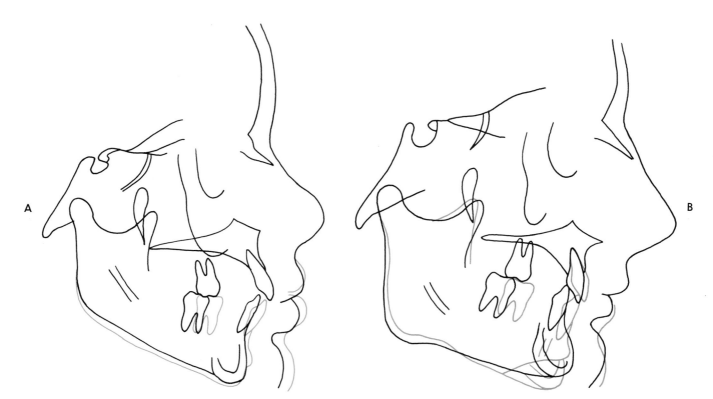

Fig. 12-17. In a mandibular-deficient patient who has a prominent chin button before treatment, and who therefore needs the mandibular dentition advanced more than the chin, a major factor in deciding between a subapical and ramus osteotomy is whether an increase in face height is desired. Subapical osteotomy is indicated only if little or no vertical change is needed. **A,** Cephalometric superimposition from presurgery *(black)* to 6 months postsurgery *(red)* in a patient who had a subapical osteotomy to advance the mandibular dentition. Note that the chin remained in approximately the same AP and vertical position. Face height was increased by rotating the mandible downward, which tends to be unstable. **B,** Cephalometric superimposition from presurgery to 6 months postsurgery *(solid red)* in a patient who had ramus osteotomy. Note the rotation of the mandible to advance the dentition more than the chin and the use of an inferior border osteotomy to increase face height while decreasing AP chin prominence. The dentition was advanced with this ramus osteotomy but the chin was not advanced.

Whether the arches will be leveled by extrusion or intrusion also determines both whether this should be done before or after the jaw surgery and the type of orthodontic mechanotherapy. Extrusion is done more easily and efficiently after the ramus surgery, and so leveling by extrusion is postsurgical leveling; but intrusion must be done before surgery. Extrusion is accomplished best with continuous arch wires, whereas intrusion requires segmented arch mechanics (see Chapter 5 and standard orthodontic texts for more details).

One thing that is not different between the two methods for leveling the lower arch is that arch length is required to accomplish it. When the arch is leveled, either the molars must be moved posteriorly (which occurs only to a very limited extent), or the incisors must go forward (Fig. 12-18). Because space is needed for leveling as well as for alignment, extraction is more

likely to be necessary when a severe curve of Spee is combined with some degree of lower incisor crowding.

The AP position of both the upper and lower incisors also is an important consideration. If the lower incisors are positioned lingually relative to the chin, which frequently is the case, obviously it is better to move them forward. The extra space needed for leveling then would help improve the incisor position. The more the incisors are moved forward, the greater the chance of gingival stripping unless there is a good band of attached tissue, so a gingival graft may be required before nonextraction orthodontics. But if the lower incisors are crowded and well positioned or protrusive, extraction will be necessary, and frequently this is the case. If the upper incisors are extremely flared, premolar extraction to gain space for retraction may be needed, but this is rare. Even when there is some crowding in the upper arch, nonextraction treatment usually is possible. Some additional space is provided by the lateral expansion across the premolars that is needed to accommodate the mandibular arch when it is advanced. Extraction of lower but not upper premolars, therefore, is a common orthodontic plan in preparation for mandibular advancement.

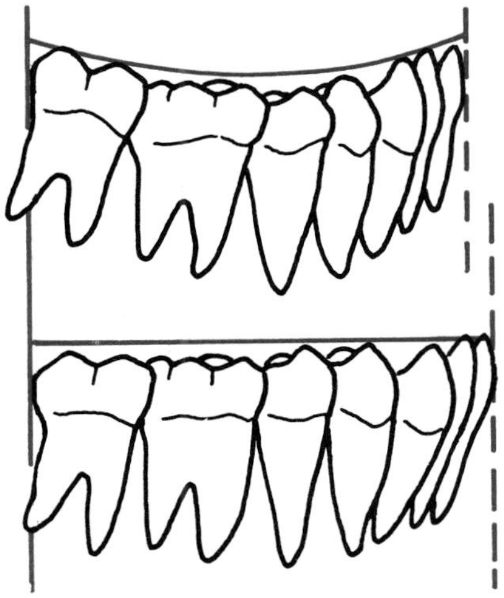

If the mandible is advanced more than a few millimeters at surgery, a tendency toward posterior crossbite is almost inevitable (Fig. 12-19). Orthodontic expansion of the maxillary arch can correct this to a limited extent, but it is unrealistic to expect to maintain more than approximately 4 mm of increased intermolar width. Expanding by opening the midpalatal suture usually requires surgical assistance in patients beyond their late teens. It may be necessary to choose between accepting a mild crossbite tendency and maxillary surgery solely to increase arch width. In that case, the benefit of surgically involving the maxilla versus cost and risk must be carefully considered. Accepting the maximum orthodontic expansion that can be obtained often is the best judgment, but sometimes surgery for transverse expansion is required.

Fig. 12-18. When the lower arch is leveled, the geometry requires additional space—the shortest distance between two points is a straight line. In practice, this means that unless an extraction space is present, leveling the arch will throw the lower incisors forward. Moving the molars back is not a realistic option, and transverse expansion rarely provides enough space.

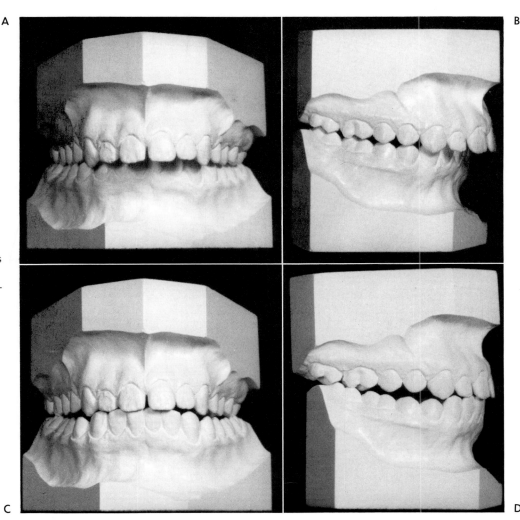

Fig. 12-19. In a mandibular-deficient patient, there is nearly always a crossbite tendency when the lower arch is moved forward, as these casts indicate. **A** and **B,** Pretreatment occlusion. **C** and **D,** Occlusion with the mandibular cast advanced, showing the posterior crossbite tendency.

In summary, the orthodontic approach to these patients usually has several elements. (1) Lateral expansion of the maxillary arch to deal with the otherwise inevitable posterior crossbite tendency after the mandibular advancement. For this reason, extraction in the upper arch rarely is necessary, even if there is moderate crowding. (2) Postsurgical leveling of the lower arch by extrusion of premolars rather than depression of incisors. This means that, although the lower teeth will be aligned before surgery, the arch will not be leveled then. Instead, the orthodontist will maintain the existing curve of Spee. Last, (3) extraction or nonextraction treatment of the lower arch. This will depend on the extent of crowding, how much additional space will be needed to level the arch, and the AP position of the incisors. Extraction of lower but not upper premolars will be needed in a significant number of patients.

Informed Consent

The procedure for obtaining informed consent outlined in Chapter 6 should be followed. Patients need to be aware of the benefits of treatment and of its risks and costs. For these patients, who have mandibular deficiency with a deep overbite and at least a tendency toward short facial proportions, the following points are important:

1. A major benefit of treatment will be improved dental and jaw function. Elimination of the deep overbite provides normal incisor function. It also reduces the chance of soft-tissue problems because of lower incisors impinging against the palate. If TM joint symptoms are present, they may be improved but are likely not to be totally eliminated.

2. Facial proportions also will be changed as the jaw is moved forward and downward. The change in appearance often is subtle, but patients usually are pleased with it. The patient can approximate the esthetic change just by holding the jaw forward.

3. There are three main risks of the orthodontic phase of the treatment: root resorption, enamel decalcification, and recession of gingival tissue. Each of these has a 5% to 10% probability of occurring but only a very small chance of being severe enough to become clinically significant, unless there are unusual risk factors such as preexisting resorption.

4. There are three types of risks associated with the surgery: a small but not zero chance of catastrophe; a 5% to 10% chance of intraoperative complications that might modify the procedure, lengthen the hospital stay, or alter the method of fixation; and a 10% to 20% chance of a long-term sensory deficit of the lower lip.

5. There will be a limitation of jaw movement following the surgery. Physical therapy will be necessary postsurgically, 6 to 12 months will be needed to attain the maximum return of movement, some long-term loss of mobility should be expected, and (as is true for any patient) there is a chance that TM joint problems will arise in the future.

In addition, the costs of treatment—orthodontic, surgical, hospital, other—should be presented clearly and discussed to prevent any misunderstanding. This type of review with the patient should be carried out before the presurgical orthodontics begins. It is not necessary at this stage to discuss all the details of the surgical experience. That is better deferred until just before the patient enters the hospital.

PRESURGICAL ORTHODONTICS

In this discussion, we assume that any necessary preparation for the orthodontic-surgical treatment (e.g., gingival grafts to the lower incisor area, appropriate restorations, and premolar, third molar, or other extractions) has been completed. We also assume that a contemporary edgewise appliance has been placed.

The goals of presurgical orthodontics for these patients are to (1) align irregular teeth, (2) establish AP and vertical incisor position, and (3) establish compatible arch forms. The steps in treatment follow this sequence.

The preferred approach to alignment depends on the degree of crowding. For most patients, the initial arch wire should be 16-mil super-elastic (austentitic) NiTi. If there is good alignment initially, a less flexible wire is acceptable. Extremely irregular teeth, particularly if one tooth is far out of line, may still be an indication for bending loops in 14-mil steel (see Case 2 below).

The keys to the presurgical treatment of these patients are the second and third items in the sequence, particularly the vertical placement of the incisors. As pointed out above, for most of these patients the approach to leveling will be extrusion post-surgically, which means that the excessive curve of Spee in the lower arch must be maintained before surgery. In conventional orthodontic treatment, it is almost routine to begin leveling the arches after preliminary alignment is completed. In these presurgical patients, a reverse curve in the upper arch usually is eliminated, but the lower arch is not leveled.

For patients who will be treated with postsurgical leveling, the second set of arch wires usually should be 16-mil steel, flat in the upper arch and with an accentuated rather than reverse curve of Spee in the lower. A sequence of heavier arch wires, still maintaining the curve of Spee in the lower arch, then is employed to gain arch compatibility and position the teeth in the AP plane of space.

Some patients do require intrusion of the lower and/or upper incisors presurgically to partially or completely level the arches. The only way to obtain significant intrusion is with a segmented arch approach, and it is better to use this from the beginning. For intrusion of the maxillary incisors, anchorage control in the form of a transpalatal lingual arch is mandatory. If more than a small amount of lower incisor intrusion is needed, a lower lingual arch also should be used. The preliminary alignment is done with flexible wires within the segments of the arch (e.g., with separate wires posteriorly and from canine to canine). An auxiliary depressing arch is used to produce the force system needed for intrusion (see Chapter 1, Case 3). Once the desired vertical position is achieved, a series of heavier continuous arch wires is used to establish AP incisor position and obtain compatible arch forms, exactly as with the more usual approach.

If lower premolars were extracted, the extraction space should be closed (or nearly so) at this stage. More specifically, if the lower arch was leveled presurgically, the space should be closed. If it was not, it may be desirable to leave 1 to 2 mm of space so that AP incisor position does not have to be changed during the postsurgical leveling (see Chapter 6, Fig. 6-19).

The culmination of presurgical orthodontic treatment is the placement of the arch wires that will be used for stabilization during surgery. These should be full-dimension rectangular wires—17×25 steel with the 18-slot appliance, or 21×25 with the 22-slot appliance. In the 22-slot appliance, either steel or TMA wires are acceptable for stabilization. Just before surgery, unless the appliance has integral hooks on the brackets, hooks or soldered spurs (with TMA wire, welded spurs) are added to the arch wires for use in maxillomandibular fixation. Even if RIF will make long-term maxillomandibular fixation unnecessary, it is needed in the operating room, and so these attachments still are required.

FINAL PRESURGICAL PLANNING

At the point that the orthodontist feels the patient is ready for surgery, complete records are taken. These include panoramic and lateral cephalometric radiographs; a PA cephalometric radiograph if needed, as for instance if asymmetry is present; facial and intraoral photographs; and dental casts for use in the model surgery and splint construction. When mandibular ramus surgery alone is planned, it is not necessary to mount the casts on a semiadjustable articulator.

No further tooth movement should occur after these records are taken, particularly after the impressions for the model surgery. Otherwise, planning errors may occur and the splints may not fit properly. At a minimum, the stabilizing arch wires should have been in place for 24 to 48 hours before the final presurgical impressions are made. A better sequence is to place the stabilizing wires a few weeks before the records appointment. Then, a week or so before surgery, the final impressions can be taken while the arch wires have been removed to have the fixation spurs added. If these

wires are replaced with no other alterations, they will be passive.

Before the surgery, the surgeon should do a cephalometric prediction using the current cephalometric radiograph and complete the model surgery. For these patients, the model surgery requires only that the casts be repositioned on an arbitrary articulator, but exactly how they are placed is important, and the orthodontist should review and approve this before the surgical splint is made. The dental relationships established at this time will largely determine the prolongation and difficulty of the postsurgical orthodontics. Guidelines for positioning the casts at this stage (Fig. 12-20) are:
1. Keep things symmetric in the transverse plane of space. Usually, there is a posterior crossbite tendency that the postsurgical orthodontics will correct. It is much easier to do this with small bilateral movements of posterior teeth.
2. Bring the incisors into an ideal relationship, correcting but not over-correcting the overjet and overbite. Avoid bringing the mandible so far forward that an anterior crossbite is produced.
3. Keep the skeletal midlines correct, even if this means that the dental midlines are slightly off. Dental midlines can be corrected during the postsurgical orthodontics, but there is little or nothing the orthodontist can do later about incorrect skeletal midlines.
4. If wire osteosynthesis and maxillomandibular fixation is planned, it is acceptable to bring the incisors to almost an edge-to-edge position and to separate the posterior teeth by up to 2 mm (but remember that the thicker the splint, the greater the chance of a significant error in positioning the jaw, which will make the finishing orthodontics more rather than less difficult) (see Case 2 below). If RIF is planned, even minimal over-correction of the incisors should be avoided, and the splint should be as thin as possible without making it too fragile (see Fig. 12-20). We recommend uniform splint thickness for RIF cases—avoid greater separation of the posterior teeth.

When the model surgery is satisfactory to all concerned, the surgical splint is fabricated as shown in detail in Chapter 7. When RIF is used, the patient may be allowed to function into the splint soon after the surgery. Even with wire fixation, a period of function into the splint for 2 to 4 weeks after maxillomandibular fixation release seems to help the patient regain jaw function. Incorporating ball clasps into the splint when it is fabricated initially enables the patient to remove it for cleaning, and we suggest this modification.

SURGERY

The surgical procedure is matched to the patient's problem list and selected to solve his or her particular

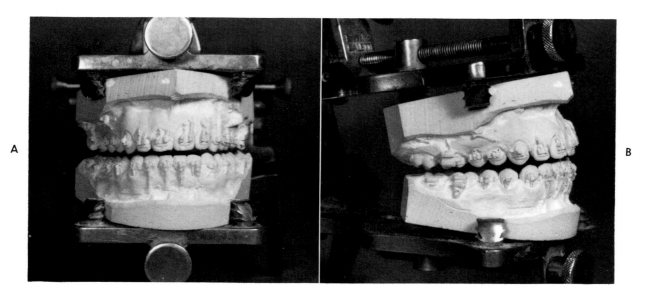

Fig. 12-20. Casts positioned before splint construction (same patient as Fig. 12-19). Note the limited amount of vertical separation. There is no advantage in making the splint thicker than the minimum necessary to provide adequate strength.

set of problems. When several surgical options exist, they should be presented to the patient, with a preferred approach indicated. Obviously, the final decision belongs to the patient. Usually the patient will accept the surgeon's recommendation.

Bilateral sagittal split osteotomy currently is the procedure of choice for lengthening a deficient mandible. The surgery is predictable, performed intraorally, and allows both lengthening of the mandible and an increase in face height with minimal alteration in the length of the elevator muscles of the mandible. It is quite compatible with RIF, minimizing the duration of maxillomandibular fixation. Inferior border osteotomy may be combined with the sagittal split osteotomy, either to provide additional mandibular length or (more frequently in this group of patients) to control what otherwise would become excessive AP or vertical prominence of the chin (see Fig. 12-17).

The technique for the bilateral sagittal split osteotomy for these patients is exactly the one described in detail in Chapter 9. The position of the maxillary and mandibular incisors controls the amount the mandible can be advanced and the face height after surgery. Both the orthodontist and the surgeon must agree on the orthodontic positioning of the incisors before treatment begins. The exact position of the incisors cannot always be achieved, but a goal for incisor position should be set.

The decision about inferior border osteotomy along with sagittal split osteotomy need not be made until the presurgical orthodontics is complete. If this is anticipated from the outset, it should be mentioned to the patient before any treatment. Often the decision is

more clear after the presurgical cephalometric prediction tracing. Most patients can make a decision regarding inferior border osteotomy even though the advantages and disadvantages are presented to them just before surgery. Details of this procedure are described in Chapter 10.

Lengthening the mandibular lower border via inferior border osteotomy is a predictable procedure to influence lip function and improve esthetics. Alloplastic augmentation (see Chapter 10) is less desirable but may be necessary in some cases. Particularly in this group of patients, where a large chin and deficient lower lip are high on the problem list, AP reduction of the inferior border of the mandible may be needed. This procedure can improve lip function, but after bony reduction, the soft tissue does not necessarily follow the bony support, so esthetic results are less predictable.

The surgeon must decide whether mandibular erupted or impacted third molars should be removed in advance of sagittal split osteotomy. The teeth are in the surgical site and occupy space that would be filled with bone if no third molars were present. The third molars can be removed at the time of sagittal split osteotomy, but this approach increases the chance of a poor split. Early removal may make it easier to use RIF. Often the best site for lag or position screws is in the third molar area, and it may not be possible to place a screw in the area where a third molar was just removed. The decision regarding third molar removal should be made by the surgeon before or very early in the presurgical orthodontic phase of treatment, more than 6 months before anticipated jaw surgery.

Many patients with mandibular deficiency have had

a long-standing habit of posturing their lower jaw forward to improve their function and esthetics. These patients pose special problems. In the planning stages, photographs, cephalometric radiographs, and occlusal records should all be taken with the mandible in the most retruded contact position. In some instances, the orthodontist and surgeon do not recognize that the patient is postured forward. In other patients, it is difficult for the patient to abandon the forward posture, and a consistent retruded contact position cannot be obtained. In this group of patients where only mandibular surgery is contemplated, planning can proceed if a position close to retruded contact position can be obtained.

Additional problems can arise during sagittal split osteotomy. Jaw lengthening and fixation is predicated on the surgeon being able to seat the condyle in the fossa as the ramus segment is positioned against the advanced tooth-bearing segment. Accurately positioning the condyle at surgery—it usually positions forward in the fossa in these patients—may not be possible. After surgery, if the condyle moves posteriorly the entire mandible will appear to shorten, usually 1 to 3 mm with an occlusal discrepancy of a similar magnitude. If a patient has this habit of posturing the mandible forward, the possibility of not being able to position the condyle properly at surgery and the consequences must be discussed with the patient. In most circumstances, the orthodontist can compensate for this minor shift in occlusion after surgery.

In some instances, mandibular subapical osteotomy is the procedure of choice, primarily when there is a deficiency in the position of the mandibular dentition but a very prominent chin. This surgical technique is quite effective in decreasing the labiomental fold and reducing the relative prominence of the chin—but remember that anterior face height is altered minimally with subapical osteotomy. Face height must be close to normal proportions if this approach is taken. The surgical technique is illustrated in detail in Chapter 10. To cut beneath the mandibular posterior teeth, the mandibular neurovascular bundle must be exposed, displaced laterally, and protected, which is increasingly difficult in the second molar region where the bundle lies deeper within the bone. Despite the potential difficulty in managing the nerve and vessels, neurosensory disturbances are no worse with this procedure than with bilateral sagittal split osteotomy.[11] Adequate bone also must exist beneath the teeth to maintain the integrity of the inferior border of the mandible after subapical bone cuts are made.

When there is significant asymmetry or it is necessary to lengthen the mandible more than 15 mm, an extraoral mandibular ramus procedure may be indicated. This circumstance is quite rare in a patient with a normal or deficient face height. The technique is illus-

trated (though for a patient with a somewhat different problem) in Chapter 9.

In addition to mandibular advancement, maxillary surgery occasionally is required in mandibular-deficient patients, primarily to widen the maxilla. A transverse deficiency greater than 4 to 5 mm, which is the maximum that can be handled with postsurgical orthodontics, is the usual indication for maxillary surgery. Although the surgical expansion can be accomplished with posterior segmental osteotomies, the preferred approach is LeFort I osteotomy with two (occasionally three) segments. With the LeFort I osteotomy, surgical access is better, the results are more predictable, and morbidity is no worse than with the isolated segments.

Moving the entire maxilla down without rotation as a way to deal with short anterior face height in mandibular-deficient patients almost never is indicated. If the upper incisors need to be brought down relative to the lip to give them greater exposure, LeFort I osteotomy allows rotating the maxilla down anteriorly without bringing it down posteriorly.

Surgical techniques for combining maxillary and mandibular surgery are described in Chapter 11.

POSTSURGICAL ORTHODONTICS

The goals of postsurgical orthodontics are to bring the teeth into excellent occlusion, correcting any discrepancies that exist after surgical repositioning of the jaw. Typically, in a mandibular-advancement patient whose lower arch is to be leveled postsurgically, vertical spaces will exist between some maxillary and mandibular teeth when the patient returns from the surgeon and the splint is removed (Fig. 12-21). Depending on the extent of the postsurgical leveling, there also may be a small amount of mandibular extraction space remaining to be closed, and a mild crossbite tendency may exist in some areas.

In our opinion, the surgical splint should not be removed until the patient is ready to resume finishing orthodontics. The patient should wear it at all times until the stabilizing arch wires also can be replaced by the postsurgical working arch wires. With RIF, the patient functions into the splint, removing it only for cleaning (which is possible if it is retained by clasps). There is no problem with functioning into the splint, for several weeks if desired, except that the patient might feel more comfortable without it. The price of that comfort can be major difficulties in the finishing orthodontics.

The reason the splint is so important is that mandibular-advancement patients who are to be leveled postsurgically typically make a "three-point landing" occlusally immediately after the surgery, hitting only on the incisors and on a single molar bilaterally. With the splint in place, there is no problem in knowing where to bite. Without it, there is no solid occlusion, and pa-

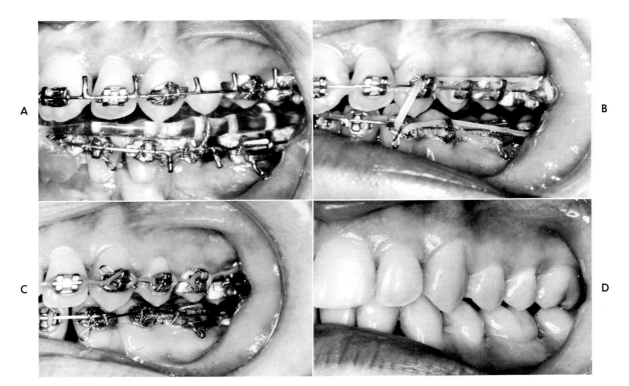

Fig. 12-21. Steps in the finishing orthodontics sequence for a typical mandibular-deficient, deep-bite patient who was planned for postsurgical leveling of the lower arch. **A,** Patient functioning into the splint after release of maxillomandibular fixation (which in this rigid fixation case occurred 3 days postsurgically). **B,** Occlusal relationships immediately after removal of the splint and stabilizing arch wires (at 4 weeks postsurgically). Note the vertical separation in the premolar-first molar region—the second molars and incisors are in contact. **C,** Occlusal relationships 8 weeks later. At that point, the box elastics were discontinued and 17×25 TMA arch wires were placed for final positioning of the teeth. **D,** Occlusal relationships 6 months postsurgically, 4 weeks after appliance removal. Even with greater leveling than this patient required, the teeth typically come into good occlusion by the third postsurgical appointment.

tients tend to develop mandibular shifts to maximize occlusal contact. If the shift persists for even a few weeks and healing progresses, the resulting centric relation-centric occlusion discrepancy can be quite difficult to eliminate later.

Orthodontic treatment should resume only when the surgeon thinks bony healing allows it (complete bony healing takes 6 months or more). Typically, this is 6 weeks with conventional wire and maxillomandibular fixation, a bit less with RIF. At that point, the splint and the stabilizing arch wires are removed, any loose bands or broken bonds are replaced, light working arch wires are placed, and light vertical elastics are continued. Typically, the initial working arch wires are 16 steel, with a reverse curve of Spee in the lower arch and an accentuated curve in the upper, and the elastics are ⅜-inch light latex worn in a box pattern (see Fig. 12-21 and Cases 2 and 3, below). If desired, a flexible rectangular wire can be used in the upper to maintain better torque control of the incisors, or the stabilizing wire can remain there for absolute control. The princi-

ple is that as function without the splint resumes, the teeth must be free to move into their final occlusion. Settling into occlusion will occur more quickly, of course, if the teeth in both arches can move.

We recommend that, following isolated mandibular advancement, the posterior box elastics should be worn full time for the first 3 or 4 weeks, including during eating. Anterior elastics would be removed for eating. At the second postsurgical appointment, the arch wires are adjusted if necessary, and elastic wear during eating can be eliminated. By the third appointment (i.e., 2 months after orthodontic treatment was resumed) the teeth almost always have settled into a solid occlusion with good centric occlusion-centric relation harmony. At this point, the settling elastics are no longer necessary and final arch wire adjustments to correct individual tooth positions are made. If a heavier rectangular wire is needed in the lower arch, this is the time to place it. For many of these patients, the orthodontic appliance can be removed at the fourth postsurgical appointment, 3 months after the finishing orthodontics began.

If there is a posterior crossbite tendency, two approaches are possible. Crossbite elastics can be employed, or an auxiliary expansion arch wire can be used (see Case 1, below). At the time they return for the finishing orthodontics, mandibular-advancement patients nearly always have limited opening, and this can make placing cross elastics difficult. A heavy labial auxiliary arch wire (36- or 40-mil steel) placed in the headgear tubes often is an attractive alternative.

A tooth positioner can be used in a postsurgical patient if desired—after the jaw has healed, the muscle stimulation created by the positioner would do no harm and might even help in regaining function. It must be kept in mind, however, that whether or not they have had surgical treatment, patients with a deep overbite tend to relapse in that direction, and tooth positioners tend to deepen the bite anteriorly. In addition, a positioner may not be tolerated well in a patient who still does not have normal sensation in the lower lip and gingiva. An alternative approach for finishing is to remove the appliance (after segmenting and partially removing the arch wires to allow final settling, if desired)[12] and go directly to a maxillary retainer with a biteplate behind the upper incisors, so that overbite control is maintained. The design of the lower retainer is determined by the original malocclusion. In most instances, a canine-to-canine clip-on retainer is satisfactory. The retainers need to be worn full-time except during eating for 3 to 4 months, then part-time for another 6 to 8 months. It should be possible to discontinue retention within 12 months for essentially all of these adult patients.

RESPONSE TO TREATMENT
Postsurgical Recovery

Neurosensory alterations, particularly over the distribution of the inferior alveolar nerve, are a predictable sequelae of sagittal split osteotomy, whether or not visible damage to the neurovascular bundle at surgery was observed. Numbness of the lip usually lasts for several weeks, then gives way to a patchy recovery that includes tingling sensations. Often there are transient areas of hyperesthesia that are painful or produce an electrical shock sensation when touched. It appears that recovery of sensation occurs over a full year for many patients. Beyond that time, some additional recovery is possible, but not predictable. Patients are counseled regarding neurosensory changes before surgery and they usually can accept sensory deficits that exist. Zaytoun and colleagues attribute this acceptance to the overall positive result of surgery, including function and esthetic improvement.[13]

Following lengthening of the mandible with sagittal split osteotomy, there is a limitation of opening when jaw function resumes. Most patients return to good jaw function within 3 months following surgery, but some experience a degree of permanent limitation.

With RIF, the period of limited function is shortened for many patients. Having 25 mm of vertical opening at the incisors at the third postsurgery week is not unusual. There is some evidence that regaining jaw movement after surgery is facilitated by physical therapy[14] as well as by limiting the duration of immobilization. A discussion of jaw rehabilitation following osteotomy and a suggested physical therapy regimen for patients having difficulty is presented in Chapter 6. We recommend that this rehabilitation schedule be followed to reduce the amount of change that occurs.

Physiologic Response
Lip Pressure

When the mandible is moved forward, and especially when the mandibular body is rotated downward anteriorly to correct deep overbite and increase face height, the lower incisors are tipped forward into the lip. The expected result would be an increase in lip pressure against these teeth and a tendency for the incisors to upright lingually. Clinically, crowding of lower incisors after mandibular advancement has not been a major problem, and recent measurements of lip pressure before and after the surgery indicate the reason.

Proffit and colleagues placed small pressure transducers in a thin plastic carrier, so that the surface of the measuring devices remained within approximately 2 mm of the incisor surface, and measured lip pressures before and 6 months and 1 year after mandibular advancement.[15] Lip pressures did not increase as expected. It appears that there is a surprisingly large degree of adaptation in lip function following surgery, and this contributes to the posttreatment stability of incisor position that commonly is observed.

Biting Force

The jaws are a classic lever system, with the jaw muscles interposed between the point of force delivery (the teeth) and the fulcrum (the TM joint). Increasing the distance between the muscle attachments and the teeth, as by an osteotomy to move the mandible forward, therefore should reduce biting force, or at least would do so if the geometry of the jaws were a major influence. Because the amount of advancement is small relative to the total length of the jaw, however, the change in biting force should be small, about 10%.[16]

In fact, advancing the mandible in patients with short or normal face height often changes occlusal force considerably in either direction.[17] Some patients have little or no change; others bite significantly harder after this surgery or have a considerable decrease in bite force. About a third of the patients fall into each category, and on the average there is no change. In this as in many other situations that clinicians have to deal with, the unchanged average is misleading. The variability is the clinically relevant item (see Chapter 13, Fig. 13-18).

Occlusal force is a physiologic measure of what the patient will do, influenced to an unknown extent by what he or she can do. The effect of jaw geometry easily could be overcome by physiologic feedback mechanisms, and obviously this is what happens. For instance, when bite force increases after mandibular advancement, it is possible that the patients' improved occlusion allows them to bite harder without discomfort, or that a degree of sensory deficit in the periodontal ligament reduces the inhibitory feedback from pressure receptors that modulates bite force and prevents damage. Decreased bite force could be related to the change in geometry, but also to increased inhibition from sore teeth that recently experienced orthodontic tooth movement or from TM joint receptors.

Feedback into the physiologic control system can come from higher levels as well as from peripheral receptors. A patient who believed that his or her jaw was fragile after surgery would be understandably reluctant to bite hard, whereas one who thought that with screws in place it was stronger than ever, might really crunch down on the measuring device. Previous studies of influences on biting force have suggested that the patient's mental state does have an effect.[18] It is interesting to note in the data that maximum biting force and the force for simulated chewing change almost exactly in parallel, whereas the force with which the teeth are brought into contact during swallowing (which is less voluntary) changes in a slightly different pattern. This suggests that what the patient thinks really may be an important factor in how hard he or she is willing to bite.

In summary, at this point we do not know how to predict the effect of mandibular advancement on biting force. Despite the geometry, which predicts that it should decrease, it is as likely to increase.

Temporomandibular Joint Function

It is all but impossible to carry out mandibular ramus surgery without changing the position of the mandibular condyle in the TM joint. Even if the center of the condyle is maintained precisely in its presurgical location—which is possible, but small changes of 1 to 2 mm in any of the three planes of space are likely—the condyle nearly always rotates in either or both of two planes, around and across the condylar axis.

Rotation around the condylar axis will occur if the ramus inclines forward after the osteotomy. Keeping the ramus upright may improve postsurgical stability,[19] but there is no evidence that this type of rotation has any long-term effect on joint function or is related to the development of TM joint problems. Rotation in this plane always occurs when the maxilla is moved superiorly and the mandible rotates upward and forward in response, again without apparent effect on function (see Chapter 13).

Rotation across the condylar axis occurs when the condyle is twisted as the ramus and body fragments are reapproximated. Any change in the thickness of the ramus requires some reorientation of the football-shaped condyle. This occurs to a larger degree when the mandible is set back and the ramus and body fragments are overlapped (see Chapter 14), but some rotation is inevitable with advancement. Again, there is no evidence that this is related in any way to the development of TM joint problems at a later time.

The fact that long-term problems do not arise does not mean that there are no short-term effects. After sagittal split advancement, as we have described above, patients experience a considerable limitation of opening. In part, this is related to the surgical incisions and detachment of muscles at surgery, but in part it probably is related to the postsurgical orientation of the condyle. Remodeling of the joint (changes in bony contour on both the temporal and mandibular sides) would be expected as a response to the surgery, and there is evidence the remodeling does occur.[20,21] Patients regain jaw opening at a rate that is more compatible with the speed of bone remodeling than with resolution of soft-tissue wounds, and understanding the necessity of condylar remodeling makes it easier to understand what is happening in this regard.

With RIF, it is possible to torque the condyle medially or laterally or move the condyle in the transverse plane when the screws are placed. This does have the potential to cause both TM joint pain and severe limitation of jaw movement. This technical problem can be overcome with proper technique (see Chapters 7 and 9 for a more complete discussion).

Stability

Following mandibular advancement, changes potentially can occur in three important time frames: (1) during the first 6 weeks postsurgically (stabilization, initial healing); (2) during the first year (completion of healing, postsurgical orthodontics); and (3) long-term (beyond 1 year posttreatment). These are examined in turn.

1. *The first 6 weeks postsurgically.* McNeill and co-workers at the University of Washington[22,23] were the first to document that after mandibular advancement with wire fixation at the osteotomy sites and maxillomandibular fixation, there is a short-term tendency for the mandible to slip posteriorly, even though the occlusion is maintained. A number of subsequent investigations, including a recent report from our clinic,[24] have confirmed that changes occur during fixation. Orthodontic tooth movement, in response to the light but steady pressure from stretched soft tissues, makes this skeletal relapse possible: as the lower teeth move forward slightly and the incisors tip labially, while the upper teeth are retracted slightly and the incisors tip lingually, the chin can slip back. The effect on the dentition is remarkably similar to that of Class II elastics (see Chapter 5, Fig. 5-13).

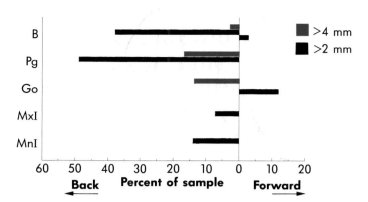

Fig. 12-22. The percentages of the group of patients with wire fixation after mandibular advancement who had changes during the period of maxillomandibular fixation. Note that about a third of the patients had no AP change at pogonion, whereas 50% had 2 to 4 mm and 18% had more than 4 mm of change. The majority of patients had less than 2 mm change at other landmarks.

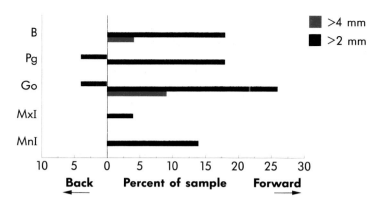

Fig. 12-23. The percentages of the group of patients with screw fixation after mandibular advancement who had changes during the first 6 weeks postsurgically. Note that in this group, most of the patients had no change, but pogonion and point B came forward in about 15%. The overall pattern of change is quite different from the wire fixation group shown in Fig. 12-22.

At first the relapse tendency was blamed on the suprahyoid muscles, and myotomy of the anterior belly of the digastric and the geniohyoid was proposed to control it. Recent work with monkeys supports the concept,[25] but evidence in humans indicates that this does not improve stability.[26] The changes seem to be due to the gentle but constant pull of the stretched soft tissues around the mandible. All other things being equal, the greater the advancement, the greater the relapse tendency, presumably because there is more soft-tissue stretching with larger advancements. This relationship only becomes clear when the advancement is greater than 8 to 10 mm. There also is a relationship between the time that it takes for healing and the amount of relapse because changes continue until the the osteotomy site becomes strong enough to resist the soft-tissue pull. McNeill and coworkers[22] suggested that taking head films at 1-week intervals and observing whether changes occurred was one way to evaluate healing. When the changes stopped, clinical healing had occurred, usually at 5 to 6 weeks. Patients who have some complication that delays healing nearly always have more short-term relapse, which would be expected. More frequent clinical and radiographic examination is indicated in the these patients.

Although the general description above is accurate, the amount of individual variation in this response also is impressive. By no means do all patients show the typical response (Fig. 12-22). Surgical technique undoubtedly is an important variable and was the most important one in Schendel and Epker's early study.[26] How accurately the surgeon can position the condyles after the osteotomy probably contributes to the difference in techniques.[27] Nevertheless, there are no good data to demonstrate that stability is significantly better with, for instance, the sagittal split osteotomy as opposed to another design. Why some patients show better stability than others is not as clear as we might wish.

If relapse during initial healing is due to the inability of the teeth to resist sustained soft-tissue pressure, skeletal fixation should produce better stability. In monkeys, Ellis and coworkers[28] have demonstrated that maxillomandibular fixation alone after mandibular advancement produced the same pattern of short-term relapse seen in human patients, but either RIF without wiring the teeth together or supplementing dental with skeletal fixation (piriform aperture and circummandibular wires) was effective in maintaining the advancement. In humans, there is evidence that short-term stability is better when screws are used for RIF after mandibular advancement.[29,30]

Recent data from the UNC Dentofacial Program allow a comparison of stability after mandibular advancement with wire osteosynthesis and RIF (Fig. 12-23). The results in a series of 76 mandibular-deficient patients with deep or normal bite who underwent sagittal split advancement with wire fixation confirm the general picture described above.[24] On the average, the mandible slipped back and rotated downward during the first 6 weeks, while the patients were in maxillomandibular fixation. The incisors were elongated in compensation; the upper incisors tipped back and the lowers forward (Fig. 12-24). In a comparable group of RIF patients,[31] the tendency for the mandible to slip down and back was lessened by the screws (Fig. 12-25).

With rigid as with conventional fixation, there is impressive variability among the patients (see Fig. 12-23). It is true that average relapse is less, but many rigid fixation patients have significant changes. In fact, the data indicate that with RIF during the first 6 weeks, the mandible is as likely to go forward as to slip posteriorly. The reason is not known with certainty. With RIF

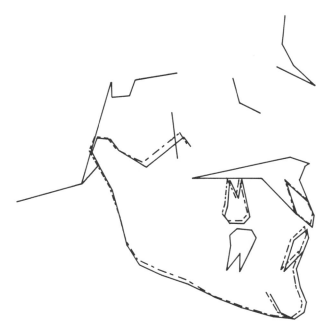

Fig. 12-24. Composite tracing, UNC patients with wire fixation after mandibular advancement (N = 76). On the average, the chin slipped back and down while the teeth were in maxillomandibular fixation *(dashed red)*. The relationship of the lower to the upper incisors was maintained (i.e., the lower incisors were proclined relative to the chin). A tracing of this type illustrates the mean changes—but the variability in the sample illustrated in Fig. 12-22 must be kept in mind.

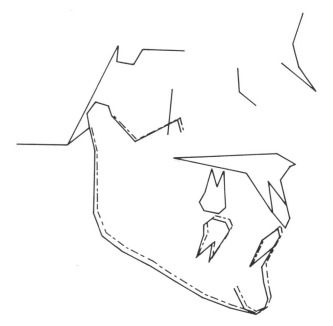

Fig. 12-25. Composite tracing, UNC patients with rigid (screw) fixation after mandibular advancement (N = 35) (immediate postsurgery, *solid red;* 6 weeks postsurgery, *dashed red*). Note that average changes in both the AP and vertical planes of space were smaller than the average changes in the wire group (compare with Fig. 12-24).

the surgeon is able to force the condyle back into the temporal fossa as he or sher could not with wire osteosynthesis. It seems reasonable that if this were overdone, the patient would posture the mandible further forward, particularly in the first few weeks after surgery. Obviously, patients who had a habit of posturing forward for years might also have this tendency after surgery, particularly with early maxillomandibular fixation release.

2. *Stability from 6 weeks to 1 year.* Although Bhatia and coworkers[32] suggested that steady changes occurred for the first year postsurgically, it seems clear now that this is not the case. Instead, although changes continue after the initial healing is complete, the pattern tends to be quite different from 6 weeks to 1 year than it was during the first 6 weeks after surgery.

In the UNC patients who had traditional wire fixation, the mandible often stopped slipping posteriorly after the first 6 weeks. On the average, it moved forward instead (Fig. 12-26). In contrast, patients who had rigid fixation tended to have the mandible slip slightly more posteriorly after the first 6 weeks (Fig. 12-27). In the UNC sample, there was a statistically significant difference in the AP position of the chin between the traditional and rigid fixation groups at 6 weeks, but it disappeared at 1 year.

In comparing the two groups, it was apparent that the pattern of change was different for the vertical and AP planes of space. During initial healing, the mandibular plane tended to rotate down anteriorly and up posteriorly for the wire fixation group, but much less so for the rigid fixation group. This was due in part to the chin slipping downward and in part to remodeling resorption at the gonial angle. For the wire fixation group, these vertical changes stabilized after the first 6 weeks. For the RIF group, the vertical chin position stabilized, but remodeling at the gonial angle continued. The result is interesting and unexpected: with RIF, the ramus was shorter at 1 year than in the traditional group (i.e., there was less rather than more stability in that area). There was a trend toward slightly better vertical stability at the chin in the RIF group, but the greater change at the gonial angle with RIF was the only statistically significant difference at 1 year postsurgery.

As with the changes during initial healing, the relatively large individual variations must be kept in mind (Fig. 12-28). Note that some patients in the wire group had the mandible move further back between 6 weeks and 1 year, whereas some in the rigid fixation group had it come forward, opposite from the general trend. Most patients—about two-thirds—had little or no change, whereas one-third had more than 2 mm of change.

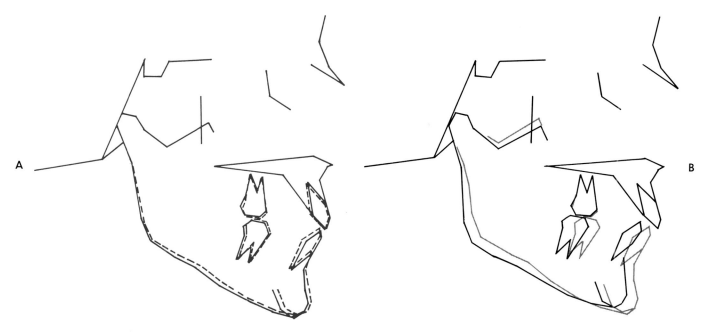

Fig. 12-26. Composite tracings, wire group. **A,** Six weeks to 1 year *(dashed red).* **B,** Presurgery to 1 year. Note the tendency for the mandible to come forward again between 6 weeks and 1 year *(pink).*

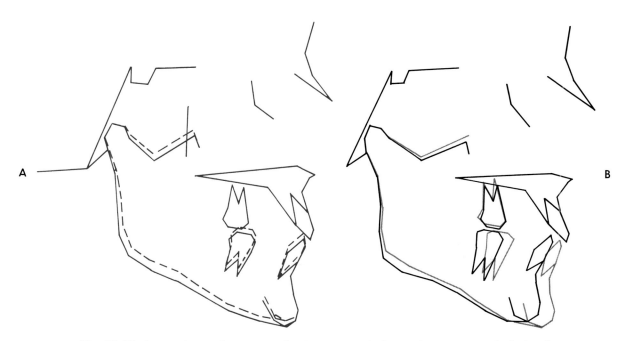

Fig. 12-27. Composite tracings, screw fixation group. **A,** Six weeks to 1 year *(dashed red).* **B,** Presurgery to 1 year *(pink).* Compare these tracings with Fig. 12-26. Although the average tracing for the wire and screw groups looked quite different at 6 weeks postsurgically, the differences had almost totally disappeared at 1 year. By then, the only statistically significant difference was the slightly higher gonial angle in the screw group.

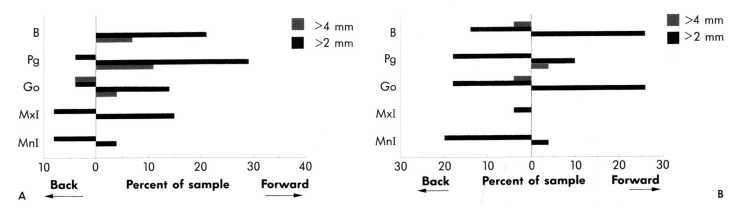

Fig. 12-28. The percentages of patients with changes from 6 weeks to 1 year postsurgically. **A,** Wire group. **B,** Screw fixation group. Note the relatively large number of wire fixation patients in whom the mandible came forward again after fixation was released. For the most part, these were the same patients who had the greatest backward movement during fixation. But in the screw group, fewer patients came forward, and more showed relapse changes. This differing pattern of medium-term response explains why the wire and screw groups looked different at 6 weeks but almost identical at 1 year.

Why the changes at the gonial angle are greater with RIF is easier to explain than why the mandible tends to come forward again when conventional maxillomandibular fixation is released. Some loss of bone at the gonial angle is inevitable when the mandibular elevator muscles are detached from the bone during the surgery (see Chapter 2 for a discussion of the muscle-bone relationship). All other things being equal, the greater the stripping of the muscles, the more net shortening of the ramus will occur. It seems reasonable that more muscle detachment is needed to place screws than to put in a superior border wire. If so, greater long-term bone remodeling would be the inevitable side effect.

The position of the mandible is established to a considerable extent by the musculature, even with the condyles "seated" in the temporal fossa. It is possible that while a patient is in maxillomandibular fixation and jaw movements are prevented, tonic innervation diminishes and the muscles are unusually passive. This would allow the mandible to be pulled more posteriorly by the stretched soft tissues. When jaw movements are resumed after maxillomandibular fixation release, some degree of anterior repositioning may occur. At the moment, this is only a plausible hypothesis—there is no direct evidence as to what really happens.

The changes that occur in patients postsurgically by no means indicate poor treatment results. Reasonable criteria for clinical success in these patients might be acceptable facial esthetics, correction of excessive overjet (postsurgical overjet 3 mm or less), and correction

of deep overbite (postsurgical overbite 3 mm or less). In the UNC group of 76 patients who had traditional wire fixation, 73 (96%) met these criteria for success.[24] Of the three who were considered failures, two had previously sustained bilateral condylar fractures and one experienced bilateral nonunion, which subsequently required a bone graft. Similar results (>90% successful) were obtained with RIF.[31] The combination of sagittal split osteotomy with orthodontic preparation and finishing is remarkably effective in correcting mandibular deficiency and the associated malocclusion.

3. Long-term stability. Although there are anecdotal reports of a few patients who experienced relapse several years after mandibular advancement, remarkably little data on long-term stability are available at this time. It is possible that a patient who had seemed quite stable, but who had been consistently posturing the mandible forward, might suddenly experience change when a disclusion splint was placed. We have had one such experience more than 2 years after surgery (Figs. 12-29 to 12-31). It also is possible that remodeling of the condylar process could continue over a long period, leading to a gradual loss of bone at the condyle and relapse in chin position. This has been observed,[33] but rarely. Clinical observation suggests that the great majority of mandibular-advancement patients are quite stable in the period from 1 to 5 and 10 years postsurgically. Data for a carefully studied sample of reasonable size will be available in the near future.

A   B   C

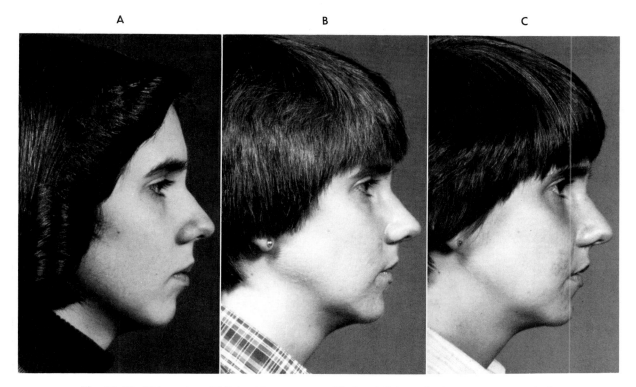

Fig. 12-29. This patient (C.D.) with severe mandibular deficiency had surgery to superiorly reposition the maxilla and advance the mandible, with a good occlusal and facial result. Two years postsurgery (18 months after removal of the orthodontic appliances), she lost her upper retainer; a new one was placed, and almost immediately she went from ideal occlusion to a half cusp Class II occlusion with 4 mm overjet. The new retainer turned out to be an inadvertent disclusion splint: the lower incisors contacted the retainer behind the upper incisors, which took the posterior teeth out of occlusion. The result was "instant relapse" as the mandible seated posteriorly in the patient, who had been posturing the mandible forward previously. Postural changes of this type are the most probable explanation for long-term changes when they occur. **A,** Pretreatment. **B,** Posttreatment. **C,** Immediately after the new retainer.

A   B   C

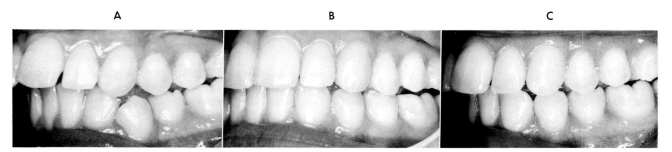

Fig. 12-30. Patient C.D., occlusal views. **A,** Pretreatment. **B,** Completion of treatment. **C,** After the new retainer.

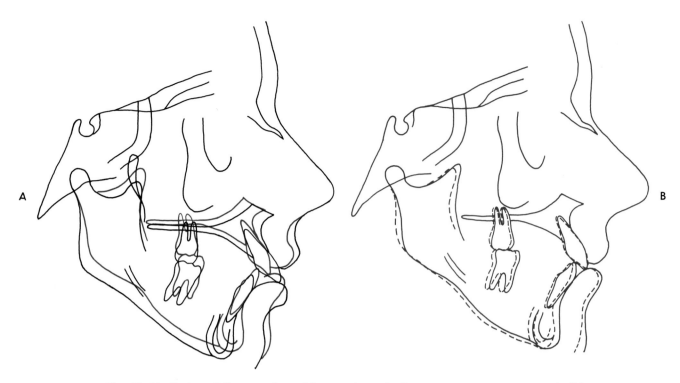

Fig. 12-31. Patient C.D., superimposition tracings. **A,** Presurgery to posttreatment *(solid red)*. **B,** Before/after *(dashed red)* new retainer.

CASE REPORTS

Case 1

J.W., age 48 years, 10 months, and a businessman, sought orthodontic consultation after being told by his family dentist that he was in danger of losing his maxillary central incisors because of his impinging overbite and that restorative replacement would be almost impossible unless his occlusion were corrected. His chief complaint was the deep overbite and the maxillary central diastema, which he reported had become larger in the last few years. He had no facial esthetic concerns. His medical history revealed hypertension that had been controlled with medication over the previous 3 years.

On clinical examination, the periodontal condition was good except for moderate inflammation lingual to the maxillary incisors. Numerous teeth had been restored. Maximum opening was 48 mm, with normal protrusive and lateral movements and no TM joint sounds. Lower face height was short, with a strong chin button, retrusive lower lip, and exaggerated labiomental fold (Fig. 12-32). The occlusion was full cusp Class II on the right and half cusp Class II on the left, with 8 mm overjet and a deep overbite (Fig. 12-33). The mandibular incisors were moderately crowded.

Panoramic and bitewing radiographs confirmed good alveolar bone levels in all areas and numerous restorations that generally were satisfactory. Cephalometric analysis (Fig. 12-34) showed AP mandibular deficiency and skeletal deep bite, with the mandible rotated upward and forward and relative undereruption of posterior teeth. The lower incisors were protrusive relative to the mandible.

J.W.'s problems were summarized as (1) skeletal deep bite with short anterior face height, (2) mandibular deficiency, and (3) flared and spaced maxillary incisors, with crowded and moderately protrusive mandibular incisors. The preferred solution to the first and second problems was bilateral osteotomy of the mandibular ramus, advancing the mandible and rotating it to increase the mandibular plane angle. Correcting the third problem would require extraction in the mandibular but not in the maxillary arch.

The treatment plan was as follows:
1. Extraction of mandibular left and right first premolars.
2. Placement of a complete fixed edgewise appliance (18-slot), with bands on molars and bonded attachments anteriorly.
3. Alignment and space closure in both arches, retracting the lower incisors about 2 mm, but with no effort to depress the incisors and without leveling the lower arch.

Case 1—cont'd.

4. Maxillary and mandibular 17×25 steel stabilizing arch wires with soldered intermaxillary hooks in final preparation for surgery. The presurgical phase of treatment was estimated to require 12 months.
5. Bilateral sagittal split osteotomies, with maxillomandibular fixation for 6 weeks and function into the splint for an additional 2 to 3 weeks.
6. Finishing orthodontics, with postsurgical leveling of the lower arch.
7. Orthodontic retainers full-time for 3 to 4 months, then on a decreasing part-time basis for the next year.
8. Replacement of posterior restorations postsurgically as needed and desired. Ideally, following completion of postsurgical orthodontics, the existing restorations would be replaced with new ones coordinated to the new occusal relationships.

The orthodontic treatment began with 16-mil nickel-titanium (16 NiTi) arch wires. These were followed by 16 steel, then 16×22 closing loops in the lower arch. After space closure was completed, 17×25 nickel-

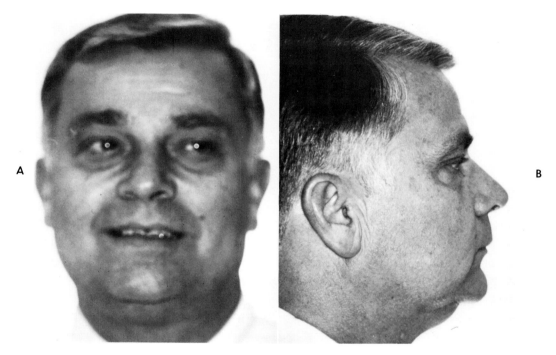

Fig. 12-32. J.W., age 48 years, 10 months, pretreatment facial photographs.

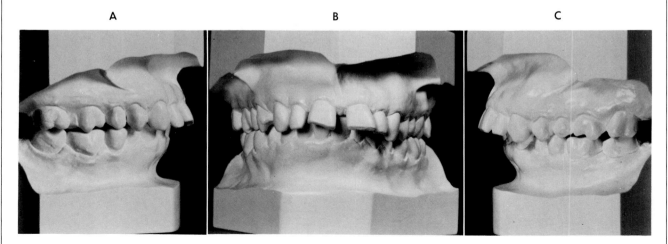

Fig. 12-33. J.W., pretreatment dental casts. Note the anterior deep bite and overjet.

Continued.

Case 1—cont'd.

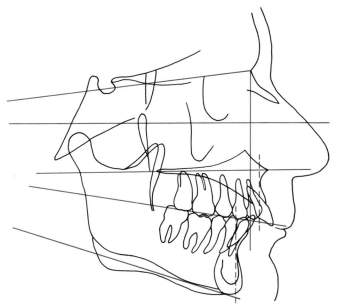

Fig. 12-34. J.W., pretreatment cephalometric tracing. Cephalometric measurements: N perp to A, 5 mm; N perp to Pg, −5 mm; AB difference, 12 mm; UFH, 54 mm; LFH, 68 mm; mand plane, 17 degrees; MxI to A vert, 6 mm, 31 degrees; MnI to B vert, 9 mm, 38 degrees. The maxillary dental protrusion and mandibular deficiency can be seen readily in the relative positions of the upper incisors and chin, respectively, to the anterior vertical reference line. Note that anterior face height is somewhat short.

titanium wires were used in both arches, and then 17×25 steel wires were placed for final arch coordination. After these had been in place long enough to be passive, lugs were added, and these wires were used for surgical stabilization. As planned, the lower arch was not leveled (Fig. 12-35), but the upper and lower incisors were retracted during the presurgical preparation (Fig. 12-36, *A*).

Fourteen months after the presurgical orthodontics began, J.W. was admitted to NC Memorial Hospital, and the sagittal split osteotomies were carried out uneventfully. Postoperative films showed the condyles were seated in

the fossa with the mandible advanced to the predetermined position (Fig. 12-36, *B*). He was discharged 2 days postsurgically in maxillomandibular fixation. Fixation was released 6 weeks postsurgically. He functioned into the splint for an additional 3 weeks, guided with ⅜-inch, 2-oz elastics for the initial week. Then the splint and stabilizing arch wires were removed, 16-mil steel wires were placed, and ⅜-inch, 3½-oz latex elastics were placed in a box pattern posteriorly, to be worn full time, and anteriorly, to be worn at night only. Three weeks later, a 36-mil steel wire was placed in the headgear tubes on the maxillary molars for slight max-

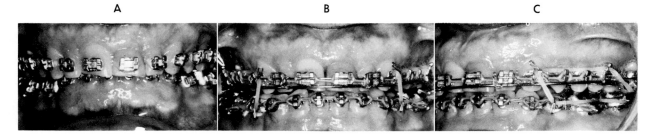

Fig. 12-35. J.W. **A,** Occlusal relationships just before surgery. At this point the 17×25 stabilizing arch wires, which had been placed 3 weeks earlier, were in the laboratory having the lugs needed for maxillomandibular fixation soldered. Note that the lower arch has not been leveled. The splint impressions are taken while the arch wires are out. **B** and **C,** Occlusal relationships at the time orthodontic finishing was resumed. The stabilizing arch wires were removed, maxillary and mandibular working arch wires were placed (16 steel), a maxillary auxiliary wire for additional expansion (40 steel) was placed in the headgear tubes, and posterior box elastics (⅜-inch light) were worn full-time.

Case 1—cont'd.

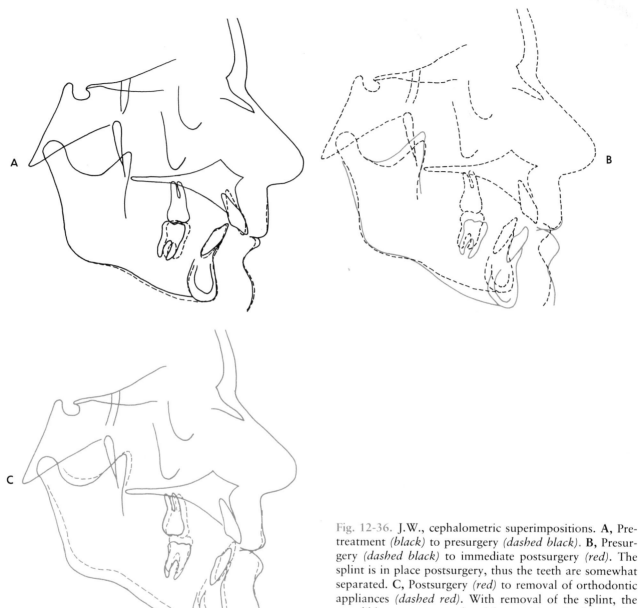

Fig. 12-36. J.W., cephalometric superimpositions. **A,** Pretreatment *(black)* to presurgery *(dashed black).* **B,** Presurgery *(dashed black)* to immediate postsurgery *(red).* The splint is in place postsurgery, thus the teeth are somewhat separated. **C,** Postsurgery *(red)* to removal of orthodontic appliances *(dashed red).* With removal of the splint, the mandible rotates upward and forward into the final occlusion.

illary expansion, and the settling elastics were continued (see Fig. 12-35, *B* and *C*).

The orthodontic appliances were removed 3 months after postsurgical orthodontics was resumed, and an immediate positioner was used for 3 weeks. Then maxillary Hawley and mandibular canine-to-canine clip-on retainers were placed. He did not tolerate the maxillary re-

tainer well, complaining of interference with speech and a tendency toward gagging. Two months later, a bonded wire was placed between the maxillary central incisors, and the upper retainer was discontinued.

At 6 months postsurgery (when the retainers were placed), facial proportions showed somewhat greater face height accompanied by greater prominence of the lower lip

Continued.

Case 1—cont'd.

(Fig. 12-37). The deep overbite and excess overjet were corrected. Posterior occlusion was improved and would be better when new restorations were placed (Fig. 12-38). The cephalometric tracing (see Fig. 12-36, C) showed that the mandible rotated upward and forward when the splint was removed, without other major changes from the postsurgical position.

On 5-year recall, the postsurgical facial proportions were well maintained (Fig. 12-39). The overbite and overjet remained ideal, and new posterior restorations had led to improvements in occlusion (Fig. 12-40). On cephalometric superimposition, no changes from removal of appliances at 6 months postsurgery to 5 years could be demonstrated. He was quite pleased with the overall re-

sult, but complained that full sensation in the lower lip had never returned.

Comments. The most stable mandibular advancement occurs when the mandible is rotated downward anteriorly to increase anterior face height, as it was in this patient, so that the dentition is advanced more than the chin. In these patients, how much face height increases is determined by the position of the lower incisors. Usually, it is more effective (because this prevents intrusion of the incisors) and more efficient (because the tooth movement proceeds more quickly) to level the lower arch postsurgically, as was done here.

At the time this patient was treated, RIF had not come into regular use, and positioners were used for finishing

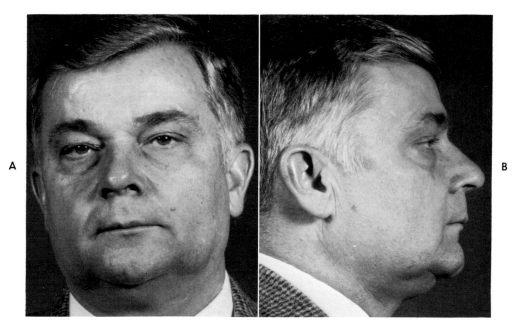

Fig. 12-37. J.W., facial photographs, completion of treatment.

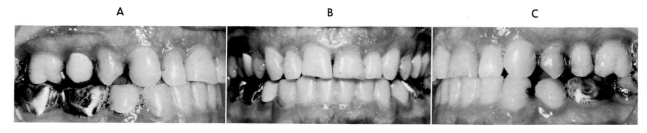

Fig. 12-38. J.W., intraoral photographs, completion of treatment.

Case 1—cont'd.

much more than at present. If he were treated now (1990), J.W. would have rigid rather than wire fixation and 1 week of settling elastics without posterior arch wires at the end of orthodontics rather than the positioner—but otherwise the treatment would be essentially the same.

On careful neurosensory testing, the majority of patients who undergo sagittal split osteotomy can be shown to have decreased long-term sensation in the lower lip. Only a minority indicate that this bothers them, as did this patient. There is some evidence that older patients are more likely to have neurosensory loss and more likely to complain about it than are those who are under 30 years old at the time of operation. For the older patients, a warning about the possibility of neurosensory changes is particularly important.

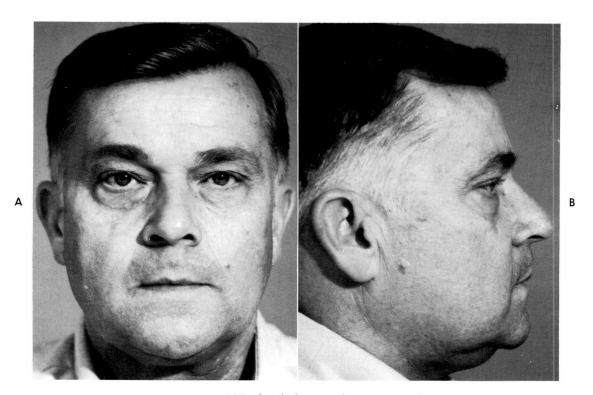

Fig. 12-39. J.W., facial photographs, 5-year recall.

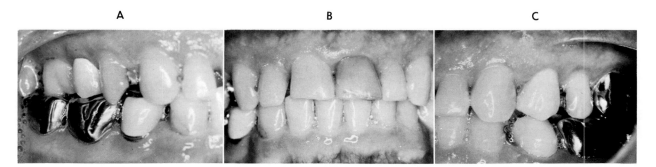

Fig. 12-40. J.W., intraoral photographs, 5-year recall.

Case 2

R.D., age 18 years, 5 months, was referred from his orthodontist in a distant city after enrolling in a nearby university. He had had orthodontic treatment of 2½ years' duration beginning at age 10 and then wore retainers for 2 to 3 years. After it had been decided that surgery would eventually be needed and should be delayed until growth had been completed, he had been followed without further active orthodontic treatment. He was aware of his chin deficiency and desired treatment to correct this and his bite.

The medical history revealed removal of tonsils and adenoids in early childhood, removal of a lung cyst at age 10, and cardiologic evaluation for a heart murmur in childhood that was no longer present. Present health was reported to be excellent.

On clinical examination, facial proportions showed a tendency toward maxillary hyperplasia with a large nose and extreme retrogenia and mandibular deficiency (Fig. 12-41). Teeth and intraoral tissues were healthy, but there was minimal attached gingiva on the mandibular canines, and periodontal consultation was obtained. Jaw opening and TM joint functions were excellent. The molar and canine relationships were Class I, but the canines were Class II. There was severe mandibular incisor crowding, 8 mm overjet, and deep bite anteriorly (Fig. 12-42).

The panoramic radiograph revealed mesioangular impacted mandibular third molars, with otherwise normal and healthy teeth and good alveolar bone levels. Cephalometric analysis (Fig. 12-43) confirmed severe man-

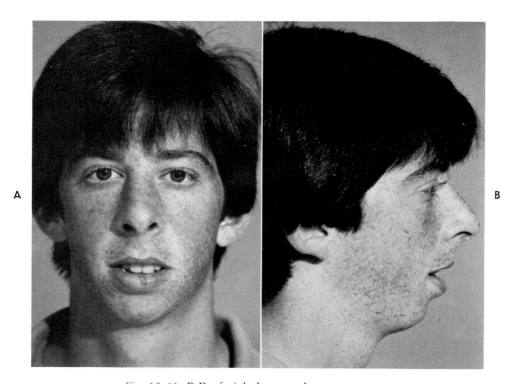

Fig. 12-41. R.D., facial photographs, pretreatment.

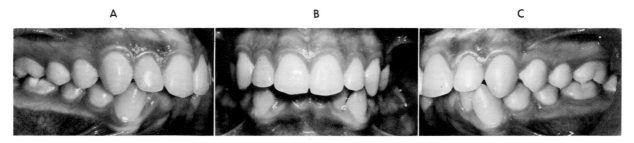

Fig. 12-42. R.D., intraoral photographs, pretreatment.

Case 2—cont'd.

dibular deficiency with a moderately steep mandibular plane angle due to a shortened ramus. The lower incisors were extremely protrusive relative to the mandible, whereas the upper incisors were well related to the maxilla. The nasolabial angle was excessive, due more to the prominence of the nose and an underdeveloped upper lip than to a posterior position of the maxilla.

His problems were summarized as follows: (1) severe mandibular deficiency and retrogenia, somewhat compensated dentally by previous orthodontic treatment; (2) severe crowding of mandibular incisors; and (3) lip incompetence and a tendency toward excessive vertical development of the maxilla.

It seemed clear that successful treatment for the first problem would require both mandibular advancement and chin augmentation. The mandibular crowding would require extractions in that arch, but maxillary extractions were not needed. The periodontist felt that if the mandibular incisors were retracted rather than advanced, gingival grafting would not be needed. The lip incompetence could be improved somewhat by an infe-

rior border osteotomy to elevate as well as advance the chin; further correction would require maxillary as well as mandibular surgery.

Based on these considerations, the treatment plan was as follows:

1. Extraction of the mandibular right and left first premolars and third molars.
2. Presurgical orthodontics to align and retract (to the extent possible) the mandibular incisors, estimated to require 10 months.
3. Orthodontic stabilization.
4. Mandibular ramus and inferior border osteotomies for advancement of the mandible and chin, with further consideration of maxillary osteotomy.
5. Finishing orthodontics, estimated to require 4 to 6 months.
6. Orthodontic retention.

Following extraction of the teeth, bands with 18-slot edgewise attachments were placed on upper and lower first molars and lower second molars and bonded brackets were placed on premolars, canines, and incisors. In the maxillary arch, a 16 NiTi arch wire was used for initial alignment; in the lower arch, a 14 steel arch wire with loops was used to retract the canines while the incisors were being aligned (Fig. 12-44). Then a 16×22 TMA wire was placed in the upper, and

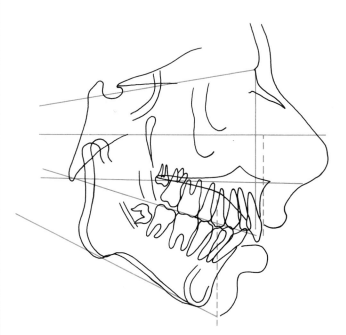

Fig. 12-43. R.D., pretreatment cephalometric tracing. Cephalometric measurements: N perp to A, 2 mm; N perp to Pg, −25 mm; AB difference, 23 mm; UFH, 61 mm; LFH, 69 mm; mand plane, 26 degrees; MxI to A vert, 2 mm, 8 degrees; MnI to B vert, 15 mm, 45 degrees. Note the tendency toward midface protrusion (not just maxillary protrusion) and the extreme mandibular deficiency and retrogenia. Despite the relatively steep mandibular plane angle and short mandibular rami (the antegonial notching indicates some restriction on ramus growth), anterior face height was approximately normal. The upper lip was quite short and underdeveloped.

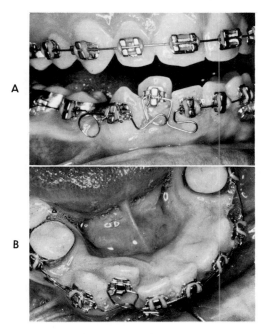

Fig. 12-44. R.D., alignment in the maxillary arch was accomplished with a continuous 16 NiTi wire. Because of the severe crowding in the mandibular arch, it was desired to tip the canines distally into the extraction site as the incisors were aligned, and a "drag loop" in 14 steel wire was used.

Continued.

Case 2—cont'd.

16×22 closing loops were used to complete mandibular space closure. Finally, 17×25 steel wires (Fig. 12-45, *A*) were placed for stabilization at surgery, and presurgical records were obtained.

Cephalometric superimposition at this stage (Fig. 12-46, *A*) showed that the lower incisors had been retracted while upper incisors were slightly flared labially. Prediction tracings showed that the mandible could be advanced straight along the mandibular plane without increasing posterior face height and stretching the pterygomandibular sling (i.e., maxillary surgery was not necessary to prevent the instability associated with "wrong-way rotation" in mandibular advancement). In consultation with the family, it was decided to perform only mandibular advancement with sagittal split osteotomy and inferior border osteotomy, accepting the midface features that were familial characteristics.

Ten months after presurgical orthodontics was begun, surgery was performed uneventfully. Because of the relatively steep mandibular plane, the mandible was advanced to an end-to-end incisor relationship (see Fig. 12-45), and he was placed in maxillomandibular fixa-tion in an occlusal splint. Fixation was maintained for 6 weeks, and he functioned into the splint guided by ⅜-inch, 2-oz elastics for another 2 weeks before postsurgical orthodontics was resumed.

Eight weeks postsurgically, the stabilizing arch wires and the splint were removed, 16 steel wires were placed, and ⅜-inch light latex elastics in a posterior box pattern were worn full time initially. Four weeks later, steps were placed in the wires in the upper premolar regions and the elastics were continued. Three weeks later, 17×25 TMA wires were placed in the mandibular arch and elastics were worn only at night. The appliances were removed 4 months postsurgically, and maxillary Hawley and mandibular anterior clip-on retainers were placed the same day.

Cephalometric superimposition (Fig. 12-46, *C*) showed that from immediately postsurgery to completion of treatment, the mandible repositioned posteriorly and rotated upward and forward as the splint was removed. Chin prominence and overall facial proportionality was improved, but some lip incompetence remained (Fig. 12-47). Good occlusal relationships were obtained (Fig. 12-48).

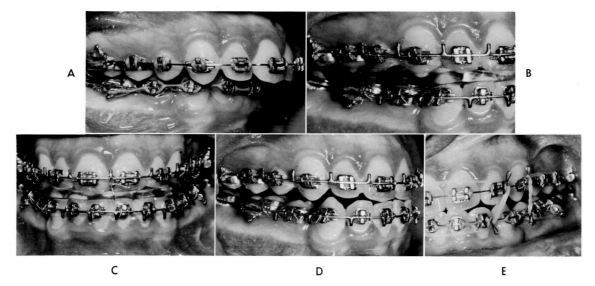

Fig. 12-45. R.D. **A,** The 17×25 steel arch wires that would serve for surgical stabilization were placed 4 weeks before the surgery date, with light activation. **B,** One week before surgery, splint impressions were made while the wires were removed for addition of soldered brass lugs; then the wires were replaced with no bends or changes, which guaranteed they would be passive so the splints would fit. This postsurgical view with the splint in place demonstrates the separation of the casts at splint construction that was used for this patient. **C,** Six weeks postsurgery, the splint was tied to the upper arch wire (note the ligature in the midline—there is another on each side) so the patient could function into the splint. **D,** The occlusion after splint removal, 8 weeks postsurgery. The stabilizing arch wires were removed at the same appointment as the splint and were replaced with 16 steel working arch wires. **E,** Working arch wires and box elastics in place, at the beginning of postsurgical orthodontics (same appointment as **C** and **D**).

Case 2—cont'd.

On recall 18 months later (2 years postsurgery), facial proportions had been maintained (Fig. 12-49) and occlusal relationships had improved with further settling (Fig. 12-50). Cephalometrically, no changes from the previous film were apparent. Sensation over the lip and chin area was within normal limits.

Comments. Whether to surgically involve both jaws or limit the surgery to one can be a difficult decision. In this case, our judgment was that a stable result could be achieved by mandibular advancement along the mandibular plane and chin augmentation and that the esthetic changes produced by repositioning the maxilla were not desirable enough for this patient to warrant the additional treatment. Maxillary surgery, LeFort I osteotomy to elevate the posterior maxilla, would have been required if the vertical position of the maxilla had produced wrong-way rotation of the mandible when it was advanced, as often is the case when the mandibular

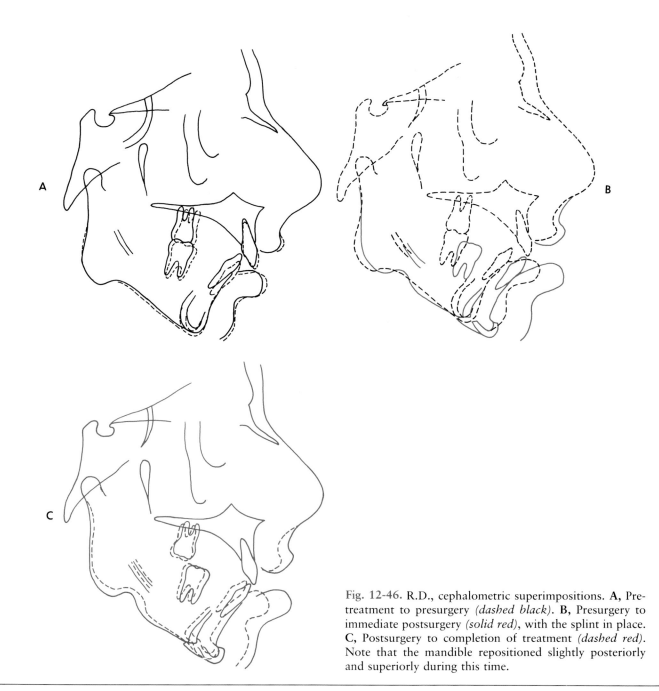

Fig. 12-46. R.D., cephalometric superimpositions. **A,** Pretreatment to presurgery *(dashed black).* **B,** Presurgery to immediate postsurgery *(solid red),* with the splint in place. **C,** Postsurgery to completion of treatment *(dashed red).* Note that the mandible repositioned slightly posteriorly and superiorly during this time.

Continued.

Case 2—cont'd.

plane angle is steep. Moving the maxilla upward would have reduced the lip incompetence that still was present postsurgically but might have made the midface and nose even more prominent. Decisions of this type must be made in consultation with the patient and family, with the alternatives presented as clearly as possible.

The position of the mandible in the splint for this patient illustrates the maximum overtreatment in mandibular advancement that we would recommend. In this regard, it is significant that he was planned for maxillomandibular fixation rather than RIF. If RIF were planned, we would not advance the mandible quite so far, nor separate the teeth as much in the splint.

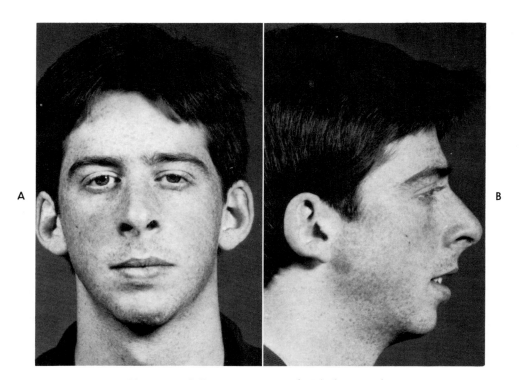

Fig. 12-47. R.D., posttreatment facial photographs.

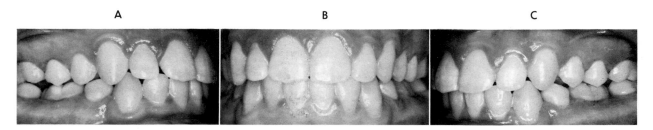

Fig. 12-48. R.D., postreatment occlusal relationships. With premolar extraction in the mandibular but not the maxillary arch, canine relationships are Class I but molars are Class III, which is functionally satisfactory.

Case 2—cont'd.

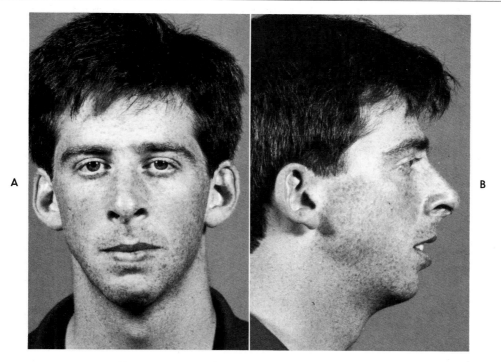

Fig. 12-49. R.D., facial photographs, 2-year recall.

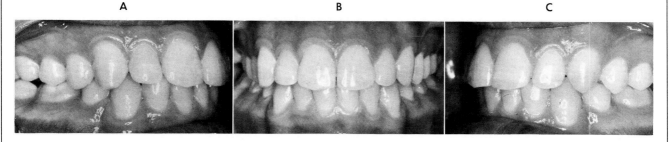

Fig. 12-50. R.D., occlusal relationships, 2-year recall.

Case 3

B.Y., age 23 years, 4 months, and a teacher, sought orthodontic consultation relative to her protruding maxillary incisors. She had always wanted orthodontic treatment and could afford it now that she was employed. Except for hospitalization in early childhood for respiratory infection, the medical history was unremarkable. She reported her general health as excellent. She was surprised to be told that her problem appeared to be due more to mandibular deficiency than to maxillary dental protrusion. Although she was taken aback at the suggestion that surgery might be required for treatment, she agreed to further diagnostic evaluation knowing that this might be the recommendation.

On clinical examination, teeth and oral tissues were healthy. Jaw opening and TM joint function were normal. On full-face examination, the chin was deviated

Continued.

Case 3—cont'd.

about 4 mm to the right. There was moderate but obvious mandibular deficiency (Fig. 12-51). The occlusion was a full cusp Class II bilaterally, with 7 mm overjet, anterior deep bite, and mild irregularity of the maxillary incisors (Fig. 12-52). The panoramic radiograph revealed three impacted third molars (two upper, one lower). Cephalometric analysis confirmed Class II malocclusion due almost entirely to mandibular deficiency, with a good relationship of the maxilla to the cranium and of the maxillary and mandibular teeth to their respective jaws (Fig. 12-53).

At the case presentation, it was emphasized that her prob-lem was almost entirely due to mandibular deficiency. Two alternative treatment plans were presented. The first, orthodontic treatment only, would involve extraction of maxillary first premolars and retraction of the upper incisors, with an estimated treatment time of 27 months. She was told that this would improve the dental occlusion but would not produce a favorable esthetic change and in fact probably would make facial esthetics worse. The second plan, surgical-orthodontic treatment, would involve nonextraction orthodontic preparation for surgical mandibular advancement; sagittal split advancement, more on the right than left side so as to

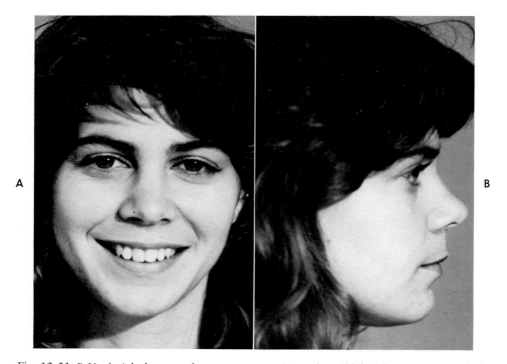

Fig. 12-51. B.Y., facial photographs, pretreatment. Note the mild facial asymmetry with the chin somewhat off to the right, in addition to the mandibular deficiency and moderately decreased face height.

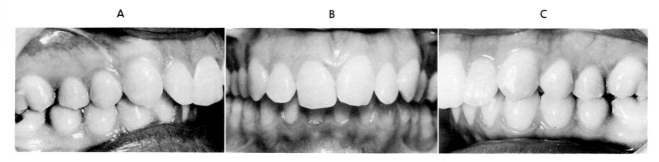

Fig. 12-52. B.Y., intraoral photographs, pretreatment.

Case 3—cont'd.

bring the chin to the midline; and finishing orthodontics, with an estimated total treatment time of 15 months. This approach would produce good occlusion and improved facial esthetics. The relative risks and costs of surgical-orthodontic versus orthodontic-only treatment were reviewed in detail, and she was encouraged to think this over carefully before making a decision.

Soon after the case presentation, the third molars were removed (by the surgeon with whom she had discussed orthognathic surgery), and she sought out other patients who were undergoing surgical-orthodontic treatment to learn of their experiences. Eight months later, having become engaged to be married in the meantime and with the support of her fiancee, she decided to proceed with surgery.

Following the placement of a complete fixed appliance (18-slot edgewise), a sequence of 16 NiTi, 16 steel, 17×25 TMA, and 17×25 steel arch wires was used over a 7-month period in preparation for surgery. RIF was planned, and lugs for maxillomandibular fixation were placed on the stabilizing arch wires (Fig. 12-54). These are necessary to hold the teeth in place at surgery while screws are placed and also are a safety measure in case RIF proves impossible for some reason.

On the day following hospital admission, a bilateral sagittal split osteotomy was carried out, and the mandible was advanced 8 mm into the previously prepared surgical splint. The teeth were held in the splint with four 26-gauge wire loops, and RIF was accomplished with a lag screw technique, employing three screws on each side (Figs. 12-55 and 12-56). The maxillomandibular fixation then was released in the operating room, and the lower jaw rotated into the splint without difficulty. She was discharged on the second postoperative day, with guiding elastics allowing some mandibular function but bringing the mandible firmly into the splint.

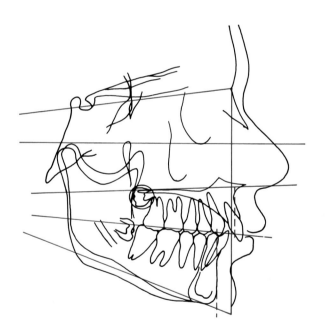

Fig. 12-53. B.Y., initial cephalometric tracing. The face is vertically well proportioned, with a deficient mandible. Cephalometric measurements: N perp to A, 1 mm; N perp to Pg, 7 mm; UFH, 53 mm; LFH, 65 mm; mand plane, 21 degrees; MxI to A vert, 2 mm, 20 degrees; MnI to B vert, 5 mm, 34 degrees.

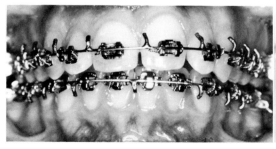
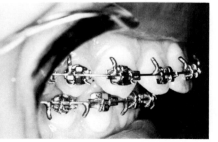

Fig. 12-54. B.Y., occlusal relationships immediately before surgery, with 17×25 stabilizing arch wires in place.

Continued.

Case 3—cont'd.

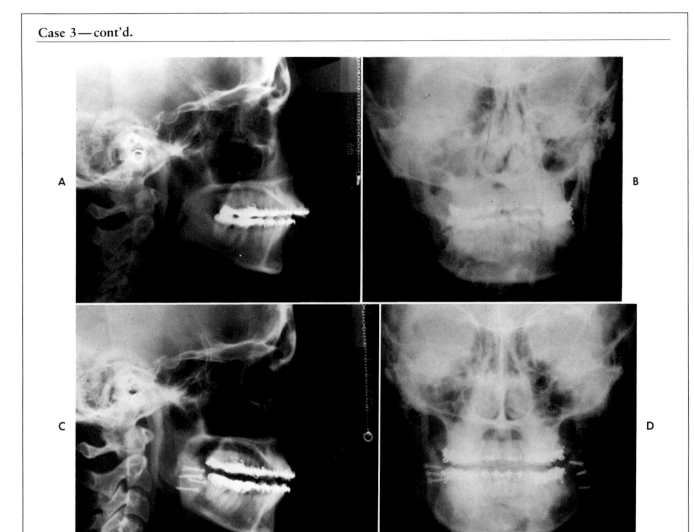

Fig. 12-55. B.Y. **A** and **B**, Lateral and PA cephalometric films immediately before and **C** and **D**, immediately after bilateral sagittal-split osteotomy. Note the use of screws placed from within the mouth for RIF.

Case 3—cont'd.

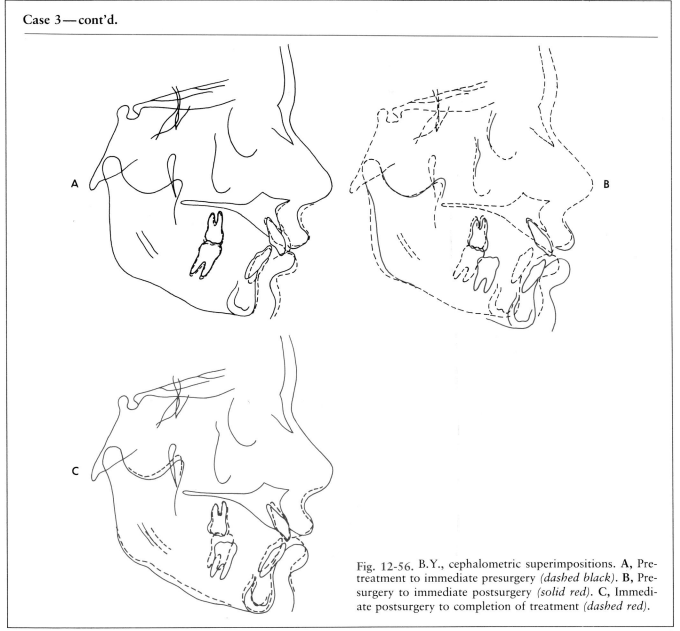

Fig. 12-56. B.Y., cephalometric superimpositions. **A,** Pretreatment to immediate presurgery *(dashed black).* **B,** Presurgery to immediate postsurgery *(solid red).* **C,** Immediate postsurgery to completion of treatment *(dashed red).*

Continued.

Case 3—cont'd.

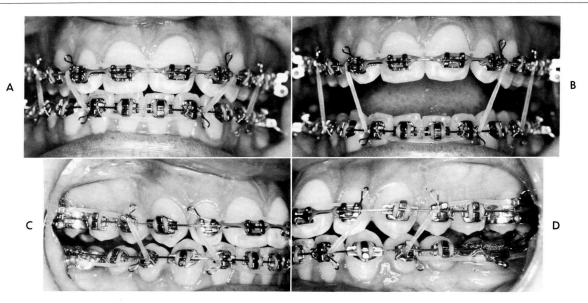

Fig. 12-57. B.Y. **A** to **D**, Occlusal relationships at the beginning of postsurgical orthodontics. At this initial postsurgical orthodontic appointment, the splint and stabilizing arch wires have been replaced by light working arch wires (16 steel). Note the vertical space between the posterior teeth. It is important for the patient to wear full-time posterior box elastics (typically ⅜-inch, 3½-oz) that are light enough to allow good jaw motion but provide a settling force until the teeth settle into occlusion. An anterior box elastic usually is worn 12 hours/day.

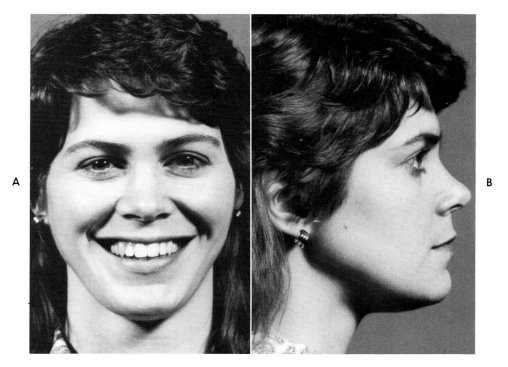

Fig. 12-58. B.Y., facial photographs 1 year after removal of the orthodontic appliances (18 months postsurgically).

Case 3—cont'd.

At 3 weeks postsurgery, the splint was adjusted so the patient could remove it to clean it. Light elastics with function into the splint were continued. At 6 weeks, the splint and the stabilizing arch wires were removed, 16 steel arch wires were placed, and ⅜-inch posterior box elastics were placed (Fig. 12-57). Two and a half months later (with no further arch wires being employed), the appliances were removed and retainers were placed. Soon thereafter, the patient reported some TM joint symptoms on the right side, which subsided after balancing contacts on the left first and second molars were equilibrated.

One year later, full-face and profile esthetics were excellent and appeared stable (Fig. 12-58). Occlusal relationships were excellent (Fig. 12-59). Retention, which had been tapered from full-time for the first 3 months to nights only after 5 months, was discontinued. Full sensation had returned to the lower lip.

Comments. Correcting a moderate mandibular asymmetry by advancing one side more than the other is not difficult with bilateral sagittal split osteotomies. In the planning, it is critically important that the skeletal midlines be determined. When the jaw comes forward, the chin must be placed in the center of the face even if the dental midline is not correct at that point. During the postsurgical orthodontics, the dental midline usually can be corrected. If a compromise is required, having the mandibular dental midline slightly off does not create a major functional or esthetic problem. But patients often are acutely aware of facial symmetry or its lack, and if the chin is not positioned correctly at surgery, there is no way to correct it later without further surgery.

When screws for RIF are used as they were in this case, early mobilization of the mandible provides greater patient comfort and earlier resolution of edema. We recommend, however, that the patient function into the splint until the surgeon is ready for postsurgical orthodontics to resume. The orthodontist, not the surgeon, should remove the splint, because the stabilizing arch wires should be replaced with light working arch wires at the same time.

A   B   C

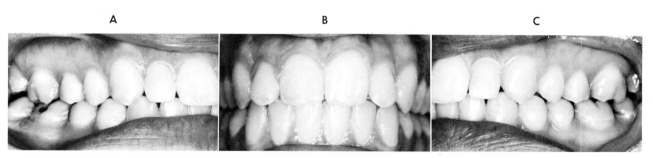

Fig. 12-59. B.Y., intraoral photographs, 1 year after completion of postsurgical orthodontics.

REFERENCES

1. Proffit WR, Phillips C, Dann C IV: Who seeks surgical-orthodontic treatment? The characteristics of patients evaluated in the UNC Dentofacial Clinic, Int J Adult Orthod Orthognath Surg [in press].

2. Riolo ML, Brandt D, TenHoeve TR: Associations between occlusal characteristics and signs and symptoms of TMJ dysfunction in children and young adults, Am J Orthod Dentofacial Orthop 92:467-477, 1987.

3. Mohlin B, Thilander B: The importance of the relationship between malocclusion and mandibular dysfunction and some clinical application in adults, Eur J Orthod 6:192-204, 1984.

4. Egermark-Eriksson I, Ingervall B, Carlsson GE: The dependence of mandibular dysfunction in children on functional and morphologic malocclusion, Am J Orthod 83:187-194, 1983.

5. Egermark-Eriksson I, Carlsson GE, Magnusson T: A long-term epidemiologic study of the relationship between occlusal factors and mandibular dysfunction in children and adolescents, J Dent Res 66:67-71, 1987.

6. Bjork A: The face in profile, Sven Tandlak Tidskr 40(Suppl), 1947.

7. Baumrind S, Kom EL, Issacson RJ, et al: Quantitative analysis of the orthodontic and orthopedic effects of maxillary traction, Am J Orthod 84:384-398, 1983.

8. Righellis EG: Treatment effects of Frankel, activator and extraoral traction appliances, Angle Orthod 53:107-121, 1983.

9. Behrents RG: A treatise on the continuum of growth in the aging craniofacial skeleton, Ann Arbor, 1984, University of Michigan Center for Human Growth and Development.

10. McCollum AGH, Reyneke JP, Wolford LM: An alternative for the correction of the Class II low mandibular plane angle, Oral Surg Oral Med Oral Pathol 67:231-241, 1989.

11. Terry BC: Neurosensory changes after four different mandibular procedures, Proc Eur Soc Oral Maxillofac Surg, 1982 (abstract).

12. Steffen JM, Halton FT: The five cent tooth positioner, J Clin Orthod 21:528-529, 1987.

13. Zaytoun HS, Jr, Phillips C, Terry BC: Long term neurosensory deficits following transoral vertical ramus and sagittal split osteotomies for mandibular prognathism, J Oral Maxillofac Surg 44:193-196, 1986.

14. Bell WH, Gonyea W, Finn RA, et al: Muscular rehabilitation after orthognathic surgery, Oral Surg Oral Med Oral Pathol 56:229-235, 1983.

15. Proffit WR, Phillips C: Adaptations in lip posture and pressure following orthognathic surgery, Am J Dentofacial Orthop 93:294-302, 1988.

16. Throckmorton GS: Biomechanics of differences in lower facial height, Am J Orthod 77:418-421, 1980.

17. Proffit WR, Turvey TA, Fields, HW, Phillips, C: The effect of orthognathic surgery on occlusal force, J Oral Maxillofac Surg 47:457-463, 1989.

18. Fields HW, Proffit WR, Case JC, et al: Variables affecting the measurement of vertical occlusal force, J Dent Res 65:118-122, 1986.

19. Epker BN, Wolford LM, Fish LC: Mandibular deficiency syndrome. II. Surgical considerations for mandibular advancement, J Oral Surg 45:349-363, 1978.

20. Boyne PJ: Osseous healing after oblique osteotomy of the mandibular ramus, J Oral Surg 24:124-133, 1966.

21. Boyne PJ, Matthews FR, Stringer DE: TMJ bone remodelling after polythylene condylar replacement, Int J Oral Maxillofac Implants 2:29-33, 1987.

22. McNeill RW, Hooley JR, Sundberg RJ: Skeletal relapse during intermaxillary fixation, J Oral Surg 31:212-227, 1973.

23. Ive J, McNeill RW, West RA: Mandibular advancement: skeletal and dental changes during fixation, J Oral Surg 35:881-886, 1977.

24. Phillips C, Turvey TA, McMillian A: Surgical-orthodontic correction of mandibular deficiency by sagittal osteotomy: clinical and cephalometric analysis of one year data, Am J Orthod Dentofacial Orthop 96:501-506, 1989.

25. Ellis E III, Carlson DS: Stability two years after mandibular advancement with and without suprahyoid myotomy: an experimental study, J Oral Maxillofac Surg 41:426-437, 1983.

26. Schendel SA, Epker BN: Results after mandibular advancement surgery: an analysis of 87 cases, J Oral Surg 38:265-282, 1980.

27. Will LA, Joondeph DR, Hohl TH, et al: Condylar position following mandibular advancement: its relationship to relapse, J Oral Maxillofac Surg 42:578-588, 1984.

28. Ellis E, Reynolds S, Carlson DS: Stability of the mandible following advancement: a comparison of three postsurgical fixation techniques, Am J Orthod Dentofacial Orthop 94:38-49, 1988.

29. Van Sickels JE, Larsen AJ, Thrash WJ: Relapse after rigid fixation of mandibular advancement, J Oral Maxillofac Surg 44:698-702, 1986.

30. Thomas PM, Tucker MR, Prewitt JR, et al: Early skeletal and dental changes following mandibular advancement and RIF, Int J Adult Orthod Orthognath Surg 1:171-178, 1986.

31. Watzke I, Turvey TA, Phillips C, et al: Stability of mandibular advancement after sagittal osteotomy with screw or wire fixation: a comparative study, J Oral Maxillofac Surg 48:108-121, 1990.

32. Bhatia SN, Yan B, Behbehani I, Harris M: Nature of relapse after surgical mandibular advancement, Br J Orthod 12:58-69, 1985.

33. Phillips RM, Bell WH: Atrophy of the mandibular condyles after sagittal ramus osteotomy: report of case, J Oral Surg 36:45-49, 1978.

CHAPTER 13

Long-Face Problems

William R. Proffit
Raymond P. White, Jr.

NEED AND DEMAND

Excessive face height was noted as a clinical problem long before anything substantial could be done about it. The subject received little attention from clinicians until treatment possibilities were developed. It was not until Sassouni's description of "skeletal open bite" in the 1960s[1]—which by no coincidence appeared at about the time high-pull headgear offered a way to treat it—that excessive vertical development of the face began to receive any emphasis in cephalometric diagnosis. Even then, the focus on open bite concealed for a while the fact that the long-face condition can occur in patients who have normal or deep-bite incisor relationships. With the development of surgical techniques for vertically repositioning the maxilla in the 1970s, the term *long-face syndrome* was coined and delineated.[2]

To this date, no good epidemiologic data exist for long-face problems because the surveys have concentrated on dental occlusion rather than on facial proportions. As the discussion in Chapter 1 points out, if we assume that 25% of those with more than 3 mm anterior open bite have too long a face, there would be about 220,000 affected individuals of appropriate age for treatment in the United States, and about 6,000 new cases would be added yearly (see Table 1-4). Not all long-face individuals have open bite, so the estimates based on that characteristic can be misleadingly low. Unfortunately, an analysis of vertical facial proportions was eliminated from the 1989-1990 NHANES III survey of the U.S. population, so good data are not likely to be forthcoming any time soon.

Although population estimates are difficult, the number of patients with excessive face height who seek surgical-orthodontic treatment is known. Of 1139 patients evaluated through the Dentofacial Program at the UNC in the 1980s, 342 (30%) were noted at their initial clinical examination to have a long lower third of the face, and another 57 (5%) had a long middle third (3% had both). Of the 739 patients who were not in orthodontic treatment at their first examination, 13% had more than 6 mm of the upper incisor exposed at rest, and 31% had an anterior open bite of at least 1 mm. A combination of excessive face height and mandibular deficiency was noted in 20% of the total sample. These data suggest that long-face individuals make up a third of the dentofacial deformity group who seek clinical treatment, almost twice as many as would have been expected from the presumed population incidence.[3] Because the long-face condition often is combined with other problems, especially mandibular deficiency, it is hard to be certain exactly what as-

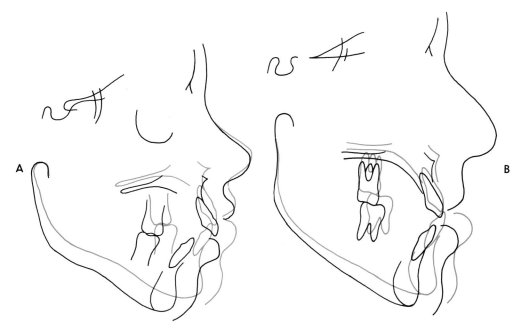

Fig. 13-1. Vertical-horizontal interactions in long-face patients. **A,** Class I (normal) rotated to Class II (the black tracing shows the patient's present condition with the mandible rotated down and back, the red shows the jaw relationships with only the vertical dimension corrected). **B,** Class III rotated to Class I (the black tracing shows the patient's present condition with the mandible rotated down and back so that there is no AP discrepancy, the red shows that correcting the vertical dimension would produce a Class III problem). The anteroposterior effects of mandibular rotation make normal AP relationships almost impossible in long-face patients. If there is no AP problem when the long-face condition is present (Class III rotated to Class I), there will be when it is corrected. Conversely, correcting the long face may also correct a mandibular-deficient Class II problem as the mandible rotates up and forward.

pects of the deformity are most important in leading a patient to seek treatment. But the chief complaint often includes the "gummy smile" and/or anterior open bite that are the hallmarks of the long-face condition. The combination of esthetic and functional problems in the long-face condition seems to be harder to live with than, for instance, mandibular deficiency without excess face height.

DIAGNOSTIC CHARACTERISTICS

A long face is just that: the primary distinguishing characteristic is a large total face height that is manifest almost entirely in elongation of the lower third, leading to disproportions on the facial height and width indices (see Chapter 4, Tables 4-3 and 4-4). A major component of the problem nearly always is an inferior rotation of the posterior maxilla. As face height increases and the maxillary palatal plane and posterior teeth are more inferior, the mandible tends to rotate downward and backward. For this reason, the vertical disproportion also affects AP jaw relationships. It is almost impossible for the patient to have excess face height but no problem in the AP plane of space. Either there is an

AP problem when the excess face height is present before treatment, or there will be when it is corrected; that is, a long-face patient can be described as skeletal Class I rotated to Class II, or as skeletal Class III rotated to Class I (Fig. 13-1). All other things being equal, excess face height makes AP mandibular deficiency worse and prognathism better (Fig. 13-2).

As the mandible rotates down and back during the development of the long-face condition, the lower incisors tend to become more upright and therefore more crowded than they would have been otherwise. Mandibular rotation throws the incisors forward relative to the chin, and it seems reasonable to presume that resting lip pressure is responsible for the uprighting. The rotation also separates the incisors vertically, creating an open-bite tendency. If the incisors erupt enough to compensate for the growth pattern, the bite can stay closed or even deep; if they do not, there will be an anterior open bite. Even in patients with open bite, excessive incisor eruption almost always occurs.

Whatever the tooth relationships, one sign of excessive face height is lip incompetence, defined as excessive separation of the lips at rest. Some normal individ-

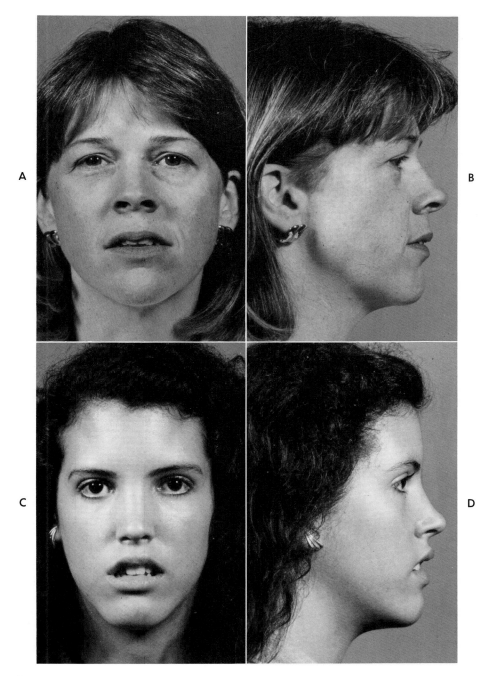

Fig. 13-2. A series of long-face patients with increasingly severe problems. Note the increasing lip incompetence and downward rotation of the mandible as face height increases.

Continued.

uals have their lips completely in contact at rest, but usually there is 1 to 3 mm of lip separation. Four mm of separation at rest can be considered the outer limit of normal—only beyond that should a patient can be considered lip incompetent.

From one perspective, the extent of lip separation might seem a more sensitive indicator of excessive face height than are linear measurements, which obviously must be adjusted for the overall size of the individual.

Unfortunately, lip separation by itself can be terribly misleading because it is strongly influenced by the length of the lips themselves, particularly the upper lip. Lip incompetence due to excessive face height must not be confused with lip separation due to a short upper lip.

A short upper lip is particularly likely to be encountered in a patient with severe mandibular deficiency who has never had normal lip function during develop-

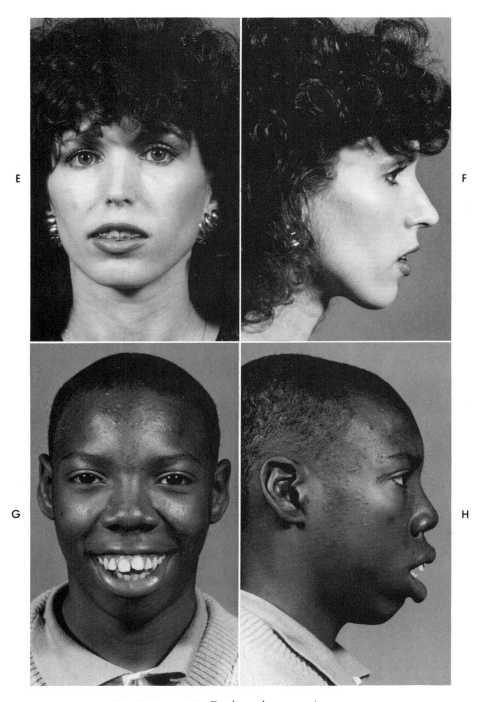

Fig. 13-2, cont'd. For legend, see previous page.

ment. Such patients achieve an oral seal by elevating the lower lip against the protruding maxillary incisors. The result is a well-developed, almost excessive lower lip, but a thin, short upper lip that has little musculature and does not cover the incisors (see Chapter 12, Figs. 12-9 to 12-14). Moving the maxilla up to achieve a normal relationship of the incisors to such a lip would shorten the face too much and should be avoided.

In summary, on clinical examination long face patients are characterized by:
- Excessive anterior face height, particularly in the lower third.
- Lip incompetence (resting lip separation >4 mm). This judgment must be made with soft tissues at rest, not in a smile. Lip elevation during smiling is quite variable, and exposure of gingiva then may be neither abnormal nor unesthetic.

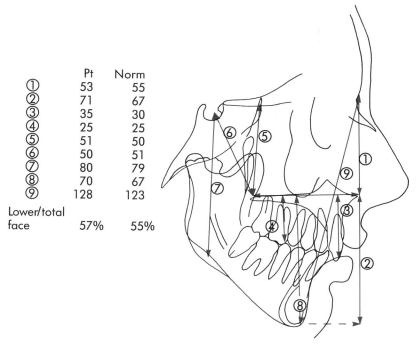

	Pt	Norm
①	53	55
②	71	67
③	35	30
④	25	25
⑤	51	50
⑥	50	51
⑦	80	79
⑧	70	67
⑨	128	123
Lower/total face	57%	55%

Fig. 13-3. Linear measurements can be helpful in establishing the presence of a long-face deformity, as shown in this tracing from Case 3 (Figs. 13-45 to 13-54). The measurements indicate that the maxilla is down more posteriorly than anteriorly and that the maxillary incisors but not molars are supraerupted (see Chapter 4, Table 4-6, for additional reference data).

- A tendency toward anterior open bite—but only two-thirds of the patients have this type of malocclusion. Deep bite may occur in the others.
- A tendency toward mandibular deficiency and Class II malocclusion—but the AP relationship can be anything from severe Class II to mild Class III. A severe Class III problem puts the patient into a different category (see Chapter 14).
- A tendency toward more lower- than upper-incisor crowding.
- A tendency toward a narrow maxilla and posterior crossbite, a finding in about half the patients.

Cephalometrically, long-face patients nearly always have:

- Rotation of the palatal plane down posteriorly (i.e., the maxilla has descended posteriorly more than anteriorly). This is shown clearly by the inclination of the palatal plane to the other horizontal reference planes. The linear distance from the cranial base to posterior landmarks (e.g., PNS) usually is increased (Fig. 13-3).
- Excessive eruption of maxillary posterior teeth (i.e., the distance from the palatal plane to the cusps of the upper teeth is increased).
- Rotation of the mandible down and back, giving an increased mandibular plane angle. To a large extent, this is secondary to the maxillary rotation and elongation of the maxillary molars, but the

mandibular ramus often is short, so many patients have skeletal changes in the mandible as well as in the maxilla. The rotation usually is not related to excessive eruption of mandibular posterior teeth: linear distances from the lower border of the mandible to the cusps of the lower molars nearly always are normal.

- Excessive eruption of maxillary and mandibular incisors in partial compensation for the jaw rotation. Even patients who have anterior open bite have this finding, but it is greatest in those with a deep bite.

Although a number of investigators have tried to find a single cephalometric criterion that would reliably indicate the long-face condition, this has proved impossible. Fields and colleagues[4] have demonstrated that three cephalometric criteria in combination are necessary to quantify the condition observed by skilled clinicians—not a surprising finding, perhaps, when the disturbed proportional jaw and tooth relationships of these patients are considered. Several combinations of characteristics are diagnostic, but the best result is based on a combination of increased mandibular plane angle, increased total anterior face height, and decreased percentage of upper face height. If a patient has all three, he or she can be considered to have a long-face deformity with very high confidence.

Because of the variable presence of AP and transverse problems in addition to the basic vertical problems and the frequent presence of more crowding in the lower than the upper arch, it is particularly important for those clinically assessing long-face patients to use a systematic diagnostic approach such as that outlined in Chapter 4 to be sure that no important points have been overlooked.

ETIOLOGIC CONSIDERATIONS

These patients often have the facial appearance characterized many years ago as the "adenoid facies": the cheeks are narrow, the nostrils are narrow and pinched, the lips are separated, and often there are exaggerated shadows beneath the eyes (see the case reports below). The label is unfortunate because it implies that the adenoids are the cause of the problem and—at least most of the time—that is not correct. Long-face patients often look as if they were breathing through their mouth, but this may not be the case. Laboratory studies (see Chapter 2 for more details) indicate that most children and adults with the long-face condition breathe perfectly normally through the nose.[5,6] On the other hand, more long-face than normal children and adults have an increased oral and decreased nasal airflow (i.e., an increased oral/nasal ratio). It appears, therefore, that for some patients, difficulty with nasal respiration may play a role in the development of the long-face condition, but this is not the only or the major cause.

In a number of muscle weakness syndromes, the facial appearance produces an exaggeration, almost a caricature, of a typical long-face patient (e.g., see Chapter 2, Fig. 2-31). This clinical finding led to the idea that weak mandibular elevator muscles might cause the long-face condition. In theory, if the muscles were weak, biting force would decrease, allowing the posterior teeth to erupt too much and the mandible to rotate downward. Although adult long-face patients do have below-normal occlusal forces,[7] preadolescent children who already can be recognized as long-face types do not.[8] The long-face patients appear not to gain muscle strength during adolescence, at least in the mandibular elevators, as do normal individuals. How that fits into the etiology of this condition is not clear at present.

Long-face patients with an anterior open bite are very likely to be labeled as having a tongue thrust because they place the tongue tip into the opening, where it is obvious during swallowing and speech. The position of the tongue is a necessary physiologic adaptation to the open bite, not its cause. When the incisors overlap normally, the tongue can be placed behind them to create the anterior seal necessary for successful swallowing or articulation of several consonant sounds. With an open bite, the tongue must protrude to seal against the lips, so tongue thrust is a reasonably accu-

rate description. As with adenoid facies, the harm in the tongue thrust label comes in wrongly supposing cause and effect. It is easy to demonstrate that tongue position during swallowing and speech adapts to the position of the teeth, rather than the other way around. In fact, the best clinical demonstration is the patients' response to orthognathic surgery to correct open bite, which nearly always eliminates tongue thrust as it corrects the malocclusion.

The role of tongue posture in the etiology of malocclusion is explored in some detail in Chapter 2. Two points are worth special emphasis with regard to long-face patients: (1) although resting tongue posture can be a significant etiologic factor in dentofacial deformity, tongue position during speech and swallowing is much less important; and (2) the patients in whom tongue posture is most likely to be significant are not the long-face types who are the subjects of this chapter. Instead, certain Class III problems (see Chapter 14) are most likely to develop when tongue posture is abnormal.

Previous family studies have made it clear that vertical facial proportions have a strong inherited component, but the prevalence of long-face deformity among the close relatives of those who seek treatment has not yet been determined. There is a racial difference—long-face, open-bite problems seem to be proportionately more frequent in blacks than in whites or Orientals. Presumably, this is related to the same slightly different facial proportions that make short-face, deep-bite problems less frequent in blacks (see Chapter 12, Fig. 12-3). For any individual patient, it seems likely that both environmental influences and inherited tendencies have played a role as the long face developed. Environmental factors (largely unknown at present) probably push individuals who are susceptible because of their inherited facial proportions outside the normal range of variation.

TREATMENT PLANNING
Preadolescents with Growth Potential

Although the growth pattern that leads to the long-face condition is complex, excessive vertical growth of the maxilla, particularly the posterior maxilla, is its major characteristic. The primary objective of treatment in a growing child with a long-face problem, therefore, must be to restrain and control that area. If vertical movement of the posterior teeth (which is due to a combination of jaw growth and eruption) could be controlled well enough, downward and backward rotation of the mandible could be prevented, and it might even be possible to produce upward and forward rotation of the mandible as growth continued.

The treatment goal may be reasonably obvious, but methods for accomplishing it have been remarkably difficult to work out. The long-face growth pattern is

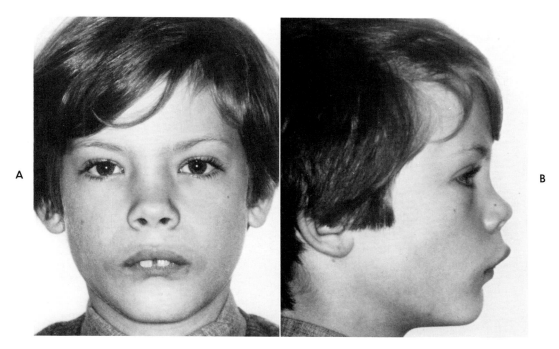

Fig. 13-4. I.H., pretreatment facial photographs. (Courtesy Harry Orton, Kingston Hospital, England.)

hard to modify, and it persists until late in the teens, so treatment must continue over many years. There has been significant progress in recent years toward effectively modifying and controlling long-face growth, with little or no success in shortening the duration of treatment.

The two traditional methods for impeding excessive vertical growth have been (1) high-pull headgear to a complete or partial maxillary fixed appliance or (2) a functional appliance that incorporates bite blocks between the teeth. The headgear applies a direct external force to oppose vertical maxillary develoment; the functional appliance does this indirectly, by stretching the musculature and other facial soft tissues to create a reactive force, which then is applied to the occlusal surfaces of the teeth via the bite blocks.

A functional appliance with bite blocks can control the vertical position of the maxillary and mandibular teeth if the patient cooperates well (i.e., if the appliance is worn 14 to 16 hours per day), and skeletal effects can be observed. More significant alteration in the growth pattern of the maxilla can be obtained with headgear—provided, of course, the child wears it consistently and at least 12 to 14 hours per day. The biggest problem with high-pull headgear is that a purely vertical pull is almost impossible to achieve. Instead, the force has a significant backward component. For some patients with excessive AP growth, this is desirable. But for the majority of long-face patients, the maxilla is not protrusive and only vertical force is

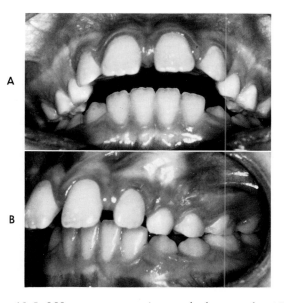

Fig. 13-5. I.H., pretreatment intraoral photographs. (Courtesy Harry Orton, Kingston Hospital, England.)

needed. In addition, it can be difficult to control the entire dentition with headgear to a fixed appliance, especially in younger (mixed dentition) children where a complete fixed appliance cannot be placed.

These difficulties can be overcome to a considerable extent by combining the functional and headgear approaches (Figs. 13-4 to 13-9). One significant improve-

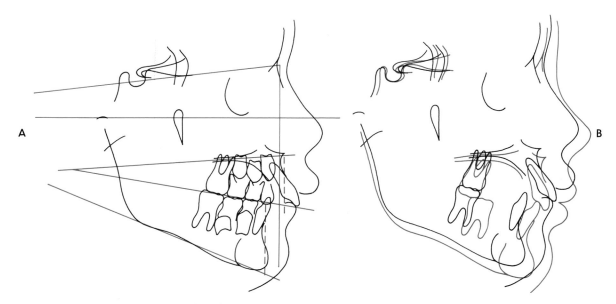

Fig. 13-6.I.H. **A,** Initial cephalometric tracing. Note the maxillary dental protrusion, mandibular deficiency with upright mandibular incisors, tipped palatal plane and long face tendency. Cephalometric measurements: N perp to A, 3 mm; N perp to Pg, −4 mm; AB difference, 10 mm; UFH, 50 mm; LFH, 63 mm; mand plane, 23 degrees; MxI to A vert, 10 mm, 31 degrees; MnI to B vert, 4 mm, 20 degrees. **B,** Superimposition showing the response to combined headgear and functional appliance treatment (following treatment, *solid red*). (Courtesy Harry Orton, Kingston Hospital, England.)

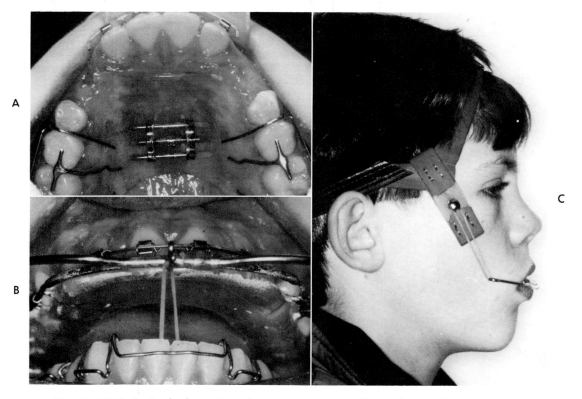

Fig. 13-7.I.H. **A,** At the beginning of treatment a removable appliance (shown here after expansion had been completed) was used to expand the maxillary arch. **B,** After expansion, high-pull headgear was worn to a maxillary splint, and an elastic to a lower removable appliance was used to posture the mandible forward, producing a functional appliance effect. **C,** An anteriorly positioned head cap was used with a short outer bow, providing as vertical a direction of pull as possible. (Courtesy Harry Orton, Kingston Hospital, England.)

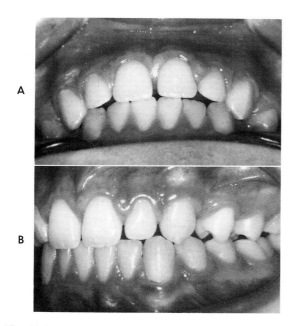

Fig. 13-8.I.H., intraoral photographs, completion of phase 1 treatment. (Courtesy Harry Orton, Kingston Hospital, England.)

ment comes from using a full arch splint to deliver force to the maxilla (see Fig. 13-7), rather than a partial fixed appliance. With a splint, all the teeth are controlled, not just those with bands or bonded attachments. Perhaps more important, the headcap can be altered to bring the line of force more anteriorly, closer to the center of resistance of the maxilla. With headgear to the first molars, if the line of force is too vertical or too far anteriorly, it will pass in front of the center of resistance of these teeth, and the molars will tip forward. With a splint, the center of resistance is that of the entire maxilla, and a more vertical pull is possible.

Although headgear to a maxillary splint gives good control of maxillary growth and eruption of maxillary teeth, there is nothing to prevent eruption of the lower teeth. To shorten face height, the mandible must rotate upward and forward as growth continues, and that will not happen unless lower eruption also is prevented. The maxillary splint also can incorporate bite blocks to control the vertical position of the lower teeth (Fig. 13-10). Such a splint needs only a construction bite that alters mandibular position to be described as a functional appliance.

Headgear to a functional appliance with bite blocks, therefore, appears theoretically to be the best approach to controlling the long-face pattern of growth. In a

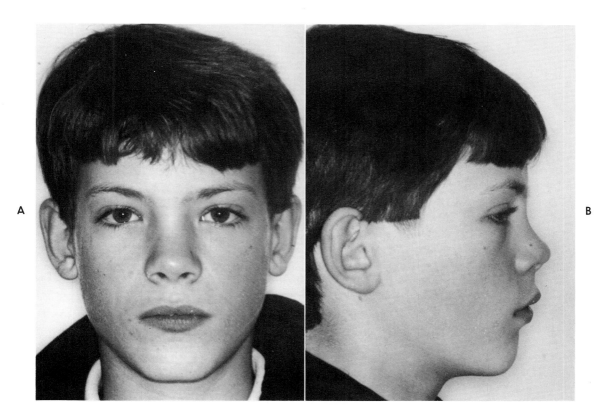

Fig. 13-9.I.H., facial photographs, completion of phase 1 treatment. (Courtesy Harry Orton, Kingston Hospital, England.)

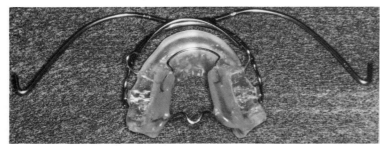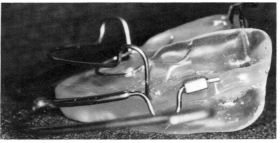

Fig. 13-10. **A,** Occlusal view and **B,** lateral view of a bionator with bite blocks fitted with headgear tubes. The effect of this appliance on the maxilla is similar to that of a maxillary splint, but it also controls the vertical position of the lower teeth.

mandibular-deficient patient, it would be advantageous to advance the mandible when the functional appliance impression was taken, whereas in a patient with a normal-size mandible and a largely vertical problem, the blocks would be positioned without any mandibular advancement. Clinically, the theory seems to be borne out rather well: the combination of headgear and a functional appliance, in a cooperative child, can produce a significant improvement in long-face growth during the mixed dentition years.

Adolescents with Questionable Growth Potential

In evaluating orthodontic patients, it is easy to focus on AP problems. As we have pointed out, long-face patients almost always have an AP jaw discrepancy—the majority are mandibular deficient and Class II. Often the chief complaint is that the upper incisors are too prominent. An occasional teenager or parent is perceptive enough to describe the gummy smile as a problem that should be corrected, but most know only that they do not like the prominence of their upper incisors, without differentiating its vertical and horizontal components. A camouflage treatment plan based on retraction of the upper incisors may be suggested if the orthodontist views the problem as Class II primarily, without recognizing the skeletal vertical problem. This conclusion is more easily reached if no anterior open bite is present.

Correcting the overjet in that way in long-face adolescents is ineffective at best and disastrous at worst. Extraction of premolars does nothing to help correct the vertical problem. As the upper incisors are retracted, it is difficult to keep from elongating them further. The nasolabial angle will increase. If Class II elastics are used, the mandible likely will rotate further down and back, making the long face worse. Before surgery to vertically reposition the maxilla was available, the negative effect on facial esthetics was accepted as inevitable. There is no excuse for that attitude at present.

If extraction for camouflage is to be avoided, are there any orthodontic alternatives for the long-face adolescent? The fact that growth in these patients continues into the late teens is both a problem and a potential opportunity. A problem exists because the growth pattern in long-face patients is poor—an opportunity is present because growth can be modified only when it is occurring, and at least some growth potential usually is present.

The best plan for adolescents with questionable growth potential follows logically: attempt growth modification, using headgear to a functional appliance as described above or to a fixed appliance, and counsel the patient and parents that if this conservative approach does not succeed, surgical treatment will be needed. Unlike attempts at camouflage, growth modification treatment does no harm, and it can improve the vertical and AP relationships sometimes in patients who otherwise would have been labeled "too old" for conservative treatment.

Patients who are treated with this nonextraction orthodontic approach may end up on an uncomfortable borderline. Their occlusion has been corrected reasonably well, but both facial esthetics and long-term stability are questionable. The lower incisors are too protrusive relative to the chin for good stability, and the chin is still deficient. Moderate lip incompetence remains—all of which add up to much less than the optimal treatment result. Viewing the nonextraction treatment as unsuccessful and retreating the patient with extractions will only make things worse.

In the borderline situation, an angled inferior border osteotomy in the mandible to bring the chin upward and forward can produce a tremendous improvement[9] (Fig. 13-11; see also Case 1, Figs. 13-21 to 13-30). The lower lip relaxes and moves up as the chin is elevated. The change in lip position reduces the lip incompetence and should reduce pressure against the lower incisors, improving their stability (the latter point is under investigation now; definitive data for lip pressures and incisor stability after this type of inferior border osteotomy are not yet available). The inferior border osteot-

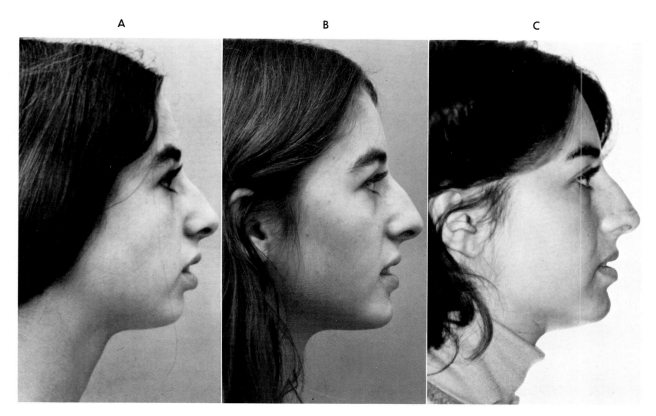

Fig. 13-11. In this 14-year-old girl, nonextraction orthodontic treatment had resulted in excellent occlusion but an undesirable degree of protrusion of the lower incisors, a deficient chin, and moderately long face height with lip incompetence. The upper teeth were well related to the maxilla, so orthodontic retreatment with premolar extraction and retraction of the incisors in both arches would not help and probably would harm facial esthetics. Inferior border osteotomy to elevate and advance the chin solved the esthetic problem. **A,** Facial profile after completion of orthodontics, before inferior border osteotomy. **B,** Three months later, after inferior border osteotomy. **C,** Long-term recall.

omy (see Chapter 10) is not a complicated sugical procedure. It can be done on an outpatient basis, without overnight hospitalization. The result is immensely preferable to the more traditional orthodontic camouflage approach.

Adults with Little or No Growth Potential

For long-face patients with no prospect for successful growth modification, there is no real alternative to surgery. As we have noted above, orthodontic camouflage simply does not work when the problem is primarily vertical. For the patients with anterior open bite, it might be possible to use vertical elastics to pull the anterior teeth together. That is not a good idea for two reasons: (1) relapse into open bite nearly always occurs, and (2) elongating the already prominent incisors makes things worse esthetically rather than better. A patient who has a genuine long-face problem, and who refuses to consider surgical correction, is better left untreated.

PLANNING SURGICAL-ORTHODONTIC TREATMENT
Surgical Approach

Excessive lower-face height is the primary distinguishing clinical characteristic of long-face patients. It follows logically that surgery to decrease the vertical separation of the chin and nose is the key to treatment of this problem. A decrease in face height can be accomplished in three ways:

1. Superior repositioning of the maxilla, or at least the posterior part of the maxilla, via total or segmental maxillary osteotomy. When the maxilla moves up the mandible rotates around the horizontal condylar axis to move up with it, so that the chin moves upward and forward. Indirectly, the maxillary surgery repositions the mandible.
2. Mandibular surgery to bring the lower jaw forward and upward, which could be accomplished in an open-bite patient by tilting the body of the mandible up after a ramus osteotomy. The posi-

tion of the maxilla would not be altered at all, so this treatment approach implies that the problem is largely in the mandible.

3. Superior repositioning of the chin via a mandibular inferior border osteotomy. Rarely is this procedure adequate by itself in an adult, but it is a useful adjunct to either of the other two surgical possibilities.

The guideline for choosing between maxillary and mandibular surgery is quite clear: in patients whose face height should be reduced, maxillary surgery is the primary procedure. A mandibular ramus osteotomy is recommended only as a secondary procedure, after the maxilla has been repositioned vertically. Note that this is just the opposite of the guideline for short-face patients discussed in the previous chapter: for them, mandibular surgery is preferred when face height must be increased, and a maxillary osteotomy is a secondary procedure if required.

The maxilla is the focus of surgical treatment in long-face patients for two major reasons. First, the maxilla nearly always has excessive vertical development, whereas the mandible may not be involved beyond the indirect rotation that maxillary surgery corrects. Neither normal jaw function, lip function, nor good esthetics can be achieved without correcting the maxillary deformity for most patients. Second, moving the maxilla up produces a stable surgical correction. Rotating the mandible at the ramus osteotomy site in a counterclockwise direction stretches soft tissues posteriorly and is notoriously unstable (see the section on treatment possibilities in Chapter 5 for a more complete discussion).

More specifically, in patients with a normal mandible that has been rotated downward and backward (i.e., who could be characterized initially as Class I rotated to Class II) (see Fig. 13-1), superior repositioning of the maxilla to correct the vertical discrepancy also corrects the AP problem because the mandible rotates at the horizontal condylar axis. If the mandible is both small and rotated, a ramus osteotomy for further advancement is needed in addition to superior repositioning of the maxilla. In patients with a large but rotated mandible (who might have been characterized initially as Class III rotated to Class I), correcting the vertical position of the maxilla causes the mandible to rotate into a prognathic position, and a ramus osteotomy to shorten it is required.

Many long-face patients have excessive eruption of the lower incisors (i.e., the distance from the incisal edge to the chin is too great). In addition, the incisors tend to be flared forward, which produces poor chin-lip balance. Both of these problems can be addressed with a mandibular inferior border osteotomy. The bony cuts are angled up anteriorly, allowing the chin to be moved up and forward.

During the maxillary surgery, with the maxilla in the downfractured position, dentoalveolar segments can be created readily. The usual indication for two segments, created by a parasagittal osteotomy, is to allow the maxilla to be widened as it is moved superiorly. Three segments, two posterior and one anterior, usually are employed to correct a vertical step in the arch, typically by moving the posterior segments up more than the anterior. Simultaneously, the posterior segments can also be widened. Isolated posterior maxillary segmental surgery produces the same clinical result as a three-segment total osteotomy with no movement of the anterior segment. Although this approach can be used quite successfully in the treatment of some long-face patients with significant anterior open bite, the LeFort I osteotomy with three dentoalveolar segments gives the surgeom more flexibility to reposition dentoalveolar segments and is often a more logical choice. If necessary, the anterior segment also can be split in the midline, producing four segments and allowing the intercanine distance to be widened.

In summary, the surgical approach to long-face patients almost always includes a LeFort I osteotomy to superiorly reposition the maxilla. Maxillary segments, mandibular ramus osteotomy to advance or set back the mandible, and inferior border osteotomy to reposition the chin are added as the requirements of the individual case dictate.

Orthodontic Approach

As with any surgical-orthodontic case, the orthodontic approach is oriented toward positioning the teeth presurgically in all three planes of space so their position will facilitate the surgical plan and the teeth will fit appropriately when the surgery is completed. To accomplish this goal, the orthodontist must know the general surgical plan and two things quite specifically: (1) whether the maxilla will be kept in one piece or segmented transversely or into anterior and posterior dentoalveolar segments, and (2) whether the chin and inferior border of the mandible will be repositioned, or whether chin-lip balance is to be achieved by orthodontically repositioning the incisors.

Long-face patients rarely have a severely exaggerated curve of Spee in the mandible, even if a deep overbite is present. As a general rule, it is preferable to level the lower arch before surgery. Again, this guideline is in sharp contrast to the one for short-face patients, whose leveling often is done postsurgically. The reason is the same, however. Postsurgical leveling makes it easier to increase face height, whereas presurgical leveling is better when decreased face height is the goal.

On the other hand, a long-face patient with severe anterior open bite often has an extreme curve of Spee in the upper arch, to the point that vertical steps exist in the arch (Fig. 13-12). Usually, the steps are distal to

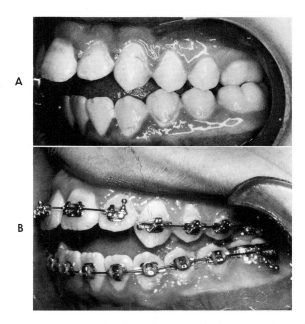

Fig. 13-12. **A,** In this long-face open-bite patient, there is a distinct step in the maxillary arch distal to the lateral incisors. The treatment plan called for surgical leveling via three-segment osteotomy, with the canines in the posterior segments. **B,** From the beginning of treatment, segmental arch wires were used within the segments, avoiding continuous arch wires that would level across them. Note the use of separate NiTi wire segments from lateral to lateral and from canines to molars.

the canines, but they may occur between the lateral incisors and canines. The more severe the steps, the more advantageous it is to segment the maxilla during the surgery and level the arch by repositioning the dentoalveolar segments rather than by moving the teeth orthodontically. The orthodontist's role when surgical segments are planned is to see that there is enough space between the roots of the involved teeth to allow interdental osteotomies and to level presurgically within the segments but not across the osteotomy sites.

Similar thinking guides the decision as to whether to expand a narrow maxillary arch with dental expansion (arch wires only) or orthopedic separation of the midpalatal suture (jackscrew appliance or equivalent), or to defer this for segmental osteotomy. The more severe the narrow maxilla and the older the patient, the better the decision to expand surgically. If the patient is young enough that it is possible to open the suture orthopedically, presurgical expansion with a jackscrew appliance is acceptable. We do not recommend surgically assisted palatal expansion to widen a narrow maxilla in a patient who will be scheduled for LeFort I osteotomy later. A two-segment LeFort I osteotomy is a better choice than two anesthetics and two surgical procedures. Nor is there any reason to expand orth-

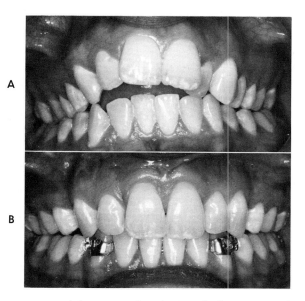

Fig. 13-13. If there is inadequate attached gingiva in the upper arch, there is a risk of gingival recession following LeFort I osteotomy to superiorly reposition the maxilla. **A,** Pretreatment. **B,** Completion of treatment involving premolar extraction and three-segment LeFort I osteotomy. Note the recession around the maxillary central incisors. Gingival grafts before the orthognathic surgery probably could have prevented this complication.

odontically if the dentoalveolar segments can be created with LeFort I osteotomy.

Decisions on these points must be made before the orthodontist can set the detailed plan for the presurgical and postsurgical orthodontics. Careful joint planning between the surgeon and orthodontist to establish the general approach to treatment and make these critical decisions is essential before any treatment begins. Informed consent requires a discussion of these issues (see Chapters 6 and 12).

PRESURGICAL ORTHODONTICS

The selection of the appliance and the general principles of alignment, leveling, and positioning of incisors have been covered in some detail in Chapter 12. Three points are of special interest for long-face patients.

1. A LeFort I osteotomy requires a long incision in the maxillary vestibule. If an inferior border osteotomy is part of the surgical plan, an incision in the mandibular anterior vestibule also will be necessary. These incisions tend to stress the gingival attachment of adjacent teeth, presumably because scar contraction during healing pulls the attachment apically. It is much easier to prevent stripping of gingival tissues and unsightly exposure of roots than it is to correct this if it occurs (Fig. 13-13). When the gingival attachment is questionable, the attachment should be augmented by placing gingival grafts in doubtful areas at least 2 to 3 months

before the orthognathic surgery (preferably, before the orthodontic treatment begins). Gingival stripping is most common around lower incisors in patients who have orthodontics and mandibular inferior border osteotomy, but loss of gingival attachment around the upper incisors can and does occur in patients having maxillary osteotomy, and there it can be an esthetic problem.

2. In a patient with an anterior open bite whose plan calls for a segmental maxillary osteotomy with anterior and posterior dentoalveolar segments, it is important not to level the upper arch during the presurgical orthodontics. Instead, the orthodontist should level within the segments (see Fig. 13-12). Although continuous arch wires with steps at the planned osteotomy sites can be used until just before surgery if desired, usually it is easier and better to use separate arch-wire segments throughout the presurgical treatment. The size of the arch-wire segments and their sequence would be the same as the continuous wires for any other patient (see Chapter 6, Table 6-4), culminating with full-dimension rectangular stabilizing segments. An auxiliary arch wire fitted to the model surgery casts is placed in the headgear tubes at surgery.

It is a mistake to level the upper arch presurgically in the severe open-bite patients because this produces a potentially important relapse tendency. The leveling would occur primarily by elongating the upper incisors. When the orthodontic appliance is removed postsurgically, the incisors would tend to relapse apically to some extent—and of course that would lead to reopening of the bite anteriorly. If the incisors have been elongated during the presurgical orthodontics, the continuous arch wire should be removed and replaced by an anterior segment several weeks before the surgery, so that any relapse tendency can express itself before the final surgical planning is done.

3. Similar considerations guide the approach to maxillary width. If the arch will be expanded orthodontically, this should be done at the very beginning of the presurgical orthodontics, so the expansion can be maintained as long as possible before the expansion appliance is eventually removed. If a LeFort I osteotomy with separate posterior dentoalveolar segments is planned and the expansion will be accomplished surgically, the orthodontist should be careful not to produce any orthodontic expansion. Indeed, in these patients any transverse tooth movement should be contraction rather than expansion of the arch. The surgical segments inevitably will relapse somewhat toward the midline, and teeth tend to move back toward the midline after dental expansion. There is nothing to be gained but something to lose by combining the two relapse tendencies.

FINAL PRESURGICAL PLANNING

Complete records—panoramic and lateral cephalometric radiographs, other radiographs if indicated (e.g., periapical radiographs in areas where interdental osteotomy for segmental surgery is planned), facial and intraoral photographs, and dental casts—are required immediately before surgery. Because these long-face patients will have maxillary surgery, a facebow transfer to a semiadjustable articulator is necessary.

The planning at this stage is largely a repetition of what was done before treatment started. The goals are to verify the original plan, precisely quantify the movements needed at surgery, and complete the model surgery so that occlusal splints can be made. The first step is a cephalometric prediction. From this, the measurements that are necessary for model surgery are taken, and the casts are repositioned on the articulator (see Chapter 5, Fig. 5-27; Chapter 6, Fig. 6-24; Chapter 7, Figs. 7-10, 7-27, and 7-28; and Chapter 11, Figs. 11-1 and 11-2).

There are two critical elements in the planning at this stage: (1) how far the maxilla is moved up, and (2) if there would be residual overjet with a straight vertical movement of the maxilla, whether the maxilla is moved forward or back to correct overjet or the mandible lengthened or shortened by ramus osteotomy.

Moving the maxilla up too far is as harmful to facial esthetics as leaving the long face uncorrected. In the 1970s when LeFort I surgery was first done, many patients were overtreated, largely because it was not appreciated that a few millimeters of lip incompetence is normal. It is a mistake to elevate the maxilla enough to bring the lips into contact at rest, although that was the guideline 2 decades ago. Younger patients can tolerate more upward movement of the maxilla (esthetically and psychologically) than can older ones.

As a general rule, it is better to leave approximately 4 mm of lip separation in the younger patients, perhaps even more in those over age 30. When the maxilla is moved up, the soft tissues of the cheeks are relaxed. That is great for stability but bad for esthetics. The wrinkles that inevitably accompany aging are accentuated, and not many patients beyond their early twenties appreciate suddenly looking older. An additional consideration is the amount of maxillary incisor exposed with the lips at rest. Generally, exposing 30% to 40% of the clinical crown of the maxillary incisor beneath the lip is esthetically pleasing, whereas completely covering it is not.

Long-face patients who have a moderate degree of mandibular deficiency can be a treatment planning dilemma. The mandible rotates forward as it rotates upward—which means that if the maxilla were moved up enough, the mandible could come forward to a normal AP position. Or, if the maxilla were moved back as it

A   B   C

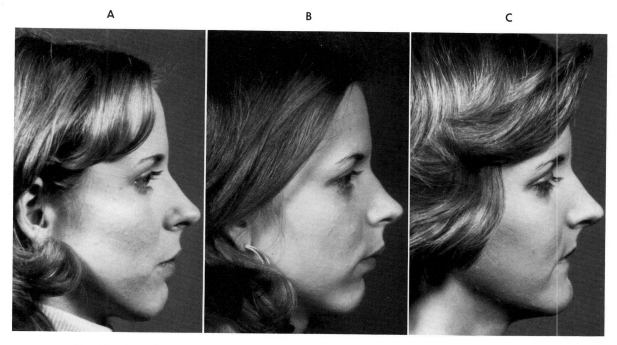

Fig. 13-14. In this patient, a long-face problem with mandibular deficiency even after the mandible rotated up and forward was treated with maxillary surgery alone. To achieve normal overjet, the anterior maxilla was retracted, at considerable cost to support of the upper lip. **A,** Pretreatment. **B,** Immediately before surgery. **C,** Completion of postsurgical orthodontics, 6 months postsurgery. Retracting the maxilla to correct residual overjet can create esthetic problems; mandibular advancement in addition to the maxillary surgery usually is a better option.

moved up, the overjet could be corrected without so much vertical movement. For many patients, moving the maxilla just a little more could prevent having to operate on both jaws.

All other things being equal, one-jaw surgical procedures have less morbidity, better stability, and lower cost as compared with two-jaw surgery. In this clinical situation, however, all other things are emphatically not equal—moving the maxilla up too much is bad esthetically, and moving it back is worse. Often the maxilla should be advanced somewhat to obtain the best lip support and esthetics. Almost never should it be retracted. It is much better to accept the need to do two-jaw surgery to obtain a good result than to significantly compromise esthetics to keep the surgery within one jaw (Fig. 13-14).

The planning is even more of a problem in a patient who habitually postures the mandible forward, so that there is more than 1 to 2 mm difference between intercuspal position (centric occlusion) and retruded contact position (centric relation). Because articulator mountings and the rotation of the mandible around the horizontal condylar axis are predicated on a clinically repeatable retruded contact position of the mandible,

planning cannot be accurate if this repeatable position cannot be found. Fortunately, after patients have been under orthodontic treatment for some months, the dental cues that lead to repeatable forward shifts of the mandible usually are disrupted. It is easier to obtain an accurate mounting just before surgery than at the beginning of treatment.

In the planning stage, it sometimes appears that a patient with a long face can be corrected with mandibular ramus surgery alone. The maxilla adequately supports the upper lip, the maxillary occlusal curve is not steep, and prediction tracings show that bone contact after bilateral sagittal split osteotomy would be sufficient for adequate healing. But if the prediction tracing also demonstrates that the tooth-bearing segment of the mandible must rotate in a counterclockwise direction to produce a satisfactory occlusion, mandibular surgery must be done very cautiously. Even with RIF, the surgical movement in a counterclockwise direction is not stable and the result is not predictable. Postsurgical orthodontics also is exacting. Any elongation of maxillary posterior teeth must be avoided. Too often, the end result is an open bite that can be corrected only by maxillary surgery.

Often, mandibular inferior border osteotomy is added to maxillary surgery with or without mandibular ramus surgery to correct long-face problems. In the prediction tracings, it is apparent that better facial balance can be achieved by lengthening the mandible at the inferior border and removing bone to decrease vertical height in the lower third of the face. Addition of this short surgical procedure produces little risk of additional morbidity and provides stable and predictable results.

The reappraisal of these critical factors when the presurgical records are available may lead to a change in the original surgical plan for some patients. It is wise in the beginning to present the treatment in a way that acknowledges this possibility. If there is any doubt about the need for both LeFort I and mandibular surgery as the plan for treatment is being developed, the orthodontist and surgeon should discuss the possible need for two-jaw surgery with the patient. Patients appreciate candor and full disclosure and would rather learn just before surgery that only LeFort I surgery is needed than a shift in plans from LeFort I surgery to two-jaw surgery. But if any change is decided on immediately before surgery, the reasons for change must be communicated to the patient carefully and tactfully, being sure that he or she understands what is being done and why. A good approach is to present the revised plan as a desirable alternative, showing the patient why and requesting approval.

The final step in the presurgical planning is preparation of the splint or splints. If two-jaw surgery is planned, it is helpful to have an intermediate splint that fits the result of the first (maxillary) stage of surgery as well as a final one. The technique for producing these is illustrated in Chapter 11, Fig. 11-3.

SURGERY

To correct the vertical discrepancy in the long-face patient, the maxilla must move up with LeFort I surgery. Positioning the maxilla to support the lip may dictate that it should move anteriorly or posteriorly as well. With LeFort I surgery, a movement up and forward is not difficult technically. But a movement up and back can be quite a challenge.

To move the maxilla to a posterior position as well as up, bone must be removed from the posterior maxilla, the tuberosity area, and the junction with the palatine bone. Often this bone is dense, access is limited, and the descending palatine vessels (which should be preserved) lie just where bone must be removed. Removing sufficient bone is a critical and important step (see Chapter 8, Fig. 8-16). Otherwise, the maxilla cannot be repositioned and the planned occlusion and lip support will not be achieved. If there is serious question in the planning stages about the feasibility of repositioning the maxilla, two-jaw surgery with mandibular

advancement should be carried out (see description of LeFort I surgery technique, Chapter 8, and two-jaw surgery, Chapter 11).

In some patients, LeFort I osteotomy and mandibular autorotation around the horizontal condylar axis allow correction of the skeletal imbalance in the long face with good esthetic results. The surgeon must take great care in the operating room to position the maxilla as close to the planned position as possible. Both reference marks on the bone and the occlusal splint are used as guides in accomplishing this task. When the maxilla has been freed so that it can be repositioned, the mandible is fixed to the maxilla with maxillomandibular wires and the intervening occlusal splint. With pressure beneath the inferior border of the mandible just anterior to the angles, the maxilla should move easily into its planned new position. Even minor bony interferences in the posterior maxilla can affect its position and displace mandibular condyles (see Chapter 8, Fig. 8-17).

At this stage, with RIF, the malposition of the maxilla is detected before wound closure. After removing maxillomandibular wires, the mandible will not occlude into the occlusal splint, usually hitting prematurely in the molar region. If that happens, the screws holding bone plates in place must be removed, maxillomandibular fixation reapplied, the bony interferences located and eliminated, and rigid fixation reapplied. With only wire fixation in the maxilla, malposition may not be noticed for several weeks. When maxillomandibular fixation is released, the patient will not occlude into the splint. If only a small (1 to 2 mm) discrepancy exists, elastic traction with the splint removed may correct the problem. Occasionally, the discrepancy is greater and reoperation is required. At that point, the surgeon has the option of correcting the position of the maxilla or lengthening the mandible.

As often as not, LeFort I surgery must include several dentoalveolar segments. Widening a narrow maxilla is easily accomplished after the maxilla is downfractured. Parasagittal cuts extended through a midline osteotomy between the maxillary central incisors allow transverse expansion of 5 to 8 mm in the molar region without compromising the soft-tissue pedicle on the palate, which maintains blood supply to the segments (see Chapter 8, Fig. 8-20). Additional expansion is often difficult and may require carefully planned incisions in palatal mucosa. Once the dentoalveolar segments are positioned laterally and into the occlusal splint, an auxiliary arch wire (40-mil steel) prepared before surgery and inserted into the headgear tubes on first molar bands stabilizes the segments well.

When an excessive occlusal curve exists in the maxilla, presurgical orthodontics will position the maxillary teeth so three or four dentoalveolar segments can be created after the maxilla is mobilized. Enough space, 3 to 4 mm, must exist between teeth (usually anterior or posterior to the canine) for interdental vertical bone cuts. The available space should be confirmed just before surgery with periapical radiographs. Occasionally, root proximity exists in a critical area where interdental osteotomy is planned in spite of the best attempts of the orthodontist. Delaying surgery while the orthodontist opens more space is preferred to the risk of severe periodontal defects developing around the maxillary canine or other teeth adjacent to interdental bone cuts.

Surgery in the mandibular ramus is indicated along with LeFort I osteotomy in many long-face patients. When the mandible must be lengthened, the bilateral sagittal split osteotomy is the choice of most surgeons. If the mandible must be shortened to achieve the planned occlusion with the repositioned maxilla, sagittal split or transoral vertical ramus osteotomy will produce comparable results. The technical difficulty in applying RIF after transoral vertical ramus osteotomy has limited its use, and many surgeons will select the sagittal split procedure as their preference. Patients prefer the jaw function soon after surgery that RIF in the mandible allows.

POSTSURGICAL ORTHODONTICS

As with all orthognathic-surgery patients, we recommend for long-face patients that the orthodontist, not the surgeon, remove the splint when the patient is ready for postsurgical orthodontics. The splint should not be removed until the patient is ready to have the stabilizing arch wires removed so that finishing orthodontics can proceed. It is the surgeon's judgment as to when that step is appropriate. With maxillary surgery only and RIF, orthodontic treatment probably can resume as early as 4 or even 3 weeks postsurgically. With two-jaw surgery, a longer healing time seems prudent, even with the use of RIF. When the stabilizing wires are removed, they should be replaced at the same appointment with working arch wires and light vertical elastics, as described in detail in Chapters 6 and 12.

One difference in the postsurgical orthodontics for long-face patients, particularly those who had a maxillary anterior segment osteotomy, is that torque control of the upper incisors may be needed during the initial finishing. Torque requires a rectangular arch wire—but flexibility is needed to align between the segments. The best solution to this dilemma usually is a full-dimension NiTi or braided rectangular arch wire in the upper arch and the typical 16 steel working arch wire in the lower. For patients with 22-slot brackets, 21×25 NiTi usually is better than a similar-sized braided wire because the braided wire may be too stiff. For patients with 18-slot brackets, a braided 17×25 wire usually is better, for the same reason—the smaller NiTi wire often has too little torsional stiffness for effective torque.

With these arch wires, light posterior and anterior box elastics are worn (see Chapter 6 and the case reports below).

The trickiest part of postsurgical orthodontics for long-face patients is maintaining transverse maxillary expansion, particularly surgical expansion. If the maxillary buccal segments relapse medially following the surgery, not only is there relapse toward crossbite, but also the bite tends to open anteriorly because of cuspal interferences posteriorly. It takes at least 6 months following surgery for the maxillary dentoalveolar segments to stabilize transversely, so they must be held in their expanded position during the finishing orthodontics. The easiest way to do this is to use a heavy labial auxiliary wire in the headgear tubes along with the light working arch wires (see Chapter 12, Fig. 12-35). If segmental surgery was done, this can be the same auxiliary wire that was used at surgery (see Chapter 8). If dental expansion was done presurgically, it may be wise to make a new labial auxiliary wire for use at the postsurgical stage.

An alternative for maintaining width is a transpalatal lingual arch. (Although a removable palate-covering appliance also might be possible, this tends to interfere with finishing, and we do not recommend it.) The lingual arch recently has become more practical, and in fact it may now be the appliance of choice over the labial auxiliary wire because of the introduction of lingual brackets that accept 36-mil square wire.[10] A lingual arch would interfere when segmental surgery is done, so it cannot be in place at surgery, and with previous systems it was difficult to add one after surgery. The new system makes that relatively easy, and it has the significant advantage of excellent torque control.

Because the arches were leveled either presurgically or during the surgery, postsurgical orthodontics for long-face patients often is accomplished quickly. The teeth usually fit quite well when the patient returns from surgery, and it is only necessary to settle them into position before going to retainers. Keep in mind that the patients who had transverse expansion must wear the maxillary retainer diligently—full-time for several months at least.

RESPONSE TO TREATMENT
Physiologic Response
Respiration

The possible role of respiratory factors in the etiology of long-face problems has been alluded to above (and discussed in more detail in Chapter 2). To many observers, it has seemed reasonable that nasal obstruction was a major cause of the deformity and that surgery to move the maxilla up would make it worse. The palate also is the floor of the nose, so moving that part of the maxilla up inevitably decreases the volume of the nasal cavity. If the nasal passages were deficient initially, it would seem that they should be even more so after maxillary surgery.

Technically, it is possible to design a LeFort I osteotomy so that the center of the palate is moved up less than the periphery where the teeth are located, and modifications of this type are common in contemporary surgery (see Chapter 8). But even if these modifications are not used, there is no evidence that nasal obstruction is worsened by LeFort I osteotomy. In fact, most patients can move air through the nose better postsurgically than they could before.

The best data are those of Turvey and colleagues.[11] Nasal resistance was measured in 52 patients before and after LeFort I osteotomy to superiorly reposition the maxilla. Two findings are of particular interest. First, the majority of these long-face patients did not have nasal obstruction before surgery—two-thirds had normal resistance to nasal airflow (Fig. 13-15). It is of interest that one-third had elevated resistance to air flow. In a control population with normal facial dimensions, the corresponding figure would be 10% to 15%. In other words, patients with elevated nasal resistance appear to be over-represented in a long-face population who seek and receive surgical-orthodontic treatment.

Second and more important, the effect of the maxillary surgery was the opposite of what might have been expected. None of the patients with normal nasal resistance presurgically had significantly elevated resistance postsurgically (i.e., no normal patient developed even moderately high resistance to air flow as a result of the maxillary repositioning). Ten of the twelve individuals with moderately high nasal resistance presurgically had normal resistance postsurgically; one stayed the same; and one showed an increase but remained in the same range. Six of the seven patients with very high nasal resistance presurgically, for whom nasal respiration would have been all but impossible, had normal resistance to air flow postsurgically; one was unchanged. These data indicate a better than 80% chance that long-face patients who have trouble moving air through the nose presurgically will have normal air flow postsurgically, even if the resistance was very high initially.

The explanation for this effect is deceptively simple. The nostril is described physiologically as the "liminal valve" of the nasorespiratory system. In most people, it is the limiting factor in nasal air flow. When there are difficulties in nasal breathing, clinicians tend to focus on obstructions more posteriorly along the airway. Engorged nasal mucosa, large turbinates, a deviated septum, and/or enlarged adenoids frequently are cited as the cause. Those structures may indeed cause obstruction, but a narrow, pinched nostril also can be a potent limiting factor. Surgery to move the maxilla up tends to open the nostrils by widening the alar base, which is

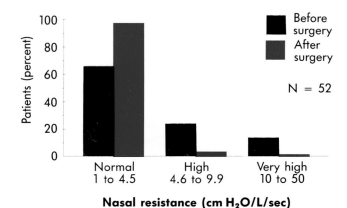

Fig. 13-15. Nasal resistance before and after LeFort I osteotomy for superior repositioning of the maxilla. Note that resistance was normal in two-thirds of these long-face patients before surgery, whereas one-third had resistance high enough to cause some increase in mouth breathing. After surgery, 6 of the 7 patients with very high resistance were normal, with 1 unchanged; 10 of the 12 with moderately high resistance were normal, with 2 unchanged; and none of the normals developed elevated resistance. (Data replotted from Turvey TA, Hall DJ, Warren DW: Alterations in nasal airway resistance following superior repositioning of the maxilla, Am J Orthod 85:109-114, 1984.)

desirable esthetically most of the time because the long-face patients usually have narrow nostrils (see Case 3 below). And the change in nostril shape seems to explain the changes in nasal resistance and air flow.

If nasal resistance is high enough, it is a safe assumption that the patient largely breathes through the mouth. On the other hand, low nasal resistance only makes nasal respiration possible; it does not indicate how the patient breathes. Instrumentation to totally account for nasal and oral airflow has been developed in recent years,[12,13] though it is not yet widely used outside research laboratories. Only a small data set is yet available for patients having LeFort I surgery, but this suggests that most of these patients do have a greater percentage of nasal respiration after their surgery.[14]

Jaw Posture

What dentists refer to as the rest position of the mandible is really its postural position. The difference can be illustrated readily by observing what happens when an individual totally relaxes—the jaw drops. Typically, in the true rest position (minimum electromyographic activity), the jaws are separated by 8 to 10 mm at the molars,[15] whereas the postural position is at 2 to 3 mm of separation.

The role of the teeth in determining the postural position of the mandible often is obscured by prosthodontic concepts based on edentulous patients. When the teeth have been lost, dentures must be fitted within

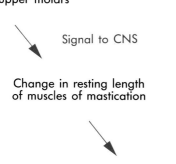

Change in vertical position
of upper molars

Signal to CNS

Change in resting length
of muscles of mastication

Change in posture of mandible

Fig. 13-16. Diagrammatic representation of the physiologic mechanism that alters jaw posture when the maxilla is repositioned superiorly. The nature of the signal from the upper posterior teeth to the central nervous system is unknown. Because the adaptive mechanism is lost when the teeth are extracted, it probably is based on (pressure?) receptors in the periodontal ligament.

the space between the jaws that the musculature establishes, and that space is relatively fixed. It is influenced only slightly by where the prosthodontist places the denture teeth. If the vertical dimension is opened or closed too much, the jaw posture does not adapt—hence the concept of an unchangeable mandibular rest position (remember, really the postural position).

When the natural teeth are present, however, there is a strong feedback between their vertical position and the posture of the mandible. If the posterior teeth erupt too much, the mandible rotates down and back in accommodation—which is exactly what happens in the development of long-face problems, except that we do not know what is cause and what is effect. One might expect, therefore, that if the natural maxillary posterior teeth were moved superiorly, whether by surgery or orthodontics, the mandible would rotate upward in response. Indeed, this occurs following superior surgical repositioning of the maxilla. Studies of patients show that the interocclusal space postsurgically is essentially the same as it was before treatment. In some way that is not understood at present, the central nervous system monitors the position of the jaw when the teeth come into contact and adjusts the postural position accordingly (Fig. 13-16).

Lip Pressure

When the maxilla is moved up and the mandible rotates upward in response, the lower lip follows the teeth upward and forward, and the protrusion of the lower incisors relative to the chin is reduced. One might predict, therefore, that pressure by the lower lip against the incisors would be reduced. If so, the stabil-

ity of the incisors in their new position should be improved.

When pressure transducers are used to measure lip pressures in long-face patients before and after surgery, this hypothesis is borne out—the resting pressure of the lower lip does decrease.[16] Upper and lower lip pressures during speech and swallowing are essentially unchanged, which indicates good functional adaptation, but short-duration pressures are irrelevant for tooth position. The decreased resting pressure of the lips probably contributes to the stability of mandibular incisors that usually is observed in long-face patients, even when the lower arch was expanded with nonextraction orthodontic treatment before surgery.

When a ramus osteotomy is used to lengthen the mandible, the lower incisors are moved forward into the lip, and one might expect that resting lip pressures would increase, with a consequent tendency toward incisor crowding after the treatment was completed. Surprisingly, this does not occur. In our patients who had a mandibular ramus osteotomy for advancement, with or without simultaneous maxillary surgery, lip pressures in function and at rest were maintained at presurgery levels. Good stability of incisor position is observed in most of the long-face patients who have mandibular lengthening as well as maxillary surgery. The adaptation in resting lip pressure undoubtedly contributes to this stability.

Biting Force

The geometry of the jaws suggests that as the maxilla rotates down (as in the long-face growth pattern), the mechanical advantage of the elevator muscles decreases, and biting force in long-face patients therefore should be lower than normal. Surgery to reposition the maxilla superiorly should increase mechanical advantage and biting force, by about 10% with typical surgical changes.[17,18] When we measured occlusal force in 15 patients who had maxillary surgery to correct their long-face condition, we observed that on the average, occlusal force did increase following this surgery.[19] Changes occurred not only in maximum biting force (MBF) but also for forces in simulated chewing and for tooth contact in swallowing, which suggests that this is a true physiologic adaptation, not just a change in how hard the patient is willing to bite. It is more accurate to say, however, that in 10 of the 15 patients the increase in force was greater—for many patients, much greater—than would have been expected from the geometry alone. Two of the 15 patients showed a decline rather than an increase in occlusal force (Fig. 13-17). At this point, there is no explanation for the variability in response. Nearly all patients feel that they have better jaw function following orthognathic surgery (see Chapter 3), and the measurements of occlusal force provide some physiologic evidence that this is correct.

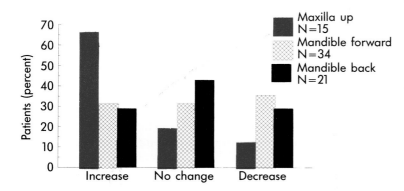

Fig. 13-17. Changes in maximum biting force related to orthognathic surgery. Note that the increase in MBF predicted by geometrical considerations did occur in 10 of the 15 patients who had superior repositioning of the maxilla—but the increase was considerably greater than can be explained as a geometric effect, and did not occur in a third of the group. Patients who had mandibular advancement or setback, alone or in combination with maxillary surgery, often had surprisingly large changes in biting force in either direction.

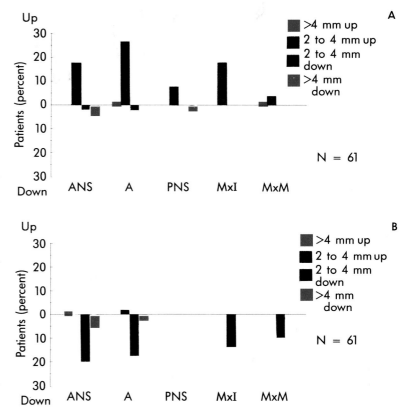

Fig. 13-18. **A,** The percentages of the UNC sample of patients undergoing superior repositioning of the maxilla who had changes in the vertical position of the maxilla during the first 6 weeks after surgery. Note that the majority of the sample were stable, whereas about 20% showed 2 to 4 mm further upward movement of maxillary landmarks. **B,** The percentages of patients who had changes in the vertical position of the maxilla between 6 weeks and 1 year postsurgery. Note that about 20% showed some downward movement of maxillary landmarks, whereas the majority were stable. Downward movements were observed almost exclusively in the patients who had upward movement immediately postsurgery (i.e, the long-term pattern was stability in the majority of the patients, with some upward movement postsurgically and then recovery in almost all the others).

Stability

When surgery to superiorly reposition the maxilla was first carried out, there was concern that the maxilla would relapse downward, leading to return of the open bite and/or gummy smile. Fortunately, elevating the maxilla has proved to be one of the most stable of the orthognathic surgical procedures.

At this point, the most extensive data for stability after superior repositioning of the maxilla are from the UNC data base,[20] but other data sets[21] give the same general picture. The UNC data for 61 patients who had a LeFort I downfracture with the maxilla moved superiorly at least 2 mm, no mandibular surgery except

for inferior border osteotomy, and wire osteosynthesis (no RIF) are the basis for the report here.

In these patients, when the maxilla was moved superiorly, there was little or no tendency during the first 6 weeks for it to move back down. On the average, there was a slight further upward movement. A better way to look at the data, however, is by examining the percentage of the patients who had varying degrees of change. From Fig. 13-18, *A* it can be seen that about 80% of the patients had little or no vertical change during this period, whereas 20% showed 2 to 4 mm of further upward movement.

In the period from 6 weeks to 1 year, the mean

change was a slight downward movement (i.e., relapse), but again this is misleading. Fig. 13-18, *B* shows that during this time, approximately 80% of the patients had no change, whereas 20% had landmarks that moved down. The remarkable finding is that the 20% who had downward movement of landmarks after 6 weeks were the same patients who had further upward movement during the first 6 weeks. In other words, those who were vertically stable remained so, whereas in those who had further upward movement soon after surgery, the maxilla moved back down to its original postsurgical position. As a result, from immediate postsurgery to 1 year, only 3 patients (5%) had significant net relapse—95% were vertically stable. In the one of those three who had the greatest change, complications during and immediately following the surgery interfered with stabilization of jaw segments.

Stability was not as good in the AP plane of space. The primary reason for the maxillary surgery in all these patients was the superior repositioning, but about half the patients had the maxilla moved anteriorly or posteriorly 2 to 4 mm at surgery. During the first 6 weeks postsurgically, there was about one chance in three of partial relapse in the horizontal plane after the maxilla was moved forward or backward respectively. From 6 weeks to 1 year, AP changes seemed primarily related to postsurgical orthodontic tooth movement and to remodeling around the anterior nasal spine. After the first 6 weeks, the changes were not related to the direction of AP movement at surgery.

The data were analyzed to see if any discernible effects on stability could be traced to clinically important factors. For instance, it seems reasonable that stability might be less in younger patients because excessive vertical growth could continue postsurgically, ultimately producing relapse. A third of the patients in this sample were age 18 or younger, but the youngest were 14. All were chosen for surgery because they were judged to be past the adolescent growth spurt and therefore not to have a great deal of growth remaining. Perhaps it is not surprising then that no differences in stability emerged between the younger and older groups. If surgery had been done on patients who still had significant growth remaining, the result might have been different, so it would be incorrect to say that age does not matter. Once a long-face patient is beyond the adolescent growth spurt, however, it appears that there is no reason to delay surgery.

It also has been suggested that segmenting the maxilla after LeFort I downfracture leads to instability. In some quarters, this is an argument for orthodontic or surgically assisted maxillary expansion, so that a one-piece osteotomy can be done when the maxilla is moved vertically. Of the UNC group, 36 had a one-piece LeFort I osteotomy and 25 had LeFort I with segments. No difference in AP or vertical stability existed

between the groups. (Transverse stability as a function of the type of surgical treatment is discussed in detail in Chapter 16.)

It might seem reasonable that the greater the movement at surgery, the greater the relapse tendency. Within the UNC sample, the range of vertical movement was 2 to 12 mm, with a mean of 4 mm. There was no correlation between stability and the distance of surgical movement. Also, no difference was detected between the patients who did or did not have mandibular inferior border osteotomy.

These data support the conclusion that LeFort I osteotomy to superiorly reposition the maxilla produces remarkably stable results, particularly in the context of overall change from surgery to 1-year follow-up. Segmenting the maxilla or adding mandibular inferior border osteotomy to the procedure does not decrease stability, nor does increasing the amount of vertical movement, at least up to approximately 10 mm.

Data also are available from UNC for an additional group of 53 long-face patients who had both the maxilla moved up and a ramus osteotomy for mandibular lengthening, with conventional (not RIF) wire fixation.[22] Stability following mandibular advancement alone has been discussed in some detail in Chapter 12. The postsurgical changes in landmark locations in the patients who had both surgical procedures were similar in some ways to those in patients with each type of one-jaw surgery, but the combination produced some unique features.

In the patients with two-jaw surgery, during the first 6 weeks postsurgically there was a strong tendency for the mandible to slip posteriorly, just as with mandibular advancement alone. As Fig. 13-19, *A* shows, in nearly half the patients, pogonion moved posteriorly 2 to 4 mm, and in 15% it moved more than 4 mm. The maxilla was more stable horizontally, but in 15% point A moved posteriorly 2 to 4 mm. The lower incisors showed much less change than did pogonion, which reflects compensatory forward movement of the incisors. But incisor position also was considerably influenced by the rotation of the jaws that occurred at the same time. The maxilla tended to tip up posteriorly (in 20% of the patients the upper molar moved up 2 to 4 mm) (Fig. 13-19, *B*), and the mandibular plane angle increased, largely because the gonial angle moved upward.

After the first 6 weeks, the vertical response of the maxilla was quite different in the patients with two-jaw surgery that it had been with LeFort I osteotomy alone. There was no tendency for the posterior maxilla to come back down in the patients in whom it moved further superiorly during the first 6 weeks, but there was a strong tendency for the upper incisors to move upward (80% had 2 to 4 mm intrusion during this time) (Fig. 13-20, *B*). In only 30% did the lower inci-

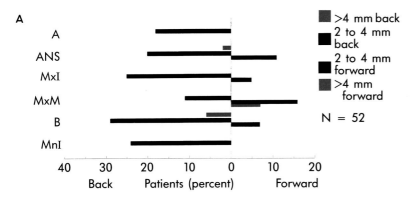

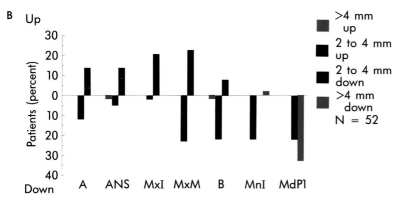

Fig. 13-19. The percentages of the UNC patients with **A,** horizontal and **B,** vertical changes following two-jaw surgery to reposition the maxilla superiorly and advance the mandible. In the first 6 postsurgical weeks, the changes were similar to a combination of those from isolated maxillary and mandibular surgery (compare with Fig. 13-18 and Chapter 12, Fig. 12-28, respectively).

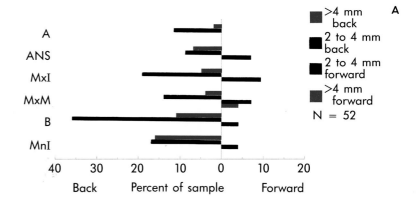

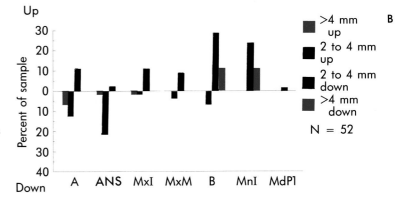

Fig. 13-20. The percentages of patients with **A,** horizontal and **B,** vertical changes 6 weeks to 1 year following two-jaw surgery. Note that, unlike the patients who had isolated maxillary or mandibular surgery, there was little or no tendency to recover the changes that occurred in the first 6 postsurgical weeks during fixation.

sors also move up 2 to 4 mm, which meant that there was a tendency for the bite to open somewhat in many of these patients.

The AP changes from 6 weeks to 1 year were more variable than with isolated surgery in either jaw. Nearly half the patients had continued backward movement of pogonion (Fig. 13-20, *A*), and there was 2 to 4 mm of backward movement of the maxillary incisors and molars in 30% of patients. On the other hand, about 10% of the sample had 2 to 4 mm forward movement of the mandibular landmarks. In the UNC sample with mandibular advancement alone, there was a strong tendency for the mandible to slip back during maxillomandibular fixation, then come forward again between 6 weeks and 1 year (see Chapter 12). That happened to a much lesser extent with the two-jaw patients.

Patients who require two-jaw surgery have more severe problems initially than those who can be treated with surgery in the maxilla or mandible alone, and so it must be kept in mind that the patient groups are significantly different. This probably is the major reason that not only was there less stability in the two-jaw group, there also was a lower percent of clinical success. With either mandibular advancement or maxillary elevation alone, more than 90% of the patients were judged to have an excellent clinical result (i.e., they had correct molar and canine relationships, absence of open bite or deep overbite, and improved facial esthetics). In the long-face two-jaw group, using the same criteria, 32 (60%) were judged to have an excellent clinical result; 10 (19%) had a good result (not more than half-cusp Class II, no open bite); and 11 (21%) had a poor result (more than half-cusp cusp Class II and/or open bite). Ten of the eleven patients with a poor result had a severe open bite before treatment. The intrusion of upper incisors that occurred in most of the patients between 6 weeks and 1 year contributed to bite opening, but why this occurred is less clear.

The impact of RIF on stability after mandibular advancement has been discussed in Chapter 12. Because of the excellent stability of maxillary elevation, one could hardly expect significant improvement from substituting RIF; isolated maxillary surgery often still is done with wire osteosynthesis. In the two-jaw cases, however, the improved stability of RIF should improve the situation in both jaws, lessening the tendency for the mandible to slip back and tip the maxilla back with it. Recent reports from the University of Washington[23] and from Baylor University[24] show that RIF does indeed improve vertical and AP stability after simultaneous maxillary elevation and mandibular advancement. With rigid fixation of the maxilla, the tendency to rotate up posteriorly is almost completely eliminated. The data are not yet adequate to differentiate the pattern of change during healing (the first 6 weeks) from later changes.

There is no reason to believe that major changes occur in long-face patients after 1 year postsurgically, but at this point individual case reports are the only thing available. There simply are no long-term data for groups of reasonable size. Five- and ten-year data will be forthcoming from the longitudinal studies now being carried out.

CASE REPORTS

Case 1

J.W., age 7 years, 11 months, was seen on referral from her pediatric dentist because of concern over her excessive overjet, increased face height, and lip incompetence. Her medical history revealed only occasional upper respiratory infections and a fall that knocked out one primary incisor. Her father was noted to have a long-face appearance, and the maternal grandmother also was reported to have this problem.

On clinical examination, she was a thin girl, small for her age, with obviously increased anterior face height (Fig. 13-21). There was mild crowding in both arches, a V-shaped maxillary arch with posterior crossbite, and 6 mm overjet (Fig. 13-22). Cephalometric analysis (Fig. 13-23) confirmed a developing long-face condition, with the mandible rotated down and back. She was placed on observation and recall, with treatment deferred until more active skeletal growth could be expected.

A second cephalometric film was obtained at age 10 years, 3 months, and additional diagnostic records at age 10 years, 9 months (Figs. 13-24 and 13-25). Over this period, her growth pattern had been unfavorable (Fig. 13-26, *A*), and the overjet had become worse. High-pull headgear was considered, but because she was a cooperative patient and because maximal mandibular growth and maxillary transverse expansion were desired, it was decided to use a Frankel appliance initially, then change to a different appliance for better vertical control. A construction bite was taken with 6 mm advancement and 2 mm opening. She responded very well to the Frankel appliance. During 4 summer months she wore it nearly full-time, overjet reduced from 11 mm to 6 mm, and facial proportions improved noticeably. A second Frankel appliance was made after 6 months, advancing to ideal overjet, which she wore regularly but only part-time. Progress was noticeably slower. After 10

Continued.

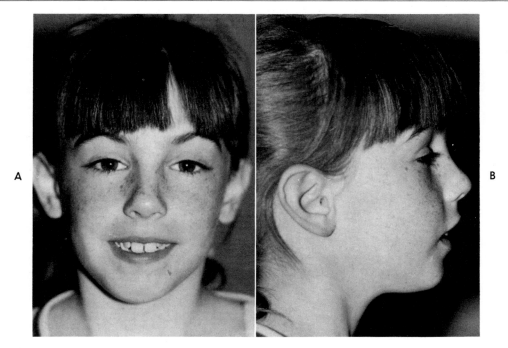

Fig. 13-21. J.W., age 7 years, 11 months. Note the excessive face height and lip separation at rest.

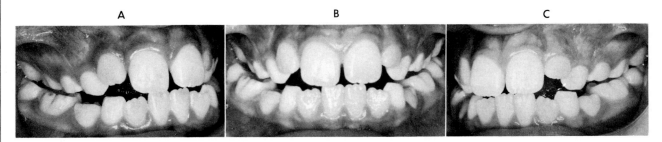

Fig. 13-22. J.W., age 7 years, 11 months.

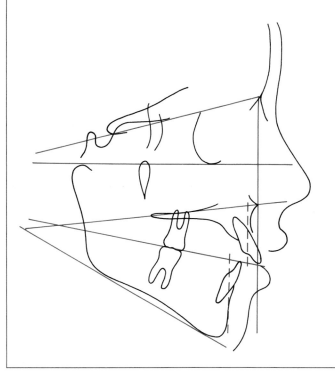

Fig. 13-23. J.W., initial cephalometric tracing. Note the tipped palatal plane, increased mandibular plane, and posteriorly-positioned maxilla. Cephalometric measurements: N perp to A, −5 mm; N perp to Pg, −13 mm; AB difference, 9 mm; UFH, 53 mm; LFH, 65 mm; mand plane, 31 degrees; MxI to A vert, 5 mm, 31 degrees; MnI to B vert, 4 mm, 27 degrees.

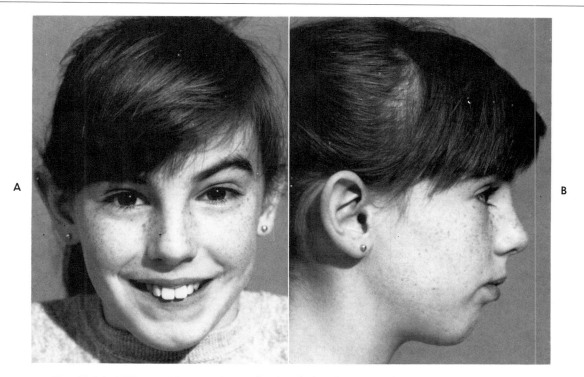

Fig. 13-24. J.W., age 10 years, 9 months, just before beginning functional appliance treatment.

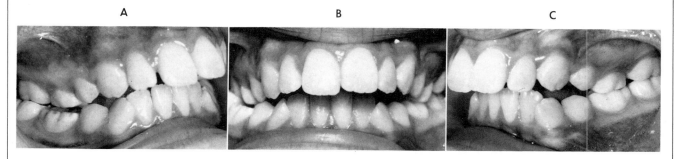

Fig. 13-25. J.W., age 10 years, 9 months.

months, cephalometric superimposition suggested that much of the clinical improvement was due to a headgear effect on the maxilla rather than to favorable mandibular growth (Fig. 13-26, *B*), but the occlusion and face continued to look better (Fig. 13-27). A third Frankel appliance was made at age 12 years, 2 months, which she did not wear well. Functional appliance treatment was discontinued at age 12 years, 8 months. Cephalometric superimposition over the period of functional treatment (see Fig. 13-26, *B*) indicated that differential mandibular growth had been obtained, with evidence of both a headgear effect on the maxilla and a Class II elastic-like effect on the maxillary and mandibular teeth. Dental occlusion (Fig. 13-28) and facial appearance (Fig. 13-29, *A* and *B*) were improved, but further treatment was needed.

At age 12 years, 10 months, a second phase of fixed-appliance orthodontic treatment was begun, with the goal of completing alignment, correcting the residual posterior crossbite tendency, and reducing the overjet to ideal. The plan was to treat without extractions, avoiding camouflage that would make surgical correction impossible if the orthodontic treatment were unsuccessful. An 18-slot edgewise appliance with bands on first molars and bonded brackets elsewhere was placed. As alignment was obtained with 16 NiTi, 16 steel, and then 17×25 TMA arch wires, the mandible rotated slightly down and back and overjet increased. In consultation with the parents, it was decided to use interarch elastics to bring the teeth together and then surgically reposition the chin upward and forward. Elastics without the inferior border osteotomy would produce an unstable

Continued.

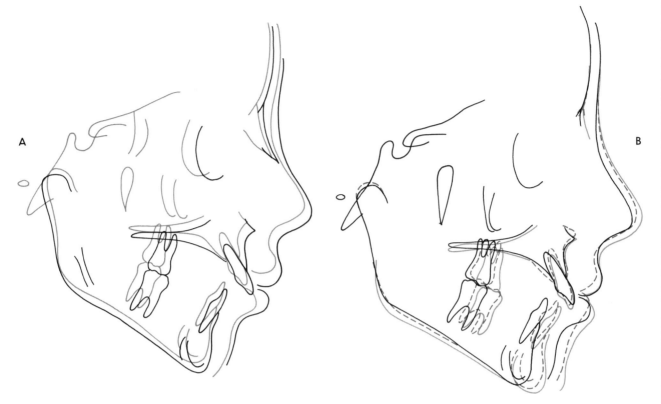

Fig. 13-26. J.W., cephalometric superimpositions. **A,** Ages 7 years, 11 months *(red),* to 10 years, 3 months *(black):* observation without treatment. **B,** Ages 10 years, 3 months, to 11 years, 7 months, to 12 years, 8 months: response to Frankel appliance treatment.

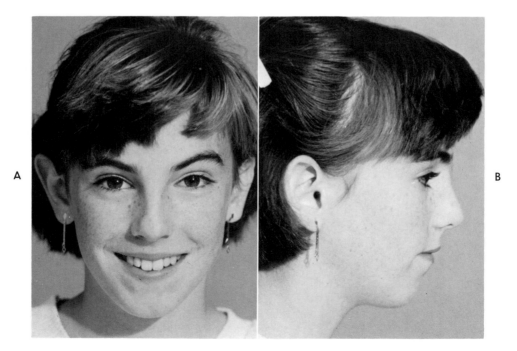

Fig. 13-27. J.W., age 12 years, during functional appliance treatment. At this point, the second Frankel appliance was discontinued and a third one was placed.

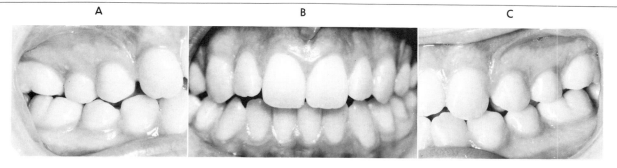

Fig. 13-28. J.W., age 12 years, 8 months, dental relationships before beginning fixed-appliance treatment.

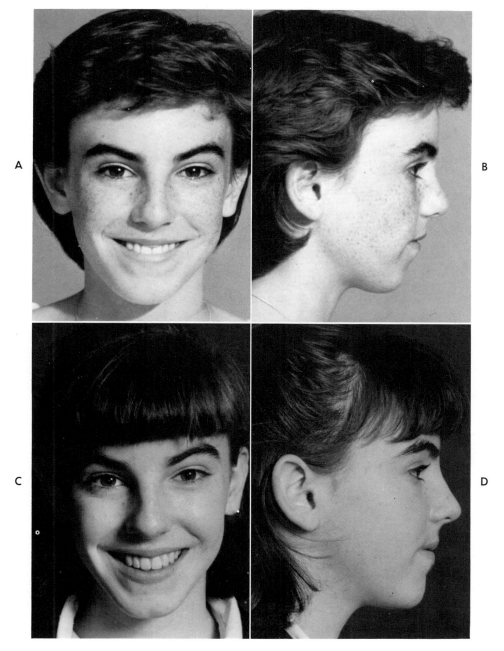

Fig. 13-29. J.W. A and B, age 12 years, 8 months, before and C and D, age 14 years, after inferior border osteotomy to reposition the chin.

Continued.

Case 1—cont'd.

result, and the only other alternative was LeFort I osteotomy, which was felt to be overtreatment for this patient. In anticipation of an incision in the mandibular anterior vestibule, periodontal consultation was obtained relative to the attached gingiva in the incisor region; no grafts were recommended.

At age 13 years, 9 months, with the occlusion slightly overtreated with elastics that were discontinued at that point, mandibular inferior border osteotomy to bring the chin upward and forward was done as an outpatient procedure (i.e., the patient was admitted to the hospital in the morning, the procedure was carried out under general anesthesia in the special surgical facility for patients scheduled in this way, and she was discharged on

the same afternoon). The chin was approached via an incision in the anterior vestibule, a submucosal dissection was carried out, and a reciprocating saw was used to free the lower border segment that was pedicled lingually. The inferior border segment was repositioned and stabilized, and the wound was closed. She was discharged with a pressure dressing in place (see Chapter 10 for details of the surgical procedure).

Three months later, at age 14 years, 2 months, the orthodontic appliances were removed, and removable retainers (maxillary Hawley, mandibular canine-to-canine clip-on) were placed. Facial proportions were considerably improved (Figs. 13-29, 13-33, *B*), and occlusal relationships were good (Fig. 13-30).

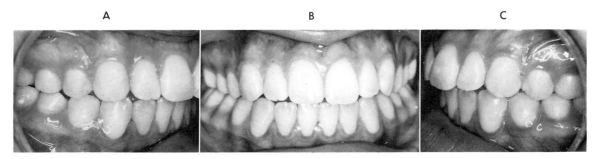

Fig. 13-30. J.W., age 14 years, 3 months, dental relationships 3 months after removal of the fixed appliance. With conventional retainers, the mandible was beginning to rotate downward again, and at this point a bionator as a retainer was begun.

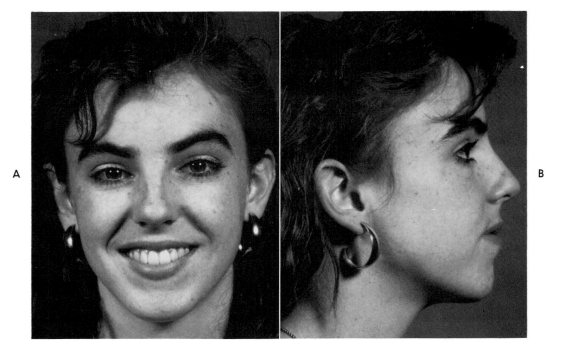

Fig. 13-31. J.W., age 16 years, 6 months, 2½ years after appliance removal.

Case 1—cont'd.

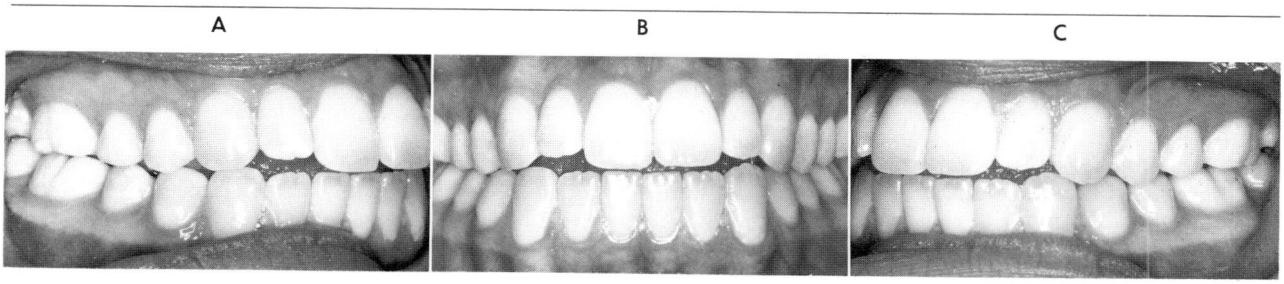

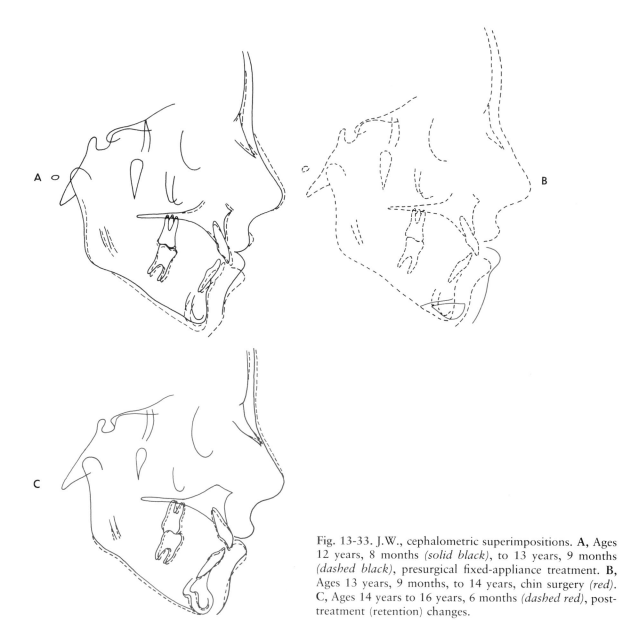

Fig. 13-32. J.W., dental relationships, age 16 years, 6 months. At this point, she was still wearing the bionator at night to control the tendency for bite opening as growth was completed.

Fig. 13-33. J.W., cephalometric superimpositions. **A,** Ages 12 years, 8 months *(solid black)*, to 13 years, 9 months *(dashed black)*, presurgical fixed-appliance treatment. **B,** Ages 13 years, 9 months, to 14 years, chin surgery *(red)*. **C,** Ages 14 years to 16 years, 6 months *(dashed red)*, post-treatment (retention) changes.

Continued.

Case 1—cont'd.

Almost immediately, the bite began to open slightly anteriorly. After 4 months, the traditional retainers were replaced with an open-bite bionator, which incorporates bite blocks to control posterior eruption. The occlusion stabilized. On recall at age 16 years, 6 months, the patient and her parents were quite pleased with the facial proportions (Fig. 13-31). Also, occlusal relationships were good, but with 2 mm anterior open bite (Fig. 13-32). Cephalometric superimposition (Fig. 13-33, C) showed that further vertical growth had occurred between ages 14 and 16.

Comments. This patient illustrates the difficulties in orthodontic treatment caused by the long-face pattern of growth. She responded well initially to a functional appliance, then progressed much more slowly. There is no way to know how much of the result was due to decreasing cooperation and how much to unfavorable growth, but the cephalometric superimpositions illustrate the downward-rotating growth pattern that is characteristic of long-face patients. In J.W.'s case, the long-face pattern was expressed except when treatment to control it was being used.

Surgery to reposition the mandibular inferior border often is not thought of as an adjunct to orthodontic treatment in the same way that extractions can be, but it can be extremely beneficial to patients of this type. Twenty years ago, this girl probably would have been treated with premolar extractions. That would have made both the maxillary and mandibular dentitions less prominent, but would not have improved the excessive face height or helped the open-bite tendency. In contrast, repositioning the inferior border of the mandible improves facial balance vertically and anteroposteriorly, as the chin is brought upward and forward. It also improves lower incisor stability (we think) by decreasing lip pressure against these teeth. The surgery itself is straightforward, and the results are quite predictable.

Vertical growth in long-face patients usually continues until the late teens, which means that relapse due to further growth can occur after treatment is completed. The standard orthodontic retainers hold teeth in alignment but do not control unfavorable growth. As the tendency toward posttreatment bite opening demonstrates, it would have been wiser in this patient to use a bionator as the retainer from the time of debanding. Once growth has been completed, the tendency toward bite opening almost always disappears (which is further evidence that tongue thrust, on which the problem traditionally has been blamed, is not the culprit). But retention must be maintained to that point. Even in girls, this often is not until age 18, and may be the early twenties in boys.

Case 2

J.M., age 13 years, 1 month, was referred for consultation and assistance in planning treatment by an orthodontist in a nearby city because of concerns about the patient's severe open bite, underdeveloped maxilla, and probable need for surgical-orthodontic treatment. Her medical history revealed that at birth, both hips were dislocated, there was a minor defect in the trachea, and a heart murmur was noted that disappeared later. The obstetrician reported that the umbilical cord was wrapped around the neck but apparently had not caused major difficulties. The dislocated hips were treated between ages 3 and 9 months with no residual problems.

On clinical examination, slightly excessive anterior face height and a tendency toward maxillary deficiency were noted. There was severe maxillary and moderate mandibular crowding, with a 5 mm anterior open bite. The teeth and soft tissues appeared healthy, except for questionable quality of the attached gingiva in the mandibular anterior area. TM joint function was normal. A mild problem with speech articulation existed. It appeared that some of the midline muscle of the uvula was missing or deficient, and a submucous cleft of the palate was suspected. She was referred for laboratory examination and evaluation by the cleft palate team. Pressure-flow analysis showed that she could completely close off the nose during speech, and soft-palate function was normal, so a submucous cleft was ruled out. The speech pathologist felt that the articulation problems were compatible with the severe open-bite malocclusion. Extraction of maxillary and mandibular first premolars, with orthodontic treatment to align teeth and gain arch compatibility in preparation for maxillary surgery, was suggested.

Nearly 2 years later, at age 14 years, 10 months, (Figs. 13-34 to 13-36), with no treatment having being done in the meantime, she returned to the university, requesting treatment. The clinical findings were essentially the same as previously. The maxillary canines were completely blocked out of the arch, and moderate mandibular incisor crowding existed. There was a 5 mm anterior open bite with no tooth contacts forward from the lower first molars and a bilateral posterior crossbite. Cephalometric analysis (see Fig. 13-36) confirmed maxillary deficiency, with excessive eruption of the maxillary posterior teeth, downward-backward rotation of the mandible, and excessive lower-face height. Her problems were summarized as (1) severe underdevelopment of the maxilla anteroposteriorly and transversely, but with excessive vertical development; (2) anterior open bite, skeletal, related to the rotation of maxilla

Case 2—cont'd.

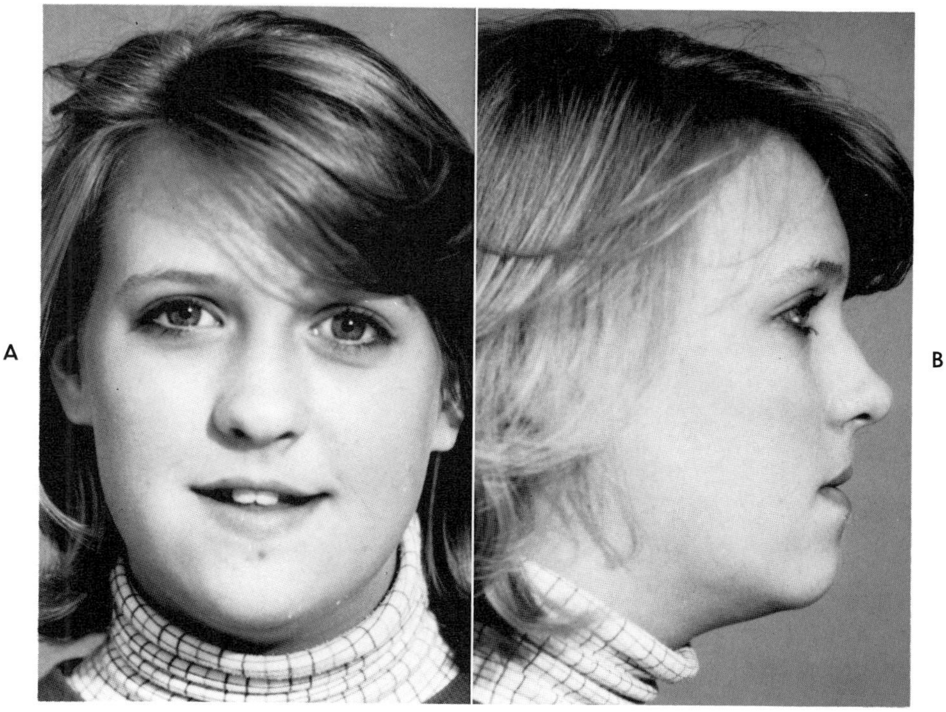

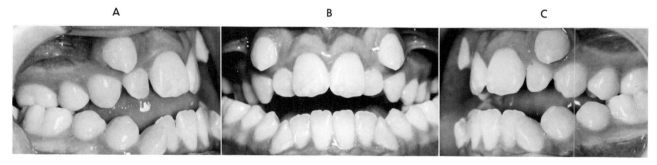

Fig. 13-34. J.M., age 14 years, 10 months.

Fig. 13-35. J.M., dental relationships, age 14 years, 10 months.

and mandible; and (3) severe maxillary and moderate mandibular crowding.

The treatment plan called for:

1. Extraction of maxillary first and mandibular second premolars.
2. Orthodontic treatment to align the teeth and obtain arch compatibility.
3. Orthognathic surgery to widen the upper jaw, bring it forward, and rotate it up posteriorly. Possibly, mandibular surgery would be needed at the same time. The timing of the surgery would depend on whether she showed significant continuing growth during the presurgcial orthodontics, which would take at least 12 months.

4. Postsurgical orthodontics, to bring the teeth into their final position.
5. Orthodontic retainers, full-time initially and then part-time until growth was complete.

Following the extractions, bands were placed on molars and bonded brackets (18-slot edgewise) on other teeth. Alignment was accomplished with 16 NiTi followed by 16 steel arch wires. In the maxilla, there was almost no residual space after alignment. In the mandible, elasto-meric modules on the 16 steel arch wires were used to close the remaining extraction space (an approach calculated to minimize retraction of the incisors); then 17×25 NiTi, TMA, and steel arch wires were placed sequentially. In the maxillary arch, 17×25 TMA, then

Continued.

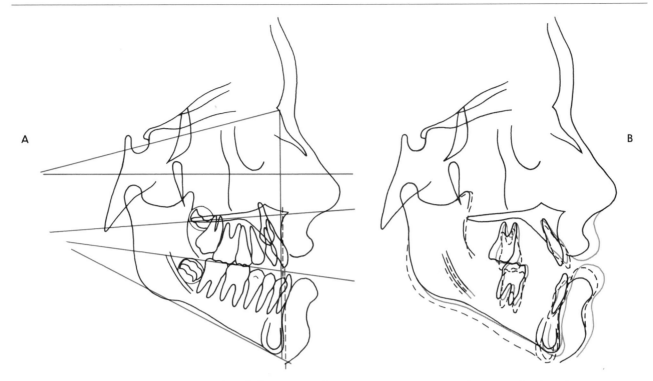

Fig. 13-36. J.M. **A,** Initial cephalometric analysis, age 14 years, 10 months. Note the tipped palatal plane, lip incompetence, and tendency toward a Class III jaw relationship. Cephalometric measurements: N perp to A, 1 mm; N perp to Pg, 1 mm; AB difference, 1 mm; UFH, 43 mm; LFH, 59 mm; mand plane, 28 degrees; MxI to A vert, 1 mm, 22 degrees; MnI to B vert, 2 mm, 17 degrees. The maxillary unit length (Harvold) is mm; mandibular unit length, mm; max-mand difference. **B,** Superimposition, ages 13 years, 1 month *(black)*, to 14 years, 10 months *(solid pink)*, observation without treatment, to 15 years, 9 months *(dashed black)*, ready for surgery.

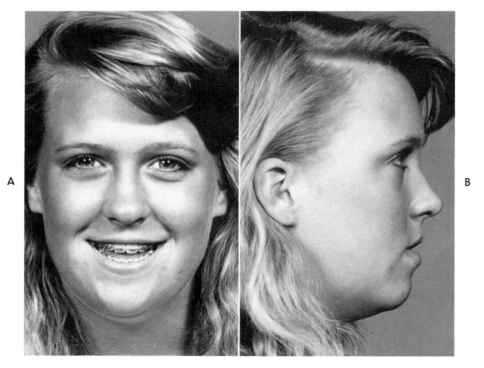

Fig. 13-37. J.M., age 16 years, 1 month, just before surgery.

17×25 steel was used. After the 17×25 steel wires had been in place for 3 weeks, the final presurgical impressions on which the splints would be made were taken, and lugs were added to the arch wires.

A cephalometric film taken at age 15 years, 9 months, showed little or no growth during the previous year. The patient very much wanted the surgery as soon as possible, and it was decided that it would be acceptable to proceed with it the next summer. From cephalometric prediction, it was determined that the best result would be achieved from a combination of LeFort I osteotomy of the maxilla, bilateral sagittal split osteotomy, and inferior border osteotomy of the mandible to reposition the chin. Cephalometric prediction showed

that without setting the mandible back, the maxilla would have to be advanced too much—the result would be bimaxillary protrusion. Repositioning the chin was needed to improve both vertical and AP relationships with the mandibular teeth. A bone graft to the maxilla would be needed, and it was planned to obtain cranial bone from the parietal region for this purpose. At age 16 years, 1 month, 12 months after the orthodontic preparation began, she was admitted to UNC Hospitals for the surgery (Figs. 13-37, 13-38, and 13-39, A).

In the initial part of the surgical procedure, after preparation of the right parietal region, a full-thickness incision was made to bone and a 3 × 3-cm square area of bone

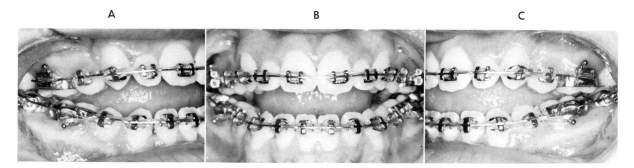

Fig. 13-38. J.M., age 16 years, 1 month, dental relationships at the completion of presurgical orthodontics. At this appointment, the 17×25 steel wires were removed, splint impressions were taken while they were in the laboratory having soldered spurs attached, and the arch wires then were replaced with no activation.

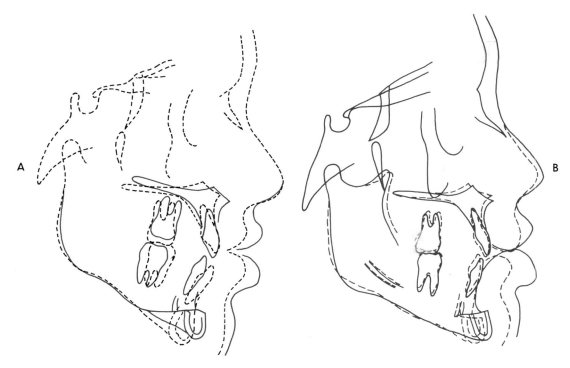

Fig. 13-39. J.M., cephalometric superimpositions. **A,** Age 16 years, 1 month *(dashed black),* to 16 years, 2 months *(red),* presurgery to postsurgery. **B,** Age 16 years, 2 months *(red),* to 16 years, 11 months *(dashed red),* postsurgery to completion of treatment.

Continued.

Case 2—cont'd.

was outlined by bony cuts through the outer diploic table only, using rotary instrumentation. This bone was divided into three 1 cm strips, which were removed using chisel and mallet. Hemorrhage was controlled with bone wax, and the wounds closed.

After the harvest of cranial bone, LeFort I osteotomy was performed under hypotensive anesthesia as described in Chapter 8. The maxilla was moved upward 4 mm posteriorly, 3 mm anteriorly, and forward 3 mm. The strips of calvarial bone were secured in place on the anterior maxilla. With maxillomandibular fixation released and the splint in place, the position of the maxilla was checked by rotating the mandible into the splint. Next, the sagittal split osteotomies (see Chapter 9 for details) were performed and the mandibular right and left third molars were identified and removed. With the teeth in MMF and the splint intervening, three 2.0-mm position screws were placed bilaterally. When fixation was released to check the jaw position, the mandible rotated into the splint without interference.

After the sagittal split incisions were closed, the chin was approached via an incision in the anterior vestibule, an inferior border osteotomy advanced the chin 3 mm, and two 2.0-mm position screws were placed for stabiliza-

tion (see Chapter 10 for details) (Fig. 13-39, *B*). Finally, the maxillary incisions were closed. A pressure dressing was placed in the operating room.

The patient did well postoperatively. She received one unit of autologous blood on the day following her surgery and was discharged on the morning of the third day. At that point, she was in maxillomandibular fixation. After 3 weeks, the fixation was released and she functioned into the splint, guided by ⅜-inch elastics.

Six weeks postoperatively, the splint and stabilizing arch wires were removed and 16 steel arch wires were placed. Posterior box ⅜-inch elastics were worn full-time, with an anterior box elastic added at night only (Fig. 13-40). Six weeks later, with the posterior teeth settling into occlusion nicely, 17×25 TMA arch wires were placed in the maxilla and mandible, and ⁵/₁₆-inch triangular Class II elastics were used to reduce overjet. Six months after orthodontics resumed, she was debanded to an immediate positioner, and 3 weeks later, maxillary Hawley and mandibular canine-to-canine clip-on retainers were placed. Facial esthetics (Fig. 13-41) and occlusal relationships (Fig. 13-42) were good.

The retainers were worn full-time for 3 months, then only at night. On 2-year follow-up, facial proportions had

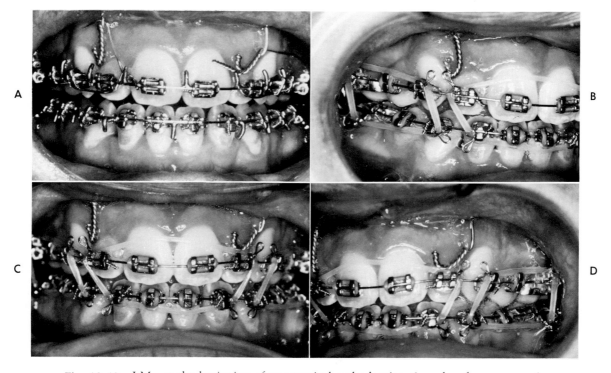

Fig. 13-40. J.M., at the beginning of postsurgical orthodontics, 6 weeks after surgery. **A,** Occlusal relationships immediately after removal of the splint. Note the use of skeletal suspension wires to the maxillary orthodontic stabilizing arch wires. After MMF was released 2 weeks postsurgically, she had been functioning into the splint. **B to D,** Same appointment, stabilizing arch wires replaced by 16 steel working arch wires, ⅜-inch box elastics in place.

Case 2—cont'd.

been maintained nicely (Fig. 13-43), but the bite was slightly open anteriorly (Fig. 13-44), and additional orthodontic treatment to close it was offered.

Comments. Maxillary deficiency often involves only one or two of the three planes of space rather than all three. Three-dimensional maxillary deficiencies occur almost exclusively in patients with repaired cleft lip and palate. Excessive vertical development accompanies transverse deficiency as often as not (see Chapter 13 for further discussion). For J.M., the rotation of the maxilla down posteriorly was the major cause of the open bite. Although she had bilateral posterior crossbite initially, this was due mostly to the AP position of the maxilla

rather than to an absolute width deficiency. Thus her maxillary deformity could be described best as a combination of AP deficiency and vertical excess with rotation down posteriorly, an unusual but by no means unheard of combination.

Following maxillary surgery, adaptations in the velopharyngeal closure mechanism are required to maintain a palatal seal. Leakage of air through the nose produces cleft-palate speech, which would be a serious complication of LeFort I osteotomy. In the absence of a preexisting cleft, this almost never happens. In a patient with a cleft, however, even a mild submucous cleft that previously was not recognized, there is a risk of cleft-palate

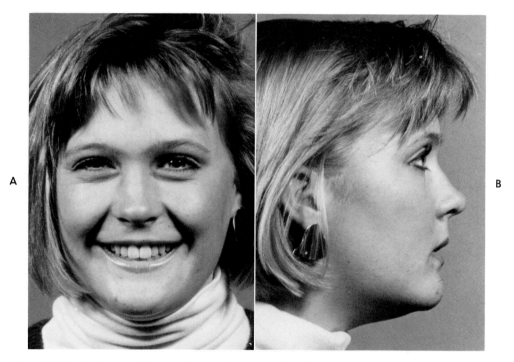

Fig. 13-41. J.M., age 17 years, 5 months, 6 months after completion of postsurgical orthodontics and 15 months postsurgery.

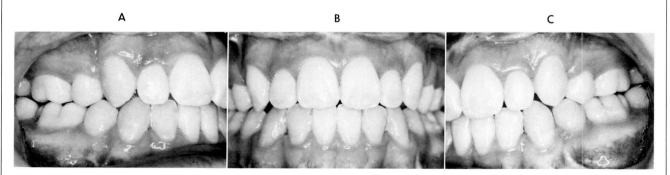

Fig. 13-42. J.M., age 16 years, 11 months, dental relationships at completion of treatment.

Continued.

speech if the maxilla is repositioned. Presumably, this occurs because the patient already was at the limit of physiologic adaptation in producing normal speech presurgically. J.M. and her parents were warned that there was a small chance of this complication, and that pharyngeal-flap surgery as a secondary procedure might be required if it occurred, but there were no posttreatment speech problems.

The staging of the four separate procedures employed for this patient was typical: where all are required, it usually is better to harvest the bone for grafting first; reposition the maxilla, using an intermediate splint to assist in locating it; reposition the mandible to the stabilized maxilla; and finally reposition the inferior border of the mandible. Using cranial bone as the graft source has the considerable advantage of reduced postsurgical morbidity. Note that the hospitalization with the combined procedures was 1 day longer than the typical stay for one-jaw surgery.

With surgery in the midteens, there is always the possibility of some relapse due to additional growth, and J.M. had a mild open bite at age 18 because a small amount of additional vertical growth occurred. This may be related to tongue posture, and it has been suggested recently that postsurgical relapse can be controlled by forcing a change in tongue posture.[25] Once growth has ended, however, the position of the teeth appears to be stable after orthodontic correction, so the tongue is not the sole cause of instability in the occlusion.

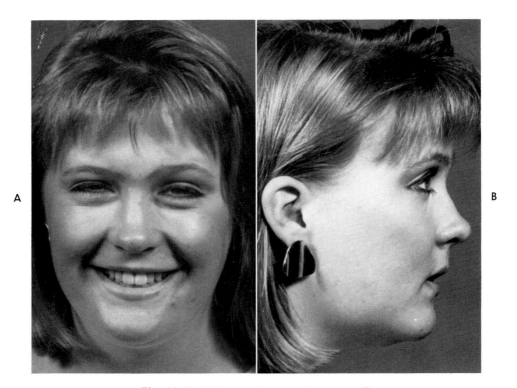

Fig. 13-43. J.M., age 18 years, 2-year recall.

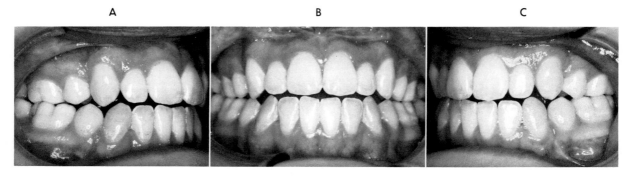

Fig. 13-44. J.M., age 18 years, dental relationships at 2-year postsurgery recall. At this point, she was still wearing retainers at night, but the bite had opened anteriorly.

Case 3

S.D., age 23 years, 8 months, and now employed as a computer programmer in the area, was referred by her home-town orthodontist for treatment of her long-face condition. Her chief concern was the appearance of her maxillary anterior teeth and gingiva when she smiled.

The medical history revealed a fracture of the left condylar process of the mandible at age 9. Radiographically, there was an obvious distortion of the form of the left condyle, but no limitation of motion or significant facial asymmetry existed. She appeared very slender, almost frail.

On clinical examination, TM joint function was good. Severe gingivitis was present around a crown on the maxillary left central incisor, which contributed to the unsightliness of the exposed gingiva when she smiled. Oral tissues otherwise were healthy. Anthropometric mea-surements confirmed the excessive length of the face compared with its width, with the vertical excess in the lower third (Fig. 13-45). There was a full-cusp Class II malocclusion, with a Class II, division 2 pattern in the incisor relationship and an anterior deep bite (Fig. 13-46). Cephalometric analysis confirmed that the Class II relationship was entirely due to downward-backward rotation of the mandible in response to excessive vertical development of the maxilla. The maxillary teeth were well related to the maxilla, and the mandibular incisors were protrusive and supraerupted relative to the mandible (Fig. 13-47; also see Fig. 13-3).

Her nondevelopmental problems were summarized as: (1) frail physical condition, (2) old mandibular fracture with good healing and normal function despite some condylar distortion, and (3) inadequate restorations re-

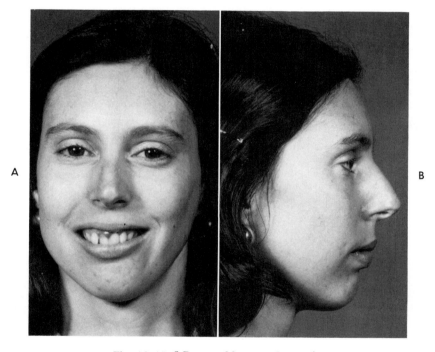

Fig. 13-45. S.D., age 23 years, 8 months.

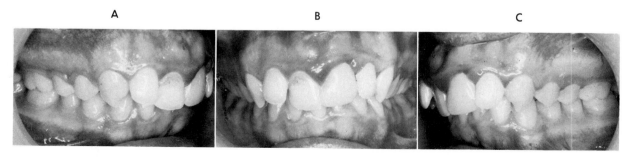

Fig. 13-46. S.D., age 23 years, 8 months, dental relationships.

Continued.

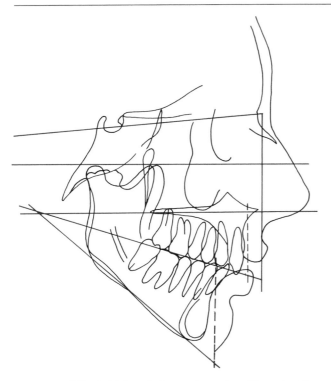

Fig. 13-47 S.D., initial cephalometric tracing. Note the bimaxillary retrusion, steep mandibular plane, retroclined maxillary incisors and proclined mandibular incisors. Cephalometric measurements: N perp to A, −7 mm; N perp to Pg, −26 mm; AB difference, 17 mm; UFH, 54 mm; LFH, 71 mm; mand plane, 41 degrees; MxI to A vert, −2 mm, −4 degrees; MnI to B vert, 11 mm, 35 degrees (also see Figure 13-3 for additional measurements).

sulting in marginal gingivitis, particularly around the crown on the maxillary left central incisor. Developmental problems in priority order were: (1) vertical maxillary excess, with exposure of maxillary gingiva; (2) downward-backward rotation of the mandible, producing Class II malocclusion; (3) crowded maxillary and protrusive mandibular incisors; and (4) deep bite anteriorly.

The treatment plan called for:

1. Temporary replacement of the defective crown presurgically (permanent replacement later), and periodontal treatment to bring gingivitis under control.
2. Nonextraction orthodontic treatment to align the crowded maxillary incisors and produce arch compatibility.
3. LeFort I osteotomy to elevate the maxilla and bring it slightly anteriorly, and mandibular inferior border osteotomy to elevate and advance the chin.
4. Postsurgical orthodontics to bring the teeth into final interdigitation.
5. Orthodontic retainers, full-time initially, then part-time on a decreasing basis.

After the preliminary restorative and periodontal treatment was completed, brackets (18-slot edgewise) were bonded from second premolar to second premolar in both arches, and bands were placed on first molars. Alignment was begun with 15-mil multistrand steel wires, which were followed by 17.5 multistrand, 16 steel, and 17×22 steel arch wires. During the presurgical orthodontics, she was seen at regular intervals by the periodontist. At the point that she was almost ready for orthognathic surgery, she was hospitalized twice in 2 months for a collapsed lung and underwent thoracotomy for treatment of associated problems, after which her general health improved considerably.

At the time of hospital admission for orthognathic surgery, 10 months after the presurgical orthodontics be-

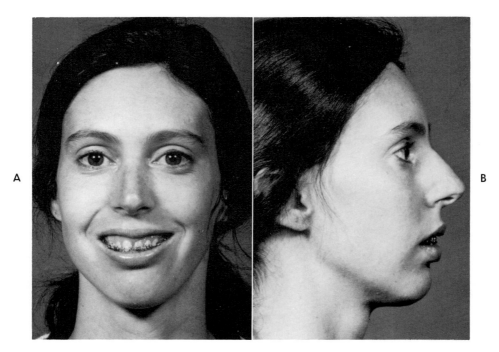

Fig. 13-48 S.D., age 24 years, 6 months, just before surgery.

gan (and after a 4-month delay related to the thoracotomy), facial proportions were essentially unchanged and overjet had increased significantly (Figs. 13-48 and 13-49). Cephalometric superimposition showed that the maxillary incisors had been advanced and that the mandible had rotated slightly further down and back in response to the orthodontic mechanotherapy (Fig. 13-50, *A*).

LeFort I osteotomy, with removal of a 5-mm wedge of bone, was performed to move the maxilla upward and slightly anteriorly to its predetermined position. Transosseous wires were placed for stabilization. Inferior

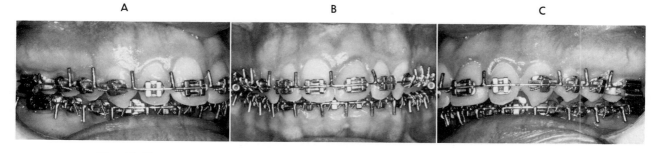

Fig. 13-49.S.D., age 24 years, 6 months, with 17×25 steel stabilizing arch wires in place just before surgery.

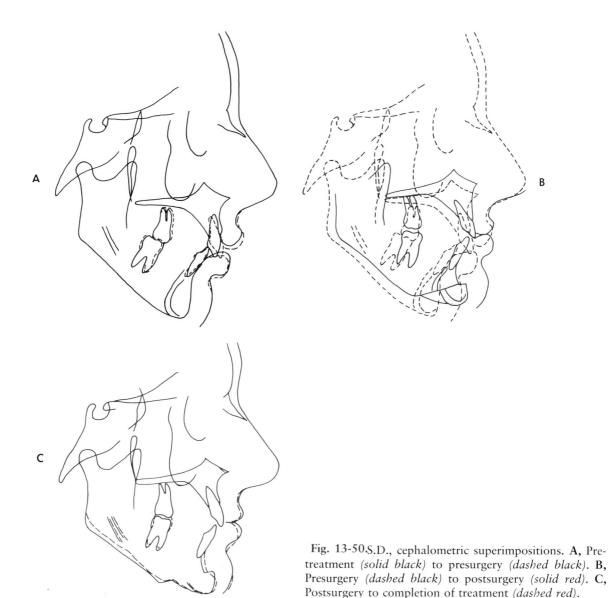

Fig. 13-50.S.D., cephalometric superimpositions. **A,** Pretreatment *(solid black)* to presurgery *(dashed black).* **B,** Presurgery *(dashed black)* to postsurgery *(solid red).* **C,** Postsurgery to completion of treatment *(dashed red).*

Continued.

Case 3—cont'd.

border osteotomy to reposition the chin was performed uneventfully, and the patient was placed in maxillomandibular fixation. After extubation, as the patient was awakening, vigorous jaw activity that moved the maxil-

lary and mandibular teeth despite the fixation were observed. These continued in the recovery room, and the transosseous wires in the maxilla broke. On the following morning, the patient was reexplored under IV con-

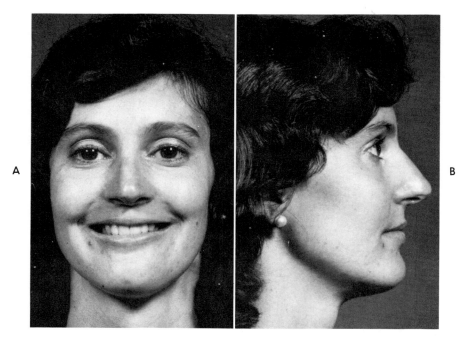

Fig. 13-51. S.D., 26 years, 7 months, 2 years postsurgery.

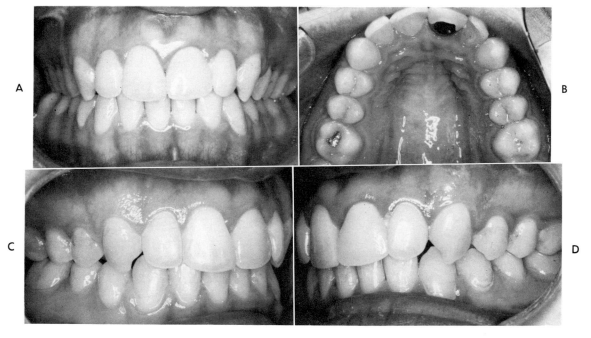

Fig. 13-52. S.D., age 26 years, 7 months, dental relationships 2 years postsurgery. A permanent crown on the maxillary left central incisor has replaced the temporary one used during the surgical-orthodontic treatment. At this point, retention was discontinued.

Case 3—cont'd.

scious sedation, the transosseous wires were replaced, and skeletal suspension wires were added. The remainder of the hospital course was uncomplicated, and she was discharged 4 days postsurgically in maxillomandibular fixation. The cephalometric changes produced by surgery are shown in Fig. 13-50, *B.*

Six weeks postsurgically, the stabilizing arch wires, occlusal splint, and skeletal suspension wires were removed, and 16 steel working arch wires were placed. She wore ⅜-inch light posterior box elastics full-time and a ⅜-inch light anterior box elastic at night only. Eight weeks later, the occlusion had settled into almost ideal interdigitation. A 17×25 braided steel arch wire was placed in the maxillary arch for 3 weeks to improve incisor positioning; then the appliance was removed and maxillary and mandibular removable retainers were

placed. These were worn full-time initially, then only at night after 4 months. One year later, a porcelain-faced metal crown was placed on the left central incisor and retainer wear was discontinued.

Facial esthetics were dramatically improved (Fig. 13-51), and dental occlusion was excellent (Fig. 13-52). Cephalometric superimposition showed that the mandible had rotated further up and forward from the immediate postsurgical position when the occlusal splint was removed, but the maxilla remained almost exactly where it had been placed at surgery (Fig. 13-50, C). On 7-year recall (5 years after retention was discontinued), there was mild incisor irregularity reminiscent of the pretreatment positioning, but facial proportions were unchanged (Figs. 13-53 and 13-54). No changes could be discerned on cephalometric superimposition.

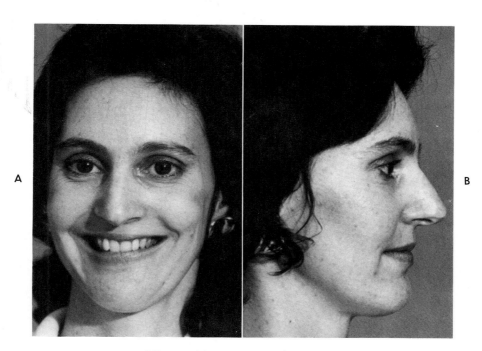

Fig. 13-53. S.D., age 31 years, 4 months, 7 years postsurgery.

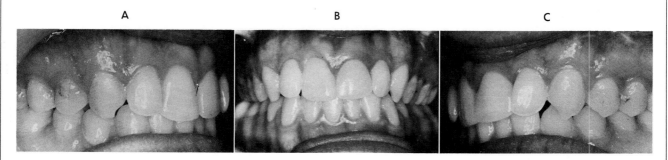

Fig. 13-54. S.D., age 31 years, 4 months, dental relationships after retention was discontinued.

Continued.

Case 3—cont'd.

Comments. Most long-face patients have anterior open bite, but a significant minority (perhaps a third) have deep bite instead. As the mandible rotates down and back during growth, the erupting maxillary incisors are likely to be impeded by contact with the lower lip. If that occurs, an open bite will result. But if the maxillary incisors can slip behind the lower lip, they continue to erupt, producing the paradoxical situation seen in S.D., a deep bite in a patient who has skeletal open-bite jaw relationships.

Both superior repositioning of the maxilla and mandibular inferior border osteotomy to reposition the chin produce remarkably stable results. The combination, as employed for this patient, is ideally suited for treatment of the type of problem that can be described succinctly as "Class II rotated from Class I" (see Fig. 13-1).

Case 4

D.M., age 22 years, 9 months, and a secretary at a nearby college, was sent for consultation by a faculty member who knew about previous surgical-orthodontic treatment for students there. The patient was concerned about the appearance of her teeth and face, particularly the protrusion of upper incisors and chin deficiency. The medical history was noncontributory to the dentofacial problem. She reported her present health as excellent.

On clinical examination, mandibular deficiency was obvious. Lower face height was mildly excessive and there was lip strain on closure and excessive display of gingiva on smiling. Throat form was poor (Fig. 13-55). There was 15-mm overjet; incomplete overbite, with an exaggerated curve of Spee; and moderate crowding and irregularity in the maxillary arch but reasonably good tooth alignment in the mandibular arch (Fig. 13-56). All maxillary teeth were present, but the mandibular right first molar and the mandibular left second premolar were missing. Attached gingiva in the mandibular anterior area was minimal; the periodontal consultant felt that gingival grafting would be necessary if the incisors were to be advanced but might not be needed if they would be retracted or left in the same position. TM joint function was normal.

On cephalometric evaluation (Fig. 13-57), a small mandible was obvious. Severe maxillary dental protrusion was evident. The 15-mm overjet appeared to be about equally due to these two causes. The mandible was rotated somewhat downward and backward, and moderate maxillary vertical excess was present. The mandibular teeth were well related to the mandible.

Her problems were summarized as: (1) severe mandibular deficiency, (2) vertical maxillary excess, (3) maxillary

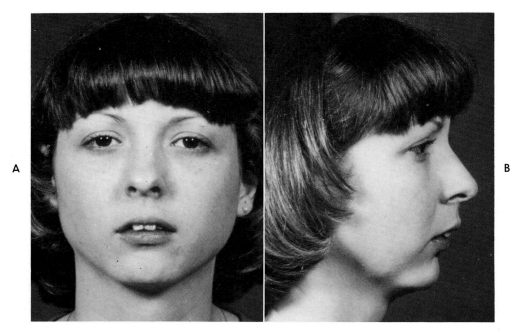

Fig. 13-55.D.M., age 22 years, 9 months.

Case 4—cont'd.

A   B   C

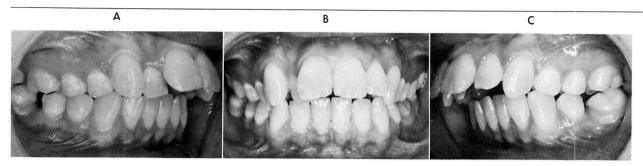

Fig. 13-56.D.M., dental relationships, age 22 years, 9 months.

dental protrusion and crowding, and (4) multiple missing teeth in the mandibular arch. Although there was no crossbite initially, she would be in posterior crossbite if the mandible were in the correct AP position.

The treatment plan was:

1. Extraction of maxillary right and mandibular left third molars and maxillary right and left first premolars.
2. Orthodontic treatment to align and retract the maxillary incisors and level the mandibular arch, closing the right first molar and left second premolar spaces.
3. LeFort I osteotomy to elevate, widen, and somewhat advance the maxilla, and bilateral sagittal split osteotomy to advance the mandible.
4. Postsurgical orthodontics.
5. Orthodontic retention.

At age 23 years, orthodontic treatment was begun with bands on molars and bonded attachments (18-slot edgewise) on all other teeth. Initial alignment was accomplished in the maxillary arch with loops in a 14 steel arch wire and in the mandibular arch with a 17.5 multistrand arch wire. After alignment was completed with 16 steel wires, 16×16 loop arches were used for space closure, and 17×22, then 17×25, steel arch wires were placed.

At age 23 years, 9 months, she was very anxious to proceed with the surgery, for personal reasons. Although leveling and space closure were not quite complete, particularly at the old extraction sites in the lower arch, the AP position of the incisors was satisfactory (Fig. 13-57, *A*). Soldered spurs were added to the mandibular 17×25 arch wire. A new 17×25 maxillary arch wire, to be placed in the operating room, was fitted to the model surgery casts, and the previous wire was removed to allow for the maxillary segmental osteotomy. At age 23 years, 10 months, she was admitted to UNC Hospitals for two-jaw surgery.

At surgery, the mandibular rami were approached initially, and the bone cuts for sagittal split osteotomy were made, but the splits were not completed. Next, the maxilla was approached; bone was removed as planned in the posterior region and set aside for future bone grafting if needed; the maxilla was downfractured, and

parasagittal osteotomies were made bilaterally and connected in the midline anteriorly. The maxillary segments were widened approximately 4 mm in the canine region and 6 mm at the second molars. At that point, an orthodontist in the operating room tied in the maxillary stabilizing arch wire. The maxilla then was placed into the intermediate splint and repositioned superiorly as

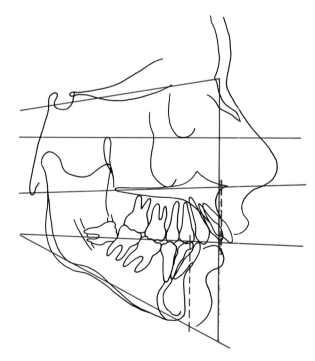

Fig. 13-57.D.M., initial cephalometric tracing. Note the severely deficient and rotated mandible, lip incompetence, and elongated maxillary posterior teeth relative to the palatal plane. Cephalometric measurements: N perp to A, 1 mm; N perp to Pg, −12 mm; AB difference, 13 mm; UFH, 45 mm; LFH, 56 mm; mand plane, 28 degrees; MxI to A vert, 6 mm, 36 degrees; MnI to B vert, 5 mm, 33 degrees; Mx molar to palatal plane, 21 mm.

Continued.

Case 4—cont'd.

planned. The patient was placed in MMF, and wires were placed through previously prepared holes in bone and ligated tightly to hold the maxilla in position. Osteotomes were used to complete the sagittal splits, the patient again was placed in MMF with the mandible in the final splint, and wire ligatures were tightened between the condylar and body fragments. The patient tolerated the procedure well and was discharged on the third postsurgical day. The cephalometric changes are shown in Fig. 13-57, C.

Six weeks postsurgically, the splint and stabilizing arch wires were removed. A 17×22 wire was placed in the maxillary arch and a 17.5 multistrand wire in the mandibular arch; ⅜-inch posterior box elastics were worn. Four weeks later, a 17×22 arch wire was placed in the mandibular arch, and Pletcher springs were used for space closure while posterior box elastics were continued. The appliances were removed 3 months after postsurgical orthodontics resumed, and maxillary and mandibular retainers were placed. At that point, both facial esthetics (Fig. 13-58) and occlusal relationships (Fig. 13-59) were greatly improved. The cephalometric changes are illustrated in Fig. 13-60.

From the beginning, there were problems with the lower retainer, which was not worn well. Spaces reopened at the old lower extraction sites, and the premolars were not in occlusion. Ten months after the initial debanding, a bonded appliance was placed again, and over a period of 8 months, light round, then 17×25 TMA and 17×25 steel arch wires were used to bring the teeth into ideal occlusion. This time retainers were worn uneventfully, gradually being decreased to nights only.

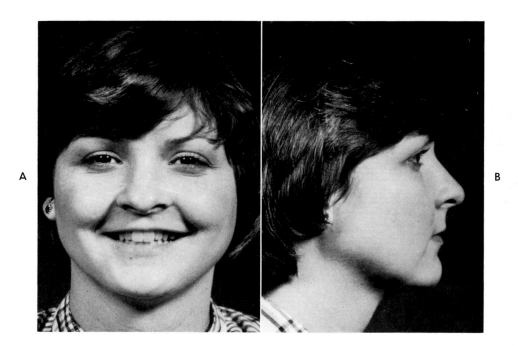

Fig. 13-58. D.M., age 24 years, 1 month, at completion of treatment.

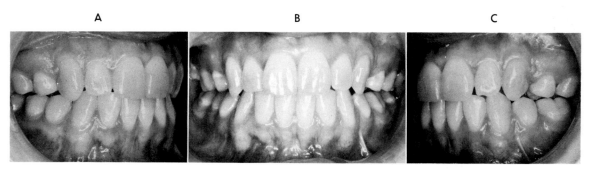

Fig. 13-59. D.M., age 24 years, 1 month, dental relationships at completion of treatment.

Case 4—cont'd.

On 6-year recall, excellent facial proportions and occlusion had been maintained (Figs. 13-61 and 13-62). Cephalometric superimposition showed no changes from the postsurgical jaw positions.

Comments. This patient's major problems were in the AP plane of space, but mandibular advancement alone would have produced an unstable and unesthetic result—unstable because of the wrong-way rotation of the mandible that would have resulted, unesthetic because the secondary but nonetheless significant vertical maxillary excess would not have been corrected. This patient is quite different from Case 3 above, in that she would be Class II mandibular-deficient whether or not the maxillary vertical excess were present; thus maxillary surgery alone would be inappropriate. Moving the maxilla back to meet a mandible that does not rotate forward far enough creates a severe esthetic problem. Two-jaw surgery is the only solution.

In two-jaw surgery of this type, it is almost always better to reposition the maxilla, then the mandible. The sequence employed in this patient is a subtle variation to the one described in Case 2 above. Here, the surgeon made all the preparatory cuts in the mandible before carrying out the maxillary osteotomy, the preferred approach to minimize displacement of the maxilla while mandibular osteotomy is completed (see Chapter 11).

A continuous orthodontic stabilizing arch wire cannot be placed presurgically when a segmental osteotomy is planned. There are two alternatives: (1) a full-dimension rectangular stabilizing wire can be fabricated on

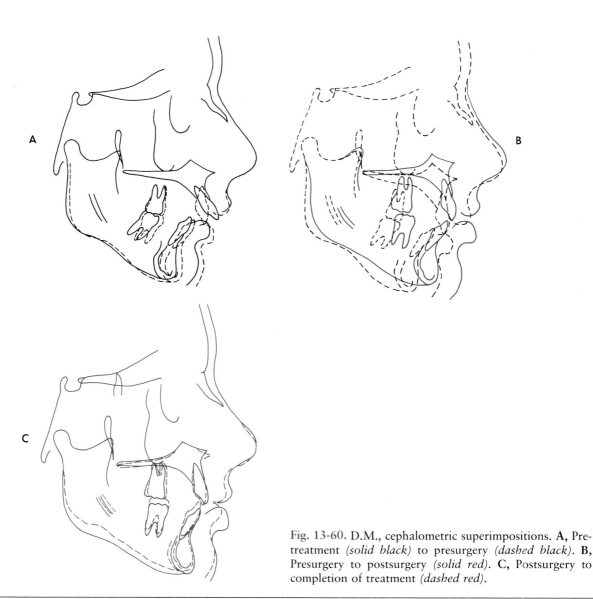

Fig. 13-60. D.M., cephalometric superimpositions. **A,** Pretreatment *(solid black)* to presurgery *(dashed black)*. **B,** Presurgery to postsurgery *(solid red)*. **C,** Postsurgery to completion of treatment *(dashed red)*.

Continued.

Case 4—cont'd.

the model surgery casts and placed by the orthodontist in the operating room, as was done for this patient, or (2) rectangular stabilizing segments can be tied into the bracket slots presurgically, and a heavy round auxiliary wire that was prepared from the model surgery casts can be placed in the headgear tubes at surgery. It can be difficult to engage a precisely fitting arch wire after the osteotomy cuts have been completed, and the orthodontist has to be present to accomplish that fit. The round wire can be fitted much more easily, by the surgeon if desired, so that approach usually is employed.

With 20/20 hindsight, the problems experienced with orthodontic instability after the hurried treatment that was done initially are not surprising. The surgery date was rushed, and the postsurgical time was the absolute minimum, so stable occlusal relationships were not present when the appliance was removed. With poor compliance, a difficult retention situation then became impossible. D.M.'s impatience contributed to these problems but was not solely responsible. She accepted with good grace the period of retreatment with fixed appliances that was the only way to produce a good long-term result.

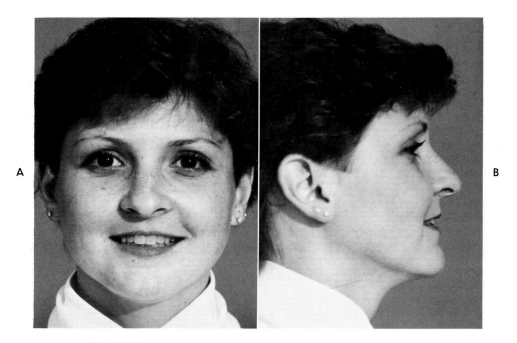

Fig. 13-61. D.M., age 30 years, 2 months, 6 years postsurgery.

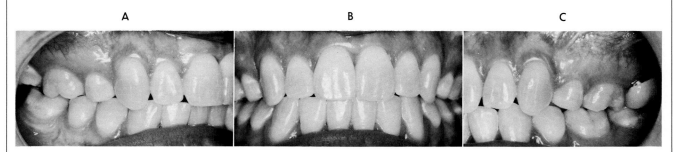

Fig. 13-62. D.M., age 30 years, 2 months, 4 years after final removal of orthodontic appliances. At this point, she still wore a mandibular retainer at night.

REFERENCES

1. Sassouni VA: A classification of skeletal facial types, Am J Orthod 55:109-123, 1969.
2. Bell WH, Creekmore TD, Alexander RG: Surgical correction of the long face syndrome, Am J Orthod 71:40-67, l977.
3. Proffit WR, Phillips C, Dann C IV: Who seeks surgical-orthodontic treatment? The characteristics of patients evaluated in the UNC Dentofacial Clinic, Int J Adult Orthod Orthognath Surg, in press.
4. Fields HW, Proffit WR, Nixon WL, et al: Facial pattern differences in long-faced children and adults, Am J Orthod 85:217-223, 1984.
5. Warren DW, Hinton WA, Seaton D, et al: Relationship of size of the nasal airway and nasal-oral breathing, Am J Orthod Dentofacial Orthop 93:289-293, 1988.
6. Fields HW, Warren DW, Black BK, et al: Relationships between vertical dentofacial morphology and respiration in adolescents, Am J Orthod Dentofacial Orthop [in press].
7. Proffit WR, Fields HW, Nixon WL: Occlusal forces in normal and long face adults, J Dent Res 62:566-570, 1983.
8. Proffit WR, Fields HW: Occlusal forces in normal and long face children, J Dent Res 62:571-574, 1983.
9. Proffit WR, Turvey TA, Moriarty J: Augmentation genioplasty as an adjunct to conservative orthodontic treatment, Am J Orthod 79:473-491, 1981.
10. Burstone CJ: Precision lingual arches: active applications, J Clin Orthod 23:101-109, 1989.
11. Turvey TA, Hall DJ, Warren DW: Alterations in nasal airway resistance following superior repositioning of the maxilla, Am J Orthod 85:109-114, 1984.
12. Keall CL, Vig PS: An improved technique for the simultaneous measurement of nasal and oral respiration, Am J Orthod Dentofacial Orthop 91:207-212, 1987.
13. Warren DW, Hinton VA, Hairfield WM: Measurement of nasal and oral respiration using inductive plethysmography, Am J Orthod 86:480-484, 1986.
14. Lints RM: The effect of maxillary respiration, master's thesis, 1989, University of Michigan.
15. Rugh JD, Drago CJ: Vertical dimension: a study of clinical rest position and jaw muscle activity, J Prosthet Dent 45:670-675, 1981.
16. Proffit WR, Phillips C: Adaptations in lip posture and pressure following orthognathic surgery, Am J Orthod Dentofacial Orthop 93:294-304, 1988.
17. Throckmorton GS, Finn RA, Bell WH: Biomechanics of differences in lower facial height, Am J Orthod 77:410-420, 1980.
18. Throckmorton GS, Johnston CP, Gonyea WS, et al: A preliminary study of biomechanical changes produced by orthognathic surgery, J Prosthet Dent 51:252-261, 1984.
19. Proffit WR, Turvey TA, Fields HW, et al: The effect of orthognathic surgery on occlusal force, J Oral Maxillofac Surg 47:457-463, 1989.
20. Proffit WR, Phillips C, Turvey TA: Stability following superior repositioning of the maxilla, Am J Orthod Dentofacial Orthop 92:151-163, 1987.
21. Bishara SE, Chu GW, Jakobsen JR: Stability of the LeFort I one-piece maxillary osteotomy, Am J Orthod Dentofacial Orthop 94:184-200, 1988.
22. Turvey TA, Phillips C, Zaytoun HS, et al: Simultaneous superior repositioning of the maxilla and mandibular advancement: a report on stability, Am J Orthod 94:372-383, 1988.
23. Hennes JA, Wallen TR, Bloomquist DS, et al: Stability of simultaneous mobilization of the maxilla and mandible utilizing internal rigid fixation, Int J Adult Orthod Orthognath Surg 3:127-141, 1988.
24. Satrom KD, Sinclair PS, Wolford LM: The stability of double jaw surgery: a comparison of rigid versus wire fixation, Am J Orthod Dentofacial Orthop [in press].
25. Denison TF, Kokich VG, Shapiro PA: Stability of maxillary surgery in open bite vs non-open bite malocclusions, Angle Orthod 59:5-10, 1989.

CHAPTER 14

Class III Problems: Mandibular Excess/Maxillary Deficiency

Peter M. Sinclair
William R. Proffit

NEED AND DEMAND

Skeletal Class III malocclusion has long been recognized as difficult and intractable to manage with orthodontic treatment alone. In 1907, Edward Angle first suggested that a combined orthodontic and surgical approach was the only way to correct a true mandibular prognathism once it was fully developed.[1] Before the 1970s, the literature portrayed Class III problems as being primarily mandibular prognathism, with little attention being paid to the maxilla. More recent studies indicate that isolated true mandibular prognathism occurs in only about 20% to 25% of Class III cases.[2] The remainder involve some degree of maxillary skeletal deficiency, either alone (again in about 20% to 25% of the Class III population) or in combination with mandibular prognathism (50% to 60% of the Class III population). Thus as many as three-quarters of the Class III patients have some degree of maxillary skeletal deficiency.

Since the classic studies of the Hapsburg monarchy,

a definite familial tendency toward mandibular prognathism and Class III malocclusion has been recognized. The inherited factors include not only the size of the mandible, but also the size of the maxilla, the length and angulation of the cranial base, and the position of the glenoid fossa. The point at which anteriorly divergent but harmonious facial proportions (see Chapter 4) become a disproportionate facial deformity must be viewed against a racial, ethnic, and familial background. For instance, a degree of chin prominence that is quite appropriate in Pacific islanders is inappropriate and a problem in northern Europeans.

The extent to which environmental influences on growth can produce mandibular prognathism is unknown. If the mandible is postured forward continuously, growth at the condylar processes to maintain the articulation with the skull is known to occur. Harvold's experiments with impaired nasal respiration in monkeys suggest that positioning the mandible forward to facilitate mouth breathing causes a prognathic tendency.[3] In the same way, a large tongue or reduced pharyngeal dimensions could make it necessary for a child to posture the mandible forward in order to breathe and thus could contribute to excessive growth. It is conceivable but less likely that a functional shift accompanying early incisor interference (the "built-in activator" hypothesis) could lead to increased mandibular growth (i.e., the dental interference created by mildly excessive mandibular growth could in turn lead to more excessive growth, an unfortunate example of positive feedback). Effects on growth are produced by constant posturing, and the functional shift is present only when teeth are brought into occlusion, so the theoretic basis for this positive feedback is questionable.[4]

Environmental contributions to maxillary deficiency are difficult to discern. Impaired growth in cleft-palate patients is well recognized, and the special problems of these patients are discussed in Chapter 18. The suggestion in the functional matrix theory (see Chapter 2), that function of the respiratory passages is important for maxillary growth, led to some speculation about mouth breathing causing decreased growth. No evidence supports such an effect. The animal experiments suggest that morphologic changes in response to mouth breathing are almost entirely in the mandible. Nevertheless, it is possible that growth changes secondary to some as yet undiscovered environmental influence may be important. As with other developmental deformities, skeletal Class III malocclusion probably arises when an individual who is susceptible because of inherited facial proportions is tipped into the deformity category by some alteration in the growth pattern.

Although Class III problems due to mandibular prognathism/maxillary deficiency are much less prevalent in Caucasian populations than are Class II problems due primarily to mandibular deficiency (see Chapter 1), the frequently unacceptable esthetics of severe Class III malocclusion leads a high percentage of these patients to seek surgical treatment. Slightly more than a third of the nearly 1200 patients evaluated through the Dentofacial Program at the UNC in the 1980s were skeletal Class III, although they compose less than 2% of the general population. Of the 739 patients who were not in orthodontic treatment at their initial evaluation, 28% had negative overjet. Skeletally, 17% were judged to have anteroposterior maxillary deficiency, 20% mandibular protrusion, and 10% both. Half the Class III patients are male, although two-thirds of the total patient group seen in the Dentofacial Clinic are female.[5]

Excessive vertical as well as AP growth of the mandible is common in prognathism, and 6% of the patients had both vertical and AP mandibular excess. If the maxilla is vertically deficient, the mandible rotates upward and forward and becomes more protrusive; 3% of the patients had this combination (i.e., could be considered Class I rotated to Class III). If the maxilla is vertically excessive, an otherwise prognathic mandible could be rotated to a normal AP position (Class III rotated to Class I); only 1% of the patient population showed this condition.

DIAGNOSTIC CHARACTERISTICS
Frontal Facial View

On frontal facial examination, patients with a significant component of mandibular prognathism often present a "flat" appearance in the lower third of the face with little or no prominence of the chin button, a thin lower lip, and a reduced labiomental fold. The tight soft tissue seems to be related to soft-tissue stretch as throat length increases (Fig. 14-1). Conversely, in a mandibular-deficient patient with a reduced lower anterior facial height, the lower lip will often be large and everted due to redundant soft tissue, and the patient often has a strong, pointed chin (see Chapter 12, Fig. 12-2). If there is a question as to whether relative mandibular prognathism due to deep bite with a reduced lower anterior facial height is present, the clinician can have the patient rotate the mandible open to see if the lower facial height can be brought back to normal (Fig. 14-2).

Profile View

From the profile view, the determination of true mandibular prognathism often can be aided by evaluating neck form in addition to throat length. A normal neck-chin angle of about 120 degrees along with a well-defined inferior mandibular border is often seen in true prognathism, whereas in relative prognathism, where the maxilla is at fault, the neck-chin angle often is poorly defined and the submental area may show some layers of excess connective and adipose tissue

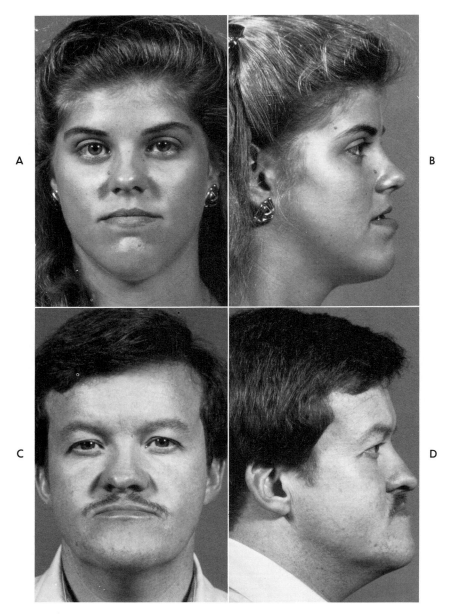

Fig. 14-1. **A-D,** Two examples of the "flat" appearance of the lower third of the face often associated with the Class III malocclusion.

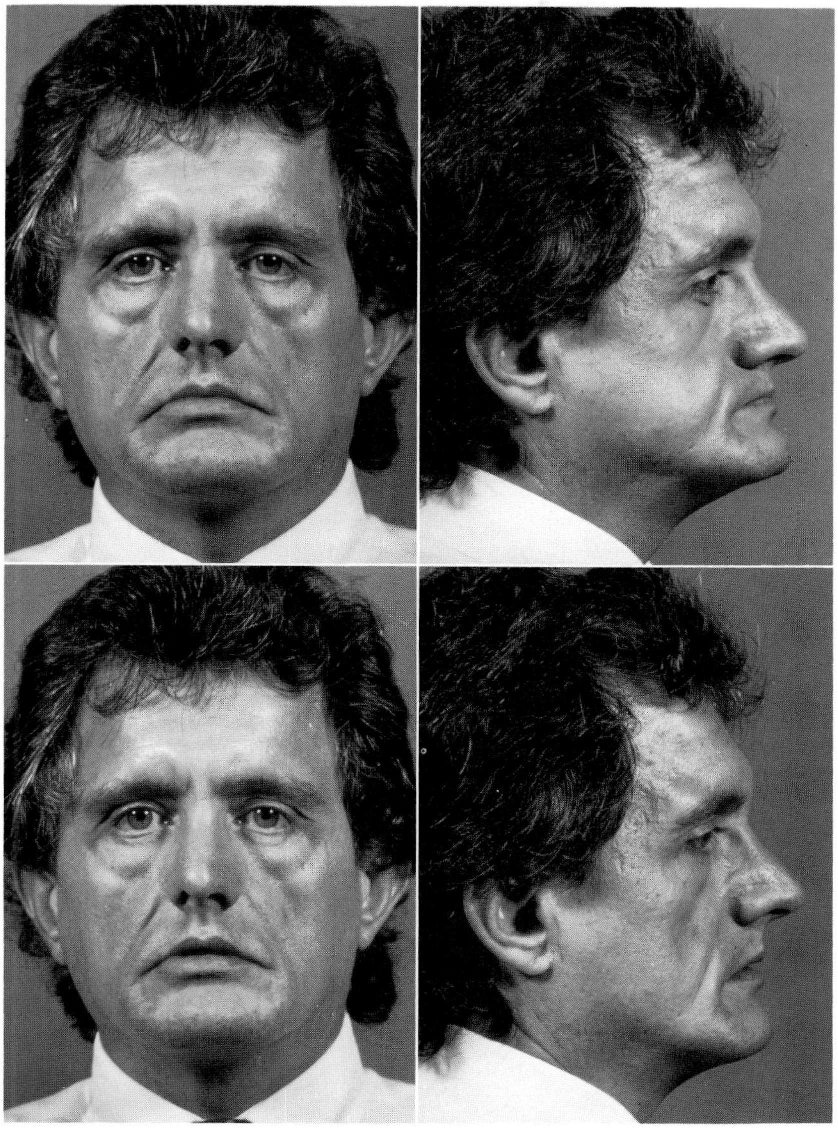

Fig. 14-2. In a patient with a deep bite and reduced lower face height, rotating the mandible open until normal vertical proportions are achieved can assist with the diagnosis of relative mandibular prognathism. **A** and **B,** Occlusal vertical position. **C** and **D,** Opened to normal face height. Note the reduction in the apparent prognathism.

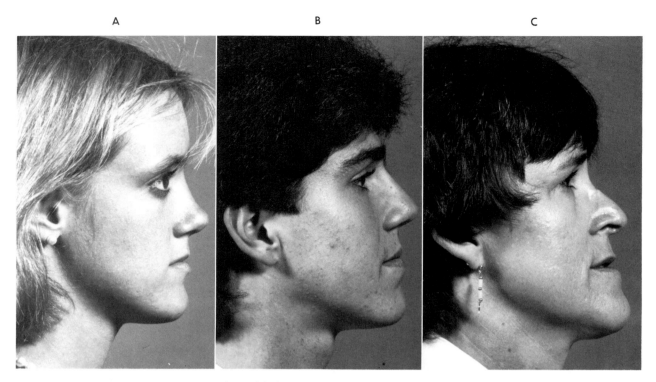

Fig. 14-3. A-C, A series of mandibular prognathic patients of increasing severity. As severity becomes great enough, two-jaw surgery must be considered.

(Fig. 14-3). Surgically setting back the mandible in patients with apparent or relative prognathism may cause redundant tissue in the submental area and produce less than ideal esthetic results.

A Class III patient with midface deficiency often displays a "sunken in" or flat appearance of the upper lip along with a thin vermilion border and reduced maxillary incisor exposure at rest. Upper lip length (subnasale to stomion) is often reduced below its normal of 20 to 24 mm. Frequently there is an acute nasiolabial angle, with the columella of the nose oriented more horizontally than is normal due to reduced nasal growth (Fig. 14-4). Other major characteristics of midface deficiency include a narrowed alar base and deficient zygomatic, paranasal, and infraorbital areas, the latter frequently resulting in a margin of sclera showing below the pupils of the eyes (see Fig. 14-19).

Differential diagnosis of the facial characteristics can be aided by blocking out the mandible and then the maxilla with a hand or card (Fig. 14-5). In this way the relationship of each jaw individually to the cranium can be evaluated, putting their relative contributions to the total discrepancy in better perspective.

Dental Characteristics

Intraorally, many Class III patients present with minimal attached gingival tissue over their lower anterior teeth. Such a deficiency, which can affect both the height and the thickness of the attached gingiva, is an important factor in planning treatment.

Another frequent dental characteristic is absent or small maxillary lateral incisors in patients with a significant component of maxillary deficiency. Conversely, patients with mandibular prognathism may present with considerable generalized interdental spacing and flared incisors, which should raise the suspicion of a large and/or anteriorly positioned tongue. Further evidence of a large tongue includes an even, generalized open bite, with indentations (crenations) reflecting the mandibular teeth present on the lateral margins of the tongue (Fig. 14-6).

Cephalometric Characteristics

Two areas are of prime importance in evaluating the cephalometric characteristics of Class III patients. First, it must be determined whether one jaw is primarily at fault, or, if the malocclusion is a combination of maxillary deficiency and mandibular excess, how much each jaw contributes to the overall anteroposterior problem. Second, the strong interaction between the vertical development of the maxilla and the AP position of the mandible must be carefully evaluated. Cephalometric evaluation of Class III patients is made more complex by the variations that often are present in the cranial base. The cranial base (S-N distance) has

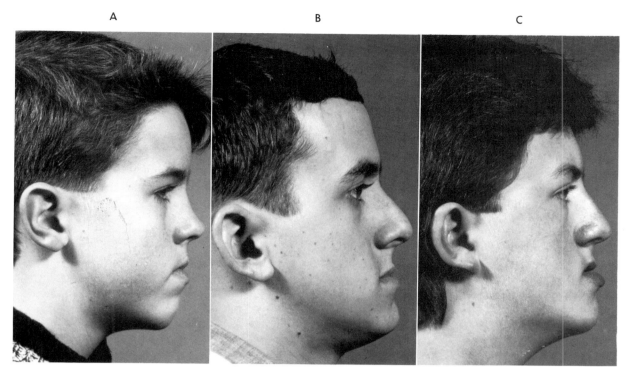

Fig. 14-4. A-C, A series of midface-deficiency patients of inceasing severity.

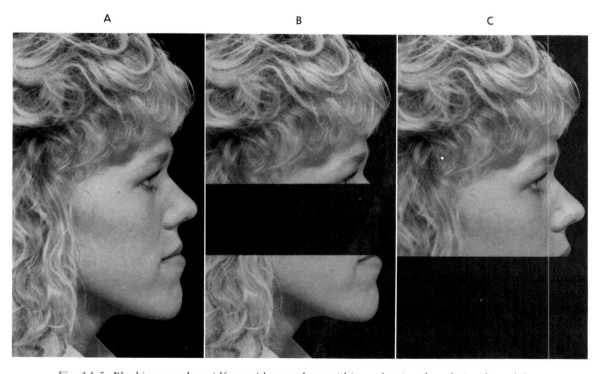

Fig. 14-5. Blocking out the midface with a card can aid in evaluating the relationship of the mandible to the cranium; blocking out the mandible can help in evaluating the position of the midface. Note that with the mandible blocked out, it is more apparent that this patient's Class III problem has a large component of maxillary deficiency. With the maxilla blocked out, it can be appreciated that the mandible is only slightly prognathic.

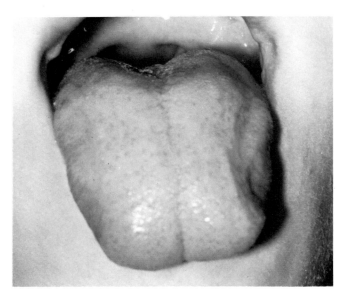

Fig. 14-6. Crenations (indentations) present on the lateral margins of the tongue can reflect a large tongue resting against the teeth.

been reported to be shorter in Class III patients and may in addition show a reduced cranial base angle (nasion-sella-basion), both of which would tend to result in a more anterior glenoid fossa and hence anterior mandibular position.[6]

With the objective of determining both the absolute size of each jaw and its AP and vertical positions relative to the cranial base, the diagnostic approach outlined in Chapter 4 should be utilized. If template analysis is selected, the tendency toward a short cranial base should be kept in mind when selecting a reference template. If the measurement approach is used, the short cranial base also can affect the analysis. It is important to keep in mind that maxillary retrognathism may be masked in angular and linear analyses that use nasion because its position is abnormal when the anterior cranial base is short. A key determination is whether AP chin prominence is due to an absolute increase in mandibular length or is caused by some combination of a forward glenoid fossa and an upward-forward mandibular rotation. If the latter is suspected, then template analysis is especially helpful in evaluating the position of the glenoid fossa, which rarely is taken into account in measurement analyses (Wylie's AP dysplasia being the prominent exception).[7] The case reports at the end of this chapter further illustrate these points.

If there is a significant component of maxillary deficiency in the malocclusion, maxillary dental crowding is frequently present, particularly in the canine/premolar area. Even if the widths of the maxilla and mandible are normal, the AP discrepancy produces a cross-

bite tendency. If the maxilla is narrow (surprisingly, often this is not the case even when AP and vertical deficiency is present) or the mandible is wide (which occurs frequently), the crossbite is likely to be bilateral. If width dimensions are normal, the crossbite is more likely to be unilateral, with or without a CO-CR slide. In either case, often there is a significant degree of buccal crown tip in the maxillary molars, which of course is a dental compensation for the transverse skeletal discrepancy. Recognizing this characteristic, and the fact that correcting it by uprighting the molars during presurgical orthodontics would worsen the crossbite, is important in determining the severity of the transverse skeletal component of the Class III malocclusion.

TREATMENT PLANNING
Preadolescent Children with Growth Potential
Diagnostic Characteristics

The most difficult problem in planning treatment for young children with Class III malocclusion is establishing the seriousness of the problem and thereby the prognosis for conservative treatment. In the normal (i.e., Class I) pattern of development, the mandible is small at birth but grows more rapidly than the maxilla thereafter. Many a dentist has been struck by how mandibular-deficient his or her (normal) newborn child was, and moderate deficiency remains the norm throughout the mixed dentition years. A 6-year-old with a mild anterior crossbite and a strong chin that is within normal limits for adults is at risk of increasingly severe Class III malocclusion as growth continues. On the other hand, some children do have a relatively prominent chin at an early age without ever developing a Class III problem. Certain morphologic characteristics have been recognized that, if evident on the lateral cephalogram in the preadolescent years, may indicate a developing skeletal Class III malocclusion.[8] These include an increased gonial angle, antegonial notching, a backward direction of condylar growth when the tracings are superimposed on the mandibular symphysis, and a thin mandibular symphysis (Fig. 14-7).

Dentally, a young patient with a developing Class III malocclusion almost always has compensations in the positions of upper and lower incisors in response to the disproportionate jaw growth. The mandibular incisors frequently are retroclined, and, as the child becomes older, their roots tend to press against the labial plate, producing a "washboard" effect (Fig. 14-8). Conversely, the maxillary incisors usually flare anteriorly, and spacing often appears as the malocclusion worsens.

When evaluating a child with an apparent Class III malocclusion, it is first necessary to eliminate the possibility that the patient may be posturing forward into a reverse overjet. This "pseudo" Class III is often initiated by displaced permanent incisors. If the patient can

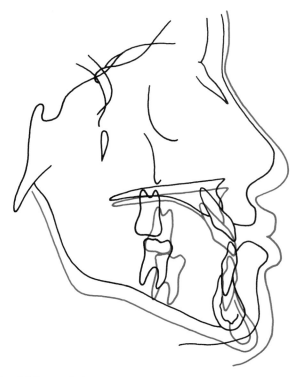

Fig. 14-7. Cephalometric superimposition showing an unfavorable Class III growth pattern *(solid red)* with anteroposterior mandibular growth exceeding that of the maxilla.

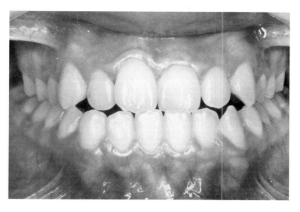

Fig. 14-8. The "washboard" effect produced by prominent mandibular incisor roots pressed against the labial plate is a common finding in developing Class III malocclusions.

achieve a edge-to-edge incisal occlusion, a true skeletal Class III malocclusion is less likely to be present, and the prognosis for orthodontic treatment is much better.

Treatment Approaches

As with any skeletal malocclusion, modification of growth to correct the problem is the ideal treatment. For a child with a developing Class III malocclusion, the objective would be to stimulate maxillary growth, particularly in those in whom it is markedly deficient, and restrain excessive mandibular growth, especially when it is largely at fault. Unfortunately, at the present state of the art in orthodontics, our capability for either type of growth modification is small. A complete correction of skeletal Class III malocclusion is much less likely to occur than with an apparently equivalent Class II problem; or to put it differently, 2 mm of reverse overjet presents approximately the same orthodontic challenge as 8 to 10 mm of excessive overjet. Further, several phases of treatment may be required in the Class III patient due to the strong tendency for disproportionate mandibular growth to continue into the late teens. This probably is due to the greater genetic and smaller functional component to the malocclusion than in most Class II cases.

One way of estimating the possibility of correcting a Class III problem with orthodontic growth modifica-

tion is to apply the envelope of discrepancy (see Chapter 1). The greater the discrepancy and the older the patient, the less the chance of a successful result. Prolonged orthodontic treatment that has little or no chance of success can be frustrating for the child, parents, and orthodontist. On the other hand, if there is a reasonable hope of intervening successfully, it would be foolish not to make the attempt. Making this determination from the initial evaluation of a young child can be very difficult. Direct observation of the growth pattern, via serial cephalometric radiographs, helps in estimating the prognosis and planning the treatment approach. Sometimes the only way to know whether a child would respond well or poorly to growth modification treatment is to try it—which is perfectly acceptable if the parents understand that the treatment may or may not succeed.

In recent years, it has become apparent that stimulation of deficient maxillary growth is more possible than had been thought previously, but only if treatment is begun at an early age.[9] Restraint of mandibular growth, though theoretically possible, remains more problematic and less successful. Because most patients have a combination of deficient maxillary and excessive mandibular growth, treatment aimed at both may be needed. For convenience, treatment aimed at the maxilla and the mandible is discussed separately below.

Treatment of Maxillary Deficiency

Many patients with AP maxillary deficiency and Class III malocclusion also present with problems in the transverse and vertical planes of space. Absolute transverse deficiency probably occurs in less than half these patients, but maxillary crowding is common, and a relative transverse deficiency (i.e., posterior crossbite) is found in nearly all for the reasons described above. The prevalence of vertical deficiency is similar (but has not been studied carefully, so the possibilities of error in this estimate must be acknowledged).

The objectives of treatment for a preadolescent child with maxillary deficiency are to correct the relative transverse discrepancy and to translate the maxilla forward and downward to the extent that this is possible. Transverse expansion of the maxillary arch, by opening the midpalatal suture, is the only practical approach to the transverse problem even if the crossbite is largely due to the AP position of the jaws. Forward and downward traction, displacing the maxilla as much and the teeth as little as possible, is the preferred approach to the AP and vertical components of the deficiency (see Case 1).

In a preadolescent child, transverse expansion by opening the midpalatal suture can be achieved by a variety of techniques. In the early mixed dentition only 1 to 2 pounds of force are required to open the suture.[10] This can be achieved easily by any palatal expansion appliance (see Chapter 16) or even by a lingual arch (quad-helix or W-arch) designed primarily for dental expansion. In the late mixed dentition, greater force levels (i.e., 4 to 6 pounds) often are required.

Transverse expansion improves not only posterior but also anterior crossbite because the mandible rotates down and back in response to the dental interferences created by the expansion. Forward displacement of the maxilla as a side effect of lateral expansion has been reported, but this cannot be relied on to occur routinely.[11] Rotation of the mandible with an increase in face height is the primary reason for the AP improvement in almost every case. In patients with a high mandibular-plane angle and open-bite tendency, these characteristics may worsen during the expansion phase.

An alternative approach for transverse deficiency is the use of the Frankel functional regulator. This removable appliance relies on buccal shields in an attempt to stretch the periosteum enough to produce expansion at the suture as well as buccal movement of the molars. It is quite effective in producing expansion. The amount of skeletal versus dental change is debatable, but in younger children, some sutural expansion probably does occur.

The FR-III version of the Frankel appliance also has been used in the mixed dentition in attempts to stimulate anterior maxillary growth while restraining the mandible (see Case 1). The FR-III rotates the mandible down and incorporates plastic shields in the maxillary vestibule that are intended to stimulate forward maxillary growth. Although some successes have been reported,[12] only modest maxillary growth usually is observed.

The most effective method at present to improve the position of the maxilla is the Delaire face mask, which was developed in France by a surgeon interested in the growth problems of cleft-palate children (see Chapter 2).[13] The appliance consists of a simple mask with rests on the forehead and chin that can be used to provide forward and downward traction to the maxilla. A fixed or removable splint to the maxillary teeth is employed to minimize tooth movement. The key to the Delaire appliance is not so much its design, although that clearly is an advance, as its use at quite young ages. As a general guideline, forward traction to the maxilla can produce anterior and downward displacement, but only up to approximately 8 years of age. After that, tooth movement occurs, but the amount of skeletal change is disappointing. Whenever the maxilla moves down, the mandible rotates down and back, so use of this appliance can also result in lengthening of face height and reduction of relative mandibular prognathism.[14]

The problem with maxillary traction in older children seems to be not so much that the maxilla cannot be displaced, as that tooth movement overwhelms the desired skeletal change. Moving the maxillary teeth forward relative to the maxilla only increases an undesirable dental compensation. Another way to apply force to the maxilla is needed, avoiding the teeth. Recent developments in bony implants now offer this possibility. Preliminary work with primates shows the maxilla can be displaced by force applied to implants placed in the supra-alveolar bone,[15] and experience with the first human subjects is being gained at this writing. If successful, the implant approach should offer the chance of much improved orthodontic protraction of the maxilla in the future.

Treatment of Mandibular Excess

Controlling excessive mandibular growth in preadolescent children can be remarkably difficult. Animal studies have demonstrated that mandibular growth can be restrained,[16] but equivalent clinical success in humans rarely is achieved, perhaps because the force magnitudes and durations required are too much for children to tolerate. The major effect of force directed against the mandible is to rotate it downward and backward, not to reduce the amount of growth (see Case 1). Given this somewhat discouraging situation, the selection of appropriate patients for growth modification treatment is particularly important. Positive indicators include a low mandibular-plane angle with normal or short anterior face height, anterior crossbite produced in part by a functional shift, symmetric mandibular growth, a relatively mild skeletal discrepancy (e.g., ANB less than −2 degrees), and no familial history of prognathism.[17] In these circumstances, treatment can be aimed at producing a backward rotation of the mandible in order to reduce its relative prominence and increase lower facial height to a normal value.

Two methods are available to accomplish this goal:

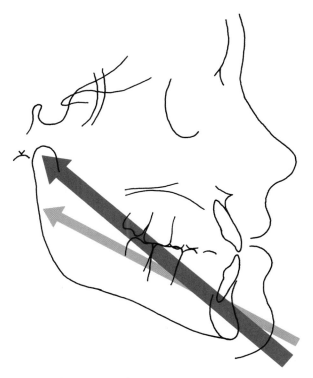

Fig. 14-9. One approach to chin-cup therapy is to aim a strong force directly at the mandibular condyle; the other approach is to use a lighter force, directed below the condyle, so that the mandible is rotated down and back. (Reprinted with permission from Proffit WR: Contemporary orthodontics, St. Louis, 1986, The CV Mosby Co.)

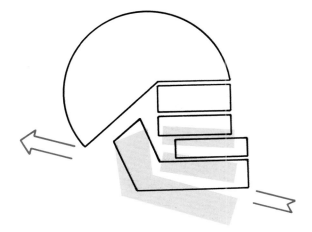

Fig. 14-10. The typical response to chin-cup therapy includes downward and backward mandibular rotation, and it seems most efficient to deliberately induce this with a lower direction of pull. (Reprinted with permission from Proffit WR: Contemporary orthodontics, St. Louis, 1986, The CV Mosby Co.)

(1) a chin cup to place backward force against the mandible—if the direction of force is on a line that passes below the condyle, rotation is facilitated (Figs. 14-9 and 14-10), or (2) a Class III functional appliance, the construction bite for which is taken with the mandible rotated down. The appliance leaves posterior teeth free to erupt, so that an increase in face height and mandibular plane angle is produced. To the extent that a chin cup might actually reduce mandibular growth, it should be more effective than a functional appliance, but in practice the two approaches seem about equally effective—or ineffective, as neither produces major changes.

In mandibular prognathism, any early skeletal correction may show considerable relapse because of the continuing disproportionate growth in many prognathic patients (as Case 1 demonstrates). When preadolescent treatment is undertaken, all concerned should understand that a second phase of treatment at a later time is almost certain to be required. Despite this in children with the characteristics described above, early treatment still is indicated in many instances to alleviate potential psychosocial problems, prevent the problem from becoming too severe, and perhaps reduce the need for surgery.

By the same token, for a preadolescent Class III patient with mandibular excess combined with a divergent facial pattern (including such characteristics as a high mandibular plane, anterior open bite, and increased lower facial height), there are no good nonsurgical treatment solutions. Such a child is outside the range of orthodontic treatment from the beginning. As we have pointed out, it is almost impossible to stop excessive mandibular growth even with long-term chin-cup therapy, and rotating the mandible posteriorly and increasing anterior face height makes things worse, not better, in this type of malocclusion.

Early surgery is one possible alternative solution, but surgical intervention in the maxilla in a young child has the potential to reduce growth that already is likely to be somewhat deficient, whereas mandibular surgery does not prevent subsequent excessive mandibular growth.[18] The net result is that if surgery is done at an early age, almost certainly additional surgery will be necessary after growth is completed. Occasionally, because of the psychologic impact of extremely severe deformity, early surgery is the best choice for an individual child, but in most cases it is better to wait.

For patients of this type, the obvious presence of orthodontic appliances provides a positive signal that some care is being provided, which can be important psychologically. The unspoken message, "We're working on it" is more acceptable than a problem that appears ignored. The appropriate orthodontic treatment often is limited to the alignment of anterior teeth and the avoidance of any treatment (such as tooth removal) that might compromise a future combined surgical and orthodontic solution. Some treatment of the maxillary incisors is frequently indicated. This usually is done best with fixed appliances in the form of molar bands and incisor bonded attachments (a "2 × 4" setup) in order to achieve maximum control for correction of crowding and rotations. Labial crown torque for maxillary incisors can help reduce the appearance of maxillary deficiency.

Adolescents with Questionable Growth Potential
Diagnosis and Prognosis

The critical questions in evaluating adolescents with Class III malocclusion are (1) the severity of the problem, and (2) the amount and direction of future growth. The key decision in planning treatment is whether to attempt to treat the patient with orthodontics alone or to start on a plan that leads to surgery at a later date. If the case is borderline, the orthodontic approach must not compromise a future surgical solution if this becomes necessary. This means that tooth removal for camouflage and AP displacement of incisors should be used only after extremely careful consideration of the severity of the malocclusion.

The more severe the underlying skeletal discrepancy, particularly if the patient still has considerable growth potential remaining, the less the likelihood that camouflage will produce a satisfactory result. This is particularly true if the patient also has increased lower facial height and anterior open bite. The more dental crowding the patient exhibits, particularly if correcting it will interfere with the required movements of the incisors, the more difficult camouflage treatment becomes. Maxillary incisors that already are flared, severely retruded mandibular incisors, and a Class III canine relationship can all be regarded as indicators of increasing severity of the Class III malocclusion. These findings suggest decreasing potential for successful camouflage treatment.

Our present ability to predict facial growth is not very good in any circumstances, but it is particularly weak for adolescents with skeletal Class III malocclusions (Fig. 14-11). Those with true mandibular prognathism demonstrate disproportionate sagittal and vertical growth that may continue for several years beyond puberty. Basic techniques such as evaluating height and weight, recent growth history, and the stage of ossification in the hand/wrist film are notoriously inaccurate. TM joint tomography, MRI, and CT, while allowing a clear view of the size and shape of the condyle, provide few clues as to future growth potential. Skeletal scintigraphy, utilizing radioactive isotopes (technetium-99) to evaluate cellular activity in the mandibular condyles, is useful for identifying abnormal asymmetric growth as in hemimandibular hypertrophy (see Chapter 15), but currently does not provide quantitative information as to future growth potential.[19] Therefore continuing mandibular growth must be as-

sumed until two lateral cephalograms taken at least 1 year apart show no demonstrable growth occurring over that period. In general, the more severe the presenting skeletal problem and the greater the period of growth remaining, the poorer the prognosis for a nonsurgical resolution of the problem.

Treatment of Maxillary Deficiency

In an adolescent patient, transverse maxillary deficiency is much more amenable to treatment than is AP or vertical deficiency. Opening the midpalatal suture is still feasible after puberty, although considerably higher forces are necessary than in preadolescents, and the downward and backward rotation of the mandible that usually results will improve the AP relationships—at the cost of increasing anterior face height. In contrast, the chances of producing significant forward or downward movement of the maxilla are significantly reduced as compared with the mixed dentition period. Presumably this is due to increased bony interlocking in the posterior and superior maxillary sutures. Some reports of successful displacement of the maxilla with reverse-pull headgear (face mask) therapy have appeared,[20] but in adolescents these appliances are much more likely to merely procline the teeth than produce significant skeletal change.

Further complicating the treatment planning at this stage is the fact that maxillary growth tends to stop 1 to 2 years before mandibular growth, making it very difficult to camouflage maxillary deficiency. Camouflage therapy usually would involve treating the maxilla nonextraction, advancing the maxillary incisors to achieve normal overjet, and overbite. Tooth removal in the mandibular arch, to allow for retraction of the mandibular incisors and the use of Class III elastics, could be included in this camouflage option. It is not uncommon to produce a good occlusal and facial result with such a plan, only to see late mandibular growth produce a relapse into reverse overjet and relative chin prominence. And if that happens, the displacement of teeth created by the orthodontic extraction and mechanics patterns will severely limit the skeletal correction that could be achieved surgically. Thus, although significant changes can be induced at this age, long-term stability and the possibility of compromising a future surgical-orthodontic treatment plan should be carefully assessed.

Treatment of Mandibular Excess

Treatment with a chin cup or functional appliance has the same limitations in adolescents as in younger children—rotation of the mandible can be produced, but restricting excessive growth is unlikely. If face height is short, the facial pattern convergent, and the prognathic tendency mild, a chin cup or a removable appliance to rotate the mandible can be successful.

A

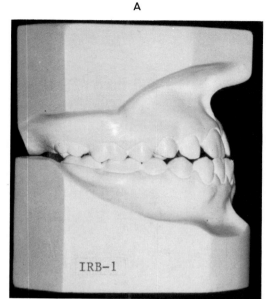

Fig. 14-11. **A** and **B**, 13-year-old girl with a mild Class III dental relationship and a straight profile. **C**, The same patient at age 15 after undergoing a significant amount of mandibular growth. **D**, The patient's profile following mandibular setback surgery. (Courtesy of the Orthodontic Department, University of Washington.)

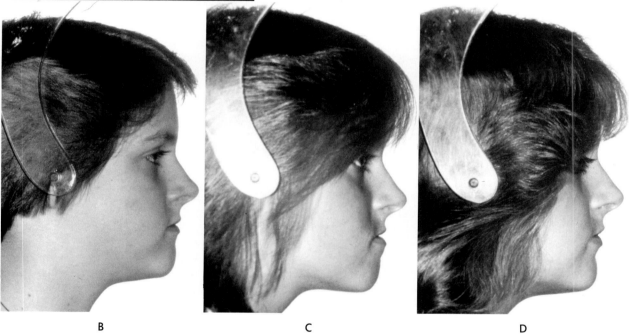

B   C   D

Otherwise, these approaches will be ineffective.

A camouflage treatment plan might include removal of the lower first premolars only, to allow for maximum mandibular incisor retraction. Alternatively, the removal of maxillary second and mandibular first premolars would facilitate the achievement of Class I molar and canine relationships. Class III elastics usually are needed to aid in this correction. Not only do the elastics assist in retracting the lower incisors and proclining the uppers, they also elongate the upper molars, producing some downward rotation of the mandible (see Figs. 14-9 and 14-10).

The limitations of orthodontic camouflage, however, are even more severe in patients with excessive mandibular growth than in those with maxillary deficiency. If tooth removal and elastics are used to maintain the occlusion as mandibular growth continues, the lips are flattened but the chin becomes more prominent. Only a small amount of lower incisor retraction is compatible with reasonable facial esthetics. The worse the growth pattern, the greater the chance that lower incisors could be retracted too much. Extraction for camouflage in patients with excessive mandibular growth must be considered a high-risk orthodontic treatment plan from two points of view: it may not succeed, and if it does not, the chances of successful surgical treatment have been compromised.

Timing of Surgery in Class III Adolescents

Adolescents with problems severe enough to require surgery understandably want to have definitive treatment as soon as possible. For social and psychologic reasons, early treatment is desirable. On the other hand, if the surgery is done before mandibular growth is completed, relapse is likely. When the problem is primarily maxillary deficiency, the termination of growth may be reached at age 15 or even 14, but in mandibular prognathism, growth may continue into the early twenties. Many patients are unwilling to wait that long and elect to have surgery earlier to correct their mandibular prognathism, recognizing that a second, later surgery may well be necessary. In the patients with the most severe problems, two-jaw surgery with combined maxillary advancement and mandibular setback is likely to be needed. If this is done at an early age, the second operation usually involves only the mandible (see Chapter 5, Fig. 5-18).

If early surgery is to be performed for maxillary deficiency, a small amount of anteroposterior overcorrection may be indicated if normal continued mandibular growth is expected.[16] Following surgery, any remaining maxillary growth is redirected vertically; almost certainly, there will be no further anterior movement of the maxilla. The difficulty lies in dealing with excessive mandibular growth that also may be a part of the developmental problem. In general it appears that, unless there is an overwhelming psychosocial need, surgery in Class III adolescents should be postponed until there is reasonable certainty that growth has ceased and only one definitive surgery will be required.

Adults with Little or No Growth Potential

The key question in planning treatment for an adult patient with Class III malocclusion is whether or not camouflage treatment is a realistic option. The answer must be based on the orthodontic movements required, the stability of the orthodontic changes, and whether the probable esthetic result would be acceptable to the patient. With the uncertainties about future growth removed, in many ways the decision is easier than in an adolescent. On the other hand, psychosocial factors are more complex in adults, and it is extremely important to have a clear picture of the patient's desires and expectations. In some instances the patient may be so out of touch with reality that psychologic counseling rather than (or at least preceding) orthodontics and surgery is the best choice.[21]

For all the reasons discussed above, orthodontic camouflage is a realistic option to surgery only if the jaw discrepancy is relatively mild. As a general guideline, a reverse overjet greater than 3 mm, or an A-B difference (projected to the true horizontal line) greater than −2 mm, indicates a problem too severe for orthodontic treatment alone. It also is true for adults as for younger patients that the more divergent the facial pattern (i.e., the more there is a skeletal open-bite tendency), the poorer the prognosis for only orthodontic treatment. Conversely, the more convergent the pattern, the greater the opportunity for orthodontic camouflage.

For orthodontic treatment alone to be successful when no improvement in jaw relationship is possible, the clinician must first be able to advance the maxillary incisors and/or retract the mandibular incisors so as to achieve a normal overjet. The treatment must result in incisor inclinations that suggest a reasonable chance for occlusal stability both statically and during excursive movements. The incisor position at the end of this treatment also must be esthetically satisfactory from the context of the amount of incisor displayed at rest and the angulation of their labial surfaces to the face.

In the vertical plane of space, for camouflage treatment to be deemed successful, the clinician should achieve normal anterior facial proportions (i.e., a 1:2 ratio in the subnasale/stomion versus stomion/soft-tissue menton distances) (see Chapter 4, Fig. 4-6 and Table 4-4) while correcting the incisor overbite. This is much more likely to be possible in a patient with mild maxillary deficiency, low mandibular plane angle, and deep bite, in whom some degree of backward rotation of the mandible and increase in lower facial height would be acceptable.

In the transverse plane many Class III patients have a component of maxillary deficiency with significant posterior crossbite and crowding. In the postpubertal patient where palatal expansion is not a viable option, dental expansion with either a removable appliance or arch wires is the only orthodontic possibility. Careful consideration should be given as to whether these changes are achievable while maintaining buccal segment torque and preventing the production of balancing interferences in lateral excursions.

Other factors of importance in evaluating the possibility of camouflage are the likely effects of the projected tooth movement on the patient's periodontal health and jaw function and the potential for increased root resorption when heavy forces are applied over long treatment periods in an attempt to produce dental compensations for a skeletal problem. Finally, careful consideration should be given as to whether the overall esthetic changes will result in a significant improvement in the patient's facial appearance, particularly if this was the chief complaint. If not, a plan including surgery may be warranted for this reason alone.

In summary, in evaluating a patient on the border for surgical versus camouflage treatment, the relative

Fig. 14-12. Changes in neck and throat form from a large mandibular setback (done in 1969). **A**, Before surgery (the patient is masking the extent of his prognathism by posturing the mandible downward, which he did habitually). **B**, Following 15 mm mandibular set-back. Note the prominence of the tongue mass in the floor of the mouth. One indication for two-jaw surgery, partially correcting the jaw discrepancy by advancing the maxilla, is to prevent the development of a double chin, or "turkey gobbler," as a result of soft-tissue adaptation to mandibular setback (see Fig. 14-24 for a cephalmetric illustration of the change in tongue position). (Courtesy of the University of Kentucky.)

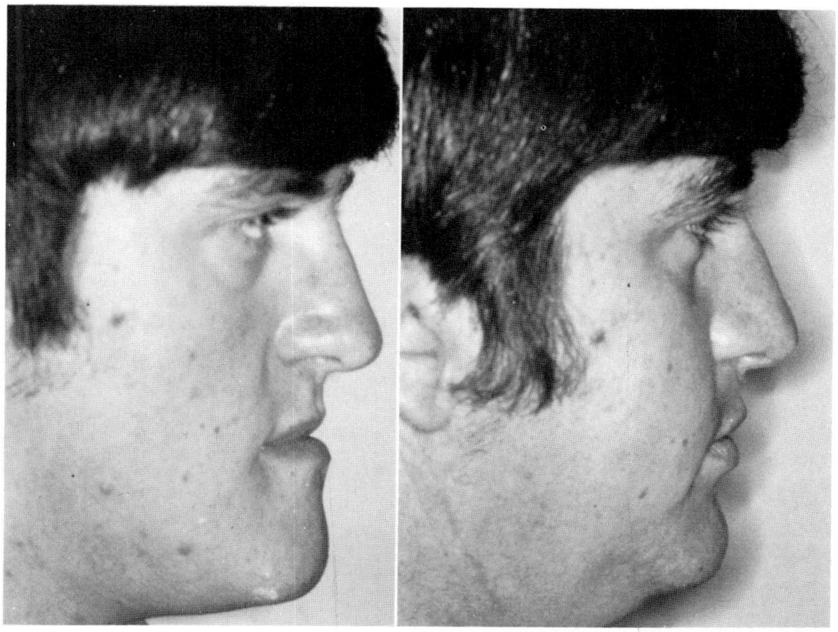

risks and benefits must be considered carefully. All other things being equal, camouflage treatment is likely to be more prolonged and more demanding in cooperation than surgical treatment, but the surgery will be more expensive and may carry greater risk. The risk-benefit considerations are influenced by the patient's concerns. It is imperative for the clinician to present the pluses and minuses of each method, so that the patient understands and makes an informed decision (see Chapter 6).

PLANNING SURGICAL-ORTHODONTIC TREATMENT

Once a decision for surgical-orthodontic treatment has been made, the general surgical and orthodontic approaches must be decided, in that order, before the final detailed treatment plan can be established.

Surgical Approach

The surgical methods appropriate for correcting skeletal Class III problems are ramus osteotomy to set back a prognathic mandible (with occasional consideration for mandibular subapical osteotomy or body ostectomy); LeFort I osteotomy to advance a deficient maxilla, often with segments to allow transverse expansion; and mandibular inferior border osteotomy to reduce chin height and/or prominence.

The clinical keys outlined earlier in this chapter, along with the cephalometric analysis described in detail in Chapter 4, provide an organized way to decide which jaw is primarily at fault. If the patient presents with an isolated true prognathism, mandibular setback surgery alone should be considered, but the decision may not be that simple. If a patient has a throat length that is normal or short to begin with, setting the mandible back a significant distance may produce an unesthetic neck form with poor definition of the neck/chin angle and the appearance of excessive submental tissue (sometimes called the "turkey gobbler" appearance) (Fig. 14-12). This situation is worsened if the patient already has redundant submental tissue before treatment. Although a submental lipectomy and/or platysma muscle plication may alleviate the problem,[22] it may be better to carry out part or all of the AP correction in the maxilla.

In mandibular prognathism with a divergent facial pattern (increased face height), two further treatment planning considerations apply. First, if a significant open bite is present, a mandibular setback alone might require some counterclockwise rotation to close the

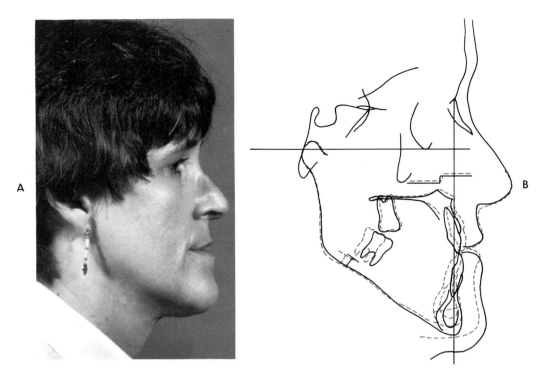

Fig. 14-13. A, Class III patient with increased lower facial height. **B,** Cephalometric prediction of the changes in lower face height that might be achieved with maxillary advancement combined with a mandibular setback and an inferior border osteotomy and wedge reduction *(dashed red)* to reduce face height.

open bite. This stretches the suprahyoid and mandibular elevator muscles, which in turn produces an increased potential for relapse.[23] The presence of an open bite, therefore, may signify the need for maxillary surgery, with consideration for both esthetic and stability reasons to limiting the surgery to the maxilla alone.

Second, as described earlier in this chapter (see Fig. 14-1), many long-face Class III patients have an increase in the stomion/soft-tissue menton distance and also have little or no chin projection (Fig. 14-13). Either of these factors can be considered as an indication for inferior border osteotomy in conjunction with the mandibular ramus surgery. The increased lower facial height can be reduced by removing a wedge of bone above the chin. If increased anterior chin projection is required, the bony cut at the mandibular inferior border can be angled to allow this projection. Therefore a common solution for isolated mandibular prognathism is a ramus osteotomy to set back the mandible combined with an inferior border osteotomy to advance and elevate the chin.

If AP maxillary deficiency exists, maxillary advancement via LeFort I osteotomy is the preferred plan. If the amount of advancement needed is large (i.e., >10 mm) then, to increase the potential for long-term stability, consideration should be given to achieving part of the sagittal correction with ramus osteotomy. Maxillary advancements of more than 5 mm frequently require the use of bone grafts to enhance their stability. If the anterior cuts of the LeFort I osteotomy are placed high along the lateral wall of the nose, the surgery has the potential to significantly improve the midfacial flatness frequently seen in these patients.

If the patient has AP and vertical maxillary deficiency with relative mandibular protrusion due to upward and forward rotation, moving the maxilla forward and down with bone grafting could produce a satisfactory solution not only to the sagittal but also the vertical problems by rotating the mandible down and back to its proper position.[24] Because moving the maxilla down can be unstable, this plan should be adopted only after careful consideration. Special methods for stabilization (e.g., bone plates or vertical wire struts for skeletal fixation and bone grafts, allogeneic or autogenous) will be required to maintain the increased face height.

In contrast, moving the maxilla up to correct vertical maxillary excess is one of the most stable orthognathic surgical procedures (see Chapter 13). In a patient with a Class III tendency, however, maxillary impaction may cause the mandible to rotate forward to the point that compensatory maxillary advancement would be neither stable nor esthetically pleasing. The plan for such a patient should include ramus osteotomy to set back the mandible in addition to the maxillary advancement.

In summary, although restricting the surgery to one jaw is preferred if feasible, two-jaw surgery often is required to correct severe Class III problems. The decision to employ two-jaw rather than one-jaw surgery may be necessitated by one or more of the following factors:

1. A severe anteroposterior skeletal deformity, the correction of which in one jaw alone might be beyond the probable limits of stability (e.g., a 10 mm maxillary advancement).
2. The need to correct a transverse discrepancy (e.g., maxillary constriction).
3. The need to correct a vertical discrepancy (e.g., anterior open bite and/or excessive incisor exposure; some short-face problems).
4. A soft-tissue morphology (e.g., mandibular throat length) that would preclude an esthetic result if the surgery was limited to one jaw.

Facial asymmetries, such as a canted maxillary occlusal plane combined with asymmetric mandibular growth, also are indications for two-jaw surgery. These problems are discussed in detail in Chapter 15.

Orthodontic Approach

The orthodontic approach to treatment of severe Class III problems is shaped by the need to properly position the maxillary and mandibular incisors, in both the AP and vertical planes of space, so that the surgeon can achieve the optimal skeletal and esthetic correction without being inhibited by dental interferences. This approach necessitates adoption of what Jacobs called the "two-patient" concept, whereby the maxillary and mandibular arches are treated independently, almost as though they belonged to different patients.[25] The objective is to position the incisors as ideally as is practical, relative to their own jaw, but without reference to interarch occlusion. In order to achieve these objectives, significant retraction of the maxillary incisors usually is required, and this may necessitate tooth removal in the maxillary arch (Fig. 14-14). If maximum incisor retraction is required or significant crowding is present, the extraction of maxillary first premolars usually is preferred. Extraction of maxillary second premolars could be considered if there was inadequate space for alignment but little or no need to retract the incisors.

In the mandibular arch the most common presurgical requirement is to advance the lower incisors from an upright or lingually tipped position. This is compatible with nonextraction treatment even in the presence of moderate crowding—but lack of attached gingiva and a thin alveolar ridge may limit the amount of forward movement of the incisors (see Fig. 14-14). Gingival grafts are likely to be required, especially if inferior

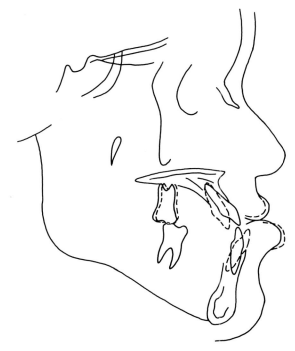

Fig. 14-14. Presurgical orthodontic preparation of a Class III malocclusion frequently involves decompensating the incisors from their current positions (*solid line*) to "ideal" presurgical inclinations (*dashed line*).

border osteotomy in addition to advancement of the incisors is planned. If the dental crowding is too great to manage nonextraction, the removal of mandibular second premolars may be the treatment plan of choice. This option also allows for the advancement of the mandibular molars into a more Class III relationship, usually desired before surgery. Therefore the most common extraction pattern in Class III cases is removal of upper first premolars only. When tooth removal is needed in both arches, the usual pattern is extraction of maxillary first and mandibular second premolars.

Before any teeth are removed, a careful Bolton tooth-size analysis should be carried out because many Class III patients have a significant tooth-size discrepancy. This is caused most frequently by small or peg-shaped maxillary lateral incisors associated with maxillary deficiency.[26] A resultant Bolton mandibular excess of greater than 3 to 4 mm, in combination with mandibular anterior crowding of sufficient severity to require tooth removal, indicates that extraction of a lower incisor should be considered. A diagnostic set-up is required to confirm that a satisfactory occlusion would be achieved.

In the transverse plane of space, the primary objective is to achieve an arch form that is compatible with each jaw's underlying shape, leaving the correction of any subsequent skeletal transverse discrepancy to the surgeon. This means if surgical changes are to be carried out in the transverse plane, the orthodontist should independently select maxillary and mandibular arch forms. The gross coordination of the arch forms will be carried out at surgery and will be refined by the orthodontist postoperatively. If no transverse expansion is to be carried out, then the orthodontist should select a maxillary arch form that is comparable with the basic underlying mandibular shape, and regular progress models should be taken to assess the degree of arch coordination when the models are positioned in a Class I relationship.

In the vertical plane, the orthodontist should not attempt a dental correction of the skeletal problem. This means not extruding incisors or using high-pull headgear to partially correct an open bite. These changes have a high potential for postoperative relapse (i.e., open bite) that could considerably reduce the success of the overall skeletal correction.

An additional consideration in Class III cases that undergo major skeletal changes at surgery is the pattern of possible relapse and the need to set up the occlusion preoperatively so as to give some flexibility should this occur. In the AP plane of space, leaving 2 to 3 mm of overjet allows for any rebound of a mandibular setback. If this rebound does not occur, the overjet could be used to further upright the maxillary incisors, an objective that is often difficult to complete preoperatively. In younger patients where late mandibular growth is possible, this approach provides a safety valve to accommodate any postoperative growth. Similarly, ensuring 2 to 3 mm of overbite at debanding would provide some flexibility in patients who originally had an open bite.

The principles of the orthodontic approach are similar no matter whether one- or two-jaw surgery is being planned. However, due to the decreased flexibility available when single-jaw surgery only is being planned, some compromise may have to be accepted. With mandibular surgery alone, it may prove difficult to advance the mandibular incisors enough to allow for the optimium amount of skeletal correction due to the limitations of the alveolus and attached tissue. Similarly, ideal retraction of maxillary incisors in cases with significant maxillary deficiency is very difficult to achieve and may limit the amount of maxillary advancement that is possible.

Informed Consent

The procedure for obtaining informed consent outlined in Chapter 6 should be followed, with patients being made fully aware of the benefits of treatment as well as its risks and costs. In Class III patients, the following points are of particular concern.

1. All patients should be made aware that continued mandibular growth beyond the end of the normal growth period is still possible, even if all the indicators mentioned previously have suggested that growth is complete. Minor changes may be compensated for by orthodontic treatment alone, but a significant late growth spurt may require additional surgical procedures.

2. A common characteristic of many Class III patients with mandibular prognathism is very thin, friable attached tissue overlying the mandibular incisors. This tissue, even if it appears to have a normal 2 mm thick band of attached gingiva, is prone to recession, particularly when the presurgical orthodontics involves the advancing of the lower incisors as is usual. A free gingival graft before orthodontics may be needed to prevent this problem.

3. Patients should be made aware that in certain cases, large mandibular setbacks may result in redundant soft tissue forming folds at the lower margins of the mouth and in the submental area. In a few cases, these folds may require secondary soft-tissue surgery for their removal (Fig. 14-15).

4. The correction of midface deficiencies involving large maxillary advancements may lead to widening of the patient's alar base and upturning of the nasal tip. Careful muscle approximation with sutures and an alar base cinch-suture procedure can minimize this side effect,[27] but the possibility of nasal changes should be mentioned to the patient (see Chapter 8).

PRESURGICAL ORTHODONTICS

The goals of presurgical orthodontics for these patients are to (1) eliminate or at least significantly reduce the dental compensations for the skeletal deformity, (2) establish appropriate AP and vertical positions of the incisors, canines, and molars, (3) provide arch forms whose widths and midlines will be compatible after the sagittal correction has been completed, and (4) align irregular teeth and deal with tooth-size problems.

Preparation for Maxillary Advancement

The key to the surgical treatment of maxillary deficiency lies in achieving complete decompensation of the maxillary incisors so as to allow for optimum maxillary advancement. This requires good AP and vertical control as well as careful anchorage management. In order to reduce the considerable incisor flaring and significant crowding often seen in maxillary deficiency cases, removal of maxillary first premolars may be indicated, alone or in conjunction with the extraction of mandibular second premolars.

Even with a first premolar extraction space, once the crowding has been alleviated, full maxillary incisor retraction and decompensation may still prove to be difficult. Excellent maxillary molar anchorage is critical if

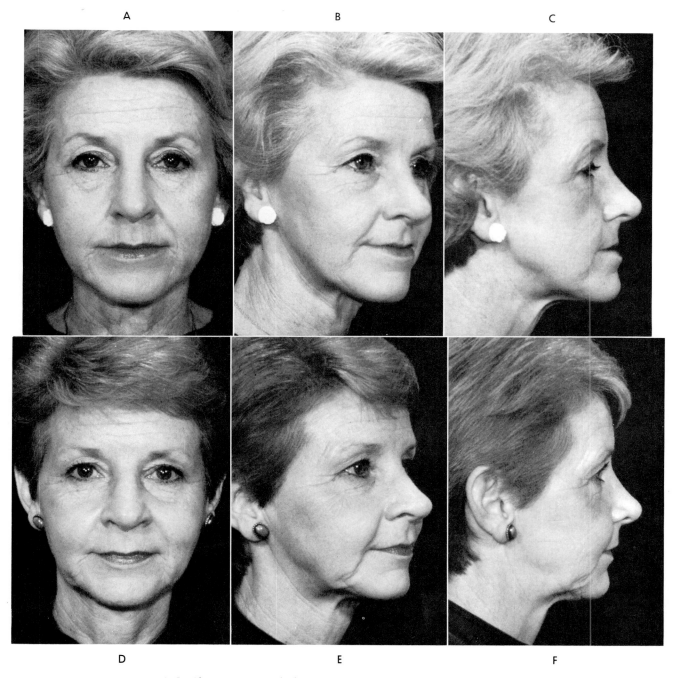

Fig. 14-15.A-C, Class III patient before maxillary advancement and mandibular setback. **D-F,** Following surgery, the soft-tissue folds at the lateral margins of the mouth and submental area are accentuated.

full incisor decompensation is to be attained. In severe cases this may involve wearing headgear at night (usually a cervical headgear in an open-bite case so as not to intrude the maxillary molars), along with other measures such as a transpalatal arch and Class II elastics.

Before placing the initial arch wire, a careful evaluation of the maxillary curve of Spee is necessary. In many patients with an open-bite Class III relationship

there is an upward anterior curve. It is then necessary to decide whether to level the arch and eliminate this curve during the presurgical orthodontics, or maintain the curve until it is removed at the time of surgery. If there is a clear "step" in the occlusal plane so that the maxillary anterior teeth (often just the four incisors, occasionally all six anterior teeth) are at a different height from the buccal segments, the maxillary arch is best treated as three segments. This can be done either by forming each arch wire with vertical steps to mirror steps in the occlusal plane so that it is passive in the vertical plane or by dividing every arch wire into three independent segments corresponding to the three occlusal planes (Fig. 14-16). Segmenting the arch wire will lead to a loss of mechanical efficiency, but failure to do so may result in significant postoperative openbite relapse as the anterior teeth that were extruded return to their original positions. In either case the vertical steps will be corrected at surgery as the maxilla is segmented.

When segmental maxillary osteotomies are planned and maxillary premolars have been extracted, the orthodontist should leave at least 3 mm of space until surgery. In a nonextraction case, in order for the surgeon to have adequate interdental access, the roots of the teeth on either side of the osteotomy sites must be actively diverged, starting with the first arch wire placed. The amount of divergence produced should be checked with periapical radiographs at least 3 months before surgery so as to allow time for any additional corrections. In a continuous arch wire, the root divergence can be gained using V bends, whereas in the three segmented wire approach, the portion of each wire involving the tooth adjacent to the future osteotomy site has to be bent to produce the required root divergence.

In the most common maxillary deficiency case where upper first premolars have been removed and a single level arch wire is to be used, the initial arch wire might be a 17.5-mil braided or 16-mil NiTi, with alignment then being completed with a 16-mil stainless steel wire. During space closure, care must be taken not to extrude the flared maxillary incisors as they are retracted. This may require the use of a closing loop with intrusive capabilities or the maintenance of a curve of Spee in the arch wire. Since good torque control is also required at this stage, a rectangular steel wire usually is needed for space closure. Segmental canine retraction can be carried out to minimize anchorage loss, although many adult patients dislike the esthetics of the large space distal to the lateral incisors that result from this technique. The final arch wire in the maxillary sequence should be as close to full size as possible (i.e., 17×25 or 21×25) so as to achieve the maximum lingual crown torque on the maxillary incisors.

If a skeletal transverse discrepancy is to be corrected surgically, then it is critical that no attempt be made to coordinate the maxillary arch form with that of the mandible. This change will be effected at surgery with maxillary segmental osteotomy and refined in the postsurgical orthodontics.

Preparation for Mandibular Setback

Just as with the maxillary advancement procedure, the principles of treatment are to eliminate the incisor

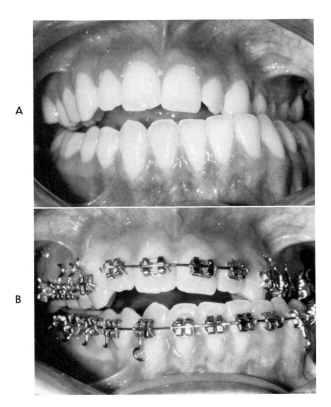

Fig. 14-16. **A,** Before treatment, this Class III patient with anterior open bite and skeletal crossbite had a step in the maxillary arch distal to the lateral incisors. **B,** Presurgical view showing the three-segment arch wire used in the maxilla before a three-piece maxillary osteotomy, placing the canines in the posterior segment.

compensations, align the teeth, and provide appropriate transverse and vertical tooth positioning. The initial arch wire might be a light braided wire or 16-mil superelastic (austenitic) NiTi to gain alignment.

Decompensation of the lower incisors then can be achieved using a 16-mil stainless steel wire with stops bent in such a way as to cause the wire to lie 1 to 2 mm in front of the incisors when it is inserted and tied in. This will advance and flare the incisors simultaneously. If more control of incisor angulation is required, then a rectangular stainless steel or TMA wire may be indicated. There is the potential for rapid loss of attached gingival tissue on the labial surfaces of the lower incisors as the teeth are aligned/advanced, and the health of these tissues should be monitored carefully. The final position and angulation of the lower incisors should be determined by the degree of negative overjet required for an adequate correction by ramus surgery shortening the mandible within the limitations of not opening up space or causing tissue recession. If some forward movement of the entire mandibular alveolus is indicated, either to increase the negative overjet or to create a Class III molar and canine relationship preoperatively, then Class II elastics may be indicated. The elastics should only be used once heavy stainless steel wires (i.e., 17×25 or 19×25) have been placed, as they may cause unwanted extrusion of the mandibular molars or maxillary incisors.

In the transverse plane, presurgical orthodontics should primarily be concerned with uprighting any teeth in the buccal segments that are lingually inclined (dental compensation for excess mandibular width). The amount of uprighting ideally should place the mandibular teeth over the center of the alveolar ridge. However, if this would result in a transverse discrepancy being present after the mandibular setback, three options should be considered: (1) not fully uprighting these teeth, thereby accepting less than ideal inclinations, function, and long-term stability; (2) uprighting the teeth fully and carrying out an osteotomy in the anterior mandibular midline to narrow the mandible (see Chapter 10)—this relatively rare and more complex procedure would require orthodontically providing some space at the osteotomy site between lower incisors, and it should be recognized that some torquing of the mandibular condyles may result from the procedure; and (3) uprighting the teeth and then correcting the crossbite by expanding the maxilla, either orthodontically or surgically, using the guidelines outlined previously.

Preparation for Two-Jaw Surgery

All the principles previously outlined apply when surgery in both jaws is being considered in Class III cases. The ability to achieve part of the change in the mandible and the remainder in the maxilla, particularly when segmental surgical procedures are being planned, tends to reduce the difficulty of the presurgical orthodontics. Less extreme orthodontic movements usually are required than when all the skeletal correction has to be carried out in one jaw.

During the presurgical orthodontics for all Class III cases, it is vital to take progress records (casts, cephalometric radiographs) to evaluate the AP and transverse corrections. The mandible cannot be postured so as to approximate the surgical correction, and there is no other way to check the dental relationships.

FINAL PRESURGICAL PLANNING

With experienced teams of orthodontists and surgeons who have been working together for some time and understand the other's role, it may not be necessary for the surgeon to see the progress records taken during the presurgical preparation of Class III cases. If there is any question, the records taken 3 to 4 months before the projected surgery date should be be reviewed by both members of the team. Thus if any additional orthodontic preparation is required it can be accomplished during this period, preventing a last-minute cancellation of the operation, as might happen if a problem were discovered only in the final presurgical records.

Ideally, the Class III patient before surgery should have his or her upper and lower incisors decompensated to the maximum amount possible within the limitations of the alveolus and periodontal attachments. The buccal segments should have been uprighted over the ridge and the roots diverged at any planned interdental osteotomy sites. All the extraction spaces should have been closed, except for 2 to 3 mm in the planned interdental osteotomy sites, and any tooth-size discrepancy dealt with by interproximal enamel reduction or by maintaining the appropriate spacing. The arches should have been set up correctly in the transverse plane, either with coordinated arch wires in place or prepared for coordination by maxillary segmental surgery. The patient should have full-dimension passive rectangular arch wires in place with fixation attachments placed for the interdental surgical wires (see Case 2).

When these orthodontic preparations have been completed correctly, the final surgical decisions can be made free of any impediments caused by incomplete or incorrect orthodontics. The final decision regarding one- or two-jaw surgery can then be based solely on the best way to achieve optimum esthetics, stability, and function for the individual patient.

SURGERY

The surgical procedures utilized in Class III treatment should be those which best solve a patient's particular set of problems. When several options exist, the one that provides the optimum in esthetics, stability, and function as well as meeting the patient's chief complaint should be chosen.

Maxillary Advancement

LeFort I osteotomy is the preferred surgical procedure for advancing the maxilla to correct AP deficiency. Vertical and transverse correction can be made also, and the maxilla can be segmented into several dentoalveolar segments to correct an occlusal plane discrepancy. The technical details of the maxillary procedures are described in Chapter 8.

In many patients with maxillary deficiency, the Class III malocclusion is combined with a midface deficiency at the level of the alar base of the nose. Additional support to the alar base area can be gained by making osteotomy cuts higher on the piriform rim of the nasal cavity or by augmenting the area with bone grafts. If the deficiency is severe, both may be done. Autogenous bone from the cranium or from osteotomy sites in the maxilla and mandible, or allogeneic bone (bank bone) can satisfactorily change the soft-tissue contours of alar base area. Some evidence exists to support the clinical

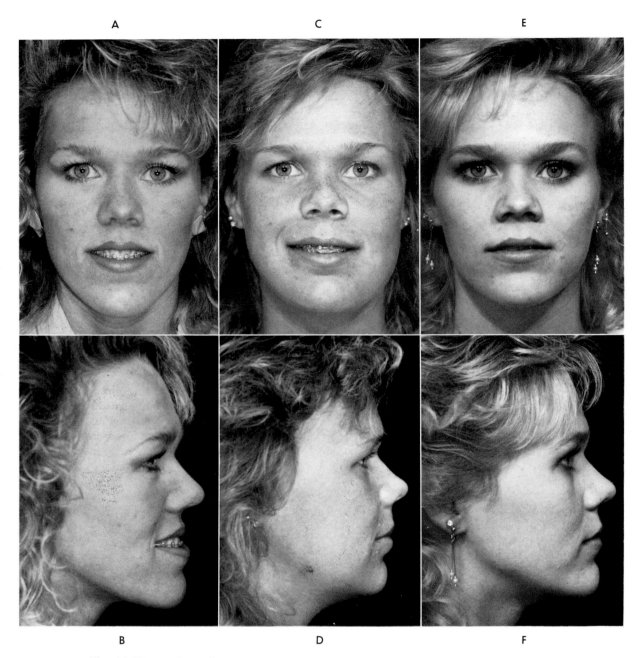

Fig. 14-17. **A** and **B,** Class III patient before maxillary advancement and mandibular set-back. **C** and **D,** Five days postsurgery demonstrating postoperative swelling. **E** and **F,** Post-treatment after resolution of facial edema. (Courtesy of the Orthodontic Department, Baylor College of Dentistry.)

impression that autogenous bone grafts from a donor site in the cranium provide more predictable long-term contour changes in the face with less resorption in the 6 to 24 months following surgery[28] (Figs. 14-17 and 14-18). Bank bone grafts contoured at surgery will provide soft-tissue support, but resorption is less predictable and the final result may feel quite firm to the touch, very different from the surrounding bone. A few

patients exhibit midface deficiency to the level of the body of the zygoma. These areas also can be augmented with bone grafts, or a modified LeFort II osteotomy can be performed. This surgical procedure is not discussed in this book—the interested reader is referred to other recent surgery texts.[29]

As has been discussed in Chapter 8, parasagittal osteotomy cuts in the nasal floor, extended through the

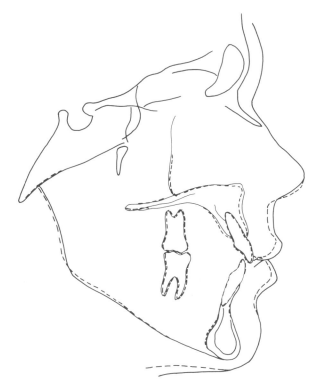

Fig. 14-18. Superimposition demonstrating the reduction in facial protrusion that occurred as postoperative swelling reduced (same patient as Fig. 14-17).

midline alveolar bone between the central incisors, provide the most effective means of widening the maxilla to correct transverse deficiency in the posterior maxilla. Increases in width of 4 to 6 mm usually are easily obtained. The orthodontist must remember that any transverse expansion must be maintained carefully for at least 4 to 6 months after surgery. Maintaining the transverse expansion does not mean that orthodontic finishing must be delayed for this length of time. Vertical settling of the teeth is compatible with a stabilizing auxiliary arch wire in the headgear tubes (see Chapter 12, Case 1). Details of the surgical stabilization are provided in Chapter 8.

Occasionally, narrowing the transverse width of the maxilla is necessary. Parasagittal osteotomy cuts in the nasal floor extended through the midline alveolar bone also allow this movement. Bone usually must be removed if more than 2 to 3 mm of decreased width is to be achieved. Special care must be taken to free palatal mucosa so this tissue is not folded and trapped in the nasal floor osteotomy sites, possibly compromising the blood supply.

If the occlusal plane is to be altered, it may be necessary to separate posterior and anterior dentoalveolar segments. The osteotomy can be extended laterally through alveolar bone anterior or posterior to the ca-

nine teeth (see Chapter 8 for details). The location of the interdental osteotomy cuts must be decided before the final stages of the presurgical orthodontics so space between teeth can be opened—or maintained if teeth were removed—for the osteotomy. Ideally this decision should be made before beginning the orthodontics, but a midcourse correction is possible if it becomes necessary.

Maxillary advancement is relatively easily accomplished with LeFort I osteotomy. Retaining the entire amount of advancement is difficult. If after repositioning the maxilla forward, minimal bone contact exists in the piriform rim and zygomatic buttress areas, bone grafts should be added for stabilization. Allogeneic bank bone is quite adequate for this purpose, but autogenous bone also may be used, particularly if this bone is placed also for alar base augmentation and if RIF (bone plates) is employed. Not all patients who have maxillary advancement require bone grafts, and the surgeon's clinical judgment is important in deciding their exact location. Some surgeons advocate porous block hydroxylapatite for maxillary stabilization because it is mechanically more stable.[30] The material has the advantage of not resorbing, but wound dehiscence is more common and the blocks may have to be removed if they become displaced into the maxillary sinus or the nasal cavity (see Chapter 8).

When an increase in the vertical height of the midface is advantageous for achieving a proper tooth-lip relationship and facial balance, the maxilla can be repositioned inferiorly with LeFort I osteotomy. There is a strong relapse tendency when the maxilla is moved down, however, particularly with conventional fixation (see below). To maintain an increase in face height with maxillary surgery, the maxilla must be properly stabilized with a combination of autogenous bone, bank bone, or even porous block hydroxylapatite and RIF (see Chapters 7 and 8). Even with the best fixation and stabilization, some degree of vertical relapse is to be expected in the first year following surgery.

Wound closure for LeFort I osteotomy is described in Chapter 8. If alar base widening is to be avoided, very careful musculoperiosteal suturing is required before the V-Y mucosal closure. These sutures can be augmented with an alar base cinch suture,[27] but this suture is not a substitute for precise closure of the periosteum, muscle, and mucosa.

Maxillary advancement produces a decrease in the nasolabial angle and raises the nasal tip, whereas inferior repositioning of the maxilla usually has the opposite effects on the nose. Thus if significant inferior movement accompanies advancement, the soft-tissue changes may at least partially offset each other. Precise prediction of the postsurgical soft-tissue contours may improve as more data are accumulated. The changes in the nose from maxillary surgery must be taken into account when rhinoplasty is planned, which makes simultaneous rhinoplasty and maxillary advancement somewhat unpredictable.

Mandibular Setback

Surgery to shorten the mandible usually is done in the ramus via bilateral sagittal split or transoral vertical ramus osteotomy. On rare occasions, total subapical osteotomy or even body ostectomy are indicated. An inferior border osteotomy may be combined with the above procedures (see Chapters 9 and 10 for details of the surgical techniques).

Today bilateral sagittal split osteotomy is most often performed to shorten the mandible, due to both the relative ease of applying RIF with this procedure as compared with the transoral vertical ramus osteotomy and the clear preference of patients for the early jaw function possible with rigid fixation. Properly executed, results with both procedures are good. Transoral vertical ramus osteotomy has a lesser incidence of neurosensory morbidity but an increased risk of poor control of the proximal condylar segment.[31] Bilateral sagittal split osteotomy clearly poses more risk to the inferior alveolar neurovascular bundle, but the neurosensory difference may not be clinically significant to the majority of patients.

With a sagittal split setback, much more care must be taken to position the proximal (condylar) segment than with mandibular advancement. Enough of the medial pterygoid muscle must be freed from the ramus to allow the distal (tooth-bearing) segment to be positioned passively in a posterior direction. If not, the proximal segment will be carried back with the distal segment. Following return to function, the muscles will tend to posture the mandible forward again, creating relapse. Positioning the segments at surgery usually is not difficult, but the position of the segments must be checked with a lateral cephalometric radiograph within the first few days following surgery. If the proximal segment is only rotated back minimally, the tendency for the patient to posture the mandible forward can be counteracted with elastics during the postsurgical orthodontics. If significant posterior displacement is obvious, reoperation to reposition the condylar segment may be required. The most difficult problems seem to arise when mandibular asymmetry also is corrected during the setback.

Repositioning the teeth in a posterior direction with total subapical osteotomy is more difficult than advancement with this procedure. A possible indication for this procedure is several missing posterior teeth and protrusive incisors. Anterior subapical osteotomy for 2 to 3 mm retraction of the anterior segment also can be considered when space can be made available distal to the canines (see Chapter 10 for details of the surgical procedures).

Body ostectomy or ostectomy in the midline may be indicated when occlusion posterior to the ostectomy sites is close to ideal or when multiple teeth are missing and the best occlusion could be obtained with ostectomy in the extraction sites. These procedures also may be indicated to decrease the transverse width of the mandible posterior to the ostectomy sites, with rotation of the mandible around the vertical condylar axis (see Chapter 10).

Mandibular inferior border osteotomy and/or augmentation of the inferior border with bone grafts, cartilage grafts, or alloplastic materials may be required along with ramus osteotomy or other surgical procedures for mandibular setback. To achieve facial balance, Class III patients may need the chin moved anteriorly, laterally, or posteriorly when the body of the mandible is moved posteriorly. Moving the chin forward provides the most predictable results. Mild degrees of asymmetry also can be corrected quite satisfactorily. Shortening the inferior border of the mandible in the AP direction with osteotomy or ostectomy is less predictable, and unesthetic results and poor lip function may ensue. If possible, alternative surgical procedures should be chosen to reduce the prominence of the chin. For instance, chin prominence relative to the dentition can be decreased by increasing the mandibular plane angle at surgery, and even if two-jaw surgery would then be required, this often is a better choice than an inferior border osteotomy to move the chin back. (See Chapter 5 for a discussion of cephalometric prediction in assessing the possibilities and Chapter 10 for details of inferior border osteotomy techniques.)

Two-Jaw Surgery

When significant AP maxillary deficiency exists along with mandibular excess, two-jaw surgery may be indicated. As has been discussed, two-jaw surgery can be performed safely if it is required, but the additional length of the surgery and the added morbidity of two surgical procedures must be outweighed by the significant benefits that will accrue to the patient with surgery in both jaws.

Vertical jaw relationships often dictate two-jaw rather than one-jaw surgery. If surgery in the maxilla only could correct the problem but the maxilla would have to be moved several millimeters downward, better stability can be achieved with simultaneous ramus osteotomy,[32] and the maxilla may not have to be moved so far in an inherently unstable direction. When surgery in the mandible only is considered, the ramus should not be significantly lengthened as a consequence of the setback procedure. If it would be, relapse into open bite is likely to occur, and it is better to rotate the maxilla up posteriorly in addition to setting the mandible back. In addition, the rotation of the mandibular

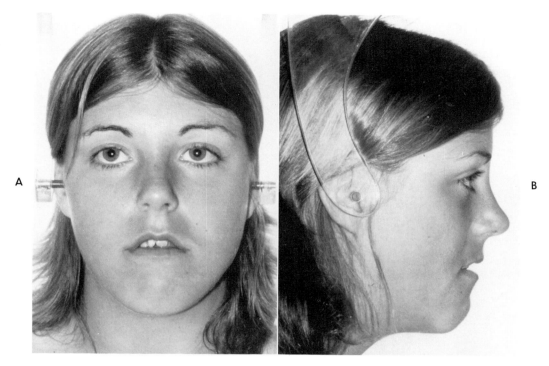

Fig. 14-19. K.I., a 17-year-old girl with severe Class III open-bite malocclusion. (Courtesy of the University of Washington.)

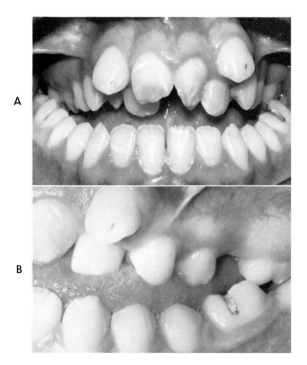

Fig. 14-20. K.I., dental relationships before treatment. Note the severe discrepancies in the transverse, AP, and vertical planes of space, in addition to severe crowding in the maxillary arch.

plane that would occur then often further decreases chin prominence in a desirable way. For these reasons, approximately half of the patients who have surgery now for Class III problems have two-jaw surgery (Figs. 14-19 to 14-23).

The details of the sequence of two-jaw surgery, fixation and stabilization, and rehabilitation are discussed in Chapter 11.

Adjunctive Soft-Tissue Procedures

Occasionally soft-tissue procedures are indicated along with osteotomy. Submental lipectomy with platysma muscle plication can eliminate excess tissue folds in the neck. If possible, jaw surgery should be planned to minimize this soft-tissue condition, but this is not always possible. Soft-tissue surgery of this type is described in several recent references.[33-37]

In rare instances the lower lip has considerable bulk and lip function and position is not satisfactory following osteotomy. Reduction cheiloplasty, though unpredictable, can be considered to possibly improve the situation. At least 6 months should pass following osteotomy, preferably also after completion of active orthodontics, before reduction cheiloplasty is planned.[38] Soft-tissue adaptation following osteotomy is not predictable for the individual patient, and the lips may

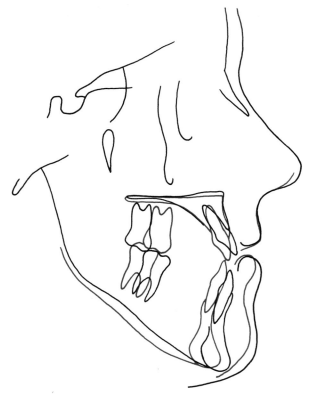

Fig. 14-21. K.I., cephalometric superimposition showing the effect of two-jaw surgery to correct her three-dimensional problems. A three-piece maxillary osteotomy was used to expand the maxilla and reposition it anteriorly, bilateral ramus osteotomies were used to set the mandible back, and a Proplast implant at the chin was used to maintain soft-tissue chin projection and improve chin-lip balance.

adapt well under function, a possibility not always easily anticipated. These soft-tissue procedures are described in standard cosmetic surgery texts.

POSTSURGICAL ORTHODONTICS

The principles of postsurgical orthodontics have been outlined in Chapter 6 and described in some detail in Chapter 12, so the discussion here focuses on additional details that are particularly pertinent to Class III patients. Routine postsurgical orthodontic treatment is very similar for all patients. The objectives are to bring the teeth into their final occlusal relationships, settling them into position and refining the static and dynamic occlusion and artistic positioning.

Following surgery and maxillomandibular release, the patient should function into the occlusal splint until the surgeon agrees that healing is adequate and active orthodontics can be resumed. Then both the splint and the stabilizing arch wires should be removed, and working arch wires and elastics should be used as described in Chapter 12.

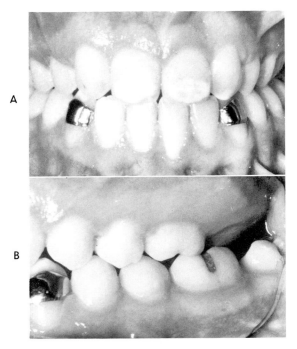

Fig. 14-22. K.I., dental relationships at the conclusion of treatment following removal of carious maxillary first molars and palatally positioned maxillary lateral incisors and the two-jaw surgery described above (Fig. 14-21). Eruption of maxillary third molars in the near future should provide improved posterior occlusion.

When segmental maxillary surgery has been performed, it may be advantageous to ligate together, underneath the stabilizing arch wire, the teeth on either side of the osteotomy sites. This should be done as soon as possible after occlusal splint removal to counteract any tendency for space to open when the first postoperative arch wire is placed. Ideally, this arch wire should not produce large differential forces between osteotomy segments and should provide some measure of incisor torque control. Both 16×22-mil stainless steel and 17×25 TMA have acceptable characteristics. A lighter round wire, typically 16 steel, could be used in the mandibular arch with light box elastics. After segmental surgery, care should be taken to attach the elastics to hooks placed on both sides of the segmental osteotomy sites, as attachment of the elastics to one segment alone may cause differential extrusion and rotation of the segment. As with all cases, finishing may require the use of zig-zag style 2-oz elastics as described by Alexander and Steffen, so as to provide the tightest possible interdigitation.[39,40]

The amount and length of the postoperative orthodontics will depend on the type of malocclusion initially present. In the open-bite Class III cases, every attempt should be made to prepare the occlusion before surgery so that only postoperative orthodontic move-

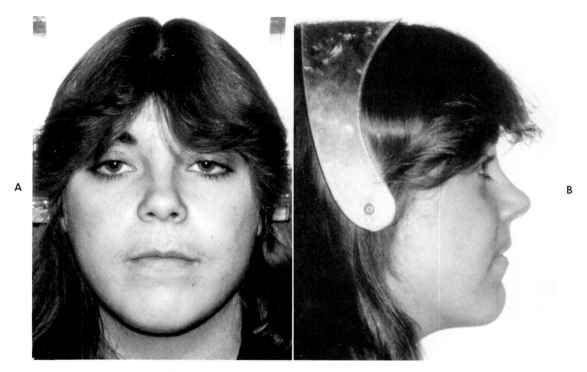

Fig. 14-23. K.I., facial proportions at the conclusion of treatment.

ments that have little potential to open the bite will be needed. Before removal of appliances, these patients should be allowed to function without elastics for 4 to 6 weeks to be sure there is no tendency for bite opening to recur. In deep-bite cases where some leveling has been postponed until after surgery, more tooth movement will be required, but the postsurgical treatment time should exceed 6 months only rarely.

If mild relapse toward a Class III relationship is observed during the postsurgical orthodontics, one of the first options that should be considered to obtain sagittal correction might be the use of moderate (200 to 300 gm) Class III elastics. With this much elastic force, a rectangular arch wire is needed in the maxilla to minimize extrusion of the molars and development of an open bite. In the presence of slightly greater relapse, flaring of the maxillary incisors, perhaps even to the extent of opening spaces, may provide effective camouflage. Another option would be interproximal reduction, retraction, and retroclination of the mandibular incisors.

Retention should be designed with the original malocclusion and its possible relapse tendencies in mind. Patients with an open-bite tendency should not have any wires crossing the occlusion, therefore a wrap-around–type maxillary retainer with C clasps soldered onto the second molars for additional retention is often the best choice. When premolars were extracted in the mandibular arch, removable retainers should be carried distal to the extraction site and may require an occlusal rest on the first molar for vertical stability. Zachrisson-type spiral wire retainers bonded to each tooth should be considered in cases with significant initial generalized spacing, maxillary diastemas, and severe lower incisor crowding.[41]

Unless the patient has further mandibular growth after surgery, the results of treatment tend to be stable (see below). If mild continuing relapse toward Class III is a problem, removable retainers can be designed with small hooks embedded in the acrylic to allow for very light Class III elastic wear. It is much easier, however, to achieve the necessary retention with a maxillary rather than a mandibular removable appliance. For posttreatment elastics to be effective, attaching the elastics to soldered cleats on the labial surface of a banded mandibular canine-to-canine retainer and using a maxillary removable stabilized by molar bands may be required.

RESPONSE TO TREATMENT
Physiologic Response
Posture

The postural response to mandibular setback is of particular clinical interest and importance because of its relationship to the maintenance of normal respiration postsurgically. The tongue is attached to the mandible, and it seems logical that when the mandible is moved posteriorly, the tongue also should move back.

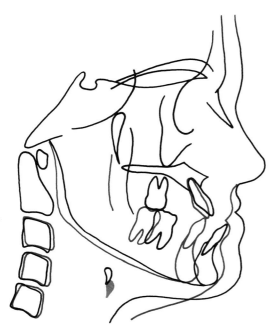

Fig. 14-24. Cephalometric superimposition of a patient before and after *(solid red)* a typical mandibular setback procedure. Note that, although the mandible moved posteriorly, the tongue moved downward (as indicated by the change in the position of the hyoid bone and the altered contour of the submental soft tissue).

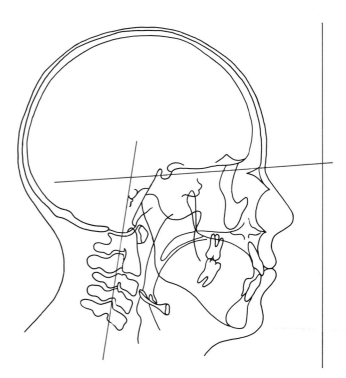

Fig. 14-25. With cephalometric radiographs taken in natural head position, changes in head posture in response to orthognathic surgery can be evaluated in two ways: craniovertical orientation, the inclination of the SN plane to a true vertical line (NSL-VER); or craniocervical orientation, the inclination of the SN plane to a line through the cervical vertebrae (usually tangent to the body of the third vertebra, as illustrated here [NSL-CVT]). Changes in these angles after different surgical procedures are shown in Table 14-1; changes in craniovertical orientation are illustrated in Fig. 14-26.

But if that happened, there would be a risk of blocking the pharyngeal airway. Concern about this led to recommendations that tongue reduction should accompany mandibular setback, and a wedge reduction of the tongue was commonly used along with body ostectomy (the standard operation for mandibular prognathism) in the 1940s and with the early ramus osteotomies of the 1950s.[42]

If it were not for postural adapation, tongue reduction would indeed be necessary, but in fact this is not needed. Fig. 14-24 illustrates the change in tongue posture that typically accompanies ramus osteotomy to set the mandible back. Note that the mandible moved posteriorly, but the tongue moved down. This can be seen not only in the position of the hyoid bone, but also in the soft-tissue contours. The greater the setback, the greater the downward movement of the floor of the mouth, which can create something of an esthetic problem with large posterior movements because of the "double chin" appearance postsurgically. The change in tongue posture means that respiration is unaffected, however, and the distance from the base of the tongue to the posterior pharyngeal wall is maintained.

Given the change in tongue posture, one would not be surprised if changes in jaw or head posture also occurred after mandibular setback or after other orthognathic surgery. Mandibular posture seems to be programmed in some way so that an approximately con-

stant distance is maintained between the maxillary and mandibular posterior teeth (i.e., freeway space is relatively constant even if the mandible is reoriented). Changes in mandibular posture when the maxilla is repositioned vertically have already been described in Chapter 13, and this occurs if vertical changes accompany anteroposterior movements, as when the maxilla is advanced to correct maxillary deficiency. The mandible rotates to a new position to compensate for the maxillary vertical changes.

Head posture is determined by a complex interaction that includes inputs from visual and labyrinthine (inner ear) receptors but is modified in response to other (presently unknown) influences. If cephalometric head films are taken in natural head position with the patient relaxed, as recommended for orthodontic-surgical patients, changes in head posture related to surgery can be determined. If the head tips upward postsurgically, the SN-true vertical angle will decrease; if it tips downward, the angle will increase (Fig. 14-25).

Mean changes in head posture for five groups of surgical patients, based on the paper by Snow and col-

TABLE 14-1 Head posture changes related to orthognathic surgery

Surgical procedure	N	Cranicovertical angle (NSL/VER)			Craniocervical angle (NSL/CVT)		
		Presurgery	Immediate postsurgery	One year	Presurgery	Immediate postsurgery	One year
Maxilla up	45	100.2 (4.5)	98.7* (4.9)	100.1 (5.3)	113.8 (7.6)	112.0 (8.1)	111.8 (8.0)
Mandible forward	78	98.6 (4.2)	95.8* (4.2)	97.7 (4.5)	108.5 (7.0)	107.1 (7.4)	107.4 (6.8)
Maxilla up and mandible forward	46	99.8 (4.4)	95.7* (4.5)	97.7* (4.1)	113.1 (7.2)	109.8* (7.0)	109.0* (6.9)
Mandible back	19	95.5 (3.9)	95.9 (2.7)	95.6 (3.4)	106.0 (6.8)	108.4 (6.0)	106.8 (7.9)
Maxilla up and mandible back	13	98.1 (5.0)	95.4 (4.4)	95.6 (3.4)	110.2 (9.2)	107.7 (10.5)	107.0 (10.0)

*p > .05.

leagues,[43] are shown in Table 14-1 and illustrated in Fig. 14-26. Note that the SN-true vertical angle is different for the patient groups initially. Those who have a long-face condition, alone or in combination with mandibular deformity, tend to have a larger angle before treatment. This does not necessarily reflect different posture at that point—the inclination of the anterior cranial base affects this angle and probably is its major determinant. But changes in the angle can be attributed entirely to changes in posture, and it is interesting to note that the response is different when the mandible is set back than when it is advanced or the maxilla is moved up. With other surgical procedures, patients tend to flex the head so that the chin goes down. Following mandibular setback there is no long-term change, and many patients have some short-term extension of the head (i.e., the chin is tipped up).

Lip and Tongue Pressure

It also seems logical on first thought that when the mandible is moved back, tongue pressure against the lower incisor teeth should increase and lip pressure should decrease. If this occurred, one would expect to observe a tendency for the lower incisors to move forward relative to their supporting bone, creating a dental relapse tendency even if the jaw position were stable. The greater the change in tongue posture, of course, the less the likelihood of increased tongue pressure, and tongue posture changes have just been discussed. In fact, both tongue and lip pressure are very little affected by surgery to reposition the jaws in the Class III patient.[44] For the tongue and the lips, both resting pressure and pressures during swallowing and speech are almost constant after the mandible is moved back. Lower lip pressure does decrease if the maxilla is

moved up and the mandible rotates up and forward, thereby relaxing the lips and decreasing lip incompetence. The adaptations in tongue and lip pressure undoubtedly contribute to the inicisor stability that usually is observed following surgical treatment.

Stability
Maxillary Advancement

From the early reports of maxillary advancement, it was recognized that there was a tendency for the maxilla to relapse posteriorly, and bone grafts were recom-

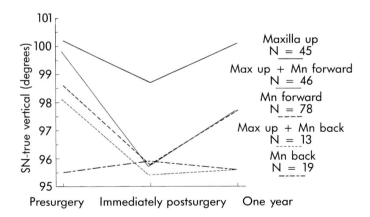

Fig. 14-26. Changes in craniovertical head posture related to the type of orthognathic surgery. Extension of the head is indicated by a decrease in the angle, flexion by an increase. Note that a tendency toward head extension occurs only with mandibular setback. Statistically significant short-term head flexion occurs with superior repositioning of the maxilla, mandibular advancement, and the combination of these procedures; the long-term change is significant only for the two-jaw procedure.

TABLE 14-2 Stability after maxillary advancement: mean changes in landmark positions (mm)						
	At surgery		First 6 weeks		6 weeks to 1 year	
	N = 38		N = 30		N = 38	
Landmark	Horiz	Vert	Horiz	Vert	Horiz	Vert
ANS	3.7	1.3	−0.1	−1.5	−1.5	−0.1
A	4.6	1.4	−0.1	−1.4	−0.9	−0.4
Mx inc	3.1	1.3	0.8	−1.7	0	−0.4
Mx molar	3.4	0.1	0.8	−1.1	−0.4	0.3
B	−0.8	0.3	1.5	−1.4	1.4	−0.8
Pg	0.5	−0.7	1.7	−1.8	0.3	0.2
Mn inc	−0.9	0.1	1.0	−1.9	1.2	−1.4
Mn plane		0.5		0.9		0.8

Horizontal: + = anterior; − = posterior
Vertical: + = down; − = up

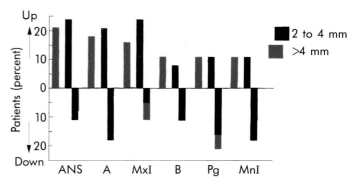

Fig. 14-27. The percentage of patients in the UNC sample with vertical changes in landmark locations associated with maxillary advancement. Note that in 20% of the patients the maxilla was moved up, whereas in 50% it was moved down, which caused a downward and backward rotation of the mandible (and therefore in 30% the maxillary movement was essentially straight forward).

mended to decrease this tendency.[45] Relapse superiorly after the maxilla was moved downward also was recognized soon after these procedures were attempted, and a number of options to improve stability were offered, involving the choice of graft materials and stabilization procedures.[46] Recently, data from reasonably large samples have become available to document and extend these clinical impressions.

Data from a sample of 39 patients at the UNC, all of whom were advanced more than 2 mm at point A, are summarized in Table 14-2.[47] From the mean changes in the table, it is apparent that the typical patient had the maxilla moved forward and downward, producing some downward and backward rotation of the mandible, but as Fig. 14-27 illustrates, this pattern of vertical change was present in only half the sample. The other patients had the maxilla moved up somewhat or maintained at the same vertical level. Twenty-two of these patients, just over half, had bone grafts, and 14 had RIF. Changes during healing (i.e., the first 6 postsurgical weeks) and from 6 weeks to 1 year were examined.

Several points are worth noting. First, during the first 6 weeks, although the mean change in the horizontal position of skeletal landmarks was almost zero and not statistically significant, changes in both directions did occur. As with much data of this type, the variation rather than the mean tendency is more important clinically. As Fig. 14-28, *A* shows, during the initial healing there was a 20% chance that the maxilla would slip posteriorly more than 2 mm and a 10% chance that it would move anteriorly. From 6 weeks to 1 year, however, there was a greater chance of posterior movement of landmarks (Fig. 14-28, *C*).

Second, there were significant changes in the vertical plane. On the average, the anterior skeletal landmarks moved up 1.5 mm and PNS moved up 0.5 mm (see Table 14-2) (i.e., there was no net downward movement of the maxilla). In this also, however, there was considerable individual variation, and Figs. 14-28, *B* and 14-28, *D* give a more clinically useful picture. In the majority of the patients the maxilla remained vertically within 2 mm of its immediate postsurgical position, but in a third of the group the maxilla moved up more than 2 mm. More importantly, the upward movement occurred almost exclusively in the patients whose maxilla had been moved down. No patients had downward movement of the maxilla.

Third, RIF improved short-term stability, more in the vertical than in the AP plane of space (Table 14-3). During the first 6 weeks, there were only small horizontal changes in both groups, but the average upward movement of the maxilla was considerably greater in the conventional wire fixation group, and that led to more upward and forward rotation of the mandible in those patients. The difference in vertical stability was statistically significnt. From 6 weeks to 1 year, there was a tendency for the anterior maxillary landmarks to be repositioned posteriorly in both groups, which was slightly but not significantly greater in the rigid fixation group. There was little or no difference in the pattern of changes in the vertical plane of space after the first 6 weeks but also no recovery of the upward movement in the wire fixation group.

Other investigators also have reported improved stability of maxillary advancement with several forms of RIF.[48-50] From a synthesis of the existing data, it appears that rigid fixation is particularly helpful if the maxilla is to be moved downward. Without it, long-term net downward movement in one-jaw surgery is unlikely.

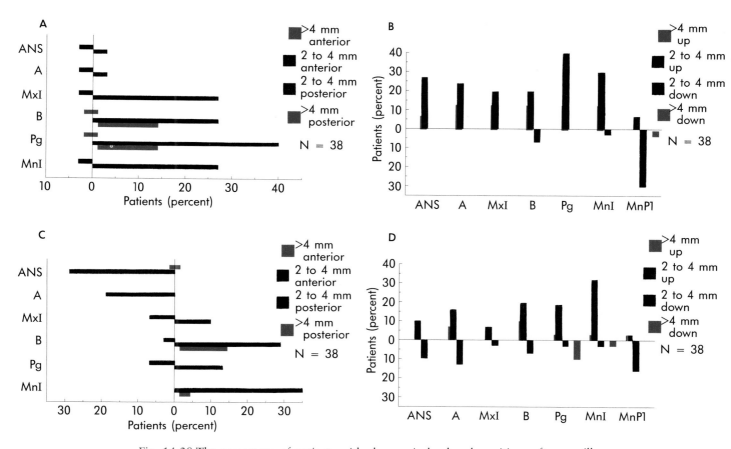

Fig. 14-28. The percentage of patients with changes in landmark positions after maxillary advancement. **A,** Horizontal and **B,** vertical changes during the first 6 weeks postsurgically. **C,** Horizontal and **D,** vertical changes from 6 weeks to 1 year.

TABLE 14-3 Stability after maxillary advancement, rigid versus nonrigid fixation: changes in landmark position (mm)

	Rigid fixation				Wire fixation			
	N = 14				N = 24			
	First 6 weeks		6 weeks to 1 year		First 6 weeks		6 weeks to 1 year	
Landmark	Horiz	Vert	Horiz	Vert	Horiz	Vert	Horiz	Vert
ANS	0.6	−0.7	−2.1	−0.7	−0.3	−1.8	−1.3	0.1
A	0.4	−0.4	−1.2	−1.5	−0.2	−1.8	−0.8	0
Mx inc	0.6	−0.9	−0.9	−0.4	0.9	−2.0	0.2	−0.4
Mx molar	0.9	−0.6	−0.6	0.2	0.7	−1.3	−0.3	0.3
B	1.1	−0.8	0.3	−0.2	1.6	−1.6	1.7	−1.0
Pg	1.2	−1.1	−0.4	1.4	1.8	−2.1	0.5	−0.2
Mn inc	1.1	−1.0	0.6	−2.3	0.9	−2.3	1.4	−1.4
Mn plane		0.4		0.4		1.1		0.9

Horizontal: + = anterior; − = posterior
Vertical: + = down; − = up

TABLE 14-4 Stability after mandibular setback: mean changes in landmark positions (mm)

| | At surgery | | First 6 weeks | | 6 weeks to 1 year | | Postsurgery to 1 year | |
| | N = 38 | | N = 11 | | N = 11 | | N = 38 | |
Landmark	Horiz	Vert	Horiz	Vert	Horiz	Vert	Horiz	Vert
Mx inc	−0.1	0.3	−0.5	−0.1	0.6	−0.2	−0.3	0.1
B	−5.8	0.2	−0.4	−0.1	2.6	−0.9	0.5	−0.6
Pg	−5.2	−0.3	−0.9	−0.1	1.2	−1.3	0.4	−0.9
Mn inc	−6.0	−0.5	−0.4	−0.6	1.7	−1.3	0.7	−1.4
Mn plane		0.6		−2.4		1.1		−2.4

Horizontal: + = anterior; − = posterior
Vertical: + = down; − = up

Another way to improve stability when the maxilla is moved forward and/or downward is to stablize the maxilla with grafts. Because bank bone is incorporated less rapidly than autogenous grafts, blocks of cadaver bone might well be advantageous in advancement or downgraft surgery. Synthetic hydroxylapatite can serve as a bone graft substitute,[51,52] and using this in combination with RIF, Wardrop and Wolford recently have reported relapse changes of 1 mm or less with both advancement and downward movement of the maxilla.[30]

Mandibular Setback

Considering that mandibular setback was the major, indeed almost the only surgical procedure of 30 years ago, it is ironic that its stability is no better characterized than maxillary advancement and other procedures. Continuing changes in surgical techniques have occurred that prevent the older data from being entirely applicable, and the more recent patients have not been studied extensively. Nevertheless, reasonable data do exist. The vertical oblique ramus osteotomy for mandibular prognathism was introduced in the 1950s. It quickly replaced the earlier horizontal ramus and body ostectomy procedures because of more predictable and presumably more stable results. In the 1970s, a relapse tendency after this ramus surgery but reasonable stability in the absence of renewed growth was well documented.[53] By 1980, surgery to set the mandible back was carried out almost entirely either with bilateral sagittal split osteotomy (BSSO) or transoral vertical oblique osteotomy (TOVRO), a considerably modified version of the older vertical ramus procedure. It is interesting to view the stability of the modern procedures in comparison with the older ones and to compare BSSO with TOVRO.

Stability data for a group of patients who underwent mandibular setback surgery, pooling patients treated with BSSO and TOVRO, are shown in Table 14-4. Note that the average setback at surgery was 6 mm at

the mandibular incisor and 5.2 mm at pogonion, with almost no vertical change. In approximately 20% of the sample, however, the mandible was rotated upward, and in another 20% it rotated down. From postsurgery to 1 year, the mean values in Table 14-4 show that on the average there was only a fraction of a millimeter of horizontal change, with somewhat greater upward and forward rotation of the mandible but no more than would be expected from splint removal. Again, this conceals some of the variation within the sample that Fig. 14-29 emphasizes. In this group, there was about a 25% chance that the mandible would move forward more than 2 mm postsurgically and an approximately equal chance that the chin would rotate upward that much.

When postsurgical changes occur, do they happen during the first 6 weeks of initial healing, or after the patient returns to jaw function? The data from a smaller UNC group who had radiographs at 6 weeks postsurgically (see Table 14-4) suggest that on the average the mandible moves slightly more posteriorly during fixation, then comes forward after fixation is released and function is resumed. This is similar to the distal positioning of the mandible that occurs in the first few weeks after mandibular advancement when patients are held in maxillomandibular fixation (see Chapter 12) and perhaps is due to a similar mechanism (related to condylar positioning in normal jaw function?). Rosenquist and colleagues[54] also noted forward displacement of the mandible after maxillomandibular fixation was released, as had the investigators of the 1970s cited above.

Is there any difference in stability with BSSO and TOVRO? Data for 19 BSSO and 20 TOVRO patients, who were similar in the degree of mandibular setback, are displayed in Table 14-5. Note that the mandible tended to move forward again in the BSSO group (i.e., there was a relapse tendency), whereas in the TOVRO group the mean change was further backward move-

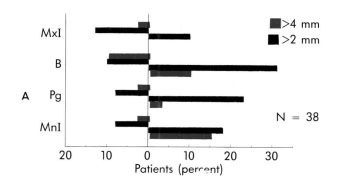

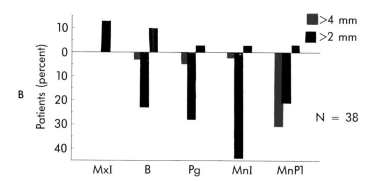

Fig. 14-29. The percentages of patients with changes following mandibular setback surgery, from surgery to 1 year. **A**, Horizontal changes. **B**, Vertical changes.

TABLE 14-5 Mandibular setback stability—BSSO versus TOVRO: mean changes in landmark positions (mm) from immediate postsurgery to 1 year

Landmark	BSSO N = 19		TOVRO N = 20	
	Horiz	Vert	Horiz	Vert
Mx inc	0.7	−0.4	−1.3	0.5
B	2.5	−0.7	−1.4	−0.5
Pg	1.3	−1.1	−0.5	−0.8
Mn inc	2.4	−2.0	−0.9	−0.8
Mn plane		−0.8		−4.0

Horizontal: + = anterior; − = posterior
Vertical: + = down; − = up

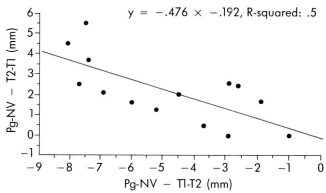

Fig. 14-30. Scattergram demonstrating the tendency for mandibular relapse postoperatively to increase as the magnitude of the setback increases. (Redrawn with permission from Franco JE, van Sickels JE, Thrash WJ: Factors contributing to relapse in rigidly fixed mandibular setbacks, J Oral Maxillofac Surg 47:451-456, 1989.)

ment. The difference was statistically significant. This does not necessarily mean that stability and outcomes are better with the TOVRO procedure. Failure to seat the condyles completely at surgery can lead to inadvertent overcorrection of the prognathism when function is resumed, which apparently did happen in some patients in the TOVRO group.

Are there other factors in stability after mandibular setback? At least three have been supported by recent studies: (1) all other things being equal, the greater the setback, the greater the relapse is likely to be (Fig. 14-30);[55,56] (2) skeletal suspension wires, so that the body of the mandible is supported by the bony maxilla rather than by the teeth, have the potential to reduce but not eliminate relapse tendencies;[57] and (3) if the proximal (ramus) segment is allowed to rotate posteriorly during surgery, greater relapse is likely to occur.[58] Interestingly, there is no evidence that RIF produces greater stability after mandibular setback,[56] and indeed one could argue from the existing data that the relapse tendency may be somewhat greater with rigid than with conventional fixation.

Two-Jaw Surgery

A combination of maxillary advancement and mandibular setback is increasingly frequent in treatment of

Class III problems. During the last 2 years, nearly 50% of the Class III patients at UNC had two-jaw surgery, whereas the remainder were divided almost equally between isolated maxillary and mandibular surgery. Nevertheless, there is no published study of stability with this combination of procedures.

Data for a relatively small North Carolina sample, all of whom had conventional fixation, are shown in Table 14-6. Note that at surgery, the amount of downward movement of the maxilla was almost as great as the forward movement, so that the mandible was rotated down and back as well as shortened. Compared with the patients who had only downward movement of the maxilla (see Table 14-2), the vertical stability is impressive. Note that in the two-jaw patients, on the average there was almost no relapse of the maxilla su-

TABLE 14-6 Stability after combined maxillary advancement-mandibular setback: change in landmark position (mm)

Landmark	At surgery N = 14		Surgery to 1 year N = 14	
	Horiz	Vert	Horiz	Vert
ANS	3.1	−2.5	−1.6	0
A	3.2	−2.7	−0.2	−0.1
Mx inc	2.9	−2.7	−0.6	−1.6
Mx molar	3.8	−3.1	0.9	−0.2
B	−0.1	−5.0	2.2	−2.0
Pg	2.1	−6.3	1.0	−1.0
Mn inc	−1.8	−4.8	2.1	−3.1
Mn molar	0.1	−2.6	3.0	−2.4
Mn plane		3.8		−0.8

Horizontal: + = anterior; − = posterior
Vertical: + = down; − = up

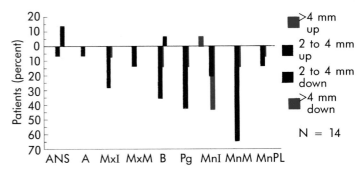

Fig. 14-31. The percentages of patients with changes in landmark positions following combined maxillary advancement and mandibular setback (from immediate postsurgery to 1-year follow-up).

periorly or posteriorly, except that ANS moved posteriorly (probably due to remodeling in that area) and the upper incisor moved superiorly. Note in Fig. 14-31 the minimal tendency for upward relapse of the maxilla. Surprisingly, the change in upper incisor position occurred during the first 6 weeks postsurgically and therefore apparently was not due to rebound after elongation during fixation, as seemed to occur in the long-face mandibular-deficient patients discussed in Chapter 13.

It has been reported previously that vertical stability after maxillary downgrafting is improved by simultaneous ramus osteotomy.[59,60] Perhaps the soft-tissue pressures that tend to displace the maxilla superiorly are reduced by the muscle detachment necessary for a ramus osteotomy. At any rate, the limited data available at present do indicate that if significant vertical change is needed, surgery on the maxilla and mandible is more likely to produce a stable long-term change.

Case 1

C.C. was first seen for orthodontic consultation at age 4 years, 3 months, because of concern about her anterior crossbite. A cephalometric radiograph was made at that time, but no treatment was undertaken. On recall at age 6 years, 5 months, a repeat cephalometric film showed considerable growth in a skeletal Class III pattern (Fig. 14-32), and treatment in the near future was suggested. At age 7 years, 1 month (Fig. 14-33), a chin cup with 16-oz force was placed, to be worn 12 hours/day. The reverse overjet reduced rapidly, and a maxillary removable appliance to procline the upper incisors was placed. After 8 months, the anterior crossbite was corrected, and a W-arch for transverse maxillary expansion was placed. Cephalometric superimposition showed the downward and backward mandibular rotation that is a typical response to a chin cup (Fig. 14-34).

Although she continued to wear the chin cup at night, there was gradual relapse toward anterior and posterior crossbite as the mandible grew but not the maxilla. At age 8 years, 8 months, a Frankel-III functional appliance (Fig. 14-35) was placed. She experienced some difficulty in adapting to the appliance originally, then wore it well. At age 9 years, 3 months, a new FR-III was placed (Fig. 14-36) after the original one had become distorted; she continued to wear it well and made good progress (Figs. 14-37 and 14-38). By age 10 years, wear was only marginal. A third appliance was made but was not worn regularly and was discontinued after being

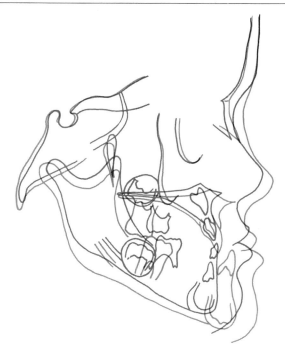

Fig. 14-32. C.C., cephalometric superimposition, ages 4 years, 3 months, to 6 years, 11 months *(solid pink)*, no treatment.

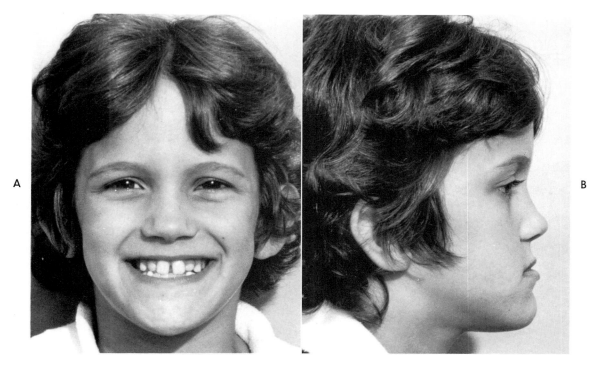

Fig. 14-33. C.C., facial appearance, age 6 years, 11 months, at the beginning of chin-cup therapy.

Continued.

Case 1—cont'd.

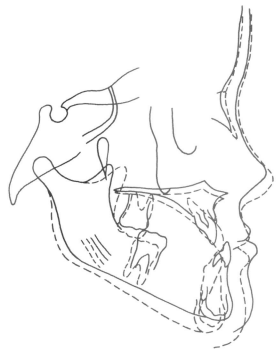

Fig. 14-34. C.C., cephalometric superimposition, ages 6 years, 11 months, to 7 years, 11 months (*dashed black*), response to chin cup.

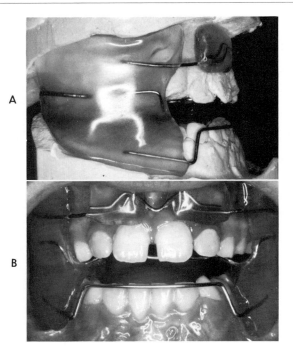

Fig. 14-35. C.C., FR-III appliance, **A,** on cast and **B,** intraorally. Note the pads in the maxillary vestibule, which are intended to stretch the periosteum anteriorly and so stimulate forward growth of the maxilla. The appliance also opens the bite, thereby rotating the mandible down and back.

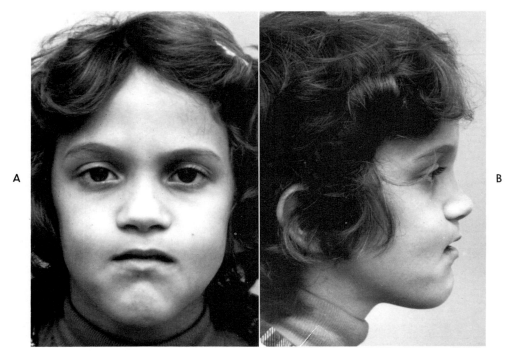

Fig. 14-36. C.C. **A** and **B,** Age 9 years, 3 months, facial appearance just after insertion of the second FR-III appliance.

Case 1—cont'd.

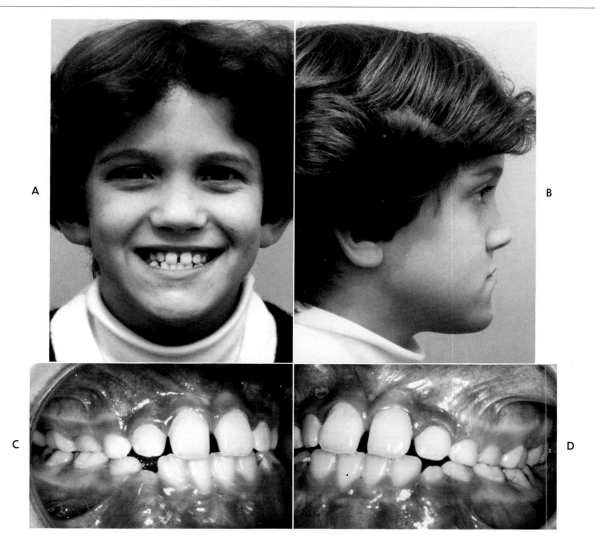

Fig. 14-37. C.C., age 9 years, 7 months, after nearly 1 year of Frankel treatment. **A** and **B**, Facial appearance, and **C** and **D**, occlusal relationships.

broken at age 10 years, 6 months. The parents were told that the difficulty of controlling the growth pattern made surgery probably necessary in the future. As she reached menarche at age 11, a spurt in mandibular growth occurred and reverse overjet returned (Fig. 14-38, *B*).

By age 14 years, 10 months, it appeared that the adolescent growth spurt had been completed. Facially, there was an appearance of midface deficiency and chin prominence (Fig. 14-39). Dentally, the teeth were well aligned, but anterior and posterior crossbite existed, and the mandibular incisors were tipped lingually in compensation for the Class III growth pattern (Fig. 14-40). Cephalometric analysis confirmed AP and vertical maxillary deficiency, with the maxillary teeth protrusive

relative to the maxilla and the mandibular teeth lingually positioned relative to the chin (Fig. 14-41).

In preparation for surgery, molars were banded and bonded brackets placed on all other teeth (18-slot edgewise). Initial alignment was accomplished with 16 NiTi; then a sequence of 16 steel, 17×25 TMA, and 17×25 steel arch wires were employed. Orthodontic preparation required 6 months (Figs. 14-42, 14-43, and 14-44, *A*).

At age 15 years, 6 months, LeFort I osteotomy to reposition the maxilla forward and somewhat downward and mandibular inferior border osteotomy to reduce chin projection were carried out (Fig. 14-44, *B*). At operation, after the maxilla had been freed and advanced, it was secured to the mandible using the prepared splint,

Continued.

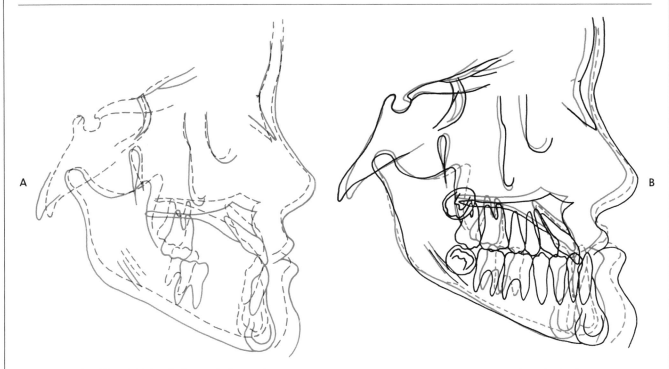

Fig. 14-38. C.C., cephalometric superimpositions. **A,** Ages 7 years, 11 months *(dashed pink)*, to 10 years, 6 months, FR-III treatment. **B,** Ages 10 years, 6 months *(pink)*, to 11 years, 6 months, to 14 years, 10 months. Note the almost total lack of maxillary growth during the adolescent growth spurt. Mandibular growth was only slightly in excess of normal but was projected more forward and less down than normal because of the lack of vertical maxillary growth.

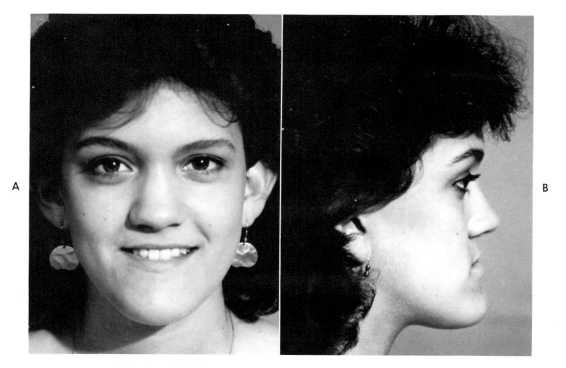

Fig. 14-39. C.C., age 14 years, 10 months, facial appearance.

A   B   C

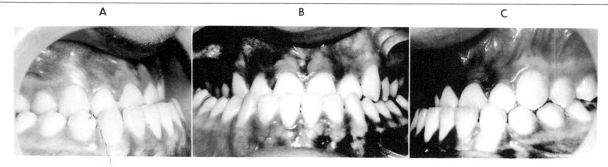

Fig. 14-40. C.C., age 14 years, 10 months, occlusal relationships.

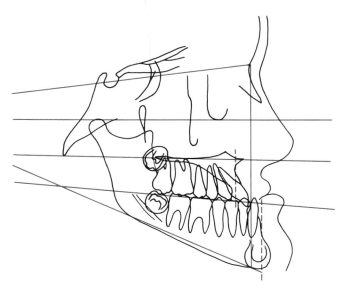

Fig. 14-41. C.C., age 14 years, 10 months, cephalometric tracing before the final phase of treatment, preparing for jaw surgery. Cephalometric measurements: **N perp to A, −8 mm; N perp to Pg, 10 mm; AB difference, −14 mm; UFH, 53 mm; LFH, 59 mm; mand plane, 23 degrees; MxI to A vert, 7 mm, 37 degrees; MnI to B vert, −4 mm, 5 degrees.**

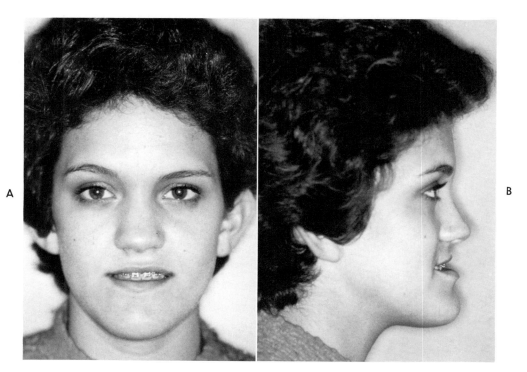

Fig. 14-42. C.C., age 15 years, 6 months, facial appearance immediately before surgery.

Continued.

Case 1—cont'd.

A   B   C

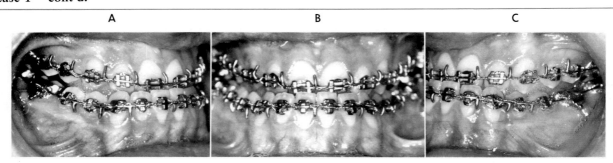

Fig. 14-43. C.C., age 15 years, 6 months, occlusal relationships before surgery.

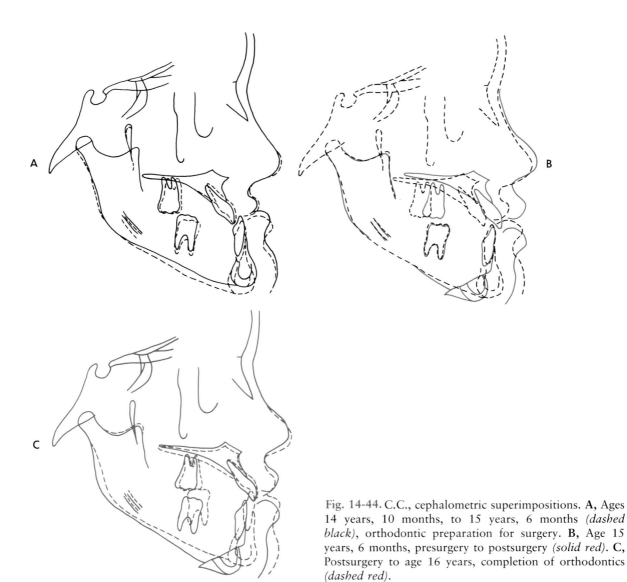

Fig. 14-44. C.C., cephalometric superimpositions. **A,** Ages 14 years, 10 months, to 15 years, 6 months *(dashed black)*, orthodontic preparation for surgery. **B,** Age 15 years, 6 months, presurgery to postsurgery *(solid red)*. **C,** Postsurgery to age 16 years, completion of orthodontics *(dashed red)*.

Case 1—cont'd.

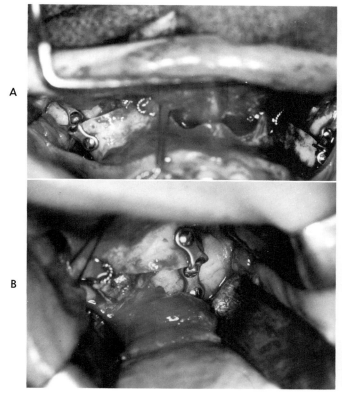

Fig. 14-45. C.C. **A,** Anterior and **B,** lateral views at surgery, showing the small bone plates for rigid fixation.

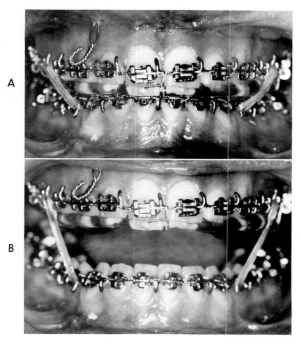

Fig. 14-46. C.C. **A,** Occlusal relationships in the splint 1 week postsurgery. **B,** Functioning into the splint, 3 weeks postsurgery.

and blocks of freeze-dried cartilage were placed in the tuberosity areas bilaterally. Two small bone plates were adapted to lie passively between the zygomatic buttress and the lateral aspect of the maxilla and were secured with two screws above and one below (Fig. 14-45). The chin was approached via an incision in the vestibule from canine to canine, well out into the lip in the mid-line; an osteotomy was performed so that the chin could be moved posteriorly; and a pressure dressing was applied after the tissues had been sutured. She was discharged on the second postoperative day in maxillomandibular fixation (Fig. 14-46). After 2 weeks, the splint was ligated to the upper arch, and she was allowed to function into the splint.

Six weeks postsurgically, the 17×25 stabilizing arch wires were replaced with 16 steel wires, and light posterior box elastics with a Class III component (Fig. 14-47)

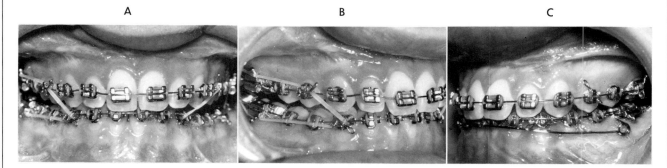

Fig. 14-47. C.C. **A** and **B,** Occlusal relationships at the resumption of orthodontics after removal of the splint. Note the Class III component to the posterior box elastics. **C,** Auxiliary depressing arch used to slightly open the bite anteriorly, just before removal of the orthodontic appliance.

Continued.

Case 1—cont'd.

were worn full-time. The round wire was later replaced in the mandibular arch only with 17×25 TMA to improve the axial inclination of the lower incisors. For 1 month before completion of treatment, a 17×22 steel auxiliary depressing arch was used to decrease overbite (Fig. 14-47, *C*). At age 15 years, 11 months, 4 months after finishing orthodontics was resumed, she was debanded to a positioner. Retainers were placed 4 weeks later. Facial proportions (Fig. 14-48) and occlusal relationships (Fig. 14-49) were much improved. At age 17 years, 2 months, occlusal relationships were well main-

tained despite a somewhat more Class III facial appearance (Figs. 14-50 and 14-51). At that point, retainers were worn only on occasional nights and no relapse tendency was observed.

Comments. This patient illustrates the difficulty of controlling a Class III growth pattern with orthodontic treatment. Although gratifying corrections were obtained during the mixed dentition, first with the chin cup and again with the FR-III after that had relapsed, the amount of disproportionate growth at puberty was too much to manage. In skeletal Class III malocclusion,

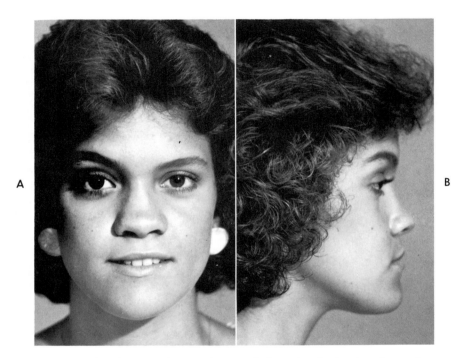

Fig. 14-48. C.C., facial proportions at the completion of orthodontics, 6 months postsurgery.

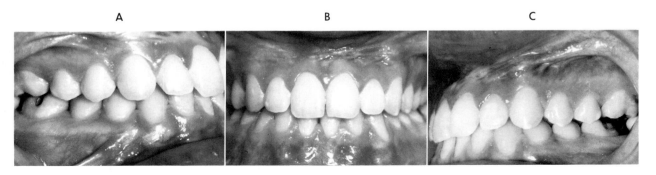

Fig. 14-49. C.C., occlusal relationships at the completion of orthodontics.

Case 1—cont'd.

whether the problem is primarily excessive mandibular or (as here) deficient maxillary growth, this is a distressingly frequent occurrence. Extraction of teeth in the mandibular arch in an attempt to maintain normal overjet during the adolescent growth spurt obviously would have been disastrous—considerable dental compensation in the form of uprighting of lower incisors occurred even without treatment.

Maxillary advancement obviously was a necessary component of the surgical treatment. Whether to set back the mandible at the same time was a matter of some debate.

Ultimately, our judgment was that profile esthetics might be better with a mandibular ramus procedure, but full-face esthetics would not and in fact might be worse because of the effect on throat form. For this reason, mandibular surgery was confined to the inferior border osteotomy, which could correct the disproportion between chin and lower lip without compromising throat form. The result, which can best be described as a harmonious but "anterior divergent" profile (see Chapter 4), is quite pleasing to the patient.

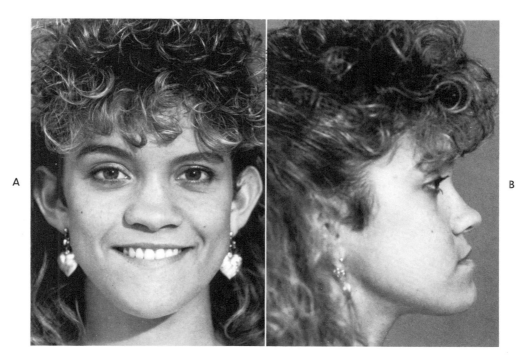

Fig. 14-50. C.C., age 17 years, 10 months, facial proportions.

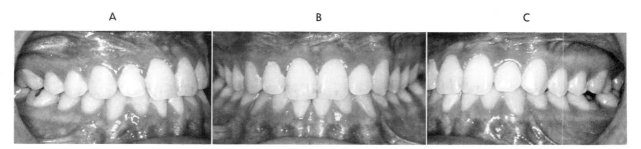

Fig. 14-51. C.C., age 17 years, 10 months, occlusal relationships.

Case 2

A.S. was seen for orthodontic evaluation at age 11 years, 11 months, because of concern about her mildly crowded and asymmetric maxillary incisors and posterior crossbite with a shift of the mandible to the left. Cephalometric analysis confirmed the clinical impression of a mild long-face, skeletal Class III pattern (Fig. 14-52). A partial fixed appliance was placed and cross elastics on the left side were used for 3 months, which eliminated the mandibular shift. After a review of the growth pattern, it was decided to defer further treatment until the adolescent growth spurt was completed.

Puberty did not occur until age 14. Disproportionate mandibular growth, partially compensated by downward rotation, reached a maximum rate at that time, then declined. Despite the jaw discrepancy, anterior occlusion remained almost normal because the maxillary incisors tipped labially and the mandibular incisors became increasingly upright, compensating for the Class III jaw relationship (Fig. 14-52, B). The patient and her parents were reluctant to consider the possibility of surgical-orthodontic treatment but were told that there were no realistic options. After talking with other patients who had had surgery, they agreed to at least consider it.

At age 17 years, 3 months, a complete diagnostic evaluation confirmed a long-face deformity with a prominent chin that was mildly deviated to the left (Fig. 15-53). There was a mild anterior open bite and anterior crossbite tendency (Fig. 14-54). Cephalometric analysis doc-umented excessive anterior face height, with a steep mandibular plane angle and downward rotation of the maxilla posteriorly (Fig. 15-55). The maxillary incisors were proclined relative to the maxilla, whereas the mandibular incisors were upright. Dental radiographs revealed partial resorption of the root of the maxillary right first premolar. This was thought to be nonprogressive and probably related to pressure from the erupting canine in previous years.

To correct the jaw discrepancies, LeFort I osteotomy to move the maxilla superiorly and slightly anteriorly and mandibular ramus osteotomy to set the mandible back were planned. Mandibular setback alone would have produced a lengthening of the pterygomandibular sling and thus a tendency to relapse into anterior open bite. To control this, surgery to elevate the posterior maxilla also was needed, and if the maxilla were to be involved anyway, bringing it slightly anteriorly would improve the overall facial balance. Because of the proclination of the maxillary incisors, extraction of the maxillary first premolars and incisor retraction were needed to decrease the dental compensation and create reverse overjet, but as in many Class III patients, the mandibular crowding would be best treated without extraction. This also had the virtue of eliminating the tooth that had experienced severe root resorption. All four third molars were present and partially impacted where they potentially could interfere with the osteotomies; these

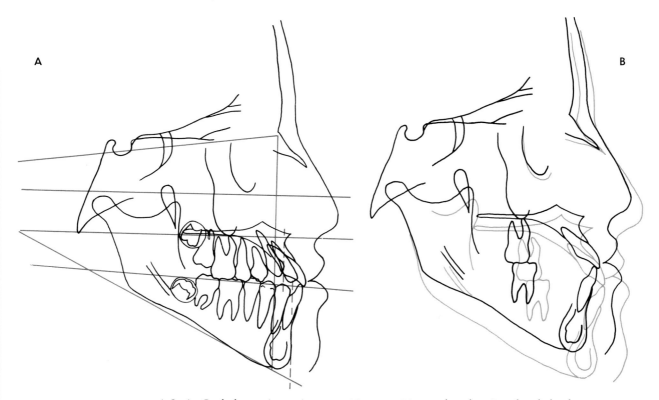

Fig. 14-52. A.S. **A,** Cephalometric tracing, age 11 years, 11 months, showing the skeletal Class III jaw relationship at that time despite the absence of reverse overjet. Cephalometric measurements: N perp to A, 4 mm; N perp to Pg, 7 mm; AB difference, −3 mm; UFH, 50 mm; LFH, 66 mm; mand plane, 27 degrees; MxI to A vert, 9 mm, 44 degrees; MnI to B vert, 3 mm, 19 degrees. **B,** Superimposition from age 11 years, 11 months, to 17 years, 3 months *(solid pink)*, showing the strong Class III growth pattern.

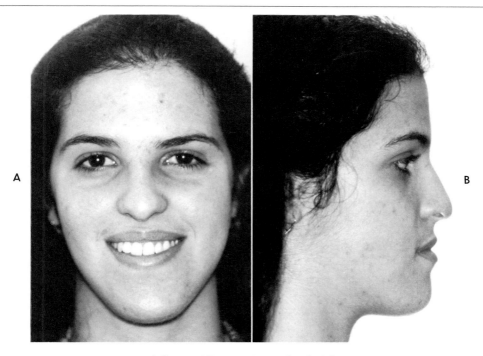

Fig. 14-53. A.S., age 17 years, 3 months, facial appearance.

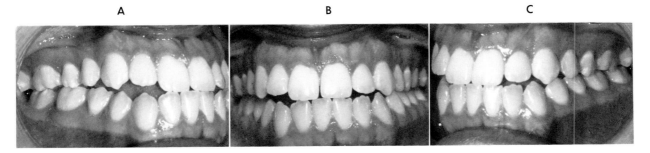

Fig. 14-54. A.S., age 17 years, 3 months, occlusal relationships.

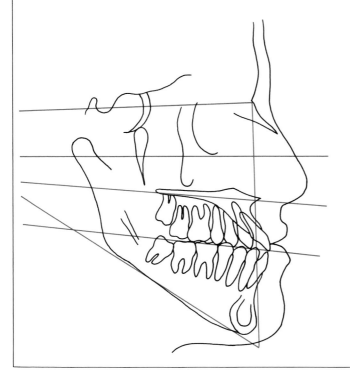

Fig. 14-55. A.S., age 17 years, 3 months, cephalometric analysis. Note the extensive dental compensations for the skeletal deformity: the maxillary incisors are proclined and elongated, whereas the mandibular incisors are upright and also elongated. Cephalometric measurements: N perp to A, −3 mm; N perp to Pg, −2 mm; AB difference, −4 mm; UFH, 53 mm; LFH, 71 mm; mand plane, 33 degrees; MxI to A vert, 9 mm, 34 degrees; MnI to B vert, 4 mm, 31 degrees.

Continued.

Case 2 — cont'd.

were scheduled for extraction at the same time as the premolars.

The recommendations for treatment were accepted after further consultation with other orthognathic-surgery patients and considerable thought by the family. After

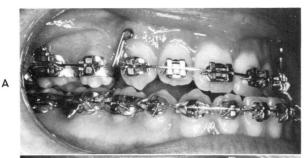

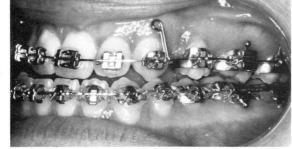

Fig. 14-56. A.S., age 17 years, 10 months, maxillary space closure nearly completed. Note the increase in reverse overjet as dental compensation is removed during the presurgical orthodontics.

alignment with 16 NiTi arch wires, 17×22 closing loops were used to retract the upper incisors and close the extraction spaces (Fig. 14-56), and 17×25 stabilizing arch wires were placed. As expected, removal of the dental compensations made the jaw discrepancy more apparent (Fig. 14-57). At age 18 years, 1 month, a one-piece LeFort I osteotomy and bilateral sagittal split ramus osteotomies were carried out (Fig. 14-58), staging the two-jaw procedure as described in Chapter 11. Transosseous wires were placed in the maxilla and mandible, and wire loops were used to complete maxillomandibular fixation. She tolerated the procedure well and was discharged on the second postoperative day.

Maxillomandibular fixation was released 6 weeks postsurgically, and she functioned into the splint for another 2 weeks. The stabilizing arch wires and splint were removed at that time; 16 steel arch wires were placed, using an elastomeric chain to close the small residual extraction spaces and Kobayashi hooks as needed for interarch elastics, and she wore light box elastics anteriorly and posteriorly full-time. As the teeth settled into occlusion, a maxillary 17×22 arch wire was used for better torque control. At age 18 years, 8 months, orthodontic appliances were removed and removable retainers were placed (Fig. 14-59). Facial proportions were greatly improved (Fig. 14-60), and the patient and her family were pleased with the outcome. On 5-year recall, both facial and occlusal relationships appeared stable (Figs. 14-61 and 14-62). Cephalometric superimposition revealed no change from 4 years previously.

Comments. Removal of dental compensations presurgically is one key to successful surgical-orthodontic treatment in general. For this patient, it was absolutely es-

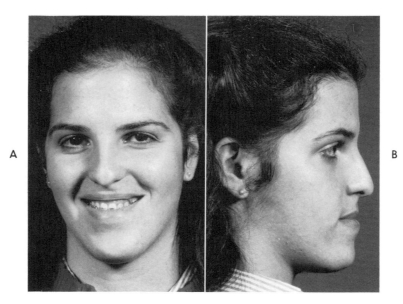

Fig. 14-57. A.S., age 18 years, 1 month, just before surgery.

Case 2—cont'd.

sential: a good result would have been almost impossible to achieve without extraction of maxillary but not mandibular premolars, so that the proclined maxillary incisors could be retracted. Although the instability produced by mandibular setback alone in a long-face patient seems not to be as severe as with mandibular advancement, relapse into open bite is a real possibility. Vertical stability is enhanced by elevating the posterior maxilla so that the pterygomandibular sling is not lengthened, and this also allows total face height to be shortened if desired.

Like many patients with excessive mandibular growth, A.S. had mild mandibular asymmetry. There is no problem in correcting this with a somewhat greater setback on one side than on the other when bilateral ramus osteotomies have been performed. In this case, there was no maxillary asymmetry, but if there had been, a modest rotation of the maxilla to correct it also would have been possible.

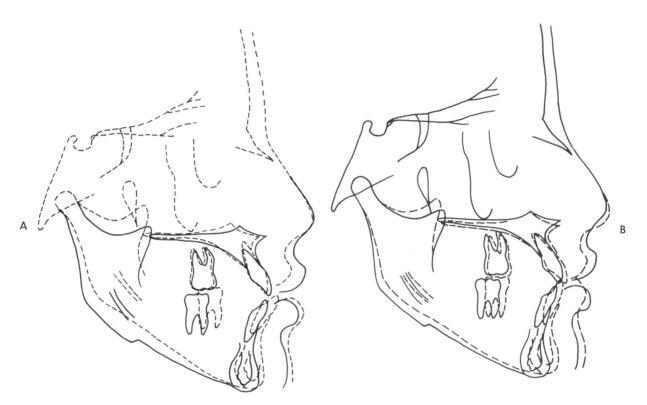

Fig. 14-58. A.S., cephalometric superimpositions. **A,** Presurgery to postsurgery *(solid red).* **B,** Postsurgery to completion of treatment *(dashed red).*

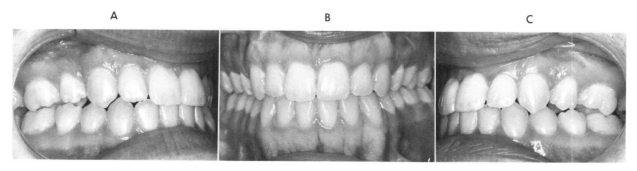

Fig. 14-59. A.S., age 18 years, 8 months, occlusal relationships at completion of treatment.

Continued.

Case 2—cont'd.

A B

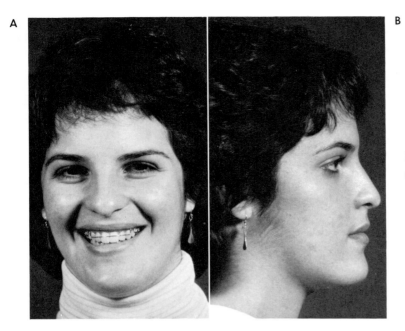

Fig. 14-60. A.S., age 19 years, 1 month, facial appearance 1 year postsurgery.

A B

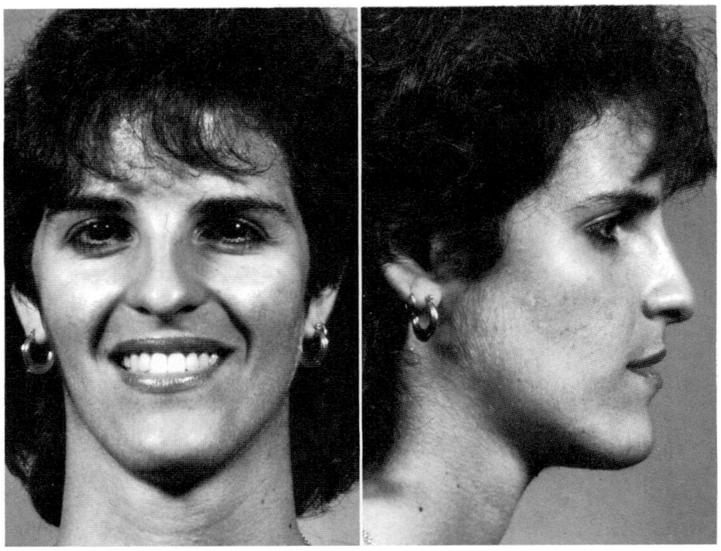

Fig. 14-61. A.S., age 23 years, 4 months, facial appearance at 5-year recall.

A B C

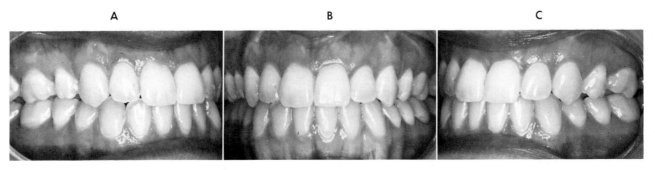

Fig. 14-62. A.S., age 23 years, 4 months, occlusal relationships at 5-year recall, nearly 3 years after retention was discontinued.

L.H. was first seen at age 39 years because of concern about his crooked teeth and the spaces between the maxillary incisors. A complete diagnostic evaluation revealed a symmetric facial appearance from the front, with the maxillary dental midline deviated 2 mm to the right of the midsagittal plane. In profile, components of midface deficiency as well as mandibular prognathism and an increased lower facial height were evident, along with a relatively short throat length and poorly defined throat form (Fig. 14-63). Cephalometric analysis documented significant anteroposterior and vertical maxillary deficiency while demonstrating relatively normal upper and lower incisor positions (Fig. 14-64). Dentally, there was considerable spacing in both arches, with the maxillary second premolars being congenitally absent (Fig. 15-65). A bilateral buccal crossbite became evident when the casts were repositioned to a normal overjet relationship.

After consultation with a prosthodontist it was decided to align the upper and lower anterior teeth but leave 1 to 2 mm of space between each tooth for future restorations. In the maxillary arch, a three-piece LeFort I osteotomy was planned to move the maxilla down and forward while simultaneously expanding to eliminate the crossbite. In preparation, premolars were to be retracted against the molars so as to provide space distal to the canines for the osteotomy cuts. In the mandible, a subapical procedure was planned to retract the anterior teeth into space that would be consolidated between the canines and first premolars. This combination of procedures met the objectives of increasing the patient's midface prominence while allowing for retraction of the

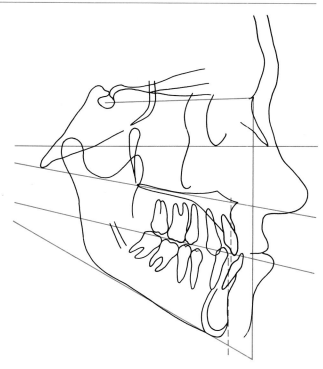

Fig. 14-64. L.H., initial cephalometric tracing. Note the maxillary deficiency and mandibular dental protrusion. Cephalometric measurements: N perp to A, −12 mm; N perp to Pg, −12 mm; AB difference, 0 mm; UFH, 59 mm; LFH, 71 mm; mand plane, 31 degrees; MxI to A vert, 3 mm, 15 degrees; MnI to B vert, 9 mm, 28 degrees.

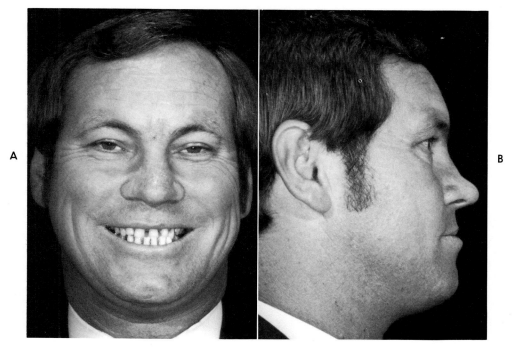

Fig. 14-63. L.H. A, Frontal and B, facial views, age 39 years, before treatment. (Courtesy of the Orthodontic Department, Baylor College of Dentistry.)

Continued.

Case 3—cont'd.

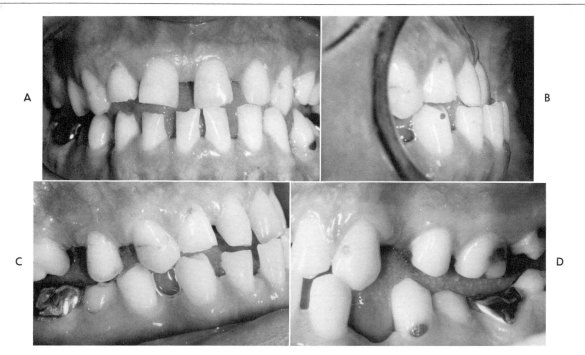

Fig. 14-65. L.H., age 39 years, occlusal relationships.

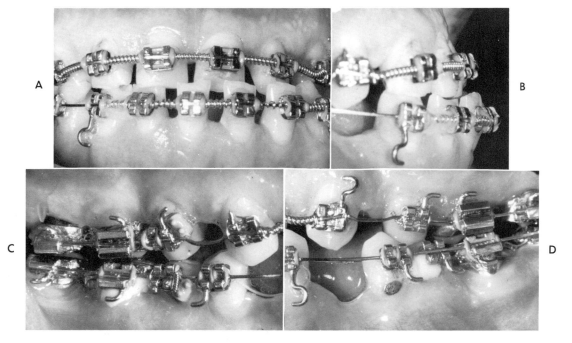

Fig. 14-66. L.H., age 40 years, 3 months, presurgical occlusal relationships.

Case 3—cont'd.

mandibular teeth without producing shortening of the patient's throat length.

After initial alignment with 17.5-mil twist arch wires followed by 16 and 18 stainless steel, 17×25 arch wires were placed to distribute space and provide anterior and buccal segment torque. Once the appropriate anterior spacing was achieved and approved by the prosthodontist, the arches were stabilized and the spaces maintained with passive segments of coil springs (Fig. 14-66). Presurgical orthodontic preparation took just over 1 year (Fig. 14-67).

At age 40, LeFort I osteotomy to position the maxilla forward (3 mm) and downward (4 mm) was carried out in three segments to allow for correction of the buccal crossbites. A mandibular canine-to-canine subapical procedure was used to retract the lower anterior segment (3 mm). After the maxilla had been freed and advanced, it was secured with four small bone plates, which were adapted to lie passively between the zygomatic buttress and the lateral aspect of the maxilla. Each plate was secured with two screws above and two screws below the osteotomy. Additional anteroposterior and vertical stability was achieved with the placement of blocks of porous hydroxylapatite at the "step-osteotomy" site in the zygomatic buttress as well as interpositionally superior to each of the three segments. Additional hydroxylapatite was placed between the segments in the palate to augment transverse stability (Fig. 14-68). The mandibular subapical segment was stabilized using two rigid fixation screws. The patient remained in maxillomandibular fixation for 48 hours, at which point he was discharged from hospital with the splint ligated to the upper arch and allowed to function into the splint.

Six weeks postsurgically, the splint was removed and 17×25 TMA arch wires were placed, along with light Class II box elastics that included all the maxillary segments. In the maxilla a 17×25 TMA wire was used for 5 months followed by a 17×25 stainless steel arch wire for 2 months before debanding. In the mandible a 17×25 stainless steel wire was inserted 1 month after surgery. After 7 months of postsurgical orthodontics to refine the buccal occlusion and detail the anterior spacing, appliances were removed and removable retainers placed within 24 hours of debanding. Facial appearance was considerably improved, with more harmonious facial proportions and a pleasant degree of incisor exposure at rest and upon smiling (Fig. 14-69). Considerable improvement in the occlusal (Fig. 14-70) and skeletal relationships were evident (Fig. 14-71).

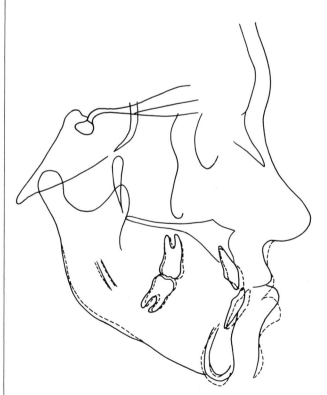

Fig. 14-67. L.H., initial to presurgical *(dashed black)* superimposition.

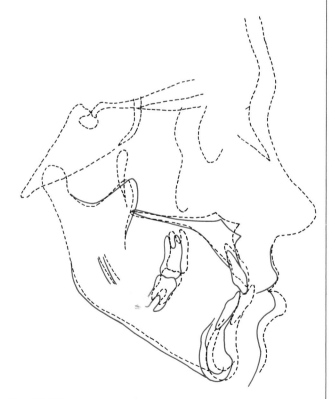

Fig. 14-68. L.H., presurgical to postsurgical *(solid red)* superimposition (40 years, 3 months, to 40 years, 6 months).

Continued.

Case 3—cont'd.

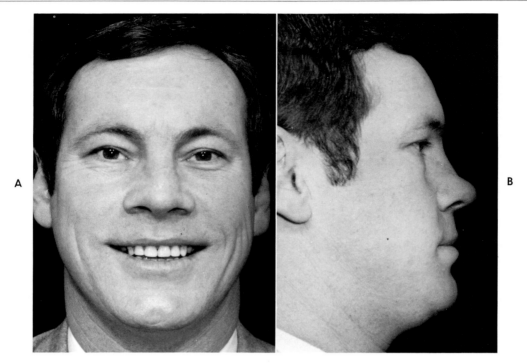

Fig. 14-69. L.H., age 40 years, 10 months, facial appearance at completion of treatment.

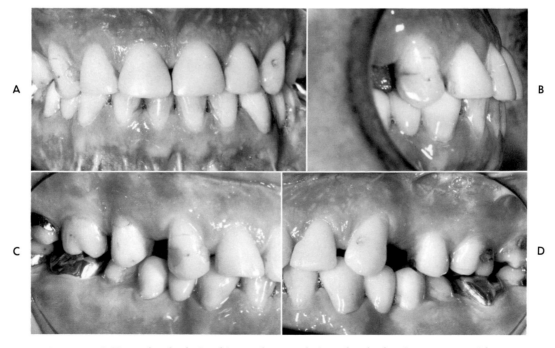

Fig. 14-70. L.H., occlusal relationships at the completion of orthodontic treatment with provisional restorations placed on the maxillary anterior teeth and the mandibular buccal segments.

Case 3 — cont'd.

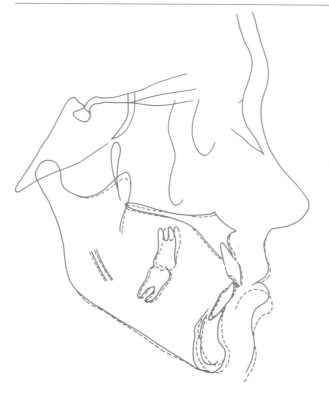

Fig. 14-71. L.H., cephalometric superimposition from postsurgery *(solid red)* to end of treatment *(dashed red)*.

Three years later, both the facial (Fig. 14-72) and skeletal changes appeared stable (Fig. 14-73) and the final restorations had been placed (Fig. 14-74).

Comments. This patient illustrates the importance of coordinated planning between the orthodontist, surgeon, and prosthodontist. With this combination of characteristics, maxillary surgery was obviously necessary, particularly as the patient's throat form precluded any significant mandibular setback. The mandibular subapical procedure was chosen as it offered the ability to improve the patient's apparent chin projection and contour while also closing some mandibular spacing and reducing the amount that the segmentalized and downgrafted maxilla would need to be advanced. The use of RIF in combination with interpositional hydroxylapatite grafts was deemed necessary to provide the maximum potential for stability in all three dimensions. (This case courtesy of the Department of Orthodontics, Baylor College of Dentistry.)

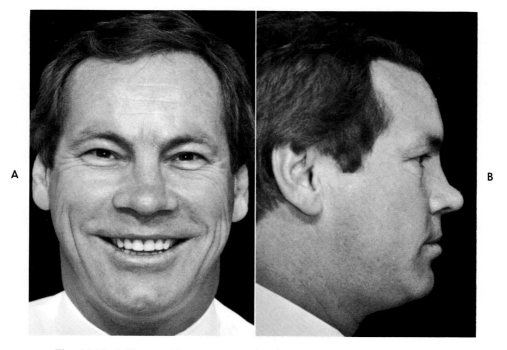

A   B

Fig. 14-72. L.H., age 43 years, 9 months, facial appearance at 3-year recall.

Continued.

Case 3—cont'd.

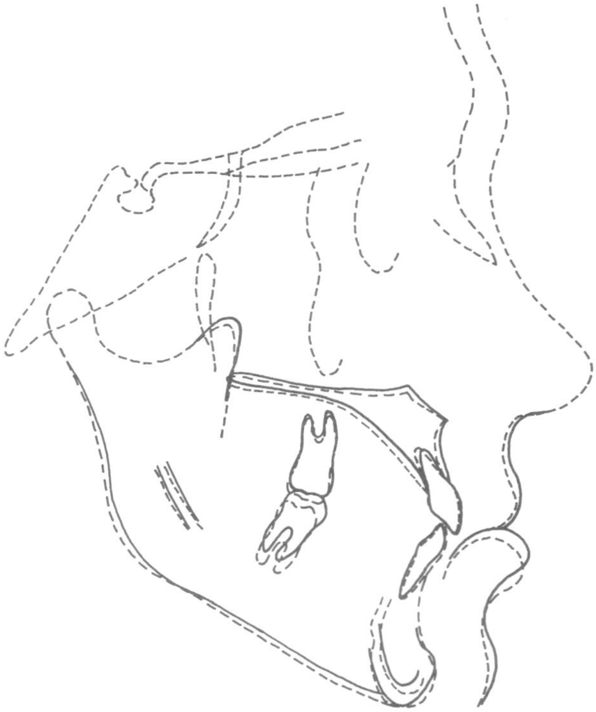

Fig. 14-73. L.H., superimposition from end of treatment, age 40 years, to 3-year recall, age 43 years, 9 months.

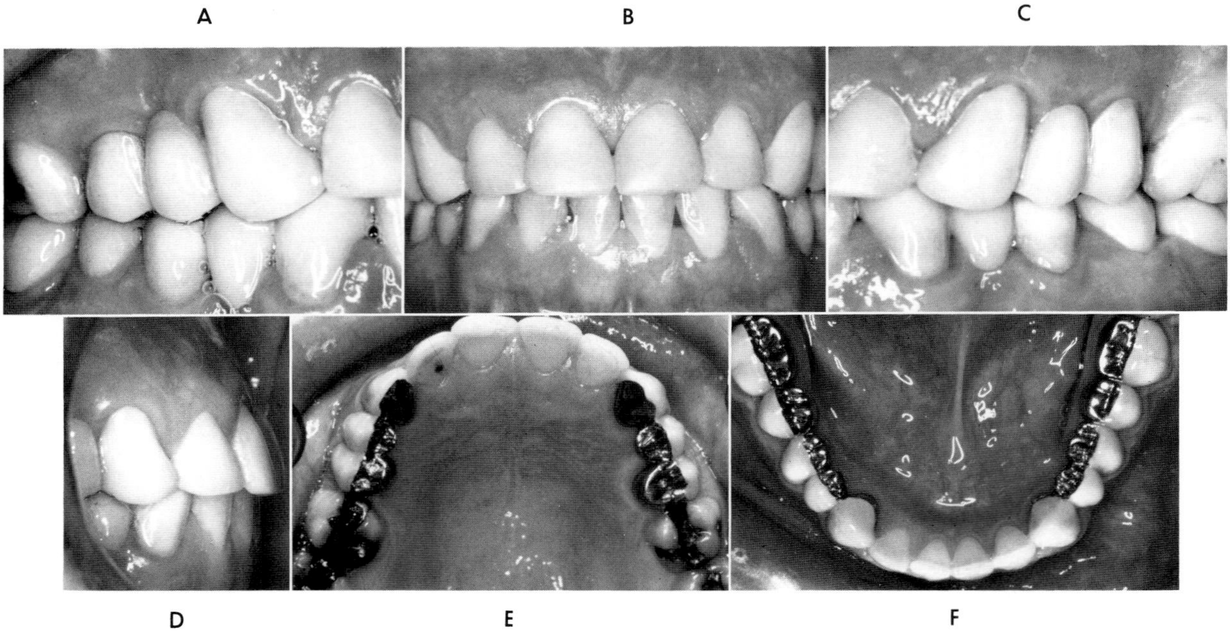

A   B   C

D   E   F

Fig. 14-74. L.H., occlusion at 3-year recall with restorative work completed.

REFERENCES

1. Angle EH: Treatment of malocclusion of the teeth, Philadelphia, 1907, SS White Dental Mfg. Co.
2. Ellis E, McNamara JA: Components of adult Class III malocclusion, J Oral Maxillofac Surg 42:295-305, 1984.
3. Harvold EP: Neuromuscular and morphological adaptation in experimentally induced oral respiration. In McNamara JA, editor: Naso-respiratory function and craniofacial growth. Monograph 9, Craniofacial Growth Series, Center for Human Growth and Development, Ann Arbor, 1979, University of Michigan.
4. Moss ML, Rankow RM: The role of the functional matrix in mandibular growth, Angle Orthod 38:95-103, 1968.
5. Proffit WR, Phillips C: The characteristics of patients seeking surgical-orthodontic treatment, Int J Adult Orthod Orthognath Surg [in press].
6. Hopkin GB, Houston WJB, James GA: The cranial base as an etiological factor in malocclusion, Angle Orthod 38:250-255, 1968.
7. Wylie W: The assessment of anteroposterior dysplasia, Angle Orthod 17:97-109, 1947.
8. Schulhof RJ, Nakamura S, Williamson WV: Prediction of abnormal growth in Class III malocclusions. Am J Orthod 71:421-430, 1977.
9. Turley P: Early management of the developing Class III malocclusion, Pacific Coast Soc Orthod Bull 60(4):32-36, 1988.
10. Bell RA: A review of maxillary expansion in relation to rate of expansion and patient's age, Am J Orthod 81:32-37, 1982.
11. Haas AJ: Palatal expansion: just the beginning of dentofacial orthopedics, Am J Orthod 57:219-255, 1970.
12. Frankel R: Maxillary retrusion in Class III and treatment with the function corrector III, Trans Eur Orthod Soc 46:249-259, 1970.
13. Delaire JP, Verdon J, Lumineau A, et al: Quelques resultats des tractions extra-orales a appui fronto-mentonier dans de tractment orthopedique des malformations maxillo mandibulaires de Class III et des sequelles osseuses des fente labio-maxillaires, Rev Stomatol Chir Maxillofac 73:633-642, 1972.
14. Petit H: Adaptations following accelerated facial-mask therapy. In McNamara JA, Jr, Ribbens KA, Howe RP, editors: Clinical alterations of the growing face. Monograph 14, Craniofacial Growth Series, Center for Human Growth and Development, Ann Arbor, 1983, University of Michighan.
15. Smalley WM, Shapiro PA, Hohl TH, et al: Osseointegrated titanium implants for maxillofacial protraction in monkeys, Am J Orthod 94:285-295, 1988.
16. Janzen EK, Bluher JA: The cephalometyric, anatomic and histologic changes in Macaca Mulatta after application of a continuous-acting retraction force on the mandibular, Am J Orthod 51:823-850, 1965.
17. Campbell PM: The dilemma of Class III treatment. Early of late? Angle Orthod 53:175-191, 1983.
18. Kokich V, Shapiro P: The effects of LeFort I osteotomies on the craniofacial growth of juvenile Macaca Nemestrina. In McNamara JA, Jr, Carlson DS, Ribbens KA, editors: The effect of surgical intervention on craniofacial growth. Monograph 12, Craniofacial Growth Series, Center for Human Growth and Development, Ann Arbor, 1982, University of Michigan.
19. Cisneros GJ, Kaban LB: Skeletal scintigraphy. A technique for analysis and prediction of growth and for monitoring effects of treatment on growth. In Bell WH, editor: Surgical correction of dentofacial deformities, vol 3, Philadelphia, 1985, WB Saunders Co.
20. Turley PK: Orthopedic correction of Class III malocclusion with palatal expansion and custom protraction headgear, J Clin Orthod 22(5):314-325, 1988.
21. Kiyak HA, McNeill RW, West RA: The emotional impact of orthognathic surgery and conventional orthodontics, Am J Orthod 88:224-234, 1985.
22. Kennedy BD: Suction assisted lipectomy of the face and neck, J Oral Maxillofac Surg 46:546-558, 1988.
23. Bell WH, Jacobs JD: Tridimensional planning for surgical/orthodontic treatment of mandibular excess, Am J Orthod 80:263-288, 1981.
24. Bell WH, Jacobs JD: Mandibular excess with vertical maxillary excess or deficiency. In Bell WH, editor: Surgical correction of dentofacial deformities, vol 3, Philadelphia, 1985, WB Saunders Co.
25. Jacobs JD, Sinclair PM: Principles of orthodontic mechanics in orthognathic surgery cases, Am J Orthod 84:399-407, 1983.
26. Woodworth DS, Sinclair PM, Alexander RG: Bilateral congenital absence of maxillary lateral incisors: a craniofacial and dental cast analysis, Am J Orthod 84:280-293, 1985.
27. Guymon M, Crosby DR, Wolford LM: The alar base cinch suture to control nasal width in maxillary osteotomies, Int J Adult Orthod Orthognath Surg 2:89-95, 1988.
28. Zins JE, Whitaker LA: Membranous vs. endochondral bone: implications for craniofacial reconstruction, Plast Reconstr Surg 72:778-784, 1983.
29. Epker BN, Fish LC: Dentofacial deformities: integrated orthodontic and surgical correction, St. Louis, 1986, The CV Mosby Co.
30. Wardrop RW, Wolford LM: Maxillary stability following downgraft and/or advancement procedures with stabilization using rigid fixation and porous block hydroxylapatite implants, J Oral Maxillofac Surg 47:326-342, 1989.
31. Phillips C, Zaytoun HS, Jr, Thomas PM, Terry BC: Skeletal alterations following TOVRO or BSSO procedures, Int J Adult Orthod Orthognath Surg 1:203-213, 1986.
32. Proffit WR, Phillips C, Patty SJ, et al: Stability after surgical-orthodontic correction of maxillary deficiency, Am J Orthod Dentofacial Orthop [pending].
33. Kinnebrew MC, Emison JW: Simultaneous maxillary and nasal reconstruction, J Craniomaxillofac Surg 15:312-325, 1987.

34. Rubens BC, West RA: Ptosis of the chin and lip incompetence: consequences of lost mentalis muscle support, J Oral Maxillofac Surg 47:359-366, 1989.

35. O'Ryan F, Schendel S: Nasal anatomy and maxillary surgery, Int J Adult Orthod Orthognath Surg 4:27-37, 75-84, 1989.

36. O'Ryan F, Schendel S, Carlotti A: Nasal anatomy and maxillary surgery. III. Surgical techniques for correction of nasal deformities in patients undergoing maxillary surgery, Int J Adult Orthod Orthognath Surg 4:157-174, 1989.

37. Turvey TA, Fonseca RJ: Management of soft tissues. In Bell WH, Proffit WP, White RP, editors: Surgical correction of dentofacial deformities, Philadelphia, 1980, WB Saunders Co.

38. Stecker FJ: Reduction cheiloplasty, Arch Otolaryngol Head Neck Surg 114:779-780, 1988.

39. Alexander RG: Countdown to retention, J Clin Orthod 211:526-527, 1987.

40. Steffen JM, Haltom FT: The five-cent tooth positioner, J Clin Orthod 21:528-529, 1987.

41. Zachrisson BU: Clinical experience with direct-bonded orthodontic retainers, Am J Orthod 71:440-448, 1977.

42. Egyedi P, Obwegeser H: Zur operativen Zungenverk-Leinerung, Deutsch Zahn Mund Kieferheilk 41:16-26, 1964.

43. Snow MD, Phillips C: Changes in head posture after orthognathic surgery, Int J Adult Orthod Orthognath Surg [pending].

44. Proffit WR, Phillips C: Adaptations in lip posture and pressure following orthognathic surgery, Am J Orthod Dentofacial Orthop 93:294-304, 1988.

45. Araujo A, Schendel SA, Wolford LM, et al: Total maxillary advancement with and without bone grafting, J Oral Surg 36:849-858, 1978.

46. Wessberg GA, Epker BN: Surgical inferior repositioning of the maxilla: treatment considerations and comprehensive management, Oral Surg 52:349-356, 1981.

47. Weiss MJ, Patty S, Phillips C: Dental and skeletal stability following maxillary advancement, J Dent Res 68:259, 1989 (abs 625).

48. Luyk NW, Ward-Booth RP: The stability of LeFort I advancement osteostomies using bone plates without bone grafts, J Oral Maxillofac Surg 13:250-253, 1985.

49. Bennett MA, Wolford LM: The maxillary step osteotomy and Steinmann pin stabilization, J Oral Maxillofac Surg 43:307-311, 1985.

50. Bays RA: Maxillary osteotomies utilizing the rigid adjustable pin (RAP) system: a review of 31 clinical cases, Int J Adult Orthod Orthognath Surg 1:275-279, 1986.

51. Kent JN, Zeide MF, Kay JF, et al: Hydroxylapatite blocks and particles as bone graft substitutes in orthognathic and reconstructive surgery, J Oral Maxillofac Surg 44:597-605, 1986.

52. Wolford LM, Wardrop RW, Hartog JM: Coralline porous hydroxylapatite as a bone graft substitute in orthognathic surgery, J Oral Maxillofac Surg 45:1034-1042, 1987.

53. Astrand P, Ridell A: Positional changes of the mandibular and the upper and lower teeth after oblique sliding osteotomy of the mandibvular rami, Scand J Plast Reconstr Hand Surg 7:120-129, 1973.

54. Rosenquist B, Rune B, Selvik G: Displacement of the mandible after removal of the intermaxillary fixation following oblique sliding osteotomy, J Maxillofac Surg 14:251-258, 1986.

55. Franco JE, van Sickels JE, Thrash WJ: Factors contributing to relapse in rigidly fixed mandibular setbacks, J Oral Maxillofac Surg 47:451-456, 1989.

56. Kobayashi T, Watanabe I, Ueda K, Nakajima T: Stability of the mandible after sagittal ramus osteotomy for correction of prognathism, J Oral Maxillofac Surg 44:693-697, 1986.

57. Komori E, Aigase K, Sugisaki M, Tanabe H: Skeletal fixation versus skeletal relapse, Am J Orthod Dentofacial Orthop 92:412-421, 1987.

58. Komori E, Aigase K, Sugiski M, Tanabe H: Cause of early skeletal relapse after mandibular setback, Am J Orthod Dentofacial Orthop 95:29-36, 1989.

59. Moser K, Freihofer HP: Long-term experience with simultaneous movement of the upper and lower jaw, J Maxillofac Surg 8:271-277, 1980.

60. LaBanc JP, Turvey T, Epker BN: Results following simultaneous mobilization of the maxilla and mandible for correction of dentofacial deformities: analysis of 100 consecutive patients, Oral Surg Oral Med Oral Pathol 54:607-612, 1982.

CHAPTER 15

Dentofacial Asymmetry

William R. Proffit
Timothy A. Turvey

Perfect facial symmetry is exceedingly rare. Mild degrees of left-right asymmetry in apparently symmetric faces can be demonstrated by special techniques—but most patients do not believe these are clinical problems (Fig. 15-1). Mild asymmetries within the dental arches also are a common finding and are accommodated by the patient without causing any particular difficulty in jaw function.

More severe asymmetries of the face and jaws, large enough to be easily noted on clinical examination, are found surprisingly frequently in patients with dentofacial deformity. In the large series of patients who were evaluated through the Dentofacial Clinic at the UNC in the 1980s,[1] 26% were noted to have an asymmetry in the position of the chin; 6% had a midface asymmetry involving only the nose, and an additional 2% had a midface asymmetry affecting both the nose and other structures; and 6% had asymmetries of both the middle and lower thirds of the face. The fact that an asymmetry is clinically present, of course, does not mean that it is of major importance to the patient. Often patients are not aware of what trained observers view as major asymmetry. On the other hand, when asymmetry is the patient's major concern, it takes on great significance, at least in part because patients can evaluate it themselves.

DIAGNOSTIC CHARACTERISTICS

The general approach to diagnosis and treatment planning is the same for patients with asymmetry as for those with other deformities. The only major difference is greater reliance on PA and other radiographs to obtain better three-dimensional information. Careful clinical examination of facial proportions in all three planes of space also is important. Because of the possibility that trauma was involved in the development of an asymmetry problem,[2,3] a careful history in this respect is needed. More often than not, a condylar fracture was not diagnosed at the time that it occurred, and indeed the trauma often has been all but forgotten.

Changes in the form of the mandibular condyles usually can be seen on the panoramic radiograph, but occasionally the diagnosis of an old condylar injury requires tomography. The presence of a clinically apparent asymmetry is the primary indication for obtaining a PA cephalogram in addition to the lateral cephalometric film.

The analysis of lateral and PA cephalometric radio-

A   B   C

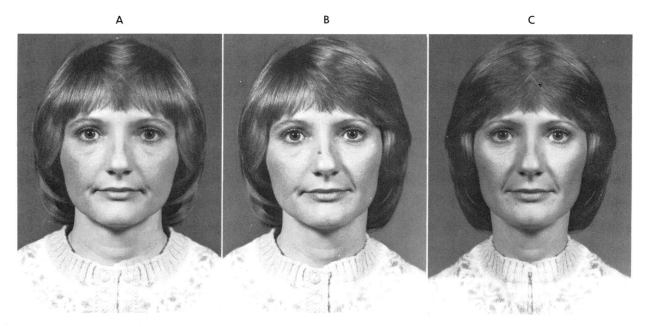

Fig. 15-1. All normal faces have a degree of asymmetry, which can be revealed most easily with a composite photograph of this type. The real face is in the center. On the left is a composite made of two left sides, and on the right a composite from the two right sides. (Reprinted with permission from Proffit WR: Contemporary orthodontics, St. Louis, 1986, The CV Mosby Co.)

graphs is discussed in detail in Chapter 4, and the application of the diagnostic and treatment planning process to a typical asymmetry problem is further illustrated in Figs. 15-2 to 15-7. The location of landmarks on PA cephalometric films is unreliable enough that small deviations may be concealed by tracing error— or minor deviations may appear to exist when in fact they do not. The PA film, therefore, is most useful to better define a problem when a rather specific area of deformity exists clinically. Sometimes, despite an obvious clinical appearance of asymmetry, the PA film does not clarify a precise location. Asymmetry, like other discrepancies, can be due to the combination of small deviations at multiple locations, and both radiographs and clinical findings are needed to define the problem.

In the lateral cephalometric film, vertical asymmetries often can be recognized by the failure of bilaterally symmetric structures to superimpose as they normally will, but of course this appearance also can be created by improper head positioning. In standard cephalometric technique, it is assumed that the ears are on the same vertical level when the patient is in natural head position—as they are unless an ear deformity accompanies the facial asymmetry, as often is the case in hemifacial microsomia. The ear rods of the cephalostat will line up the ear canals. So if the ear canals are not level with the patient in natural head position, the cephalometric radiograph must be taken without the use of ear rods. Otherwise, the head will be tilted and

the radiograph will be misleading. The target midsagittal-plane distance can be standardized when the ear rods are not used by having the patient look into his or her own eyes in a mirror, using the image of the chain that is mounted in the midline to bisect the face (see Chapter 4, Fig. 4-14).

A additional dimension can be added to the radiologic examination by taking a submental vertex film,[4] which is most useful when the mandibular ramus is severely deformed. It is possible to combine information from lateral, PA, and submental vertex films to allow a three-dimensional reconstruction of the mandibular ramus and, with less accuracy, parts of the maxilla. A three-dimensional reconstruction also can be obtained from stereometric pairs of radiographs,[5] coordinated lateral and PA films,[6] or computed tomography (CT) scans.[7] Although significantly more radiation is required, the multiple views available from CT scans make this a more versatile and generally preferred approach (see Case 1). This information tends to be more valuable for detailed surgical treatment planning than for diagnosis and is primarily indicated in patients who have missing or severely distorted skeletal areas because of congenital deformities or major trauma. For the patients with less severe developmental deformities who form the bulk of candidates for orthognathic surgery, neither a submental vertex film nor CT scan is necessary.

Orthognathic surgery for patients who are still grow-

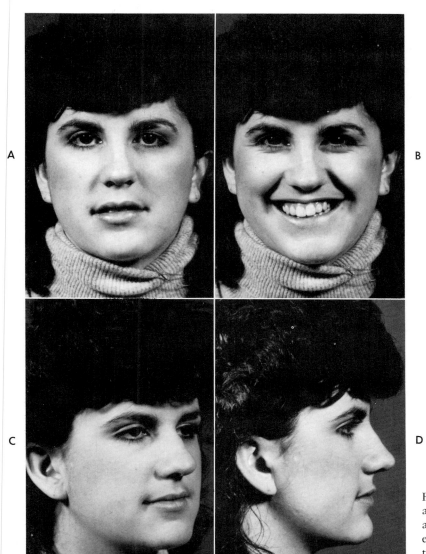

Fig. 15-2. M.B.B., age 19 years, 6 months, and a university student, was concerned about the asymmetry of her face and the lateral shift of her jaw. She had had orthodontic treatment between ages 13 and 15. Her history revealed a fall from horseback at age 12, with no serious injury diagnosed at that time.

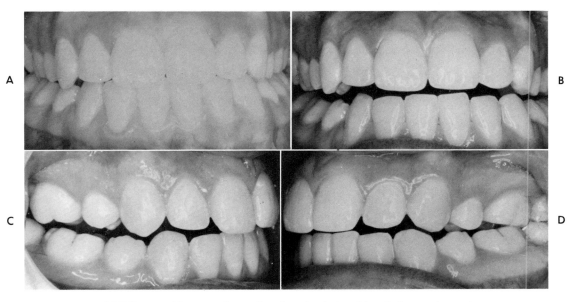

Fig. 15-3. M.B.B., age 19 years, 6 months, dental relationships **A,** in maximum intercuspation and **B-D,** at initial contact.

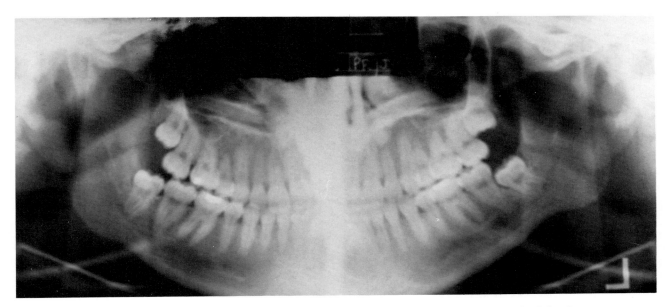

Fig. 15-4. M.B.B., panoramic radiograph. Note the small condylar process on the left, almost certainly the result of an old fracture.

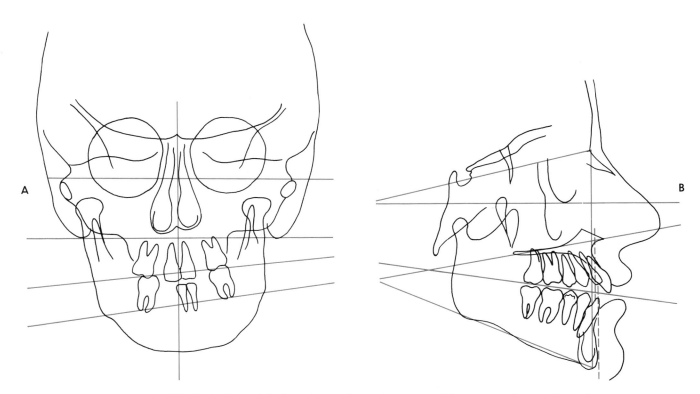

Fig. 15-5. M.B.B. **A,** PA and **B,** lateral cephalometric tracings. The cant to the maxilla and the shorter mandibular ramus on the left side can be clearly visualized. Her problems can be summarized as asymmetric mandibular deficiency due to a short ramus on the left side and a cant to the maxilla.

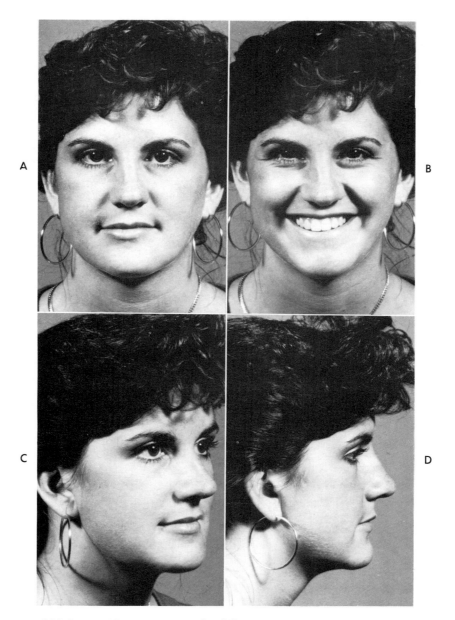

Fig. 15-6. M.B.B., age 19 years, 11 months, following LeFort I osteotomy to level the maxilla (more by elevating the right side than by elongating the left) and bilateral sagittal split osteotomy to advance the mandible on the left side. Because the teeth were well aligned initially, presurgical orthodontics required only 3 months, and appliances were removed 8 months after they were placed.

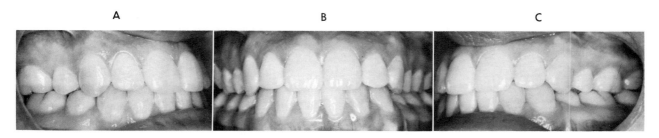

Fig. 15-7. M.B.B., age 19 years, 11 months, dental relationships after treatment.

ing rarely is necessary. But when it is, the major indication is severe and progressive asymmetry. In the discussion below, we describe the orthodontic and surgical-orthodontic approaches to asymmetry problems in preadolescent children, adolescents, and adults. Surgical intervention may be indicated in each of these age groups, not reserved for adults as in the previous clinical chapters. For that reason, case reports are at the end of each section instead of only at the end of the chapter.

ASYMMETRY IN PREADOLESCENT CHILDREN

In preadolescent children, two major problems cause severe dentofacial asymmetry: hemifacial microsomia and mandibular ankylosis due to fracture of the condylar process of the mandible. Their etiology is discussed in Chapter 2, along with other rarer causes of asymmetry. Here the focus will be on the detailed evaluation of affected patients and on the appropriate treatment procedures.

Both hemifacial microsomia and condylar fracture primarily affect the mandible, and both cause deficient growth on the affected side. In both cases, the maxilla is affected secondarily as deficient vertical growth of the mandible leads to distortion of the alveolar portion of the maxilla. However, there is a basic and important difference. In hemifacial microsomia both soft- and hard-tissue elements are missing, affecting growth potential. The magnitude of the effect depends more than anything else on how much tissue is missing. Condylar fracture may produce partial (functional) ankylosis that restricts what otherwise would have been normal growth. The effect will depend on the extent of soft-tissue scarring that restricts translation. The severe forms of both conditions are obvious, but it can be quite difficult to distinguish mild forms of hemifacial microsomia from mild functional ankylosis or to be sure that the asymmetry was not caused by some other unknown factor.

Whatever the cause of an asymmetry, the principle of treatment in growing children is, insofar as possible, to modify the expression of growth so that the child literally grows out of the deformity. That goal often cannot be reached, but it does clarify the role of early surgery: the major reason for early surgical intervention would be to improve the chances of subsequent favorable growth. At the very least surgery should be growth-neutral; that is, it should produce no deleterious effects on growth. This principle also places orthodontic growth-modification treatment in perspective: the affected patients will need continuing treatment to guide growth as long as a deviant growth pattern might continue, whether or not surgery is carried out at an early age.

Hemifacial Microsomia

Of all the causes of significant asymmetry, hemifacial microsomia is the most variable in its expression and therefore the most unpredictable in the possible response to growth modification.[8] In children with this deformity who are severely affected, reconstructive surgery at approximately age 5 often is suggested. This indeed may be the best approach if the deformity is severe enough. On the other hand, the possibility that a child with hemifacial microsomia will respond well to growth modification treatment, to the point of making some possible surgery unnecessary, argues for attempting growth modification first in all but the most severe cases.

There are two possible benefits from a period of functional appliance treatment at an early age.[9,10] First, to the extent that a favorable growth response occurs, the surgical result will be better than might otherwise have been the case. Second, the surgical reconstruction is almost entirely a reconstruction of the missing hard-tissue elements. In hemifacial microsomia the problem is that not only skeletal but also muscle and other soft-tissue elements are missing. With the stimulation provided by a functional appliance, it is possible to obtain some development of soft tissue or to at least stretch the soft tissues so that a better surgical field exists at the time surgery is carried out. In at least some mildly affected children, such favorable growth can be obtained that surgery ultimately is not necessary (Figs. 15-8 to 15-10).

Functional Appliances for Asymmetric Growth Modification

In the fabrication of a functional appliance for a child with asymmetry due to hemifacial microsomia or another cause, it is important to keep in mind that all three planes of space have become distorted. In the construction bite, it is necessary not only to bring the mandible forward and to the midline, but also to open vertically more on the affected side. This is accomplished most easily by having the bite wax soft on the unaffected side and harder on the affected side so that the ramus is torqued downward on the short side. More transverse expansion probably will be needed on one side than the other, requiring modification of the appliance design but not the construction bite.

One way to design any functional appliance is to consider it an assembly of component parts, selected from the considerable array of appliance possibilities.[11] All functional appliances reposition the mandible, so the appliance must include some component that guides the mandible to a new postural position. Other elements of the appliance control the eruption of teeth, shield the soft tissues from lip, cheek, or tongue pressures, and if desired produce orthodontic tooth movement.

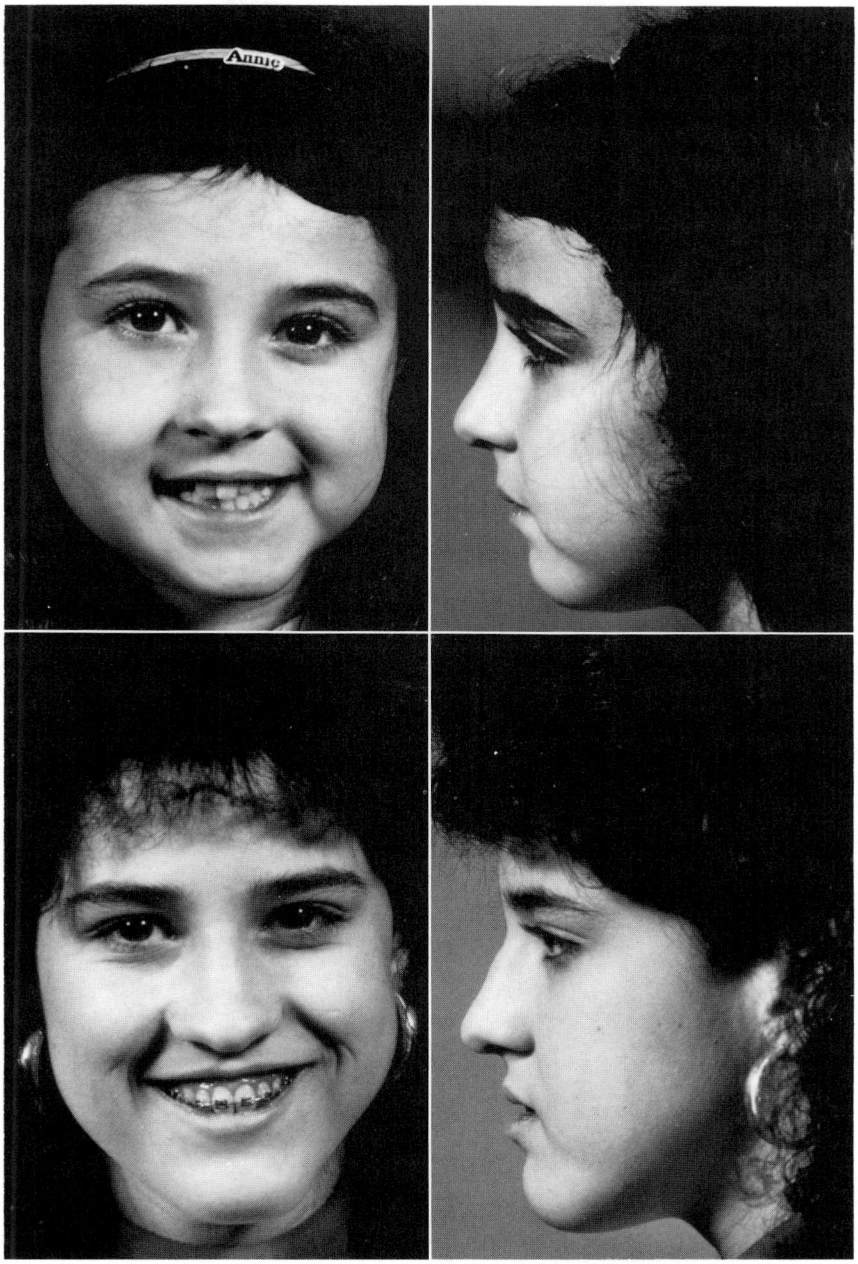

Fig. 15-8. M.B. had moderately severe hemifacial microsomia with underdevelopment of the left side of the face but a complete mandibular ramus and TM joint. **A** and **B,** age 8 years, 10 months, before beginning functional-appliance treatment (and after use of a fixed appliance for preliminary alignment of the maxillary teeth). **C** and **D,** Six years later, toward the end of orthodontics.

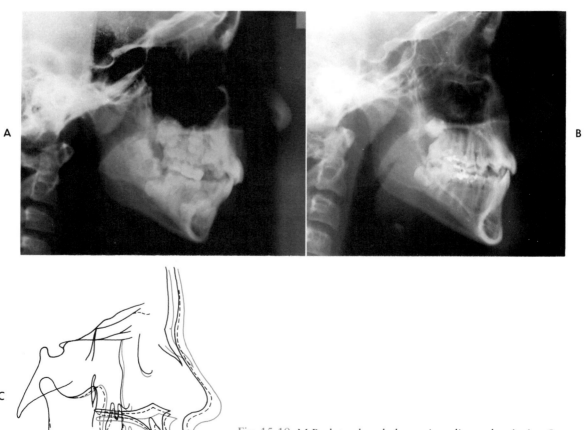

Fig. 15-9. M.B. **A,** Age 8 years, 10 months. **B,** Age 9 years, 2 months, after preliminary alignment of the incisors. **C,** Functional appliance in place. Bite blocks were used on the normal side, and the teeth were free to erupt on the deficient side. **D** and **E,** Fixed appliance used to elongate teeth on the deficient side. Note the bite block on the right side, creating a space into which the teeth can be erupted on the left.

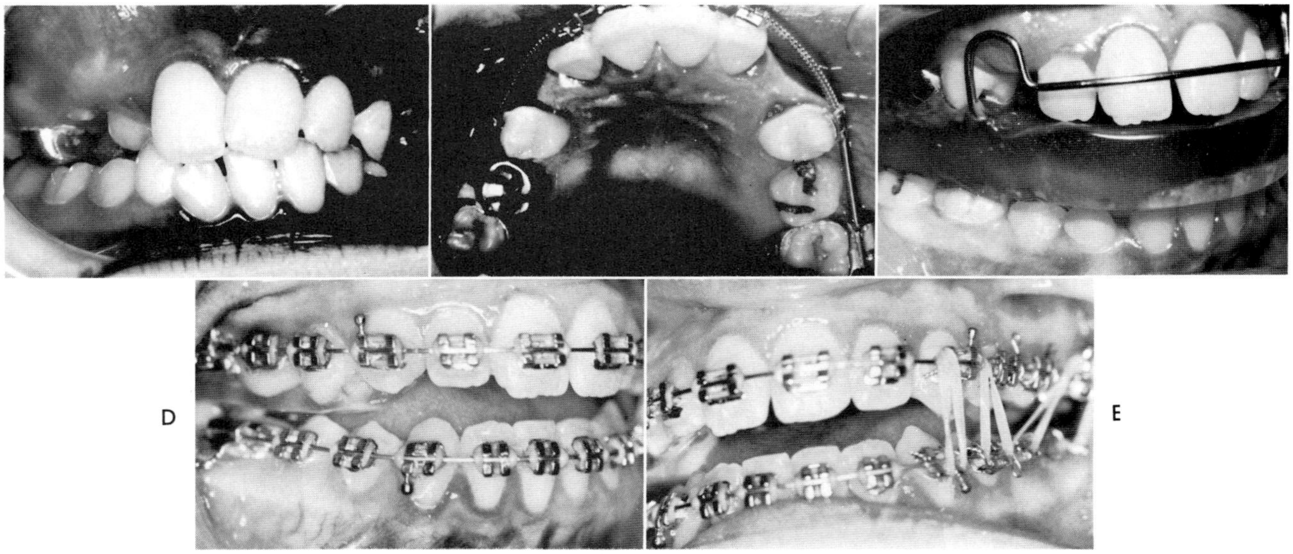

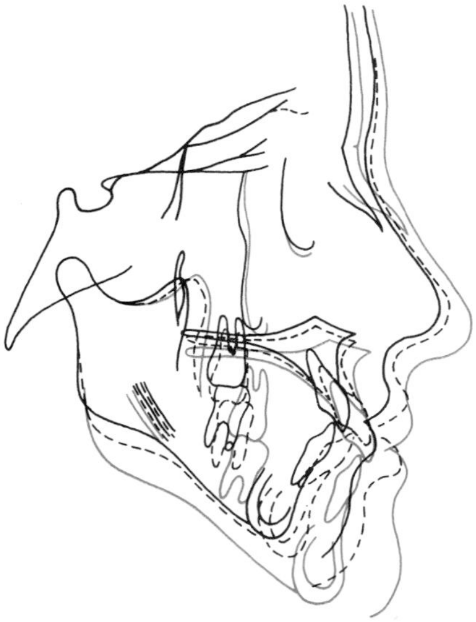

Fig. 15-10. M.B., lateral cephalometric radiographs. **A,** Age 8 years, 10 months, before treatment. **B,** Age 14 years, 5 months, orthodontic progress. **C,** Cephalometric superimposition age 8 years, 10 months *(black),* to 10 years, 6 months *(dashed black),* to 14 years, 5 months, toward the end of orthodontic treatment. She experienced such excellent growth that surgical treatment of the mandibular deficiency was not necessary.

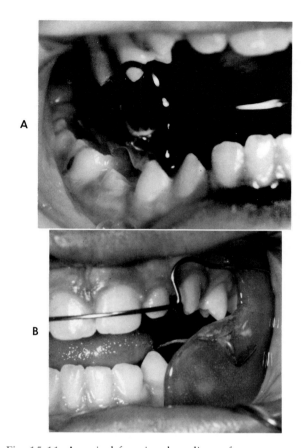

Fig. 15-11. A typical functional appliance for a severe asymmetry problem. Note the buccal and lingual shields on the affected side, where maximum development of the arch vertically and transversely is desired, and the bite block on the nonaffected side, where vertical development should be restrained to prevent canting of the maxilla. In the construction bite, the mandible is postured laterally as desired.

The "components" approach makes it much easier to design functional appliances for asymmetry patients.[12] The appliance will have to be different on the left and right sides, which simply means that different components are used on the two sides. The usual goal is to obtain as much growth as possible on the short side, facilitating tooth eruption there, while producing less growth on the normal side and impeding tooth eruption. A typical appliance to accomplish this is shown in Fig. 15-11. Note that the appliance incorporates a lingual pad to posture the mandible forward and to the more normal side, a lingual shield to keep the tongue out of the space between the teeth on the affected side, a Frankel-type buccal shield on the affected side to create transverse expansion, and a bite block to stabilize the occlusion on the more normal side, preventing eruption there. The teeth are free to erupt on the affected side. Wire elements connect these components. The design is adapted to the needs of a

specific patient. It can be modified by the addition or substitution of other component parts as needed for the problems of a particular patient.

The response to an appliance of this type will depend almost entirely on the patient's growth potential. Only if there is the potential for growth can a functional appliance guide it. In hemifacial microsomia, children who lack only a small amount of tissue are likely to respond well, whereas those who have major deficits in hard and soft tissues simply do not have the growth potential and are less likely to respond favorably. If there is doubt about the growth potential, attempting growth modification before the initial surgical reconstruction is the conservative approach and usually is a good idea. The more severe the deformity, and the more it appears to be getting worse rather than better with subsequent growth, the greater the indication for early surgical intervention. Obviously the success of presurgical functional-appliance therapy must be carefully monitored. It should be continued only as long as it is effective in producing skeletal change.

Surgery for Hemifacial Microsomia

The three stages of surgical intervention described by Converse[13] and reviewed more recently by Munro[14] and Kaban and colleagues[15] are a useful framework for discussing the treatment of hemifacial microsomia. In severely affected children, the initial surgery is at age 5 to 8 years. The goal is to replace missing skeletal elements and augment severely deficient areas to create a more favorable environment for subsequent growth of unaffected areas. At age 12 to 15, after the adolescent growth spurt, orthognathic concerns are addressed, with repositioning of both jaws as necessary. The third stage, in the late teens, is designed to enhance the contour of the skeleton and the soft tissues. The severity of the condition strongly influences both the timing and extent of surgery. By no means do all patients require all three stages of surgery, and treatment at the second and third stages is strongly influenced by the success of earlier surgery.

Initial Surgical Phase: Augmentation of Deficiencies. The missing tissue in a child with hemifacial microsomia produces transverse, vertical, and anteroposterior asymmetry, with vertical asymmetry dominant in most patients. The initial surgery is directed at augmenting deficiencies in both jaws, reconstructing missing skeletal elements, and improving three-dimensional symmetry.

If the patient has a ramus and condyle and is able to open and close the mandible, it is better to accept this articulation regardless of the joint morphology. Construction of a condyle and ramus should be reserved for grade 3 hemifacial microsomia, in which the proximal portion of the mandible is completely missing. Augmentation of a complete but severely deficient

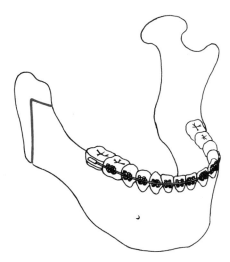

Fig. 15-12. Bony cuts in the mandibular ramus as they would be placed to allow three-dimensional correction for a hemifacial microsomia patient. An extraoral approach is needed.

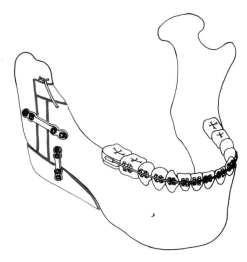

Fig. 15-13. After osteotomy in the mandibular ramus, the tooth-bearing portion of the mandible is advanced and lengthened as illustrated here. Defects in the ramus are filled with autogenous bone, and the segments are stabilized with small bone plates, screws, and wire sutures. Additional autogenous bone is added at the inferior border in the angle region.

mandible can be accomplished by an inverted L osteotomy via an extraoral approach, with the placement of grafts as appropriate (Figs. 15-12 and 15-13).

If the zygomatic arch is missing or severely deficient, one may be constructed at the initial stage. To accomplish zygoma reconstruction, both a hemicoronal incision and an incision in the maxillary mucobuccal fold are employed. In a subperiosteal plane, the dissections are made continuous to allow the bone graft to span the defect in the zygomatic arch and be securely anchored at both ends. After the jaws are stabilized and fixation is in place, skin and intraoral wounds are closed meticulously to minimize surgical scarring that might adversely affect jaw function.

A more complete discussion of reconstructive procedures at the initial stage of surgical treatment can be found in texts of facial plastic surgery.[16]

It is important for a child who has had early surgery for hemifacial microsomia to have functional appliance treatment in the immediate postsurgical period to control eruption of the teeth, minimize the tendency for canting of the maxilla to develop, and stimulate normal jaw function as much as possible. Parents and the patient must be educated on the importance of this follow-up therapy because failure to cooperate will diminish the benefit of the surgery.

Second Surgical Phase: Jaw Relationships. The second phase of surgical treatment, after the adolescent growth spurt, should address orthognathic concerns. Depending on growth, additional mandibular advancement, usually with vertical elongation of the affected ramus and the placement of a graft on that side, often is necessary. If vertical correction is not necessary but sagittal correction is, sagittal split osteotomies may be employed bilaterally.

The second stage of surgery also usually involves an asymmetric inferior border osteotomy to bring the chin to the midline, which improves both lip function and esthetics. Additional onlay bone grafting to the mandible or maxilla for contour purposes also is performed at this time if needed.

The more successful the first stage of surgery, the less the likelihood that maxillary surgery to level a canted maxilla will be required, but if a cant persists beyond age 15, a LeFort I osteotomy to correct it may be required.

Cephalometric prediction of the planned three-dimensional changes requires templates from both PA and lateral cephalometric radiographs, and visualization of the defects from computed tomography is helpful. The occlusal wafer splint constructed for surgery establishes a Class I occlusion and an open bite of at least 1 cm on the affected side.

The application of treatment of this type to a 12-year-old girl, who had had initial surgery at age 5 with limited success at that point, is illustrated in Figs. 15-14 to 15-17. The modification of orthognathic surgical techniques for a patient of this type is discussed and illustrated in more detail below.

Second-Stage Surgical Considerations. If additional elongation of the affected ramus is required, an extraoral approach is preferred, even though there is more risk to the facial nerve as compared with an intraoral approach. The extraoral approach also gives the surgeon better access for the extensive dissection

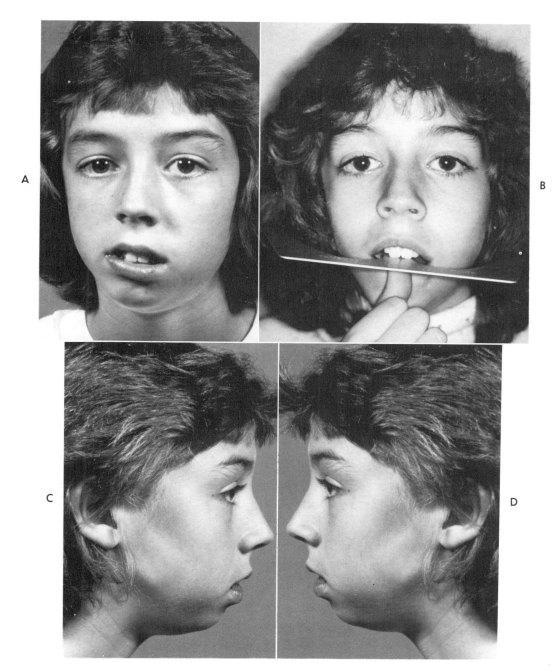

Fig. 15-14. C.R., age 12 years. **A-D,** Facial appearance on initial evaluation. **B,** Fox plane in place, demonstrating the cant to the occlusal plane.

needed to detach or stretch the tissue surrounding the mandible in order to minimize the residual soft-tissue tension. A natural skin fold low in the neck is selected to place the incision in the submandibular tissue so that when the ramus is elongated, the scar remains approximately 3 cm below the mandible. As the dissection deepens through the superficial layer of the deep cervical fascia, a hypoplastic masseter muscle usually is encountered, but occasionally the muscle is completely absent.

Once the inferior border of the mandibular ramus is identified, subperiosteal dissection of the ramus is conducted on both the lateral and medial surfaces. The normal anatomy of the ramus is always distorted. Occasionally, the inferior alveolar neurovascular bundle is observed entering the lateral cortex of the ramus. It should be preserved in all circumstances.

An inverted L osteotomy is usually made in the ramus, which allows the condyle and posterior border of the mandible to remain in place and the tooth-bearing

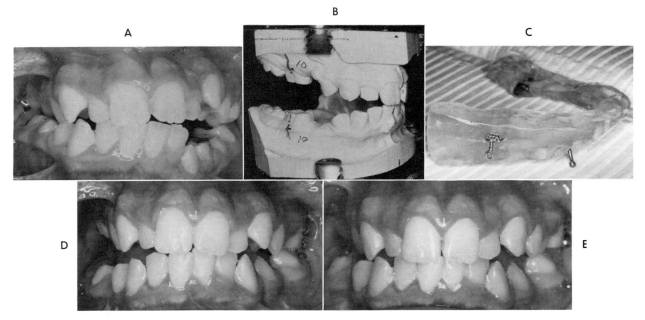

Fig. 15-15. C.R. **A**, Dental relationships at age 12 years, before treatment. **B**, Dental casts oriented at model surgery, showing the vertical elongation planned for the deficient right side. **C**, The surgical splint, which was worn for 6 months postsurgically, then progressively reduced on the right side to allow the teeth to erupt. **D**, Dental relationships postsurgically with the splint removed. **E**, Dental relationships 1 year postsurgically, at the point where the splint was discarded and fixed-appliance orthodontics begun.

segments to be repositioned (see Chapter 9). The horizontal arm of the osteotomy is made below the coronoid notch but above and posterior to the neurovascular bundle. If the coronoid process is well developed, an ostectomy should be performed to release the coronoid process and temporalis muscle. This minimizes the chance of the proximal segment becoming displaced during the postsurgical period.

A sagittal split osteotomy, as described in Chapter 9, is completed on the nonaffected side. This procedure may be carried out before or after the inverted L osteotomy. When the bilateral osteotomies have been completed, the mandible is repositioned and bone grafts harvested from the cranium or the ilium are inserted into the vertical and horizontal defects and secured with wires, bone plates, or screws. Maxillomandibular fixation including an occlusal wafer splint is applied and continued for 4 weeks while healing takes place.

Overcontouring the affected side with bone grafts helps camouflage some of the missing soft tissues. Onlay bone grafting usually is needed in both the zygoma and the body and ramus of the mandible. The donor site for this bone is usually the cranium or the ilium; rib grafts rarely are necessary at this stage.

At 4 weeks postsurgery, maxillomandibular fixation

is released and the patient is encouraged to function into the occlusal splint. It is critical for the patient to wear the occlusal splint continuously, removing it only for cleaning. This is easier if retention clasps are added to the splint. Over several weeks the mandible should return to the presurgical range of motion or improve beyond that level. Occasionally, physical therapy (active jaw exercises) may be required to assist the patient.

The occlusal splint is maintained in place for at least 6 months to retain as much of the ramus elongation as possible. Then the maxillary surface of the splint on the affected side is gradually relieved to allow the teeth to erupt. A fixed orthodontic appliance is needed to maintain control as the teeth are brought to their final position and the splint is eliminated.

If a cant to the maxilla is a prominent part of the problem, a LeFort I osteotomy, as described in Chapter 8, can be carried out simultaneously with bilateral osteotomies of the mandible. Leveling the maxilla is accomplished by a combination of shortening the normal side and lengthening the affected one.

Third Surgical Phase: Contour Modification. The third stage of surgery, in the late teens, is designed to enhance the contour of the skeleton and the soft tissues. If the other stages of surgery have been successful,

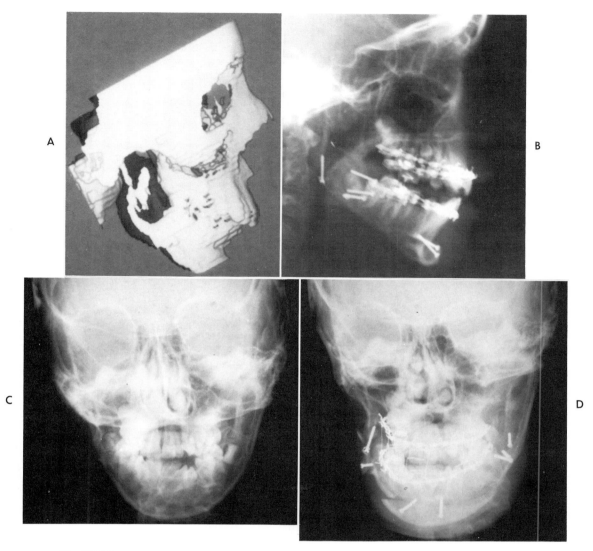

Fig. 15-16. C.R. **A,** Age 12 years, computed tomographic view of the right side before treatment. **B,** Lateral cephalometric radiograph after surgical reconstruction. **C** and **D,** PA cephalometric radiographs before and after surgery.

only minor or no changes are needed. If severe problems persist, major reconstructive surgery with placement of grafts in the zygomatic and/or mandibular ramus areas may be required (Fig. 15-18). Orthognathic surgery to reposition the jaws may be needed (see Case 1), but in most instances this has been accomplished earlier.

At this stage, soft-tissue augmentation is seldom necessary. If ear tags have not been removed or macrostomia has not been corrected previously, surgical correction is performed at this time. Occasionally, mandibular inferior border osteotomy or onlay bone grafts to augment deficient areas are planned to enhance the final result.

Ear reconstruction may be undertaken at the time of

any of the three surgical stages, but this decision depends on the degree of microtia. Because the ear may be concealed easily with hairstyling and because ear reconstruction usually requires multiple surgical procedures and distant transfer of skin or cartilage, it usually is considered less a priority than correcting defects of the more noticeable areas of the face.

Condylar Fractures: Asymmetry due to Trauma

The most frequent cause of mandibular asymmetry in children appears to be functional ankylosis secondary to trauma to the mandible at an early age.[2] Unilateral fracture of the condylar process is easy to produce with a blow to the anterior lower border of the mandible. This injury can occur readily as the result of a fall

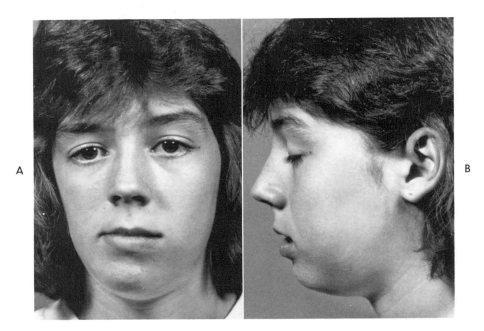

Fig. 15-17. C.R., age 13 years, 1 month, facial appearance 1 year following surgery.

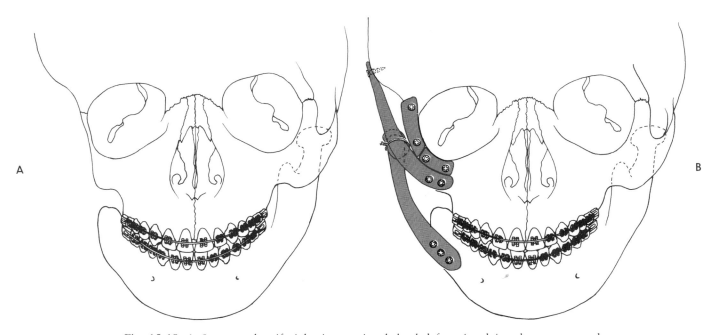

Fig. 15-18. **A,** In severe hemifacial microsomia, skeletal defects involving the zygoma and ramus may still be present in patients whose growth is essentially complete. **B,** At that stage, autogenous bone grafts stabilized with bone screws are employed to augment the deficient facial skeleton, as illustrated in this representation of reconstruction of the zygomatic arch and ramus.

or contact during sports and play. In most cases, the fractured condyle resorbs and a new ramus articulation forms.

At one time, it was thought that condylar fracture was a devastating injury because the growth center for the mandible would be lost. As has been discussed in some detail in Chapter 2, that is not correct. The condylar process regenerates,[17] and the child has a good chance of total recovery. Long-term follow-up data suggest that only about 25% of children who have an early condylar fracture will have some growth deficit on the affected side.[18] When growth restriction does occur, however, both jaws are affected. As the ramus grows more on the normal side, the chin deviates toward the affected side. Less tooth eruption takes place there. This distorts dentoalveolar development of the maxilla as well as the mandible so that a three-dimensional asymmetry affecting both jaws develops. The problem is caused by a relative lack of translation of the mandible on the affected side, which we have termed *functional ankylosis* because jaw movement and function occur but are impaired. The greater the degree of restricted motion, the more rapidly asymmetry develops and the more severe it will become as the child moves through periods of active growth.

Acute Management of Condylar Fractures in Children

Condylar fractures in children often are overlooked at the time of injury, and indeed the diagnosis can be difficult.[19] In one series, the condyle was involved in just over one-third of children who had mandibular fractures.[20] The diagnosis was missed initially in the majority of the children we have seen with asymmetry because of functional ankylosis. If only the more severe fractures are diagnosed, which seems reasonable, this may mean that the rate of recovery without subsequent growth problems is even higher than what has been reported previously.

When the diagnosis is made immediately after injury, a decision as to proper management at that time must be made. The principle of treatment is the one outlined initially: management of the patient should focus on obtaining the best possible growth subsequent to the injury. The practical question is whether surgery for open reduction of the fracture is indicated, and that relates to the importance of the condylar fragment. When the "growth center" at the head of the condyle was considered a very important part of the growth mechanism, its theoretic importance made it logical to try to maintain this special tissue in its proper position. Animal experiments and human data have shown quite clearly in recent years that the cartilage of the condyle is not necessary for normal growth (see Chapter 2). Instead, after an injury the condylar process remodels extensively and completely regenerates in the majority of patients. Open reduction, therefore, is not necessary to obtain normal growth after the injury. Because some scarring inevitably will accompany healing after any surgery, the effect of the surgical intervention can be some growth inhibition. In short, open reduction may do more harm than good. It should be avoided as a routine procedure for managing condylar fractures in children.

The recommended management for a child with a recent condylar fracture is immobilization of the jaw for

a few days, until initial soft-tissue healing can occur, followed by physiotherapy to maximize jaw movement and function into the previous occlusal relationships. If the child has difficulty coming into normal occlusion, a functional appliance to guide him or her to the proper position is indicated. The key to full recovery and normal growth is normal jaw movement and function and maintaining proper occlusion.

In rare circumstances the condylar segment can be displaced laterally or wedged between the ramus and temporal bone, preventing motion on the injured side. When this occurs, closed manipulation to free the segment should be attempted first. If this fails and mandibular motion is still restricted, an open approach must follow to free the mandible, removing the condylar head or repositioning it.[21] Postsurgical orthodontic management with a functional appliance is necessary for these patients.

Following condylar fracture with conservative management and return to function, the parents of the child should be advised that annual follow-up care is required until the child's growth is complete. The patient can be followed by a knowledgeable general dentist who can refer the patient to the orthodontist at the earliest sign of developing asymmetry.

Management of Posttraumatic Asymmetry

If an asymmetry develops following a condylar fracture, it occurs because there is more growth on the normal than on the affected side. The facial morphology of these patients can become very similar to those with a congenital problem. Indeed, it can be difficult in many instances to be certain whether an asymmetry is due to a partially healed old condylar fracture or to a mild expression of hemifacial microsomia (Figs. 15-19 to 15-21; see also Case 2). If the ramus is short and the condylar process distorted but the ear and adjacent soft tissues are normal, an old fracture usually is the problem, whether or not a diagnosis was made or specific trauma can be remembered.

Even though the diagnosis may remain in doubt, the decision as to whether surgery should be done at an early age or deferred until later can be based on definite criteria. The indication for early surgery is that the deformity is progressive (i.e., it is steadily getting worse), presumably because of functional ankylosis at the TM joint. Whether the problem is progressive can be determined with certainty by observing the child over time, but it can be estimated immediately by observing how far the child can translate the mandible forward on the affected side. If he or she can move the mandible forward reasonably freely, growth is theoretically possible and quite likely to occur. If the mandible cannot be translated forward, there is no hope for normal growth, a progressive deformity can be presumed, and early surgery should be considered.

A   B   C

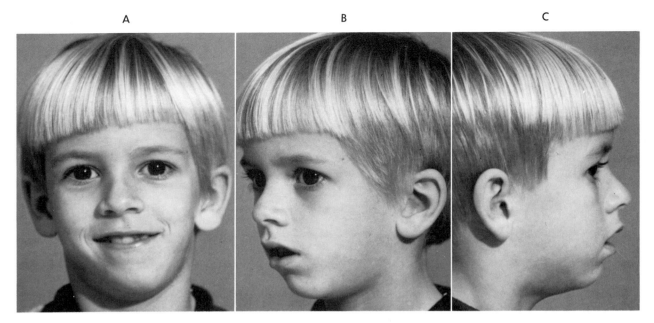

Fig. 15-19. R.S., age 8 years, was referred from a nearby military base because of their concern about his facial asymmetry. He had been evaluated at another base at age 5 because the mother had noted his chin deviating to the left, and malformation of the left condyle was noted. Additional radiographs taken there 2 years later were reported to indicate that the asymmetry was less marked and that bilateral growth had occurred. The medical history revealed only the usual childhood illnesses. There was no record of specific trauma, and no other congenital malformations were present.

A   B   C

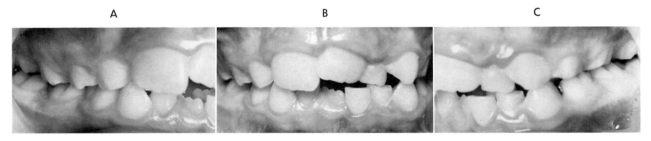

Fig. 15-20. R.S., age 8 years, dental relationships. The dental arches showed severe crowding but only mild asymmetry. On clinical examination, he deviated slightly to the left on closure. There was a mild cant to the maxillary dental arch. He had normal opening, and both condyles moved well, except that right lateral excursion was limited, indicating lack of lateral pterygoid function on that side.

To put it simply, in a child with an old fracture and asymmetry, if it is possible to bring the mandible to a normal symmetric position in the midline without undue strain, so that the construction bite for a functional appliance can be taken, treatment of this type should be attempted before any surgery (Figs. 15-22 to 15-25). If it is not possible for the child to bring the jaw to a position in which the asymmetry has been corrected, growth modification alone cannot succeed. The questions then are the timing and type of surgery.

The timing of surgery is intimately related to the choice of surgical procedure, specifically the decision as to whether the surgery should involve the damaged TM joint. Only by entering the TM joint can the surgeon hope to release ankylosis and provide for jaw movement and growth in the future. On the other hand, surgical intervention in the TM joint may lead to a decrease in the existing joint function, further compromising rather than improving long-term growth.

A more conservative type of surgical intervention would be a ramus osteotomy to bring the mandible to its approximately normal position, accepting the existing limited joint function. The initial surgery probably would be delayed until there was no other way to con-

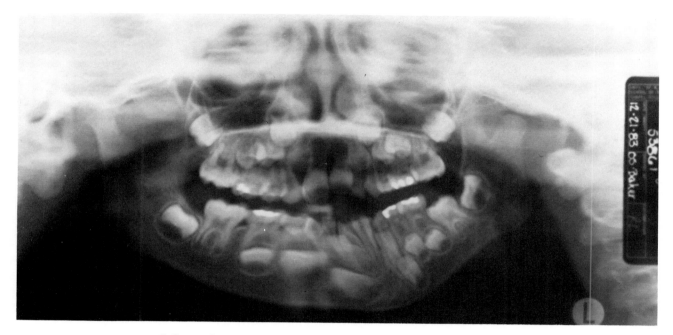

Fig. 15-21. R.S., age 8 years, panoramic film. Note the blunted condylar process on the left, almost certainly indicative of an old condylar fracture with partial healing.

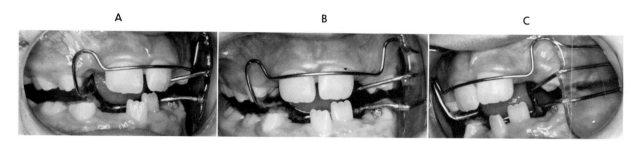

Fig. 15-22. R.S., age 8 years, 4 months. Because of the normal or near-normal jaw movements, he appeared to have reasonable growth potential. A hybrid functional appliance was placed, opening the bite on the left side and bringing the chin about 75% of the way to the midline (see Fig. 15-11 for a view of a similiar appliance with the mouth open). He wore this full-time and responded well; 5 months later a second appliance was made, further correcting the asymmetry.

trol the secondary canting of the maxilla that occurs when there is deficient vertical growth. The treatment would then be quite similar to the first stage of surgery for hemifacial microsomia, creating a vertical space between the teeth postsurgically on the affected side (see Fig. 15-15 and Case 2). This surgery can produce a significant improvement in the facial asymmetry, but of course as subsequent growth occurs the asymmetry will tend to recur because growth still will be restricted on the affected side, and a second surgical procedure later may be required. The timing of the second surgery would depend on the severity of the facial asymmetry and the child's reaction to it.

If surgical intervention in the TM joint is decided on,

there is no reason to delay. Release of the ankylosis to provide free movement involves removing soft tissue and bone within the joint. Removing bone that has been proliferated in the joint and excessive scar tissue can be technically difficult. Often the coronoid process must also be released, and in that circumstance it is better to remove it. Physical therapy following surgery is mandatory to maintain the degree of jaw motion attained at surgery. Getting compliance from the patient, who must perform regular jaw exercises over a period of months to years, is the most difficult task of all. If jaw motion is not maintained following joint surgery, additional surgery may be required to free the affected joint again.

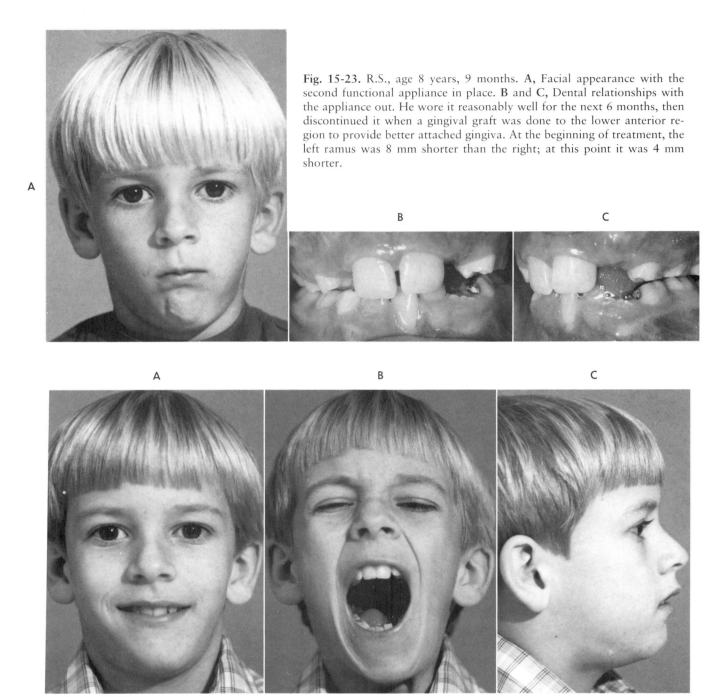

Fig. 15-23. R.S., age 8 years, 9 months. **A,** Facial appearance with the second functional appliance in place. **B** and **C,** Dental relationships with the appliance out. He wore it reasonably well for the next 6 months, then discontinued it when a gingival graft was done to the lower anterior region to provide better attached gingiva. At the beginning of treatment, the left ramus was 8 mm shorter than the right; at this point it was 4 mm shorter.

Fig. 15-24. R.S., age 12 years, 1 month, facial appearance, nearly 2 years after functional-appliance treatment was discontinued. Note the normal opening without deviation, which suggests continued normal growth.

Reconstruction of the damaged condylar process may be necessary if joint anatomy is obliterated. This may involve a costochondral junction graft,[22,23] chondroosseous iliac crest graft,[24] or perhaps a graft from another joint.[25] By far the greatest experience is with costochondral transplants. Generally good but variable results have been reported.[26-28] In young children, the data suggest that there is about a 50% chance of normal postsurgical growth when a costochondral junction transplant is done at an early age—which means that there is about a 50% chance of a poor response (due either to deficient or excessive growth) that would make further surgery necessary. Whether to accept these odds, or to use an approach that only frees up the

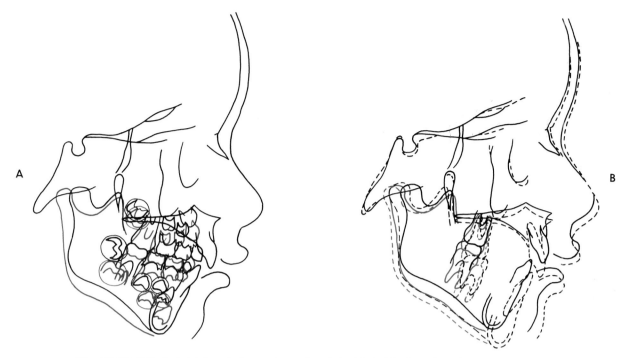

Fig. 15-25. R.S. **A,** Initial cephalometric tracing, left side in black, right side in red. **B,** Cephalometric superimposition (left sides) ages 8 years, 4 months, to 12 years, 1 month, showing the normal downward and forward pattern of growth over this period.

joint, must be a matter of individual surgical judgment. The specific patients are so different that general guidelines are difficult to formulate, but as a rule, good postsurgical growth is most likely when there is not extensive scarring in the vicinity of the TM joint already and when there is only a modest soft-tissue deficit (rather than the major loss of muscular and connective tissue elements in addition to bone that occurs in severe hemifacial microsomia).

When early surgical intervention is necessary, functional appliance treatment to guide subsequent growth almost always is needed. This should be instituted as soon as possible after the surgery to stretch the soft tissues and control any limitations on movements and growth that might occur during healing (see Cases 2 and 3). The design of the appliance, as with presurgical treatment, would be customized to the needs of each patient, along the lines described above.

Surgical Considerations in TM Joint Reconstruction in Children

As we have described above, surgical reconstruction of the TM joint may be necessary in children with both hemifacial microsomia and functional ankylosis. The possibilities are to use local tissue such as the stump of the remaining ramus or to employ a costochondral graft. If it is possible to use local tissue, this is the more conservative approach. A severe deficiency in local tis-

sue, as in grade 3 hemifacial microsomia or a severely damaged condyle, is the indication for a costochondral graft.

When the cartilage of the mandibular condyle was considered an important center for mandibular growth, it was logical to include cartilage in the graft material for a child to provide the missing growth potential. In the modern concept, all that is necessary for growth is normal translation, allowing the graft to grow. The cartilaginous cap is valuable primarily to minimize the potential for bony fusion of the mandible to the temporal bone. If cartilage is not used in reconstruction, it is necessary to have either an intact TM joint meniscus or a layer of some inert material (e.g., a silastic sheet) over the remaining bone of the condylar neck and ramus. From this perspective, particularly in a young child with missing or damaged joint structures, cartilage may be the material of choice.

Unfortunately, in children the graft sometimes behaves as if it does have growth potential independent of the mandible or its investing tissues. Excessive and uncontrollable growth is one of the major problems with costochondral grafting during childhood (see Case 2), particularly in the trauma patients with normal growth potential. Because of the unpredictable growth, adolescents and adults may be better candidates for costochondral grafts than children. Despite these potential difficulties, there is no alternative to costochon-

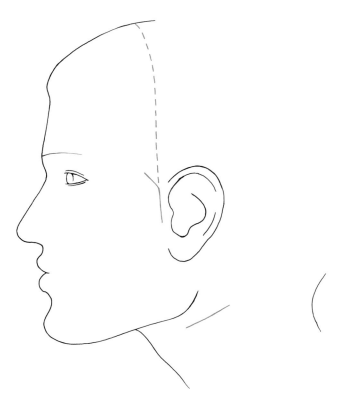

Fig. 15-26. Hemicoronal incision for reconstruction of the zygoma and TM joint.

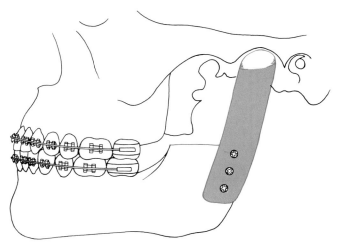

Fig. 15-27. Autogenous costochondral graft secured with bone screws to reconstruct the TM joint.

dral grafting in some severe problems in children.

When costochondral grafting is indicated, placement usually requires both a preauricular and submandibular incision. Greater access can be obtained through a hemicoronal incision if reconstruction of the zygoma or glenoid fossa is also necessary (Fig. 15-26). Normally the seventh, eighth, or ninth ribs are long enough to be utilized for graft material. If two ribs are needed, they can be harvested adjacent to each other. If more than two ribs are necessary, it is wisest to harvest two adjacent ribs, skip a rib, and harvest the next one inferiorly. This pattern prevents flail chest or paradoxical respiratory efforts.

When placing the costochondral graft it is important to carve the cartilaginous portion to fit in the glenoid fossa at rest and during function (Fig. 15-27). In severe hemifacial microsomia the glenoid fossa is absent and the graft must be carved to rest against the skull base. Some surgeons advocate fabricating a fossa from an additional cartilage graft. If this is done, the cartilaginous fossa must be secured to the base of the skull with either a wire or a screw (see Case 1).

Orienting the graft to both fit in the fossa and connect to the remaining ramus raises another surgical detail. Adding bulk to the deficient side is a goal of surgery with hemifacial microsomia. This can be accomplished by placing the graft so it overlaps the ramus laterally, which not only adds bulk but also permits the graft to be secured with several screws on the lateral side of the remaining ramus. When adding bulk to the face is not a goal of surgery, the graft may be turned 90 degrees and secured to the posterior border of the ramus with several screws. Sometimes decorticating the graft is necessary to mortice it to the remaining ramus, thus permitting the condyle to rest passively against the skull base.

Case 1

S.F., a 20-year-old woman with grade 3 hemifacial microsomia, had undergone multiple reconstructive surgical procedures previously at another insitution. These included two iliac bone grafts, augmentation genioplasty, and an abdominal fat graft to the affected side of the face. Additionally, extensive orthodontics had been performed. Her concerns focused on facial asymmetry (Fig. 15-28) and her lack of mandibular function. Although her teeth were well aligned, it was necessary for her to posture her mandible anteriorly and laterally to achieve occlusal contact (Fig. 15-29).

On clinical examination, the lack of soft tissue and muscular development on the right side of the face were apparent. Because the condyle and ramus as well as the

muscles of mastication were missing on the right side, the mandible deviated to the right on opening and protrusion, and left excursive movement was minimal. Her face animated well and there was no cant of the occlusal plane. The profile was convex. When the mandible was guided into maximum occlusal contact, her occlusion was adequate.

Three-dimensional CT images (Fig. 15-30) revealed absence of the zygoma, mandibular condyles, and ramus on the right side and hypoplasia of the orbit on that side. Previous attempts to reconstruct the mandible were evident: bone segments extended from the body of the mandible on the right. Resorption of the mandibular symphysis where a previous inferior border osteot-

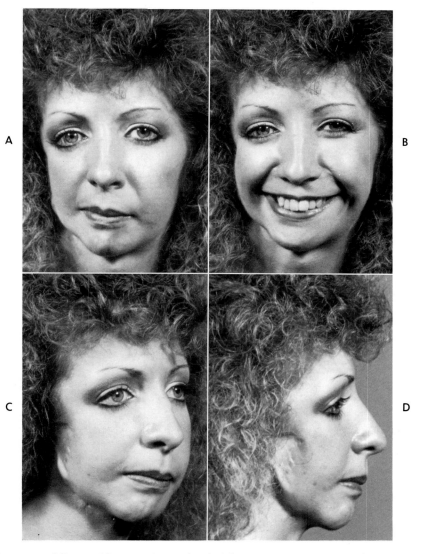

Fig. 15-28. S.F., age 20 years, 3 months, facial appearance at our initial evaluation.

Continued.

Case 1—cont'd.

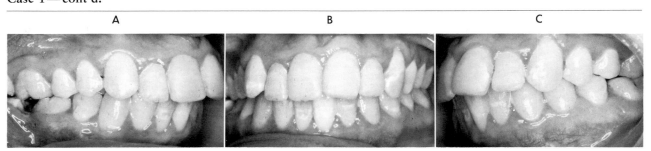

Fig. 15-29. S.F., age 20 years, 3 months, dental relationships. Previous orthodontic treatment had produced reasonable occlusal relationships.

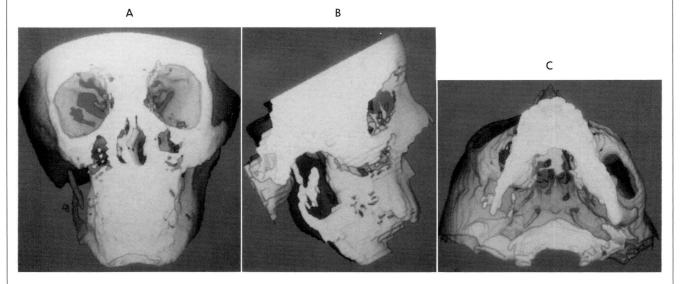

Fig. 15-30. S.F., skeletal morphology reconstructed from computed tomography. **A,** Frontal view. **B,** Right lateral. **C,** Submental vertex.

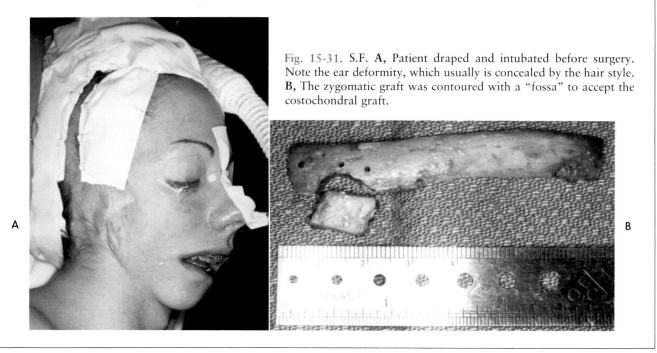

Fig. 15-31. S.F. **A,** Patient draped and intubated before surgery. Note the ear deformity, which usually is concealed by the hair style. **B,** The zygomatic graft was contoured with a "fossa" to accept the costochondral graft.

Case 1—cont'd.

omy had been performed also was noted. The patient's previous surgery had been successful in eliminating the canted maxilla and providing bulk to the right side of the face. Resorption of the chin, which is unusual after an inferior border osteotomy, probably occurred because of the severe soft-tissue limitation or because the soft-tissue pedicle left to perfuse the mobilized segment was inadequate. Because the ramus and condyle were never adequately reconstructed, the mandible had no articulation on the right side.

Before surgery, fixed orthodontic appliances were placed on both dental arches and the incisor teeth were repositioned to make the arches compatible with the canines in Class I occlusion. The surgery included construction of a zygomatic arch and glenoid fossa on the right: the ear, which was well covered by the patient's hair, was not reconstructed (Fig. 15-31). A costochondral composite graft was harvested to construct a ramus and condyle, and the fossa was lined with cartilage. The chondral portion of the rib was placed against the cartilage lining the fossa and attached to the remaining mandible laterally. To provide further bulk to the face, additional bone was harvested from the cranium and onlayed to the right body of the mandible. An inferior border osteotomy also was performed (Fig. 15-32). Hemicoronal, submandibular, and intraoral incisions were utilized for access.

Maxillomandibular fixation was placed at surgery and maintained for 6 weeks. At that point, vigorous physical therapy was employed to restore mandibular opening and range of movement. Light working arch wires and box elastics were used to settle the teeth into occlusion, and the orthodontic appliances were removed 6 months postsurgically (Fig. 15-33). Facial proportions were significantly improved (Fig. 15-34).

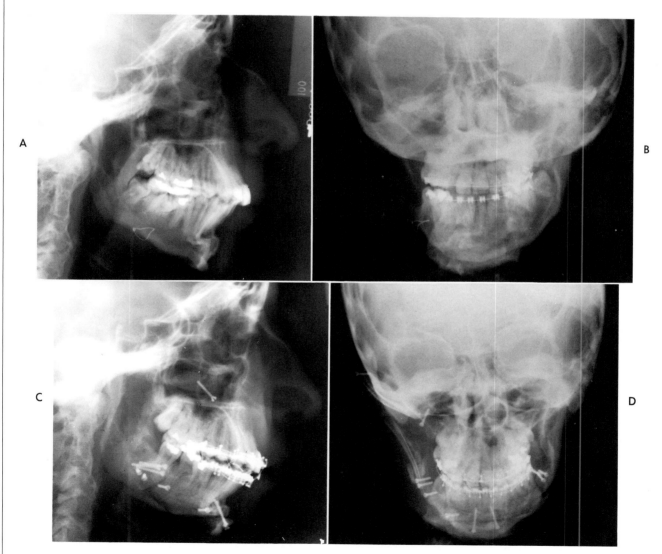

Fig. 15-32. S.F. **A**, Presurgical lateral and **B**, PA cephalometric radiographs. **C**, Postsurgical lateral and **D**, PA cephalometric radiographs.

Continued.

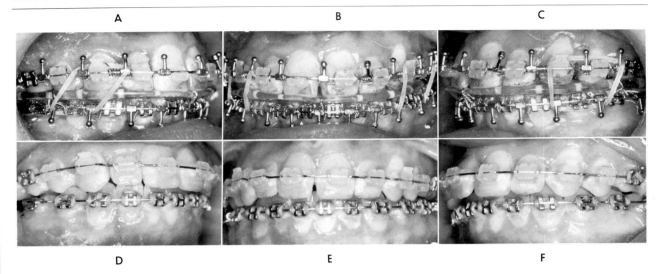

Fig. 15-33. S.F., dental relationships postsurgically. **A-C,** Functioning into the splint. **D-F,** Six months postsurgically, during the finishing orthodontics.

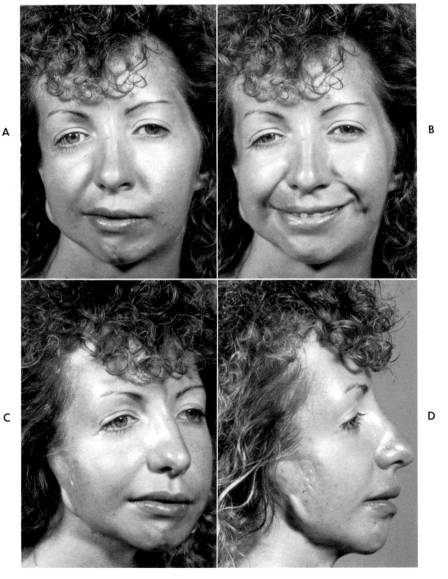

Fig. 15-34. S.F., age 23 years, 2 months, 1 year postsurgically.

Case 2

M.P. was first seen at age 8 years, 10 months, on referral from his pediatrician, who noted a facial and dental asymmetry and felt that this had developed recently, or at least was much greater now than previously (Figs. 15-35 and 15-36). On radiographs, the left ramus was shorter than the right but appeared normal (Fig. 15-37), with no evidence of an old condylar fracture. A cant to the maxilla was present (Fig. 15-38, *A*). The parents thought that an asymmetry had been present for a long time and produced a photograph from age 4 that seemed to confirm this (Fig. 15-38, *B*). The medical history was unremarkable, no congenital defects had been noted, and there was no history of trauma. Despite the absence of any ear malformations, a diagnosis of hemifacial microsomia was made, and functional appliance treatment to evaluate the possible growth response before surgery was planned.

He was assigned to the orthodontic clinic for treatment. At age 9 years, 5 months, it proved impossible to take the desired construction bite for a functional appliance. At that point, ankylosis due to an old fracture was suspected, and a series of tomographic views of the mandibular condyles demonstrated an old and partially healed fracture on the left side (Fig. 15-39). The asymmetry had become noticeably worse since the original evaluation (Fig. 15-40). On further questioning, the family still failed to remember specific trauma. They suggested that he might have been struck by a babysitter at age 2 years, 3 months, or perhaps had fallen at age 5. Because of the progressive nature of the deformity, surgery to release the ankylosis at the left condyle was planned, with reconstruction of the damaged condyle with a costochondral graft.

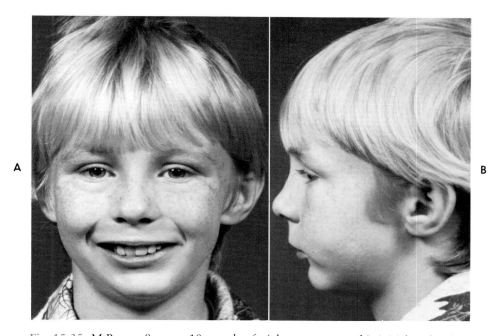

Fig. 15-35. M.P., age 8 years, 10 months, facial appearance at his initial evaluation.

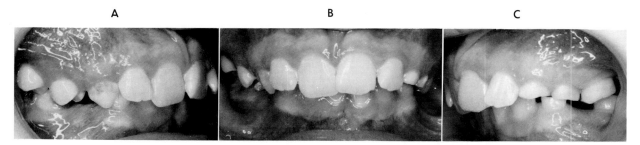

Fig. 15-36. M.P., age 8 years, 10 months, initial dental relationships. Note the tendency toward buccal crossbite on the right side, which often accompanies a deviation of the mandible to the left.

Continued.

At age 9 years, 9 months, the condyle was exposed through a preauricular incision and the damaged condylar head and neck were resected. A portion of an autogenous rib was harvested, and through a submandibular incision, a costochondral graft replacing the condyle process was placed (Fig. 15-41). A sagittal split osteotomy was carried out on the right side to allow bilateral advancement, more on the left than the right (Fig. 15-42). A thick splint on the left side was used to increase face height there, and Erich arch bars were used for maxillomandibular fixation. He tolerated the procedure well and was discharged on the fifth postoperative day in maxillomandibular fixation.

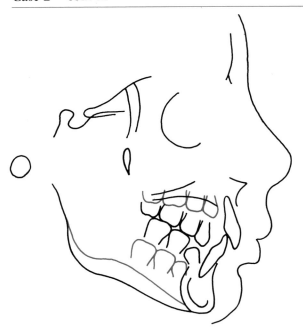

Fig. 15-37. M.P., age 8 years, 10 months, initial cephalometric tracing. The normal left side is traced in black and the affected right side in red.

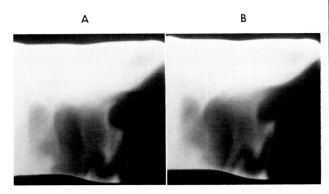

Fig. 15-39. M.P., age 9 years, 5 months. Tomographic cuts through the left condyle clearly show the old and partially healed fracture, which was not visualized in plain films.

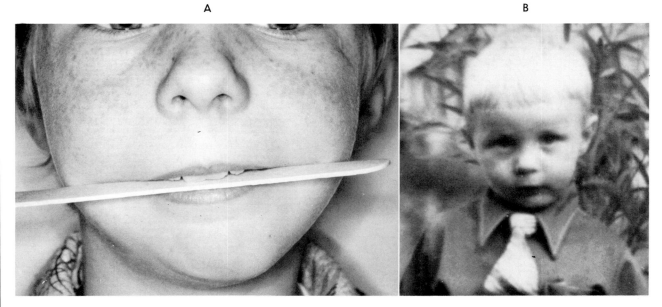

Fig. 15-38. M.P. **A,** The lack of vertical ramus growth on the left side has already produced a significant cant of the occlusal plane. **B,** A family snapshot taken at age 4 suggests that a left-side deficiency was already present (but because of the shadow pattern it is impossible to be certain).

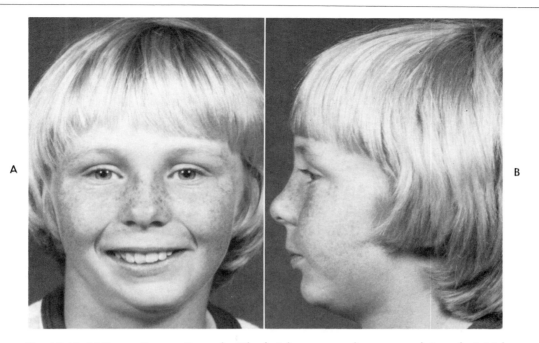

Fig. 15-40. M.P., age 9 years, 9 months. The facial asymmetry has worsened since the initial evaluation, as would be expected with functional ankylosis.

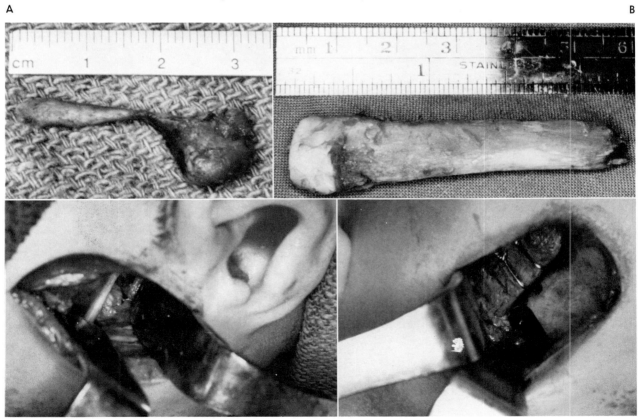

Fig. 15-41. M.P. **A,** The left condyle after resection. Note the inclination of the condylar head after the old fracture. **B,** The costochondral graft before insertion. **C,** The submandibular incision for placement of the graft (note the closed preauricular incision above, used for removal of the condyle). **D,** The costochondral graft wired into position.

Continued.

Case 2—cont'd.

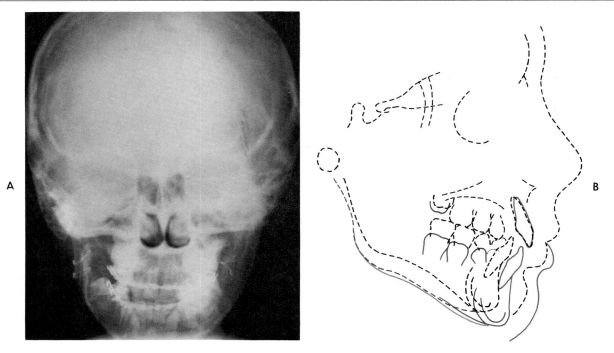

Fig. 15-42. M.P. **A,** PA cephalometric radiograph after surgery. The costochondral graft was placed on the left side, and a sagittal split advancement was done on the right side. **B,** Cephalometric superimposition from before *(dashed lines)* to after surgery *(solid lines)*. The right side is red/pink; the left side black/gray.

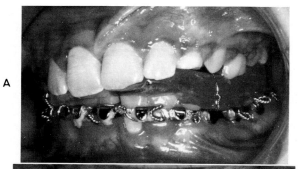

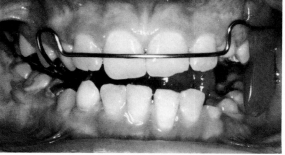

Six weeks later, the maxillomandibular fixation was released and he was allowed to function into the splint for 2 weeks (Fig. 15-43, *A*). Then it was removed and a hybrid functional appliance was placed (Fig. 15-43, *B*). At age 10 years, 11 months, an excellent growth response was noted (Fig. 15-44) and facial symmetry was much improved (Fig. 15-45), but some dental asymmetry and crowding on the left side persisted. The functional appliance was discontinued and a fixed appliance to complete the alignment of the teeth was placed.

Fig. 15-43. M.P. **A,** Splint in place 8 weeks after surgery, when he returned for postsurgical orthodontic treatment. The splint was tied to the lower arch bar so that he could function into it when maxillomandibular fixation was released at 6 weeks. **B,** The initial functional appliance. This design was quickly modified to include a lingual shield to keep the tongue from interfering with eruption on the left side, so the appliance was quite similar to the one shown in Fig. 15-11.

Case 2—cont'd.

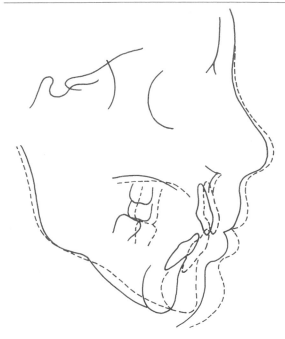

Fig. 15-44. M.P., cephalometric superimposition from immediately postsurgery *(solid line)* to 1 year later *(dashed line),* during the functional-appliance treatment. The upward rotation of the mandible was due to removal of the surgical splint.

Unimpeded jaw movement and normal growth continued for another year, but at age 11 years, 8 months, a tendency toward reankylosis was noted. At that point, facial symmetry was still quite good (Fig. 15-46) and there was good progress toward nonextraction orthodontic management of the crowding and intra-arch asymmetry (Fig. 15-47). A panoramic radiograph showed proliferation of bone in the area of the graft (Fig. 15-48, *A*). His ability to open gradually diminished. At age 12 years, 7 months, the cartilaginous portion of the graft was removed, the bony stump was recontoured, and a silastic sheet was placed to prevent bony ankylosis. By the time the orthodontics could be completed at age 13 years, 2 months, further bony proliferation was apparent (Fig. 15-48, *B*) and motion was again restricted. Cephalometric superimposition showed downward and backward rotation of the mandible (Fig. 15-49).

By age 16, he could open only 12 mm (Fig. 15-50). CT scans showed tremendous proliferation of bone on the temporal and mandibular sides of the TM joint area (Fig. 15-51). At age 16 years, 7 months, when surgery to release the ankylosis was undertaken, a massive bony and fibrous union between the mandible and zygoma was noted. The left ramus was resected and the zygoma was reconstructed. Impressions were taken in the operating room so that a modified bionator could be placed,

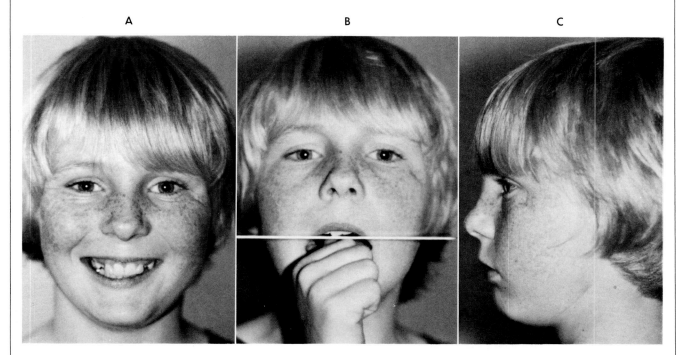

Fig. 15-45. M.P., age 10 years, 11 months, 1 year postsurgery, facial appearance at the point where functional-appliance treatment was discontinued.

Continued.

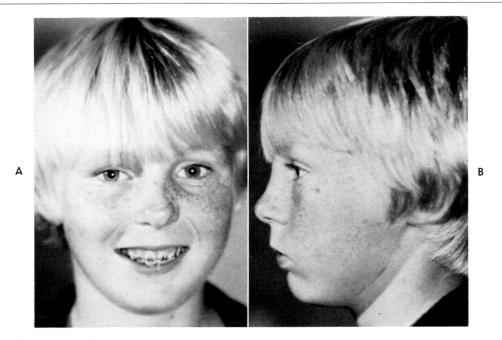

Fig. 15-46. M.P., age 11 years, 8 months, facial appearance at the point when limitation of motion again began to appear.

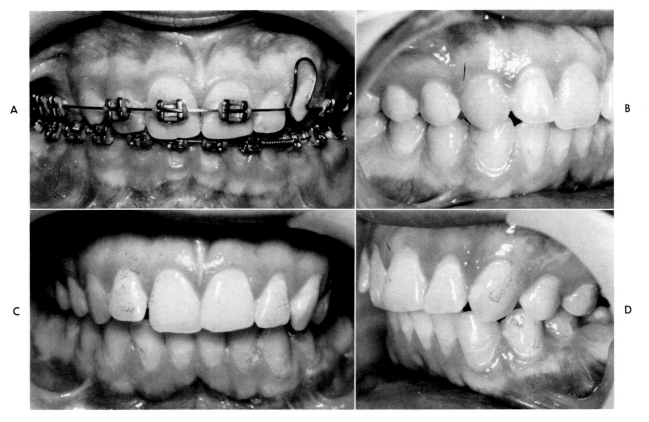

Fig. 15-47. M.P. **A**, Age 11 years, 8 months, dental relationships during the fixed-appliance orthodontic treatment. **B-D**, Age 13 years, 2 months, soon after removal of orthodontic appliances.

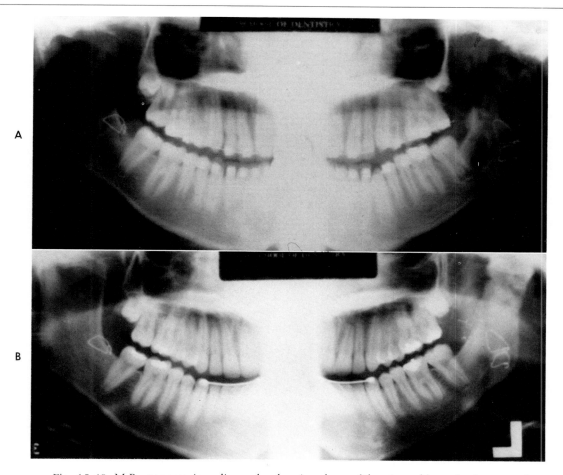

Fig. 15-48. M.P., panoramic radiographs showing the proliferation of bone in the area of the left condyle. **A,** Age 11 years, 8 months, before the second surgery. **B,** Age 13 years, 2 months, following the second surgery.

Fig. 15-49. M.P., cephalometric superimposition age 11 years, 8 months *(solid line),* to age 13 years, 2 months *(dashed line).* Note the change to downward-backward growth rather than the normal growth pattern observed in the absence of ankylosis following the initial surgery.

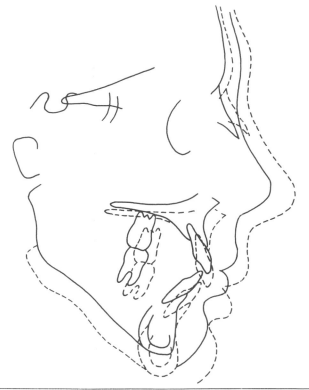

Continued.

Case 2—cont'd.

A   B   C

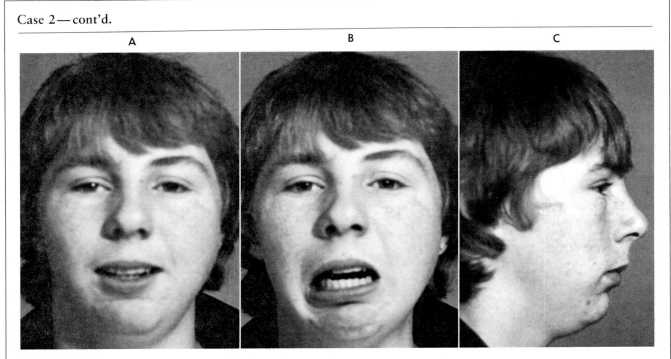

Fig. 15-50. M.P., age 16 years, 5 months, facial appearance before the third surgery. His maximal opening of 12 mm at that point is demonstrated in **B**.

and he began wearing this during the first postoperative week (Fig. 15-52). The appliance differed from the standard design only in that it incorporated the longest possible lingual flange on the right side, to maintain the jaw in the midline upon opening as far as possible. Immediately after surgery, he could open 32 mm but deviated sharply to the left. One year later, he could open 28 mm without deviation and 42 mm total (Fig. 15-53). A panoramic radiograph at age 18 revealed a considerable degree of regeneration of the ramus. Facial appearance at age 19 was quite symmetric (Fig. 15-54), and jaw function remained essentially normal.

Comments. This case illustrates a number of interesting points in diagnosis, treatment planning, and management. It can be very difficult to distinguish between mild hemifacial microsomia and functional ankylosis in the absence of a definite history of trauma, as in this case. The correct diagnosis would have been made sooner if the restriction of jaw movement had been properly appreciated in the beginning.

A key point in planning treatment is how rapidly the deformity is progressing. From the pediatrician's perspective, the asymmetry had developed recently and was rapidly progressive, implying recent injury and little or no subsequent growth. The worsening of the problem while we observed it tends to support that view and the decision to intervene in the joint. If the family was correct and the injury occurred at age 2, some growth must have been possible, strengthening the argument for conservative surgical treatment. With 20/20 hindsight, it might have been better to accept the limited TM joint function that he had rather than to reconstruct the joint at age 8. Excessive growth after a costochondral transplant has been reported previously. The surgical option would have been ramus osteotomies to reposition the jaw at age 8 with no attempt to release the ankylosis, accepting that additional surgery probably would be required at about age 14 because the normal side would continue to grow more than the affected one.

Case 2—cont'd.

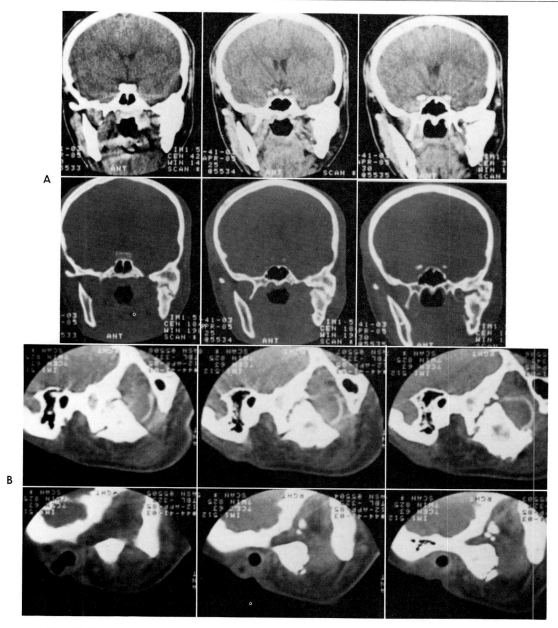

Fig. 15-51. M.P., age 16 years, 5 months, CT scans. **A,** Anterior view. Compare the amount of bone on the right (normal) and left sides. It is apparent that bone formation has occurred on both the temporal and mandibular sides of the TM joint. **B,** Lateral view of the left TM-joint area. Note the exceptionally wide area of articulation.

Continued.

Case 2—cont'd.

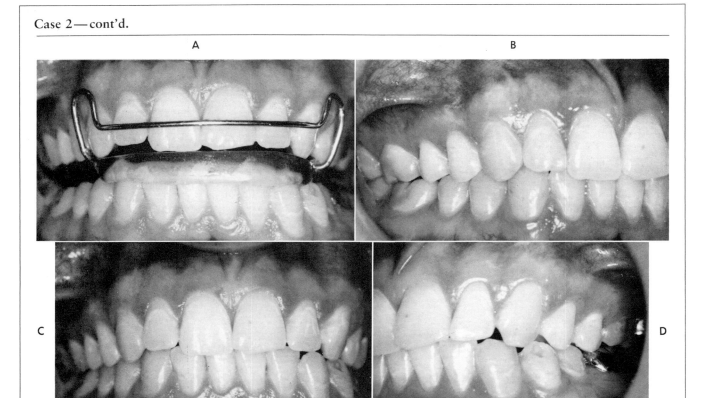

Fig. 15-52. M.P. **A,** Age 16 years, 10 months, functional appliance in place. **B-D,** Age 18 years, dental relationships.

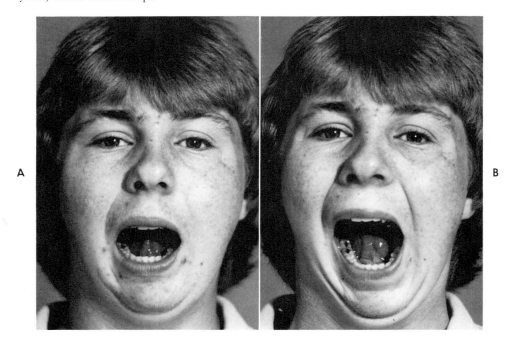

Fig. 15-53. M.P., age 17 years, 5 months. **A,** He opens to 28 mm without deviation, despite the absence of a condylar articulation on the left. **B,** On maximal opening (>40 mm), the jaw deviates to the left.

Case 2—cont'd.

It also is interesting to note the use of a functional appliance postsurgically as a training device, and how well this patient functioned after the left ramus had been resected. Experience with other patients demonstrates that normal function does not require both condyles perfectly centered in the fossae. Even if one is totally missing, essentially normal jaw function is possible as muscular guidance takes over. (Normal growth can occur in the absence of a condyle, too—see Chapter 2, Figs. 2-23 to 2-26).

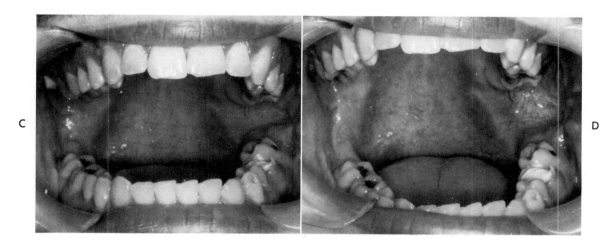

Fig. 15-53, **cont'd.** C and D, Maximum opening of 42 mm, with some deviation to the left.

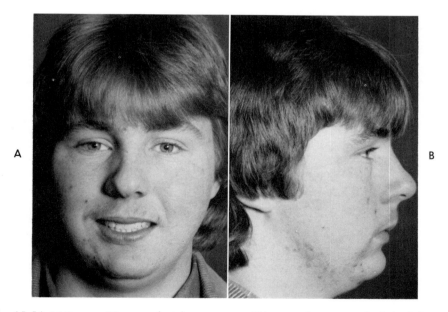

Fig. 15-54. M.P., age 19 years, facial appearance 2½ years after removal of the left ramus. Jaw function is essentially normal.

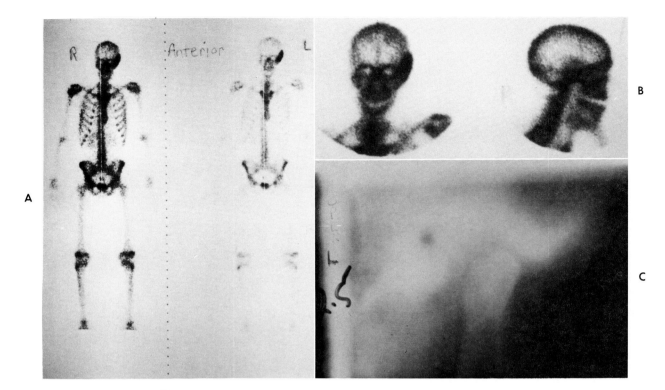

Fig. 15-55. ^{99}Tc bone scan in a patient with hemimandibular hypertrophy. Note the "hot" condyle on the left side, indicating more uptake of the isotope and therefore greater metabolic activity there.

ASYMMETRY IN ADOLESCENTS

After the adolescent growth spurt has ended, severe asymmetry is much more likely to arise because of excessive rather than deficient growth. Even if a condylar fracture restricts translation, there is not enough growth remaining to cause more than moderate mandibular asymmetry. An adolescent with a growth problem following a condylar fracture is managed best with a functional appliance until growth is complete or all but complete, to prevent the development of a maxillary as well as mandibular asymmetry if possible. This is followed by corrective surgery as necessary (see Figs. 15-2 to 15-7).

In contrast, excessive unilateral growth of the mandible can be an indication for surgical intervention in adolescents. This condition formerly was called condylar hyperplasia, but because the body of the mandible as well as the condyle and ramus are affected by the overgrowth, *hemimandibular hypertrophy* and *hemimandibular elongation* are more accurate descriptive terms.[29] The problem usually becomes apparent only after the adolescent growth spurt, when one side of the mandible continues to grow after the other has all but stopped. The condition can occur before or during the adolescent growth spurt but is extremely rare before the late teens. Although the excessive growth tends to

be self-limiting, it may continue until an extremely severe deformity has been created (see Chapter 2).

The key question when hemimandibular hypertrophy is first discovered is whether the deformity is progressive (i.e., whether excessive growth is continuing). If the asymmetric growth stops and the condition stabilizes, it is preferable to delay surgery until the patient is a young adult and to correct the asymmetry without involving the TM joint (see Case 6). If the asymmetry is already severe enough to cause a problem and is becoming progressively worse, there is no option to removing the growth site at the head of the affected condyle, even in young patients.

A ^{99m}Tc bone scan (Fig. 15-55) is the most direct way to determine whether asymmetric growth is still occurring. More uptake of the isotope on the affected than the nonaffected side is evidence that it is occurring. Unfortunately, false negatives do occur with this diagnostic approach.[30] Clinical findings may demonstrate continuing growth, and clinical judgment ultimately may indicate surgery to remove the affected condyle even though repeated bone scans do not demonstrate continued isotope uptake.

If progressive deformity requires removing the condylar growth site, the surgical options for the affected side are (1) excision of bone at the head of the

A

B

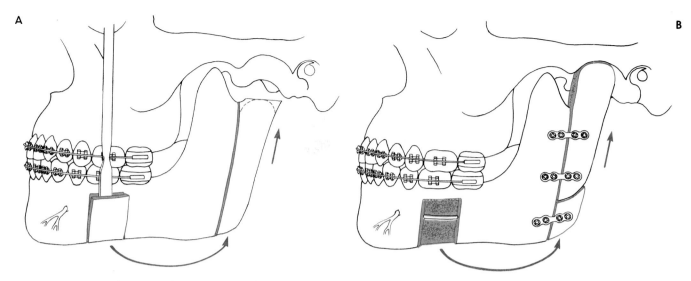

Fig. 15-56. **A,** Bony cuts in the mandibular ramus to allow superior movement after excision of the condyle. Autogenous bone is freed from the anterior mandible to fill the defect at the inferior border in the angle region. **B,** After the base of the original condylar process is repositioned superiorly to replace the condyle, the bony segments are secured with small bone plates.

condyle, then recontouring or repositioning the bony stump, or (2) removing the condyle and condylar process and reconstructing the area, either with a costochondral junction transplant as described above or with a free graft.[31] In addition, a sagittal split osteotomy on the unaffected side almost always is needed to allow proper positioning of the mandible. In an adult, if the maxilla is canted because of excessive vertical growth on the affected side, maxillary surgery also is required. In younger patients, surgery in the maxilla should be avoided if possible. When postsurgical growth can be anticipated, the maxillary cant can be corrected postsurgically by blocking further eruption of teeth on the affected side and allowing teeth to erupt on the nonaffected side (see Case 3).

Surgery for Condylar Reconstruction

Surgery to excise the head of the condyle and then to reposition the bony stump into the glenoid fossa requires both a preauricular and a submandibular surgical approach (Fig. 15-56). The preauricular incision permits access for the condylectomy and allows direct visualization of the reconstructed condyle, meniscus, and fossa. Through the submandibular approach, a vertical ramus osteotomy is performed to lengthen the remaining condylar process, and stabilizing devices are applied (see Case 3). If the contour of the inferior border of the mandible is to be altered, it may be done through this approach as well. If a posterior open bite is present on the affected side, the condylar process can be shortened as the condylar head is "shaved," thus

bringing the teeth into contact. In this circumstance, it is not necessary to perform a vertical ramus osteotomy as long as an exact amount of condyle is removed to permit the posterior teeth to contact.

The surgical technique for reconstruction of the condylar process with a graft is described in the above section on asymmetry in children.

The deformity in hemimandibular hypertrophy affects the body as well as the ramus of the mandible. Typically, a downward bowing of the mandibular body exists. This can be at least partially corrected by removing bone from the lower border on the affected side. In younger adolescents with growth remaining, we recommend delaying this surgery until approximately 1 year after the TM joint reconstruction so that postsurgical orthodontics can bring the teeth together and jaw function can stabilize. In adults, it can be done simultaneously.

Functional Appliances Following Condylar Reconstruction

In a young patient in whom the teeth on the nonaffected side were left out of occlusion at the time of surgery, so as to avoid maxillary and mandibular surgery, postsurgical functional-appliance treatment will be necessary (see Case 3). The purposes of the appliance are to guide the eruption of teeth on the nonaffected side and to control subsequent growth. The appliance design usually is a "hybrid," similar to the ones pictured in Figs. 15-11 and 15-64.

Case Reports

Case 3

J.L., age 12 years, 8 months, was seen because of his parents' concern about his increasing facial asymmetry (Fig. 15-57). They had first noted this 5 months previously and had consulted an orthodontist and surgeon, who suggested delaying treatment and observation. At this point, the asymmetry was noticeably greater than at the initial examination. Intraorally, there was no dental contact on the right side, suggesting extremely rapid vertical growth (Fig. 15-58). The panoramic and PA cephalometric radiographs showed a grossly enlarged mandibular condyle on the right side and a downward bowing of the body of the mandible (Fig. 15-59). On the lateral cephalometric film, the right ramus was 1.5 cm longer than the left (Fig. 15-60).

A ^{99}Tc bone scan showed intense activity in the right condyle (Fig. 15-61). Because of the severe and rapidly progressive deformity at this early age, right condylectomy with TM joint reconstruction via a costochondral graft, ramus osteotomy to free the left side, and postsurgical functional-appliance therapy were planned.

At age 13 years, after the left fourth rib was harvested, the right mandibular ramus was exposed via a submandibular incision and the condyle was resected. A vertical ramus osteotomy was completed on the left side, and the left coronoid process was freed. With the prepared splint in place to separate the jaws more on the left than on the right side, maxillomandibular fixation was applied, and the graft was secured into position with a

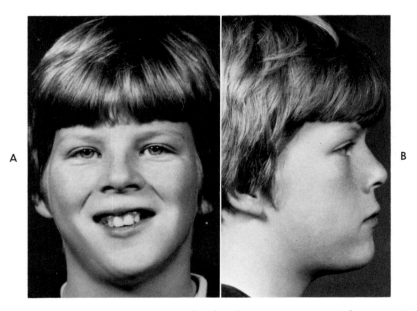

Fig. 15-57. J.L., age 12 years, 8 months, facial appearance on initial examination.

Case 3—cont'd.

A   B   C

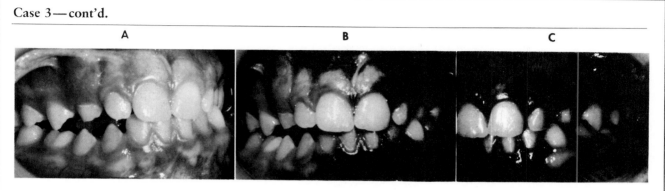

Fig. 15-58. J.L., age 12 years, 8 months, dental relationships on initial examination. Note the posterior open bite on the right side—even the molars are slightly separated, which implies vertical ramus growth at a rate tooth eruption cannot match.

A   B

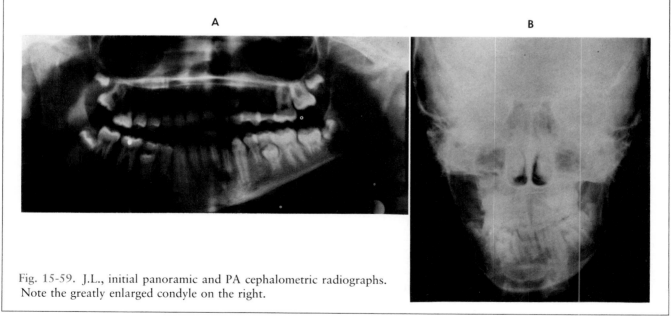

Fig. 15-59. J.L., initial panoramic and PA cephalometric radiographs. Note the greatly enlarged condyle on the right.

Continued.

Case 3—cont'd.

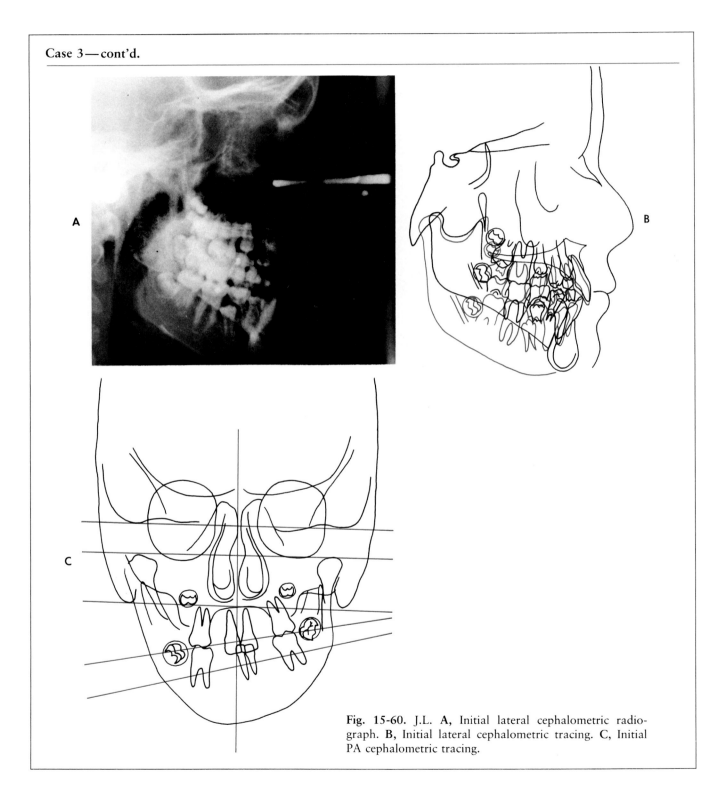

Fig. 15-60. J.L. **A,** Initial lateral cephalometric radiograph. **B,** Initial lateral cephalometric tracing. **C,** Initial PA cephalometric tracing.

Case 3—cont'd.

A   B   C

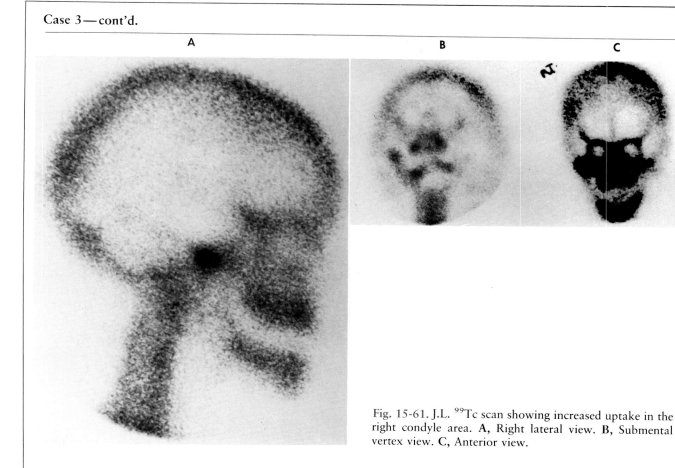

Fig. 15-61. J.L. ^{99}Tc scan showing increased uptake in the right condyle area. **A**, Right lateral view. **B**, Submental vertex view. **C**, Anterior view.

small bone plate (Fig. 15-62). He was maintained in maxillomandibular fixation for 8 weeks, then functioned into the splint for 3 weeks before returning for postsurgical orthodontics (Figs. 15-63 and 15-64).

A hybrid functional appliance, to allow teeth to erupt on the left but not the right side, was worn full-time for 3 months. At that point the teeth were in contact bilaterally. A second appliance, separating the teeth again on the left side and slightly swinging the mandible to the right, was placed at age 13 years, 6 months. After 4 months, the bite block on the right side was progressively trimmed away from the underside, and the orthodontic treatment was discontinued at age 14 years, 2

months, 12 months after the surgery (Fig. 15-65). Occlusal relationships and jaw function were excellent at that point.

At age 14 years, 5 months, a second surgical procedure to recontour the inferior border of the mandible on the right side was performed, with further improvement in facial symmetry (Fig. 15-66). He underwent a dramatic adolescent growth spurt between ages 16 and 17, but no problems arose. Both the facial proportions and occlusal relationships present at the end of active treatment were nicely maintained (Fig. 15-67). Cephalometric superimpositions showed that little or no mandibular growth occurred despite the growth elsewhere (Fig. 15-68).

Continued.

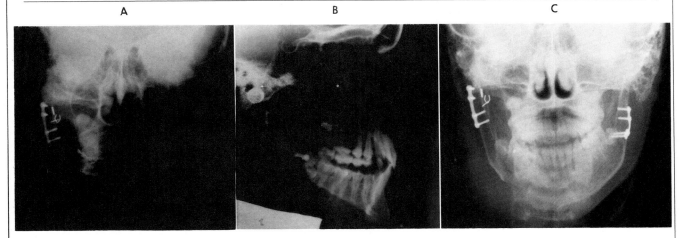

Fig. 15-62. **J.L. A, Postsurgical PA** and **B,** lateral cephalometric radiographs. **C,** Follow-up PA cephalometric film after removal of bone from the lower border of the mandible on the right side.

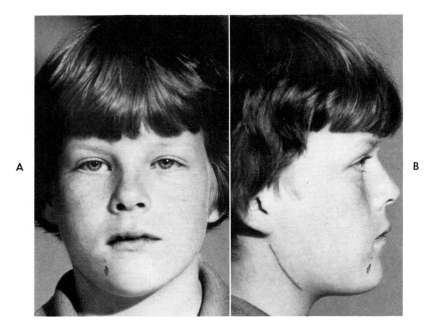

Fig. 15-63. J.L., age 13 years, 3 months, facial appearance 11 weeks postsurgically, when orthodontic treatment began.

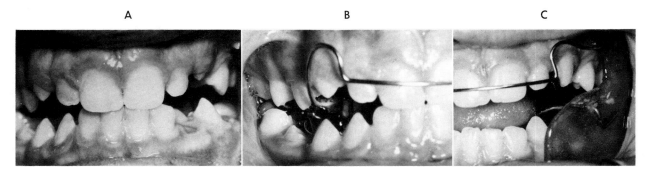

Fig. 15-64. J.L., age 13 years, 3 months. **A,** Dental relationships when the surgical splint was removed, showing the interocclusal space on the left. **B** and **C,** Functional appliance in place.

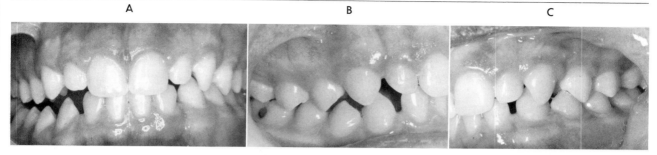

Fig. 15-65. J.L., age 14 years, 2 months, dental relationships at the discontinuation of functional-appliance treatment.

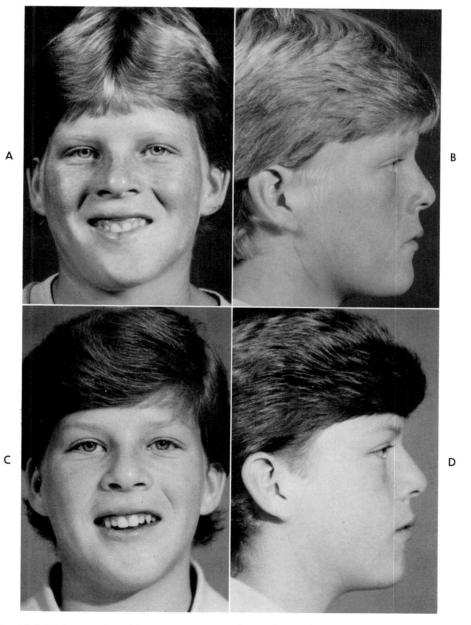

Fig. 15-66. J.L., age **A** and **B**, 14 years, 2 months, and **C** and **D**, 14 years, 7 months, before and after secondary surgery to recontour the lower border of the mandible on the right side.

Continued.

Case 3—cont'd.

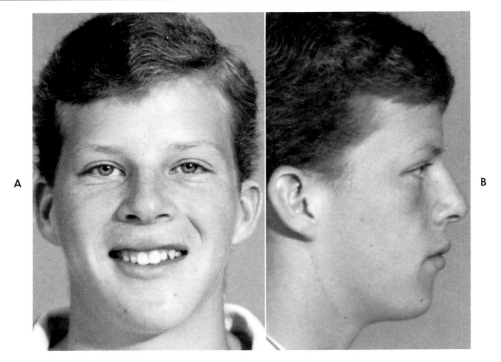

Fig. 15-67. J.L., age 18 years, 3 months, facial appearance 5 years after the initial surgery.

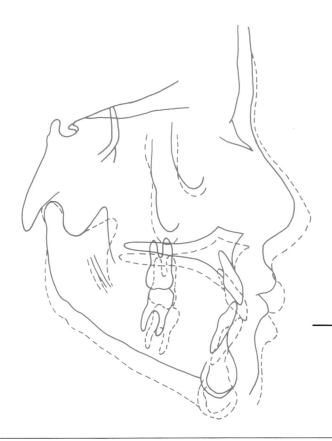

Comments. The decision to use a costochondral graft was based on the feeling that, for this young patient, cartilage would be the best long-term choice to prevent re-ankylosis. Because of his facial dimensions at the time of treatment, the affected right ramus could remain at its present length, which was approximately the adult size, while the left side was brought to the adult dimensions. In that circumstance, little or no postsurgical jaw growth was desired or expected, and that is what occurred. A similar approach with costochondral grafting has been successful in the only other preadolescent patient with hemimandibular hypertrophy (a 10-year-old girl) we have treated in recent years.

Fig. 15-68. J.L., cephalometric superimposition ages 14 years, 7 months *(solid)*, and 18 years, 3 months *(dashed)*, showing the vertical direction of maxillary and mandibular growth during the adolescent growth spurt. There was no tendency for a recurrence of disproportionate or excessive mandibular growth.

Case 4

D.R., age 19 years, 3 months, and a university student, was seen for evaluation of the facial asymmetry (Fig. 15-69) and anterior crossbite/lateral open-bite malocclusion (Fig. 15-70) that had gradually developed during the last 2 to 3 years. A panoramic radiograph showed an enlarged right mandibular condyle (Fig. 15-71), and cephalometric analysis confirmed lengthening of the right ramus (Fig. 15-72). She had had orthodontic treatment previously to correct Class II, division 1 malocclusion, with a satisfactory response at that time (Fig. 15-73). When asymmetric growth began to occur, the decision was made to wait for growth to stop before correcting it.

Because of uncertainty as to whether growth had stopped, she was placed on recall. One year later, the clinical impression was that the asymmetry had increased, but she was not eager for treatment. At age 22 years, 6 months, there was obvious progression as evidenced by the unilateral open bite and the increased facial asymmetry (Fig. 15-74), and it was decided that right condylectomy was necessary. The teeth were aligned with a fixed appliance and stabilized, without leveling the lower arch at that point (Fig. 15-75).

At age 22 years, 8 months, a condylectomy was performed on the affected side through a preauricular incision (Fig. 15-76) and a sagittal split osteotomy was

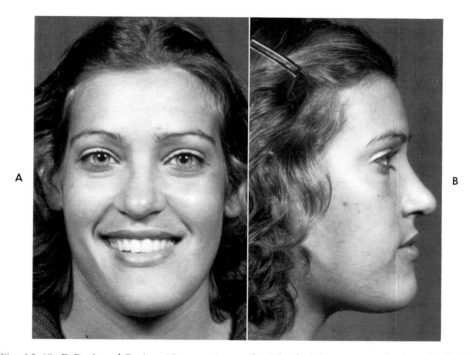

Fig. 15-69. D.R. **A** and **B**, Age 19 years, 3 months. The facial asymmetry had gradually developed since her initial orthodontic treatment (for Class II, division 1 malocclusion) was completed at age 13.

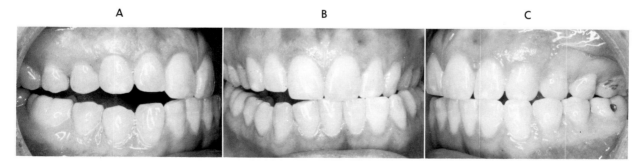

Fig. 15-70. D.R., age 19 years, 3 months. The lateral open bite had developed since her original orthodontic treatment was completed.

Continued.

Case 4—cont'd.

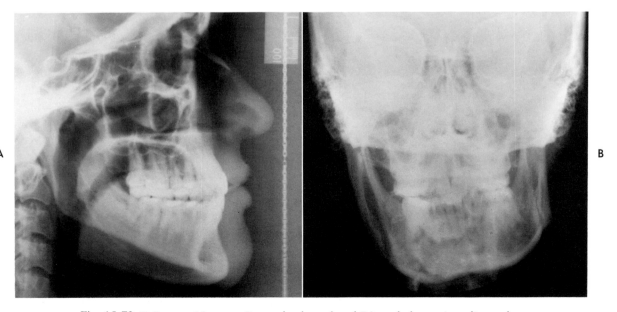

A   B

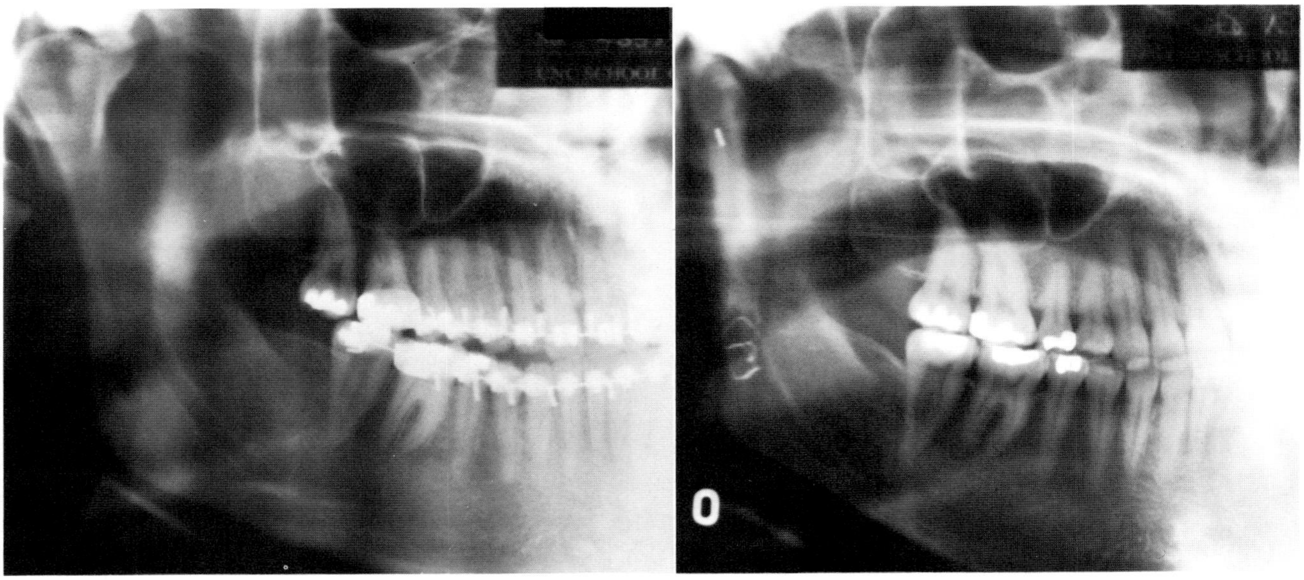

Fig. 15-71. D.R., panoramic radiographs. **A,** Presurgery. Note the enlarged condyle on the right side. **B,** Postsurgery.

A   B

Fig. 15-72. D.R., age 19 years, 3 months, lateral and PA cephalometric radiographs.

Case 4—cont'd.

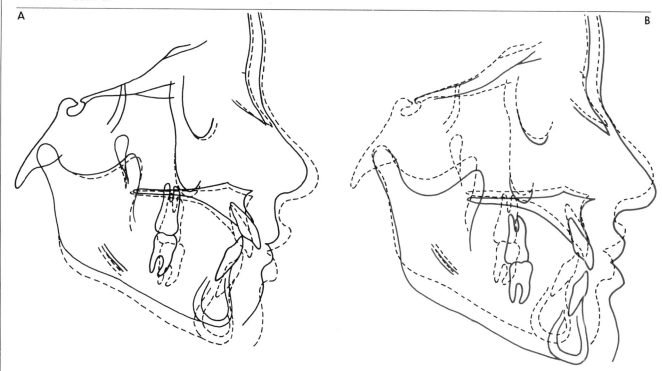

Fig. 15-73. D.R., cephalometric superimpositions. **A,** Age 11 years, 2 months, to 12 years, 9 months *(dashed black)*, during her original orthodontic treatment to correct moderate Class II, division 1 malocclusion. **B,** Age 12 years, 9 months, to 16 years, 4 months *(solid red)*, as asymmetric mandibular growth occurred.

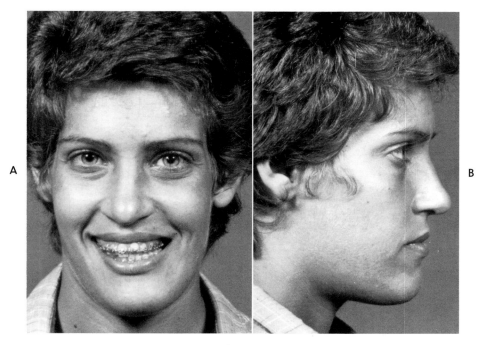

Fig. 15-74. D.R., age 22 years, 6 months, facial proportions. Note the increased asymmetry from her initial examination.

Continued.

Case 4—cont'd.

A   B   C

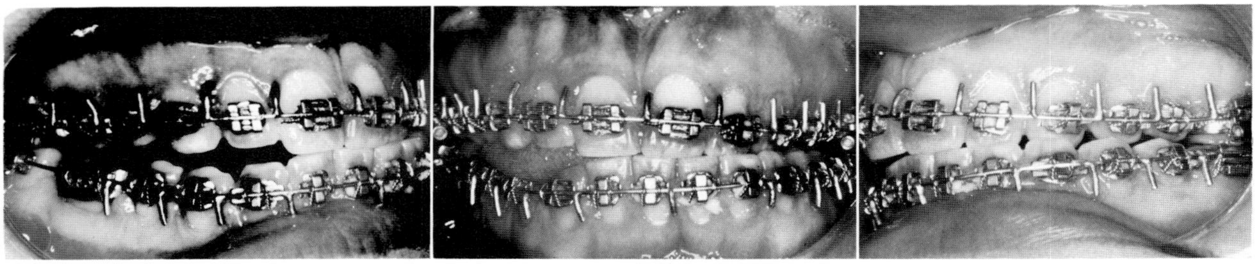

Fig. 15-75. D.R., age 22 years, 8 months, dental relationships immediately before surgery, with the stabilizing arch wires in place.

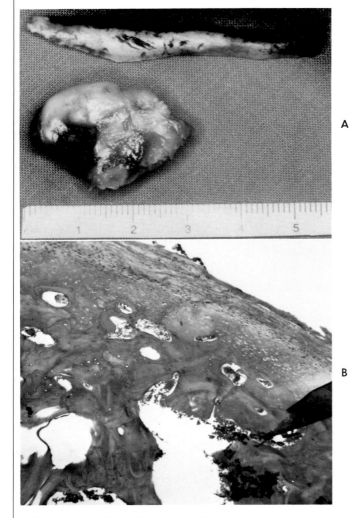

Fig. 15-76. D.R. **A,** The resected hyperplastic condyle and bone removed from the lower border of the mandible. **B,** Histologic specimen from the condyle, showing normal appearance. The problem in these patients is excessive but entirely normal growth, not a benign tumor or an obviously pathologic process.

done on the opposite side. The mandible was rotated to the midline, and maxillomandibular fixation was applied. A submandibular incision then was made on the affected side, and a vertical ramus osteotomy was performed to reconstruct the condyle. Through the preauricular incision, the stump of the ramus was guided superiorly into the glenoid fossa to articulate with the meniscus, and through the submandibular incision the proximal and distal segments were secured with wire fixation and a portion of the inferior border of the mandible on the affected side was excised to improve vertical symmetry (Fig. 15-77).

At 3 weeks postsurgery, maxillomandibular fixation was released and a forced opening of 16 mm was recorded. For the next 3 weeks, this was repeated every 3 or 4 days. At 6 weeks postsurgery, she could open voluntarily 23 mm and stretch to 26 mm. The stabilizing arch wires were replaced with 16 steel working arch wires 10 weeks postsurgery. After 2 months with light box elastics she had settled into excellent occlusion (Fig. 15-78), and the fixed appliances were replaced with full-time retainers. She opened 35 mm voluntarily and had excellent functional relationships in lateral excursions. Good facial symmetry was obtained (Fig. 15-79). Six years later, at age 29 years, 8 months, facial and dental relationships were nicely maintained, 5 years after retainers had been discontinued (Figs. 15-80 and 15-81).

Comments. In this patient, excessive growth on one side began during the late teens and continued slowly over a period of at least 7 years with a steadily worsening asymmetry and no evidence of spontaneous cessation. The fact that there is a tendency in hemimandibular hypertrophy for the excessive growth to stop certainly does not mean that it always will stop. In our (admittedly limited) experience, patients who experience asymmetric lengthening of the condylar neck on one side are more likely to stop growing spontaneously than are those, such as this patient, who have enlargement of the condylar head.

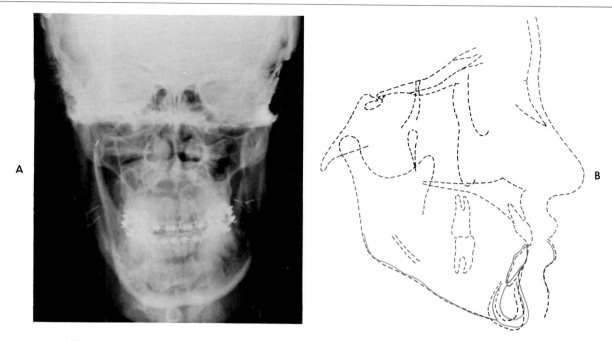

Fig. 15-77. D.R., **A,** PA cephalometric radiograph immediately after surgery. **B,** Cephalometric tracing presurgery to postsurgery *(solid pink).*

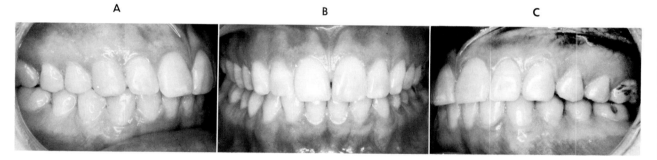

Fig. 15-78. D.R., age 22 years, 11 months, dental relationships at the completion of orthodontic treatment.

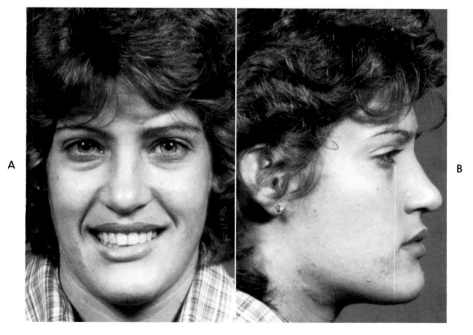

Fig. 15-79. D.R., age 22 years, 11 months, at the completion of orthodontic treatment.

Continued.

Case 4—cont'd.

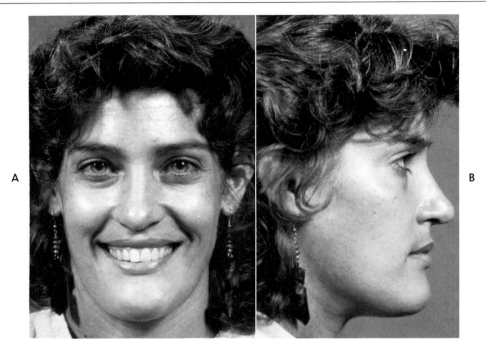

Fig. 15-80. D.R., age 29 years, 8 months, 7 years postsurgery.

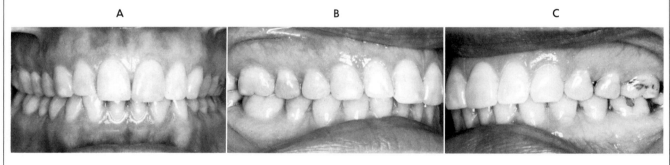

Fig. 15-81. D.R., age 29 years, 8 months, occlusal relationships 5 years after retainers were discontinued.

ASYMMETRY IN ADULTS
Treatment Planning Considerations

In adults, skeletal asymmetry cannot be managed orthodontically, and the only question is the type of surgical intervention. The general approach is the same as for any other type of surgical-orthodontic treatment: a fixed orthodontic appliance is placed a few months before surgery so that initial alignment of the teeth can be achieved, jaw surgery is done as necessary to correct the asymmetry, and the appliances are used for finishing orthodontics.

For these patients the major treatment planning decision is the extent to which surgery will be used to cor-

rect the deformity at its point of origin, as opposed to compensating for existing deformity and in essence camouflaging its existence. For example, an asymmetric mandible can be approached by surgery in the ramus, correcting the unequal ramus length that is a major cause of the deformity, or it can be managed by inferior border osteotomy to slide the chin sideways, correcting the obvious asymmetry anteriorly and leaving the gonial angles as they were. Similarly, an asymmetric maxilla could be approached by rotating the entire upper jaw, or could be camouflaged by asymmetric onlay grafts.

All patients are at least somewhat different, but

asymmetries are particularly difficult to put into distinct groups. As general guidelines in planning treatment, however, we offer the following:

1. Patients are much more aware of transverse than of vertical distortions of facial symmetry and are much more concerned about the position of the chin than of the mandibular angles. For this reason, it can be quite acceptable to leave a vertical asymmetry of the angles uncorrected and to correct a chin position that is off to one side by using an inferior border osteotomy to reposition the chin transversely—provided, of course, that dental occlusion and jaw function would be satisfactory if the entire mandible were not repositioned (see Chapter 5, Figs. 5-16 to 5-18).

2. The transverse position of the maxillary teeth is obvious and therefore esthetically important. Rarely is it acceptable to leave the maxillary dental midline uncorrected, and the easiest way to correct this in many instances is to rotate the maxilla surgically (see Case 5). In contrast, the mandibular dental midline is not obvious, and provided acceptable occlusion can be achieved, there is no reason to go to extraordinary lengths to correct dental midline deviation. For some patients an asymmetry can be corrected with a maxillary osteotomy and repositioning of the chin without concomitant mandibular ramus surgery.

3. When an asymmetry of the jaws develops, it sometimes happens that the nose deviates in the same direction as the chin. In this case, there is little or no alternative to rhinoplasty to correct the nose in addition to jaw surgery. The reason is simple: moving the jaw to a more symmetric position magnifies the deviation of the nose, and the patient is likely to be more conscious of it and dissatisfied with it. On a few occasions, patients who were not warned of this have insisted that orthognathic surgery created a nasal deviation, which in fact was present but not noticed previously. In a significant minority of patients with a developmental asymmetry, however, the jaws deviate in one direction and the nose in the other. For these patients, orthognathic surgery has the effect of improving overall facial symmetry, and often the residual deviation of the nose is esthetically acceptable.

   Rhinoplasty done simultaneously with orthognathic surgery has become more feasible with the routine use of RIF, especially if the jaw surgery involves only the mandible[32] (see Chapter 10). Particularly in asymmetry problems, we recommend that the orthognathic surgery be done first and rhinoplasty deferred for a few months after the jaw surgery—but the likelihood that rhinoplasty will be needed should be thoroughly discussed first. This approach ensures that the final soft-tissue contours can be observed when the rhinoplasty is done.

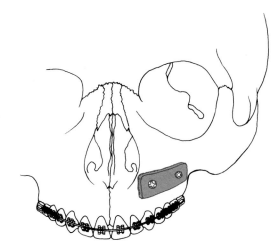

Fig. 15-82. Autogenous bone graft to augment midface contour, secured with bone screws.

4. When asymmetry affects the higher structures of the maxilla (infraorbital rims, zygomatic arch), jaw function is less affected than is facial symmetry. In this circumstance the use of onlay grafts to reposition the deficient bony areas, alone or in combination with osteotomies, is particularly advantageous (Fig. 15-82; see Chapter 10 for details of surgical technique). Typically, the grafts provide a way to augment the midface without the increased risk and morbidity of a LeFort II or III osteotomy (Figs. 15-83 to 15-87).

Orthodontic Considerations

Neither the presurgical nor the postsurgical orthodontic treatment for adults with asymmetry differs significantly from the orthodontics in other types of problems. The principles discussed in Chapter 6 and illustrated in more detail in Chapter 12 are applicable.

As with all patients, one of the goals of presurgical orthodontics is to remove dental compensations for the skeletal deformity. In asymmetries, dental compensation typically means that the dental midlines are not off as much as the skeletal midlines (i.e., if the chin deviates to the left, the maxillary dental midline often is also off to the left, but the mandibular dental midline relative to the chin is usually to the right) (see Case 6). If the dental compensations cannot be removed by the presurgical orthodontics, the surgical approach must be modified to take this into account. It is better to decompensate the dentition presurgically, to the extent this is possible.

The two approaches to transverse decompensation are (1) asymmetric extraction, so that the incisors are retracted more on one side than on the other and the midline shifts in the desired direction, and (2) asymmetric elastics, usually anterior diagonal elastics. With appropriate extractions, the midline can be shifted sev-

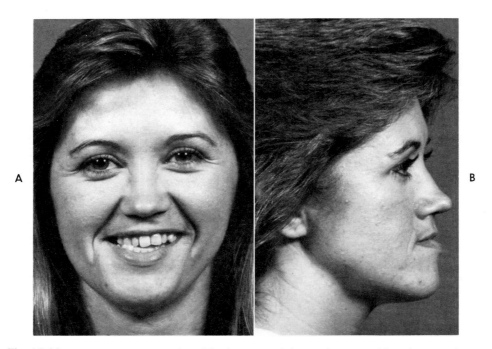

Fig. 15-83. P.M., age 28, was referred by her general dentist because of her deviating lower jaw, which she felt had become significantly worse in the previous 2 years. Her obvious facial asymmetry included an element of orbital dystopia, with the left orbit superior to the right one. The zygoma on the left was higher and more prominent, and the alar base and the smile deviated upward on the left side.

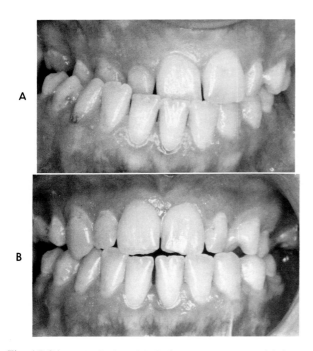

Fig. 15-84. P.M. **A,** Age 28. Before treatment, multiple posterior teeth were missing, and she had anterior and right lateral crossbite. **B,** Age 29, dental relationships after surgical treatment but before placement of partial dentures, showing the correction of asymmetry. Without orthodontics, it was not possible to totally close the open bite.

eral millimeters; without extraction or the presence of spaces in the arches, only small changes can be made with elastics alone.

For acceptable esthetics the maxillary dental midline must be close to the midline of the face. If only mandibular surgery is planned, the orthodontist must make the maxillary midline correction. If maxillary surgery is necessary anyway, the surgeon can rotate the jaw enough to change the midline 3 to 4 mm without great difficulty (see Case 5). Such a rotation will produce some occlusal interferences posteriorly, but usually these are not great enough to prevent orthodontic tooth alignment during postsurgical orthodontics. The wisest decision in a patient who will have a maxillary osteotomy, therefore, may be to minimize the presurgical orthodontics and let the surgeon correct the maxillary midline, accepting that somewhat more extensive postsurgical orthodontics will be required.

The mandibular dental midline must be considered from two perspectives: (1) its relationship to the facial and maxillary dental midlines, and (2) its relationship to the chin. At the conclusion of treatment everything should line up, but the critical elements are the chin and the maxillary teeth. It is an error to correct the dental midlines and leave the chin asymmetric—which will happen unless the transverse relationship of the lower teeth to the chin is corrected presurgically or an

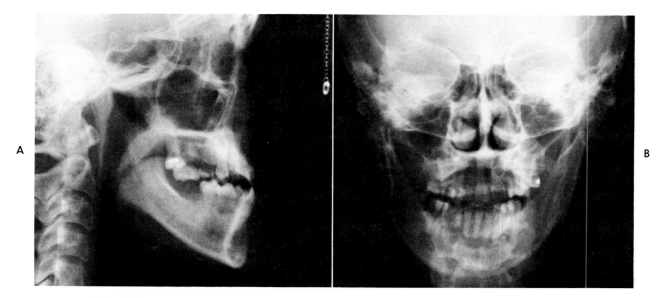

Fig. 15-85. P.M. **A,** Lateral and **B,** PA cephalometric radiographs before treatment. A ^{99}Tc scan was positive for hyperplasia of the left condyle. She was scheduled for LeFort I osteotomy, bilateral sagittal split osteotomies, left condylectomy with recontouring of the condylar stump, inferior border osteotomy to move the chin laterally, and onlay grafts of cranial bone to the infraorbital areas to reduce the appearance of asymmetry at that level.

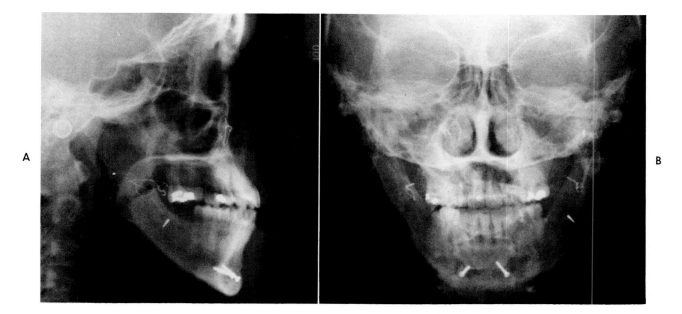

Fig. 15-86. P.M. **A,** Lateral and **B,** PA cephalometric radiographs following surgical treatment. In addition to the rigid fixation for the osteotomies, note the wires to maintain the onlay grafts in the zygomatic areas.

inferior border osteotomy to reposition the chin is planned in addition to surgery to bring the teeth together. In some patients, there may be a choice between extractions in the presurgical orthodontic preparation so that inferior border osteotomy is not necessary and nonextraction treatment in the knowledge that

chin surgery will be used to correct the residual asymmetry. The decision should be made before treatment.

Surgical Considerations

The three-dimensional changes needed for correction of asymmetry are some of the most difficult orthog-

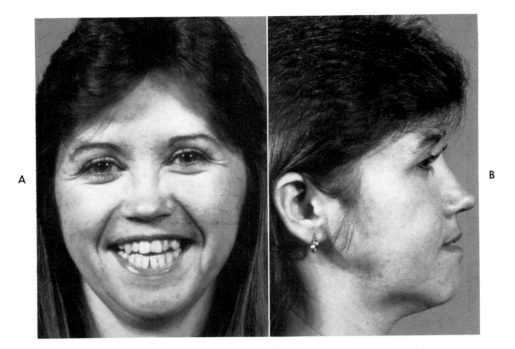

Fig. 15-87. P.M., 12 months following the completion of treatment. Lower face symmetry was greatly improved, and the onlay grafts contributed signficantly to decreasing the appearance of asymmetry higher in the face.

nathic surgical procedures to plan and carry out. Nevertheless, the treatment planning methods described in Chapter 5 and the surgical techniques discussed in Chapters 6 through 11 are applicable, with only minor modifications.

The use of CT scans to provide a three-dimensional view of asymmetric jaw structures has been described above. In orthognathic surgery, the major indication for CT scans is severe asymmetry involving the posterior maxilla and mandible. For these patients, the CT images supplement prediction tracings from lateral and PA cephalometric films.

If a vertically asymmetric maxilla is to be corrected by LeFort I osteotomy, the greater stability of superior versus inferior movement must be kept in mind. Bone grafts with autogenous or allogeneic bank bone frequently are necessary to support at least one side of the maxilla in its new position. The repositioned maxilla may be stabilized with wire fixation or RIF, with rigid fixation more indicated in patients in whom the maxilla is moved down (see Chapter 8).

Severe asymmetry in the mandibular ramus is an indication for an extraoral approach to the affected side, because of the better access and visualization it provides, and a modification of the osteotomy technique. Less extreme mandibular asymmetries can be corrected with standard bilateral sagittal split osteotomies. Asymmetric repositioning of the mandible often makes it necessary to place bone grafts in defects in the ramus osteotomy sites. Correction of three-dimensional asymmetry also makes alignment of jaw segments unpredictable so that RIF across osteotomy sites may not be sufficient to allow jaw function. These patients should be warned that they are likely to require maxillomandibular fixation for 4 to 6 weeks before jaw rehabilitation begins.

The timing of mandibular inferior border osteotomy requires good clinical judgment. For some patients, this can be carried out quite successfully at the same time as LeFort I and mandibular surgery (see Cases 4 and 6). In other cases, inferior border osteotomy is best deferred until 6 months to 1 year following LeFort I and mandibular ramus surgery (as in Case 3). As a general rule, when only moderate asymmetry will remain following maxillary and mandibular ramus osteotomy, delaying the inferior border osteotomy allows a more predictable result because soft-tissue adaptation will be obvious and future change more easily estimated.

Case Reports

Case 5

M.R., age 18 years, 10 months, and a university student contemplating a career in TV broadcasting, was concerned about the protrusion and asymmetry of her upper incisor teeth (Fig. 15-88). She had contemplated orthodontic treatment while in high school but did not want to wear braces for 2 years and inquired about the possibility of quicker treatment with surgery. Dentally, she was nearly a full-cusp Class II, with the maxillary dental midline displaced 3 to 4 mm to the left (Fig. 15-89). Cephalometric analysis confirmed moderate maxillary protrusion and dental but not skeletal asymmetry (Fig. 15-90).

The treatment options considered were extraction of one maxillary right premolar, with comprehensive orthodontic treatment, or nonextraction treatment with surgical retraction and rotation of the maxilla, which also would allow face height to be shortened slightly. The patient was enthusiastic about the surgical approach, primarily because of the presumably shorter treatment time.

After a free gingival graft to the mandibular anterior region was accomplished and all four third molars had been removed, a fixed appliance was placed and alignment was begun with 16 NiTi arch wires. She was anxious to have the surgery done during the Christmas holidays, only 2 months away. With alignment still incomplete, the upper arch was stabilized with a 17×25 arch wire incorporating numerous adjustment bends while the lower arch was left without an arch wire to minimize the chance that the surgical splint would not fit (Figs. 15-91 and 15-92).

At age 19 years, 6 months, a LeFort I osteotomy was done to retract, rotate, and slightly intrude the maxilla. The surgery was performed with a standard Lefort I downfracture technique. Because the maxilla required both rotation to the right and posterior movement (Fig. 15-93), bone was excised from the posterior maxilla and pterygoid plate regions.

At 3 weeks postoperatively, maxillomandibular fixation was released and she was allowed to function into the splint. At 4 weeks, the maxillary stabilizing arch wire was removed and maxillary 16 steel and mandibular 16 NiTi arch wires were placed. This was followed by 17×25 NiTi in the lower arch. She settled into occlu-

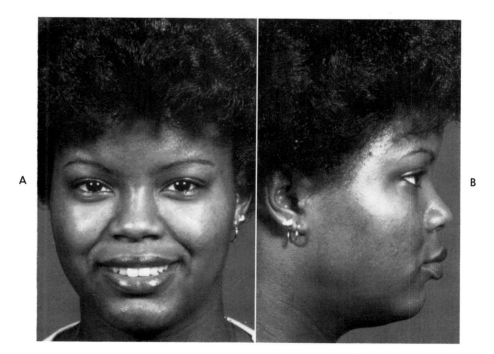

Fig. 15-88. M.R., age 18 years, 10 months, facial appearance before treatment.

Continued.

Case 5—cont'd.

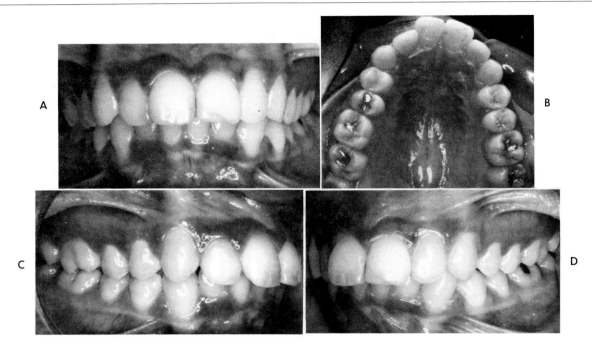

Fig. 15-89. M.R., age 18 years, 10 months, dental relationships before treatment. Note the asymmetry in the maxillary arch, with the midline off to the left.

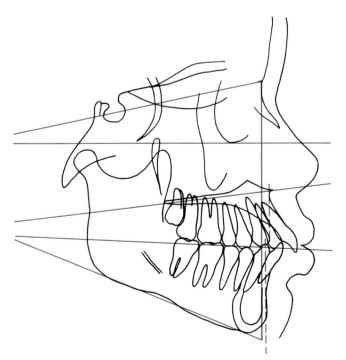

Fig. 15-90. M.R., initial cephalometric tracing. Note the maxillary dentoalveolar protrusion. Cephalometric measurements: N perp to A, 3 mm; N perp to Pg, 2 mm; AB difference, 2 mm; UFH, 53 mm; LFH, 70 mm; mand plane, 22 degrees; MxI to A vert, 12 mm, 34 degrees; MnI to B vert, 7 mm, 27 degrees.

Case 5—cont'd.

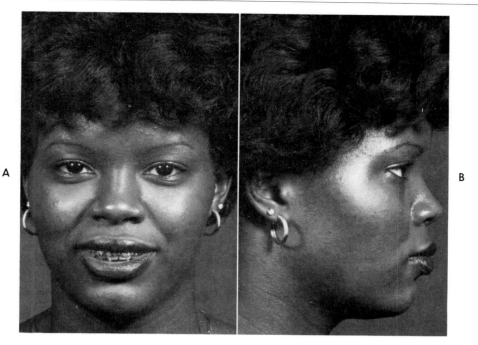

Fig. 15-91. M.R., age 19 years, 6 months, immediately before surgery.

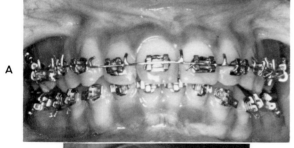

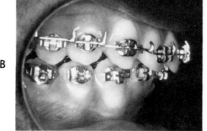

Fig. 15-92. M.R., dental relationships immediately before surgery. Preliminary orthodontic treatment has slightly accentuated the asymmetry as dental compensation was removed. A lower stabilizing arch wire was not used because of concern that it would not be passive and could cause tooth movement after the final presurgical impressions that would keep the splint from fitting.

sion nicely, and the appliances were removed at age 20 years, 2 months, 7 months after postsurgical orthodontics resumed. Retainers were discontinued at age 21 years, with excellent esthetic and functional relationships established (Figs. 15-94 and 15-95). On recall at age 24 years, 3 months, the results were nicely stable (Figs. 15-96 and 15-97).

Comments. Posterior movement of the maxilla is technically difficult because of the need to remove bone posteriorly. The surgeon must be especially careful not to displace the mandibular condyles when checking the occlusal result. Condylar displacement is a common problem when this movement of the maxilla is attempted.

Continued.

Case 5—cont'd.

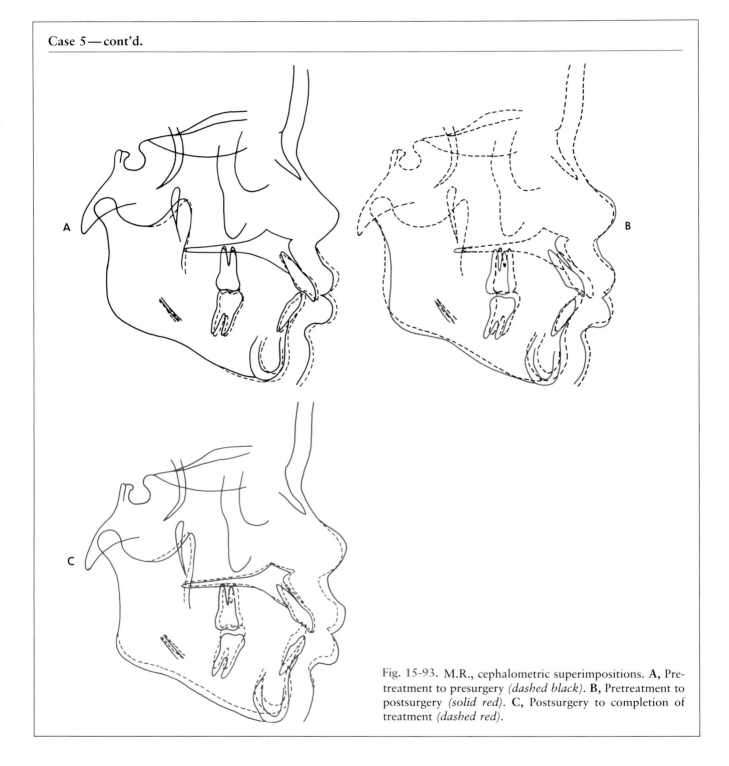

Fig. 15-93. M.R., cephalometric superimpositions. **A,** Pretreatment to presurgery *(dashed black)*. **B,** Pretreatment to postsurgery *(solid red)*. **C,** Postsurgery to completion of treatment *(dashed red)*.

Case 5—cont'd.

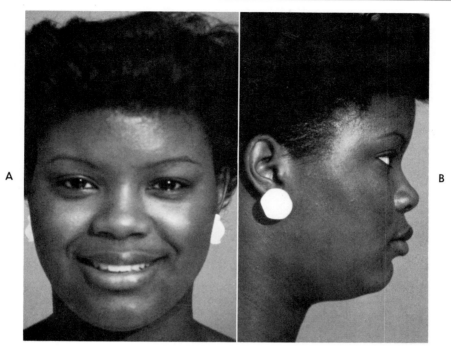

Fig. 15-94. M.R., age 21 years, at the discontinuation of retention.

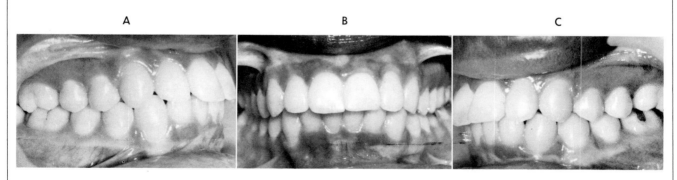

Fig. 15-95. M.R., age 21 years, dental relationships at the discontinuation of retention.

Continued.

Case 5—cont'd.

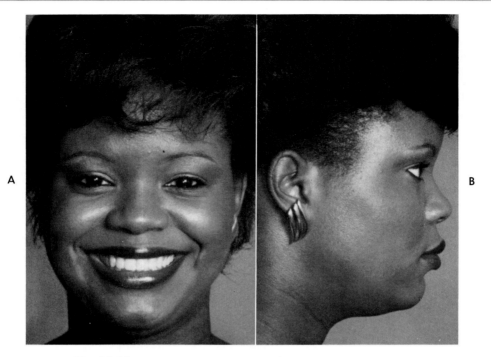

Fig. 15-96. M.R., age 24 years, 3 months, 4¾ years postsurgery.

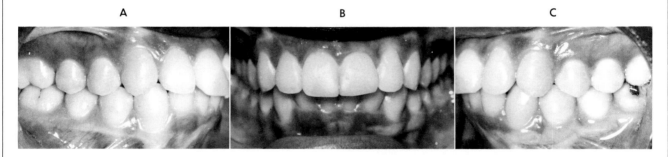

Fig. 15-97. M.R., age 24 years, 3 months, dental relationships 3 years out of retention.

Case 6

C.S., age 31 years, 11 months, sought consultation because of her intermittent TM joint symptoms and her facial asymmetry, which she thought was getting worse (Fig. 15-98). She had been evaluated 1 year previously for TM joint pain/dysfunction but did not follow up with treatment. She had been involved in two automobile accidents in recent years, without serious injury; the medical history was otherwise noncontributory. The teeth were reasonably well interdigitated, with the mandibular midline off to the left and crowding in the lower premolar areas, particularly the left (Fig. 15-99). There was no shift on closure. The panoramic radiograph showed an enlarged right condyle (Fig. 15-100), and PA and lateral cephalometric analysis confirmed excessive growth of the mandible on the right side (Fig. 15-101).

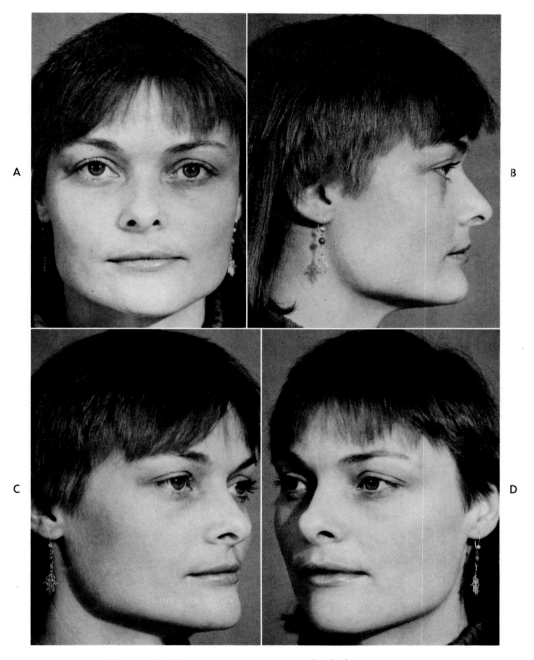

Fig. 15-98. C.S., age 31 years, 11 months, before treatment.

Continued.

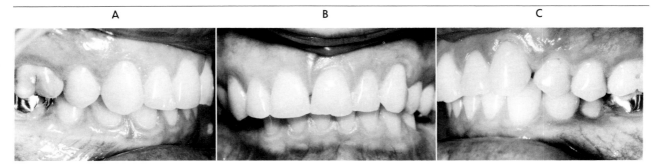

Fig. 15-99. C.S., age 31 years, 11 months, dental relationships before treatment.

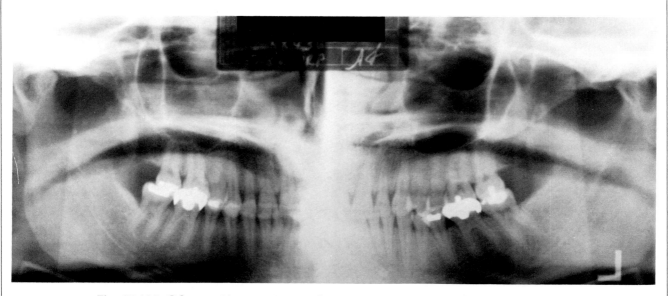

Fig. 15-100. C.S., age 31 years, 11 months, panoramic radiograph showing the enlarged right mandibular condyle.

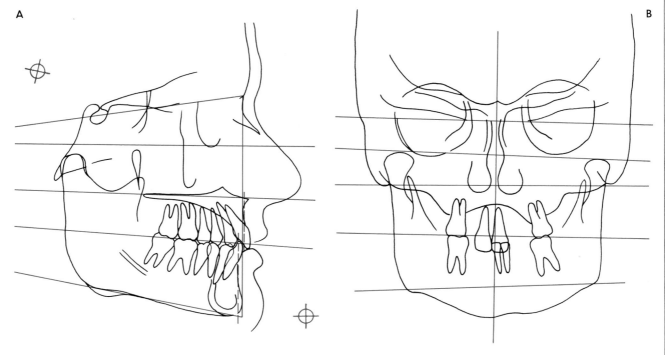

Fig. 15-101. C.S., lateral and PA cephalometric tracings. Note that the asymmetry is due primarily to lengthening of the right ramus, but with canting of the maxilla and deviation of the chin. Dentofacial relationships in the lateral tracing are normal.

Because of her impression of recent change in the asymmetry, a ^{99}Tc scan was done, which was negative for excessive activity in the right condyle. It was decided to align the arches without extraction and observe during the period of preparatory orthodontics to be certain that no further growth was occurring. After 10 months and a succession of arch wires from 16 NiTi to 17×25 steel, surgical lugs were added. No changes in the jaw relationships were observed on repeat lateral and PA cephalometric films, and it was concluded the hemimandibular hypertrophy was now quiescent. The surgical treatment plan was to accept the existing TM joint function and correct the asymmetry with LeFort I osteotomy to level the maxilla, bilateral sagittal split osteotomy to bring the mandible laterally and somewhat posteriorly, and lower border osteotomy to move the chin laterally. Because the maxilla would be moved down on the left side, a homologous bone graft would be needed there (Fig. 15-102).

At surgery, the mandibular rami were exposed and the bone cuts for the sagittal splits were made but not completed, then the maxilla was mobilized, bone was removed in the right posterior area, an intermediate splint was placed and the teeth were brought into maxillomandibular fixation, and the maxillary and mandibular units were rotated down so that the left side of the maxilla was lengthened 3 to 4 mm. Rehydrated freeze-dried allogeneic bank bone was placed bilaterally and wired at the piriform rim and buttress area, then bone plates were used for stabilization (see Fig. 15-102). With maxillomandibular fixation removed, she closed directly into the intermediate splint. The intermediate splint was then removed, the sagittal splits were completed, she was placed in maxillomandibular fixation with the final splint between the teeth, and three 15 mm screws were placed on each side of the ramus for stabilization. Then an incision in the mandibular anterior vestibule was used to approach the chin, which was moved 4 to 5 mm to the right. One unit of autologous blood was transfused postoperatively. She tolerated the surgery well and was discharged on the third postoperative day (Fig. 15-103).

After 1 week, she was allowed to function into the splint with light vertical elastics (Fig. 15-104). At 5 weeks postsurgery, the stabilizing arch wires were removed and 16 steel arch wires were used with light ³/₈-inch box elastics for settling. Appliances were removed 4 months later (Fig. 15-105). During the next year, she had episodes of intermittent TM pain/dysfunction, which gradually subsided. Excellent facial symmetry was maintained (Fig. 15-106).

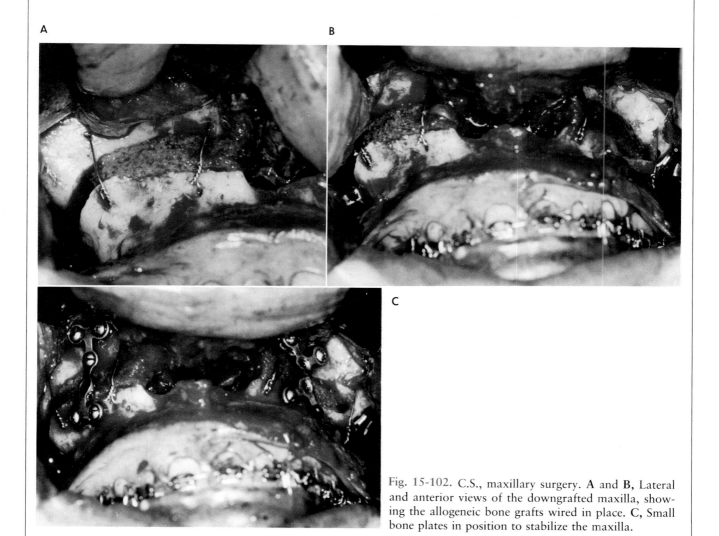

Fig. 15-102. C.S., maxillary surgery. **A** and **B,** Lateral and anterior views of the downgrafted maxilla, showing the allogeneic bone grafts wired in place. **C,** Small bone plates in position to stabilize the maxilla.

Continued

Case 6—cont'd.

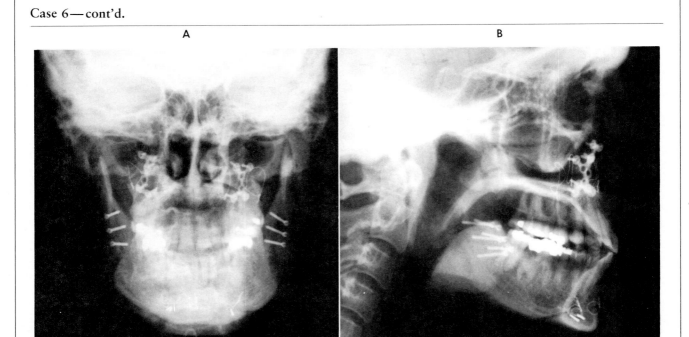

Fig. 15-103. C.S., postoperative PA and lateral cephalometric films.

Comments. Exactly when hemimandibular hypertrophy appeared in this patient is unknown, but she probably experienced additional growth in her late twenties. The enlarged right condyle undoubtedly contributed to the TM joint pain/dysfunction symptoms she experienced both before and after the jaw surgery, but growth was no longer occurring, and we felt that surgical intervention in the joint for this patient was as likely to make things worse as better. The intermittent nature of the pain/dysfunction and its gradual improvement indicate that conservative management of this aspect of the patient's problems probably will succeed (see Chapter 19 for additional discussion of the management of TM joint problems in orthognathic surgery patients).

Case 6—cont'd.

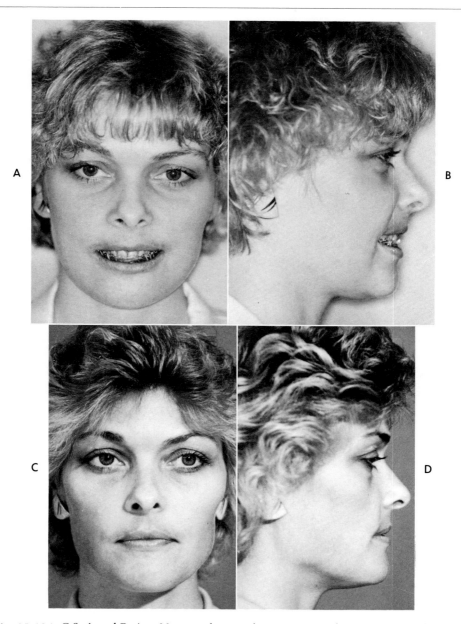

Fig. 15-104. C.S. **A** and **B,** Age 33 years, four weeks postsurgery, functioning into the splint. **C** and **D,** Age 33 years, 4 months, completion of active orthodontics.

Continued.

Case 6—cont'd.

A B C

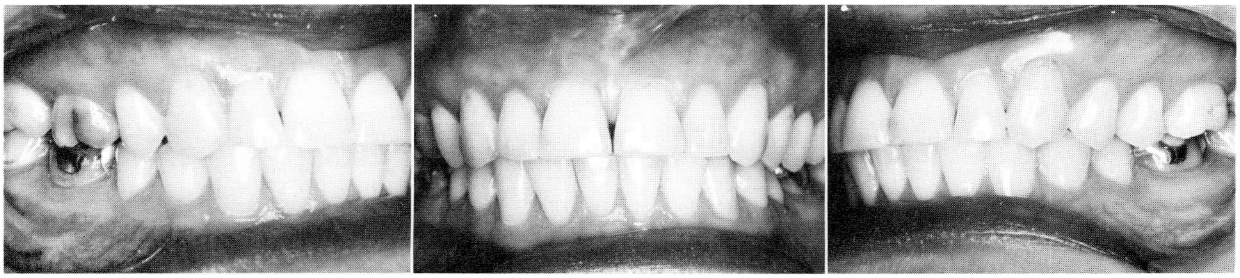

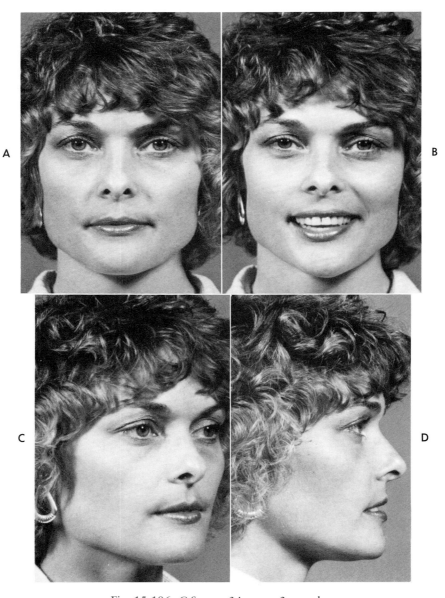

Fig. 15-105. C.S., age 34 years, 2 months, dental relationships at the discontinuation of orthodontic retainers.

A B C D

Fig. 15-106. C.S., age 34 years, 2 months.

REFERENCES

1. Proffit WR, Phillips C: Who seeks surgical-orthodontic treatment? The characteristics of patients evaluated in the UNC Dentofacial Clinic, Int J Adult Orthod Orthognath Surg [in press].
2. Proffit WR, Vig KWL, Turvey TA: Fractures of the mandible condyle: frequently an unsuspected cause of facial asymmetry, Am J Orthod 78:1-24, 1980.
3. Newton TH, Hasso AN, Dillon WP: Computed tomography of the head and neck, New York, 1988, Raven Press.
4. Forsberg CT, Burstone CJ, Hanley KJ: Diagnosis and treatment planning of skeletal asymmetry with the submental-vertex radiograph, Am J Orthod 85:224-237, 1984.
5. Rune B, Sarnas KV, Selvik G, Jacobsson S: Roentgen stereometry in the study of craniofacial anomalies—the state of the art in Sweden, Br J Orthod 13:151-157, 1986.
6. Grayson B, Cutting C, Bookstein FL, et al: The three-dimensional cephalogram: theory, technique and clinical application, Am J Orthod Dentofacial Orthop 94:327-337, 1988.
7. Donlon WC, Young P, Vassiliadis A: Three-dimensional computed tomography for maxillofacial surgery, J Oral Maxillofac Surg 46:142-147, 1988.
8. Vargervik K, Ousterhout DK, Farias M: Factors affecting long-term results in hemifacial microsomia, Cleft Palate J 23(Suppl 1):53-68, 1986.
9. Melsen B, Bjerregaard J, Bundgaard M: The effect of treatment with functional appliance on a pathologic growth pattern of the condyle, Am J Orthod 90:503-512, 1986.
10. Mulliken JB, Kaban LB: Analysis and treatment of hemifacial microsomia in childhood, Clin Plast Surg 14:91-100, 1987.
11. Fields HW, Jr: Skeletal problems in preadolescent children. In Proffit WR (editor): Contemporary orthodontics, St. Louis, 1986, The CV Mosby Co.
12. Vig PS, Vig KW: Hybrid appliances: a component approach to dentofacial orthopedics, Am J Orthod 90:273-285, 1986.
13. Converse JM, McCarthy JG, Wood-Smith D, Coccaro PJ: Craniofacial microsomia. In Converse JM (editor): Reconstructive plastic surgery, ed 2, Philadelphia, 1977, WB Saunders Co.
14. Munro IR: Treatment of craniofacial microsomia, Clin Plast Surg 14:177-186, 1987.
15. Kaban LB, Moses MH, Mulliken JB: Surgical correction of hemifacial microsomia in the growing child, Plast Reconstr Surg 82:9-19, 1988.
16. McCarthy JG (editor): Plastic surgery, ed 3, Philadelphia, 1990, WB Saunders Co.
17. Subtelny JD: The degenerative, regenerative mandibular condyle: facial asymmetry, J Craniofac Genet Dev Biol 1(suppl):227-237, 1985.
18. Lund K: Mandibular growth and remodelling process after mandibular fractures, Acta Odontol Scand 32(Suppl 64), 1974.
19. Hurt TL, Fisher B, Peterson BM, Lynch F: Mandibular fractures in association with chin trauma in pediatric patients, Pediatr Emerg Care 4:121-123, 1988.
20. Amaratunga NA: Mandibular fractures in children—a study of clinical aspects, treatment needs and complications, J Oral Maxillofac Surg 46:637-640, 1988.
21. Jeter TS, van Sickels JE, Nishioka GJ: Intraoral open reduction with RIF of mandibular subcondylar fractures, J Oral Maxillofac Surg 46:1113-1116, 1988.
22. Politis C, Fossion E, Bossuyt M: The use of costochondral grafts in arthroplasty of the TM joint, J Craniomaxillofac Surg 6:345-354, 1987.
23. Poswillo DE: Biological reconstruction of the mandibular condyle, Br J Oral Maxillofac Surg 25:100-104, 1987.
24. Kummoona R: Chrondro-osseous iliac crest graft for one stage reconstruction of the ankylosed TMJ in children, J Maxillofac Surg 14:215-220, 1986.
25. Daniels S, Ellis E, Carlson DS: Histologic analysis of costochondral and sternoclavicular grafts in the TMJ of the juvenile monkey, J Oral Maxillofac Surg 45:675-683, 1987.
26. Lindqvist C, Pihakari A, Tasanen A, Hampf G: Autogenous costochondral grafts in TM joint arthroplasty: a survey of 66 arthroplasties in 60 patients, J Maxillofac Surg 14:143-149, 1986.
27. Obeid G, Guttenberg SA, Connole PW: Costochondral grafting in condylar replacement and mandibular reconstruction, J Oral Maxillofac Surg 46:177-182, 1988.
28. Lindqvist C, Jokinen J, Paukku P, Tasanen A: Adaptation of autogenous costochondral grafts used for TM joint reconstruction: a long term clinical and radiologic follow-up, J Oral Maxillofac Surg 46:465-470, 1988.
29. Obwegeser HL, Makek MS: Hemimandibular hyperplasia—hemimandibular elongation, J Maxillofac Surg 14:183-208, 1986.
30. Matteson SR, Proffit WR, Terry BC, et al: The use of bone scanning with 99mTechnetium phosphate to assess condylar hyperplasia: a review and report of two cases, Oral Surg Oral Med Oral Pathol 60:356-367, 1985.
31. Boyne PJ: Free grafting of traumatically displaced or resected mandibular condyles, J Oral Maxillofac Surg 47:228-232, 1989.
32. Waite PD, Matukas VJ, Sarver DM: Simultaneous rhinoplasty procedures in orthognathic surgery, Int J Oral Maxillofac Surg 17:298-302, 1988.

CHAPTER 16

Crossbite and Open-Bite Problems

William R. Proffit
Raymond P. White, Jr.

In previous chapters, our focus has been on the correction of distorted jaw relationships and the malocclusion that accompanies them. This chapter, in contrast, is oriented toward two types of malocclusion, posterior crossbite and open bite, that may require surgical-orthodontic treatment even though the problem is more dentoalveolar than skeletal. More often than not, a patient with severe posterior crossbite also has an open bite or an open-bite tendency, both of which are re-

lated to an abnormal jaw relationship. Often the underlying problem is the long-face condition that is discussed in detail in Chapter 13. Unilateral crossbite is likely to reflect skeletal asymmetry, and this is covered in Chapter 15. But crossbite or open-bite problems severe enough to warrant surgical intervention can occur in patients who do not have a major skeletal problem. Our objective here is to differentiate these patients from their more common skeletal counterparts and to discuss appropriate orthodontic and surgical-orthodontic treatment for them.

For crossbite/open-bite problems, as with most developmental conditions, surgery is reserved almost entirely for nongrowing patients, but it is important to review treatment options in younger individuals to provide an appropriate background. Because crossbite and open bite are so linked during development, the discussion for children is focused on their combination. Transverse problems and the unusual open bites that are not related to the long-face condition are described separately for adults.

OPEN-BITE/CROSSBITE PROBLEMS IN CHILDREN
Etiologic Considerations

Anterior open bite combined with posterior crossbite is quite common in young children. Prolonged thumbsucking tends to create this malocclusion, and a surprisingly large number of children continue to suck a thumb, finger, or other object well into the elementary school years[1] (Fig. 16-1). The same sucking habit that impedes eruption of the incisors also facilitates eruption of the posterior teeth and narrows the upper arch. Thus a typical 8-year-old thumbsucker has a malocclusion characterized by anterior open bite, slightly excessive face height, and transverse constriction of the maxillary arch (Fig. 16-2).

This oversimplified description needs several points

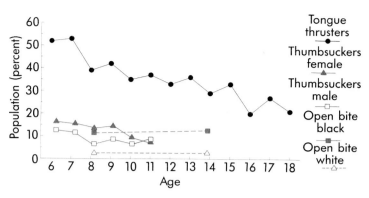

Fig. 16-1. The prevalence of tongue thrusting (whites), thumb sucking (males and females, all races), and open bite (blacks and whites) in American children. (Tongue thrusting data from Fletcher SG, Casteel RL, Bradley DP: Tongue thrust swallowing, speech articulation and age, J Speech Hear Disord 26:201-208, 1961; thumb sucking and open bite data from Kelly JE, Sanchez M, van Kirk LE: An assessment of the occlusion of teeth of children, US Public Health Service DHEW Pub No (HRA) 74-1612, Washington, DC, 1973, National Center for Health Statistics. Redrawn from Proffit WR: Contemporary Orthodontics, St. Louis, 1986, The CV Mosby Co.)

of clarification. First, not all children who suck their thumb develop malocclusion. In Fig. 16-1, compare the prevalence of thumbsucking with the prevalence of open bite and crossbite. At every age, thumbsucking is more prevalent than the problems it is said to cause. This does not mean that there is no relationship, only that a thumbsucker has about a 75% chance of developing a malocclusion, not a 100% chance. It seems most likely that children must engage in the sucking habit for more than a threshhold number of hours per day to significantly affect the position of the teeth (see Chapter 2).

Second, habit patterns are often not reported accurately to dentists, who are well known for their disapproval of thumbsucking. It should come as no surprise,

therefore, that the number of children reported as thumbsuckers differs markedly when a dentist or a neutral observer (e.g., a school nurse) inquires. Dentists are quite likely to encounter children who have an open bite but are said not to have a sucking habit. If an open bite exists, a neurologically normal child will place his or her tongue into the opening while swallowing. Essentially every open-bite child, therefore, will be observed to have a tongue-thrust swallow. That observation should carry no etiologic implication. Unfortunately, there is a strong tendency for some dentists and speech therapists to blame the malocclusion on the tongue, particularly when the parents and child deny a sucking habit. As we have discussed in some detail in Chapter 2, a tongue-thrust swallow is much more likely to be an adaptation to the open bite than the other way around, and therapy aimed at changing the swallow pattern is not indicated.

Third, if open bite/crossbite in a young child were due to thumbsucking, one would expect that the malocclusion would correct spontaneously if the etiologic agent were removed. That is not quite true. Experience has shown that the open bite has an excellent chance of correcting spontaneously, but usually it is necessary to expand the upper arch to correct the crossbite. Correcting the crossbite by expanding the maxillary arch also seems to facilitate the closure of the open bite. The treatment and response shown in Figs. 16-3 to 16-6 are typical.

Finally, it is important to differentiate the effects of thumbsucking from more general distortions of growth that produce skeletal jaw discrepancies. A child with normal growth is quite likely to recover from any dental changes produced by a sucking habit. But children with growth problems also suck their thumb, and the growth problem and its associated malocclusion will remain even if the sucking habit is stopped. The prognosis for a child with open bite/crossbite, therefore, is determined best from an examination of the skeletal relationships, not from the severity of the dental maloc-

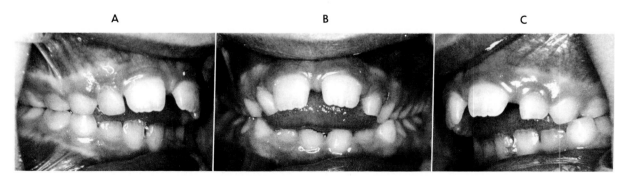

Fig. 16-2. P.C., age 8 years, 6 months, before orthodontic treatment. Note the open bite, incisor protrusion, and posterior crossbite, the classic malocclusion resulting from prolonged thumbsucking. The parents report that thumbsucking stopped a few months previously.

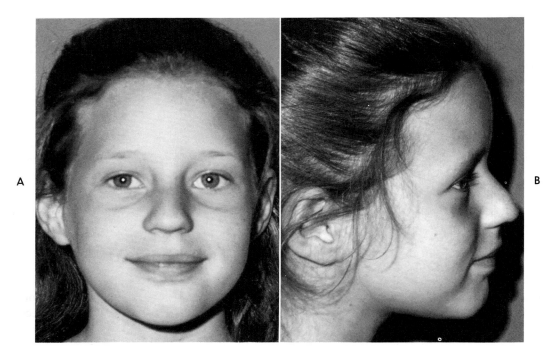

Fig. 16-3. P.C., facial appearance before treatment. Note the good facial proportions despite the malocclusion. (Courtesy of the National Institutes of Health.)

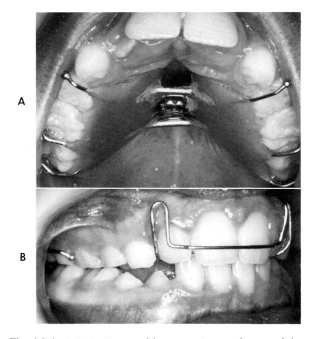

Fig. 16-4. P.C. **A,** Removable expansion appliance of the type used in her treatment (in another patient). **B,** Correction of open bite and protrusion 6 months later, after the expansion appliance was replaced by a second removable appliance to close the space between the upper incisors. In essence, the open bite corrected spontaneously when the posterior crossbite was corrected and the incisors were retracted.

clusion. Although a mild elongation of face height can be attributed to a sucking habit, if facial proportions differ significantly from normal, the problem is likely to be more than just thumbsucking.

In summary: (1) in 6- to 9-year-old children, open bite and posterior crossbite are seen together in thumbsuckers (who are likely to deny it); (2) correction of the problem often requires only transverse expansion of the narrowed maxillary arch—the open bite usually corrects spontaneously when the growth pattern is normal; and (3) the prognosis is determined by the growth pattern. There is no harm in early correction of the crossbite, and this may lead to correction of the open bite as well—but it also may not, depending on the growth pattern. Spontaneous correction does not occur when the long-face condition is present. Almost always, the long-face condition is developing in the children who do not show improvement in the open bite (see Chapter 13 for a more detailed discussion of treatment possibilities in this situation).

Treatment of Crossbite: Indications for Opening the Midpalatal Suture

A narrow maxillary arch can be expanded in two ways: dentally, by tipping (or torquing) the teeth buccally, and skeletally, by increasing the width of the palate. In the late 19th century, palatal expansion was frequently proposed as the best treatment for children with crossbite and open bite (most of whom in retrospect had a long-face problem). Its proponents felt that the procedure not only corrected the crossbite but also

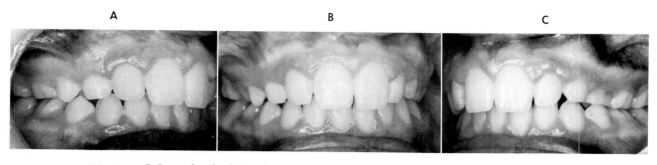

Fig. 16-5. P.C., occlusal relationships age 11 years, 9 months, 2 years after the initial treatment was completed and the retainer was discontinued.

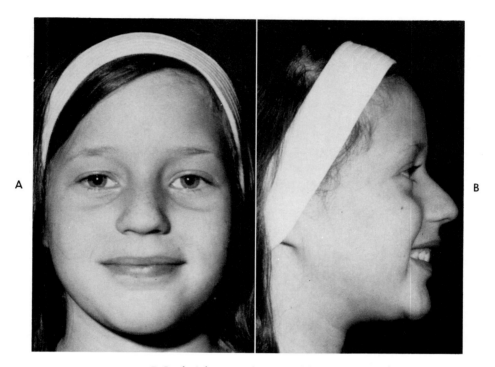

Fig. 16-6. P.C., facial proportions age 11 years, 9 months.

facilitated nasal breathing and thus attacked the root cause of the growth problem (a point of view that has reappeared recently, with no more evidence to support it now than it had then—see Chapters 2 and 13). In the United States, palatal expansion was abandoned in favor of dental expansion in the early 20th century, not because it was ineffective but because it was thought to be unnecessary. The prevailing opinion was that with proper torque, bone would grow around the teeth when dental expansion was carried out.[2] The procedure continued to be used in Europe, and was revived in the United States in the 1960s after Haas[3] and others[4,5] confirmed its clinical potential.

In modern usage, the primary indication for opening the midpalatal suture in a patient with a narrow maxilla is a simple one—transverse deficiency of the width of the palatal vault. The ideal patient would have a combination of dental and skeletal deficiency because

tooth movement always is produced by the force systems designed to open the suture. At this point, sutural expansion is widely employed, usually to correct crossbites due to a narrow maxillary arch,[6,7] but sometimes also in children who have no crossbite to create space for nonextraction treatment of dental crowding problems. This second use is highly controversial. Because it is not related to treatment of transverse problems and not relevant to surgical-orthodontic treatment, it is not included in the discussion here.

When transverse force is applied, the midpalatal suture does not open equally from the front to the back. Instead, it tends to open more anteriorly than posteriorly; typically, there is about a 3:2 ratio between expansion across the canines and the molars. For many patients, this is an advantage because the arch is relatively narrower across the canines. For others, it is a disadvantage that perhaps can be compensated with later tooth movement to change arch form. The differential movement of the palatal bony shelves is a reflection of the greater lateral buttressing of the posterior maxilla. As force is applied, it is a mistake to think only of the midpalatal suture. Changes at the lateral and superior sutures also are necessary, and these sutures contribute substantially to the resistance to the midpalatal opening. Vertically, the maxilla opens as if on a hinge from the bridge of the nose, and patients sometimes report pressure (but almost never pain) in that area.

To some extent, the amount of transversely directed force determines whether only tooth movement occurs or whether there is a combination of tooth movement and separation of the bony palatal shelves. It appears that there is an age-dependent force threshhold. Below this, only tooth movement occurs; above it, the suture opens (but of course tooth movement continues if force is applied to the teeth). As a child matures, the resistance to suture separation increases. Recent research suggests 1 to 2 pounds of force are enough to open the suture in mixed-dentition children, whereas 2 to 4 pounds are needed to accomplish this in adolescents.[8] In an adolescent, when a jackscrew is activated at the typical rate for rapid expansion, forces in the 16- to 20-pound range are generated.[9] These data provide some insight into the possibilities of accomplishing sutural expansion with various devices.

In a young child, there is every reason to believe that maxillary expansion with a lingual arch produces some expansion at the midpalatal suture.[10] The ratio between tooth movement and sutural expansion is not known, but it is unlikely that more than 50% of the expansion would be sutural in any case. As is the case with later expansion, this early expansion tends to relapse: 20% to 40% of the gain in arch width typically is lost.[11] When resistance is low, a simple expansion device such as a removable appliance with a jackscrew might also be capable of widening the palate. Frankel has suggested that with his "function regulator," even with no direct attachment to the teeth, the buccal shields stretch the periosteum enough to produce expansion at the suture as well as buccal movement of the molars.[12] Although it is hard to envision enough force to open the suture being derived from the stretched tissues, the contours of the palate do seem to change during early expansion with the Frankel appliance,[13] and it may be that even the indirect effects of this appliance can increase the rate of normal growth across the suture.

By the time a child approaches adolescence, sutural resistance has increased, and the percentage of skeletal expansion produced by orthodontic appliances decreases significantly. Only a rigidly mounted appliance across the palate offers the prospect of palatal rather than dental expansion.

Rapid versus Slow Palatal Expansion in Adolescents

Although palatal expansion does not have to be rapid, and indeed is not when it occurs naturally, the technique of rapid palatal expansion is so commonly used that the acronym *RPE* often is used to describe any sutural expansion technique. The idea behind expanding the palate rapidly was that this would maximize skeletal relative to dental change. The force to open the suture would be applied to the maxillary posterior teeth, but it would be heavy enough and applied rapidly enough that essentially all the change would be produced by opening the suture—the teeth would not have time to respond. This was true enough, as far as the analysis went. If a jackscrew across the palate is opened at the rate of 0.5 mm/day, a commonly recommended rate, 10 mm of expansion will be produced in 20 days. At that point, 75% to 80% of the total expansion will be skeletal change due to opening of the suture, whereas only 20% to 25% will be tooth movement (Fig. 16-7).[14]

When rapid expansion was popularized, the phenomenon of skeletal relapse made possible by orthodontic tooth movement had not been recognized. This pattern of relapse was first noted following surgical mandibular advancement. In these patients, although the teeth remained in the presurgical occlusion, the chin slipped posteriorly (see Chapter 12 for a more complete discussion). Only recently did clinicians realize that the same thing happens after rapid maxillary expansion. The expansion appliance is left in place for 2 to 3 months after the active expansion is completed, so that new bone can fill in—and orthodontic tooth movement occurs, allowing the lateral maxillary segments to move back toward the midline although the intermolar width is maintained. In children in the 8 to 12 years age group, the net result following treatment is approximately a half and half combination of dental and skeletal expansion; in the 12 to 18 years age range, the expansion is about two-thirds dental, one-third skeletal.[15]

When the suture is opened rapidly, histologic studies in animals have shown that the tissues are torn apart, with cell death and hemorrhage into the tissue spaces.[16] Microfractures and other evidence of disruption of the suture can be seen in humans.[17] What would happen if the suture were opened more slowly? Histologic studies suggest that expansion at the rate of 1 mm/week should be possible without tissue damage. In monkeys, expansion at this slower rate produces about equal dental and skeletal change,[18] and slow expansion seems clinically successful in children also.[8]

For slow expansion, the original recommendation was a spring activated by the orthodontist that would apply a reasonably constant force for several weeks. The amount of force on the spring was varied according to the patient's age. This method also can be used

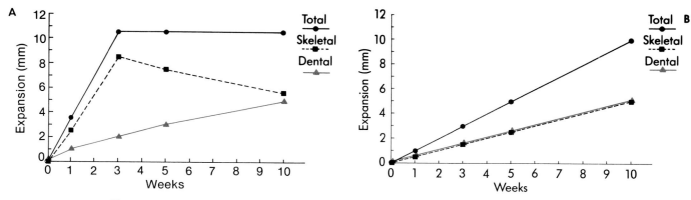

Fig. 16-7. A hypothetical plot of skeletal versus dental changes; **A**, rapid compared with **B**, slow palatal expansion. With rapid expansion, the proportion of skeletal versus dental change is large initially because the teeth cannot move more than 1 to 2 mm in the short term. After the expansion is completed, however, tooth movement while the dentition is stabilized allows the jaw segments to relapse medially even though the intermolar distance is maintained, so by the time bone continuity has been reestablished at 10 weeks, approximately equal dental and skeletal expansion is obtained. (Data from implant studies in humans suggest that in children in the 8 to 12 years age range, expansion is 50% skeletal, 50% dental; in the 12 to 18 years age group, the expansion is about 35% skeletal, 65% dental.[14]) With slow expansion in younger patients, approximately a 50-50 ratio (less in older patients, as with rapid expansion)[8] is obtained from the beginning, so the final result of rapid versus slow expansion is about the same. The long-term relapse tendency also seems to be quite similar with the two methods: 1 year after retention is discontinued, total relapse is about 40%.

with one of the standard jackscrew-based expansion appliances simply by having the patient or parent turn the screw less frequently. One turn of the screw (¼ mm) every other day produces 1 mm of expansion in 8 days, the desired rate.

Whether the expansion appliance is activated rapidly or slowly, it is preferable to distribute the expansion force over as many teeth as possible. For rapid expansion, a palatally positioned jackscrew is mounted within a heavy framework that is attached to the first molars and braced against other teeth as available (Fig. 16-8). Plastic flanges that contact the palatal mucosa

may or may not be employed. The argument for them is that this produces greater skeletal expansion by preventing or at least decreasing the amount of buccal tipping of the abutment teeth. The arguments against are that a combination of pressure against the mucosa and irritation by food trapped beneath the flanges is likely to produce tissue irritation and that the clinical results are essentially identical whether or not the flanges are used. There is no doubt that tissue irritation can be a problem, so the flanges do have a definite disadvantage, and the clinical results with or without flanges seem very similar. We conclude that for most patients,

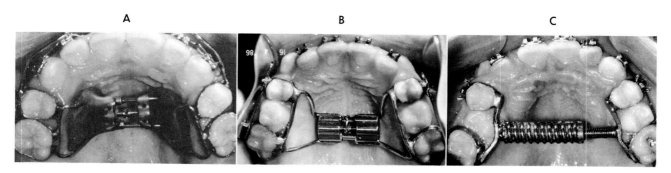

Fig. 16-8. Palatal expansion in adolescents requires a heavy framework for rigidity of the appliance against the large forces (10 to 20 pounds with rapid expansion) that will be encountered. **A**, Haas-type expander with acrylic flanges that contact the palatal mucosa. **B**, Hyrax expander with a metal framework and jackscrew. **C**, Minn expander, which incorporates a spring to smooth the force application (but still can produce quite heavy forces).

the disadvantages outweigh the advantages.

When the expansion is carried out slowly, it is reasonably stable when the active treatment is completed (i.e., the expansion device can be removed at that point, approximately 12 weeks after the expansion began, and replaced by a conventional retainer). After rapid expansion over a 2- to 3-week period, the expansion device must be left in place until new bone fills in, usually another 8 to 12 weeks. Whether expansion is rapid or slow, the total time the patient wears the rather bulky expansion device is approximately the same.

With both rapid and slow expansion, however, retention for at least another 6 months is required to control a considerable relapse tendency. One year after retention was discontinued, Timms[19] reported a mean relapse of dental (total) expansion of 41%. Implant studies suggest that about 70% of the skeletal expansion gained initially (which was not more than 50% of the total) is maintained after 1 year of retention.[15]

Growth in width of the face is essentially completed by age 16 or 17. By then, a jackscrew is increasingly likely to produce pain and, if the patient can tolerate that, only tooth movement without sutural separation. The problem is not an absolute fusion of the sutures but an increasing interdigitation at both the midpalatal and lateral maxillary sutures that causes higher and higher resistance to lateral expansion of the bony shelves.[20]

CROSSBITE PROBLEMS IN ADULTS

At this point, we must reiterate that this chapter is not oriented toward the majority of patients with posterior crossbite who have higher priority skeletal problems in other planes of space, often related to the long-face condition. Instead, the focus here is on the less frequent problems that are primarily related to the transverse plane of space. Patients who need a combination of surgery and orthodontics primarily for correction of posterior crossbite can be divided into three major categories: (1) postadolescents with a narrowed maxilla who would be candidates for palatal expansion if they were not already too old for this treatment approach, (2) patients with an excessively wide mandible, and (3) patients with all or part of the mandibular arch locked within the maxillary (i.e., the condition sometimes referred to as scissors bite or [if bilateral] Brodie syndrome).

Patients with a Narrow Maxilla

The two general possibilities for surgical treatment of a narrow maxilla in an adult are (1) a partial osteotomy to reduce the resistance to expansion so that the lateral dentoalveolar segments can be repositioned with a jackscrew (i.e., surgically assisted maxillary expansion) or (2) a total osteotomy to free the maxilla and

divide it into lateral segments that can be repositioned at the time of operation. Orthodontists often encounter a patient, typically in the late teens, who has a posterior crossbite and narrowed maxilla that would be treated with palatal expansion if he or she were younger. At this age, the chances of successful palatal expansion are slim, or perhaps there already has been an unsuccessful attempt at expansion that proves the chance is zero. If the question "Can surgery be used to make palatal expansion possible?" is asked, the answer is yes. An osteotomy in the lateral buttress area and/or in the palate significantly reduces resistance to expansion and makes widening the palate possible.[21-23] The more appropriate question is subtly but significantly different: "Should surgery be limited to making palatal expansion possible?" Then the answer often is no. It is one thing to note that surgery would be the only way to widen the palate and something else entirely to conclude that surgery to reduce resistance to a jackscrew is needed.

Surgically Assisted Rapid Palatal Expansion

In choosing between the surgical alternatives of partial or complete maxillary osteotomy, several guidelines are helpful and are discussed below.

If the patient will require orthognathic surgery for other problems after the transverse discrepancy has been corrected, there is little or no reason to do surgery twice. Patients with skeletal problems in the AP and/or vertical planes of space, as we have already pointed out, are not the focus of this chapter, but questions of surgically assisted expansion often arise. The typical example is a long-face patient with a narrow maxilla who will need a LeFort I osteotomy to superiorly reposition the maxilla. In our view, little or no reason exists to do surgically assisted expansion, then do the total maxillary osteotomy at a later time. Instead, we recommend that the transverse problem be dealt with by segmenting the maxilla at the time of the LeFort I osteotomy. Almost always a transverse discrepancy can be corrected along with vertical and AP problems in a single stage of surgery.

Two possible advantages of two-stage surgery in patients of this type have been suggested. First, if no palatal expansion were needed because it had already been accomplished, the LeFort osteotomy would be less complex and the chance of complications would be reduced. Although this might be true for the second stage, the slightly increased risk of problems with a two- or three-piece LeFort I osteotomy versus a one-piece LeFort I osteotomy is more than offset by the chance of encountering more problems in two surgical procedures than in one. Second, it is conceivable that the expansion produced with a jackscrew could be more stable than that produced via LeFort I osteotomy—but no data are available to support this conclusion.

Surgically assisted expansion is most successful in younger adults. The technique of surgically assisting palatal expansion involves reducing the resistance to expansion by making osteotomy cuts in the lateral maxillary buttress (the preferred choice) or in the palate (no longer recommended). The force from the screw then can be concentrated on the remaining suture area. Because sutures become more and more interdigitated with increasing age, the older the patient, the greater the residual resistance from areas that were not freed with an osteotomy. Surgically assisted expansion via lateral maxillary osteotomies is a reasonably predictable procedure in patients below age 25, has a greater chance of failure in the 25 to 35 years age group, and probably should not be attempted in patients over 35.

The major indication, therefore, for surgically assisted maxillary expansion is in a younger patient with only a transverse problem. In this situation, the reduced morbidity of the partial osteotomy (which can be done as an outpatient or day-operation procedure) is an advantage compared with a total maxillary osteotomy.

Unilateral or asymmetric narrowing of the maxilla also may be an indication for surgically assisted expansion (see Case 1). If osteotomy cuts are made on only one side, a differential anchorage situation is created, and activation of a jackscrew will produce more expansion on the osteotomized side. This provides almost the only way to deal with an upper arch that is severely asymmetrically narrowed. The previous guideline still applies, however: if the maxilla would require surgery for another reason, the segments can be repositioned unilaterally and that time, and there is no reason to do surgically assisted unilateral expansion as the first of two surgical stages.

If surgically assisted expansion is used, the screw should be opened rapidly rather than slowly. This guideline is based on our judgment that significant resistance from the area of osteotomy might begin to reappear after 4 to 6 weeks of healing; therefore the expansion should be completed within that time frame. To our knowledge, there are no reports of slow expansion following lateral osteotomies.

Whether the expansion involved a partial or total osteotomy, orthodontic retention for at least 12 months is needed because the risk of relapse following palatal expansion is relatively high. With surgically assisted expansion, the rigid jackscrew appliance should remain in place at least 2 months (as with any rapid palatal expansion patient), and a fixed retainer for another 6 to 12 months is a good idea. There are no good data for stability after surgically assisted expansion, except comments that it is clinically satisfactory. One would expect approximately the same stability as with nonsurgical expansion.

Osteotomy for Transverse Expansion

The alternative to surgically assisted expansion is an osteotomy to totally free the posterior maxillary segments so that the surgeon can place them in the proper position without having to overcome sutural resistance. This can be accomplished with bilateral posterior segmental osteotomies, but as a practical matter it usually is done with LeFort I osteotomy, segmenting the maxilla from the downfractured position (see Chapters 8 and 10). Stability after superior repositioning of the maxilla has been discussed in Chapter 13, and stability after maxillary advancement in Chapter 14. How stable is surgical transverse expansion?

The most complete data set currently available is from a study by Medland and colleagues[24,25] at the UNC, based on 209 patients who had orthognathic surgery between August 1985 and December 1986. Of these, 61 (29%) had segmental LeFort I osteotomy with the segments expanded surgically at least 1 mm at the first molars. The data for transverse stability are derived from the 42 patients of that group for whom follow-up dental casts could be obtained. Two segments (dividing the maxilla by parasagittal bone cuts) were created at the osteotomy for 26 patients; 13 had three segments (anterior and bilateral posterior), and 3 had four segments (bilateral anterior and posterior). RIF was used in 13 patients, 8 had bone grafts, 30 had an auxiliary labial arch wire at surgery, and 26 had the labial wire continued during the postsurgical orthodontics.

The data show a considerable relapse tendency (Fig. 16-9). The greatest expansion occurred in the second molar region, which is a necessity with a two-segment osteotomy and often occurs in multisegment cases; the greatest relapse also occurred there. Conversely, both the least expansion and the least relapse tendency were noted at the canines, which were not expanded at all in most of the three-segment patients. The mean relapse of 47% at the first molar can be compared with the 41% relapse reported in the most comparable study of orthodontic rapid palatal expansion.[19]

The variability within the sample is emphasized in Fig. 16-9, *B*, showing the number of patients who had changes of various magnitudes. Note that two-thirds of the patients had relapse at the first molars, with 20% showing more than 3 mm of transverse collapse. At the first premolars, 40% had some relapse and only 1 patient had more than 3 mm of change. Conversely, of course, the expansion was stable at the first molars in one-third of the patients and was stable at the first premolars in nearly two-thirds.

The presence of relapse does not necessarily mean that the treatment was clinically unsuccessful. In an earlier series of 103 expansion patients, Turvey[26] reported that only 7 of 103 maxillary surgery patients had "significant crossbite" at the end of treatment. In the Medland sample, 29% had at least one tooth in

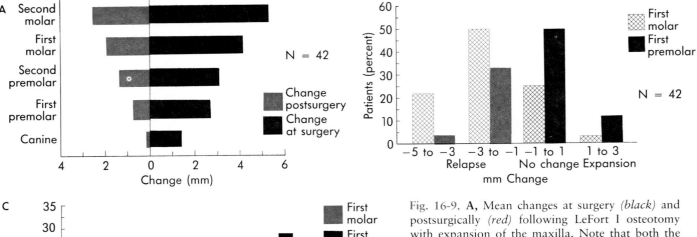

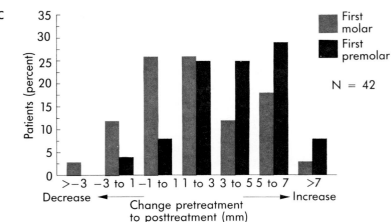

Fig. 16-9. **A,** Mean changes at surgery *(black)* and postsurgically *(red)* following LeFort I osteotomy with expansion of the maxilla. Note that both the greatest expansion and the greatest relapse occurred in the second molar region. **B,** The percent of the patients who had postsurgical changes in arch width at the first molars and first premolars. Relapse at the first molars occurred in two-thirds of the patients and was severe (> 3 mm) in 20%; at the first premolars, 40% had some relapse but only one patient had > 3 mm change. **C,** The percent of the patients with net changes in arch width at the first molars and first premolars. Because the initial expansion was greater at the molars, the net change also was greater there despite the increased relapse tendency posteriorly. Note that a few patients had a net decrease in arch width at both locations.

crossbite at the end of treatment, which might or might not be considered significant. There was a tendency for mandibular arch width to decrease during treatment, presumably as a result of the orthodontics, which helped to control crossbite tendencies.

Although one would expect that stability or relapse would be correlated with treatment variables, this was not borne out by analysis of the data. Relapse was not significantly related to the type or extent of presurgical orthodontic tooth movement, the number of segments at surgery, the amount of surgical expansion, rigid versus wire fixation, or use of an auxiliary stabilizing arch wire. Because the subsamples to test these effects were small, one cannot conclude that these factors are totally unimportant, but they do not appear to be major influences on stability.

It should be noted that the pattern of expansion with complete osteotomy usually is quite different from the expansion with a jackscrew appliance, whether or not it is surgically assisted. In the patients having an osteotomy, there was more expansion posteriorly than anteriorly. The second molars were expanded twice as much as the first premolars in the surgical group described above. In contrast, with a jackscrew appliance, more expansion occurs anteriorly than posteriorly because the resis-

tance to expansion is greater posteriorly. Perhaps a greater relapse tendency should be expected when there is major expansion across the second molars.

Without implants as markers and a series of postsurgical radiographs (a type of study that no longer can be arranged), there is no way to know what portion of the relapse was skeletal change and what was lingual movement of the maxillary posterior teeth. From these data, however, we conclude that surgical expansion via total osteotomy, like expansion with a jackscrew, is a relatively unstable movement. Overcorrection at the time of surgery to allow for some apparently inevitable relapse, surgical techniques to maximize stability, and transpalatal lingual arches as fixed orthodontic retainers are recommended.

Patients with a Wide Mandibular Arch

In planning surgical-orthodontic treatment, one key question is when a transverse discrepancy should be treated in the maxilla, and when the mandible should be the focus of treatment. Two somewhat contradictory guidelines are applicable: (1) the problem should be treated in the jaw that it is primarily at fault, but (2) if in doubt, widen the maxilla, particularly posteriorly, instead of narrowing the mandible.

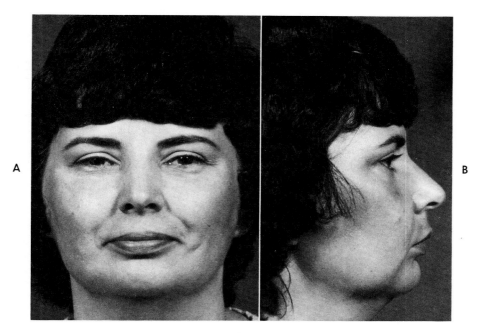

Fig. 16-10. L.D., age 40. Two years previously, she experienced severe pain upon chewing, which was partially controlled by biofeedback but was persistent enough to cause her to seek further treatment. She had no dental or facial esthetic concerns.

The reasoning is straightforward. Narrowing the mandible anteriorly is technically feasible, though difficult in some cases; narrowing it posteriorly is complicated by the fact that the condyles cannot be brought closer together. Mandibular intermolar width can be decreased surgically by a small but not a large amount. In contrast, widening the posterior maxilla surgically up to 1 cm presents no particular technical difficulties.

Although the emphasis here is on patients with a primary crossbite problem due to excess mandibular width, a comment about the width implications of surgery for other problems is necessary. Surgically, there are two practical methods to make the mandible narrower: (1) remove bone anteriorly via a step osteotomy/ostectomy near the midline—this procedure shortens the mandible somewhat but has its major impact on width, or (2) remove bone bilaterally in the premolar region via a body ostectomy (see Chapter 5, Fig. 5-4; see Chapter 10 for details of the surgical procedure). The body ostectomy procedure is used primarily to set the mandible back, but a major reason for selecting it instead of a ramus osteotomy for some prognathic patients is its effect on mandibular width. In essence, the body ostectomy offers a way to reduce intermolar width in the mandible without changing intercanine width. This pattern of change is needed only rarely in treating dentofacial deformities, but when it is, body ostectomy can be very helpful.

Anterior mandibular ostectomy near the midline requires removing one incisor (unless there is a convenient edentulous space), and that in turn is likely to

create a tooth-size discrepancy. Before committing to this procedure, we recommend a diagnostic setup to verify that the postsurgical tooth relationships will be satisfactory.

Inlocking Crossbite (Scissors Bite, Brodie Syndrome)

Inlocking crossbite problems fortunately are rare because they can be extremely difficult to treat even with surgery and orthodontics. In most patients with inlocking crossbite, the upper teeth erupt past their lower antagonists, creating severe occlusal difficulties and all but eliminating lateral excursions (Figs. 16-10 and 16-11). (Interestingly, a tendency toward maxillary buccal crossbite is found frequently in Australian aborigines who otherwise have ideal dentitions and perfect occlusion. Barrett[27] called this "X-occlusion." It is not a problem because the teeth do not erupt past each other—presumably the aborigines function equally on the two sides, chewing frequently and heavily enough to prevent supereruption.)

Unilateral Scissors Bite

Even though this is initially a transverse discrepancy with the fault in the maxilla, mandible, or both jaws, it becomes a problem because the unopposed teeth in each arch supraerupt. This creates a situation in which the elongated upper and lower posterior teeth on one side need to be intruded several millimeters as well as repositioned laterally. There is no way to accomplish that orthodontically. Segmental dentoalveolar surgery

A   B   C

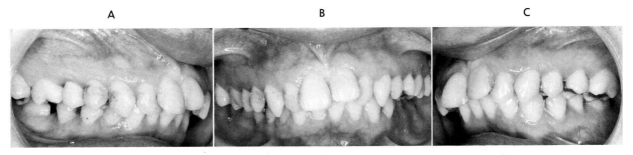

Fig. 16-11. L.D., dental relationships before treatment. She had an almost complete inlocking of the mandibular arch, the Brodie syndrome. To test the hypothesis that her myofascial pain was related to the occlusion, an occlusal splint was made. With the splint and ultrasound treatment, the pain resolved over a 6-month period, and surgical-orthodontic treatment to narrow the excessively wide maxilla and advance the deficient mandible was suggested. The plan was extraction of the mandibular left and both maxillary first premolars, alignment and space closure in the mandibular arch and segmental alignment in the maxilla with partial space closure, and a three-piece LeFort I osteotomy plus mandibular advancement.

in both jaws is the only possibility (see Chapters 8 and 10).

Stabilizing these alveolar segments at surgery can pose a major difficulty. The extreme vertical overlap on the affected side usually makes it impossible to place orthodontic attachments on the facial surface of the lower teeth presurgically. In this circumstance, after the segments are repositioned into the occlusal splint, a stabilizing wire is placed in the operating room. A heavy orthodontic arch wire (e.g., 40-mil steel) can be bonded directly to the buccal surface of the teeth, which is kinder to the tissues than a ligated fracture arch bar.

Total Inlocking (Brodie Syndrome)

The rare situation of total buccal crossbite or total inlocking is due to a combination of excessive maxillary width and mandibular deficiency. The mandibular alveolar process may or may not be narrow, but the mandibular base usually has normal width. The anteroposterior deficiency of the mandible contributes to its relative transverse deficiency. As with the unilateral scissors bite, extreme vertical overlap of the teeth exists with the mandible in its occlusal position, where often there is contact on only one or two teeth (see Fig. 16-11).

Unlike the patients with a unilateral scissors bite, however, the patients with Brodie syndrome are often quite overclosed in their occlusal position and do not have extreme supraeruption (i.e., they can be considered a variant of the short-face condition). Because of their overclosed status, patients with Brodie syndrome often can tolerate presurgical orthodontic appliances even though they are likely to be biting on brackets as soon as these are placed. Presurgical orthodontics usually is limited to the minimum alignment needed to make surgery possible, leaving relatively more to be

done postsurgically than in less severe problems. The surgery almost always involves both maxillary osteotomies to reduce width and ramus osteotomies for mandibular advancement (Figs. 16-12 to 16-16) and may include segmental dentoalveolar osteotomies in the mandible to reposition the dentition laterally. Stabilization of the resulting multiple segments can be difficult. Two-stage surgery may be needed, especially if both arches will be segmented.

Surgical Techniques: Osteotomies for Crossbite Correction

Surgical procedures useful in correcting posterior crossbite include maxillary posterior subapical osteotomy and mandibular body ostectomy, midline ostectomy, and posterior/total subapical osteotomy/ostectomy. These procedures are described in detail and illustrated in Chapter 10. In the mandible, decompression of the inferior alveolar neurovascular bundle often is required. A discussion of that procedure also is included in Chapter 10.

Lateral Buttress Osteotomy for Surgical Assistance

The lateral buttress osteotomy for assisting palatal expansion is similar to surgery for maxillary posterior subapical osteotomy (see Chapter 10), except that the palatal osteotomy and the interdental bone cuts are not made. The procedure can be performed under local anesthesia and conscious sedation, without the patient remaining in the hospital overnight. The orthodontic appliances should be in place before the procedure. Radiographs of the posterior maxillary areas (panoramic or periapical views) assist the surgeon in avoiding roots of the teeth.

Following infiltration of a vasoconstrictor (usually

2% lidocaine with 1:100,000 epinephrine) at the height of the maxillary vestibule, a mucoperiosteal incision is made from the maxillary canine area posteriorly beneath the zygomatic maxillary buttress. With a periosteal elevator, mucoperiosteum is reflected superiorly, leaving the mucoperiosteum inferior to the incision attached to bone. After exposure of the bone, a horizontal osteotomy above the teeth is made from the piriform rim to the maxillary buttress, using a bur or reciprocating saw. At this point the maxillary sinus is ex-

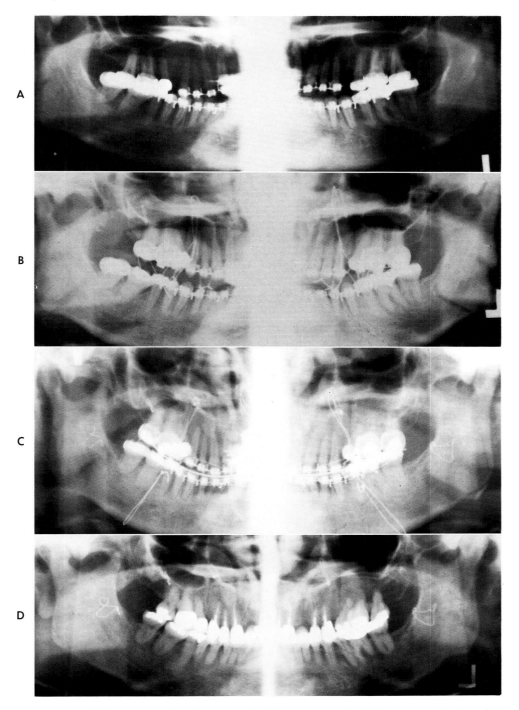

Fig. 16-12. L.D., panoramic radiographs. **A,** Before surgery. **B,** Following completion of the maxillary osteotomy. After the maxillary osteotomy was completed, reducing intermolar width 1.5 cm and premolar width 1 cm, it was difficult to stabilize the posterior segments, and mandibular advancement was deferred for 4 months until maxillary healing occurred. **C,** Four months later, after mandibular advancement. **D,** Six-year recall.

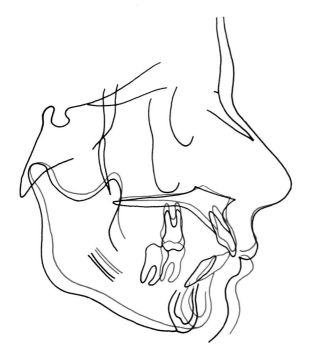

Fig. 16-13. L.D., cephalometric tracing from before to after treatment *(solid red)*.

posed. Next, the direction of the bony cut is altered as it is continued from the zygomatic maxillary buttress to the pterygomaxillary fissure. Taking care to stay above the apices of the teeth, the osteotomy is extended posterior and inferior to the pterygomaxillary fissure. As the final step, with a curved osteotome the maxillary tuberosity is separated from the pterygoid plates. The procedure is repeated on the opposite side.

Following copious saline irrigation, mucosal wounds are closed with 4-0 chromic sutures.

Significant postsurgical pain is unusual with this procedure. But facial edema can be considerable, and patients should be warned about this sequela. The edema resolves quickly, usually in 10 days. The most common complication is inadvertant damage to the teeth. Even if roots are sectioned, the teeth may retain their blood supply. Careful clinical and radiographic observation over 6 to 12 months will detect irreversible pulpal damage. Endodontic treatment usually is successful when irreversible pulpal injury has occurred.

As soon as the early soft-tissue healing is complete, 5 to 7 days, the orthodontist must activate the palatal expansion appliance. Following surgery, expansion should be rapid because clinical bony healing is complete in 4 to 6 weeks.

OPEN-BITE PROBLEMS IN ADULTS
Diagnostic Characteristics: Localizing the Deformity

In planning the treatment for unusual open-bite problems—in the context of this chapter, open bites that are not related to the long-face condition and therefore not due primarily to excessive vertical development of the maxilla—the key to success is localizing the deformity. There are three major possibilities: (1) anterior open bite due primarily to deficient eruption of the maxillary incisors; (2) anterior open bite due to deficient eruption of the mandibular incisors, perhaps coupled with excessive eruption of the mandibular posterior teeth; and (3) posterior open bite due to deficient eruption of maxillary and/or mandibular posterior teeth, unilaterally or bilaterally. Extremely rarely, a pa-

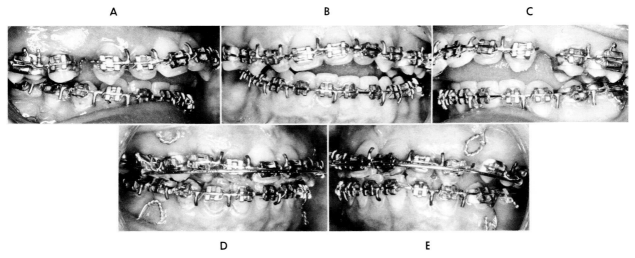

Fig. 16-14. L.D. **A-C,** Dental relationships just before surgery. **D** and **E,** Dental relationships at the completion of the two-stage surgical treatment as postsurgical orthodontics resumed. A heavy labial auxiliary arch wire was used to maintain arch form while light wires were employed for settling and final tooth positioning.

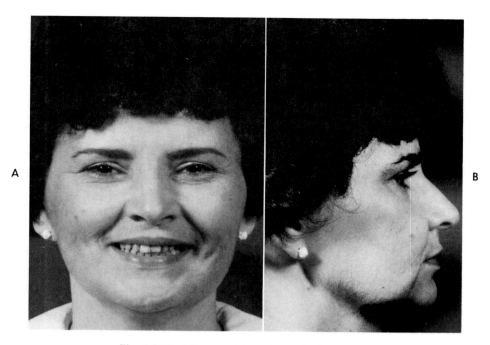

Fig. 16-15. L.D., age 44, at the end of retention.

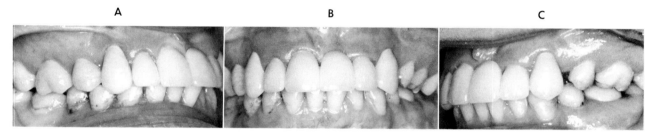

Fig. 16-16. L.D., 6-year recall, with restorations completed for anterior teeth. There were no problems with myofascial pain/dysfunction after the surgical-orthodontic treatment.

tient may be encountered in whom there is deficient eruption of all teeth in both arches. Conceptually, this can be considered a "total open bite," even though some teeth come into contact when the patient closes down far enough.

Careful cephalometric analysis is the key to distinguishing these conditions. The methods described in some detail in Chapter 4 are applicable. The preferred approach is either to use a template with both cranial base and maxillary/mandibular superimpositions — which gives a direct view of distorted relationships — or to use a series of linear measurements to locate the teeth within a coordinate system.

Anterior open bite due primarily to deficient eruption of the maxillary incisors is rare and in our experience is much more likely to be seen in black patients. A typical cephalometric tracing and analysis are shown in Fig. 16-17. Although the major component of the open

bite for this patient is the lack of eruption of the upper incisors, there is also some overeruption of the upper posterior teeth and mildly excessive face height. This finding also is typical of these patients, as is a tendency to posterior crossbite. The malocclusion, in short, is a more severe version of what is seen in younger thumbsuckers. It is tempting to think that the etiology may be similar, though from patient reports this is not always the case.

In assessing patients with open bite, it always is important to evaluate the vertical relationship of the maxillary incisors to the upper lip as well as to skeletal landmarks, keeping in mind that the lip length is quite variable. When upper incisor eruption is deficient, lack of exposure of the upper incisors is likely to be part of the chief complaint, especially when there is little or no lip elevation on smiling.

Anterior open bite also can be due primarily to a

lack of eruption of the mandibular incisors. This rare condition can be characterized more accurately as a reverse curve of Spee in the lower arch because it is produced by some excess eruption of the first molars and premolars, as well as infra-eruption of the incisors. Almost always, if the lower incisors were in occlusion, they would be supra-erupted (i.e., the distance from the incisal edge to the chin would be excessive) (Fig. 16-18). The resting posture of the tongue is a possible etiologic factor—if the tongue rested on top of the lower incisors, their eruption would be impeded—but there is no definite evidence that this is the case. In patients with a muscle weakness syndrome, the lower arch often is distorted in this way, but the patients with a syndrome also have excessive vertical development of the maxilla.

Posterior open bite can develop in three ways. (1) Excessive vertical development and excessive posterior eruption on one side. This would produce occlusion on the affected but not the normal side and would be associated with a facial asymmetry. (2) Deficient eruption of posterior teeth on one side. This would produce oc-

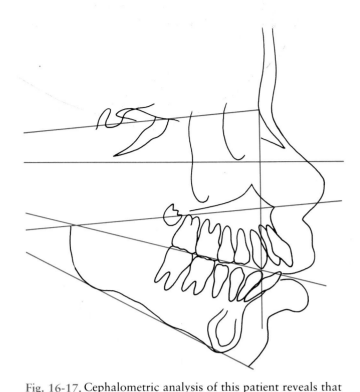

Fig. 16-17. Cephalometric analysis of this patient reveals that the open bite is primarily due to infra-eruption of the maxillary incisor segment, with a minor component of elongation of the maxillary posterior segments and downward-backward rotation of the mandible. For unknown reasons, this cephalometric pattern is most likely to be encountered in black patients. Cephalometric measurements: N perp to A, 6 mm; N perp to Pg, −10 mm; AB difference, 14 mm; UFH, 51 mm; LFH, 74 mm; mand plane, 28 degrees; MxI to A vert, 10 mm, 30 degrees; MnI to B vert, 19 mm, 52 degrees.

A

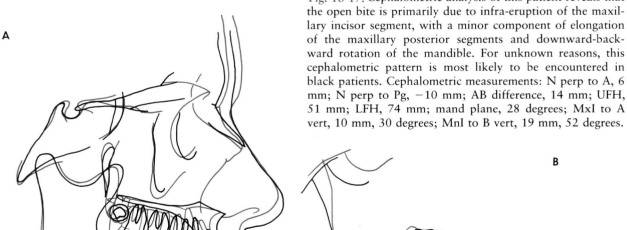

B

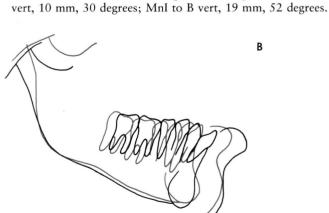

Fig. 16-18. Template superimposition can be useful in establishing the anatomic deviation in unusual open-bite cases. **A**, Cranial base superimposition of the age 18 Bolton template *(solid red)* on the initial tracing of a patient (D.C., case 3; see also Fig. 16-38). Note that the maxilla is normally oriented, not tipped, but has additional length and height anteriorly, and that the upper lip is long. Note also the downward and backward rotation of the mandible, the extreme chin deficiency, and the lower incisor protrusion. **B**, Mandibular superimposition of the same template. Note the greater eruption of the patient's mandibular posterior than anterior teeth. The patient's lower incisors are not only protrusive relative to the chin but are infraerupted relative to the posterior teeth and the lower lip.

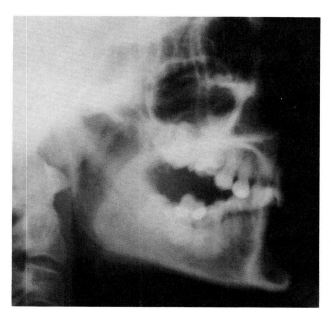

Fig. 16-19. Cephalometric radiograph of a patient with primary failure of eruption, in which posterior teeth do not erupt because of an abnormality with the eruption mechanism. Posterior open bite of this severity rarely is caused by the tongue or some other obstruction to eruption.

clusion on the normal but not on the affected side, and facial symmetry would be normal. (3) Deficient eruption of posterior teeth bilaterally. This patient would have no posterior occlusion but normal facial symmetry. All three situations occur rarely, but the first, in which the primary problem is a distortion of jaw growth leading to facial asymmetry, is by far the most prevalent. These patients have been discussed in Chapter 15. Our focus here is on the second and third groups, who do not have facial asymmetry.

Posterior open bite due to deficient eruption is recognized by template superimposition on the maxilla and mandible or by linear measurements from the palatal and mandibular planes to the molar teeth (see Fig. 16-18). There are two possible causes[28]: (1) an obstruction to eruption or (2) a problem with the eruption mechanism (Fig. 16-19). This distinction is important in planning treatment. It is made primarily from clinical examination and clinical experience, more frequently from the latter.

As with anterior open bite, patients with posterior open bite will place the tongue into the space during swallowing and may do so at rest. This does not indicate that the tongue is the etiologic agent. Unilateral posterior open bite can be caused by a distortion of tongue form (e.g., the unilateral swelling associated with a lymphangioma or hemangioma). It almost never is caused by lateral posturing of a normal tongue. The other possible etiologic factor, failure to erupt, seems to be caused by some abnormality in the periodontal ligament.[29] Teeth that are being impeded in their eruption can erupt if the impediment is removed, and they will react normally to orthodontic force to pull them into the correct position. Teeth with an abnormal periodontal ligament will not erupt on their own. They do not respond to orthodontic force, so they cannot be moved orthodontically (see Chapter 2 for a more complete discussion). A patient with posterior open bite often is seen for surgical-orthodontic consultation after orthodontic treatment has unaccountably failed—which can be a diagnostic feature of considerable significance in deciding why the posterior open bite is present in the first place (see Case 4).

In its severe forms, the rarest of all open-bite problems is total open bite, the condition in which there is deficient eruption of anterior and posterior teeth in one or both arches. This occurs in patients with cleidocranial dysplasia, whose first molars and retained primary teeth do not erupt as much as would occur under normal circumstances,[30] and also is found in individuals who have a very large tongue interposed between the teeth, whether or not there is a discernible syndrome. With the teeth in occlusion, of course, there may be no open bite. Instead, the patient will appear to have a short-face problem and somewhat prognathic mandible. The condition can be recognized in two ways: (1) by documenting the infra-eruption and upward-forward rotation of the mandible with superimpositions or measurements, and (2) by evaluating the freeway space. The postural position of the mandible is strongly influenced by the vertical position of the maxillary posterior teeth, so the increase in jaw separation at rest is likely not to be large enough to totally account for the deformity. But in severely affected individuals there is at least some increase in freeway space, and the large tongue is obvious.

Planning Treatment: Treatment Possibilities

The open-bite problems described above are more dental than skeletal (i.e., the distortions are primarily dentoalveolar rather than skeletal). For that reason, in theory they should be amenable to orthodontic treatment. In fact, surgical treatment often has to be considered in adults for two major reasons: (1) it can be quite difficult to correct a severe open bite orthodontically, and even more difficult to keep it corrected, because of the distance that teeth would have to be moved and the tendency of the elongated teeth to rebound apically after they have been brought into occlusion. There is no way to slightly overtreat an open bite orthodontically—when the teeth come into contact, they can go no further, and any relapse tendency results in a reopening of the bite. (2) Particularly in some posterior open bites, the teeth do not respond normally and cannot be moved orthodontically.

Deficient Eruption of Maxillary Incisors

The patients with deficient eruption of maxillary incisors who are seen for surgical-orthodontic consultation tend to be those with quite severe open bites who are not good candidates for orthodontic treatment alone because of the distance the teeth would have to be moved. The key decision in planning treatment is whether a maxillary anterior segemental osteotomy would be sufficient, or whether a LeFort I osteotomy with or without anterior and posterior segments should be employed (see Case 2). Even when the major component of the open bite is deficient eruption anteriorly, a component of posterior elongation often makes some elevation of the posterior segments desirable. With modern surgical techniques, the degree of difficulty and duration of LeFort I osteotomy is not much more than that of an anterior segmental procedure, and LeFort I osteotomy allows the open bite to be closed by any combination of elongation of the anterior teeth and depression of the posteriors.

Determining which teeth should be in the anterior versus the posterior segments also is important. Patients with deficient eruption of the maxillary incisors tend to have a step in the maxillary arch. The step may be mesial or distal to the canine, but often is mesial. In addition, when the lateral incisors have not erupted as much as the canines, their roots tend to be tipped mesially, which facilitates an interdental osteotomy between the canines and lateral incisors. For these reasons, often it can be easier and more effective to place the canines in the posterior segments (see Chapter 13, Fig. 13-12). The location of interdental osteotomies must be determined before orthodontic treatment begins, so the orthodontist can level the teeth within but not across segments while maintaining or creating adequate root separation at the osteotomy sites.

Reverse Curve of Spee in the Mandibular Arch

As we have noted above, patients who have a reverse curve of Spee in the lower arch often have excessive eruption of the lower posterior teeth. The distance from the lower border of the mandible to the incisal edge may be deficient or nearly normal, and the mandible usually is rotated downward so that face height is excessive. Surgically depressing the mandibular posterior segments is possible but technically difficult and rarely is indicated in the treatment of this problem. Instead, the best approach is to elevate the lower incisors and decrease face height at the same time by elevating the chin.

An anterior subapical osteotomy accomplishes both purposes, elevating the anterior segment and using bone removed from the under surface of the chin (thus reducing face height) as a graft to support the dental segment in its new position (see Chapter 10 for a description of the surgical procedure). Because the bone

cuts are anterior to the mental foramen, the inferior alveolar neurovascular bundle is avoided and there is minimal risk of neurosensory damage to the lower lip. Although the stability data are not extensive, our experience is consistent with the claim in the literature that closing an open bite in this way is remarkably stable,[31] and the esthetic results also can be quite good (see Case 3).

If necessary, the anterior subapical osteotomy can be combined with a posterior subapical osteotomy. The neurovascular bundle is protected by removing it from the bony canal while the bone cuts are made subapically (see Chapter 10). The indication for a total mandibular subapical osteotomy when the anterior segment is to be elevated usually is asymmetry or crossbite posteriorly in addition to the open bite.

Posterior Open Bite

The indication for surgical intervention in posterior open bite usually is a failure of the teeth to respond to attempted orthodontic treatment. If this is due to an obstruction to eruption, it is logical to plan surgery to remove the obstruction, so that further orthodontics can succeed. If the difficulty is an abnormal periodontal ligament, so that the teeth do not respond normally to orthodontic force, the surgery should be directed at repositioning the alveolar segments.

A large tongue sometimes produces bilateral obstruction, but failure of eruption is at least as likely to be the underlying cause of the problem. Surgical reduction of the tongue, in the hope that the teeth will erupt after this is done, should be carried out only after there is clear evidence that the tongue really is causing the open bite. Probably the best way to establish this is to place a tongue shield as part of an orthodontic appliance and observe eruption of the teeth with the appliance in place and relapse when it is removed.

In bilateral posterior open bite, it is likely that either the upper or the lower arch will be affected more. In planning surgical treatment to elongate the posterior segments, it is better to perform surgery in only one arch if possible. The preferred approach is either LeFort I osteotomy or total mandibular subapical osteotomy, with segments as necessary, to elongate the affected teeth into occlusion (see Case 4).

Total Open Bite

Total open bite is unlikely to occur in the absence of some major developmental disturbance and therefore probably will be encountered in the context of other problems. It is difficult to generalize about treatment possibilities, except to say that surgery to elongate the maxillary or mandibular dentoalveolar structures may be indicated and that tongue reduction may be necessary as a part of the overall treatment plan. Unfortunately, reducing the size of the tongue does nothing to help a patient control tongue posture, and even after surgical reduction the tongue may remain interposed between the teeth because of poor muscular control and coordination.

Surgical Procedures

Surgical procedures to reposition dentoalveolar segments in the maxilla and mandible are discussed in Chapter 10. The reader is referred to that chapter for details of the surgery, postsurgery sequelae, and common complications.

COORDINATING THE SURGICAL AND ORTHODONTIC PHASES OF TREATMENT

The guidelines for coordinating orthodontics and surgery for crossbite and open-bite patients are the same as for any other surgical-orthodontic treatment. In both situations, segmental maxillary and/or mandibular osteotomies are likely to be employed, and this must be taken into account in coordinating the treatment.

During the treatment planning phase, the surgeon and orthodontist must agree as to the location of any interdental osteotomies. During the presurgical orthodontics, the objective should be to level within but not across the segments—the surgery will level across the segments—and to maintain or create appropriate root separation at the osteotomy sites. The presurgical orthodontics should not include force to move the teeth in the direction of the surgical correction because orthodontic relapse then will compromise the total correction. In other words, cross elastics should be avoided in the presurgical treatment of patients who will have surgery to correct a crossbite; vertical elastics should be avoided in open-bite patients.

Particularly in an open-bite patient, the patient may come to surgical consultation because attempts to correct the problem orthodontically have failed. Typically, the patient has worn vertical elastics for some time, but the teeth have not been brought into occlusion. Before surgery is carried out in such a patient, we recommend replacing heavy arch wires with light ones for a few months and discontinuing all elastics. The objective is to allow any orthodontic relapse to occur presurgically. The same would be true of a patient who had worn extensive cross elastics but whose crossbite remained uncorrected. The elastics should be stopped presurgically long enough to allow any dental relapse tendency to express itself.

Postsurgically, the orthodontic finishing is no different from that of any other orthognathic surgery patient. Light vertical elastics can and should be used to settle the teeth into their final occlusion. At one time, it was feared that the dentoalveolar segments could be displaced by orthodontic elastics used postsurgically, but experience has shown that this poses no special risk.

It must be kept in mind that transverse changes, particularly when the maxilla has been expanded surgically, are unstable for a longer time than most other surgical or orthodontic movements. It takes at least 6 months to achieve solid bone continuity and stability. This means that transverse relapse is likely to occur while light arch wires and elastics are being used during the postsurgical orthodontics. Maintaining a heavy labial auxiliary arch wire in the headgear tubes during this phase of treatment is the easiest way to control arch width while the teeth are vertically settled into occlusion (see Chapter 12, Fig. 12-35). After the appliances are removed, a transpalatal lingual arch should be considered for retention, especially in a patient who might be reluctant to wear a removable retainer full-time.

CASE REPORTS

Case 1

L.A., age 16 years, 11 months, was concerned about the appearance of his upper incisors and secondarily about his bite on the right side (Figs. 16-20 and 16-21) but not about facial esthetics. The right side of the maxilla appeared slightly hypoplastic and the nose deviated slightly to the right, but facial proportions in all three planes of space were within normal limits (Fig. 16-22). The maxillary right buccal segment was lingually positioned, causing the crossbite on that side. There was no history of trauma or of any congenital anomaly. There were no mandibular shifts or signs of TM joint dysfunction.

Because of the need to differentially expand the maxillary right quadrant and the severe crowding there, extraction of the maxillary right first premolar and surgically assisted expansion with an osteotomy only on that side, followed by fixed-appliance therapy to align the teeth, was suggested. He agreed to the plan but preferred to wait to begin treatment until his participation in football had ended for the season. At age 17 years, 5 months, maxillary second premolars and first molars were banded and a palate-separating appliance was placed (Fig. 16-23). Four weeks later, under general anesthesia, all four third molars and the maxillary right first premolar were removed and a horizontal osteotomy was made in the right maxilla from the pterygo-

Continued.

Case 1—cont'd.

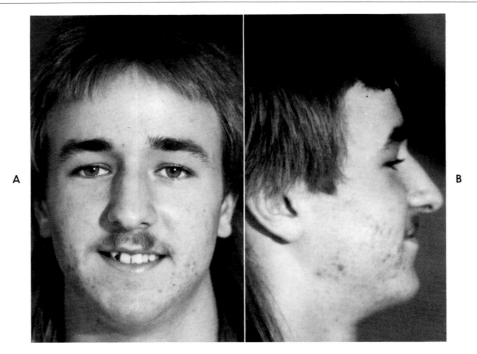

Fig. 16-20. L.A., age 16 years, 11 months. Note the mildly hypoplastic appearance of the right side of the midface, with good facial proportions otherwise.

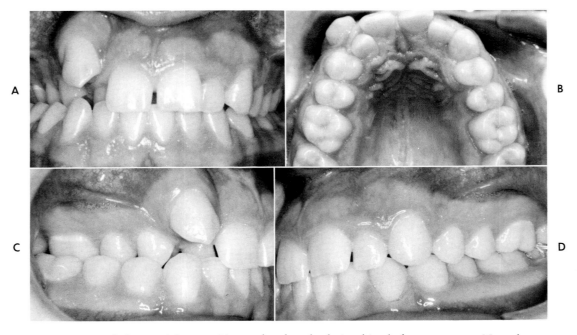

Fig. 16-21. L.A., age 16 years, 11 months, dental relationships before treatment. Note the lingual positioning of the maxillary right quadrant, with posterior crossbite on that side.

Case 1—cont'd.

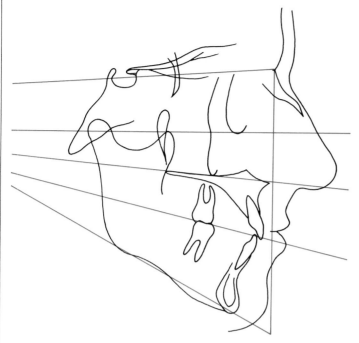

Fig. 16-22. L.A., lateral cephalometric tracing before treatment. Note the bimaxillary retrusive jaw positions, with proclined lower incisors and upright maxillary incisors compensating for the large AB difference. Cephalometric measurements: N perp to A, −7 mm; N perp to Pg, −16 mm; AB difference, 10 mm; UFH, 61 mm; LFH, 72 mm; mand plane, 30 degrees; MxI to A vert, 2 mm, 18 degrees; MnI to B vert, 9 mm, 28 degrees.

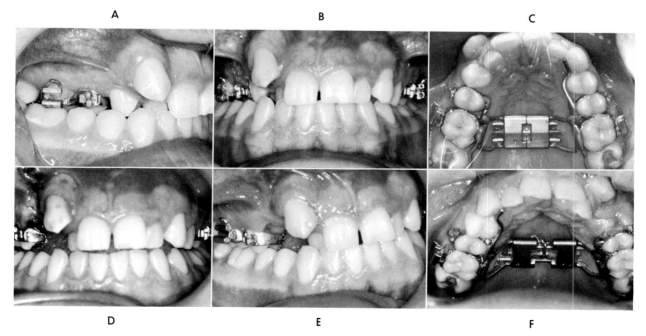

Fig. 16-23. L.A. **A-C,** Dental relationships immediately prior to surgery. Dental relationships **D,** 1 day and **E** and **F,** 1 week postsurgery, showing the 4.5 mm expansion gained initially and the total expansion.

Continued.

Case 1—cont'd.

maxillary junction anteriorly to the first premolar extraction site. An osteotome crossing the maxillary sinus was used to tap through the right palate along the line of the horizontal osteotomy. At that point, the screw of the appliance was turned to produce 4.5 mm expansion, all but correcting the crossbite. It was not necessary to totally free the segment posteriorly.

One week later, he returned for continuing orthodontic treatment. The appliance screw was turned twice more that day and once a day for another week, then was stabilized. A complete fixed orthodontic appliance was applied to the other teeth, and over the next 15 months NiTi and steel arch wires were used to align the teeth and close the extraction space, correcting the maxillary dental midline and slipping the first molar anteriorly (Fig. 16-24). Appliances were removed at age 18 years (Figs. 16-25 and 16-26).

Comments. One of the major indications for surgically assisted palatal expansion is this type of unilateral problem, in which an osteotomy that does not totally free the maxilla can alter the anchorage so that true unilateral expansion can be obtained. The surgery was made slightly less complex by not having to free the segment at the pterygomaxillary fissure and not making interdental osteotomies—but if there had still been significant resistance to turning the screw when the horizontal osteotomies were performed, an osteotomy posteriorly would have been indicated.

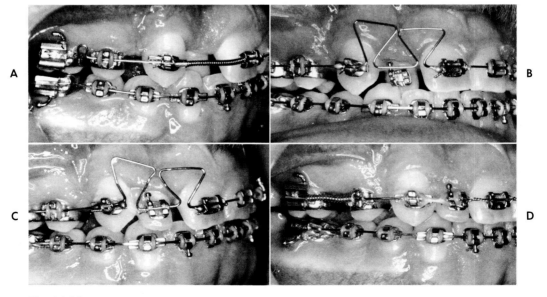

Fig. 16-24. L.A., progressive alignment and space closure after the surgically assisted expansion.

Case 1—cont'd.

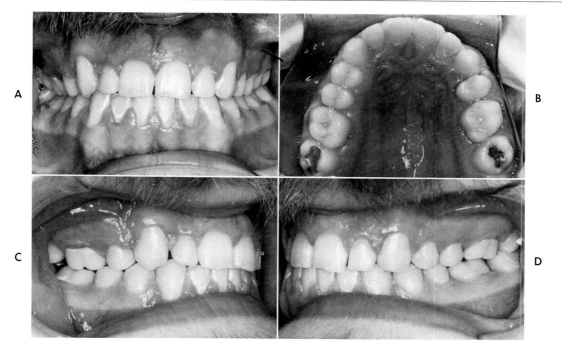

Fig. 16-25. L.A., age 19 years, 5 months, occlusal relationships at completion of active treatment.

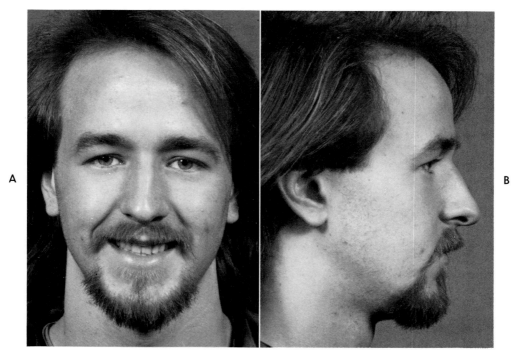

Fig. 16-26. L.A., age 19 years, 5 months, at completion of active treatment.

Case 2

S.D, age 20 years, 9 months, and a university student, was seen on referral from an orthodontist near her home. She was concerned about the appearance of her anterior teeth and her anterior open bite (Figs. 16-27 and 16-28). The medical history was benign and jaw function was normal, without any signs of TM joint dysfunction. On clinical examination, she appeared to have mild three-dimensional maxillary deficiency.

On cephalometric analysis, there was an unusual open-bite pattern with the maxilla rotated down posteriorly and the upper incisors mildly infra-erupted (Fig. 16-29). Orthodontic treatment seemed possible but difficult, prone to relapse, and unlikely to produce the esthetic changes she desired. The plan was to align the teeth without extraction and rotate the maxilla up posteriorly

and down anteriorly, closing the open bite with minimal shortening of face height.

At age 21 years, 1 month, a fixed appliance was placed and alignment was begun with 18 NiTi arch wires. Stabilizing arch wires were placed 3 months later (Fig. 16-30). For model surgery, casts were mounted on a semi-adjustable articulator, and a relatively thick splint posteriorly was fabricated, separating the molars about 4 mm. At age 21 years, 6 months, a LeFort I osteotomy was carried out. A section of bone was removed posteriorly, 3 mm thick in the buttress region and tapering to a wedge in the canine region, so that the maxilla would rotate up posteriorly and down anteriorly. The teeth were placed in the splint and the mandible was autorotated to position, measurements were checked to be

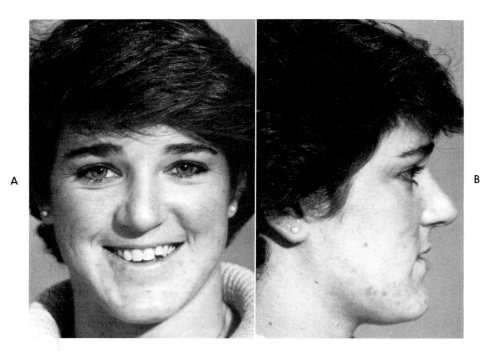

A   B

Fig. 16-27. S.D., age 20 years, 11 months.

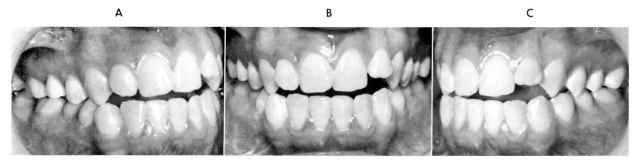

A   B   C

Fig. 16-28. S.D., age 20 years, 11 months, dental relationships.

Case 2—cont'd.

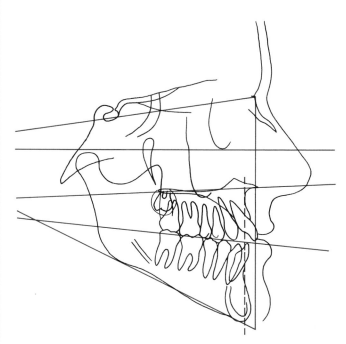

Fig. 16-29. S.D., initial cephalometric tracing. Note the normal AP position of the mandible with moderate maxillary deficiency and the rotated position of the maxilla. Cephalometric measurements: N perp to A, −6 mm; N perp to Pg, −3 mm; AB difference, 0 mm; UFH, 49 mm; LFH, 73 mm; mand plane 23 degrees; MxI to A vert, 6 mm, 23 degrees; MnI to B vert, 2 mm, 24 degrees.

sure that the maxilla was in the planned position, blocks of reconstituted allogeneic freeze-dried bone were placed in the pyriform rim and buttress areas, and transosseous wires were ligated through the bone grafts for stabilization (Fig. 16-31).

She was kept in maxillomandibular fixation for 2 weeks, then the splint was tied to the maxillary arch and she was allowed to function into it. Eight weeks postsurgically the splint and the stabilizing arch wires were removed, light working arch wires (16 steel) were placed, and she wore ⅜-inch, 3½-oz posterior box elastics fulltime. Three weeks later, the maxillary piriform suspension wires were removed under local anesthesia. A molar cross elastic (³⁄₁₆-inch) was added on the right side only, and the box elastics were continued. Two months later, the occlusion had settled nicely. Elastics were stopped, and a positioner impression was taken. Four months after postsurgical orthodontics resumed, she was debanded to a positioner; removable retainers were placed after another 3 weeks. Both facial esthetics and occlusal relationships were quite satisfactory (Figs. 16-32 and 16-33). On recall more than 1 year later, facial and dental relationships were being maintained nicely (Figs. 16-34 and 16-35).

Comments. For this patient, the open bite was corrected with a one-piece LeFort I osteotomy that rotated the maxilla down anteriorly—an infrequent procedure, but probably the most stable to accomplish this somewhat unstable movement. In this case, the maxilla was deliberately moved downward further than its expected final position, and it did move upward again during the healing phase. If bone plates had been employed for stabilization, less overtreatment at the time of surgery would have been employed, but downward movements of the maxilla tend to be unstable even with RIF. Once bony healing has occurred, however, good long-term stability can be anticipated.

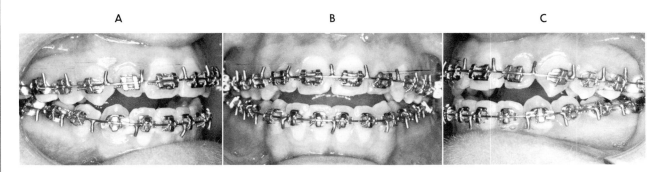

A   B   C

Fig. 16-30. S.D., stabilizing arch wires in place immediately before surgery.

Continued.

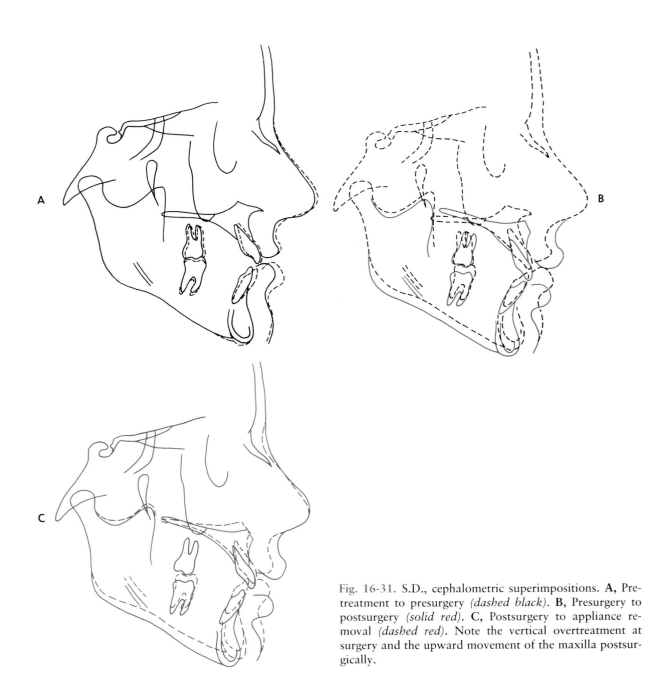

Fig. 16-31. S.D., cephalometric superimpositions. A, Pretreatment to presurgery *(dashed black)*. B, Presurgery to postsurgery *(solid red)*. C, Postsurgery to appliance removal *(dashed red)*. Note the vertical overtreatment at surgery and the upward movement of the maxilla postsurgically.

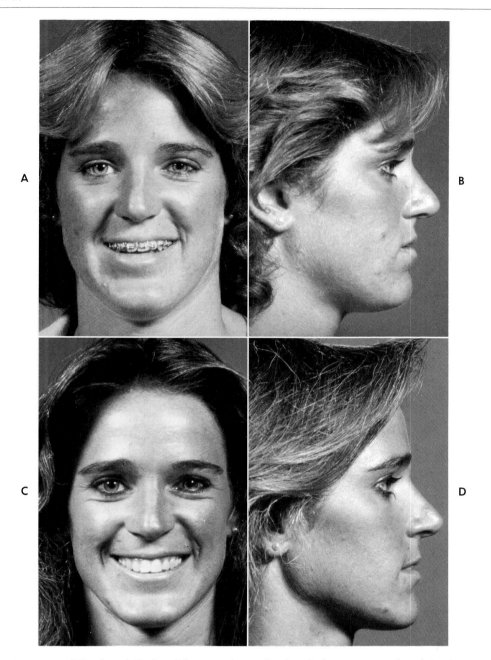

Fig. 16-32. S.D. **A** and **B,** Age 21 years, 6 months, just before surgery. **C** and **D,** Age 23 years, 7 months, at the discontinuation of retention.

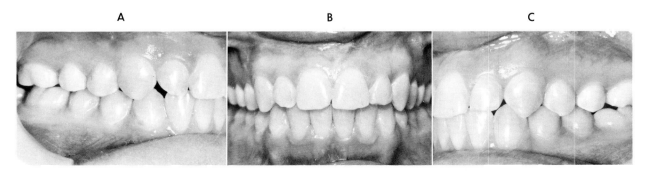

Fig. 16-33. S.D., age 22 years, at the beginning of retention.

Continued.

Case 2—cont'd.

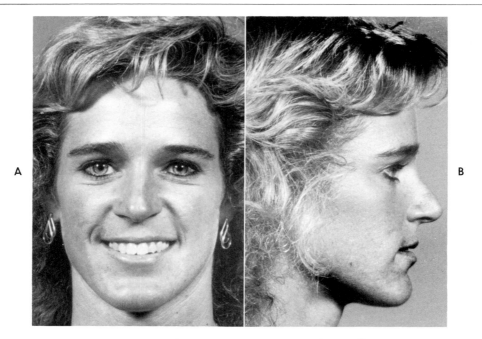

Fig. 16-34. S.D., age 24 years, 10 months, recall.

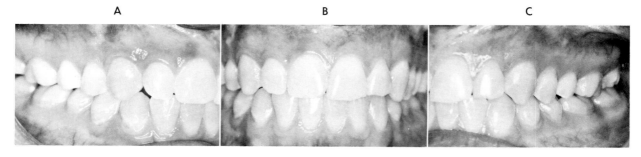

Fig. 16-35. S.D., age 24 years, 10 months, dental relationships 1 year out of retention.

Case 3

D.C., age 50, was referred by her general dentist who was concerned about her open bite, especially the possibility that she would develop TM joint problems. She had undergone orthodontic treatment between ages 15 and 18 and reported that the anterior teeth had separated again soon after this was completed. She wanted to do whatever was necessary to preserve her dentition, but was aware of her lack of chin projection and open bite and wondered what could be done about that situation (Figs. 16-36 through 16-38).

On clinical examination, the periodontal condition was normal and there were no signs of TM pain/dysfunction. Chin deficiency and poor throat form were apparent. There was a mild reverse curve of Spee in the lower arch. Cephalometric analysis confirmed good position of the maxilla and maxillary teeth, with chin deficiency and severe protrusion of the mandibular incisors relative to the mandible (Fig. 16-39; see also Fig. 16-18).

The lower face was long, entirely in the lower third. Cephalometric prediction indicated that elevating the lower anterior segment and augmenting the chin via Kole osteotomy would produce good facial balance and good occlusion.

After 6 months of preparatory orthodontics to align the teeth, the arches were stabilized with 17×25 steel arch wires. The lower stabilizing wire was separated into anterior and posterior segments between the first and second premolars immediately before surgery. An auxiliary stabilizing arch wire for the lower arch was fabricated by soldering a short extension of 17×25 wire to a 40-mil steel arch wire, so that the auxiliary wire could be fitted into the rectangular auxiliary tubes on the lower first molars. A subapical osteotomy was carried out below the apices of the lower anterior teeth and extended upward through the alveolar process between the first and second premolars. The anterior segment was

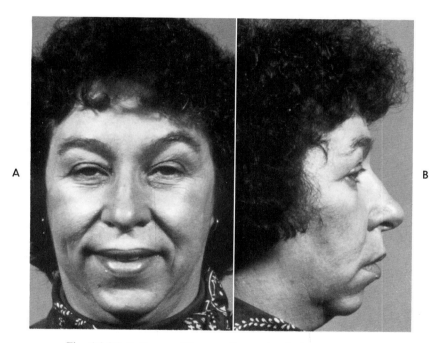

Fig. 16-36. D.C., age 50 years, 7 months, before treatment.

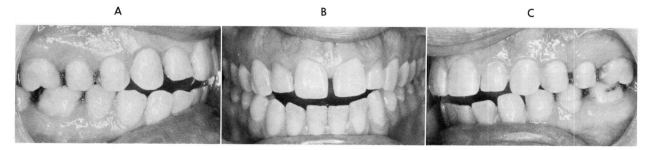

Fig. 16-37. D.C., dental relationships before treatment.

Continued.

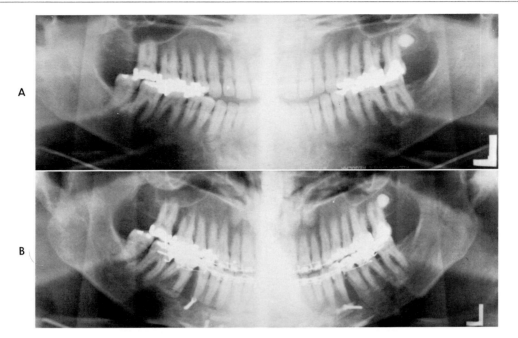

Fig. 16-38. D.C., panoramic radiographs. **A**, Before treatment. **B**, Immediately following surgery.

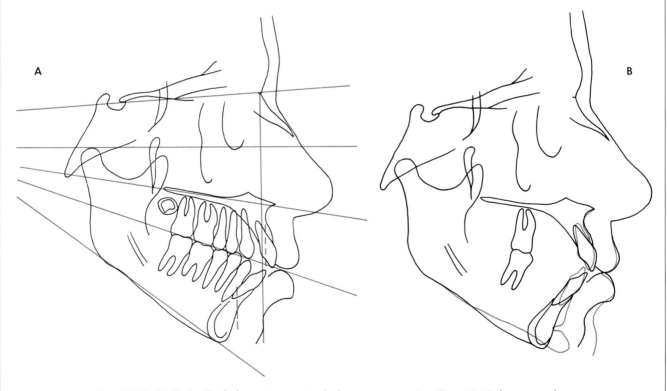

Fig. 16-39. D.C. **A**, Cephalometric tracing before treatment (see Fig. 16-18 for a template analysis of this same tracing). Cephalometric measurements: N perp to A, 2 mm; N perp to Pg, −18 mm; AB difference, 17 mm; UFH, 60 mm; LFH, 74 mm; mand plane, 35 degrees; MxI to A vert, 4 mm, 16 degrees; MnI to B vert, 15 mm, 50 degrees. **B**, Superimposition from pretreatment to completion of active treatment *(solid red)*, showing the changes produced by the combination of surgery and orthodontics.

Case 3—cont'd.

brought into the prepared splint, the teeth were placed in maxillomandibular fixation, and a 15 mm screw was placed on each side for fixation. An inferior border osteotomy then was performed. The superior portion of the osteotomized section was removed and used as a graft beneath the elevated alveolar segment; the inferior portion was advanced 14 mm, and three screws were placed in the repositioned chin to stabilize it (Fig. 16-40). After 5 days she was allowed to function into the splint.

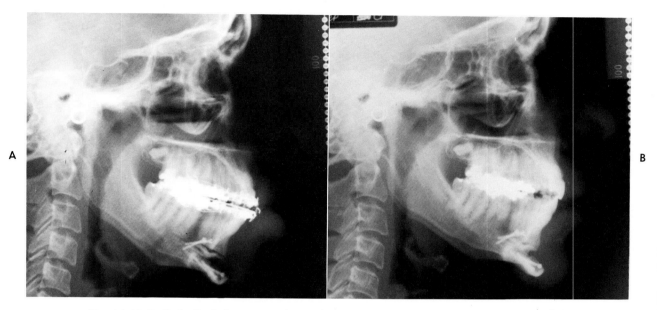

Fig. 16-40. D.C. **A,** Cephalometric radiograph immediately after surgery. Note the auxiliary stabilizing arch wire and the use of screws for RIF. **B,** Cephalometric radiograph at the completion of treatment.

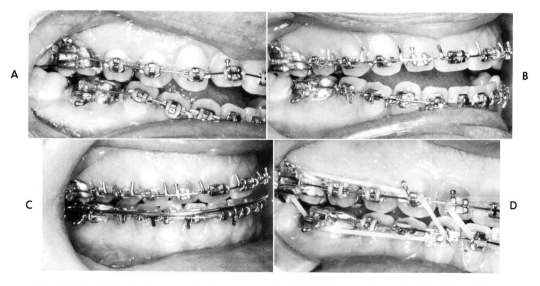

Fig. 16-41. D.C. **A,** Presurgical alignment with 16 NiTi arch wires. **B,** 17×25 stabilizing arch wires before surgery. The lower wire was sectioned between the first and second premolars immediately before surgery. **C,** Auxiliary stabilizing wire in place in the mandibular arch postsurgically. A short segment of 17×25 wire was soldered to the end of the 40-mil steel auxiliary wire so that it could fit into the auxiliary tubes on the lower first molars. **D,** ⅜-inch posterior box elastics with 16 steel arch wires, immediately after resuming postsurgical orthodontics.

Continued.

Case 3—cont'd.

At 6 weeks postsurgery, the splint and stabilizing arch wires were removed, light working arch wires were placed, and she wore posterior box elastics full-time and an anterior box elastic at night. Two months later, she had settled into excellent occlusion. Elastics were stopped but appliances were left in place for another month to be sure there was no relapse tendency, then she was debanded to retainers, 11 months after treatment began. Excellent occlusion was obtained, and she was quite pleased with the change in facial esthetics (Figs. 16-41 to 16-43).

Comments. The primary indications for the anterior subapical osteotomy are those seen in this patient: anterior open bite due primarily to a reverse curve of Spee in the lower arch, with good vertical positioning of the maxilla and excess face height only in the lower face. In those somewhat unusual circumstances, the procedure is extremely effective in closing the open bite and improving the vertical and AP position of the chin. In our series of only a few cases, stability has been excellent, and other reports of a few cases in the literature have the same conclusion.

A   B   C

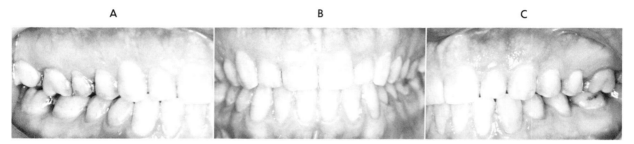

Fig. 16-42. D.C., dental relationships at the conclusion of treatment.

A

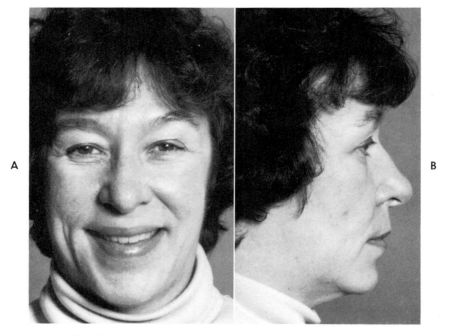

B

Fig. 16-43. D.C., age 51 years, 5 months, end of treatment.

Case 4

S.J., age 18 years, 3 months, was referred by her orthodontist because of his inability to close her lateral open bite. She had begun orthodontic treatment 2½ years previously. At that time (Figs. 16-44 and 16-45) a posterior crossbite tendency and moderate posterior open bite were noted. Mandibular second premolars were missing, and the second primary molars were retained. On cephalometric analysis, facial proportions were within normal limits with a slight tendency toward short anterior face height. She had suffered head trauma in an automobile accident at an early age without apparent sequelae. Orthodontic treatment produced some initial movement of teeth and an improvement in the crossbite, but despite elastic wear, it was impossible to bring the teeth together (Fig. 16-46). Cephalometrically, no growth had occurred. Facial proportions remained normal (Fig. 16-47).

It seemed clear that the open bite was due to failure of eruption and that surgery was the only possible way to close the open bite. The orthodontic appliances were re-moved, to give any normal teeth that had been elongated by elastics an opportunity to express any relapse tendency. Six months later (Fig. 16-48), the open bite was similar but perhaps slightly greater.

At age 18 years, 9 months, a total mandibular subapical osteotomy was carried out to elevate the mandibular teeth into occlusion, and allogeneic iliac crest bone grafts were placed to hold the alveolar segment in its elevated position. Using the procedure described in Chapter 10, the mental nerves were exposed bilaterally. Then the lateral cortical plate was removed from over the inferior alveolar neurovascular bundle to a point behind the second molars, the incisive branch of the inferior alveolar nerve was sectioned, and the bundle was carefully lifted out of its canal. Using a tunneling approach, an osteotomy was made through the lingual cortical plate and connected through at the level of the neurovascular canal, beneath the root apices of the posterior teeth. A similar osteotomy was carried out on the opposite side, and the posterior osteotomies were con-

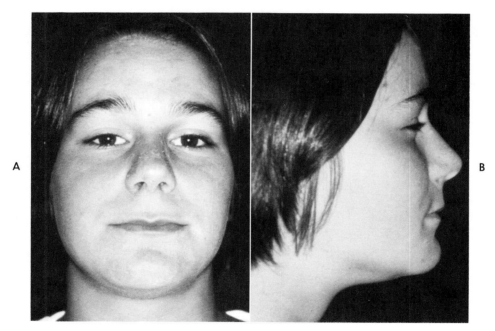

Fig. 16-44. S.J., age 15 years, 9 months, at the beginning of orthodontic treatment.

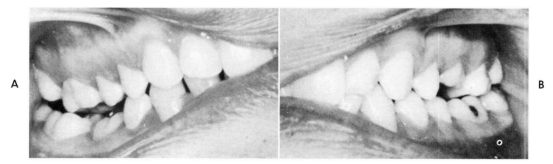

Fig. 16-45. S.J., dental relationships at the beginning of orthodontics.

Continued.

Case 4—cont'd.

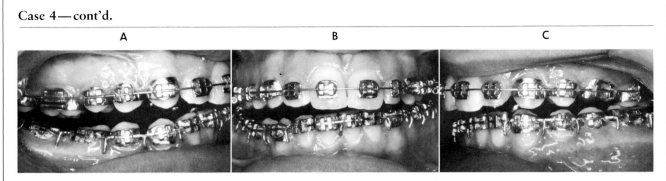

Fig. 16-46. S.J., age 18 years, 3 months, after 2½ years of orthodontic treatment.

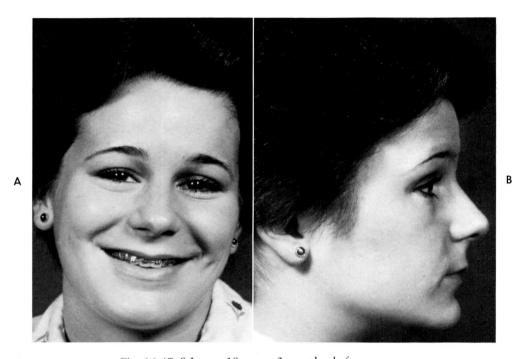

Fig. 16-47. S.J., age 18 years, 3 months, before surgery.

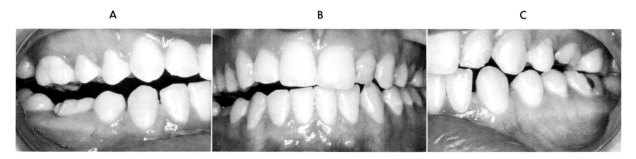

Fig. 16-48. S.J., age 18 years, 9 months, 6 months after removal of the appliances so that any relapse from the orthodontic forces could occur. Dental relationships have changed slightly.

Case 4—cont'd.

nected by an anterior subapical osteotomy. The teeth were brought into the splint and placed in maxillomandibular fixation, using Erich arch bars. Six 26-gauge

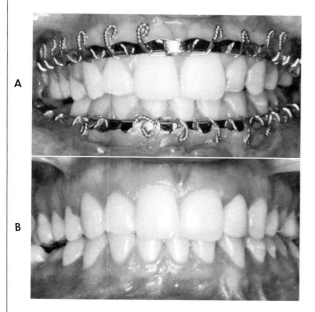

Fig. 16-49. S.J., dental relationships. **A,** Immediately following surgery to elevate the mandibular alveolar arch. **B,** Completion of treatment.

stainless steel wires were placed, two on each side and two anteriorly. Two rectangular 1 × 0.5 cm cortical cancellous bone grafts were then placed lingual to the body wires on each side, a longer and thinner rectangular block was placed anteriorly, and the wires were tightened. The defects that remained bilaterally were then packed with cortical and cancellous bone chips (Fig. 16-49).

She was maintained in maxillomandibular fixation for 6 weeks, then functioned into the splint for another 2 weeks before the arch bars were removed and active treatment concluded. At that point, all teeth were in occlusion except the retained and ankylosed second primary molars (see Fig. 16-49), and facial esthetics were quite satisfactory (Fig. 16-50). On 8-year recall, both occlusal and facial relationships had been maintained.

Comments. The only way to reposition teeth that will not respond to orthodontic forces is with subapical osteotomy. Often, as in this patient, the diagnosis is made on the basis of a failure of orthodontic therapy. Because not all teeth are affected, it is wise to remove the appliances and wait for approximately 6 months before proceeding with surgical treatment so that any teeth that did respond previously and now would relapse slightly can do so before the surgical treatment. As with anterior segmental osteotomy to elevate the lower teeth into occlusion, total mandibular subapical osteotomy is reported on the basis of only a few cases—such as this one—to be quite stable.

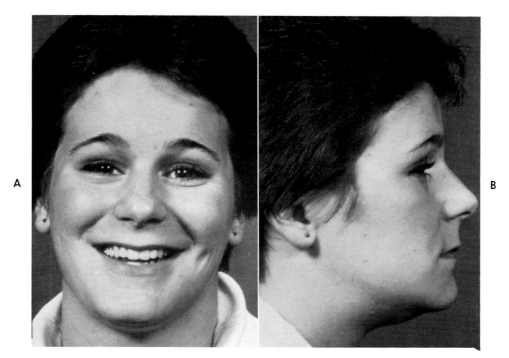

Fig. 16-50. S.J., facial appearance, age 18 years, 11 months, completion of active treatment (2 months postsurgery).

REFERENCES

1. Kelly JE, Sanchez M, van Kirk LE: An assessment of the occlusion of teeth of children, US Public Health Service DHEW Pub No (HRA) 74-1612, Washington, DC, 1973, National Center for Health Statistics.
2. Angle EH: Treatment of malocclusion of the teeth, Angle's system, ed 7, Philadelphia, 1907, SS White Dental Manufacturing Co.
3. Haas AJ: The treatment of maxillary deficiency by opening the midpalatal suture, Angle Orthod 35:200-217, 1965.
4. Wertz RA: Skeletal and dental changes accompanying rapid midpalatal suture opening, Am J Orthod 58:41-65, 1970.
5. Davis WM, Kronman JH: Anatomical changes induced by splitting of the midpalatal suture, Angle Orthod 39:126-132, 1969.
6. Bishara SE, Staley RN: Maxillary expansion: clinical implications, Am J Orthod Dentofacial Orthop 91:3-14, 1987.
7. Sarver DM, Johnston MW: Skeletal changes in vertical and anterior displacement of the maxilla with bonded rapid palatal expansion appliances, Am J Orthod Dentofacial Orthop 95:462-466, 1989.
8. Hicks E: Slow maxillary expansion: a clinical study of the skeletal versus the dental response to low magnitude force, Am J Orthod 73:121-141, 1978.
9. Isaacson RJ, Ingram AH: Forces produced by maxillary expansion. II. Forces present during treatment, Angle Orthod 34:261-270, 1964.
10. Bell RA: A review of maxillary expansion in relation to age of expansion and patient's age, Am J Orthod 81:32-37, 1981.
11. Bell R, Lecompte E: The effects of maxillary expansion using a quad helix appliance during the deciduous and mixed dentitions, Am J Orthod 79:152-161, 1981.
12. Frankel R: The theoretical concept underlying treatment with functional correctors, Trans Eur Orthod Soc pp. 223-250, 1966.
13. Owen A: Morphologic changes in the sagittal dimension using the Frankel appliance, Am J Orthod 80:573-603, 1981.
14. Krebs A: Expansion of the midpalatal suture studied by means of metallic implants, Acta Odontol Scand 17:491-511, 1959.
15. Krebs A: Midpalatal suture expansion studied by the implant method over a seven year period, Trans Eur Orthod Soc pp. 131-142, 1964.
16. Storey E: Tissue response to the movement of bones, Am J Orthod 64:229-247, 1973.
17. Melsen B: A histological study of the influence of sutural morphology and skeletal maturation on rapid palatal expansion in children, Trans Eur Orthod Soc pp. 499-507, 1972.
18. Cotton LA: Slow maxillary expansion: skeletal versus dental response to low magnitude force in *Macaca mulatta.* Am J Orthod 73:1-23, 1978.
19. Timms DJ: An occlusal analysis of lateral maxillary midpalatal suture opening, Dent Pract 18:435-441, 1968.
20. Melsen B: Palatal growth study on human autopsy material: a histological microradiographic study, Am J Orthod 68:42-54, 1975.
21. Kennedy JW, Bell WH, Kimbrough OL, et al: Osteotomy as an adjunct to rapid maxillary expansion, Am J Orthod 70:123-137, 1976.
22. Glassman AS, Nahigian SJ, Medway JM, et al: Conservative surgical orthodontic adult rapid palatal expansion: sixteen cases, Am J Orthod 86:207-213, 1984.
23. Alpern MC, Yurosko JJ: Rapid palatal expansion in adults with and without surgery, Angle Orthod 57:245-263, 1987.
24. Medland WJA: The stability of surgical orthodontic transverse expansion, master's thesis, Chapel Hill, 1989, University of North Carolina.
25. Medland WJA, Phillips C, Turvey TA: Stability after transverse surgical expansion of the maxilla with LeFort I osteotomy, J Oral Maxillofac Surg [pending].
26. Turvey TA: Maxillary expansion: a surgical technique based on surgical-orthodontic treatment objectives and anatomical considerations, J Maxillofac Surg 13:51-58, 1985.
27. Barrett MJ: Functioning occlusion, Ann Aust College Dent Surg 2:68-80, 1969.
28. Steedle JR, Proffit WR: The pattern and control of eruptive tooth movements, Am J Orthod Dentofacial Orthop 87:56-66, 1987.
29. Proffit WR, Vig KWL: Primary failure of eruption: a possible cause of posterior open bite, Am J Orthod 80:173-190, 1981.
30. Davies TM, Lewis DH, Gillbe GV: The surgical and orthodontic management of unerupted teeth in cleidocranial dysplasia, Br J Orthod 14:43-47, 1987.
31. Kloosterman J: Kole's osteotomy, a follow-up study, J Maxillofac Surg 13:59-63, 1985.

CHAPTER 17

Major Prosthodontic Problems

Raymond P. White, Jr.
Bill C. Terry
Myron R. Tucker

NEED AND DEMAND

Patients who seek surgical-orthodontic treatment fall into two major groups. The larger group, two-thirds to three-fourths of the total at present, are between their late teens and age 35. These patients want treatment to improve their jaw function and dentofacial esthetics as part of an overall strategy of improving the quality of life. In previous chapters much of the discussion has revolved around the treatment of this group of patients, most of whom have complete dentitions.

The other major group of patients seeking treatment are older, typically between ages 35 and 55. Their motivation is not so much to improve their overall life situation as to maintain what they have, which they find threatened by deterioration of their dentition. An individual who has a moderately severe discrepancy in the size or position of the jaws may decide against treatment at an early age, only to be forced to reconsider once he or she loses some teeth from caries or periodontal disease. For instance, a mandibular deficiency with deep overbite may be tolerated until the upper central incisors are lost. But if the malocclusion makes it impossible to fabricate a satisfactory prosthetic restoration as a replacement, surgical-orthodontic treatment to align the jaws becomes a necessity.

The United States and the other developed countries of western Europe and Asia in which modern surgical-orthodontic treatment is provided to large segments of the population are characterized now by declining birth rates and an aging population. On a percentage basis, the most rapidly growing segment of the population is the oldest, but this is misleading because it is not true in absolute numbers. Instead, there is a population bulge, the "baby boomers" cohort, a result of the increased birth rate of the immediate post-World War II years. The baby boomers now are in their thirties and early forties, and they will significantly expand the 40 to 55 years age group in the next decade. The implication is that the number of older patients who seek surgical-orthodontic treatment because of jaw malalignment and associated prosthodontic considerations also is likely to increase.

How many potential patients with jaw deformity and major prosthodontic problems might exist in the United States? Douglass and colleagues[1] estimated prosthodontic needs for the population based on NHANES-I data that were gathered from 1971 to 1974. Over 45% of the population ages 45 to 64 needed fixed or removable partial dentures. Meskin and colleagues,[2] in a report based on data from the National Survey of Oral Health in U.S. Employed Adults and Seniors: 1985-86, took a more definitive look at tooth-loss patterns and produced a prosthetic treatment typology (TLPT). The survey sampled employed adults representing about 100 million individuals ages 18 to 64. The data indicated that major prosthodontic problems exist in the upper arch in over 21% of the 34 to 44 years age group. This increases to about 40% in the group 45 to 54 years of age. In the lower arch, tooth-loss patterns begin to pose major problems in over 25% of individuals in the 35 to 44 years age group, increasing to over 40% in the 45 to 54 years age group. If the results of this study of the working population ages 35 to 54 can be extrapolated to the entire population in this age group, by the year 2000, 28% of 77 million individuals that age will require major prosthodontic treatment (assuming the prevalence of the problem remains stable—it is possible, of course, that tooth loss will decrease).

McLain and Proffit[3] reviewed severe or handicapping malocclusion in the U.S. population. Based on the Treatment Priority Index, 29% of adolescents were judged to have severe malocclusion, which can be compared with 25% of adult men and 34% of adult women in Swedish studies.[4,5] If 25% of individuals with major prosthodontic problems in one arch also have severe malocclusion (which seems a conservative estimate because if severe malocclusion had any effect on the rate of tooth loss, it would be more likely to increase than decrease), then over 5 million individuals in the next decade might need surgery and orthodontics to prepare them for appropriate replacement of missing teeth. Obviously, these estimates are imprecise, but they indicate in general the magnitude of the problems in the U.S. population and support the impression of clinicians that greater numbers of these individuals are actively seeking treatment.

This chapter focuses on the special problems in planning and coordinating surgical-orthodontic-periodontal-prosthodontic treatment that will be dispersed among multiple dental specialists, each with his or her own perspective and responsibility. Cohesive planning and coordination of treatment are required if the patient is to have a satisfactory result.

DIAGNOSTIC CONSIDERATIONS: COORDINATING INPUT AMONG DENTAL SPECIALISTS

A patient with major prosthodontic problems may seek treatment initially from a restorative dentist, periodontist, surgeon, or orthodontist. Although each of the dental specialists must be involved in treatment, the data base required for a problem list can be developed by any one of the dentists. Usually each contributes data based on individual expertise (e.g., the orthodon-

tist characterizes tooth-size discrepancy, and the periodontist comments on the quality of gingival tissue).

A careful assessment of the patient's health status is mandatory. Older individuals often have major health problems (e.g., hypertension) that do not preclude treatment but may require monitoring and even modifications in the approach to controlling the systemic disease. The increasing tendency toward diabetes as patients become older, and the susceptibility of diabetics to periodontal breakdown that can be exacerbated by orthodontic treatment, must be kept in mind. The implications of systemic problems for surgical-orthodontic treatment are reviewed in some detail in Chapter 6.

Before diagnostic records are made, any discrepancy between retruded contact position of the teeth and intercuspal position must be assessed. Patients with both severe malocclusion and missing teeth are particularly likely to shift the jaw to a more advantageous occlusal relationship. If more than 2 to 3 mm of discrepancy exists in any of the three planes of space, it is important to obtain all diagnostic records, not just the dental cast relationships, with the mandibular condyles in retruded contact position and the jaws at the occlusal vertical dimension (Fig. 17-1). A convenient way to position the jaws is to fabricate a wax bite registration and have it in place when photographs and radiographs are taken. In these patients, dental casts must be mounted in a semiadjustable articulator with a facebow transfer and a wax bite registration.

Often the patients already have removable partial dentures that by necessity were fabricated to match the unusual position of the jaws. Compromised jaw function and the presence of removable partial dentures often affect the health of the remaining teeth. A careful assessment of the periodontal status of the remaining teeth is particularly important, including both the degree of periodontal pocketing and a qualitative assessment of the soft tissue surrounding the teeth. In addition to panoramic and cephalometric radiographs, these patients usually require a full series of intraoral radiographs for adequate examination of periodontal and dental caries problems.

Once the data base for an individual patient is developed from a clinical interaction and diagnostic records, the problem list must be developed. The compromised dentition is always a major, high-priority item on the problem list. Other items should characterize malrelationships of the jaws and the teeth in all three planes of space. Discrepancy in the transverse and AP dimensions may be obvious, but establishing the correct occlusal vertical dimension for a patient with multiple missing teeth can be difficult. For diagnostic and planning purposes a jaw position may have to be established arbitrarily using the best clinical judgment of those involved.

After the problem list has been developed, all the

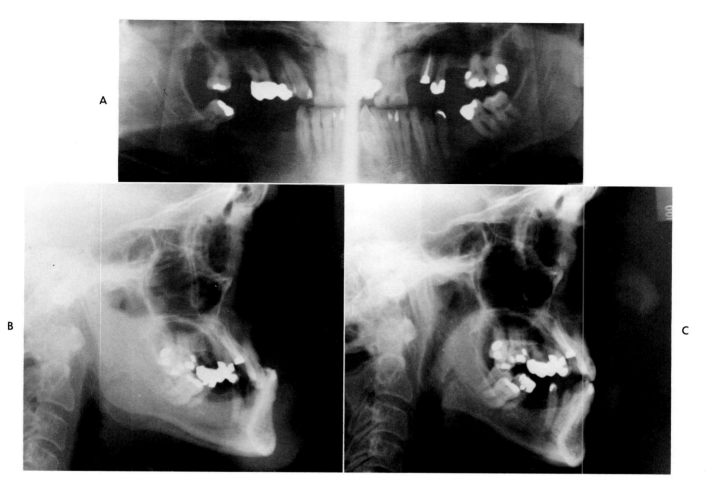

Fig. 17-1. **A,** Panoramic radiograph exhibiting multiple missing teeth. **B,** The patient has shifted the jaws forward for maximum tooth contact. This radiograph must be repeated for diagnostic purposes. **C,** The mandibular condyles are in retruded contact position, and the correct occlusal vertical dimension is established with a waxbite registration. The radiograph taken with the jaws in this position is suitable for diagnostic and planning purposes.

dental specialists who are to be involved in treatment must confer to develop the treatment plan. A major goal of the treatment planning process is to decide what periodontal-restorative-prosthodontic treatment must be done in the initial phase of treatment before orthodontics and surgery and what can be deferred until the final occlusion has been established. Each of the specialists involved in treatment must understand the entire treatment plan and the timing of treatment so that their respective roles can be coordinated.

TREATMENT SEQUENCE
Preliminary Treatment

The sequence of treatment in a patient with complex dental problems is shown in Table 17-1. In the discussion below, the particular problems of patients with multiple missing teeth are emphasized. The reader is referred to Chapter 6 for a more general discussion of the sequencing of complex treatment.

Disease Control

At the outset, active dental decay must be controlled and defective restorations repaired. Definitive restorations (i.e., precious metal or ceramic castings) should be deferred until orthodontics and surgery have been completed. But remember that definitive restorative dentistry may not take place until 2 years after the start of treatment, and dental restorations must be expected to last at least that long. Active periodontal disease also must be controlled. Obviously the patient's role in home care must be reinforced, particularly in anticipation of having orthodontic appliances in place for 18 to 24 months.

Preliminary Periodontic/Prosthetic Treatment

A major issue at the preliminary periodontic treatment stage is the usefulness of previous fixed or removable partial dentures. For both esthetics and function, the patient may need to have some replacements for

TABLE 17-1 Sequence of complex multispecialty treatment

Treatment stage	Comment
Disease control	
Systemic	Medical consultation if an ASA III risk; medication doses may have to be modified
TM-joint pain/dysfunction	Conservative initial treatment: splints, therapy
Caries	Control: endodontics, amalgam restorations
Periodontal disease	Control: scaling, curettage
Preliminary perio/restorative	
Gingival grafts	Needed if later treatment will stress gingival attachment
Treatment partial denture	Needed if original one makes treatment impossible but patient cannot get along without a replacement for missing teeth
Presurgical orthodontics	Periodontal maintenance required; may be necessary to modify partial dentures, often helpful to tie prosthetic teeth to arch wire
Orthognathic surgery	Special attention to surgical stabilization; preprosthetic surgery must be staged
Postsurgical orthodontics	Same settling procedures as other types of cases; temporary bridges immediately upon debanding often gives best stability, avoiding removable retainers
Definitive perio/restorative	
Implant placement if part of plan	Implant placement may be done while orthodontics is being completed
Osseous and soft tissue periodontal surgery	Only if absolutely necessary; conservative approach often better
Partial dentures	Fixed or removable: no need for long delay in completing treatment

missing teeth, but often it is better to minimize their use to the extent to which this is possible. The guideline is that any prosthetic replacement that is in place during the subsequent surgical-orthodontic treatment must be compatible with maintainence of the patient's oral health. If a fixed or removable partial denture is contributing to periodontal breakdown, but the patient cannot do without it, no alternative may exist to replacing it with a better temporary substitute that will minimize tissue damage.

Some periodontal surgical procedures (such as crown lengthening in anticipation of fixed restorations) should be deferred, but gingival grafting to improve the quality of supporting soft tissue should be accomplished in advance of the orthodontics. The guideline is that the preliminary periodontal therapy should include anything needed to prevent periodontal problems from becoming worse during the surgical-orthodontic treatment to follow.

Presurgical Orthodontics

A major task of the presurgical orthodontics is to align the remaining teeth over the bony base of the respective jaws. Removing dental compensations, relieving crowding of teeth, and adjusting the occlusal plane composes most of the orthodontic tooth movement. As in any presurgical orthodontic treatment, the goal is to get the patient ready for jaw surgery as expeditiously as possible, leaving some finishing orthodontics until

the postsurgical phase of treatment. Patients with multiple missing teeth pose two special orthodontic problems: (1) the management of edentulous spaces during treatment, and (2) anchorage for tooth movement when the normal anchor teeth have been lost.

Edentulous Spaces

Often the position of teeth adjacent to edentulous spaces must be altered so that a better tooth replacement can be done later, but the patient needs a replacement tooth for esthetics while this is being done. Missing maxillary incisors are the most common problem of this type, but lower incisors or upper premolars also occasionally must be supplied during the orthodontic treatment. There are three possible approaches: (1) adapt an existing fixed or removable partial denture, (2) supply the missing teeth on a new temporary removable partial denture designed to be compatible with treatment, or (3) fabricate replacement teeth that can be tied to the orthodontic arch wires.

The problem with maintaining an existing prosthetic device is that it is likely to interfere with the necessary orthodontic tooth movement. In some circumstances it may be possible to section an existing bridge between one abutment and the pontic, leaving the pontic cantilevered to the other abutment. The pontic and/or the sides of the crowns then can be reduced in size to provide space for repositioning the adjacent teeth (Fig. 17-2). The clasps of a removable partial denture may have

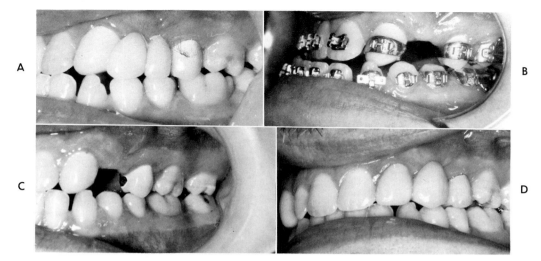

Fig. 17-2. **A,** In this patient with Class III malocclusion due to maxillary deficiency, a bridge in the maxillary left canine area made it impossible to change arch form as required for good postsurgical occlusion. **B,** Before orthodontic treatment began the bridge was sectioned and the pontic was removed, but the crowns were maintained. During active treatment, the pontic was replaced with a plastic denture tooth tied to the arch wires. **C,** Post-surgical dental relationships at the time orthodontic treatment was completed. **D,** Occlusal relationships with a new bridge in place, 1 year postsurgically.

to be adjusted to the point that its retention is severely compromised, but if this produces a situation no worse than what could be achieved with a new temporary partial denture, maintaining the old one offers economic and esthetic advantages. Maintaining and modifying what the patient already has is the best plan if it is possible.

Making a new temporary appliance to supply esthetically important teeth may be the only possibility if many teeth are missing and the abutments must be re-positioned significantly. As a general guideline, if only one or two teeth are missing, placing a bracket on a plastic denture tooth and attaching it to the orthodontic arch wire is a better alternative than a temporary partial denture. Usually it is better to supply several missing teeth with a modified orthodontic retainer, clasping teeth that will require minimal movement or changing the clasping as tooth movement proceeds. In either case the patient must accept that the replacement teeth are strictly for esthetics, and their use in function will be minimal.

One limiting factor with denture teeth tied to an orthodontic arch wire is that a full-dimension edgewise wire is needed to keep the denture tooth from rotating around the wire—but full-dimension wires are too stiff for most tooth movement. Using 18-slot attachments and flexible 17×25 arch wires (braided steel or NiTi) is one way to get around this problem. Another is to sol-der a vertical spur across a round arch wire so that it contacts the replacement tooth above and below a twin bracket.

Anchorage

Anchorage problems due to missing teeth arise most often when it is desirable to retract protruding anteriors but all the posterior teeth have been lost. Again, there are three possibilities. (1) Accomplish the retraction surgically instead of orthodontically, which is particularly feasible when surgery in the affected jaw is part of the overall plan anyway. (2) Use extraoral force to produce the tooth movement. In cooperative patients, this can be quite effective, but many adults are reluctant to wear headgear, particularly on the full-time or nearly full-time basis needed for efficient tooth movement. Remember also that lighter forces are necessary in patients who have experienced periodontal bone loss (see Chapter 6). Headgear often is contraindicated for these individuals because it is difficult to avoid heavy intermittent force. (3) Use implants as anchors for orthodontic tooth movement.

The theoretical possibility of implants as anchorage has been recognized for years, but only recently has this approach begun to be used clinically. There now is good evidence that implants will withstand orthodontic forces without becoming loose or displaced,[6-8] and tooth movement can be produced quite successfully with an implant as the anchorage. As with all implants, an important component of success is placing the implant and waiting several months for osseointegration before placing a load on it. This could mean a 6- to 9-month delay in starting presurgical orthodontics in some cases. On the other hand, with good planning the same implant that was used for orthodontic anchorage could be useful later as a prosthodontic abutment. It seems likely that implant anchorage will be used more frequently in the future.

At the completion of presurgical orthodontics, stabilization of the teeth is needed in final preparation for surgery. When multiple teeth are missing, it is particularly important to stabilize those which are present as well as is possible. This means even greater emphasis on rigid stabilizing arch wires and the recognition that the teeth alone may not be adequate for stabilization despite the most rigid attachment system (see further discussion below).

Orthognathic Surgery
Final Presurgical Planning

The steps in planning just before surgery, particularly cephalometric prediction tracing and model surgery, are described in detail in Chapter 5. In patients with multiple missing teeth the goal of the surgical phase of treatment is to properly align the jaws and the remaining teeth in anticipation of the final fixed and removable prostheses. It is necessary to anticipate the position of the replacement teeth, with special attention to occlusion and the support that the teeth would give to the soft tissues of the upper lip. If any question arises, prosthetic teeth should be waxed in place on the casts used for model surgery. At this point both the orthodontist and the restorative dentist must confer with the surgeon. Often the final position of the jaws must be altered slightly to facilitate completion of prosthetics at the end of treatment. Less than ideal facial esthetics may have to be accepted to achieve satisfactory occlusion and function.

When large edentulous spaces exist in the mandible or maxilla and alveolar bone loss is extensive, preprosthetic surgery to improve alveolar ridge contour and the quality of the covering tissue must be considered. Ridge contour augmentation can be accomplished with autogenous bone, allogeneic bank bone, or hydroxylapatite. The quantity and quality of fixed tissue over the alveolar ridges can be improved with skin or mucosal grafts. Osseointegrated implants strategically placed can improve the function and stability of final prostheses.

The problems with sequencing and combining preprosthetic surgical procedures with orthognathic surgery require coordinated planning among the orthodontist, surgeon, and restorative dentists and staging of treatment. If at all possible, the decision for preprosthetic surgical procedures and the placement of implants should be made at the same time as plans for orthodontics and surgery. This early decision may allow preprosthetic surgery during the period of presurgical orthodontics (e.g., hydroxylapatite augmentation of alveolar ridges). Early ridge contour augmentation allows for healing and consolidation of graft material

before orthognathic surgery. Preprosthetic surgery to augment alveolar bone or improve covering tissue may be done at the same time as orthognathic surgery. Implant placement usually must follow orthognathic surgery because implant position is so critical for successful final prostheses. Obviously all of these procedures may be delayed until after orthognathic surgery, but the total treatment time becomes prolonged excessively. The use of RIF also assists the surgeon and the patient because minimizing or eliminating the period of maxillomandibular fixation allows preprosthetic procedures during orthognathic surgery or in the weeks following.

Orthodontic appliances placed to aid in stabilizing the jaws at surgery are more difficult when the patient has multiple missing teeth. Rectangular arch wires with vertical lugs and bands on molar teeth should be used whenever possible. In contrast to patients with a full complement of teeth, usually orthodontic appliances alone are not satisfactory in enabling the surgeon to apply maxillomandibular fixation. At surgery the orthodontic appliances often must be supplemented with modified acrylic splints that are keyed to the new occlusion and retained with skeletal suspension wires (Fig. 17-3). The skeletal suspension wires in the maxilla usually extend from the piriform rim or zygomatic buttress. In the mandible, circummandibular wires are employed (see Chapter 7 for details of skeletal suspension wire placement). Following osteotomy the suspension wires are linked with an intermediate wire holding the maxilla and mandible into the splint(s), the new position of the jaws.

RIF across osteotomy sites can assist the surgeon greatly in managing patients with multiple missing teeth. With rigid fixation, less stress is placed on stabilizing orthodontic arch wires and the teeth that retain them. Occlusal splints need not be as complex, and skeletal suspension wires may be left in place for a shorter time or not needed at all. Figs. 17-4 to 17-16 illustrate how rigid fixation is useful in these patients. As soon as the jaws are mobilized (e.g., soon after surgery with RIF), the patient occludes into the prepared splints until jaw function is regained and bony healing has progressed to the point where orthodontics can be resumed.

Construction of the modified acrylic occlusal splint(s) is the final step in presurgical planning. The splints can be tissue borne in addition to covering the occlusal surfaces of the remaining teeth. Their design must not prevent access to surgical incisions nor compress soft tissue, which serves as the vascular pedicle to mobilized jaw segments.

Surgery and Postsurgical Management

Any of the surgical procedures described in Section III might be appropriate to align the jaws. If surgery in

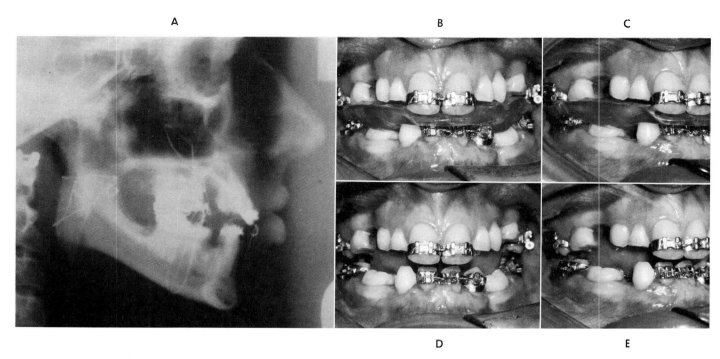

Fig. 17-3. Use of modified occlusal splints in patients with multiple missing teeth. **A,** Following jaw repositioning the splint is retained with bilateral mandibular and maxillary skeletal suspension wires. **B** and **C,** Once the jaws are released from maxillomandibular fixation and the patient begins to function, the splint is adjusted so it can be removed for cleaning and the patient functions into the splint to help retain the position of the teeth. **D** and **E,** The splint is removed just before the postsurgical orthodontics is begun or just before the patient returns to the restorative dentist for definitive restorations when no postsurgical orthodontics is necessary.

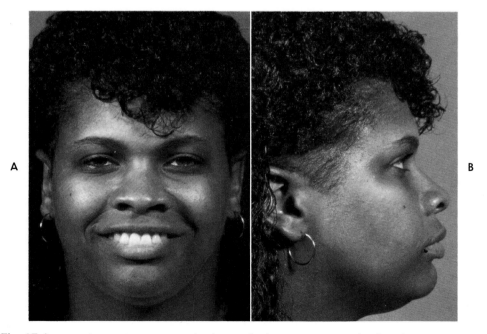

Fig. 17-4. **A** and **B,** L.S., age 30 and a hospital administrator, sought dental services to replace teeth lost to caries in her teenage years. On initial evaluation, dental caries was not active and only marginal gingivitis existed. The patient had good facial balance and no esthetic concerns.

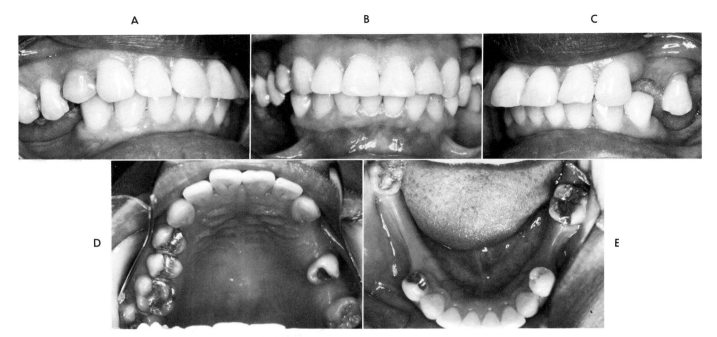

Fig. 17-5. L.S. **A-E,** Maxillary posterior teeth #2,3,4,13 had supraerupted after mandibular teeth were removed to such a degree that a mandibular removable partial denture could not be constructed. The most effective plan to replace missing posterior teeth was sought. Three options existed: (1) remove teeth #2,3,4,13,16 and replace the maxillary posterior teeth with a removable partial denture, (2) perform endodontics on supraerupted teeth #2,3,4,13, periodontal surgery to lengthen the crowns, reduce the crowns of the teeth vertically, and restore the teeth with full crowns, or (3) reposition teeth #2,3,4 and alveolar bone with a posterior maxillary subapical osteotomy and perform endodontics and crown lengthening only on tooth #13. (The patient chose the last option).

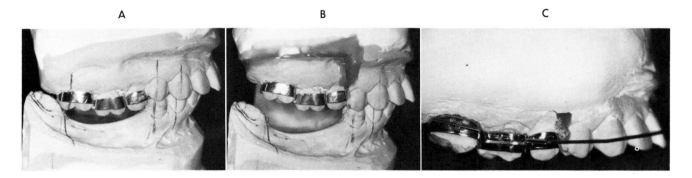

Fig. 17-6. **A-C,** Model surgery and adaptation of the stabilizing rectangular surgical arch wire. The teeth are positioned to allow space for a removable mandibular partial denture. Because the orthodontic arch wire alone would not be sufficient to stabilize the dentoalveolar segment after osteotomy, a rigid vertical wire strut was constructed using 36-mil round wire. At one end a loop was bent around a 2.0 mm screw, which would secure the strut to the bone in the zygomatic buttress at surgery. The opposite end of the strut was bent to fit into the buccal headgear tube on the molar band at surgery (see Chapter 10 for surgical technique).

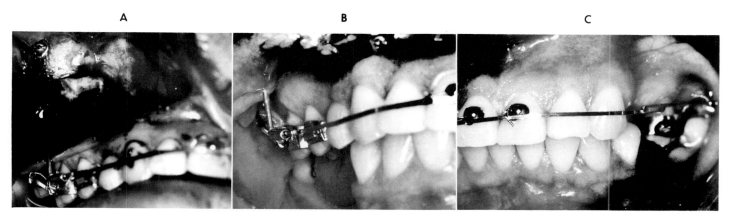

Fig. 17-7. **A,** At surgery, the dentoalveolar segment repositioned superiorly and stabilized with a rectangular arch wire. The vertical wire strut from the zygomatic buttress to the buccal tube on the molar band provided rigid fixation. **B and C,** Four weeks following surgery, the repositioned dentoalveolar segment was clinically firm.

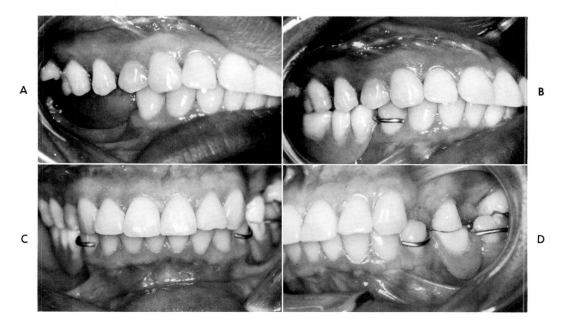

Fig. 17-8. **A-D,** A temporary removable partial denture was fabricated and placed when orthodontic appliances were removed to prevent supraeruption of teeth #2,3,4. Endodontics has been completed on tooth #13.

more than one jaw must be done, the sequence of surgery as discussed in Chapter 11 is followed. Additional surgical procedures (e.g., hydroxylapatite augmentation of edentulous areas or soft-tissue procedures to expose additional alveolar bone or improve surface tissue with mucosa or skin grafts) can be carried out at the same time as jaw surgery. Often combinations of procedures are possible. But remember that the primary purpose of the surgical procedures is to align the jaws, and this goal must not be compromised.

The healing phase to clinical bony union following osteotomy does not take longer in a patient with major prosthodontic problems. However, adequate time should be allowed for clinical bony healing, usually 8 to 10 weeks with wire fixation across osteotomy sites and maxillomandibular fixation, before returning the patient to the orthodontist. With RIF across osteotomy sites, the time frame can be reduced.

Rehabilitation of the jaws to full function is similar in these patients to those with a full complement of

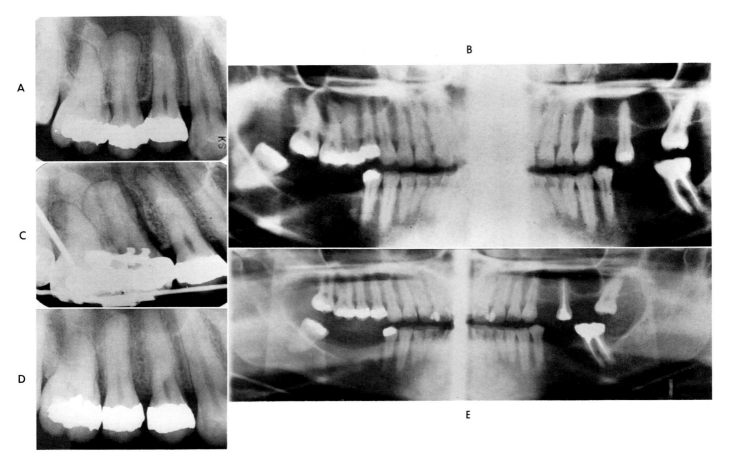

Fig. 17-9. **A** and **B**, Periapical and panoramic radiograph before treatment. **C**, Periapical radiograph immediately following surgery. **D**, At completion of surgical phase of treatment. **E**, Panoramic radiograph before definitive restorative dentistry.

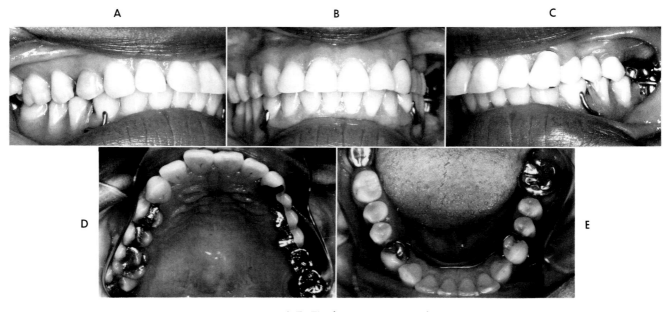

Fig. 17-10. **A-E**, Final restorations in place.

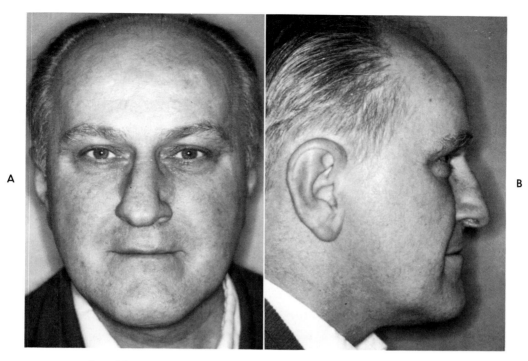

Fig. 17-11.**A** and **B**, L.A., age 54, sought replacements from his general dentist for his missing teeth. Because his jaw position would make replacing mandibular posterior teeth quite difficult, he was advised to have his lower jaw shortened. He had considered this option 10 years earlier but had decided against treatment because he could not risk sensory loss in his lower lip and did not want his teeth wired together for 6 to 8 weeks in maxillomandibular fixation.

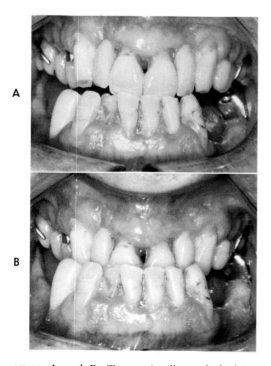

Fig. 17-12. **A** and **B**, To maximally occlude his posterior teeth, L.A. had to protrude his mandible.

teeth. Early function, within the first 2 weeks of surgery, is practical when RIF is used. Modifying the occlusal splint to allow jaw function can be difficult, but the problem is not insurmountable. Constructing the occlusal splint on a semiadjustable articulator and modifying it in anticipation of early jaw function is helpful. Often the splint must be modified again when the jaws are released following surgery if the patient is to function into it without occlusal interference or deviation of the jaws.

Postsurgical Orthodontics

The recommendation that the orthodontist remove the occlusal splint at the first return visit following surgery may have to be modified with these patients. Often the surgeon must tie the splint in place to one arch with skeletal suspension wires. It is easier for the surgeon to remove these wires and the splint in such circumstances just before the patient is to visit the orthodontist. There must be no time lag between removal of the splint and the orthodontic visit. Quite often in patients with multiple missing teeth, only a few teeth occlude after splint removal. Active orthodontics must begin very soon after splint removal or the patient may seek an intercuspal position different from the one

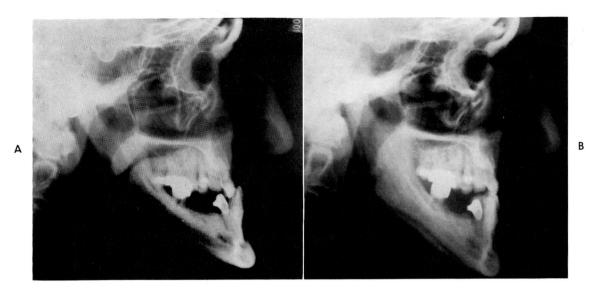

Fig. 17-13. L.A., lateral cephalometric films. **A,** With jaw positioned forward in intercuspal position for maximal occlusion and **B,** in retruded contact position.

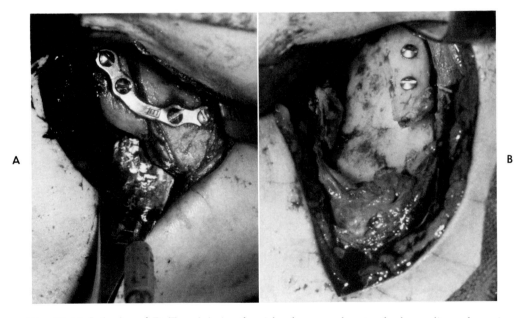

Fig. 17-14. L.A. **A** and **B,** To minimize the risk of sensory loss to the lower lip and maximize the chance that RIF could reduce the period of maxillomandibular fixation, an extraoral vertical ramus osteotomy was performed (see Chapter 9 for surgical technique). On the right side, the bone was mortised with the condyle in position (VanZile modification) and the bony segments were fixed with a semirigid bone plate. On the left side, bone was trimmed so the proximal condylar segment could overlap the distal ramus segment with the condyle still in position. Lag screws fixed the segments. The patient was in maxillomandibular fixation for 2 weeks, then was allowed minimal jaw movement with guiding elastics for an additional 4 weeks.

planned before surgery. Enough plasticity exists at the osteotomy sites at this stage of healing to allow a shift in the position of the jaws of several millimeters.

In some cases, the acrylic occlusal splint is worn for several months during the early stages of postsurgical orthodontics or even until the patient has completed orthodontics and is ready for definitive restorative dentistry (see Fig. 17-3). This implies that most or all of the postsurgical orthodontic tooth movement will be done in the arch opposite the one to which the splint is

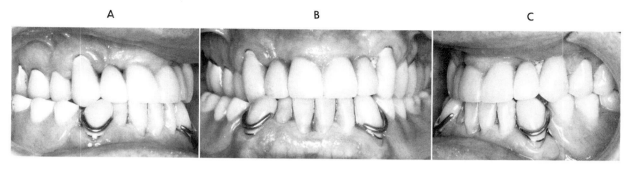

Fig. 17-15. L.A. **A-C,** Final restorations in place. Full crowns on maxillary teeth and an removable partial denture to replace missing mandibular teeth were begun 3 months following surgery and completed at 6 months following surgery.

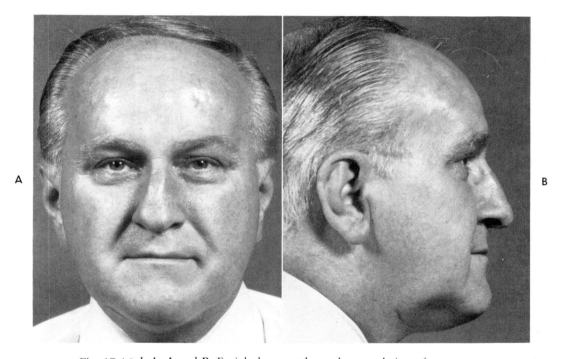

Fig. 17-16. L.A. **A** and **B,** Facial photographs at the completion of treatment.

attached. In that case, it is only necessary to modify the occlusal surface to provide a flat plane against which tooth movement can occur. For prolonged wear, the splint should be modified so the patient can remove it for cleaning, which means clasp retention instead of keeping it tied to the arch wire.

As a rule, the period of postsurgical orthodontics should be short, less than 6 months, but in some prosthodontic patients it is impossible to accomplish some necessary tooth movement before surgery and the postsurgical treatment inevitably takes longer (see Case 2). The general approach to postsurgical treatment is the same as that discussed in detail in Chapter 6. The surgical arch wires are replaced with light working arch wires and the teeth are moved as rapidly as possible to their planned positions. The major difference in prosthodontic patients is that a rectangular wire and/or

the occlusal splint is maintained in one arch to improve stability in compromised dental situations.

For these patients, the goal of retention is different and therefore the approach also is modified. Most patients with an intact dentition can eventually discontine their retainers. The typical patient wears a removable retainer full-time except for eating for 3 to 4 months until the periodontal ligament has time to reorganize, then on a gradually decreasing part-time basis until the retainer is discontinued after 12 to 24 months. In contrast, prosthodontic patients require permanent retention, at least in the areas where teeth will be replaced (see Case 1). The prosthodontic appliance becomes the orthodontist's permanent retainer.

For this reason, the major objective of retention in prosthodontic patients is to hold the teeth in the correct posttreatment position until the definitive prosth-

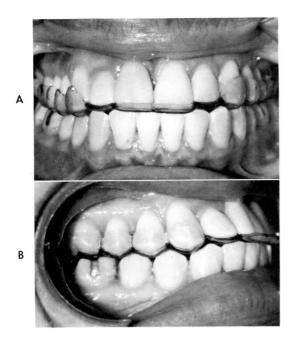

Fig. 17-17. A full-coverage plastic splint, as employed in the maxillary arch for this patient immediately after removal of appliances, is indicated instead of a conventional orthodontic retainer for patients who have a compromised periodontal situation.

odontics can be accomplished. A rigid retainer that can be worn full-time, including during eating, is needed. Sometimes the best plan is to leave the fixed orthodontic appliance in place until just before the preparations for the definitive prosthodontics are begun (see Case 2). Almost always, a long delay between removing the orthodontic appliance and beginning the final prosthodontics is undesirable. A full-time retainer must be placed immediately when the appliances are removed. When fixed partial dentures are anticipated, fixed retainers bonded to teeth adjacent to the edentulous space serve well. An alternative is a thin full-coverage splint of thermally moldable plastic (Fig. 17-17). In any event the retainers must be kept in place until the definitive restorative dentistry is begun.

Definitive Periodontics and Restorative Dentistry

Once the orthodontic phase of treatment is completed, definitive periodontic procedures can be accomplished. (This means that active tooth movement has been finished, not necessarily that the orthodontic appliances have been removed. Leaving the passive appliance as a rigid full-time retainer may be advantageous, as discussed above.) The periodontal status of remaining teeth must be reassessed at this point. Orthodontic movement of teeth often improves bony support, but occasionally the situation worsens because of an increase in periodontal pocketing or resorption of the roots of the teeth. At times the plan for periodontics

and definitive restorative dentistry must be altered because of these unanticipated changes.

If required, crown lengthening should be performed at this stage of treatment, along with periodontal flap procedures to improve the quality of the periodontal soft tissues. Preprosthetic surgical procedures (e.g., repositioning of muscle attachments, mucosa or skin grafting to the alveolar ridge, or implant exposure) are usually done at this point. If more than one of these procedures is required, often they can be combined during one surgery appointment. Usually these procedures can be done on an outpatient basis, but occasionally hospitalization overnight is necessary to manage a patient's medical problems or monitor the patient's recovery from surgery and anesthesia.

Definitive restorative dentistry, including fixed and removable prostheses, is the final step in treatment for patients with major prosthodontic problems. Often 2 years or more have elapsed since the original plan was devised. Reassessment is always required. As with any complex prosthodontic treatment, it may be wise to place the patient in provisional restorations (which also are excellent fixed orthodontic retainers) before fabricating the final fixed or removable partial dentures. The instability of the occlusal relationships without excellent retention always must be kept in mind.

RESPONSE TO TREATMENT

Results following orthodontics, surgery, and restorative dentistry are good even though multidisciplinary planning and treatment are complex, the total time for treatment is prolonged, and the patients are generally older. The surgeon and the orthodontist must see the patient frequently during the first year following completion of treatment. After that time the responsibility for follow-up generally goes to the periodontist and restorative dentist, with the surgeon and the orthodontist seeing the patient no more frequently than they would any other patient. Complications following surgery should be no greater than in any other patient having a similar surgical procedure. Obviously, patients with major prosthodontic problems have more procedures, and each has its risks.

An area of particular concern today is the potential of TM joint problems. Joint dysfunction may be a reason for the treatment initially, and of course there is the possibility that problems may arise following the treatment. Fortunately, there is no reason to expect that TM joint dysfunction will be a greater problem in prosthodontic patients than in other groups. In fact, although there are no good data to document the point, the clinical impression is that TM joint problems probably are less rather than more frequent in these patients. Special considerations in the treatment of patients with TM joint dysfunction, some of whom also will have prosthodontic problems, are discussed in Chapter 19.

Case 1

M.J., age 29, sought consultation after he was told he could not have his missing teeth replaced easily because of the position of his jaws. The patient had no esthetic concerns, but he wanted to retain his teeth and replace missing teeth so he would have good masticatory function.

On clinical examination, facial proportions were difficult to assess, but the patient appeared to have a combina-tion of midface deficiency and mandibular protrusion (Fig. 17-18). There was a Class III malocclusion, and multiple teeth were missing. Gingivitis was generalized, but no deep periodontal pocketing was present. The mandibular right canine was displaced facially and had poor-quality periodontal supporting tissue (Fig. 17-19). On cephalometric analysis, the maxilla was mildly defi-cient vertically and anteroposteriorly, with a slightly

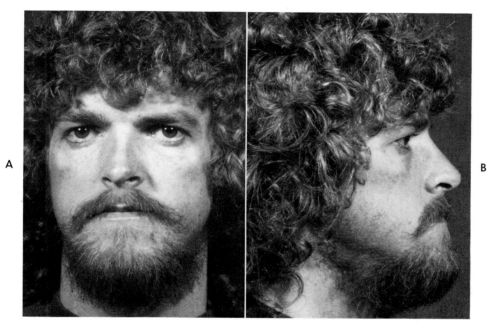

Fig. 17-18. M.J., age 29 years, 5 months. **A** and **B**, Pretreatment facial photographs.

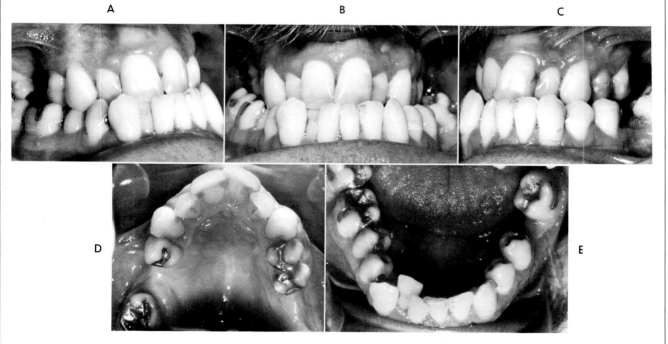

Fig. 17-19. M.J. **A-E**, Pretreatment position of the teeth. Note the missing teeth and the mal-posed mandibular right canine.

Continued.

Case 1—cont'd.

long mandible rotated upward and forward. The teeth in both arches were reasonably well related to their supporting bone (Fig. 17-20).

The treatment plan included:

1. Removal of the mandibular right canine.
2. Periodontal therapy and home care to resolve the gingivitis.
3. Replacement of several amalgam restorations on the posterior teeth.
4. Alignment of teeth and closure of the mandibular right canine space. The maxillary right second molar and the mandibular left second molar were to be moved to a more upright position, resulting in bite opening and the mandible rotating down and back.
5. Maxillary and mandibular stabilizing arch wires with soldered hooks in final preparation for surgery. Presurgical treatment including periodontics, and restorative dentistry was estimated at 18 months.
6. LeFort I osteotomy to advance the maxilla.
7. Finishing orthodontics with space maintained for final restorations replacing missing teeth.
8. Definitive periodontics with soft-tissue procedures around the mandibular left second molar before crown preparation.
9. Replacement of missing maxillary teeth with a removable partial denture and mandibular teeth with a fixed partial denture.

Twenty-one months following initial consultation, the patient was admitted for LeFort I osteotomy (Figs. 17-21 to 17-23). At 8 weeks following surgery the patient re-

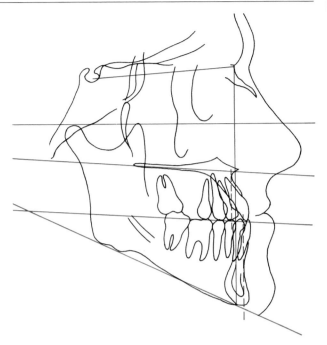

Fig. 17-20. M.J., presurgical cephalometric tracing, showing skeletal maxillary deficiency and mandibular excess. Cephalometric measurements: N perp to A, −2 mm; N perp to Pg, 6 mm; AB difference, −6 mm; UFH, 57 mm; LFH, 73 mm; mand plane, 25 degrees; MxI to A vert, 8 mm, 25 degrees; MnI to B vert, 2 mm, 12 degrees.

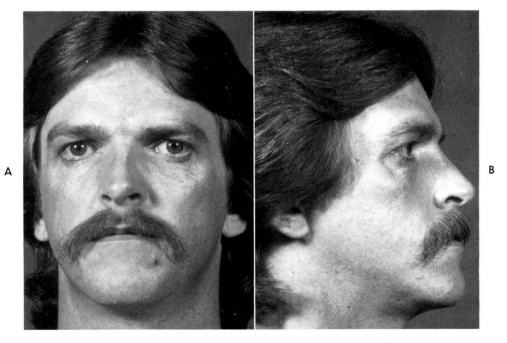

Fig. 17-21. M.J. **A** and **B,** Presurgical facial photographs.

Case 1—cont'd.

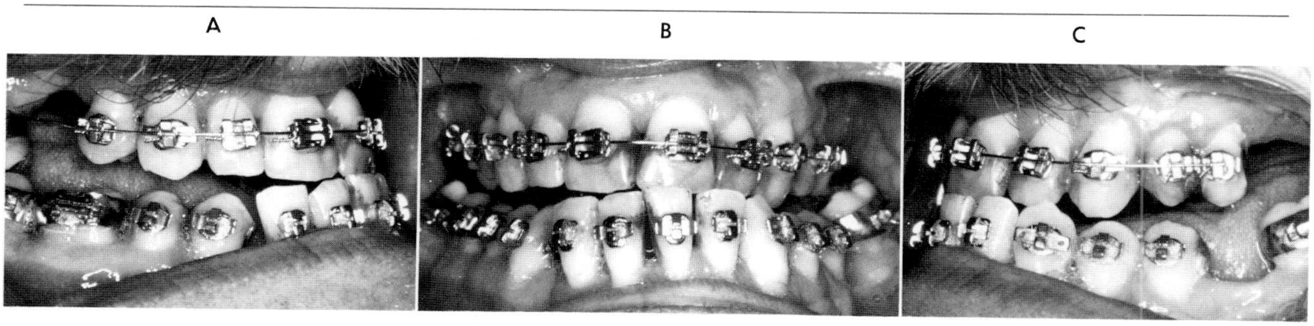

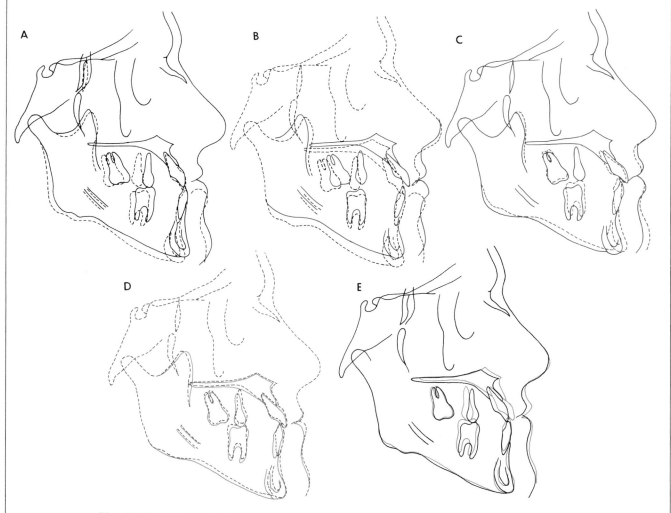

Fig. 17-22. M.J. **A-C,** Dental relationships late in the orthodontic preparation for surgery. Note that in this initial contact position, the mandibular excess is less obvious because of mandibular rotation. The space where the mandibular right canine was removed is nearly closed.

Fig. 17-23. M.J., cephalometric superimpositions. **A,** Pretreatment *(black)* to presurgery *(dashed black).* **B,** Presurgery *(dashed black)* to postsurgery *(solid red).* **C,** Postsurgery *(solid red)* to removal of orthodontic appliances *(dashed red).* **D,** Completion of orthodontics *(dashed red)* to 2 years postsurgery *(solid pink).* **E,** Pretreatment *(solid black)* to 2 years postsurgery *(solid pink).*

Continued.

Case 1—cont'd.

turned to the orthodontist for completion of tooth alignment (Figs. 17-24 and 17-25). After 6 months the patient was ready for definitive periodontics and restorative dentistry. Retainers were placed in the mandibular arch in anticipation of fixed restorations (Fig. 17-26). Two years following surgery and 14 months following completion of treatment, facial balance and the occlusion were well maintained (Figs. 17-27 and 17-28). Periodontal status was good. The retainer for the lower anterior teeth is considered permanent for this patient.

Comments. This patient sought orthodontics and surgical treatment only because his dentition was deteriorating. Before that time, he had adapted to the discrepancy in the position of his jaws. The patient was quite pleased with his result. He has maintained his periodontal status, and his occlusal function is much improved. The option existed in this patient to either shorten the mandible or advance the maxilla. Either option would have produced the same occlusion. Esthetic considerations, especially the possibility of mandibular surgery leading to a poor neck contour, led to the choice of maxillary surgery.

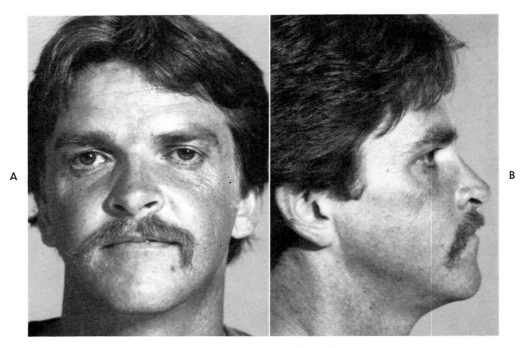

Fig. 17-24. M.J. **A** and **B**, Postsurgical facial photographs.

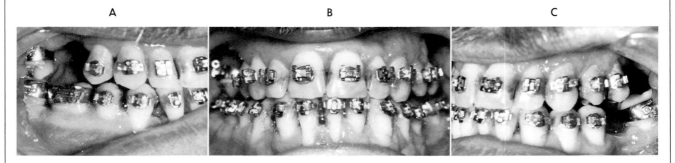

Fig. 17-25. M.J. **A-C**, Postsurgical intraoral photographs.

Case 1—cont'd.

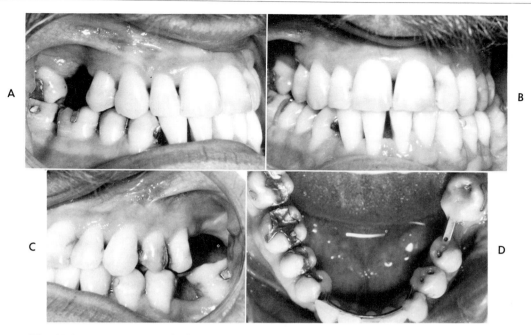

Fig. 17-26. M.J. **A-D,** Ready for definitive periodontics and restorative dentistry. Note the fixed retainers in the lower arch.

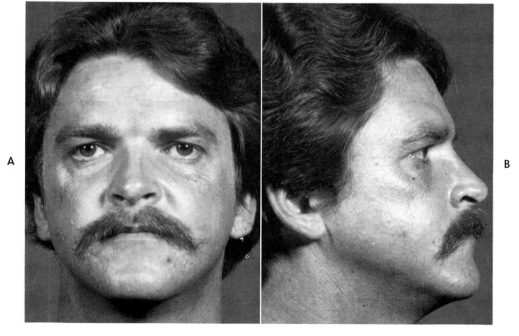

Fig. 17-27. M.J. **A** and **B,** Facial photographs 2 years following surgery (14 months following completion of treatment).

Continued.

Case 1—cont'd.

A   B   C

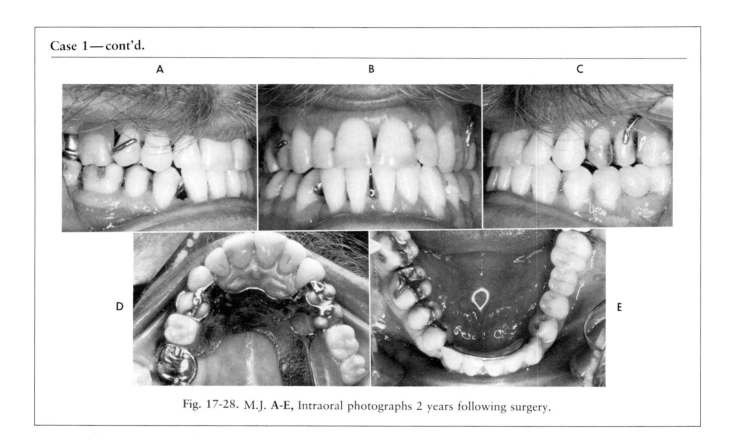

Fig. 17-28. M.J. **A-E,** Intraoral photographs 2 years following surgery.

Case 2

J.B., age 33 years, 2 months, was referred by an orthodontist in a nearby city whom he had consulted about his dependence on a prosthetic device that incorporated posterior bite blocks and replaced his maxillary incisors. Fifteen years previously, he had seen a dentist about his short face and Class II malocclusion with deep bite, which was producing soreness in his palate as the mandibular anterior teeth traumatized the palatal tissue. The treatment at that time was extraction of the maxillary incisors and replacement with a removable partial denture with a posterior splint to reposition the mandible forward and open the bite. Over the years a series of such appliances had been made, steadily increasing the thickness of the posterior bite blocks. At the initial exam the patient had no tooth contact without the appliance except that the canines touched when the mandible was advanced and moved laterally. Muscle spasms developed when the appliance was not worn full-time.

On clinical examination, face height appeared short, especially relative to his broad face width (Fig. 17-29). The ratio of zygomatic width to face height was one to one (the normal value is 0.85—see Chapter 4), the chin was prominent relative to the lower lip, and throat form and

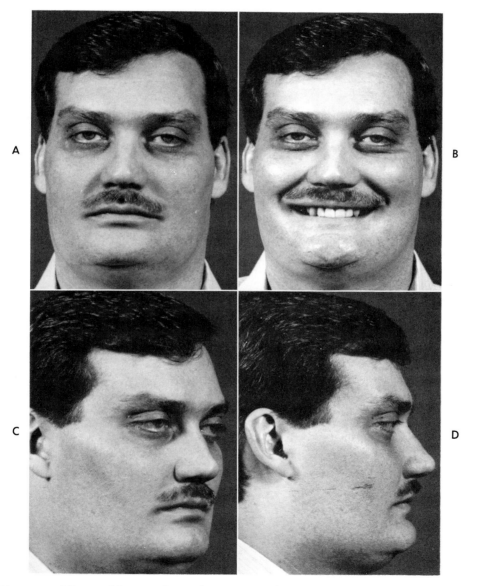

Fig. 17-29. J.B., age 33 years, 8 months. **A-D,** Facial appearance 15 years after his upper incisors had been extracted and replaced as part of a posterior bite splint.

Continued.

Case 2—cont'd.

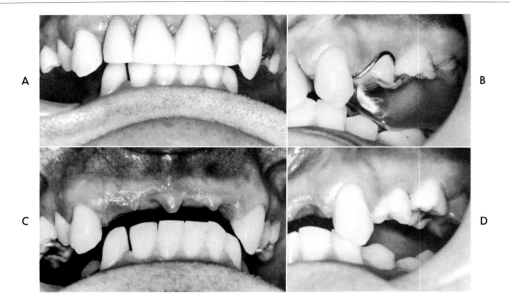

Fig. 17-30. J.B., dental relationships before treatment. **A** and **B,** Occlusion with the occlusal splint in place (in the frontal view, the lower posterior teeth cannot be seen because of its thickness). **C** and **D,** Occlusion with the splint removed. Note the elongation of the maxillary canines and the separation of the posterior teeth when the canines come into contact.

neck contour were poor. The molars were separated by more than a centimeter with the appliance in place (Figs. 17-30 and 17-31), and the maxillary canines were elongated by almost this amount relative to the maxillary posterior teeth. There was mild crepitus in the TM joints bilaterally, and the patient reported intermittent problems of pain on mastication that had become worse recently. The mandibular second premolars were missing and had not been replaced. TM joint anatomy appeared normal (Fig. 17-32). On cephalometric analysis with the prosthetic device in place, there was a skeletal deep-bite pattern and the jaws appeared overclosed; without it this condition was accentuated (Fig. 17-33).

We suggested that J.B. would benefit from orthodontic leveling of the maxillary and mandibular arches primarily by elongation of the posterior teeth, surgery to rotate the mandible downward and anteriorly to a more favorable position, and fixed prosthodontics to replace the missing mandibular posterior and maxillary anterior teeth. Four impacted third molars would need to be removed before the jaw surgery (see Fig. 17-32). The patient agreed with the plan but wished to delay treatment until some personal problems had been resolved.

At age 35 years, 1 month, the third molars had been removed and he wanted to proceed with treatment. After further consultation, the treatment plan was as follows:

1. Modification of the existing splint to relieve the coverage of the mandibular first molar and premolar to allow some presurgical leveling of the lower arch.
2. Placement of a complete orthodontic appliance, with

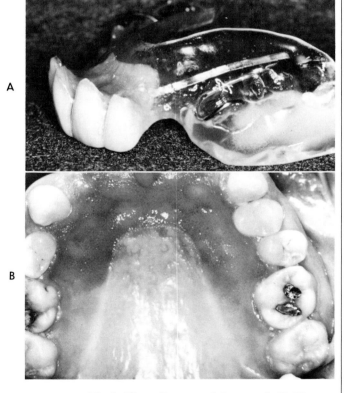

Fig. 17-31. J.B. **A,** The splint out of the mouth. **B,** Tissue irritation in the anterior portion of the palate from prolonged full-time wear of the splint.

Case 2—cont'd.

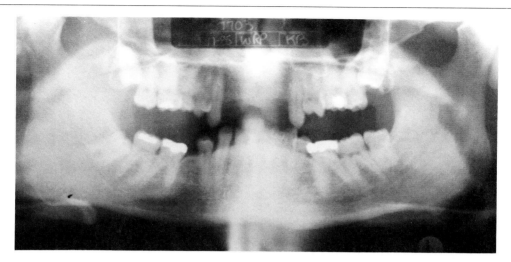

Fig. 17-32. J.B., pretreatment panoramic radiograph.

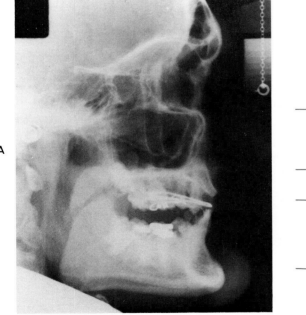

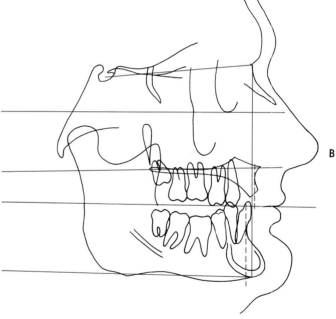

Fig. 17-33. J.B. **A,** Pretreatment cephalometric radiograph with the prosthetic appliance in place. **B,** Cephalometric tracing. Even with the splint between the posterior teeth, short facial proportions and a skeletal deep-bite pattern with parallel horizontal planes are apparent. Cephalometric measurements: N perp to A, 1 mm; N perp to Pg, 7 mm; AB difference, 5 mm; UFH, 60 mm; LFH, 63 mm; mand plane, −2 degrees; MnI to B vert, 2 mm, 13 degrees.

the prosthetic teeth removed from the splint and incorporated into the appliance. Some leveling and alignment of the upper arch also would be attempted presurgically. However, most of the orthodontic tooth movement in both arches would be done postsurgi-

cally, with the leveling to be done primarily by elongation of the posterior teeth.

3. Bilateral sagittal split osteotomy to rotate the mandible downward anteriorly and advance it slightly.

Continued.

Case 2—cont'd.

4. Finishing orthodontics to bring the posterior teeth into occlusion.
5. Mandibular posterior and maxillary fixed partial dentures to replace the missing teeth.

With a fixed orthodontic appliance in place, even with the splint relieved and the anterior teeth tied to the arch wire instead of attached to the splint, it proved almost impossible to reposition the teeth, and the decision was made to go ahead with surgery despite less-than-ideal tooth alignment. Stabilizing arch wires (17×25 steel) were placed (Fig. 17-34), and at age 35 years, 8 months, a bilateral sagittal split osteotomy was carried out, rotating the mandible down and forward (Fig. 17-35). With the teeth in the modified occlusal splint and the jaws held in maxillomandibular fixation, four 3.5 mm Richards lag screws were placed bilaterally for RIF. When fixation was released in the operating room the mandible could be rotated into the splint without difficulty. J.B. did well after surgery and was discharged on the third postoperative day, with the splint tied to the upper arch wire and light elastics to guide jaw function (Fig. 17-36).

During the next few weeks, J.B. had recurring problems with muscle spasms that were partially controlled with Flexeril. Six weeks postsurgically the splint and stabilizing arch wires were removed. A braided 17×25 arch wire, with a step to compensate for the vertical canine-premolar discrepancy, was placed in the upper arch and 16 steel in the lower, and ⅜-inch posterior box elastics

were worn full-time. With the malalignment in the upper arch and the flexible arch wire, it was difficult to control the position of the prosthetic maxillary incisors. Although good progress was made toward leveling the dental arches, problems with muscle spasms continued and TM joint popping on the right side developed. When the molars came into occlusion, it appeared that J.B. was still overclosed and needed further elongation of the posterior teeth.

After 2 months an anterior biteplate supplying the maxillary incisors was constructed so that the lower incisors contacted the appliance and the posterior teeth were separated by approximately 2 mm (Fig. 17-37). A 17×25 NiTi arch wire segment was placed in each of the upper posterior segments, giving greater flexibility in leveling the elongated canines, and vertical elastics were continued. When the posterior teeth again came into occlusion, the TM-dysfunction symptoms were better but not corrected. J.B. felt more comfortable slightly opened. The biteplate was lengthened, then remade with greater opening, and the posterior elongation was continued. The muscle spasms and joint popping disappeared (Fig. 17-38). After 8 months the posterior vertical dimension was considered approximately correct and the upper arch had been leveled, but the maxillary intercanine distance was too great for occlusion and an esthetic anterior bridge. The biteplate was discarded, and a 17×25 steel maxillary arch wire bent to ideal arch form (with prosthetic teeth tied to it) was used to

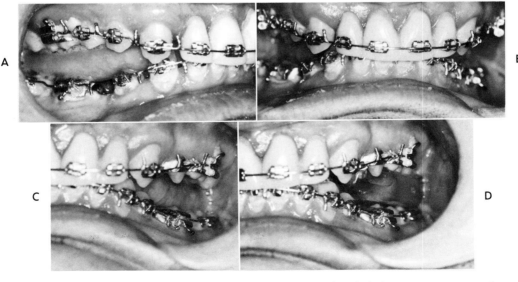

Fig. 17-34. J.B. **A-C,** Stabilizing arch wires in place immediately before surgery. **D,** He developed muscle pain if the posterior bite splint was removed, and so it had to be worn (with the anterior teeth cut off) during the presurgical orthodontics, which limited the amount of preparation that could be done.

Case 2—cont'd.

bring the canines medially (see Fig. 17-38). J.B. was considered ready for prosthodontics 12 months postsurgically (see Fig. 17-38, *D*).

The prosthodontist planned to make the two lower fixed bridges in a first phase, then fabricate the upper anterior fixed bridge after the posterior occlusion was established. Rather than make a removable upper retainer with replacement teeth, the fixed orthodontic appliance was left in place while the lower fixed bridges were constructed. The lower orthodontic appliance was re-

moved, and the crown preparations and temporary bridges were completed the same day. Three months later, with the lower fixed bridges in place, the upper orthodontic appliance was removed and a temporary bridge was placed the same day. With the prosthodontics completed (Fig. 17-39), J.B. was comfortable functionally and pleased with the changes in facial esthetics (Fig. 17-40). Cephalometric superimposition showed that face height at the conclusion of treatment was approximately the same as immediately postsurgically (see

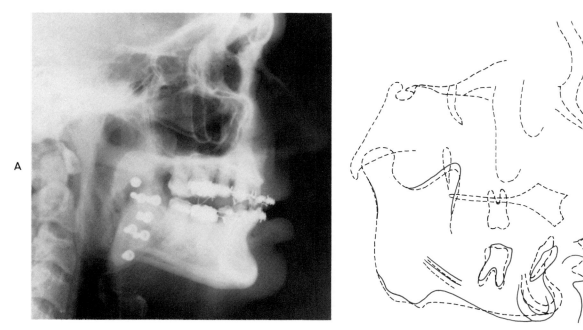

Fig. 17-35. J.B. **A,** Postsurgical cephalometric radiograph. Note the lag screws for rigid fixation. **B,** Cephalometric superimposition presurgery *(dashed black)* to postsurgery *(red).*

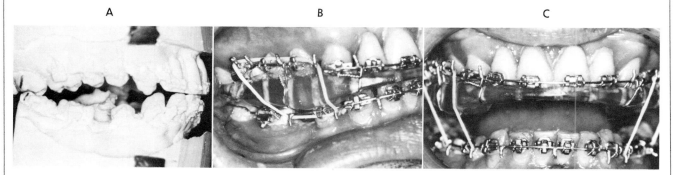

Fig. 17-36. J.B. **A,** Casts as positioned in the model surgery. Note that the second molars are almost in occlusion but the other posterior teeth are widely separated. **B** and **C,** Functioning into the splint 4 weeks postsurgically.

Continued.

Case 2—cont'd.

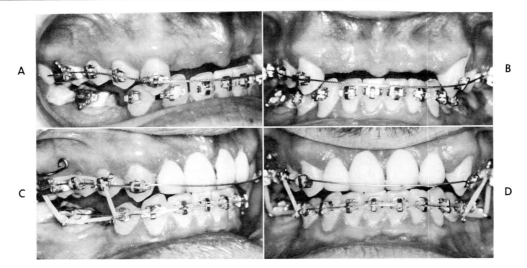

Fig. 17-37. J.B., postsurgical orthodontics. **A** and **B,** Eight weeks postsurgically, at the point that it was decided to go to an anterior bite plate. **C** and **D,** Initial anterior bite plate in place.

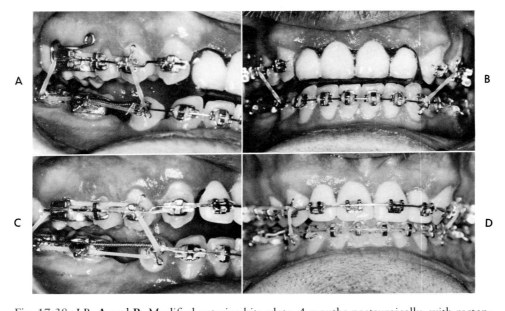

Fig. 17-38. J.B. **A** and **B,** Modified anterior bite plate, 4 months postsurgically, with rectangular NiTi segments for maxillary canine positioning. **C,** To bring the maxillary canines lingually and reduce the space for the maxillary bridge, smaller prosthetic teeth were tied to an ideal 17×25 steel arch wire (which placed a constricting force on the canines) and the spaces mesial to the canines were closed. **D,** Occlusal relationships at the conclusion of active orthodontics, 12 months postsurgically.

Case 2—cont'd.

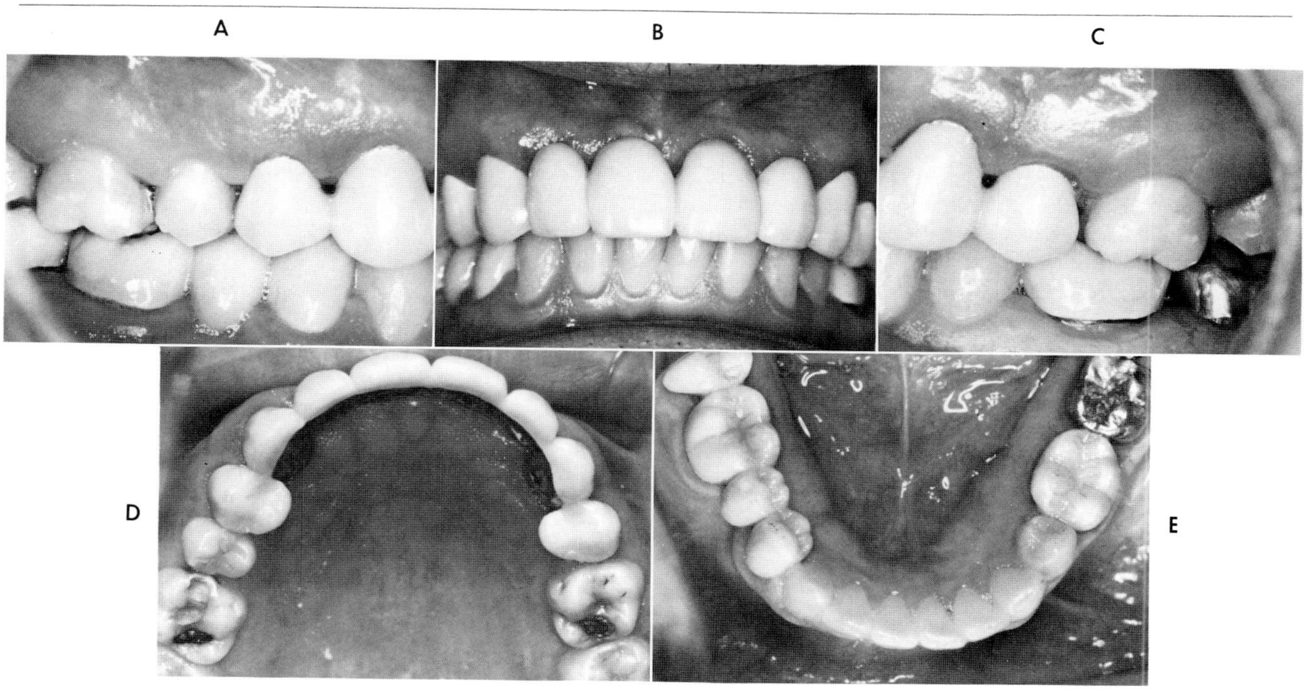

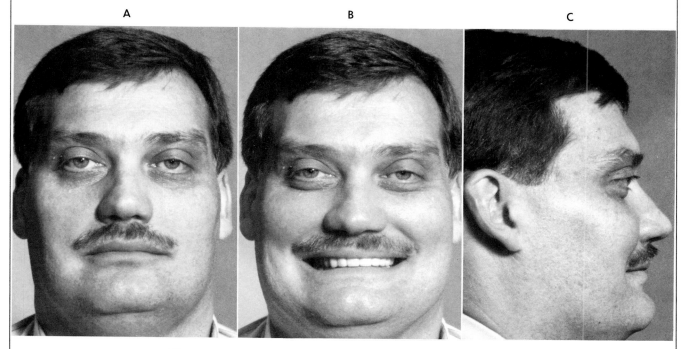

Fig. 17-39. J.B., dental relationships with prosthodontics completed.

Fig. 17-40. J.B., facial proportions at the completion of treatment.

Continued.

Case 2—cont'd.

Figs. 17-33 and 17-41) (i.e., the postsurgical orthodontic and prosthodontic treatment elongated the posterior teeth an amount equal to the thickness of the surgical splint).

Comments. Had orthodontics and orthognathic surgery been more available 15 years earlier, the patient may have been spared his difficulties with jaw function. Obviously he could have retained more of his teeth and his treatment would have been less complex and protracted. Almost certainly, he originally had a Class II, division 2 malocclusion severe enough to require orthognathic surgery. Hopefully current treatment approaches, which combine surgery, orthodontics, and restorative dentistry, will spare future patients from the complicated and protracted plan J.B. completed.

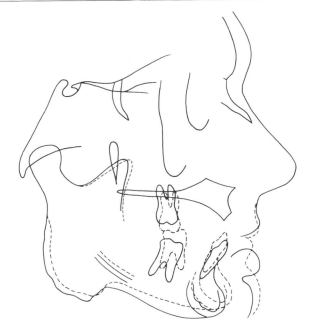

Fig. 17-41. J.B., cephalometric superimposition postsurgery to completion of treatment *(dashed red)*.

Case 3

C.C., age 56, was initially referred for preprosthetic surgery consultation. Her concerns at the time of initial evaluation were related to her inability to function properly with her current dentures. She had significant difficulty eating due to movement of the lower denture during mastication and experienced frequent denture sores. She had been told that augmenting her mandibular alveolar ridge combined with some covering soft-tissue modification might provide a more suitable base for construction of a new lower denture. After a thorough evaluation and discussion with the patient, there was agreement that implants in the lower jaw might be a viable treatment alternative. C.C. was then referred to the implant program for a complete evaluation.

At that time, full-face evaluation revealed no significant abnormalities, but the patient exposed very little of the maxillary incisor at rest or full smile. In fact the patient guarded against showing her incisor teeth during a smile. On profile evaluation, there was an obvious AP deficiency of the mandible (Fig. 17-42). Intraorally the maxilla appeared to be of reasonable size and configuration and was covered with adequate keratinized attached tissue (Fig. 17-43, *A*). The mandible was atrophic, with no attached keratinized tissue in the denture-bearing area (Fig. 17-43, *B*). The cephalometric radiograph confirmed the AP mandibular deficiency (Fig. 17-44, *A*). Despite the clinical intraoral picture of an atrophic mandible, the panoramic radiograph showed sufficient bony height for implants in both the anterior and posterior areas of the body of the mandible (Fig. 17-44, *B*).

The initial workup included mounting models on a semiadjustable articulator. At this time, the magnitude of the mandibular deficiency could be more appropriately evaluated (Fig. 17-45). A denture setup was then completed, placing the maxillary incisors in the appropriate position for proper facial esthetics. The mandibular teeth were then set in the appropriate relationship to the underlying alveolar ridge. The denture setup displayed a significant overjet, deemed unacceptable for appropriate prosthetic construction (Fig. 17-45, *B*). A simulated surgical procedure was performed on the articulated models to determine the amount of mandibular advancement necessary to create a more favorable ridge relationship (Fig. 17-45, *C*).

The problem list for C.C. included:
1. Ill-fitting lower denture.
2. Mandibular deficiency.
3. Lack of attached keratinized tissue over the denture bearing area of the mandible.

Case 3—cont'd.

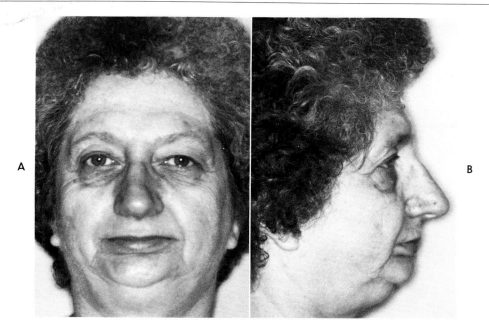

Fig. 17-42. C.C. **A** and **B**, Preoperative facial photographs. The profile view demonstrates obvious mandibular deficiency.

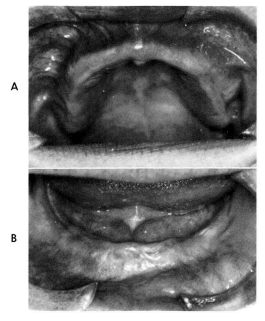

Fig. 17-43. C.C. **A** and **B**, Presurgical intraoral photographs. Note the lack of keratinized tissue in the mandibular denture-bearing area.

The recommendations and plan for treatment included:
1. Mandibular advancement by bilateral sagittal split osteotomy to create a more favorable ridge relationship.
2. A localized vestibuloplasty and split-thickness skin graft in the anterior mandible to provide fixed tissue in this area.
3. Placement of five Branemark implants in the anterior mandible.
4. Final prosthetic reconstruction with a full maxillary denture and mandibular fixed appliance borne by the Branemark implants.

In preparation for surgery, a splint was constructed to cover the mandibular denture-bearing area and secure the skin graft during a 7-day healing period (Fig. 17-46). A maxillary splint was also constructed to interdigitate with the mandibular splint, allowing the mandible to be positioned accurately after completion of the mandibular osteotomy. At the time of surgery, an anterior mandibular vestibuloplasty and a split-thickness skin graft were completed; then bilateral sagittal split osteotomies were performed and the bone segments stabilized with RIF (Fig. 17-46, C). Fixation was released at the time of surgery and the maxillary splint was removed. The mandibular splint was removed 7 days postsurgically (Fig. 17-47).

Continued.

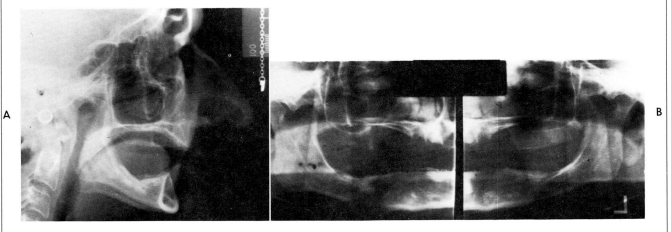

Fig. 17-44. C.C. **A** and **B**, Presurgical cephalometric and panoramic radiographs.

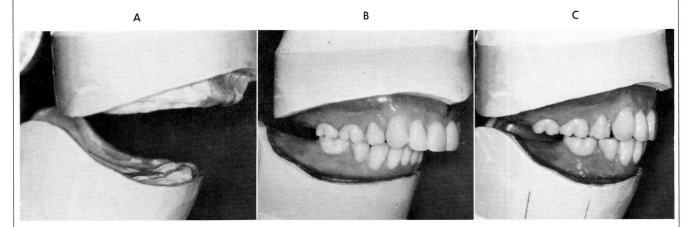

Fig. 17-45. **A,** Casts mounted on a semiadjustable articulator showing the ridge relationship abnormality. **B,** Denture setup showing significant overjet and undesirable relationship for denture construction. **C,** Position of casts after model surgical procedure to establish appropriate incisor and ridge relationships.

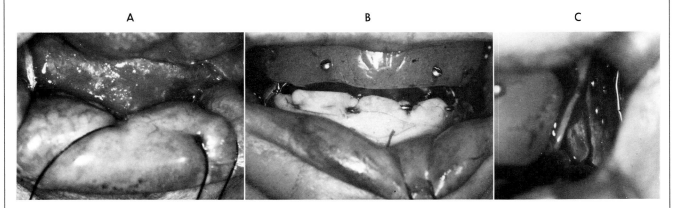

Fig. 17-46. C.C., at surgery. **A,** View of inferior positioning of the mucosa in the anterior mandible. **B,** Maxillary and mandibular splints in place. The mandibular splint secured the skin graft in place for 7 days; the maxillary splint was used only during the time of surgery to determine the appropriate position of the mandible. **C,** View of sagittal osteotomy with rigid fixation. Due to the need for access in the posterior mandibular area, the splint was modified with minimal buccal flange extension in this area to allow instrumentation for completion of the osteotomy.

Three months after the initial surgical procedure, the patient presented for placement of implants. At this stage the patient's facial balance was significantly improved by the more anterior position of the chin following mandibular advancement (Fig. 17-48). Intraorally the skin graft was well healed in the anterior mandible, providing fixed keratinized tissue in the area of implant placement. Five Branemark implants were placed in the anterior mandible without difficulty. After a 4-month healing period, the second-stage implant surgery was performed, uncovering the implants and placing the intraoral abutments (Figs. 17-49 and 17-50).

Construction of the final upper denture and lower fixed appliance was completed over a 2-month period. Figs. 17-51 to 17-53 demonstrate the final esthetic and prosthetic results.

Comments. The combined treatment for this patient resulted in a balanced facial form and good function with the prosthetic replacements for her teeth. Rigid fixation allowed the initial preprosthetic surgery to be combined with orthognathic surgery. Early jaw function possible with rigid fixation allowed implants to be placed 3 months after orthognathic surgery, decreasing further the overall treatment time. New technology (e.g., osseointegrated implants, RIF) has allowed the solution of complex problems with less inconvenience for patients. More patients will seek such treatment in the future.

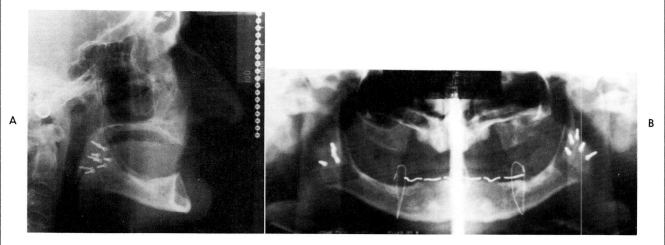

Fig. 17-47. C.C. **A** and **B**, Postsurgical cephalometric and panoramic radiographs.

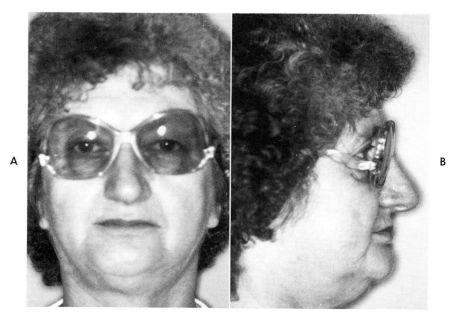

Fig. 17-48. C.C. **A** and **B**, Facial photographs after mandibular advancement before placement of implants.

Continued.

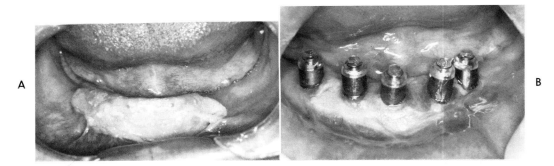

Fig. 17-49. C.C., intraoral photographs. **A,** Keratinized fixed skin-graft tissue in anterior mandible. **B,** Completion of second-stage implants with abutments in place.

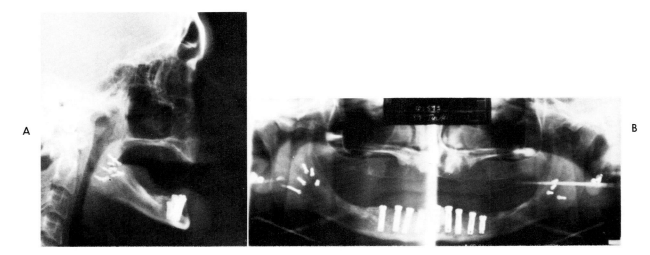

Fig. 17-50. C.C. **A,** Cephalometric and **B,** panoramic radiographs after implant placement.

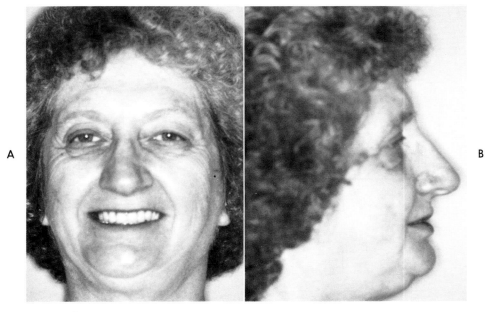

Fig. 17-51. C.C., facial photographs at the completion of treatment.

Case 3—cont'd.

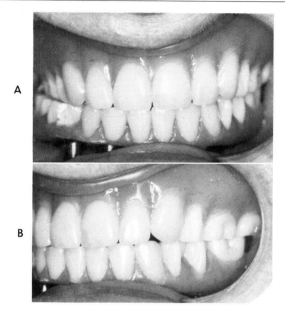

Fig. 17-52. C.C., intraoral photographs at the completion of treatment.

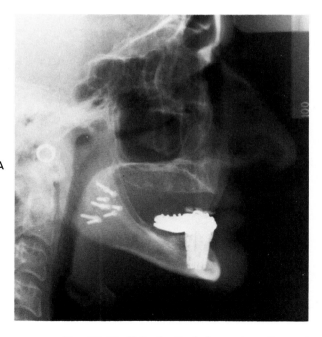
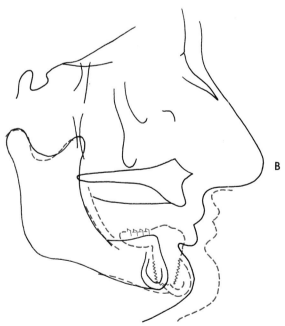

Fig. 17-53. C.C. **A,** Cephalometric radiograph at the completion of treatment, with the prostheses in place. **B,** Pretreatment to completion *(dashed red)* tracing.

Case 4

N.I., age 51, sought surgical consultation after being told that his missing posterior teeth could not be replaced unless his jaw deformity was corrected. His medical history revealed rheumatic heart disease followed by mitral stenosis. Eleven years previously he had been hospitalized for fatigue, chest pain, and mild congestive heart failure. Nine years previously he developed atrial fibrillation. After cardiac catherization confirmed severe

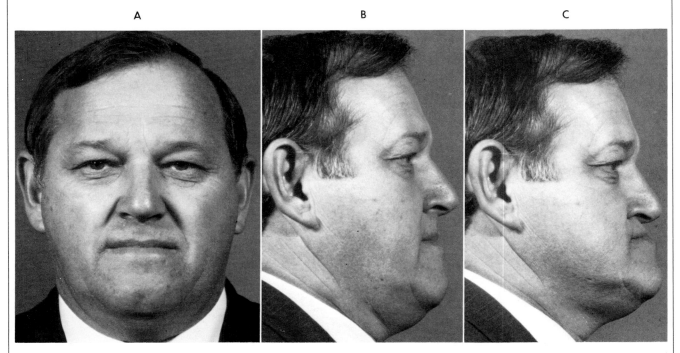

Fig. 17-54. N.I., age 51. **A** and **B,** Facial proportions with the mandible at occlusal vertical dimension. **C,** With teeth in contact.

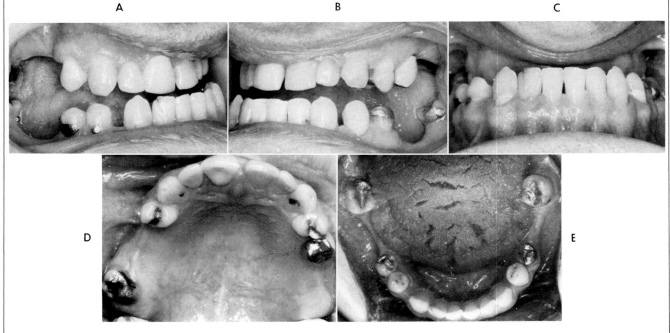

Fig. 17-55. N.I., age 51, intraoral photographs before treatment. **A** and **B,** Initial tooth contact. **C,** Occlusal relationships after his 5 mm anterior shift. **D** and **E,** Occlusal views of dental arches.

Case 4—cont'd.

mitral stenosis, N.I. underwent a closed mitral commissurotomy; 1+ mitral regurgitation was present postoperatively. Because of intolerance of side effects or inability to maintain a normal sinus rhythm, antiarrhythmic drugs were unsuccessful, and N.I. was maintained on digoxin and took warfarin (Coumadin) for prophylactic anticoagulation. At initial examination, N.I. could walk unlimited distances without difficulty and he denied chest pain, edema, or respiratory difficulties.

On clinical examination, all first and second molars were missing, along with the right second premolars and the maxillary left third molar. The other third molars were inclined mesially. On closure, N.I. had an initial contact on the right third molars, then a 5 mm forward slide with overclosure (Figs. 17-54 and 17-55). Mastication was almost impossible—the only useful occlusal contact was in the left canine-premolar region. There was a Class III jaw relationship at rest, which was magnified when he closed. To estimate the natural postural position of the mandible, face height during speech was measured (using marks on the nasal tip and chin), and a wax-bite splint was made to maintain this AP and vertical position of the mandible while the cephalometric radiograph was taken (Fig. 17-56). Cephalometric analysis indicated that the Class III problem was largely due to maxillary deficiency, once the overclosure was eliminated.

After a thorough discussion of the implications of his medical situation for elective surgery, N.I. wished to proceed with treatment. The possibility of posterior implants was discussed but was rejected in favor of conventional prosthodontics, in part because of the increased risk of complications with the additional surgery. The treatment plan was:

1. Orthodontically align the anterior teeth in preparation for maxillary advancement.
2. LeFort I osteotomy with allogeneic bank bone grafts to advance and inferiorly position the maxilla. Semirigid bone plates would help stabilize and fix the maxilla.

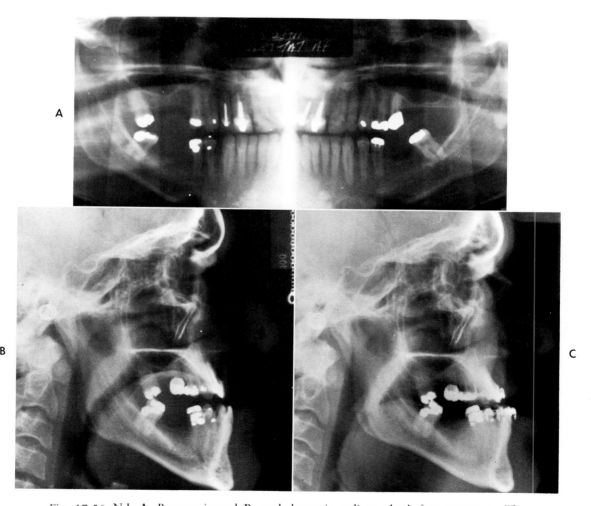

Fig. 17-56. N.I. **A,** Panoramic and **B,** cephalometric radiographs before treatment. The cephalometric film was made with a waxbite splint in place to maintain the jaw in an approximately normal vertical and AP position. **C,** Cephalometric radiograph just before surgery.

Continued.

Case 4—cont'd.

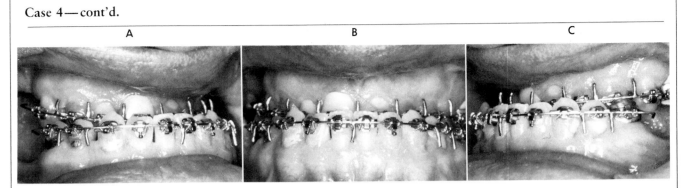

Fig. 17-57. N.I. **A-C,** Occlusal relationships just before surgery, with the stabilizing arch wires in place.

3. Postsurgical orthodontics to complete tooth alignment.
4. Construction of maxillary and mandibular fixed partial dentures after the jaw relationship had been corrected.

Special medical management at surgery would be required because of the cardiac condition and anticoagulant medication.

Bonded orthodontic attachments were placed on all teeth,

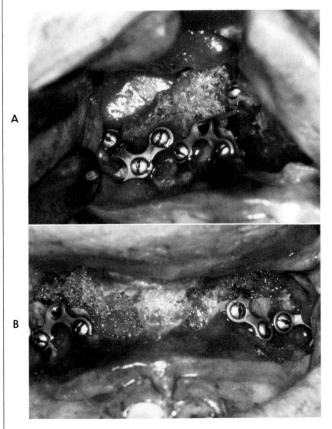

Fig. 17-58. N.I. **A** and **B,** Intraoperative photographs with bone grafts and rigid fixation in place.

and light arch wires were used to align the teeth and obtain arch compatibility. This had the effect of totally eliminating any dental occlusion. Five months after treatment began, stabilizing surgical arch wires were placed (Fig. 17-57). At the completion of model surgery, a surgical splint modified to contact the maxillary posterior alveolar ridges in addition to fitting between the anterior teeth was fabricated.

Ten days before admission, one autologous unit of packed red cells was obtained. The preadmission chest radiograph showed mild cardiomegaly without pulmonary edema. On EKG, there was atrial fibrillation with a ventricular rate of 112, normal QRS, and downsloping ST segments with T-wave inversion in inferior leads consistent with a digitalis effect. An echocardiogram indicated mild-to-moderate mitral stenosis, moderate mitral and tricuspid regurgitation, mild pulmonary hypertension, and left atrial enlargement with mild global left ventricular dysfunction. The prothrombin time (PT) was 14.5 seconds, and the accelerated partial prothrombin time (aPTT) was 25.3 seconds. Warfarin was discontinued 3 days before surgery; on admission PT was 13.1 seconds.

Immediately before surgery N.I. was given 1 million units of penicillin G and 110 mg of gentamycin intravenously for prophylaxis; he received an 80 mg dose of gentamycin 8 hours postoperatively and was maintained on 1 million units of penicillin q4h for 5 days. Modified hypotensive anesthesia was employed. LeFort I osteotomy was performed via a downfracture technique, and the maxilla was repositioned 7 mm anteriorly and 3 mm inferiorly with the aid of the modified splint and maxillomandibular fixation. Bleeding from the right descending palatine artery was controlled with hemostatic clips. Meticulous care was given to repairing tears in the nasal mucosa. RIF was accomplished with 2.0 mm semirigid bone plates in the zygomatic buttress and piriform regions bilaterally; then maxillomandibular fixation was released and the occlusion was checked. After verifying that the mandible could be rotated into the splint, allogeneic corticancellous iliac crest grafts were contoured and wedged into place and demineralized bone was

Case 4—cont'd.

packed around them (Fig. 17-58). The modified splint was secured to the maxilla, and a single light guiding elastic was applied bilaterally (Fig. 17-59).

Postoperatively, the plan was to treat sustained or symptomatic rapid ventricular rates with incremental doses of IV verapamil after pretreatment with calcium chloride to avoid hypotension. In the recovery room, N.I. was given 2.5 mg verapamil for a ventricular rate of 140 to 150, then was admitted to a cardiac telemetry unit, where no rapid ventricular rates or instability of vital signs were noted. He received his daily dose of digoxin. Forty hours postsurgically, a heparin bolus was given and a continuous heparin infusion was begun to achieve a target aPTT of 48 to 55 seconds. On the evening of the third postoperative day, N.I. was given warfarin, 5 mg PO. No loading was employed because of the brief hiatus from the drug and his essential lack of dietary vitamin K. The plan was to discontinue the heparin infusion as a therapeutic effect of warfarin was established and his PT approached 16 to 18 seconds, the desired maintenance level.

In the early morning of the fourth postoperative day, moderate nasal bleeding and right midfacial swelling occurred. The heparin infusion was discontinued, and the bleeding was controlled with nasal packs. Coagulation studies revealed a PT of 14.8 seconds and aPTT of 46.2 seconds. There was no evidence of heparin-in-duced thrombocytopenia. That evening he received warfarin, 5 mg PO. The nasal packs were removed after 24 hours, with no further episodes of bleeding, and he was discharged on the fifth postoperative day on continuing warfarin therapy.

N.I. functioned into the splint for 5 weeks. When it was removed, the occlusion was largely on the central incisors. The stabilizing arch wires were replaced with a maxillary 17×25 braided wire and a mandibular 16 round wire. A cross elastic was placed to correct the relationship of the third molars on the right, and triangular elastics in a Class III pattern were worn anteriorly to elongate the canines and first premolars and correct the anterior occlusion (Fig. 17-60). The teeth settled into occlusion nicely, and orthodontic appliances were removed 5 months postsurgically. Facial proportions were significantly improved (Fig. 17-61). Fixed partial dentures were fabricated soon thereafter, without difficulty (Fig. 17-62).

Comments. Atrial fibrillation frequently follows rheumatic heart disease, especially when the mitral valve is involved. Although it often is clinically well tolerated by patients, the condition is not benign. There is a decrease in cardiac reserve, and patients tend to develop pulmonary or peripheral emboli.[9,10] Mortality rates are increased.[11] Anticoagulant medication commonly is employed.

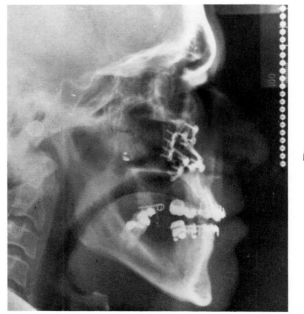
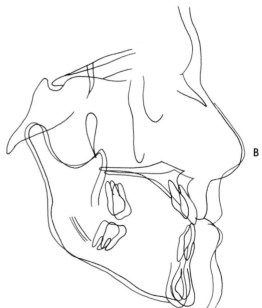

Fig. 17-59. N.I. **A,** Cephalometric radiograph immediately after surgery, showing the rigid fixation in place. **B,** Cephalometric superimposition from presurgery to postsurgery *(solid red).*

Case 4—cont'd.

Several considerations apply with regard to orthognathic surgery for a patient of this type. First, a medical evaluation of the patient's condition should be made, along with an assessment of risk for surgery and general anesthesia, so the patient can make an informed decision whether or not to pursue surgical-orthodontic treatment. If the decision is to proceed, the simplest surgical intervention that will produce a satisfactory result is indicated, and care should be taken to limit soft-tissue dissection and obtain mechanical hemostasis. Allogeneic bone is preferred to stabilize osteotomy sites, to decrease operative time and eliminate the possible increased morbidity of a harvest site for autologous bone.

The timing of reinstituting anticoagulant therapy after surgery depends on the type and extent of surgery and the patient's risk of an embolic episode. Although coumarin derivatives such as warfarin are the drug of choice for long-term anticoagulation, when patients are "rewarfarinized" it is important first to fully anticoagulate them with heparin and gradually build up the other drug. The primary complication of warfarin or heparin is an exaggeration of its effects, resulting in hemorrhage. With warfarin, the timing of the anticoagulant effects is primarily dependent on the half-life of the drug (24 to 48 hours) and the half-life of previously synthesized clotting factors (6 to 100 hours). Heparin has a half-life of approximately 90 minutes, and its effects are easily reversed by administration of protamine, making it ideal in the acute setting of initial anticoagulation. If a bleeding episode does occur, it is important to check platelet levels. Heparin-induced thrombocytopenia is an infrequent complication, but it is not necessarily a dose-related phenomenon.

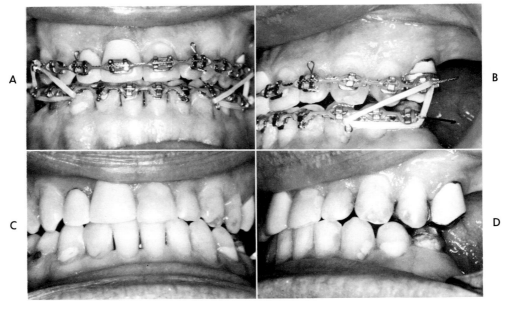

Fig. 17-60. N.I., occlusal relationships **A** and **B,** immediately after removal of the stabilizing arch wires and **C** and **D,** 4 months later.

Case 4—cont'd.

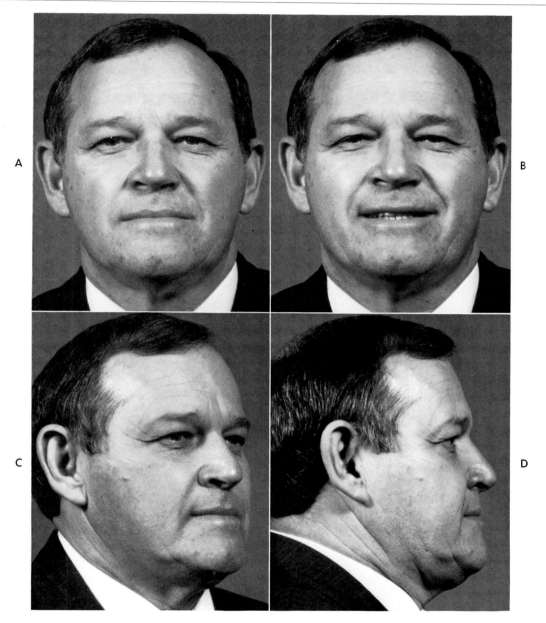

Fig. 17-61. N.I., facial proportions at the completion of postsurgical orthodontics, 5 months postsurgery.

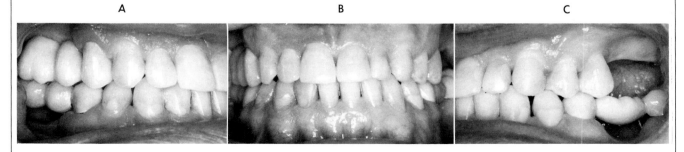

Fig. 17-62. N.I., age 52, occlusal relationships with fixed partial dentures in place.

REFERENCES

1. Douglass CW, Gammon MD, Atwood DA: Need and effective demand for prosthodontic treatment, J Prosthet Dent 59:94-104, 1988.
2. Meskin LH, Brown LJ, Brunelle JA, Warren GB: Patterns of tooth loss and accumulated prosthetic treatment potential in U.S. employed adults and seniors, 1985-86, Gerodontics 4:126-135, 1988.
3. McLain JB, Proffit WR: Oral health status in the United States: prevalence of malocclusion, J Dent Educ 49:386-396, 1985.
4. Ingervall B, Mohlin B, Thilander B: Prevalence and awareness of malocclusion in Swedish men, Community Dent Oral Epidemiol 6:308-314, 1978.
5. Mohlin B: Need and demand for orthodontic treatment in a group of women in Sweden, Eur J Orthod 4:231-242, 1982.
6. Turley PC, Kean C, Schur J, et al: Orthodontic force application to titanium endosseous implants, Angle Orthod 58:151-162, 1988.
7. Odman J, Lekholm U, Jemt T, et al: Osseointegrated titanium implants—a new approach in orthodontic treatment, Eur J Orthod 10:98-105, 1988.
8. Roberts WE, Helm FR, Marshall KJ, et al: Rigid endosseous implants for orthodontic and orthopedic anchorage, Angle Orthod 59:247-256, 1989.
9. Hurst JW, Paulk EA, Jr, Proctor HD, et al: Management of patients with atrial fibrillation, Am J Med 37:728-741, 1964.
10. Kadish SL, Lazar EJ, Frishman WH: Anticoagulation in patients with valvular heart disease, atrial fibrillation, or both, Cardiol Clin 5:591-628, 1987.
11. Kannel WB, Abbott RD, Savage DD, et al: Epidemiologic features of chronic atrial fibrillation, N Engl J Med 306:1018-1022, 1982.

CHAPTER 18

Special Problems in Cleft-Palate Patients

William R. Proffit
Timothy A. Turvey

OVERVIEW OF CLEFT-LIP/PALATE TREATMENT

Clefting of the primary and/or secondary palate leads to a series of distortions in dentofacial development. The affected individual requires prolonged treatment by a multidisciplinary team. At this point, there are well-organized cleft-palate teams in almost all areas of the United States and in the developed countries, so treatment can be coordinated among the team members from the beginning. If only the lip is involved, the problems are primarily cosmetic and surgical. If the cleft affects only the posterior part of the secondary palate, the problems are likely to be primarily speech, with perhaps a tendency toward posterior crossbite. If the cleft affects the entire dental arch, and especially if it involves both the primary and secondary palates, the patient will require treatment procedures coordinated among plastic surgery, speech therapy, oral and maxillofacial surgery, orthodontics, and prosthodontics, with potential involvement from several other practitioners as well. The coordinating function of a well-managed cleft-palate team is essential in order to obtain optimum treatment results.

Because of its complex interdisciplinary nature, an all-inclusive review of cleft-palate treatment is beyond the scope of this chapter. Here, we provide an overview of the treatment sequence in a typical cleft-lip/cleft-palate patient and focus on the two major areas of interaction between orthodontics and oral and maxillofacial surgery: (1) alveolar grafting in the preteen years and (2) orthognathic surgery in the late teens or early twenties.

Treatment for a typical patient with both cleft lip and cleft palate follows the sequence outlined in Table 18-1. Not all patients need all of these stages of treatment. Infant orthopedics is done infrequently now. Cleft surgery, speech therapy, and orthodontics are needed in each case. Bone grafts to the dental alveolus were not done routinely until relatively recently but now are considered to be indicated in the majority of cleft patients. Only a minority of cleft patients require orthognathic surgery, but the percentage is much higher than in the population at large, and the surgical-

TABLE 18-1 Stages in cleft-lip/palate treatment

Stage	Age	Comment
Presurgical infant orthopedics	1 to 4 weeks	Repositioning palatal segments can facilitate lip repair; done less frequently now
Lip closure	8 to 12 weeks	May be preceded by preliminary lip adhesion as an alternative to presurgical orthopedics
Palate closure	18 to 24 months	Closing only the soft palate initially is an alternative, but one-stage closure of the hard and soft palate is the usual procedure
Speech therapy	6 to 11 years	Articulation errors often develop as child tries to compensate for cleft
Early orthodontics	7 to 8 years	Usually incisor alignment and maxillary transverse expansion
Alveolar grafting	6 to 10 years	Needed before permanent canines erupt; timing determined by stage and sequence of dental development
Comprehensive orthodontics	11 to 14 years	Class III elastics often very helpful
Pharyngeal flap surgery	9 to 19 years	Only if required to overcome nasal air leakage during speech; sometimes needed after loss of lymphoid tissue in the nasopharynx at adolescence or following maxillary advancement
Orthognathic surgery	17 to 19 years	Maxillary advancement, perhaps combined with mandibular set-back; not done until growth completed except in rare instances of severe psychosocial impact; needed infrequently
Fixed prosthodontics	17 to 19 years	Replacement of missing lateral incisors: consider temporary bonded bridge when fixed orthodontic appliance removed, comprehensive treatment only after growth completed

orthodontic treatment involves special considerations in timing surgical and orthodontic procedures and in maintaining velopharyngeal function.

EARLY STAGES OF TREATMENT
Infant Orthopedics

In a child with a cleft lip and palate, particularly if the cleft of the primary palate is bilateral, the maxillary alveolar segments are displaced at the time of birth. In a unilateral cleft, the premaxillary segment is likely to be displaced facially adjacent to the cleft (Fig. 18-1). If the cleft is bilateral, the premaxilla usually is displaced significantly forward, with the posterior segments collapsed medially behind it (Fig. 18-2). The displacement of the bony segments emphasizes the separation of the soft-tissue segments and makes lip repair more difficult.

Burston[1] in Liverpool followed up McNeill's suggestion to use removable orthodontic appliances to reposition the segments in early infancy, before the initial lip closure. Their impressive results, first published in the late 1950s, led to widespread enthusiasm for infant presurgical orthopedic procedures. Repositioning the segments before the initial lip surgery made it easier to produce an esthetic lip with the first operation, and

there was no doubt that the patients looked better at an early age. In addition, it was thought that the children benefited from the obturation of the palatal cleft produced by a palate-covering orthodontic appliance (Fig. 18-3). With a "feeding plate" in place, it seemed reasonable that the child would be able to swallow more correctly and more efficiently, and there was hope that oral adaptive mechanisms that could produce malocclusion later would not develop. In the 1960s it became common practice to use an active plate to reposition the segments before surgery and a passive plate for some time afterward,[2] typically until the infant developed enough manual dexterity to remove it (at about age 8 months).

As the first patients became older, however, it became obvious that the differences produced by presurgical infant orthopedics decreased with each passing year. The infant who had this treatment looked much better; the 2-year-old looked better; the 4-year-old tended to look a bit better; by age 8 or 9, the concern often was deficiency rather than protrusion of the previously displaced segment.[3] The short-term advantage, it turned out, was not necessarily a long-term advantage.[4]

For this reason, the popularity of presurgical infant

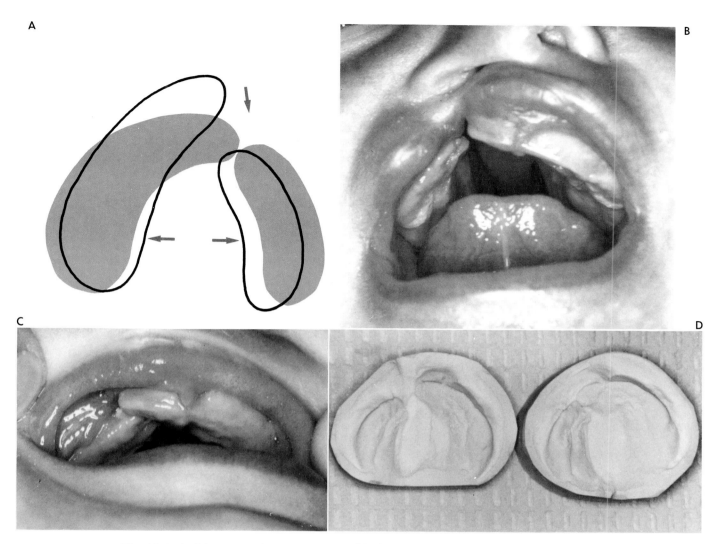

Fig. 18-1. **A,** Diagrammatic representation *(black)* of the typical position of alveolar segments at birth in a patient with a unilateral cleft, and *(red)* the changes produced by presurgical expansion and lip closure. **B,** A unilateral cleft infant before and **C,** after lip closure without presurgical orthopedic repositioning of the segments. **D,** Dental casts of the same patient before and after lip closure, showing the molding effect of the lip on the segments.

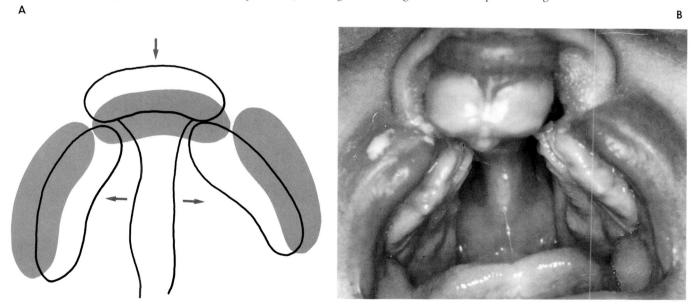

Fig. 18-2. **A,** Diagrammtic representation *(black)* of the displacement of segments in a bilateral cleft, and *(red)* the changes produced by presurgical orthopedics and lip closure. **B,** An infant with bilateral cleft before treatment.

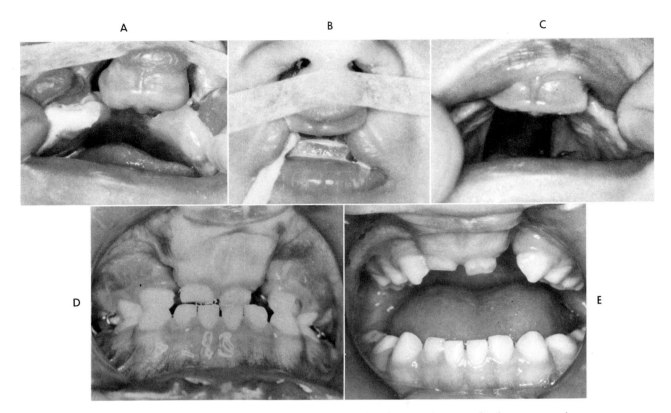

Fig. 18-3. Presurgical orthopedics in a bilateral cleft infant. **A,** Segment displacement at the time arch expansion was begun. The expansion appliance can be seen covering the gum pads. **B,** Progress 2 weeks later. **C,** Segment alignment following lip closure. **D** and **E,** Follow-up showing crossbite tendency as the teeth erupt.

orthopedics began to decline in the 1970s, and the procedure is done much less frequently now than at the height of its popularity. For a cleft-palate child who has displacement of the alveolar segments that would complicate lip closure, the typical sequence of treatment now is to do the initial lip closure in two stages, first an adhesion of the deeper tissues of the lip with no attempt to produce definitive closure of the skin, and a secondary procedure for final closure.[5] For a while after active plates were largely discontinued, passive plates continued to be used to stabilize the segments during and following the lip adhesion, but this too has largely been discontinued because it gives no apparent long-term advantage. At this point, with the exception of a few centers that continue to use the method extensively,[6] presurgical infant orthopedics is reserved for a small minority of patients with exceptionally severe displacement of segments, so that even lip adhesion is difficult or almost impossible.

Lip Closure (Primary Palate)

Surgical closure of a cleft lip is done as early in infancy as is compatible with a good long-term result. The contemporary consensus is that this is at 10 to 12 weeks of age (a common guideline is age 10 weeks,

weight 10 pounds, hemoglobin 10 grams). Correcting the lip earlier than this (immediately after birth) offers some psychologic advantages to the mother and was briefly popular in the 1960s for that reason. But it involves a greater risk of surgical morbidity, and the long-term esthetic results tend not to be as good. Allowing the nose and lip to grow before lip closure makes the surgery technically easier; after 10 to 12 weeks other problems are more likely to have been identified if they exist; and the immune system will be better developed and the risk of infection therefore less.

Many surgical techniques have been developed for primary lip and nose closure. In the United States, the rotation-advancement technique of Millard[7] is most popular. The technique preserves the lip tissue, restores the anatomically distorted lip elements, and allows the nasal base to be narrowed (Fig. 18-4).

Secondary Palate

The timing of closure of the secondary palate (hard and soft palate) is controversial because it is influenced by two opposing considerations. It seems clear that the acquisition of normal speech is aided by an intact palate at the time that speech is developing rapidly, early in the second year of life.[8] For ideal speech, therefore,

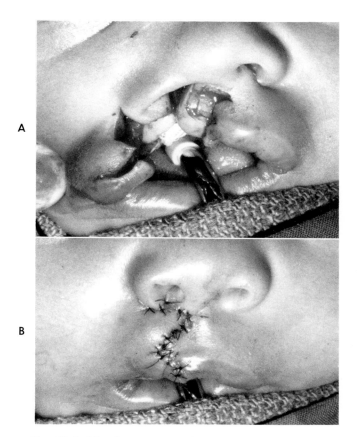

Fig. 18-4. Lip closure using the Millard rotation-advancement procedure. **A,** The flaps outlined for repair of a unilateral cleft lip. **B,** The medial flap has been rotated inferiorly, and the lateral flap has been advanced into the base of the columella. Note the good nasal symmetry.

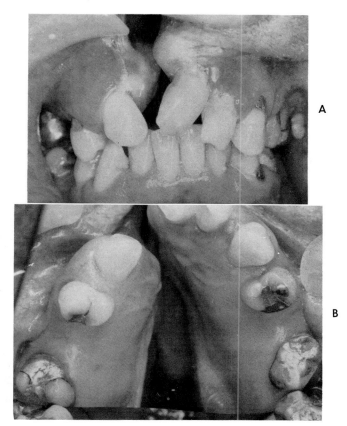

Fig. 18-5. An unrepaired cleft in a 51-year-old man. Note the absence of posterior crossbite (maxillary arch width is normal) and the width of the open cleft, which are typical of patients who never had a surgical repair.

palate closure by age 12 months would be recommended. On the other hand, it seems equally clear that all other things being equal, the later the secondary palate is closed, the less tendency toward maxillary underdevelopment in all three planes of space that commonly is seen in children with surgically repaired palatal clefts.[9] Observation of patients with untreated cleft palate (Fig. 18-5) demonstrates that underdevelopment of the maxilla is rare in the absence of surgical correction. The maxilla seems to grow downward and forward quite normally in the presence of a unrepaired cleft and is more likely to be too wide than too narrow.[10] In contrast, patients with repaired clefts almost always have a tendency toward posterior and anterior crossbite because of deficient maxillary growth. In the best cases, the deficiency is so minimal as to be negligible; in others, it can be quite severe (see Case 3).

These opposing requirements have caused the timing of palate closure to oscillate back and forth between a minimum of 10 to 12 months and a maximum of 9 to 12 years. Early surgery was popular in the World War II era; the reaction against severe malocclusions related to the early surgery led to delaying it until relatively late in growth in the 1950s and 1960s; and recent improvements in surgical techniques have led to a decrease again in the age of palate closure. There is good evidence that as surgical techniques have improved, the impact on maxillary growth has declined, but probably it is impossible to devise techniques for surgical palate repair that do not stretch soft tissue and impede subsequent maxillary growth to at least some extent.

How much of an increase in malocclusion would one accept in order to maximize the acquisition of speech? Or conversely, how much of an increase in speech difficulty would one accept in order to minimize the development of crossbite and Class III malocclusion? At this point, the policy of cleft-palate teams varies nationally and internationally, depending on their judgment on these points. It has been suggested that a rational compromise between the opposing demands of speech and growth would be to surgically close only the soft palate, doing this at approximately 12 months of age, and defer closure of the hard palate until age 4 or 5.[11] It appears that closing only the soft palate pro-

A   B   C

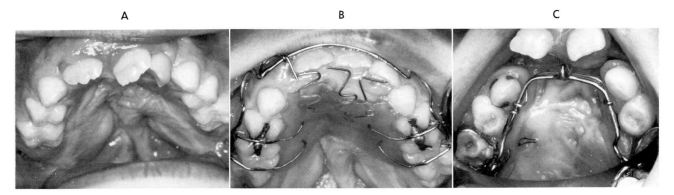

Fig. 18-6. **A,** The rotation of permanent maxillary incisors often seen upon eruption in a patient with a repaired unilateral cleft. **B,** Removable appliance being employed for initial alignment (same patient as **A**). **C,** Incisor displacement in a bilateral cleft patient, with a lingual arch being used for preliminary alignment.

vides an advantage in speech acquisition compared with doing nothing, but it may not be as good in this regard as total palatal closure. There seems to be little or no growth retardation with early closure of only the soft palate, but this has not yet been fully evaluated. At most centers, a one-stage palatal closure is done, and the average age at this procedure continues to decline as concerns about growth inhibition decrease. Most children with a cleft palate now have it repaired between ages 18 and 24 months.

The objectives of surgery for palate closure are to join the cleft palatal edges, lengthen the soft palate, and repair the levator palatini muscle. As with cleft-lip surgery, many techniques for palate closure have been described, and these have been reviewed recently by Randall and LaRossa.[12] Most surgeons now utilize modifications either of the von Langenbeck technique or of the V-Y pushback procedure. In both methods, the cleft edges along the margin are excised and the nasal edge is elevated into the nasal cavity on either side of the cleft. The nasal surface of the palate is undermined so that the mucosa can be opposed and a nasal floor can be constructed. In very wide clefts, mucosal flaps elevated from the vomer are required to facilitate nasal floor construction. The palatal tissue is incised along the entire length of the hard palate about 5 mm from the teeth, and the mucoperiosteum is elevated and mobilized medially so that it can be approximated in the midline. The trauma and soft-tissue tension associated with this probably accounts for the long-term effects on growth. These can be minimized but probably not totally eliminated by careful technique.

Early Orthodontics

In cleft-palate children, malocclusion in the primary dentition is relatively rare. When it does arise, the problem usually is posterior crossbite related to insufficient width of the developing maxilla. The presence of posterior crossbite already at that stage is ominous in terms of the severity of future crossbite problems. Crossbite at this age can be corrected with either removable (split plate) or fixed (lingual arch) appliances. Whether the effort is worth it is debatable, for crossbite problems certainly will continue and will require additional treatment in the mixed and permanent dentitions. Deferring treatment until the eruption of the first molars and permanent incisors usually is the better option.

Fortunately, most cleft-palate children who have had modern surgery do not ever have the kind of narrowing of the maxillary arch that occurred so often many years ago. Moderate crossbite tendencies often begin to appear in the mixed dentition, however. In addition, almost all children who have had a cleft-palate repair have irregularity and rotation of the maxillary permanent incisors as they begin to erupt. It appears that the soft-tissue tension developed as flaps are repositioned to close the cleft affects the eruption path of the incisors (Fig. 18-6). Quite often, when a unilateral cleft has been closed, the central incisors are rotated in the direction of the cleft. In bilateral clefts, the incisors often are tipped lingually in addition to being rotated, but other patterns of displacement also are seen. What is not likely to be present is normal alignment. In addition, the maxillary lateral incisors are likely to be affected by the cleft itself. Often these teeth are missing or reduced in size, but supernumerary teeth in the line of the cleft are relatively common. A preliminary stage of orthodontic treatment in the early mixed dentition therefore is almost always necessary.

The goals of treatment at this stage are to correct the incisor malalignment, rotating them into proper position and bringing the teeth out of anterior crossbite if this is present, and to expand the maxillary arch to correct posterior crossbite if this is necessary. Before the advent of bonded fixed appliances, removable ap-

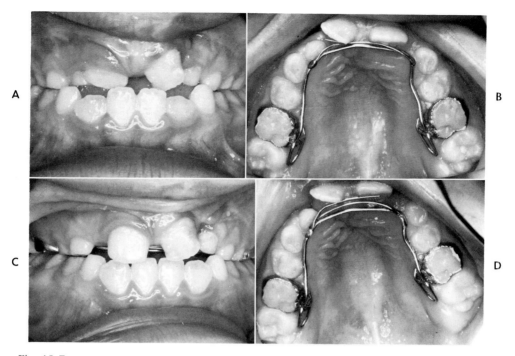

Fig. 18-7. Incisor alignment in the early mixed dentition. **A** and **B,** Lingual arch to advance the maxillary incisors and correct anterior crossbite. **C** and **D,** Six months later.

pliances often were used to accomplish this, and this approach still has advantages if good patient cooperation is present. A partial fixed appliance with bands on first molars and bonded attachments on incisors, with a lingual arch for expansion and a labial arch for incisor alignment, offers increased flexibility without great reliance on patient cooperation, and therefore it is usually employed at present (Fig. 18-7).

Whatever the mode of treatment at this stage, retention of both posterior expansion and incisor alignment is important. There is a pronounced tendency for posterior expansion to collapse in cleft patients. The tendency for teeth to rerotate is similar in cleft patients and those with no cleft. After the first phase of treatment, a removable retainer, at least at night, usually is needed until the next phase of active orthodontic treatment begins. Posterior crossbite tends to recur even if the expansion is maintained because of normal mandibular and deficient maxillary growth.

Speech Therapy

As they begin elementary school, nearly all cleft-palate children benefit from speech therapy. In most cases, this is not just to help with "cleft-palate speech," which is characterized by inappropriate nasal emission of air on some consonant sounds. Because the relatively large tonsils and adenoids of childhood reduce pharyngeal space, the majority of cleft children can achieve velopharyngeal closure at this age. Compensatory activity of the pharyngeal constrictor muscle also

helps in closing off the nose when this is needed. The therapist can help a child to accomplish this if it has not been learned spontaneously. The major speech problem, however, usually is articulation errors because of the child's compensation for the cleft.[6] Tongue position and the timing of air release on consonant sounds both are likely to be different in cleft children who have learned to speak despite a palatal cleft. The goal of the initial speech therapy is to correct the articulation errors while maintaining and reinforcing velopharyngeal adaptive mechanisms to prevent nasal escape of air.

In some children, malpositioned maxillary incisors may make correct tongue positioning more difficult, and this becomes another reason for orthodontic treatment at age 7 to 8 years. This is especially true when the central incisors are severely displaced lingually in a bilateral cleft patient. For most, however, speech therapy and orthodontics have minimal interaction, although they are being carried out at the same time.

Speech therapy may be needed later in the course of cleft treatment, particularly if velopharyngeal function begins to be deficient at puberty as the adenoid tissue decreases in size while the pharynx enlarges. Adenoidectomy and/or tonsillectomy can result in cleft-palate speech that was not present previously.[13] If adaptive measures cannot be taught, pharyngeal flap surgery to reduce the pharyngeal space (see below) may be needed, followed by speech therapy to teach the patient to use the altered structures.

ALVEOLAR GRAFTING
Background and Indications

A complete cleft of the secondary palate penetrates through the dental alveolus in the vicinity of the permanent lateral incisors, either unilaterally or bilaterally. Surgical repair consists of joining soft-tissue flaps over the bony defect, but this does not result in the formation of bone to unite the separated segments. The only way to accomplish that is to place some material into the defect that induces bone formation (i.e., a graft of autogenous or allogeneic bone, or perhaps a synthetic bone-inducing material).

The defect in the anterior alveolus is a part of the cleft of the primary palate, and in theory there is no reason why a bone graft in this area could not be placed at the time of primary palate repair at a few weeks of age. One could argue that establishing bone continuity at that point would produce an improved environment for further growth. Based on this logic, early grafting of the anterior bony defect gained some popularity in the 1960s and at some centers has been carried out for many years. Although the procedure still is defended by its most ardent proponents,[14] the current consensus is that very early grafting, at the time of lip repair, is contraindicated because of the effect on future growth.[15,16] Placing a bone graft at the time of the secondary palate repair at about age 18 months also seems to produce long-term growth deficits.[17] The graft requires more extensive surgery than only doing a soft-tissue closure, and the surgical manipulation itself rather than exactly how the graft is done probably is the culprit in reducing growth. Although early grafting still has adherents who insist that the difficulties have been due to technical problems they can overcome, this procedure has been abandoned by almost all the centers that once employed it.

On the other hand, if the alveolar defect is not corrected, there is a tendency for loss of bone on the surface of roots close to the defect. Over a period of time, unless the alveolar defect is repaired, the central or lateral incisor and the canine adjacent to the cleft are at risk of periodontal pocketing and ultimate loss. The widening defect has the potential to claim other teeth as the patient becomes older.[18] The question is not whether an alveolar graft is needed—it is—but when to do it.

Any bone graft serves merely as a matrix for the induction of new bone and is replaced as the area is remodeled and new bone is formed. The bone in the path of an erupting tooth must be resorbed to allow the tooth to pass through the area. The erupting tooth is a potent stimulus for bone formation—an erupting tooth brings its supporting apparatus with it. But after tooth eruption is complete, it can be very difficult to induce the formation of new bone along the side of an existing tooth. Placing a graft to overcome a periodontal defect has been a major goal in therapy for periodontal disease for many years, without much success to this point. The same difficulties are encountered when a graft to a congenital defect in the alveolus is attempted after tooth eruption is completed. The chance of obtaining a normal amount of interdental bone is much greater when the grafting is done before the canines erupt.[19] It appears, therefore, that the ideal time for an alveolar graft would be as late as possible in maxillary growth but before the eruption of the teeth adjacent to the cleft area.

Experiments with alveolar grafting in 8- to 10-year-old children began in the 1970s.[20] The results have shown consistently that erupting canines would move through the graft area and that, in the aftermath, excellent bone continuity and essentially normal bony anatomy were obtained[21,22] (see the case reports below). By the time the permanent canines erupt, growth in width of the maxilla is essentially complete but some anteroposterior and vertical growth remains. It does not appear that significant growth deficits accompany grafting above age 9.[23] Certainly problems of the type seen with alveolar grafts in infancy do not develop.

With the vindication of the idea that alveolar grafts before canine eruption would be of considerable net benefit to the patient, there has been a tendency to decrease the age at which these grafts are placed. If permanent lateral incisors are missing, there is no great impetus to graft before their time of eruption, but if these teeth are present, there would be a potential advantage in achieving arch continuity before they erupt at age 7 or 8. The clinical questions would be whether better bony continuity of the alveolar process could be achieved if the graft were present before the lateral incisor erupted (assuming of course that it is not congenitally missing) and whether the improvement in this regard would be overbalanced by greater growth deficits from the earlier surgery. If a defect exists alongside the lateral incisor but a graft is placed before the canine erupts, the bone remodeling accompanying eruption of the canine through the grafted area may be enough stimulus to bone formation to partially correct the problem. At the moment, the issue of the best timing still is not totally resolved.

Surgical Technique

For grafting of an alveolar defect to be successful, nasal mucosal coverage as well as oral mucosal coverage over the bone graft is necessary. To accomplish this, it is necessary to utilize the mucosal lining of the cleft to construct the nasal floor and either advance or rotate tissue from the oral cavity to cover the oral side of the graft. Figs. 18-8 and 18-9 illustrate a typical alveolar defect and the surgical technique to correct it.

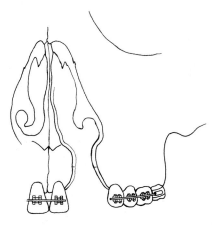

Fig. 18-8. Diagrammatic representation of a typical cleft through the maxillary alveolus, with missing bone and soft tissue and an associated oral-nasal fistula.

The bony margins of the cleft must be completely exposed up to the level of the nasal floor to ensure good osseous consolidation. The mucosal edges are approximated with an inverted horizontal mattress suture that is tied in the floor of the nose. It is important to carry the dissection of the cleft to the level of the nasal floor so that a piriform rim can be constructed. This provides a firm base for the nasal cartilages.

Cancellous bone then is densely packed into the defect. Because the margins of the cleft are hypoplastic, overpacking the bony edges is suggested. Cancellous bone chips are superior to cortical-cancellous chips or blocks of bone because of their greater osteogenic potential and speed of revascularization.

The ilium has been the standard source of autogenous cancellous bone for grafts. The abundance of bone, coupled with its relative accessibility and excellent potential for regeneration, makes the ilium an attractive site for harvesting bone. More recently, the cranium has been utilized as a source of cancellous bone to fill cleft defects.[24] The lack of pain following harvesting is a definite advantage, and rapid revascularization and embryologic similarity to alveolar bone (both are membraneous bone) also are advantageous.

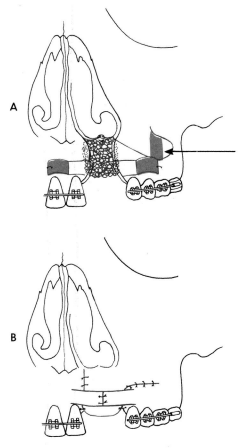

Fig. 18-9. Surgical technique for alveolar cleft repair. **A,** After exposing the bony margins of the alveolar cleft defect by reflecting both nasal and oral mucosa, the nasal mucosa is closed with an inverted horizontal mattress suture and tied in the floor of the nose. Cancellous bone is packed into the defect. Mucosal flaps are outlined in anticipation of oral closure. The arrow indicates the portion of the flaps deepithelialized before rotation. **B,** The mucosal flap then is rotated and sutured over the bone graft. Keratinized gingival tissue is closed over the de-epithelialized surface of the mucosal flaps.

Case Report

Case 1

S.N. had undergone repair as an infant of a unilateral cleft of the primary palate on the right side (Fig. 18-10). At age 7, the cleft penetrated the alveolar ridge but did not involve the secondary palate (Fig. 18-11). The right lateral incisor was displaced toward the cleft, and there was a supernumerary tooth in the line of the cleft (Fig. 18-12). Little bone was available on the cleft side of the lateral incisor to align it without producing a periodontal defect. The decision was made to proceed with a graft in advance of orthodontic treatment to reposition the incisors.

At surgery, cancellous particulate bone was harvested from the ilium. Mucoperiosteal flaps were raised, and the soft tissues lining the cleft defect were elevated, everted into the nasal cavity, and sutured to form a nasal floor. The particulate bone was packed into the defect, and a mucosal flap was elevated from the cheek and rotated to cover the grafted bone.

Two weeks following the surgery active tooth movement was begun, using a partial fixed appliance on the upper arch with bands on the first molars and bonded brackets on the incisors. Within 4 months the anterior teeth were aligned, the patient was debanded, and a maxillary retainer was placed. By age 9 the canine had erupted through the bone graft (Figs. 18-13, *E*, and 18-14). Because of a lack of fixed gingival tissue around the

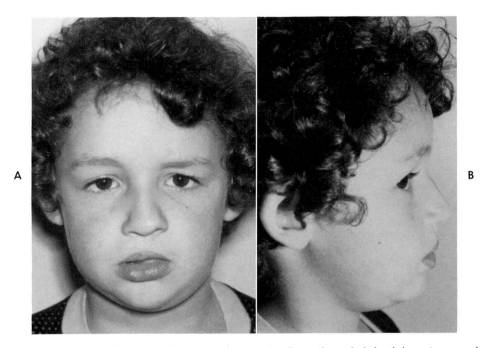

Fig. 18-10. S.N., age 7 years, 5 months, after repair of a unilateral cleft of the primary palate at age 1 month.

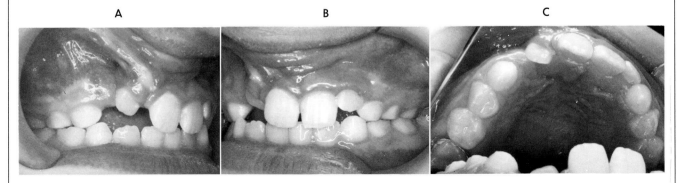

Fig. 18-11. S.N., age 7 years, 5 months. Note the displacement of the maxillary right lateral incisor toward the cleft, which did not involve the secondary palate.

Case 1—cont'd.

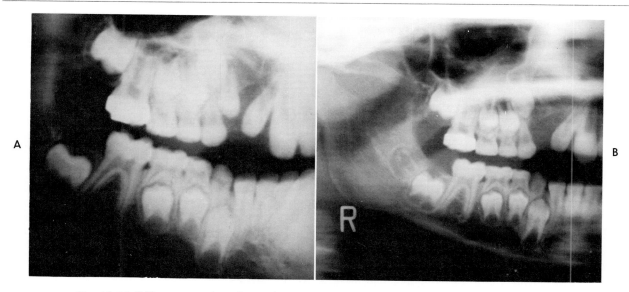

Fig. 18-12. S.N., panoramic radiographs. **A,** Age 7 years, 5 months, before alveolar grafting. Note the supernumerary tooth in the line of the cleft. **B,** Age 7 years, 6 months, immediately after extraction of the supernumerary tooth and placement of the alveolar graft.

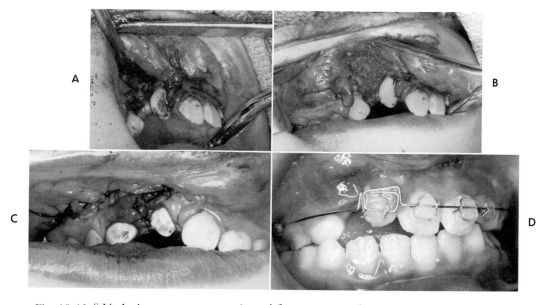

Fig. 18-13. S.N. **A,** At surgery, mucoperiosteal flaps were raised, repositioning the soft-tissue lining of the cleft. **B,** Particulate bone from the ilium packed into the cleft. **C,** Following surgery, the graft was covered by rotating a buccal mucosal flap. **D,** Active orthodontic treatment to align the incisors was begun 2 weeks postsurgically.

Continued.

Case 1—cont'd.

tooth, a free gingival graft was placed. At age 11, when a second phase of fixed-appliance orthodontic therapy was initiated to gain final alignment and interdigitation of the teeth, interdental bone in the previous cleft area was entirely normal, and an excellent orthodontic result was obtained (Figs. 18-15 and 18-16).

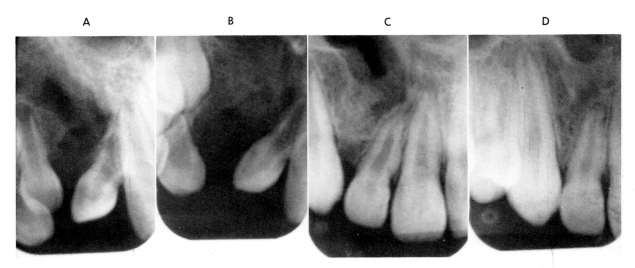

Fig. 18-14. S.N., periapical radiographs showing the bony response as the graft was placed and the canine erupted. **A** and **B**, Age 7 years, 5 months. **C**, Age 9 years, 7 months. **D**, Age 11 years, 9 months.

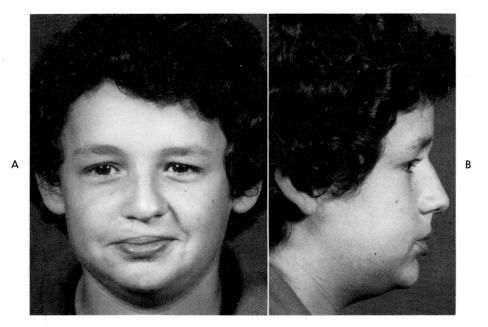

Fig. 18-15. S.N., age 13 years, 9 months.

Case 1—cont'd.

A   B   C

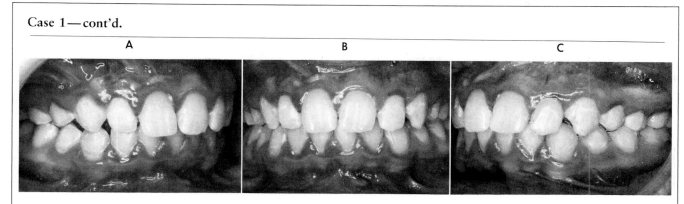

Fig. 18-16. S.N., age 13 years, 9 months, dental relationships 2 years after completion of the second phase of orthodontic treatment. The canine in the cleft area now is in normal position with good periodontal support.

LATER STAGES OF TREATMENT
Comprehensive Orthodontics

As the last of the permanent teeth erupt, cleft-palate patients nearly always require a stage of comprehensive orthodontic treatment with a full fixed appliance. The goals are to achieve alignment and arch form, which almost always are distorted in the cleft area, and to resolve any tendencies toward posterior and/or anterior crossbite.

The frequency of missing or peg lateral incisors in cleft patients means that a decision about the best way to deal with this often is required. As in any patient with small or missing lateral incisors, there are two possibilities. (1) Close the lateral inicisor space, substituting canines for the laterals. This would mean bringing the posterior segments into a Class II relationship or making compensatory extractions in the mandibular arch. (2) Maintain or create space for prosthetic build-up or replacement of the missing lateral incisors. This would imply a Class I molar relationship and a nonextraction approach to the lower arch. There is no one correct decision. Cleft palate can be superimposed on any other set of orthodontic problems. If the child would have had severe crowding in both arches and has a crowded mandibular arch but missing or diminuitive upper lateral incisors, the decision to extract in the mandibular arch and close the space of the missing upper laterals is easily made. If there is plenty of room in both arches but an upper lateral incisor is missing, the decision for its eventual prosthetic replacement is straightforward.

The situation becomes more complex when there is a jaw discrepancy in addition to alignment problems. Most but by no means all cleft-palate patients have a tendency toward Class III malocclusion, due to deficient anteroposterior and vertical maxillary growth. Because the mandible rotates upward and forward, if vertical development of the maxilla is deficient, both AP and vertical growth contribute to the development of anterior crossbite and a Class III dental relationship. If the growth deficiency is mild, it can be alleviated by orthodontic treatment, but if it is severe, orthognathic surgery at the end of growth is likely to be needed. Almost never in a cleft-palate patient is it a good idea to attempt Class III camouflage treatment (i.e., maintain space for prosthetic replacement of upper lateral incisors while extracting in the lower arch so that the lower incisors can be retracted to correct anterior crossbite).

A surgically repaired lip is likely to be tighter and less adaptable to the dentition than is a normal one. Because of the lip contours, it may be all but impossible to procline the upper incisors in some cleft patients, even though this would be desirable for overall facial esthetics. This too must be taken into account in planning the comprehensive orthodontic treatment. Retrusive upper incisors that are difficult to advance orthodontically, however, are not an argument for compensatory extraction in the lower arch. It is better to accept the limitations of orthodontic camouflage and look to orthognathic surgery to eventually correct the jaw discrepancy than to attempt orthodontic camouflage when it would be unlikely to benefit the patient.

It must be kept in mind that true mandibular prognathism can be present in a patient who also, and presumably coincidentally, has a palatal cleft. In a patient with a large mandible, all of the comments made about treatment for mandibular prognathism in Chapter 14 would apply. Controlling excessive mandibular growth in a cleft patient is no easier than in a noncleft one.

The tendency toward diminished maxillary growth in all three planes of space that is produced by palatal surgery, however, is the major factor in the posterior and anterior crossbite tendencies for most cleft patients.

In the AP and vertical planes of space, the growth deficiencies result from soft-tissue tensions that limit the normal downward and forward movement of the maxilla. Not all cleft patients have vertical as well as AP deficiency, but in those who do, the orthodontist has more freedom to use Class III elastics than would be the case if vertical growth were normal. The major side effect of Class III elastics is elongation of the upper molars, which can lead to downward and backward rotation of the mandible. In a Class III patient with normal or long vertical dimensions, that would be undesirable, but the majority of cleft patients have short anterior face height, and increased face height is needed. During the comprehensive orthodontic treatment, therefore, relatively heavy (200 to 300 gm/side) Class III elastics are likely to be helpful. They may need to be worn for many months to produce as much downward and forward movement of the maxilla and maxillary teeth as possible. Elongation of the lower incisors remains an undesirable side effect, so the best possible stabilization of the lower arch with a heavy rectangular arch wire is needed.

Two things are different about the posterior crossbite in cleft patients. First, previous surgical intervention has produced tight palatal tissue that limits the orthodontist's ability to produce successful dental expansion. Second and more important, there is no equivalent of a midpalatal suture in cleft patients, so the techniques of orthopedic maxillary expansion cannot be applied. The only way to correct a posterior crossbite is to produce dental expansion despite the unusually large resistance from the stretched palatal tissues, with full awareness of the extreme relapse tendencies. In practical terms, because of the soft-tissue limitations, not all posterior crossbites in cleft patients can be corrected, orthodontically or surgically. Any lateral expansion that is created must be maintained carefully on a long-term basis, which means either a lingual arch as a long-term retainer or excellent wear of a removable retainer.

If bone grafts to the dental alveolus are successful now in creating continuity around the dental arch, why not bone grafts to the defective midpalatal area? In theory, one could create bony continuity, but of course it would be extremely undesirable to do this before growth had been completed. The midpalatal suture is an important adjustment area in allowing normal growth and width of the maxilla to take place, and obliterating it at an early age would totally destroy any further potential for growth in width. Records from a few patients who were treated in the 1930s by fusing

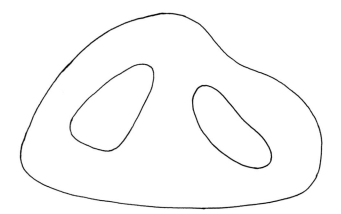

Fig. 18-17. The typical nasal deformity associated with cleft lip, as seen from below. The nostril is partially collapsed on the affected side, due to distortion of the lateral alar cartilages, and the nasal tip deviates. Secondary reconstruction usually is delayed until adolescence.

the palate at an early age demonstrate the tremendous restriction of maxillary growth that early bone continuity across a midpalatal defect can cause.[25] On the other hand, by the time growth in width is essentially complete, the palatal defect has been repaired for some time, and it is difficult to successfully place a graft in the poorly vascularized tissue that spans the palatal defect at that point. If orthognathic surgery is needed in the late teens and the maxilla will be downfractured, it may be possible to place bone in the midline cleft (see below).

Retention problems in cleft-palate patients are similar to but perhaps even worse than those in noncleft Class III patients. Any transverse expansion of the maxilla must be retained indefinitely. When Class III elastics have been used during the active treatment, there will be no further forward movement of the maxilla or maxillary teeth once the treatment ends, and in fact there may be mild relapse, but mandibular growth is quite likely to continue. If transverse stability is not a major concern, using a modified functional appliance as a retainer (typically an open bionator, to allow and encourage further eruption of posterior teeth) can be helpful. If mandibular growth continues vigorously enough, what looked like satisfactory orthodontic treatment at age 14 or 15 may lead to orthognathic surgery after all at age 19 (see Case 2).

Secondary Plastic Procedures
Nose/Lip Revision

With even the best primary closure of the lip in infancy, there is a distortion of the base of the nostril on the cleft side, and almost always the nostril on the affected side is partially collapsed and configured abnormally (Fig. 18-17). Some surgeons recently have advocated cartilaginous nasal surgery at the same time as

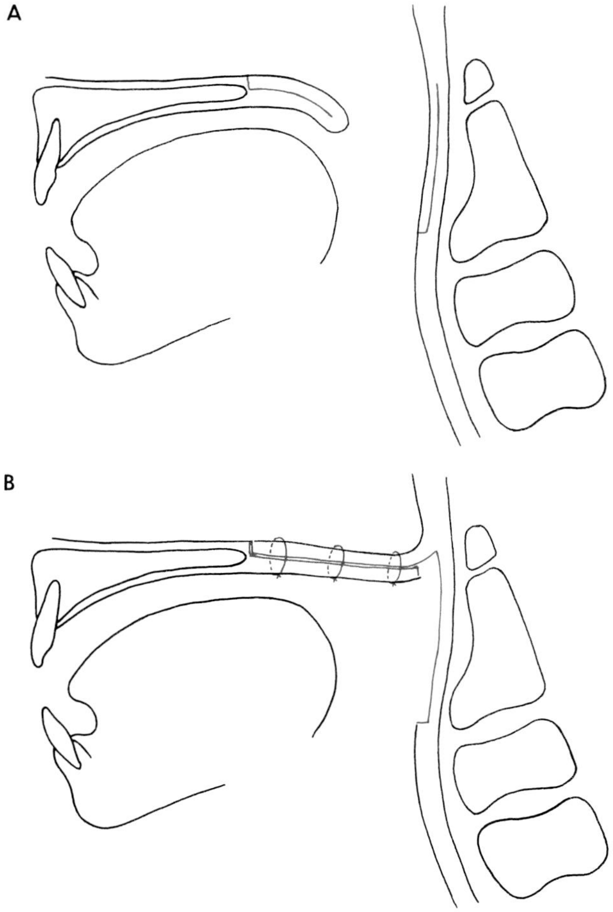

A

B

Fig. 18-18. Superiorly based pharyngeal flap lined with mucosa from the soft palate. **A,** Incisions outlined in the posterior pharyngeal wall and soft palate. **B,** Mucosal flaps mobilized and sutured in place.

primary lip closure,[26] but it remains to be seen whether this will reduce the need to revise the nose at a later date. For most patients, a secondary nasal procedure is needed.[27,28] It is tempting to perform soft-tissue revisions throughout childhood, but although this produces an immediate cosmetic improvement, further growth is likely to produce changes that require further revision. Under ideal circumstances, secondary nasal surgery would be done in adolescence, often at the same time as the comprehensive orthodontics or later.

Pharyngeal Flap

After palate repair, most children with cleft palate are able to achieve velopharyngeal closure so that they do not have the escape of air through the nose that produces cleft-palate speech. The muscles of the lateral pharyngeal wall compensate to some extent for the short and hypomobile soft palate. The reduction in pharyngeal space created by relatively enlarged tonsils and adenoids also helps cleft children prevent nasal leakage of air.

During the adolescent growth spurt, two things happen that can disrupt velopharyngeal closure mechanisms and produce cleft-palate speech. First, as a concomitant of normal growth, pharyngeal dimensions enlarge; second, as part of the same normal growth pattern, there is a tendency toward shrinkage of the lymphatic tissues. As a result, a marginal but adequate velopharyngeal mechanism can become inadequate and the patient no longer is able to avoid leakage of air and distortion of speech.

When this occurs, the preferred treatment now is the creation of a flap from the posterior pharyngeal wall to the soft palate.[29] It partially obstructs the nasal pharynx, making it easier for the soft palate and lateral pharyngeal walls to seal off the nasal from the oral pharynx during speech. After surgery, the patient must be taught to use the flap, and although it usually is successful, this is not always the case. The obstruction can produce a problem with nasal drainage for some patients, but most patients tolerate it.

The flap is elevated from the posterior pharyngeal wall along the prevertebral fascial layer and is brought forward to attach to the soft palate. Most surgeons prefer to base the flap superiorly in the nasal pharynx (Fig. 18-18). It is preferable to line the flap with mucosa, as this will minimize shrinkage. The mucosal lining is taken from the nasal surface of the soft palate and rotated posteriorly to cover the raw surface of the flap.

ORTHOGNATHIC SURGERY
Indications for Surgical-Orthodontic Treatment

Orthognathic surgery in cleft patients is almost never indicated until the conclusion of active facial growth, which often does not occur until age 18 or 19. At that point, surgery is needed when a jaw discrepancy too great to correct with orthodontics alone is a functional and esthetic problem. Occasionally, surgery to reposition the maxilla is indicated before growth is completed to help manage psychosocial problems associated with severe deformity, even though a second orthognathic procedure later almost certainly would be needed.

In essentially every instance, the cleft patients who are candidates for orthognathic surgery have had extensive previous orthodontic treatment. At one time, they had their occlusion corrected or all but corrected, only to have problems reappear in the late teens because of disproportionate growth of the lower jaw. In the absence of AP and vertical maxillary growth, normal mandibular growth can produce a significant jaw discrepancy, particularly when growth is projected almost directly forward because of the absence of vertical growth of the maxilla.

From a review of the cleft-palate patients at the UNC, it appears that only 5% to 10% have severe enough residual deformity in the late teens to need orthognathic surgery. For all other types of dentofacial deformity, about twice as many females as males seek and receive treatment, but in the cleft-palate group the sex ratio is approximately equal. This probably reflects the greater tendency in males toward prolonged mandibular growth so that a more severe jaw discrepancy develops after active orthodontic treatment is discontinued in the early teens. When orthognathic surgery is required in cleft patients, it almost always involves moving the maxilla forward. Mandibular setback at the same time may be required (see Case 3), but isolated mandibular setback is rarely indicated or performed.

Special Problems in Coordinating Surgical-Orthodontic Treatment
Interaction with Velopharyngeal Function

In a cleft-palate patient, the decision to reposition the maxilla anteriorly carries with it a risk of producing postsurgical cleft-palate speech. In noncleft patients, the velopharyngeal mechanism has enough adaptive capacity that speech problems almost never arise as a consequence of maxillary advancement. In cleft patients, however, the mechanism often is already at or near its limit of adaptation. Because of this, orthognathic surgery must be considered a potential two-stage procedure, the first stage being the repositioning of the jaws and the second stage a pharyngeal flap to bring nasal air leakage back under control.

In a few patients, a severe jaw discrepancy in the late teens indicates orthognathic surgery and a pharyngeal flap already is in place. Because the flap limits the surgeon's ability to reposition the maxilla, there is little option in this circumstance but to remove the original flap, carry out the orthognathic surgery, and then surgically create a new flap. Because shrinkage of the flap could produce force on the maxilla that would displace it, the secondary flap procedure should be delayed until 6 months after the orthognathic surgery.

Surgical Techniques: Special Considerations in Cleft Palate

There are two limiting factors in surgery for cleft-palate patients. First, most have undergone multiple surgical procedures on both the lip and palate before orthognathic surgery, and the effect of residual scarring must be considered when developing a treatment plan. Lip scars may restrict the amount of maxillary advancement and the position of the teeth. Palatal scars not only limit the amount of advancement of the maxilla, but they also reduce revascularization and bone healing after surgery.

Second, in noncleft individuals the velopharyngeal mechanism has sufficient compensatory reserve to tolerate even massive amounts of maxillary advancement (up to 15 mm) without postsurgical speech problems. In contrast, the amount of further compensation possible for cleft patients is highly variable and somewhat unpredictable. We have observed complete deterioration of velopharyngeal competence following minimal maxillary advancement (3 mm) in a cleft patient, which is testimony to the fragility of the velopharyngeal mechanism in these patients.

Both of these factors limit the amount of maxillary advancement available in cleft patients. We suggest that if the amount of reverse overjet is greater than 8 to 10 mm, even if the problem is almost entirely maxillary deficiency, simultaneous maxilla advancement and mandibular setback should be undertaken. In some individuals this may result in less than ideal facial esthetics. However, onlay grafting of the middle face is another effective means of improving midface projection in these individuals and should be considered in cases of this type.

In some cleft-palate individuals, the alveolus and palate have never been reconstructed, and this can be accomplished at the time of maxillary advancement. With the maxilla downfractured, the palatal edges can be exposed from the nasal side along the entire cleft up to the alveolus. Similarly, tissue should be removed from the bony edges of the alveolar defect and sutured on the oral cavity side. Cancellous bone chips then may be placed into both the palatal and alveolar defects, and the nasal mucosa sutured. If needed, the alar aspect of the piriform rim also can be constructed with a bone graft at the time the maxilla is downfractured and accessibility is maximal.

Surgical-Orthodontic Coordination

In orthognathic surgery for cleft-palate patients, coordination between the orthodontist and the surgeon is essentially identical to what it is for any other patient. Three points are worth special comment:

1. The timing of orthognathic surgery for these patients is critical. The problem leading to the need for orthognathic surgery is continuing growth of the lower jaw, which is disproportionate because no growth of the upper jaw is occurring. The only way to evaluate whether mandibular growth is continuing is to obtain serial cephalometric films and wait until growth has stopped. For the males who are experiencing late and prolonged mandibular growth, often there can be a considerable delay. As in other Class III patients, operating too soon carries with it a considerable risk of relapse because of continued growth, and that complication should be avoided if at all possible. If early maxillary advancement is indicated for psychosocial reasons, a second orthognathic procedure later should be anticipated.

2. The only difference in the orthodontic preparation for surgery in cleft patients is that removing the dental compensation usually is not a major goal and almost never requires extraction of teeth. The tight upper lip prevents the kind of extreme proclination of upper incisors that occurs naturally in some non-cleft patients and is produced by over-enthusiastic orthodontic treatment in others. In the cleft patients, some use of Class II elastics before the jaw surgery may help create a more stable environment postsurgically, particularly if there has been recent active orthodontics involving Class III elastics.

3. Moderate overcorrection of anterior crossbite, to

the extent of perhaps 2 mm excess overjet immediately after surgery, can be advantageous (see Case 2). This provides some compensation for the relapse that is likely to occur while leaving the occlusion within the reach of short-term orthodontic therapy if the initial dental and skeletal relationships prove stable. Excessive overcorrection can cause major difficulties in postsurgical orthodontics and should be avoided. The postsurgical orthodontics consists of settling the patient into occlusion with vertical elastics, using a Class II or Class III direction if desired, exactly as in any other surgical-orthodontic patient.

CASE REPORTS

Case 2

G.W. was seen initially by our cleft-palate team at age 7 after undergoing surgical treatment elsewhere for closure of his unilateral cleft lip at age 6 weeks and palate closure at age 2. There was a facial appearance of mild maxillary deficiency (Fig. 18-19). The maxillary right lateral incisor in the line of the cleft was missing, and the right central incisor was severely displaced toward the cleft and was hypoplastic (Fig. 18-20). As the maxillary incisors erupted, a removable appliance was used to correct the posterior crossbite tendency and gain alignment, but difficulties with both repositioning and restoring the hypoplastic right central incisor led ulti-

mately to its extraction at age 9. After the extraction, he wore a maxillary retainer, but posterior crossbite returned as the mandibular (but not the maxillary) arch widened with growth.

At age 12 years, 1 month, a complete fixed appliance was placed, and coil springs were used to open the maxillary right central-lateral spaces and shift the midline to the left. With the use of anterior diagonal and parallel Class II-Class III elastics, good interdigitation was obtained, and he was debanded to a retainer with replacement teeth at age 13 years, 6 months. Cephalometric superimposition showed a downward direction of growth

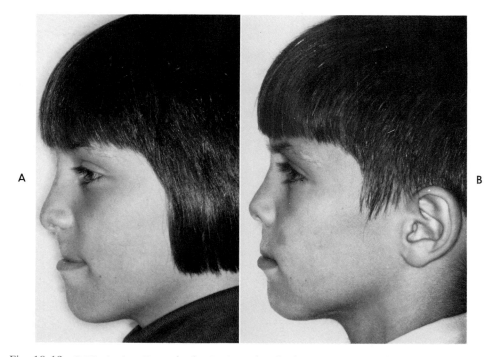

Fig. 18-19. G.W. **A,** Age 7, at the beginning of orthodontic treatment, following earlier lip and palate surgery. **B,** Age 9. Note the mild maxillary deficiency at that stage.

Continued.

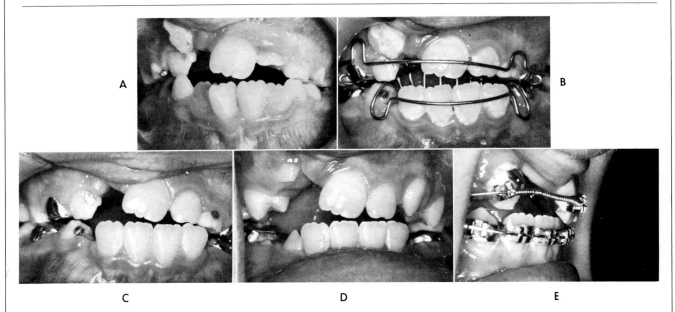

Fig. 18-20. G.W. **A,** Age 7 years, 6 months, before treatment. **B,** Age 8 years, 5 months, removable appliance with palatal expansion spring, crib for finger habit, and auxiliary springs to attempt to reposition the maxillary right central incisor. **C,** Age 9 years, 9 months, after extraction of the right central incisor. **D,** Age 10 years, 11 months. Note the return of posterior crossbite even though he had been wearing a maxillary palate-covering retainer. **E,** Age 12 years, 10 months, fixed appliance being used to correct the maxillary midline and open space for the missing central and lateral incisors.

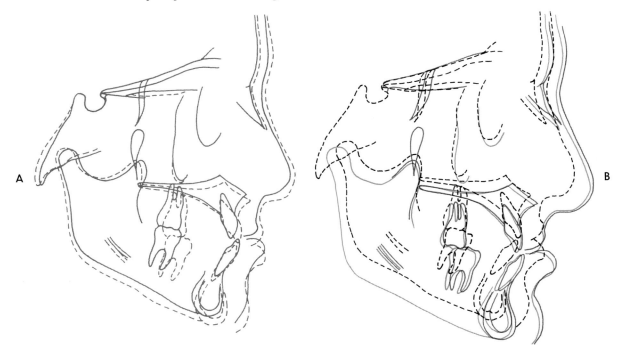

Fig. 18-21. G.W. **A,** Cephalometric superimpositions ages 11 years, 9 months, to 13 years, 6 months *(dashed black)*, during fixed-appliance treatment. **B,** Superimpositions ages 13 years, 6 months, to 16 years, 5 months *(pink)*, to 17 years, 11 months *(gray)*. Note the favorable growth pattern during the orthodontic treatment, which also had been present earlier, then the strong expression of forward mandibular growth during his relatively late adolescent growth spurt.

during the period of treatment and good facial proportions at its conclusion (Fig. 18-21). Within a few months he was tending toward anterior crossbite, and a chin cup with 16-oz force per side was placed. Over the next year, he wore the chin cup only intermittently, and the Class III growth pattern continued. Between ages 15 and 16 he grew nearly 6 inches and the Class III relationship worsened noticeably. By age 17, speech problems due to nasal escape of air were beginning to appear, presumably related to loss of adenoid tissue; at age 18 it appeared that growth had all but ceased, and surgery to advance the maxilla was suggested (Figs. 18-22 to 18-24).

He was initially quite reluctant to have further surgery, then decided suddenly in the middle of the summer that it had to be done before school started for the fall term. The molar teeth were banded and bonded attachments were placed anteriorly, but no arch wires were placed presurgically because with no time for orthodontic preparation, there was no way to be sure they would be passive. At age 18 years, 6 months, a Lefort I osteotomy was performed to advance the maxilla, bringing it forward and down (Fig. 18-24, *B*). Cancellous strips of autogenous bone from the iliac crest were used to stabilize the maxilla, and particulate cancellous bone chips were placed in the alveolar defect. Circumzygomatic wires were tied to the mandibular arch wire, providing skeletal suspension for further stabilization, and he was placed in maxillomandibular fixation.

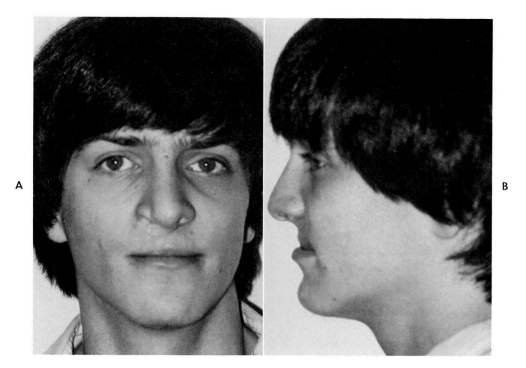

Fig. 18-22. G.W., age 18 years, at the completion of adolescent growth.

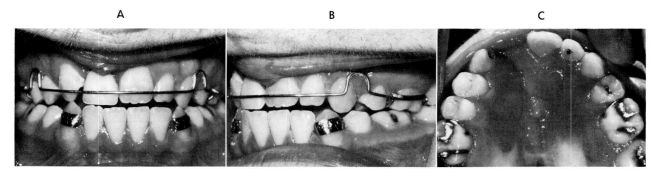

Fig. 18-23. G.W., age 18 years, dental relationships before orthognathic surgery. The missing maxillary central incisor was supplied with the maxillary retainer.

Continued.

Case 2—cont'd.

Six weeks postsurgically, fixation was released, the splint and stabilizing arch wires were removed, and prosthetic teeth were tied to a maxillary 18×25 braided arch wire. A 16 round wire was placed in the mandibular arch, and he wore ⅜-inch box elastics bilaterally. The teeth settled rapidly into occlusion, and he was debanded to a retainer with replacement teeth 4 months after finishing orthodontics was begun. Nine months later an initial maxillary fixed bridge was placed (Fig. 18-25) and other retention was discontinued. Although further deterioration in speech had been expected in the aftermath of the maxillary advancement, there was little or no change, and he did not wish pharyngeal flap surgery. The possibility of collagen injections into the pharyngeal wall as an alternative way to improve velopharyn-

geal competence was discussed, but he also rejected that. On recall 3½ years postsurgery, a permanent bridge had been placed. Both occlusal and facial relationships were being maintained nicely (Figs. 18-26 and 18-27), and he was quite pleased with the result.

Comments. The late mandibular growth in this patient that was not matched by corresponding maxillary growth is typical of the cleft-palate patients who eventually require orthognathic surgery. His diminished vertical maxillary growth was as significant as the deficient AP growth because the mandibular growth was projected anteriorly rather than vertically.

It is unusual to proceed with orthognathic surgery without stabilizing arch wires, but no arch wire is better than one that is not passive. The presence of orthodontic at-

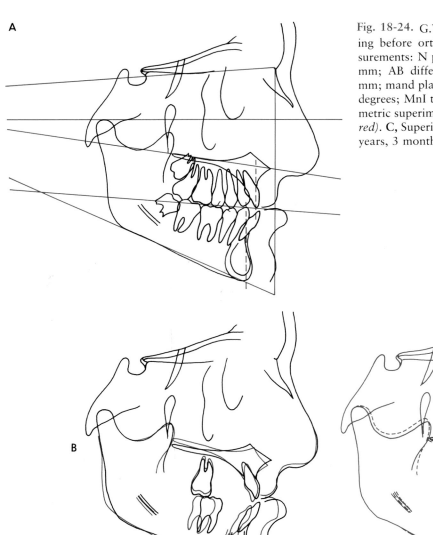

Fig. 18-24. G.W. **A,** Age 18 years, cephalometric tracing before orthognathic surgery. Cephalometric measurements: N perp to A, −10 mm; N perp to Pg, −13 mm; AB difference, 6 mm; UFH, 60 mm; LFH, 67 mm; mand plane, 24 degrees; MxI to A vert, 1 mm, 19 degrees; MnI to B vert, 8 mm, 35 degrees. **B,** Cephalometric superimposition presurgery to postsurgery *(solid red).* **C,** Superimposition postsurgery to recall at age 21 years, 3 months *(dashed red).*

Case 2—cont'd.

tachments only (sometimes referred as a "band splint") provided a means to achieve maxillomandibular fixation, and coupled with the interocclusal wafer splint, this offered adequate stabilization. Because the teeth were already reasonably well aligned from the previous orthodontics, no change in arch form or other major preliminary orthodontics was necessary.

This patient had not previously received a bone graft to the alveolar defect. Although most of the bone placed in a large defect of this type after the permanent teeth have

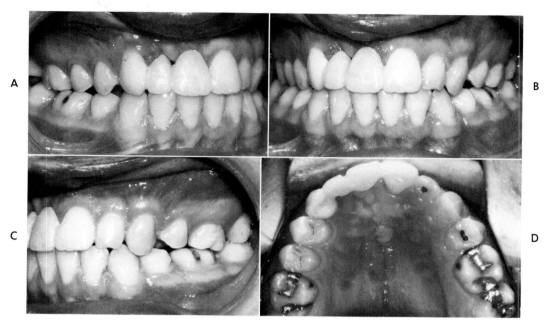

Fig. 18-25. G.W., dental relationships, age 19 years, 11 months, after the maxillary temporary fixed bridge was placed and other retention discontinued.

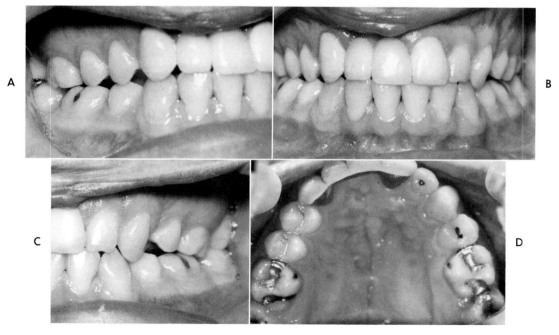

Fig. 18-26. G.W., dental relationships, age 22 years, 2 months.

Continued.

Case 2—cont'd.

erupted will be lost, even a late graft has some tendency to stabilize the defect so that it does not progressively involve adjacent teeth over time, as happens without grafting.

Advancement of the maxilla has the potential to produce velopharyngeal incompetence in cleft patients who were only marginally competent presurgically. Pharyngeal flap surgery secondary to the orthognathic surgery often is required. For this patient, a moderate but tolerable degree of incompetence was present presurgically and did not change appreciably. He saw no reason for further surgery to improve speech that was acceptable to him.

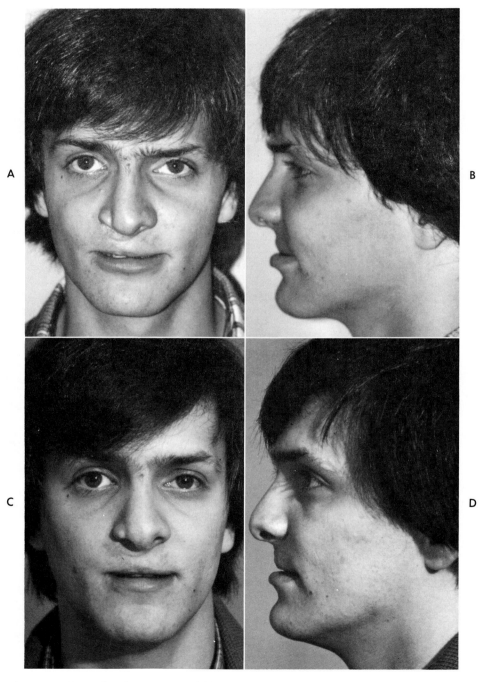

Fig. 18-27. G.W., facial appearance following orthognathic surgery. **A** and **B**, Age 19 years, 11 months. **C** and **D**, Age 22 years, 2 months.

Case 3

S.C. was first seen by our cleft-palate team at age 5, after her bilateral cleft of the lip and palate had been surgically repaired elsewhere. A panoramic radiograph at that time (Fig. 18-28) showed that the maxillary left lateral incisor was missing and the left central incisor was severely rotated, with a large alveolar defect present on the left. At age 8 years, 4 months, an autogenous graft (using bone from the ilium) was placed in the alveolar defect, with the plan that orthodontic treatment would start soon thereafter. At age 8 years, 5 months, facial proportions were mildly long and mildly mandibular-deficient (Figs. 18-29 and 18-30). Anterior but not posterior crossbite was present, with the maxillary dental midline shifted to the right (Fig. 18-31). A fixed appliance with bands on the central incisors and first molars was used over a 5-month period to advance the incisors, then a maxillary removable retainer was placed. The maxillary left canine erupted through the grafted area, stabilizing that area.

At age 11 years, 9 months, a maxillary fixed appliance was placed again for alignment and crossbite correction. To obtain room for alignment in the maxillary right quadrant and balance the occlusion with the left lateral incisor missing, the first premolar was extracted.

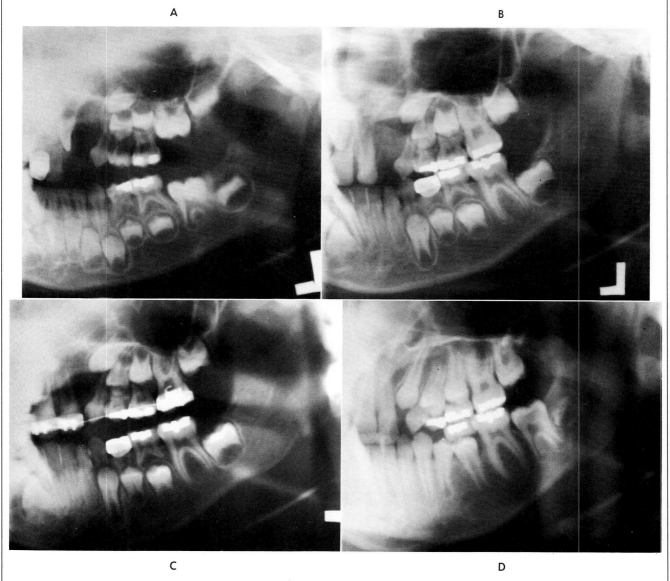

A

B

C

D

Fig. 18-28. S.C., panoramic radiographs. **A,** Age 5 years, 9 months. **B,** Age 8 years, 5 months, just after placement of the alveolar graft. **C,** Age 9 years, 2 months. **D,** Age 11 years, 8 months, with the canine erupting through the grafted area.

Continued.

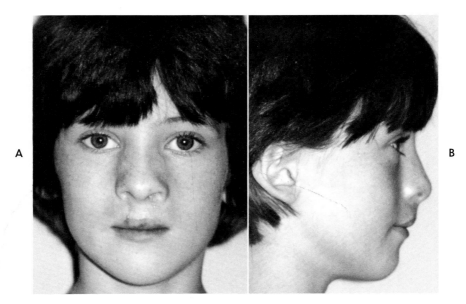

Fig. 18-29. S.C., age 8 years, 5 months.

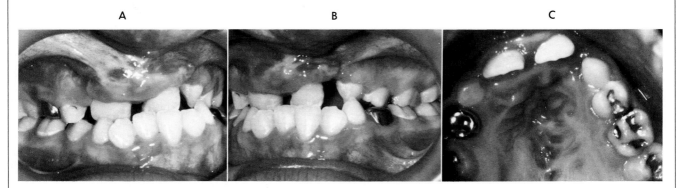

Fig. 18-30. S.C., age 8 years, 5 months, dental relationships soon after placement of the alveolar graft.

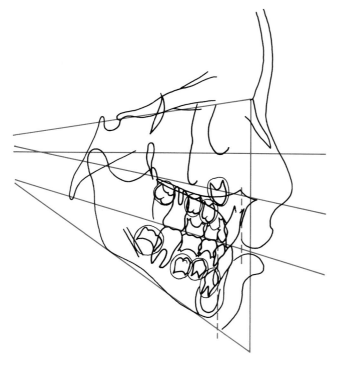

Fig. 18-31. S.C., cephalometric tracing age 8 years, 5 months. Note the moderate skeletal Class II jaw relationship, with the upper incisors tipped lingually into anterior crossbite in spite of this relationship. Cephalometric measurements: N perp to A, −2 mm; N perp to Pg, −12 mm; AB difference, 12 mm; UFH, 48 mm; LFH, 57 mm; mand plane, 36 degrees; MxI to A vert, −6 mm, −15 degrees; MnI to B vert, 7 mm, 21 degrees.

Case 3—cont'd.

Eighteen months later, the lower arch was banded and interarch elastics were used. There was no forward growth of the maxilla, and the mandible rotated down and back, producing the jaw relationship best described as Class III rotated to Class I (Fig. 18-32). By age 14, it was apparent that the jaw discrepancy was too great to manage nonsurgically.

At age 15 years, 4 months, maxillary deficiency was apparent in the facial proportions (Fig. 18-33), and she had anterior crossbite and open bite (Fig. 18-34). Surgery to advance the maxilla, rotate it up posteriorly, and augment the deficient paranasal areas with onlay grafts was planned. At surgery, a cross-cut fissure bur was used to cut through the outer cortex of the cranium

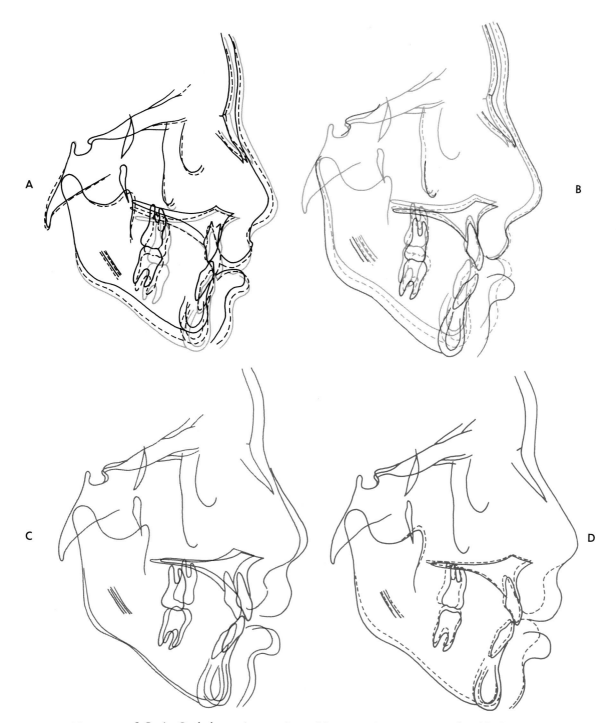

Fig. 18-32. S.C. **A,** Cephalometric superimpositions age 8 years, 5 months *(black),* to 10 years *(dashed black),* to 11 years, 8 months *(pink).* **B,** Superimposition age 11 years, 8 months *(pink),* to 13 years, 4 months *(dashed pink),* to 15 years, 6 months *(black).* **C,** Superimposition presurgery to postsurgery *(solid red),* age 15 years, 6 months. **D,** Superimposition age 15 years, 6 months, to 15 years, 10 months *(dashed red),* postsurgery to completion of treatment.

Continued.

Case 3—cont'd.

into the diploic space in the right parietal area, and strips of cranium were removed with a spatula osteotome. The remaining diploic bone was harvested using a curved osteotome. A LeFort I osteotomy then was performed to free the maxilla for advancement. When the alveolar graft area was visualized, the bone was not discernably different from the bone of the surrounding area. With the maxilla in the downfractured position, a sagittal osteotomy along both sides of the nasal crest and extended between the left canine and first premolar was performed to provide for transverse expansion. The maxilla was placed in the prepared splint and rotated to position, then stabilized with two titanium bone plates. The corticocancellous strips of cranial bone were placed in the anterior maxillary defect as grafts. Additional cortical and cancellous material was placed in the paranasal regions for further augmentation. The cancellous

bone was placed in the palatal defects created by the expansion.

Maxillomandibular fixation was maintained for 6 weeks, then the splint and stabilizing arch wires were removed, mandibular 17×25 NiTi and maxillary 18×22 arch wires were placed, and she wore posterior box elastics. The teeth settled rapidly into occlusion, and the appliances were removed 3 months later. The importance of full-time wear of a maxillary retainer, which incorporated a replacement tooth that improved its chances, was stressed (Fig. 18-35). At age 16 years, 7 months, the improvement in facial proportions produced by the surgery was being maintained (Fig. 18-36).

Comments. The timing of the alveolar graft for this patient was close to ideal; the canine began to erupt into the grafted area almost immediately. Unlike most cleft patients, she had AP but not vertical maxillary defi-

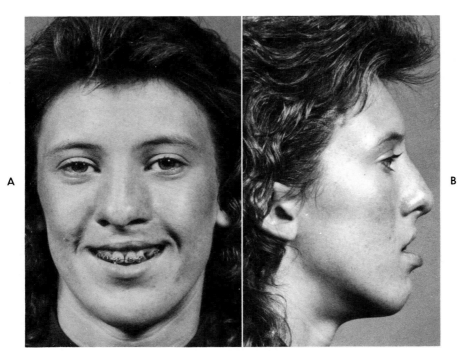

Fig. 18-33. S.C., age 15 years, 4 months, before surgery.

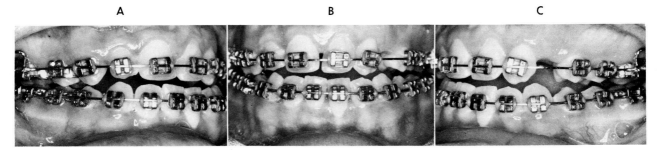

Fig. 18-34. S.C., age 15 years, 4 months, dental relationships before surgery.

Case 3—cont'd.

ciency, and in fact vertical maxillary growth was excessive, but there was no way to obtain either good dental occlusion or satisfactory facial esthetics without repositioning the maxilla. The orthognathic surgery was done somewhat earlier than usual, based on her desire to complete the treatment, early maturation, and lack of excessive mandibular growth. Even in mature girls, early maxillary advancement does carry with it some risk of relapse into anterior crossbite because of late mandibular growth.

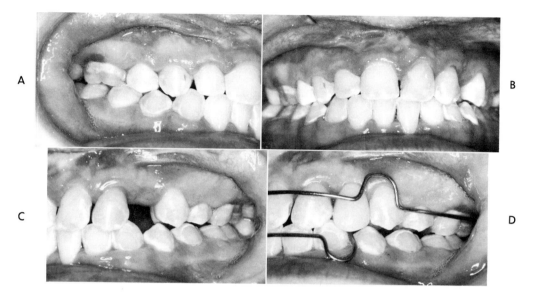

Fig. 18-35. S.C., dental relationships, age 15 years, 9 months, with the maxillary canine in the lateral incisor position and a canine pontic on the retainer.

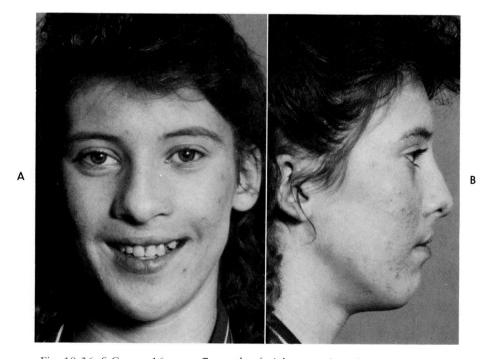

Fig. 18-36. S.C., age 16 years, 7 months, facial proportions 1 year postsurgery.

Case 4

D.P. was seen at age 8 years, 9 months. His unilateral cleft lip had been repaired elsewhere at age 3 months, and his cleft palate was closed in an initial procedure followed by three revisions between ages 4 and 5. At age 5 he was hospitalized for treatment of idiopathic thrombocytopenic purpura, and at age 8 a bone biopsy revealed a septic right hip, which was treated with incision and drainage and a full-body cast. The primary concerns now were speech and the contours of the nose (Fig. 18-37). The maxillary left lateral incisor was missing, the maxillary arch was collapsed anteriorly (Fig. 18-38), and cephalometric analysis indicated severe maxillary deficiency (Fig. 18-39). During the next year, dental restorative care was provided and a maxillary removable appliance was used to tip the central incisors anteriorly. At age 10 years, 9 months, an autogenous bone graft to the alveolar defect on the left side was placed (Fig. 18-40), and a maxillary fixed appliance was placed for transverse expansion and alignment. Reverse-pull headgear was instituted to attempt to translate the maxilla forward, but there were compliance problems, particularly in the aftermath of surgery to revise the contours of the nose. The maxillary incisors tipped forward, but no forward growth of the maxilla occurred (Fig. 18-41). After 16 months, treatment was discontinued and a maxillary retainer was placed, awaiting further eruption of teeth and skeletal maturation. He failed to wear the retainer, and most of the arch expansion gained in the initial treatment was lost.

At age 14 years, 11 months, in preparation for orthognathic surgery, a complete fixed appliance was placed, and over the next 9 months a series of arch wires were used to align the arches in preparation for surgery (Fig. 18-42). Severe maxillary deficiency was evident in the

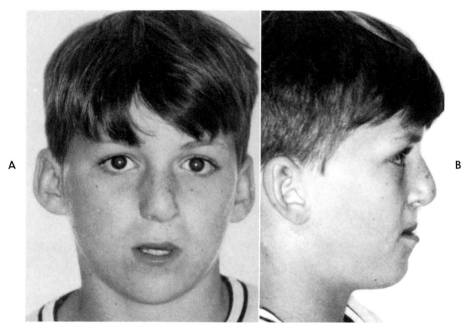

Fig. 18-37. D.P., age 8 years, 9 months.

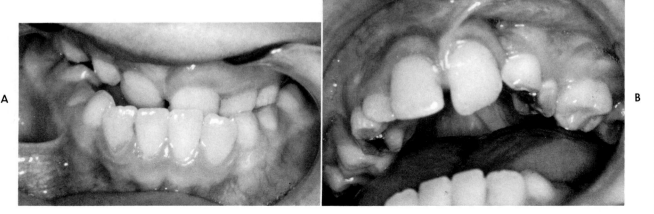

Fig. 18-38. D.P., dental relationships, age 8 years, 9 months. Note the severe collapse of the maxillary arch anteriorly.

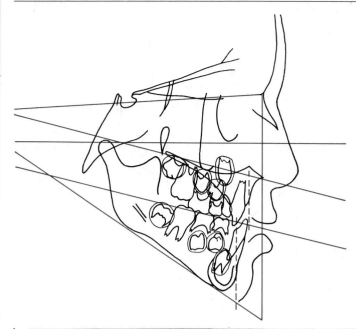

Fig. 18-39. D.P., cephalometric tracing, age 8 years, 9 months. The A-B difference projected to the true horizontal and the ANB angle are normal, but the maxillary incisors are severely tipped lingually and the palatal plane is rotated up posteriorly, indicating deficient vertical growth of the posterior palate. Cephalometric measurements: N perp to A, −4 mm; N perp to Pg, −12 mm; AB difference, 5 mm; UFH, 45 mm; LFH, 72 mm; mand plane, 34 degrees; MxI to A vert, −7 mm, −12 degrees; MnI to B vert, 7 mm, 22 degrees.

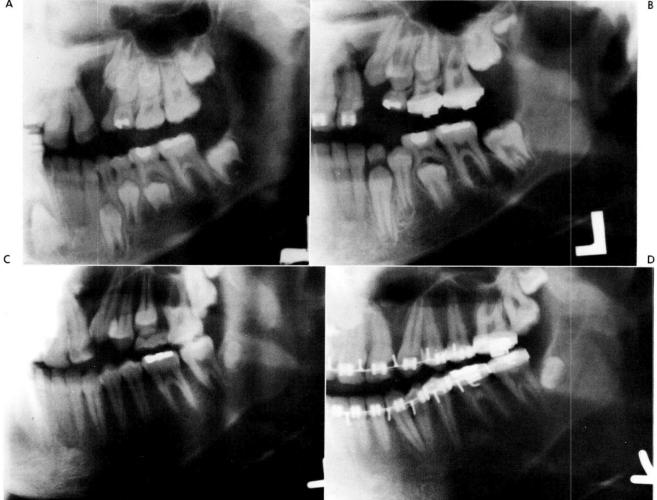

Fig. 18-40. D.P., radiographs following the grafted alveolar defect on the left side. **A,** Age 10 years, 9 months, just before the alveolar graft. **B,** Age 12 years, 6 months, showing the canine erupting through the grafted area. **C,** Age 14 years, 9 months, with the canine nearly erupted. **D,** Age 15 years, 8 months, with the canine at the occlusal level and the defect filled with bone.

Continued.

Case 4—cont'd.

facial proportions (Fig. 18-43). The plan was to surgically move the maxilla down and forward, placing an iliac bone graft, and to simultaneously mobilize the mandible, more to improve the stability of the maxillary downgraft than to retract it significantly.

At surgery, bone was harvested from the iliac crest; the osteotomies for the mandibular sagittal splits were performed, but the splits were not completed; the maxilla was freed, brought into maxillomandibular fixation in the intermediate splint, positioned properly, and stabilized with graft bone and transosseous wires, with onlay grafts added in the perinasal area; and then the mandibular sagittal splits were completed, the teeth were placed in maxillomandibular fixation in the final splint. superior border wires were placed, and circummandibular wires were attached to the maxillary suspension wires (Figs. 18-44 and 18-45, *A*). He was maintained in maxillomandibular fixation for 7 weeks, then functioned into the splint for another 2 weeks before the splint and stabilizing arch wires were removed and finishing orthodontics begun.

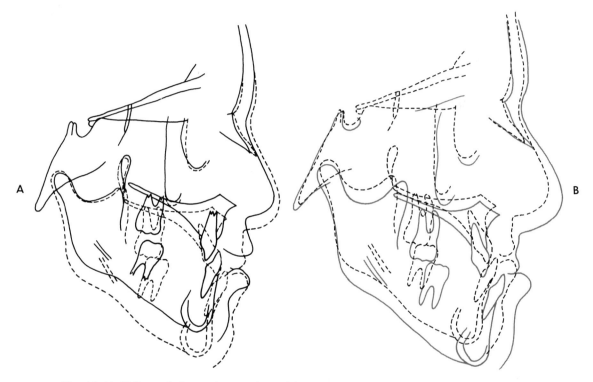

Fig. 18-41. D.P., cephalometric superimpositions. **A,** Age 8 years, 9 months, to 12 years, 9 months *(dashed black)*, when reverse-pull headgear was discontinued. **B,** Age 12 years, 9 months, to 14 years, 9 months *(solid gray)*, showing further vertical but not anterior maxillary growth.

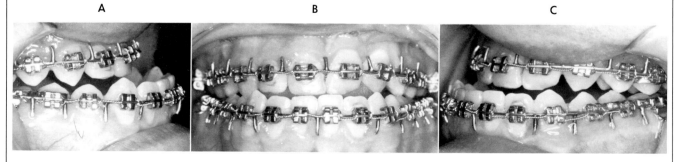

Fig. 18-42. D.P., age 15 years, 8 months, stabilizing arch wires in place before surgery.

Case 4—cont'd.

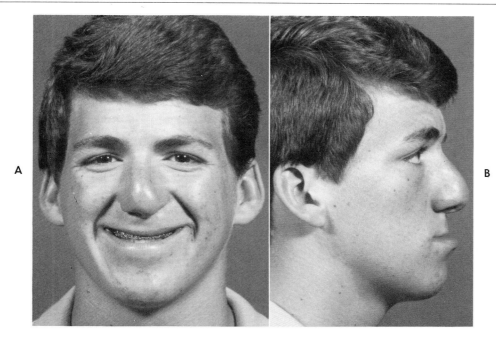

Fig. 18-43. D.P., age 15 years, 8 months, before orthognathic surgery.

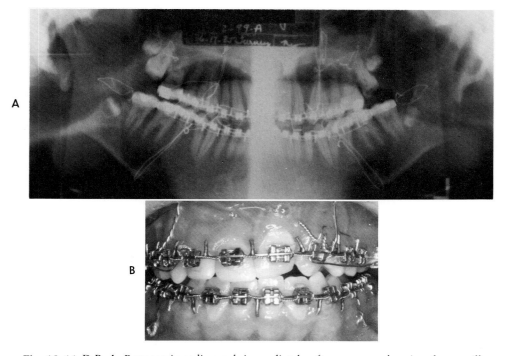

Fig. 18-44. D.P. **A,** Panoramic radiograph immediately after surgery, showing the maxillary and mandibular skeletal suspension wires. **B,** Occlusal relationships at the time of splint removal, just before removing the stabilizing arch wires. Note that the maxillary and circummandibular suspension wires are still in place. These will be removed by the surgeon.

Continued.

Case 4—cont'd.

As he settled into occlusion, an anterior crossbite tendency appeared. Cooperation with elastics waned rapidly. Appliances were removed after 11 months with good but not perfect occlusion (Fig. 18-46) and an excellent improvement in facial esthetics (Fig. 18-47). Three years later, despite some continuing mandibular growth (Fig. 18-45, *B*) and early discontinuance of retainers, both occlusal relationships (Fig. 18-48) and facial proportions (Fig. 18-49) had been maintained well.

Comments. Given this patient's prolonged and involved treatment, difficulties in cooperation with orthodontic elasics and removable appliances would have to be expected. It can be quite frustrating to apparently make progress with orthodontic treatment, only to lose much of the correction when a patient does not wear retainers, as happened in the first phase of treatment here, but that is a frequent occurrence in the treatment of cleft patients.

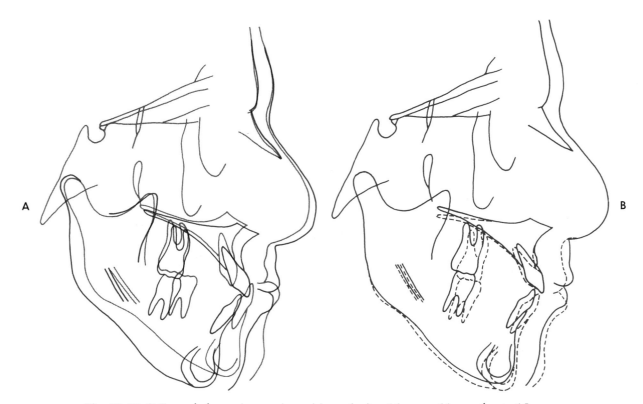

Fig. 18-45. D.P., cephalometric superimpositions. **A,** Age 14 years, 11 months, to 15 years, 11 months *(solid red),* showing the change at surgery. **B,** Age 15 years, 11 months, to 19 years, 2 months *(dashed red).* Note the late mandibular growth.

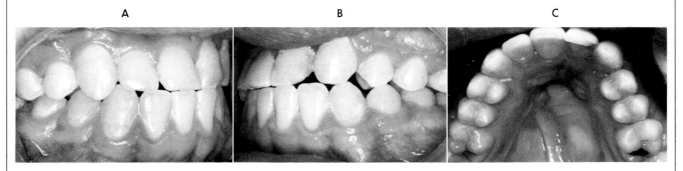

Fig. 18-46. D.P., dental relationships at age 16 years, 8 months, at the conclusion of orthodontic treatment.

Case 4—cont'd.

The choice of two-jaw surgery for this patient was influenced by three considerations: (1) the tightness of the repaired lip, which would limit the amount of maxillary advancement, (2) the need to improve vertical stability of the downgrafted maxilla: as we have discussed in Chapter 14, the current data show clearly that downward movements of the maxilla are more stable in pa-

tients who have two-jaw surgery than in those who have maxillary surgery alone, and (3) the patient's adequate velopharyngeal closure. Rather than advancing his maxilla the required amount, splitting the difference between maxillary advancement and mandibular setback minimized the risk of developing velopharyngeal inadequacy.

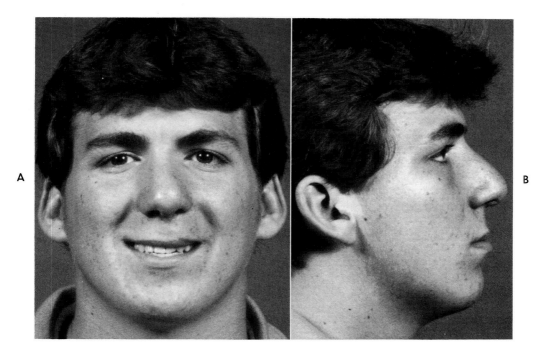

Fig. 18-47. D.P., age 16 years, 8 months, at the conclusion of treatment.

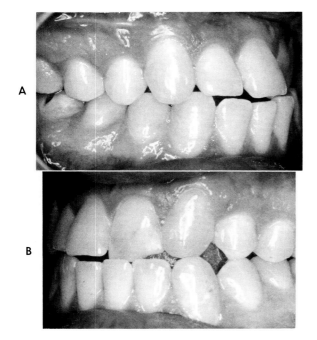

Fig. 18-48. D.P., dental relationships at age 19 years, 2 months, 2 years after retainers were discontinued.

Continued.

Case 4—cont'd.

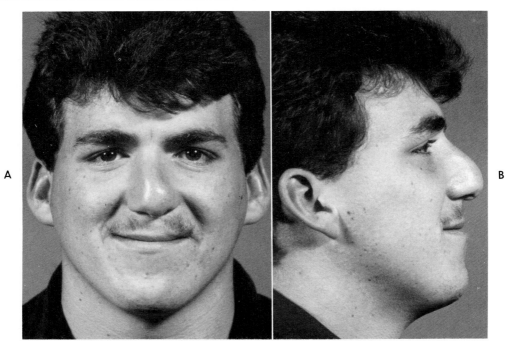

Fig. 18-49. D.P., age 19 years, 2 months.

REFERENCES

1. Burston WR: The early orthodontic treatment of cleft palate conditions, Dent Pract 9:41-56, 1958.
2. Hellquist R: Early maxillary orthopedics in relation to maxillary cleft repair by periosteoplasty, Cleft Palate J 8:36-55, 1971.
3. Friede H, Pruzansky S: Long-term effcts of premaxillary setback on facial skeletal profile in complete bilateral cleft lip and palate, Cleft Palate J 22:97-105, 1985.
4. Cooper HK, Long RE, Sr, Long RE, Jr, et al: Orthodontics and oral orthopedics. In Cooper WE, Harding RL, Krugman WH, et al (editors): Cleft palate and cleft lip: a team approach to clinical management and rehabilitation of the patient, Philadelphia, 1979, WB Saunders Co.
5. Hamilton R, Graham WP, Randall P: A lip adhesion operation in cleft lip surgery, Cleft Palate J 5:1-9, 1971.
6. Resiberg DJ, Figueroa AA, Gold HO: An intraoral appliance for management of the protrusive premaxilla in bilateral cleft lip, Cleft Palate J 25:53-57, 1988.
7. Millard DR: Cleft craft: the evolution of its surgery, Boston, 1980, Little, Brown & Co, Inc.
8. Riski JE, Millard RT: The processes of speech: evaluation and treatment. In Cooper WE, Harding RL, Krugman WH, et al (editors): Cleft palate and cleft lip: a team approach to clinical management and rehabilitation of the patient, Philadelphia, 1979, WB Saunders Co.

9. Mazaheri M, Harding RL, Nanda S: The effects of surgery on maxillary growth and cleft width, Plast Reconstr Surg 40:22-29, 1967.
10. Johnston MC, Ross RB: Cleft lip and palate, Baltimore, 1972, Williams & Wilkins.
11. Perko MA: Two-stage closure of cleft palate, J Maxillofac Surg 7:76-80, 1979.
12. Randall P, LaRossa D: Cleft palate. In McCarthy JG (editor): Plastic surgery, vol 4, Cleft lip and palate and craniofacial anomalies, New York, 1990, WB Saunders Co.
13. Witzel MA, Rich RH, Margar-Bacal F: Velopharyngeal insufficiency after adenoidectomy: an 8-year review, Int J Pediatr Otorhinolaryngol 11:15-20, 1986.
14. Rosenstein SW, Monroe CW, Kernahan DA: The case for early bone grafting in cleft lip and palate, Plast Reconstr Surg 3:297-309, 1982.
15. Lynch JB, Wisner HK, Evans RM, et al: Cephalometric study of maxillary growth five years after alveolar bone grafting of cleft palate infants, Plast Reconstr Surg 46:564-567, 1970.
16. Friede H, Johanson B: Primary early bone grafting in complete clefts of the lip and palate, Scand J Plast Reconstr Surg 8:79-87, 1974.
17. Johanson B, Ohlsson A, Friede A, Ahlgren J: A follow-up study of cleft lip and palate patients treated with orthodontics, secondary bone grafting and prosthetic rehabilitation, Scand J Plast Reconstr Surg 8:121-135, 1974.

18. Boyne PJ, Sands NR: Combined orthodontic-surgical management of residual alveolar cleft defects, Am J Orthod 70:20-37, 1976.

19. Bergland O, Semb G, Abyholm FE: Elimination of the residual alveolar cleft by secondary bone grafting and subsequent orthodontic treatment, Cleft Palate J 23:175-205, 1986.

20. Boyne PJ, Sands NR: Secondary bone grafting of residual alveolar and palatal defects, J Oral Surg 30:87-92, 1972.

21. Abyholm FE, Bergland O, Semb G: Secondary bone grafting of alveolar clefts, Scand J Plast Reconstr Surg 15:127-140, 1981.

22. Turvey TA, Vig K, Moriarty J, Hoke J: Delayed bone grafting in the cleft maxilla and palate: a retrospective multidisciplinary analysis, Am J Orthod 86:244-256, 1984.

23. Semb G: Effect of alveolar bone grafting on maxillary growth in unilateral cleft and palate patients, Cleft Palate J 25:288-295, 1988.

24. Turvey TA: Donor site for alveolar cleft bone grafts [letter], J Oral Maxillofac Surg 45:834,878, 1987.

25. Slaughter WB, Brodie AG: Facial clefts and their management in view of recent research, Plast Reconstr Surg 4:203-224, 1949.

26. Salyer KE: Primary correction of the unilateral cleft lip and nose: a 15-year experience, Plast Reconstr Surg 77:558-566, 1986.

27. Tschapp HM: The "open sky rhinoplasty" for correction of secondary cleft lip nose deformity: technique and recent results, Scand J Plast Reconstr Surg 22:153-158, 1988.

28. Jackson IT, Fasching MC: Secondary deformities of cleft lip, nose, and cleft palate. In McCarthy JG (editor): Plastic surgery, vol 4, Cleft lip and palate and craniofacial anomalies, Philadelphia, 1990, WB Saunders Co.

29. David JD, Bagnall AD: Velopharyngeal incompetence. In McCarthy JG (editor): Plastic surgery, vol 4, Cleft lip and palate and craniofacial anomalies, Philadelphia, 1990, WB Saunders Co.

CHAPTER 19

Temporomandibular Dysfunction: Considerations in the Surgical-Orthodontic Patient

Myron R. Tucker
William R. Proffit

Pain and dysfunction related to mandibular function and the temporomandibular (TM) joint, often referred to as the *TMJ syndrome,* have received increased emphasis recently. Reports of research findings, continuing education courses, and greater emphasis at the undergraduate and graduate levels in dental schools have played a major role in professional awareness of these problems. Widespread media exposure has increased the public's awareness, which also has resulted in more potential patients presenting for evaluation of pain or dysfunction related to the TM joint or muscles of mastication. Even if there were no relationship between dentofacial deformity and TM joint dysfunction, orthodontists and surgeons evaluating and treating these patients would see an increase in TM joint complaints. With many dentists convinced that malocclusion is a major cause of pain and dysfunction, it is not surprising that TM joint signs and symptoms are a major reason for the referral of a significant number of surgical-orthodontic patients. In addition, the possibility exists that surgical and/or orthodontic treatment can be related to the development of TM joint or muscular problems where none existed previously.

The goals of this chapter are to review the relationships between malocclusion and TM joint dysfunction; discuss diagnosis, treatment planning, and treatment of patients who have both a dentofacial deformity and TM joint problems; and describe the interaction between dentofacial treatment procedures and muscle/TM joint adaptations. The focus is on TM joint considerations in the treatment of patients with developmental problems, not on treatment of TM joint pain/dysfunction per se, but the guidelines for treating pain/dysfunction are remarkably similar whether or not a dentofacial deformity also is involved.

THE RELATIONSHIP BETWEEN TM JOINT PROBLEMS AND DENTOFACIAL DEFORMITY
What Constitutes Temporomandibular Dysfunction?

Patients presenting for orthodontic-surgical treatment may have a history of occasional signs or symptoms related to TM joint dysfunction or pain. One of the problems currently facing practitioners is the lack of consensus as to what actually constitutes a pathologic condition of either the TM joints or muscles of mastication.

The presence of signs or symptoms does not necessarily mean that the patient has a problem requiring treatment. In Agerberg and Carlsson's classic study[1] of Swedish people, half of all subjects examined between the ages of 15 and 44 had at least one clinical sign or symptom related to TM joint dysfunction. A third had at least two signs or symptoms. Other surveys of normal populations report the prevalence of at least some indicators of TM joint dysfunction to range from 28% to 86%.[2,3] The wide disparity is the result of disagreement about what signs and symptoms should be included. Helkimo's criteria[4] for evaluation of TM joint dysfunction, which includes limited range of motion, masticatory muscle pain, TM joint pain, crepitus or clicking of the TM joints, pain on jaw movement, and deviation on opening, are the best established and most widely used. Other studies, however, have included symptoms that may or may not be related to TM joint dysfunction, such as a variety of headache complaints[5] or even dental attrition.[6] Differences in evaluation techniques undoubtedly have contributed to the large discrepancies in the reported prevalence of TM joint problems.

It is generally accepted that symptoms of TM joint pain or dysfunction are less frequent in children than in older populations.[7,8] Williamson[9] reported the incidence of TM joint dysfunction to be as high as 35% in adolescent patients presenting for orthodontic treatment. The time at which clinical signs and symptoms begin to increase is not clear. In a 5-year longitudinal study of children who were age 8 to 11 initially, de Boever and van den Berghe[10] found no increase in clinical signs and symptoms. In an evaluation of a large group of children and adolescents, Riolo and colleagues[11] demonstrated increased signs and symptoms of TM joint dysfunction in older adolescents. By the late teens, it appears that the incidence of signs and symptoms in a nonpatient population is similar to adult populations.[12,13]

Interestingly, the prevalence of TM joint signs and symptoms does not increase steadily as the population ages. Instead, the prevalence peaks in the 25 to 40 years age group and decreases thereafter. These data make it clear that TM joint problems are not progressive in the usual sense of the word. It is unlikely that patients totally recover from internal-joint pathology, but many probably do adapt to disk displacement well enough to regain near-normal function. Problems due to muscle hyperactivity would be expected to subside if the patient ceased the causative activity over time, and that too seems to happen. Even so, the percentage of the population with TM joint signs and symptoms at all ages is impressively large.

It is clear that the number of patients who seek treatment because of complaints related to mandibular pain/dysfunction is much smaller than the number who are reported to have signs or symptoms, but the precise percentage is difficult to determine.[14] Gender and age are important variables in complaints. Females between the ages of 20 and 35 constitute a 3:1 majority of those who view their problem as severe enough to need treatment. Why treatment need is so much greater in this segment of the population remains a mystery.

What Causes TM Joint Pain/Dysfunction?

The most common causes of masticatory pain, limitation of opening, and other mandibular dysfunctions include (in the probable order of importance) myofascial pain related to muscle hyperactivity, disk displacements that may or may not be reducible, degenerative joint disease (arthrosis, osteoarthritis), and traumtic injuries to the joint. Less frequently, systemic arthritic conditions such as rheumatoid or lupus arthritis, hyperplastic or neoplastic processes of the mandibular condyle, and infections of the TM joint may be involved (Table 19-1).

Muscular pain is often widely distributed over the muscles of mastication. It arises from spasm due to hyperactivity in these muscles. This is the most common cause of TM joint pain/dysfunction. The muscle hyperactivity, in turn, is most often due to nocturnal or daytime bruxism or to pernicious habits in posturing the jaw. Constantly posturing the jaw forward to conceal mandibular deficiency can produce muscle symptoms. Clenching or grinding the teeth is exacerbated by stress,[15,16] which explains why stress is so frequently related to TM joint problems.

Disk displacement, the second most common cause of TM joint problems, leads to pain because of inflammation in the capsule, disk, or retrodiskal area. Trauma to the joint often is the precipiting factor in disk displacement problems. One of the great difficulties in establishing the etiology of TM joint pain/dysfunction is that muscle pain, though usually due to hyperactivity, also can be related to disk displacement

TABLE 19-1 Causes of TM joint pain/dysfunction

Cause	Comment
Muscle spasm/limitation	From hyperactivity (clenching, grinding, posturing jaw) and stress-related; also seen secondarily in patients with other problems listed below, complicating diagnosis
Disk displacement	Allowed by stretching or tearing of posterior ligaments, often initially produced by trauma; ? sometimes produced by hyperactivity
Degenerative joint diseases (e.g., osteoarthritis)	Older patients primarily; can be quite advanced with minimal symptoms
Systemic arthritis (e.g., rheumatoid, lupus)	Rarely affects TM joint alone; involvement of other joints, laboratory tests are diagnostic
Hyperplastic or neoplastic processes	Rare; distortion of facial form rather than pain/dysfunction usually is initial complaint

and internal-joint pathology. The joint itself may be painful, but muscle pain related to altered function often is superimposed on this—and of course there is nothing to prevent patients with joint derangement from also clenching or grinding their teeth. Symptoms related to muscle hyperactivity also are likely to be present in patients with degenerative disease or the other, rarer causes of internal-joint pathology, whose pain is primarily related to the bony degeneration. As a result, the best summary of etiology is to say that it is influenced by muscle function and the joint structures; for most patients, multiple factors are involved.

Relationship of Malocclusion to TM Joint Pain/Dysfunction

Malocclusion has frequently been cited as a cause or contributing factor in the occurrence of TM joint pain or dysfunction. This relationship, however, remains extremely controversial. The key questions would be whether malocclusion caused bruxing or clenching that could lead to muscle pain, whether problems would be more likely to arise if a patient with maloccclusion did clench or grind, and whether internal-joint pathology would be more likely to arise if malocclusion were present.

Summarizing the available data, Greene and Marbach[17] suggest that any relationship between malocclusion, morphology, and dysfunction is greatly exaggerated. They failed to document an increased percentage of Class II or III malocclusions among patients presenting for evaluation in two TM joint pain programs. Many reports document the lack of correlation between any type of malocclusion and TM joint dysfunction in children and adolescents.[10,18] The lack of a relationship between malocclusions and TM joint dysfunction symptoms has been documented in several other evaluations of adult populations.[19-21] Roberts

and colleagues[22] evaluated a large group of patients undergoing arthrography to evaluate internal-joint pathology but were unable to demonstrate a relationship between joint pathology and any type of occlusal pattern.

The increase in parafunctional habits associated with certain types of malocclusions also has been proposed as a mechanism for an increase in joint and muscle symptoms among patients with malocclusions. Clarke,[23] however, found no occlusal factors that appeared to contribute to myofascial pain/dysfunction or TM joint symptoms. Seligman and colleagues[24] showed no prevalence of any occlusal pattern among patients with dental attrition due to bruxism. They further found that signs of internal-joint pathology such as clicking and crepitus were not increased with any specific occlusal pattern.

Several studies, however, have indicated a positive relationship between some types of malocclusion and TM joint pain or dysfunction. In Seligman's previously cited study documenting no increased joint noise or attrition with any particular occlusal pattern, they did find that there was increased tenderness to palpation of the TM joints in the Class II, division 2 group.[24] Some other studies also have shown an association between Class II, division 2 malocclusion and joint or muscle signs and symptoms.[7,25] Mohlin and colleagues[26,27] reported increased mandibular dysfunction in patients with Angle Class III relationships, reverse overjets, and anterior open bite. In these and similar studies, correlation coefficients were statistically significant but small, never higher than 0.3-0.4.

Cadaver studies have frequently been cited as evidence of a positive relationship between malocclusions and abnormal joint morphology. Hansson and Oberg[28] documented increased intercapsular pathology in joints that they felt were more suspectible to increased bio-

	All initial	Had surgery	No surgery
Parameter	N = 1092	N = 237	N = 352
TM joint noises	22	23	23
TM joint/myofascial pain	12	15	13
History of trauma	8	9	5
Trauma plus TM joint symptoms	3	3	2

TABLE 19-2 Prevalence of TM joint problems (percent of sample)

Twelve percent with TM joint symptoms had history of trauma; 37% with history of trauma had TM joint symptoms.

mechanical loading as a result of malocclusions or loss of posterior support. Solberg and colleagues[29] found an increased deviation in the morphology of condyles in young adult specimens with increased anterior over-jet. There are problems with potential overinterpretation of this type of data. First, no history of symptoms or documentation of clinical signs is available to correlate with the postmortem findings. In addition, the abnormality or deviation in form found in some condyles may not represent pathology but merely normal adaptive changes that produce neither clinical signs nor symptoms of joint dysfunction. O'Ryan and Epker[30] suggested that morphologic differences in the structure of condyles may be associated with alterations in biomechanical loading. They presented several examples of morphologically different condyles that they felt represented the spectrum of normalcy rather than pathologic conditions.

Specific attention to the prevalence of muscular or joint pain and dysfunction in patients with facial skeletal abnormalities is generally lacking in the literature. Laskin and colleagues[31] surveyed oral and maxillofacial surgery training programs to determine the incidence of TM joint complaints in patients presenting for orthognathic surgery evaluation. This study was conducted by a questionnaire with little more than 50% response, and it is likely that the responses were not formulated from detailed record reviews, so the results must be viewed cautiously. For all the responding programs, the mean percent of patients presenting for orthognathic surgery evaluation who also had a TM joint complaint was 10%, but the range was from 0 to 75%. From a retrospective analysis, Upton and colleagues[32] reported that 53% of patients who underwent orthognathic surgery at the University of Michigan from 1978 to 1981 also had signs or symptoms of TM joint dysfunction. In a detailed review of over 1000 patients evaluated in the Dentofacial Clinic at the UNC, Proffit and coworkers[33] noted that TM joint signs or symptoms were found in approximately the same proportion as in the general population (Table 19-2). Two-

thirds of the total sample was female, but 88% of those with TM joint findings were female. Of those with a history of trauma that might have contributed to their jaw deformity, 37% had TM joint findings; 12% of those with TM joint findings had a history of potentially significant trauma to the jaws.

In summary, it appears that some types of malocclusion may slightly predispose patients to TM joint problems, but the relationship is weak enough to be questionable. The malocclusion types that have been indicated as potentially significant—Class II, division 2; Class III with anterior interference—seem to be those most likely to cause mandibular shifts on closure. There is no evidence that this triggers bruxism, but that outcome is possible. An obligatory shift on closure could increase muscle strain, lowering the threshold for hyperactivity. Whether this could lead to internal derangement of the joint remains unknown. In short, if there is a relationship between malocclusion and TM joint problems, the malocclusion probably makes it easier for a patient to hurt himself or herself while clenching or grinding. It is impossible to totally rule out the other mechanisms as well.

EVALUATION OF PATIENTS WITH TM JOINT AND DENTOFACIAL PROBLEMS

The diagnostic and treatment planning process for patients who have both severe malocclusion and TM joint pain/dysfunction follows the same general approach outlined in Chapter 4: a data base is developed from interviewing the patient, clinical examination, and evaluation of diagnostic records; the patient's problems are separated into pathologic and developmental components; and a treatment plan is established to produce maximum benefit to the patient, taking into consideration both the patient's chief complaint and the doctor's evaluation of the problem. For these patients, the process differs in two important ways: (1) additional diagnostic information is required, and (2) feedback from an initial phase of reversible treatment often is needed to develop the final treatment

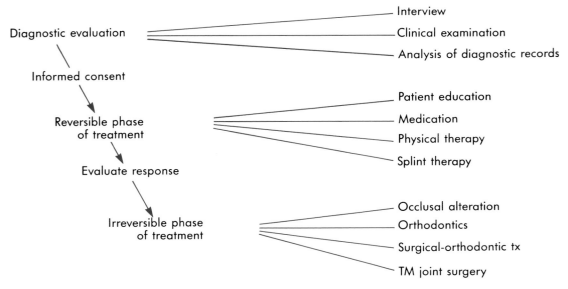

Fig. 19-1. Diagram of the process of evaluation and treatment sequencing for patients with TM joint disorders and dentofacial deformities.

plan. The process is outlined in Fig. 19-1. In the next section, we focus on the additional diagnostic information. The reversible treatment phase, which has both diagnostic and therapeutic goals, is discussed in the following section.

Interview Data

In addition to the chief complaint and the patient's desires and expectations, the historical progression of any TM joint pain or dysfunction should be investigated in detail. Important items in this history include the time of onset of symptoms; any traumatic or other etiologic events which may have contributed to the problem; the description of symptoms at the time of onset, including quality or type of pain or dysfunction, frequency, severity, and duration; and progression of symptoms since the time of onset. Any treatment which has been attempted, successfully or unsuccessfully, should be noted. Finally, detailed documentation of the current status of the symptoms and clinical signs known to the patient is necessary.

It is important to evaluate whether the patient's behavior is consistent with pain as a major life component. Whether the problem is chronic back pain, headaches, TM joint symptoms, or something else, chronic-pain patients frequently become dependent on the attention that they receive as a result of their complaints of pain and often use this attention to manipulate others with whom they interact.[34] The pain can become a necessary part of an individual's psychologic makeup so that he or she cannot afford to give it up.[33,35]

In order to gain insight into behavioral changes that may be associated with pain, an appropriate history should focus on these concerns. Important questions include any functional limitation that may result from the patient's pain or dysfunction, including modifications in occupation and social or recreational activity. If the functional limitation appears to be excessive when compared with the patient's physical findings or if the patient appears to be depressed, further psychologic evaluation may be warranted.[36] Tests to gain insight into the patient's perception of his or her problem may be helpful at this stage,[37] but for patients who are thought to have psychologic problems, there is no substitute for an interview by a well-trained examiner.

Triage by Chief Complaint

When patients present for any type of treatment, it is important to determine their chief complaint and their goals for anticipated treatment. In no group of patients is this more critical than in those who present with both a dentofacial deformity and TM joint dysfunction. They can be quickly divided into two separate groups who require different approaches.

The first group are those who present with a primary concern of malocclusion or dentofacial deformity and have as a secondary concern signs or symptoms of TM joint dysfunction. These patients usually have dentofacial esthetics or dental function as a primary concern. Even if they are experiencing pain, they place less emphasis on dysfunction than on other aspects of their problem. They frequently elect to undergo orthodontic and surgical treatment knowing that this may not affect their TM joint signs or symptoms.

The second group are those who are primarily concerned with TM joint pain or dysfunction and regard

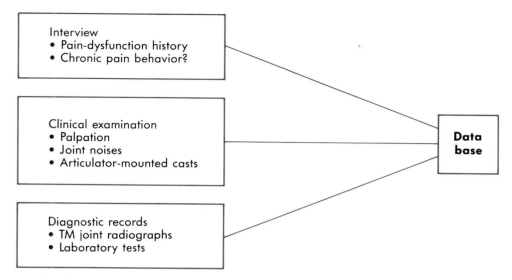

Fig. 19-2. Phases of data collection for diagnosis of TM joint pain and dysfunction.

their malocclusion or dentofacial deformity as a potential cause or contributing factor. They often state that their main reason for consulting an orthodontist and/or surgeon regarding correction of their malocclusion is to improve or eliminate their pain or dysfunction. These patients frequently exhibit the psychologic or behavioral characteristics associated with chronic pain and dysfunction. They often pursue orthodontic and surgical treatment in the hope that this finally will be the solution to their pain problem, only to be extremely disappointed.

The diagnostic evaluation for both groups of patients must thoroughly cover both the TM joint problems and dentofacial deformity, but gathering further diagnostic information during an initial phase of conservative and reversible TM joint therapy is particularly important for the second group. When chronic-pain behavior is suspected, additional interview data from psychologic interviews and/or testing (see below) may be required.

Clinical Evaluation

In addition to the detailed facial and intraoral examination that would be carried out for any dentofacial patient, a patient who has TM joint problems also requires clinical evaluation of that aspect (Fig. 19-2). The information needed for these patients goes beyond the minimum TM joint examination recommended for all patients (see Chapter 4).

Clinical Examination

The clinical examination for patients with TM joint symptoms should include palpation of the upper cervical muscles, muscles of mastication, and TM joints. This palpation should attempt to elicit tenderness to

manipulation of the muscles, as well as their texture or tone. The TM joints should be palpated laterally and posteriorly through the external auditory meatus, in both the static position and during function. This palpation should attempt to elicit pain to slight digital pressure and should evaluate joint signs of clicking or crepitus. The degree of condylar translation can also be evaluated by palpation.

The occurrence of clicking or crepitus should be noted, and the location in the opening cycle or millimeters of opening and closing at which these occur should be recorded. A stethoscope or other instrumentation such as an electric sound amplification device (i.e, doppler) can help the clinician detect joint noise—but at the risk of detecting noises from outside the TM joint and recording false positives that do not necessarily document joint pathology.

One of the most important aspects of the examination is the evaluation of functional movements. This should include recording both the maximum interincisal opening that occurs voluntarily and the maximum opening that can be produced with gentle stretching by the examiner. The presence of deviation or pain on opening should also be noted. Protrusion and left and right lateral excursions should also be recorded. A concise form for recording the pertinent information is shown on page 666.

Articulator Mounted Casts

Some controversy exists regarding the need for articulator mountings and the need for centric occlusion and centric relation bite registrations. As a general guideline, these are more helpful in planning treatment than in diagnosis—but feedback from the initial reversible therapy phase, which usually requires articula-

---

TM Joint Evaluation Form

Name _____   Chart no. _____

Age _____   Date _____   Sex _____

History

Primary complaint: Pain _____   Dysfunction _____   Malocclusion _____
    Duration _____
    Events associated with onset _____
    _____

    Characteristics and frequency of pain _____
    _____

    Changes in lifestyle (occupational, recreational, social)   Yes _____ No _____

Exam

Muscular Pain on Palpation (+,−)	R	L
Sternocleidomastoid	___	___
Masseter	___	___
Med. pterygoid	___	___
Trapezius	___	___
Temporalis	___	___
Lat. pterygoid	___	___

TM Joint Pain on Palpation (+,−)	R	L
Lateral—static	___	___
—motion	___	___
Posteriorly—static	___	___
—motion	___	___

Function

Max. voluntary opening _____ Dev. _____ Pain _____
Max. forced opening _____ Dev. _____ Pain _____
Protrusion _____ L lat. _____ R lat. _____
R click Open _____ Close _____ Crepitus _____
L click Open _____ Close _____ Crepitus _____
TM joint radiographs—interpretation _____
_____

Working DX _____

---

tor-mounted casts, often is an important element in the final diagnosis. For most of these dentofacial/TM joint patients, mounted casts eventually will be needed.

Assuming that an accurate centric relation bite registration can be taken and reproduced on articulated mounted models, these can be particularly helpful in determining the presence of occlusal interferences and the effect on condylar position when the patient functions into a centric occlusion position. Modification of these occlusal relationships with techniques such as splint construction, prosthetic reconstruction, orthodontics, or surgery can be documented and followed in an accurate manner with articulated mounted casts.[38] Mounted casts may also be helpful in following progressive occlusal changes that may take place with active condylar remodeling in the disease processes of degenerative joint disease (osteoarthritis) and rheumatoid arthritis.

Because most surgical planning is done from the "centric relation" position, this is obviously an impor-tant part of the presurgical planning phase. In patients with TM joint pain and dysfunction, the centric occlusion position should also be documented, and the presence of gross centric relation/centric occlusion discrepancies and working and balancing interferences should be recorded. For surgical planning, occlusal relationships at the end of the reversible treatment phase, not the beginning, will be most useful.

Evaluation of Diagnostic Records
Radiographic Evaluation

The radiographic evaluation of a patient with TM joint dysfunction and dentofacial deformity should be based on the patient's signs and symptoms rather than on routine orders for a set of radiographs. With TM joint films, as with any radiographs, the amount of radiation required to obtain a given view must be balanced against the importance of the information that might be gained. Cephalometric and panoramic radiographs are generally required as a portion of the dent-

TABLE 19-3 Relative radiation exposure

Radiograph	Approximate exposure*	Comment
Panoramic	13 mR	Rare earth screens
Lateral cepalometric	18 mR	Rare earth screens/filters
Standard periapical series	350 mR	For comparison—absence of intensifying screens greatly increases exposure
Transcranial		
Standard (long cone)	150 mR	Headholder increases image quality at the cost of greatly increased radiation
Head holder (Accurad)	990 mR	
Laminogram (tomogram)		
No grid	300 mR	Varies considerably with equipment; compare with standard cephalometric exposure
Grid	150 mR	
Computerized tomography (CT) scan	7000 mR	Very approximate, varies with duration of study, movement, etc.

*To maximally exposed area.

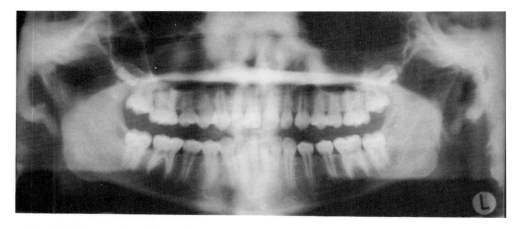

Fig. 19-3. Panoramic radiograph showing degenerative changes of the left TM joint. Resorption with flattening of the condylar head is apparent.

ofacial deformity evaluation. As Table 19-3 shows, with modern intensifying screens and film, the amount of radiation for either of these views is remarkably small. The radiation dosage of other views is much greater. In many cases, the panoramic film serves quite satisfactorily as the only radiograph necessary to evaluate the TM joints (Fig. 19-3). Additional radiographs are needed only if the TM joints are not adequately visualized or if pathology is suspected that would not be apparent on the panoramic radiograph (e.g., soft-tissue abnormalities such as disk displacements or perforations).

Transcranial radiographs can be produced with routine dental radiographic equipment and can be repro-

duced to a reasonable degree when a headholder device is used to position the patient (Fig. 19-4). Although this projection will not allow detailed examination of the medial surfaces of the condyle, excellent evaluation of the lateral poles can be accomplished when proper radiographic technique is used. Because a majority of TM joint pathology may involve the lateral pole, this technique can be helpful in diagnosing internal-joint pathology[39] (Fig. 19-5). Due to the limitations of this technique, some internal pathology may be missed. One report states that only 78% of morphologic abnormalities occurring in the TM joint can be visualized on transcranial radiographs.[40]

The radiation exposure of transcranial compared

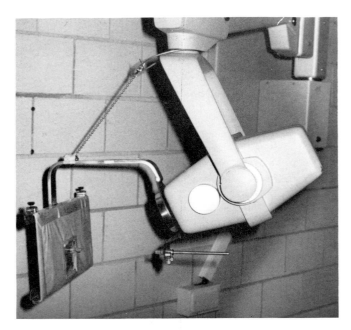

Fig. 19-4. Headholder used to reproduce transcranial radiographic projections.

with panoramic films (see Table 19-3) makes it difficult to justify their use for routine screening, and they have significant limitations as supplements to panoramic views. As a general rule, if a panoramic film is inadequate, a transcranial view also may not be satisfactory.

Tomographic evaluation allows for a more detailed view of the TM joint[41] (Fig. 19-6). Because the technique focuses on different levels of the condyle, the entire condyle can be visualized from the medial to the lateral pole (Fig. 19-7). The equipment available for this type of examination is becoming less expensive and more available for office use. Tomographic capabilities are currently being incorporated in cephalometric radiographic machines such that a cephalometric laminogram or tomographic view of the TM joint can be produced with the patient oriented similar to the position used for obtaining cephalometric radiographs. The tomographic evaluation can then be completed at the same time using the same occlusal position that is used for cephalometric evaluation—but additional radiation exposure still is involved, and these radiographs should be made only if specifically indicated.

The primary indications for tomography are suspected degenerative changes not visualized in the panoramic film and possibly more accurate assessment of position of the condyle within the fossa (this can only be predictably reproduced when done using a machine that can exactly reproduce the patient's head position). Condyle position can be assessed serially to evaluate the effects of treatment to change occlusal relationships (prosthodontic, orthodontic, or surgical-orthodontic).

Arthrotomography involves the injection of dye into the inferior or inferior and superior joint space. This allows indirect visualization of the disk tissue[42,43] (Fig. 19-8). Although proponents of more advanced radiographic techniques have advocated the use of computerized tomography (CT) or magnetic resonance imaging (MRI) for visualization of disk tissue, many consider the arthrotomogram to be the "gold standard"

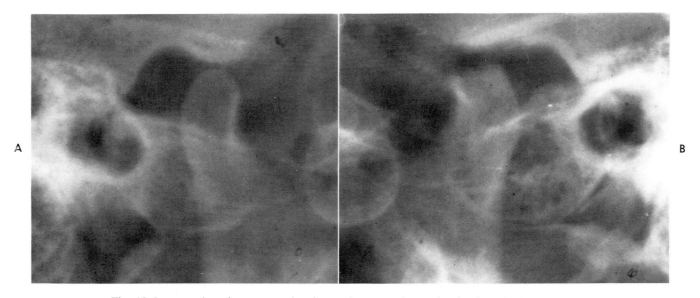

Fig. 19-5. Examples of transcranial radiographs. **A,** Radiograph of right side shows normal anatomy of the fossa and condyle. **B,** Left side view demonstrates degenerative changes of the condyle.

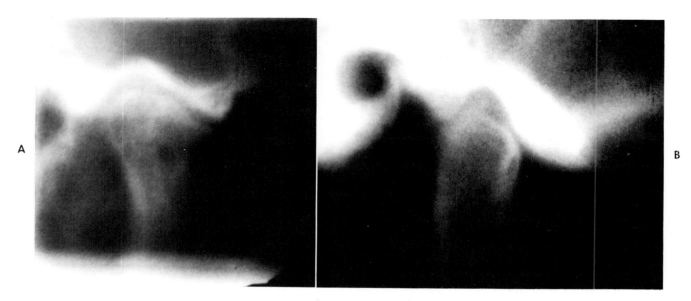

Fig. 19-6. Tomographic projections of TM joints. **A,** Typical degenerative changes with loss of a well-defined joint space, absence of cortical outline of the condylar head, and anterior condylar lipping. **B,** Ankylosis with bony-fibrous fusion in the posterior aspect of the condyle and fossa.

for evaluation of intraarticular soft-tissue pathology. This type of study should be obtained only after routine radiographic evaluation of the joint has been completed.

Following injection of dye into the inferior joint space, the anatomic relationships of the condyle and disk can be studied in a dynamic fashion under fluoroscopy. Static radiographic images can then be taken using either a transcranial or a tomographic approach to document anatomic relationships at specific points in the functional cycle. By knowing the pattern of dye associated with internal disk displacements, several pathologic problems can be identified, including anterior disk displacement with or without reduction, perforation, or adhesions.

Arthrotomography was the key to an improved understanding of disk displacement problems. Although it can be used to document disk position abnormalities and to assist in construction of an anterior repositioning splint by verifying that the disk is in the appropriate position, this information now can be obtained more directly. The primary indication at present for ar-

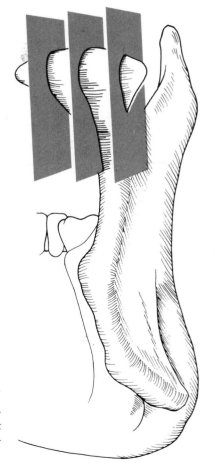

Fig. 19-7. Tomographic evaluation allows radiographic "slicing" of the condyle. Focusing of the radiographic image at different levels of the condyle allows for sequential examination of different areas of the TM joint.

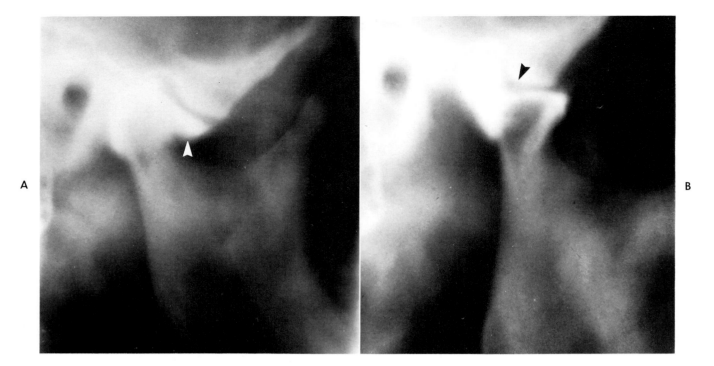

Fig. 19-8. Example of arthrotomogram showing anterior disk displacement with reduction. **A,** Closed position with accumulation of dye anteriorly *(arrow).* **B,** In the open position with the disk properly reduced, the posterior band of the disk can now be indirectly visualized in the proper position *(arrow).*

throtomography is for presurgical planning when joint surgery is required.

CT utilizes the advantages of both tomographic technique and computer enhancement to produce images of hard and soft tissue within the TM joint[44] (Fig. 19-9). This technique can be extremely useful for evaluating a wide variety of hard- and soft-tissue pathologies in the TM joint.[45] CT images of the bony structures within the TM joint provide the best accuracy in evaluating bony morphology. Using CT scan reconstruction capabilities, images can be obtained in one plane of space (i.e., axial) and reconstructed so that the images can be viewed from another plane (i.e., sagittal). This allows multiple detailed evaluations of the TM joint with a single radiation exposure.

One of the most important uses of CT scanning is the direct evaluation of bony and soft-tissue relationships within the joint. CT images allow for visualization of disk tissue and a determination of disk position in relation to the condyle and fossa. Although dynamic studies are not readily available using CT scanning, multiple still images can be obtained to assess joint function.

Indications for CT scanning are a need for detailed visualization of bony architecture, including reconstructed views in planes not obtainable with routine radiographic techniques; and images of disk-condyle re-

lationships. In many applications, CT scans now can replace arthrotomograms.

The most recent advance in imaging techniques for TM joints is the use of MRI.[46,47] Although MRI provides less distinct images of bone morphology than do radiographic techniques, the excellent images of intraarticular soft tissue makes it extremely desirable for visualizing disk position in many cases (Fig. 19-10). The fact that this technique does not use ionizing radiation is also an advantage. The disadvantages include the length of time necessary to produce the images and the claustrophobia that some patients encounter during this evaluation procedure. The significant expense of these studies is also a relative disadvantage.

The indication for MRI is a need for detailed views of disk position in the TM joint. When available, it replaces arthrotomography in most circumstances.

Nuclear imaging of the TM joint has somewhat limited applications but may be extremely useful in certain cases. Typically, this is done by injection of ^{99}Tc, a gamma-emitting isotope that is strongly concentrated in areas of active bone metabolism. Images then are obtained with a gamma camera some hours later. Single photon emission computerized tomography (SPECT) can be used to determine if active areas of bone metabolism are present.[48,49] This may help document the presence of condylar degeneration or hyperplastic growth

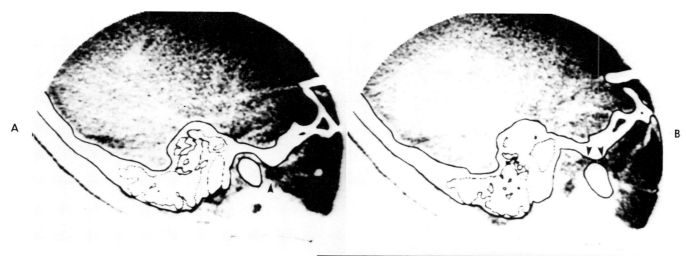

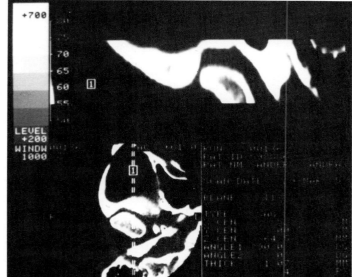

Fig. 19-9. CTs of the TM joint. **A,** Sigma mode for soft-tissue enhancement showing anterior disk displacement *(arrow).* **B,** Disk reduced after maximum opening *(arrows).* **C,** Sagittal reconstruction produced from axial images. The sagittal reconstruction is from the area indicated by the dotted lines on the axial view.

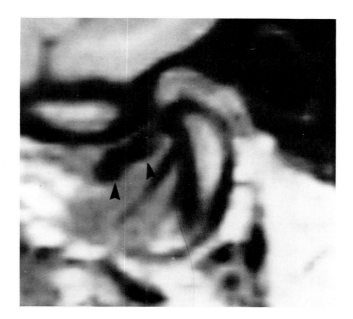

Fig. 19-10. MRI clearly demonstrating anterior disk displacement. The anterior and posterior bands of the disk are identified by the arrows.

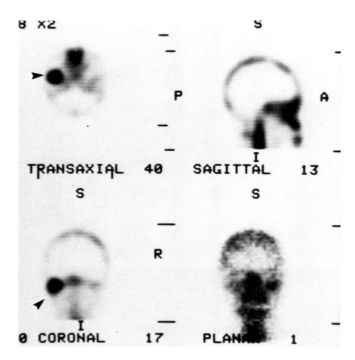

Fig. 19-11. Single photon emission CT. The area of increased activity is apparent in the TM joints *(arrow)*.

(Fig. 19-11). Although this technique is extremely sensitive, the nonspecific information obtained from this technique (there is no way to differentiate regeneration from degeneration) must be weighed cautiously in combination with clinical findings. In cases where degenerative disease within the joint has occurred, resulting in a malocclusion, it may be useful to obtain a SPECT scan to determine whether or not this process is ongoing or has ceased.

Indications for bone scanning are to evaluate bony hyperplasias or growth abnormalities to determine if bone activity (i.e., growth or proliferation) is continuing and, in cases of degenerative processes, to document continuing bone activity, which may include resorption, remodeling, or repair. In both cases, the information is important in deciding whether surgical treatment will have to involve reconstruction of the TM joint. Indications for the use of various radiographic techniques are summarized in Table 19-4.

Laboratory Evaluation

Laboratory evaluation may be important in cases where systemic illnesses are suspected of contributing to TM joint pain or dysfunction (i.e., systemic arthritis

---

TABLE 19-4 TM joint visualization: indications

View	Indicators	Comment
Panoramic radiograph	Routine screening	Adequate in the absence of specific indications for other views
Transcranial radiograph	Suspected degenerative changes (?)	Problems with image clarity are frequent; at best shows lateral pole only; rarely diagnostic by itself if panoramic film was not
	Evaluate movement (?)	Open/closed views show movement but the amount of change is of limited diagnostic value
Laminogram (tomogram)	Suspected degenerative changes	Gives clear views of bony anatomy if multiple cuts are used
	Assessment of condyle	Limited diagnostic value; can be assessed serially to evaluate treatment response
Arthrotomography	Indirect visualization of the articular disk, verifying displacement	Invasive; primarily for presurgical planning after other testing completed
Computed tomography (CT) scan	Evaluate hard- and soft-tissue pathology	Best accuracy for hard-tissue morphology; can directly visualize disk
Magnetic resonance imaging (MRI)	Detailed views of disk position	Best accuracy for soft tissue (disk); no radiation
Single photon emission computed tomography (SPECT)	Document bony metabolic activity, primarily in degenerative processes	Nonspecific; cannot distinguish degeneration from regeneration
Scintigraphy (isotope uptake)	Document bony metabolic activity, primarily in hyperplasia/neoplasia	False negative rare but false positive possible

may be involved). When rhematoid arthritis is suspected, laboratory information such as sedimentation rates and the presence or absence of rhematoid factors and antinuclear antibodies may be of value in confirming a diagnosis. Other systemic diseases such as lupus erythematosus, which may produce lupus arthritis of the TM joint, can be confirmed through laboratory analysis.

Principles in Planning Combined TM Joint and Surgical-Orthodontic Treatment

Treatment planning for patients with severe malocclusion and TM joint pain/dysfunction is unusual in the context of dentofacial deformity more generally in that the response to an initial phase of treatment often is incorporated into the diagnostic data base and used in the final treatment planning. Such an application of "therapeutic diagnosis" is by no means unique in the treatment of severe malocclusion and so is quite familiar to orthodontists. The response of a growing child to various treatment procedures often becomes part of the decision to continue with conservative (growth modification, nonextraction) treatment or to proceed to more aggressive procedures (extraction, orthognathic surgery).[50] The general scheme for patients with combined dentofacial and TM joint problems is outlined in Fig. 19-12.

The importance of an initial triage of patients by chief complaint has already been discussed above. Treatment planning for the TM joint problems can be further aided by separating two subgroups of patients, those whose pain/dysfunction is primarily related to muscular problems and those who have internal-joint pathology. The flow of treatment through a reversible to an irreversible phase will be similar for the two subgroups, but the details will differ.

For both groups of patients, treatment should begin with a phase of reversible treatment aimed at reducing TM joint symptoms and confirming the diagnosis. In many cases, the cause of the pain or dysfunction can be easily elicited, which allows a projection of the long-term course and prognosis. In addition, in those patients whose primary concern is pain or dysfunction symptoms, the reversible phase may be used to evaluate the effects of altered occlusal relationships on pain and dysfunction symptoms. For these patients, irreversible treatment such as permanent occlusal alteration (prosthodontics, orthodontics, orthognathic surgery) or TM joint procedures (arthroscopy, open surgery) should be carried out only when reversible treatment confirms the diagnosis and indicates that definitive treatment will result in a reduction in the patients' pain or dysfunction symptoms. If reversible treatment to change occlusal relationships does not reduce symptoms, further aggressive treatment probably will not either. In that circumstance, irreversible treatment should

be pursued only if the patient understands that symptoms are likely to persist even after occlusal and skeletal relationships are improved. Consent to pursue treatment in spite of this information should be recorded.

REVERSIBLE TREATMENT PHASE

Once a patient who has a combination of dentofacial deformity and TM joint dysfunction has given informed consent after a detailed discussion of his or her problems (see Chapter 6), initial reversible treatment can begin. The goals of this treatment phase are to gain further diagnostic information and minimize or alleviate the pain/dysfunction symptoms. A major objective is to clarify whether the malocclusion/skeletal deformity has any relationship to the pain/dysfunction complaints, either through direct cause and effect or as a secondary aggravating factor. The initial treatment phase should consist of patient education, medication, physical therapy, and splint therapy.

Patient Education

Patients who are made aware of causative factors can participate in their own improvement. Myofascial pain often is related to a parafunctional habit or muscle hyperactivity secondary to stress. Making patients aware of this often motivates them to control the activity reducing the discomfort or dysfunction. Feedback devices to remind the patient about harmful activity can help. For instance, the output from surface electrodes over the masseter or temporalis muscles can be used to indicate clenching or grinding during daytime activity.[51] The use of electromyographic (EMG) recordings for patient evaluation in monitoring treatment progress is well documented. Solberg and colleagues[52] demonstrated the value of EMG recordings in evaluating nocturnal bruxism and associated pain and used this method to show the effectiveness of splint therapy and medication during times of muscle hyperactivity. Other forms of stress control—physical exercise, reducing exposure to highly stressful situations—also can be explored. Once the patient is aware of the relationship between their own actions and the pain/dysfunction symptoms, behavior modification can follow.

In some instances, knowing the prognosis can help considerably. Pain/dysfunction problems of all types often stabilize or improve, but some patients, particularly the most anxious ones, are concerned that things will get inexorably worse. It is reassuring to know that muscle pain usually improves and that even though symptoms may recur on occasion, they can be controlled in the future as well. This is true in many degenerative situations as well. An example would be pain associated with early degenerative joint disease, but with relatively little dysfunction. Explaining that the long-term outcome of this problem is likely to be that the pain or dysfunction will eventually subside, allow-

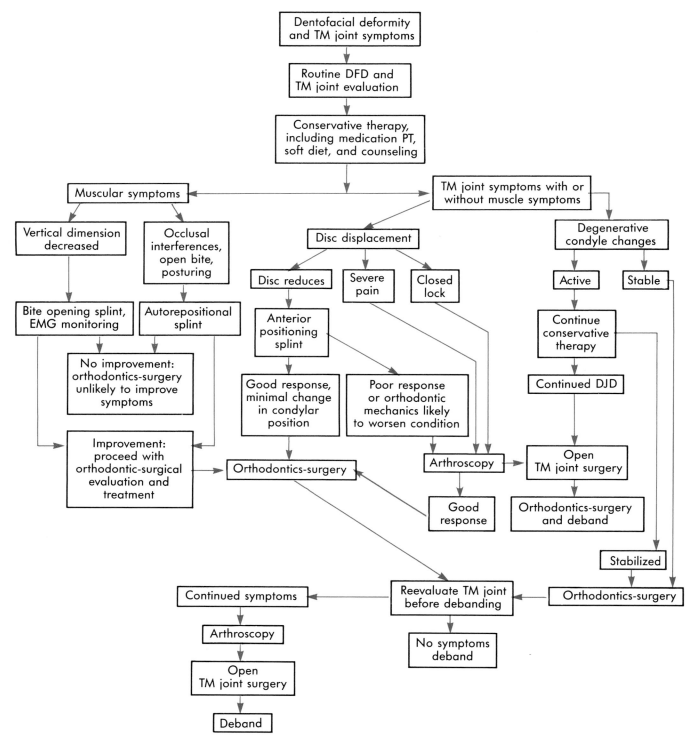

Fig. 19-12. Flow diagram for sequential treatment integrating reversible treatment for TM joint disorders, TM joint surgery, and surgical-orthodontic correction of TM joint deformities. (Adapted from Tucker MR, Thomas PM: Temporomandibular pain and dysfunction in the orthodontic surgical patient: rationale for evaluation of treatment sequencing, Int J Adult Orthod Orthognath Surg 1:11-22, 1986.)

ing function without pain, can help such patients tolerate the present situation and may convince them that no treatment is necessary now. The signs of further deterioration, so that the patient could detect any need for future treatment, should be emphasized in the educational process.

The appropriate modification of diet and home exercises are also an important part of the patient education phase. Patients who are experiencing TM joint or muscle pain frequently find that this is most apparent while chewing hard food. Temporary alteration of the diet to include only soft foods often will provide significant improvement in symptoms. This can begin with a "nonchew" diet made up of items such as blenderized food, mashed potatoes, and soup that the patient could swallow with little if any chewing. A gradual progression to a more normal diet over 3 to 6 weeks may be sufficient to reduce TM joint or muscular symptoms.

While the patient is attempting to reduce the functional load placed on the joint and muscles of mastication, some efforts should be made to maintain a normal range of motion. Home exercises may be helpful in maintaining normal function. This includes gentle stretching exercises (done only to pain tolerance) with either passive jaw opening or active finger pressure. Monitoring the amount of maximum incisal opening provides the patient with immediate feedback regarding maintenance and improvement of jaw function.

Medication

For patients who are experiencing significant muscle and joint discomfort, both acute and chronic medical management is generally appropriate. Three types of medications generally are useful: analgesics of various sorts, nonsteroidal antiinflammatory drugs, and muscle relaxants.

Analgesic medication for these patients may range from acetaminophen or aspirin to potent narcotics. An important principle of treatment for all pain/dysfunction patients is that the problem may become chronic, so medication that could produce long-term addiction should be avoided if at all possible. Due to the sedative and depressive action of narcotics as well as their potential for addiction, narcotics should be restricted to short-term use in patients with severe acute pain. In that instance, medication such as acetaminophen (Tylenol) with codeine is sufficient. This should not be used for longer than 10 days to 2 weeks.

Fortunately, the second group of medications, nonsteroidal antiinflammatory drugs (NSAIDs), not only reduce inflammation but also serve as excellent analgesics. Some examples of NSAIDs are ibuprofen (Motrin), diflunisal (Dolobid), naproxen (Naprosyn), and piroxicam (Feldene). These can be effective in reducing long-standing inflammation in both muscles and joints, and in most cases they also provide satisfactory pain relief. Because these drugs are not associated with severe addiction problems, use of this type of medication is strongly preferred over opioid drugs. One important fact regarding NSAIDs is that they work best when administered on a timetable rather than a pain-dependent schedule. Initially, patients should be instructed to take the medicine on a regular basis to obtain an adequate blood level, which should then be maintained for 10 to 14 days. Discontinuation or tapering of the medicine can then be attempted.

The final group of medications, muscle relaxants, generally have a significant potential for depression as well as sedation and again should be avoided if possible. In patients with acute pain or exacerbations of muscle hyperactivity, muscle relaxants for short periods such as 10 days to 2 weeks may be acceptable. The lowest effective dose should be used. Generally, diazepam (Valium), 2 to 5 mg, or cyclobenzaprine (Flexeril), 10 mg, is sufficient.

Physical Therapy

Several physical therapy modalities can be extremely helpful in the evaluation and treatment of the TM joint pain/dysfunction patient. The most common are EMG biofeedback and relaxation training, ultrasound, spray and stretch, and friction massage. All assist in controlling pain and in reducing limitation of jaw function.

Relaxation training, though perhaps not physical therapy in the strictest sense, can be very effective in reducing symptoms due to muscle hyperactivity. In essence, the patient needs to find out what he or she is doing to cause the problem—typically, clenching or grinding the teeth—and then stop doing it. Because the muscle hyperactivity so often occurs in response to stress, or at least is exacerbated by it, stress control becomes an important part of the therapy.

EMG monitoring of the patient's muscle activity can be used as an effective teaching tool in relaxation training therapy. An instant "feedback" of the muscle activity is used to develop effective methods to reduce muscle hyperactivity and the associated muscle pain.

Physical therapy also can relieve pain and improve function more directly by altering blood flow, relieving muscle spasm, and breaking up fibrous adhesions within the muscles. The primary advantage of ultrasound is that the ultrasonic waves can produce tissue heating, and thereby alter blood flow and metabolic activity, at a level deeper than that provided by simple surface moist-heat applications.[53] The postulated effects of ultrasound include increase in tissue temperature, increase in circulation, increase in uptake of pain-producing metabolic byproducts, and disruption of collagen crosslinking, all of which may result in more comfortable manipulation of muscles in a wider range of motion. In addition, intraarticular inflammation may also be reduced with ultrasound applications. The

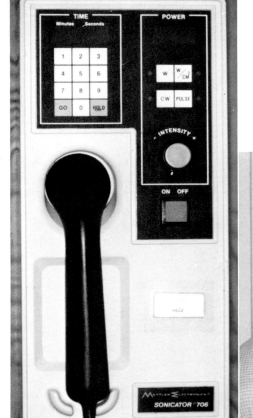

A

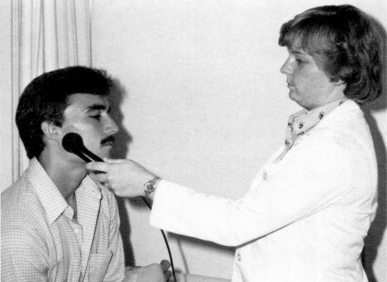

B

Fig. 19-13. **A,** Ultrasound unit for TM joint/facial pain physical therapy. **B,** Application of ultrasound to masseter muscle area.

normal routine for application of ultrasound is 0.7 to 1.0 watts/cm^2 applied for approximately 10 minutes (Fig. 19-13). The treatments are most effective when repeated every other day for several consecutive sessions.

Another technique that may be useful in improving range of motion is the use of a spray vapocoolant and simultaneous stretching of the muscles, "spray and stretch."[54] The theory behind spray and stretch is the concept that stimulating larger cutaneous nerve fibers can override pain input from smaller fibers that originate in the muscles and joints (i.e., the "gate control" theory of pain awareness). By spraying a cooling material such as fluoromethane over the lateral surface of the face, the muscles of mastication can be passively or actively stretched with a reduced level of pain input (Fig. 19-14).

Friction massage is a technique involving the application of firm cutaneous pressure, progressing to a degree where ischemia may temporarily occur. Travell[54] describes the use of friction massage, and the resulting ischemia and rebound hyperemia, as a method for inactivating trigger points or areas responsible for pain referred to muscles in the head and neck area. This technique may also be useful in disrupting small fibrous connective-tissue adhesions within the muscles.[55]

All of the above physical therapy modalities can be combined with range-of-motion exercises. These can be completed by or in the presence of the physical thera-

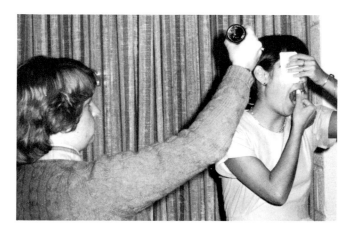

Fig. 19-14. Spray and stretch technique. A vapocoolant is applied while attempting to increase range of motion with active stretching.

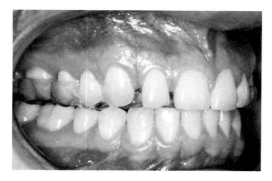

Fig. 19-15. Autorepositional splint. The splint is designed to eliminate occlusal interferences while providing point contact for all teeth in both arches.

pist, as well as continued at home by the patient.

Physical therapy can be extremely useful in the initial attempts to reduce TM joint pain and increase or restore normal range of motion. The relatively low cost as compared with other medical treatment, and the likelihood that some benefit will occur, are strong arguments for frequent use of physical therapy for pain/ dysfunction patients.

Splints

The use of splints is generally considered a reversible, and therefore conservative, type of treatment for TM joint pain and dysfunction patients. Although there are many variations on splint designs, most splints for TM joint dysfunction can be classified into two groups.

The first group, autorepositional splints (also called anterior guidance splints, superior repositioning splints, or muscle splints) are most frequently used to treat muscle problems or eliminate TM joint pain when no specific internal derangement or other joint pathology can be identified. Splints can be fabricated for the maxilla or mandible and have a wide variety of designs. The general principle, however, is essentially the same. The splint is designed to provide full arch contact without working or balancing interferences and without ramps or deep interdigitations forcing the mandible to function in any one specific occlusal position (Fig. 19-15). A typical use for a splint of this type is in a patient who has muscle pain and a significant discrepancy between centric occlusion and centric relation.

An example of the use of this type of splint in surgical-orthodontic treatment would be in a patient with a Class II malocclusion and significant overjet who continually postures forward to obtain incisor contact during mastication and improve appearance at rest. Many of these patients complain of muscle symptoms and a feeling that they do not have a definite place to bite. Wearing an autorepositional splint allows full arch dental contact with the condyles in their more poste-

rior retruded position. If the muscle symptoms are due to hyperactivity related to the forward posturing, a splint of this type usually eliminates them.

In addition to the potential therapeutic effect, it often is easier to establish the retruded contact position of the mandible after some muscular relaxation has occurred following this proprioceptive deprogramming. Vertical as well as AP changes may occur in mandibular positioning, aiding in the final evaluation of the malocclusion/dentofacial deformity (Fig. 19-16). In addition, if this type of therapy provides significant reduction in the pain or dysfunction experienced by the patient, there is reason to expect that a surgical procedure that would allow the mandible to function in a more anterior position, while maintaining the condyles in their more posterior and retruded position, would have a positive long-term effect on reduction of the symptoms. In this case, the splint is not only therapeutic but is also of significant aid in the diagnostic process and provides some information about the prognosis of anticipated orthodontic-surgical treatment.

In addition to use in Class II patients, this type of splint can also be used to temporarily and reversibily eliminate gross occlusal interferences and to alter vertical dimension in other types of malocclusion. Patients with short lower facial height, particularly those with Class III malocclusions, minor interferences, and muscle or joint pain, will frequently benefit from this type of splint.

The second type of splint is the anterior repositioning splint. It is constructed so that there is an anterior ramping effect, forcing the mandible to function in a protruded position (Fig. 19-17). This type of splint is used to provide temporary relief and in some cases a long-term cure for internal TM joint derangements. The classic use of anterior repositioning splints is in the treatment of anterior disk displacement with reduction. In this case, the anterior position is determined by the protrusion necessary to produce the proper disk/ condyle relationship (Fig. 19-18). Generally, the splint must be worn 24 hours a day for several months. In theory, after disk repositioning for a prolonged period, the posterior ligaments will shorten, maintaining the disk in the proper relationship to the condylar articulating surface when the splint is withdrawn and the mandible repositions posteriorly. Even when these splints are not curative long-term, they often provide significant relief of discomfort in the acute stages of TM joint dysfunction (i.e., even though clicking or other joint noises may continue after the splint is discontinued, pain may be significantly reduced).

One of the main objectives of splint therapy is to use this type of appliance to test the response to mandibular repositioning in a reversible way. In other words, no irreversible changes should take place as a result of splint therapy. An improperly constructed splint may

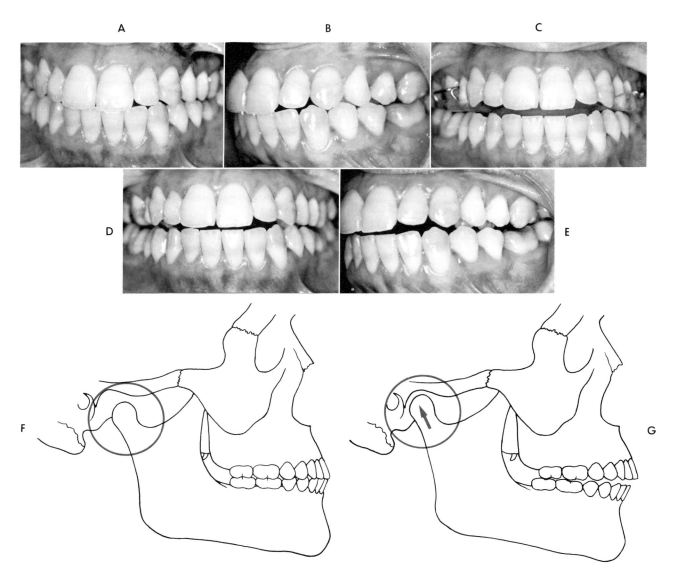

Fig. 19-16. Changes in mandibular position after deprogramming with autorepositional splint. **A** and **B**, Centric occlusion position at the time of initial evaluation. **C**, Splint in place. **D** and **E**, Occlusal relationship following deprogramming with splint. **F**, Diagrammatic representation of maximum interdigitation obtained with the condyle slightly down and forward. **G**, After deprogramming occlusal proprioception and muscle function, the change in condyle position results in retrusion of mandibular position and a slight open bite.

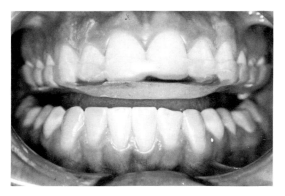

Fig. 19-17. Anterior repositioning splint. Anterior portion of splint constructed with a ramp, which postures the mandible forward when in maximum interdigitation. The posterior portion of the splint provides point contact only for molar teeth.

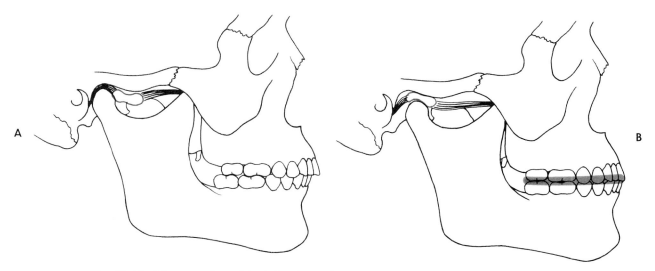

Fig. 19-18. Diagram of condyle/disk relationship. **A,** Disk displaced anteriorly. **B,** Disk interposed between the condyle and articular eminence with anterior repositioning splint in place. Anterior position of mandible allows functioning with the condyle in the appropriate relationship to the disk.

produce iatrogenic malocclusion by allowing some teeth to erupt relative to others. The major offenders are splints that do not provide full arch coverage or that are improperly adjusted (Fig. 19-19).

Splint therapy in general is temporary treatment. In the case of patients with TM joint pain/dysfunction and dentofacial deformity, this may compose only a small portion of the total treatment, and it should not be inappropriately expensive. Splint therapy should be reversible, inexpensive, and an aid in establishing the diagnosis; often it is therapeutic as well.

IRREVERSIBLE TREATMENT PHASE

The irreversible phase of treatment consists of all types of therapy that permanently change the morphology or function of the masticatory system. This includes occlusal equilibration, prosthetic restoration, orthodontics, orthognathic surgery, TM joint surgery

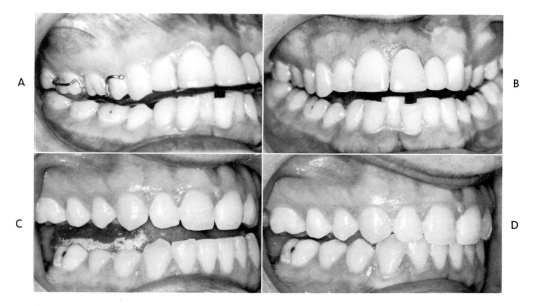

Fig. 19-19. Examples of undesirable occlusal changes resulting from inappropriate splint construction. **A,** Splint constructed without coverage of second molar teeth, allowing for slight supraeruption. **B,** Open bite resulting from passive extrusion of second molars. **C,** Splint covering posterior teeth only. **D,** Intrusion of posterior teeth resulting in posterior open bite.

or any combination of the above. If a patient has responded well to reversible treatment and it seems clear that changing the occlusion could help long-term, a malocclusion too severe to correct satisfactorily in other ways is an indication for surgical-orthodontic treatment. Failure to respond to reversible treatment may indicate a need for TM joint surgery. This portion of the chapter focuses on the implications of surgical-orthodontic treatment and its relationship to TM joint surgery.

As stated previously, when considering the sequencing of treatment for dentofacial deformity/TM joint pain/dysfunction patients, it is useful to place patients into subgroups based on their symptoms, clinical signs of pain and dysfunction, and response to the initial reversible treatment phase (see Fig. 19-12). This grouping is particularly helpful in the important decision as to which problem should be receive definitive treatment first, the malocclusion or the TM joint dysfunction. In our opinion, patients with severe malocclusion who have signs and symptoms of muscle problems or TM joint pain but who do not have obvious evidence of internal-joint pathology should be considered for surgical-orthodontic treatment before invasive joint therapy. This is especially true of those who have had significant improvement in symptoms through temporary modification of their occlusion with splint therapy.

Patients who have stable internal-joint derangements that have responded well to conservative therapy, are not particularly painful, and do not grossly interfere with function may also be considered for orthognathic surgery before TM joint treatment such as arthroscopy or open joint surgery. On the other hand, those who have internal-joint pathology that has not responded to reversible therapy may be considered candidates for TM joint surgery before surgical-orthodontic treatment is undertaken. The long-term efficacy for this sequencing, however, has not been extensively documented.

Surgical-Orthodontic Treatment First

The rationale for surgical-orthodontic treatment of the malocclusion before TM joint surgery in this select group of patients is based on several factors that may affect joint and muscle function. These include postsurgical condylar positioning, occlusal relationships, neuromuscular balance, biomechanics of the masticatory system, and altered postoperative function in the postoperative period.

Postsurgical Position of the Condyles

When orthognathic surgery is performed in the ramus of the mandible (sagittal split or vertical subcondylar osteotomy), rotation of the condyles and AP changes in condylar position are likely to occur. As the body of the mandible is advanced or set back, the ramus segment must rotate to maintain contact with the

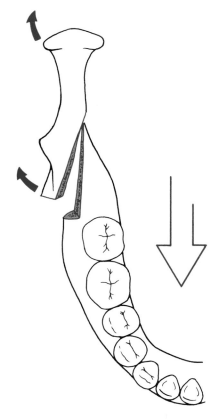

Fig. 19-20. Diagram showing axial condylar rotation resulting from advancement of the mandible after sagittal osteotomy.

repositioned tooth-bearing segment. This results in a change in the longitudinal axis of the condyle within the fossa (Fig. 19-20). Small AP changes are almost inevitable and may be introduced deliberately. Unless RIF is used, some additional spontaneous adjustment in condyle position will occur in response to muscle pull and soft-tissue pressures. These rotational and minor AP changes, which are a consequence of the geometry of the jaw and cannot be avoided, should be clearly distinguished from gross changes due to poor surgical technique that obviously would result in postoperative malocclusion and might contribute to further dysfunction (see Chapter 9).

Improvement in TM joint pain and dysfunction does occur in some patients after mandibular ramus surgery, and one possible explanation is related to these changes in condylar position. Two separate series have been reported documenting significant improvement in pain and dysfunction in TM joints following ramus osteotomies in which the jaw was not repositioned.[56,57] In these cases, high vertical subcondylar osteotomies were used to allow the condyles to be repositioned passively within the fossa, their positions dictated by postoperative muscle pull on the condylar segments. A similar effect can occur when the jaw is moved to improve occlusal and facial relationships.

The improvement in the occlusion may also play a role in improvement of symptoms. Full arch contact, anterior guidance, and posterior occlusal support have the potential to produce significant improvement in both pain and dysfunction symptoms, particularly if parafunctional activity is reduced. This is more likely to occur in patients who enjoyed similar reduction in symptoms with a splint; thus the importance of a reversible phase of therapy in planning this type of treatment.

A case illustrating the sequencing of reversible treatment followed by orthognathic surgery is shown as Case 1 below (see Figs. 19-27 through 19-33). This patient had a Class II malocclusion accompanied by anterior mandibular posturing, TM joint pain without obvious signs of internal derangements, and muscle pain. Insertion of a splint, to allow the jaw to function with the condyles in a more retruded position while providing full arch stabilized contact, resulted in significant improvement in the patient's symptoms. Orthodontic therapy was then instituted, and a mandibular advancement was eventually performed. The patient has been without symptoms for over 3 years.

Another possible factor in the improvement of TM joint symptoms following orthognathic surgery is the changed biomechanical efficiency that may result.[58] Changes in occlusal force occur that go beyond the amount that would be predicted by the changes in geometry alone,[59] indicating that neuromuscular adaptation is an important component.[60] For example, in patients with the short-face syndrome or vertical maxillary deficiency, it can be hypothesized that the shortened lower face height results in abnormal resting-muscle lengths and inefficient jaw position, both of which may be contributing factors in producing symptoms.[61,62] Restoration of lower face height often decreases or eliminates symptoms; the importance of biomechanical factors remains unclear.

Case 2 below (see Figs. 19-34 through 19-39) demonstrates this type of case. This patient initially presented with a long history of myofascial-type pain as well as TM joint pain but had no specific evidence of internal-joint pathology. He had been treated with a number of splints in the past and actually found it most comfortable when he wore two splints (one for the upper arch and one for the lower arch) simultaneously. After initial evaluation, patient education, the use of nonsteroidal inflammatory agents and physical therapy, including EMG biofeedback and muscle relaxation training, a new splint was made to allow the patient to function with a significant increase in lower face height. After a 6-month trial in this position, the patient remained totally pain-free. EMG recordings were completed using nocturnal measurements with

and without the splint. The significant differences in muscle activity readings were correlated with increased pain when the splint was removed and reduction in symptoms when the splint was worn. The final treatment plan included downgrafting the maxilla to produce the vertical face height that had been created temporarily using splint therapy. He has remained symptom-free since that time.

Both of these patients received extensive reversible treatment before definitive irreversible correction of their problem. In some cases, correction of the skeletal and dental malocclusion without an intensive course of prior reversible treatment can be considered. The primary indication is when the patient is concerned about the dentofacial deformity and malocclusion and is unaware of or not concerned about TM joint dysfunction despite the presence of some clinical signs.

The irreversible treatment phase also can be accelerated in patients who are aware of TM joint pain and dysfunction but who have as a higher priority the correction of their malocclusion or skeletal deformity. As we have described earlier in this chapter, these patients frequently will pursue orthodontic or surgical treatment knowing this may provide no benefit for their TM joint pain or dysfunction symptoms. Their interest in the correction of their malocclusion, however, is great enough that this possibility is acceptable to the patient. It must be emphasized that these patients must be aware that irreversible treatment of the dental occlusion may not produce improvement in their TM joint symptoms. Even when patients experience a significant improvement during the reversible treatment phase, no guarantee can be given regarding the long-term outcome of pain and dysfunction.

TM Joint Treatment First

Patients who must be considered for more aggressive TM joint treatment before orthognathic surgery fall into two groups: (1) those who have continuing severe pain or dysfunction despite initial reversible treatment, which is a significant problem for the patient, and (2) those who have ongoing degenerative changes that either result in loss of ramus height and a consequent rotation of the mandible into anterior open bite or lead to significant joint pathology such as ankylosis.[63]

Severe symptoms requiring early surgical treatment are most likely to be related to an acute or chronic closed lock, with the disk permanently displaced. These patients may have significant pain in both the joint area as well as the muscles of mastication and often have significant limitation of opening. In these cases, an attempt at reversible treatment, including patient education, medication, physical therapy, and splint therapy, is indicated as an initial treatment regime. Failure of these methods, however, generally indicates a need for surgical treatment.

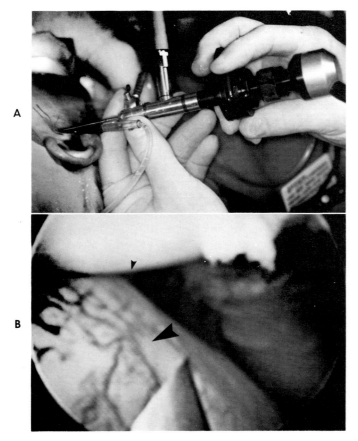

Fig. 19-21. **A,** Arthroscope placed in superior joint space. **B,** Arthroscopic view of internal derangement/anterior disk displacement without reduction. Note vascular bilaminar zone *(large arrow)* in view beneath and extending anterior to the articular eminence *(small arrow)*. The tip of the irrigation outflow needle can also be seen in this view.

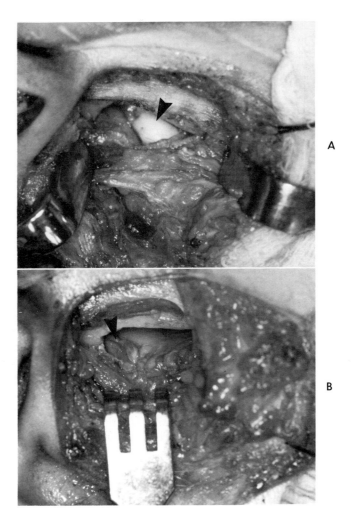

Fig. 19-22. View of open surgical approach for correction of anterior disk displacement. **A,** Disk displaced anteriorly *(arrow)*. **B,** After surgical repositioning. Note area of suture line in bilaminar zone area *(small arrow)*.

Several surgical techniques are effective in reducing or eliminating pain and dysfunction due to disk displacements. The most conservative surgical approach, and the topic of current interest, is the technique of arthroscopy.[64] This involves the placement of a small arthroscope in the superior joint space (Fig. 19-21). Exploration of the joint space is accompanied by lavage of fluid in the superior joint space and often produces lysis of any adhesions that may be found in the joint. With more sophisticated operative techniques, it is possible to reposition the disk tissue during arthroscopic visualization. Although the disk position may not be totally corrected anatomically, this intervention seems to improve symptoms for many patients.

If an arthroscopic technique fails or if the situation is deemed severe enough initially, open TM joint surgery is indicated. The surgical approach can be either preauricular or postauricular. Although there are several modifications of surgical technique, the primary goal is to remove or fold posterior attachment tissue, which

generally has been stretched or disrupted, and then suture the disk back to the correct relationship with the condylar articulating surface (Fig. 19-22). Following this type of surgical correction, patients usually require a course of physical therapy, home exercises, and diet modification. Arthroscopy or open arthrotomy are effective in alleviating pain and dysfunction symptoms from disk displacement in over 80% of operated patients.[63,65]

Following this type of surgical correction, we recommend a waiting period of 6 months to 1 year before beginning active orthodontic or surgical-orthodontic treatment. This is particularly true when treatment might involve transmitting pressure to the repaired joint, as would occur with the use of Class III elastics or in response to surgical mandibular advancement.

The second group of patients who may need surgical treatment of the TM joint before orthognathic surgery are those who have active degenerative processes occurring within the joint. In addition to the pain and dysfunction experienced by the patient, the decrease in ramus height and the consequent change in posterior vertical dimension will have a significant impact on surgical-orthodontic treatment. Successful treatment of dentofacial deformities depends on establishing the proper relationship of the condyle in the glenoid fossa at the time of surgery and maintaining it thereafter. Relapse will occur if pathologic conditions such as degenerative joint disease or rhematoid arthritis produce further changes in condylar height.

In some cases, these conditions are self-limiting, and an initial course of reversible treatment may result in an improvement in patient symptomatology and stabilization of the degenerative changes. If the active degenerative process ceases within a reasonable period, surgical treatment of the joint itself may not be necessary. Case 3 (see Figs. 19-40 through 19-49) demonstrates this principle. This 52-year-old patient presented with a progressive malocclusion and significant right TM joint pain. Radiographic examination and a bone scan confirmed active degenerative changes within the TM joint that were the obvious cause of her anterior and left-sided open bite. A splint was constructed that provided bilateral occlusal contact. The patient's symptoms subsided after a course of medication and physical therapy. Six months after cessation of symptoms, a bone scan was repeated, showing minimal metabolic activity in the bone of the joint area. At this point, orthodontic treatment was initiated with leveling and alignment of the maxillary and mandibular arches in preparation for maxillary surgery. The choice of maxillary surgery would eliminate further trauma to the mandible and the period of limitation of movement postsurgery that probably would occur with mandibular surgery. In addition, it was felt that the slight canting that would result from correction of the occlusion in the maxilla would not be unesthetic for this patient. The patient has done extremely well, with a very stable occlusion. Final prosthetic restorations were completed after no changes in the occlusal relationship had occurred. A 1-year waiting period following the surgical correction elapsed before placement of definitive prosthetic restorations.

If orthognathic surgery is performed in patients with TM joint degeneration to correct the occlusion before changes in ramus height stabilize, significant postoperative occlusal changes may result. In some cases, this can be predicted from the clinical signs, symptoms, and radiographic findings apparent in the joint before surgery. However, significant condylar resorption after orthognathic surgery has been reported in patients who had no evidence of active condylar resorption, clinical signs, or pain symptoms before orthognathic surgery.[66,67] The best guess is that these cases represent patients who had subclinical pathology present within the joints that was exacerbated by the adaptations necessary after surgery and resulted in condylar resorption and the postoperative malocclusion.

As a general rule, degenerative changes within the joint are associated with perforation of the disk and erosion of the condylar bone as well as the temporal fossa articulating surfaces. Surgical correction when the vertical change is minimal often can be accomplished by repairing the disk with a dermal graft[68] or replacing disk tissue with autogenous grafts or alloplastic implant materials.[69,70] When more severe condylar resorption is apparent, autogenous replacement of the condyle with a technique such as costochondral grafting or alloplastic joint replacement may be indicated.[71,72] In these cases, many malocclusions can be corrected by altering the length of the ramus at the time of costochondral grafting or placement of total joint replacements. The details of surgical treatment to correct the degenerative process are beyond the scope of this chapter, and the reader is referred to other sources for the specifics of TM joint surgery.[68]

When patients with malocclusion and pain/dysfunction are treated with orthodontics and orthognathic surgery first, the joints and muscles must be evaluated critically following surgery. A final reevaluation must be performed before debanding of the patient. If for any reason it is determined that secondary TM joint surgery must be performed, the orthodontic appliances should be left in place. TM joint surgery occasionally results in small open bites or other occlusal discrepancies that can be corrected with orthodontics. Likewise, patients who have undergone TM joint surgery followed by orthognathic surgery should be critically reevaluated for the stability of both procedures before orthodontic debanding.

Simultaneous Orthognathic and TM Joint Surgery

Although it is possible, when orthognathic and TM joint surgery are necessary, to perform these procedures at the same operating session, there are several reasons why this may not be indicated. First, there are problems in sequencing the two procedures within the same session. Correction of the joint problem first would seem the most logical sequence, restoring the normal condylar height and anatomy before correcting the occlusion. Intraarticular swelling and hematoma formation, however, may make it difficult to position the condylar fragments accurately when the orthognathic procedure is done. In addition, the stretching and manipulation of the joint required during orthognathic surgery may be detrimental to the surgical repair just performed within the joint. The reverse sequence presents the problems of changing condylar vertical dimension after a proper occlusal relationship has been established (i.e., there may be an instant change in occlusion, a relapse of the orthognathic correction as condyle position shifts in TM joint surgery). Second, there is significant potential for cross-contamination between a sterile TM joint and an intraoral surgical site. Finally and probably most important, immediate postoperative rehabilitation is a major factor in improving the outcome of joint surgery. If for any reason the patient must be left in maxillomandibular fixation to obtain healing at the osteotomy sites, any movement of the TM joint would obviously be eliminated. This may result in significant scarring and limitation of motion postsurgically, as well as changes within the joint. Even when RIF is used, the discomfort following the orthognathic procedure may be limiting to a point that the patient cannot adequately exercise the TM joints. Stretching exercises that require significant pressure on the jaws may also compromise healing of the osteotomy sites. For these reasons, we prefer that orthognathic and TM joint surgery be separated by several months at a minimum.

TM JOINT PROBLEMS RELATED TO SURGICAL-ORTHODONTIC TREATMENT

The chance that TM joint pain/dysfunction can arise as a result of surgical-orthodontic treatment is always of concern. The best perspective comes from considering four points of view:

1. The incidence of TM joint pain/dysfunction in patients with dentofacial deformity is approximately the same as in the rest of the population. This means that there is some chance a patient who had no problems before treatment will develop them postsurgically, quite independently of his or her surgical-orthodontic treatment. The longer the interval between the active orthodontic treatment and the appearance of a problem, the less the chance that it is directly related to the treatment. Patients who develop TM joint pain/dysfunction months after the treatment is concluded should be treated like any others who have acute problems without severe malocclusion, including treatment with the reversible modalities described above.

2. Some aspects of orthodontic treatment have the potential to cause TM joint pain/dysfunction during the presurgical or postsurgical phases of treatment. Although it has been suggested that Class II or class III elastics can lead to TM joint problems, there is no evidence to support that contention in patients with no preexisting joint pathology (but these elastics should be avoided in patients with TM joint degeneration or systemic arthritis). Problems related to orthodontic tooth movement arise primarily when a gross interference arises because of tooth movement. Second molar interferences seem particularly likely to produce a patient reaction, but even

these cause problems only in the minority of patients who clench or grind against the interference enough to cause muscle symptoms. If a problem arises during active orthodontic treatment, adjusting the appliance to relieve interferences and reassuring the patient almost always are sufficient.

3. Several factors related to surgical correction of dentofacial deformities can be associated with postoperative TM joint pain. Limitation of motion postsurgically is observed at least transiently in all patients who have mandibular ramus surgery and in a significant number long-term. Immobilization of the jaws during healing is a major contributor to postsurgical limitation of motion and may contribute to other effects as well. The effect of immobilization through the use of maxillomandibular fixation and the associated need for postoperative physical rehabilitation to restore normal function after orthognathic surgery has been described.[73] Prolonged muscle immobilization may be responsible for short-term functional problems and may actually have significant long-term implications. In addition, jaw immobilization can produce degenerative changes within the TM joints.[74,75]

The use of RIF allows jaw immobilization to be reduced or totally eliminated. The patient can begin rehabilitation exercises and physical therapy at an earlier date after surgical correction. Theoretically, the effects of immobilization on the joints and muscles of mastication should be reduced with earlier function, and the available data suggest that normal range of motion is achieved more completely and more quickly with RIF.[76]

There are some hazards for TM joint function associated with the use of RIF, primarily its effect on condylar position after mandibular ramus osteotomy. As we have described earlier, condylar rotations occur when the tooth-bearing segment of the mandible is moved forward or backward. The rotations occur whether RIF or conventional wire fixation is used. With wire fixation, some spontaneous adjustment in condyle position usually occurs after surgery, but this does not happen with RIF. In both instances, remodeling in the condyle and fossa occurs postsurgically, and the rotation usually causes no long-term problem. The beneficial effect of earlier function with RIF seems to faciliate TM joint remodeling that might be required.

A more important hazard than condylar rotation is that improper RIF of the ramus can also increase intercondylar width, placing the condyle in a more lateral position in the fossa.[77] As the body of the mandible moves forward in a sagittal ramus osteotomy, its posterior portion tends to impinge on the condylar segment, and flaring of the most anterior portion of the proximal condylar segment results.

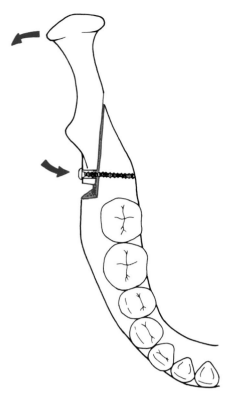

Fig. 19-23. Lateral displacement of the condyle resulting from closure of the anterior gap created as the mandible is advanced. When RIF is placed, this results in an overall increase in intercondylar width.

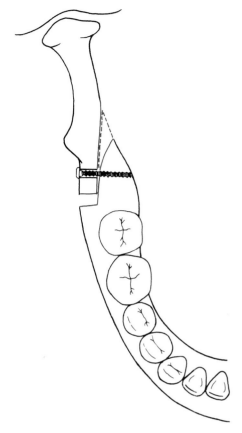

Fig. 19-24. Recontouring of the distal segment to facilitate passive positioning of the proximal segment before placing RIF.

This produces a gap in the anterior portion of the osteotomy. If screws are placed without modifying the bony segments, the proximal condylar segment shifts around a fulcrum resulting in lateral displacement of the condyle (Fig. 19-23). Joint pain and severe limitation of motion may follow.

Several techniques can be used to minimize or eliminate this problem. When minor gaps occur as a result of this flaring at the osteotomy site, recontouring of the distal segment is the easiest method (Fig. 19-24). This is done by eliminating the fulcrum point. The inferior alveolar nerve must be protected as it enters the proximal portion of the distal segment while this is being done, using a bur or bone file to remove bony projections. Once the proximal segment can be passively placed against the lateral aspect of the distal segment, a conventional lag screw or position screw technique can be used to approximate the bony segments.

When a larger gap occurs or when simple recontouring does not eliminate the flaring, other measures must be taken to prevent the condylar displacement. The use of a position screw (as described in Chapter 7) in the anterior portion of the osteotomy site can be effective in maintaining the intra-

bony gap. This will prevent the lateral displacement of the condyle and proximal segment (Fig. 19-25). If a lag screw is to be used when a bony gap remains in the anterior portion of the osteotomy, some type of shim must be placed to maintain this gap in the anterior portion of the osteotomy (Fig. 19-26). Bone removed from the proximal segment or other local areas or allogeneic graft material can be used. In cases of severe asymmetry when excessive rotation and flaring may occur on one side, a combination of all three techniques may be necessary.

Pain symptoms in the TM joint in the immediate postoperative period are rare, and if present are highly likely to be related to rigid fixation producing changes in condylar width. As the condyles remodel, the symptoms tend to decrease and disappear, so the patient can be reassured that this difficulty is likely to be transient. Reoperation to correct the fixation is an option that should be considered if pain is severe and persistent. Interestingly, if the condylar position in the AP or vertical planes is improper, pain is quite unlikely—the patient simply repositions the mandible, producing some occlusal changes (see Chapter 12 for a description of postsur-

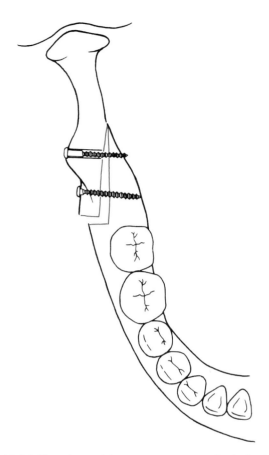

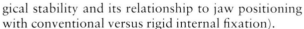

Fig. 19-25. Use of a position screw to engage both the lateral and medial cortex, preventing closure of the anterior gap.

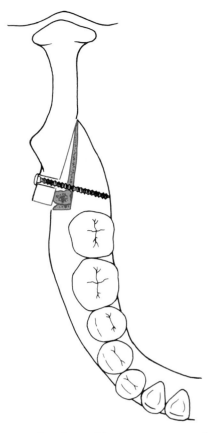

Fig. 19-26. Use of a shim of bone to maintain the anterior space prevents lateral displacement as the lag screw is tightened.

gical stability and its relationship to jaw positioning with conventional versus rigid internal fixation).

Although condylar remodeling occurs to some extent in every patient postoperatively (and indeed occurs in adults, whether treated or not), this is rarely associated with significant changes in the height of the condylar process or length of the ramus. In the presence of presurgical degenerative changes, however, there is a risk of continuing degeneration following orthognathic surgery. As we have discussed above, there are reports of posttreatment condylar resorption, which probably represents an exacerbation of previous degenerative tendencies. Patients who have any sign of degenerative changes or who have a history of trauma to the TM joint (including old condylar fracture) should be warned of this possible complication.

4. The final occlusal result can predispose to TM joint pain/dysfunction problems. In this regard, the significant factors are not different from what would

be looked for in untreated patients: interferences that produce a lateral shift on closure, balancing interferences in lateral function, or a locked occlusion anteriorly, forcing the mandible distally in function. In the absence of postsurgical orthodontics, such imperfections in the occlusion are likely to be present. A major goal of the postsurgical stage is to eliminate them. The best indicator of the success with which this can be done is the low incidence of posttreatment TM joint problems, less than 5% in current reports.[76]

In summary, although TM joint pain/dysfunction can arise from a number of things related to surgical-orthodontic treatment, this is unlikely to occur with good surgical and orthodontic technique. The combined treatment procedures, used correctly, have the potential to improve TM joint problems in many patients who have this initially, without any great likelihood of creating problems where none existed previously.

CASE REPORTS

Case 1

B.S., a 43-year-old white female, presented with a chief complaint of facial pain in the area of the muscles of mastication, primarily the masseter and temporalis, occasionally accompanied by TM joint pain. This pain had been present in varying degrees for several years but had increased in severity and frequency at the time of presentation for evaluation. There was no history of any specific etiologic event that she could associate with the onset of her symptoms. She described intermittent dull, throbbing pain in the masseter and temporalis areas bilaterally with some occasional sharp pain in the TM joint areas themselves. She complained of limitation of jaw opening, which seemed to be worse during times of severe pain, and also described difficulty chewing due to the limited opening as well as the pain. Her dental history revealed previous orthodontic treatment with four premolar extractions as a teenager. Her medical history was essentially noncontributory. There were no other symptoms of muscle or joint pain in other areas.

On facial evaluation, the patient had no obvious facial asymmetries. The patient exhibited mandibular deficiency as well as lack of chin prominence (Fig. 19-27, *A* and *B*). Examination of the muscles of mastication and TM joints revealed pain to palpation over masseter, temporalis, and lateral pterygoid areas bilaterally. There was also mild pain to palpation over the lateral and posterior aspects of the TM joints. No click or crepitus was noted at the time of initial evaluation. Maximum opening was 33 mm, which could be stretched to 39 mm with production of pain in both the muscles and joint areas. Protrusion, left and right lateral excursions, were approximately 7 mm. Examination of the occlusion revealed a centric occlusion position with Class II molar and canine relationships and slight anterior crowding in both arches (Fig. 19-27, *C-E*). Due to discomfort and significant muscle activity, it was difficult to manually position the patient's mandible; however, a more retruded position could be achieved with gentle posterior superior manipulation at the angles of the

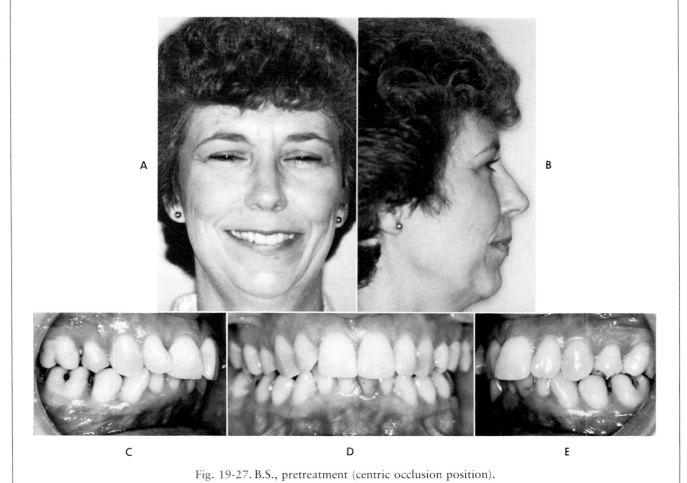

Fig. 19-27. B.S., pretreatment (centric occlusion position).

Continued.

Case 1—cont'd.

mandible. Radiographic evaluation revealed no obvious abnormalities of the TM joints or any other pathology in the jaws.

The problem list generated for B.S. included:

1. Chief complaint of pain in the muscles of mastication and TM joints.
2. Class II mandibular deficiency.
3. Crowding in both arches.
4. CR-CO discrepancy, the magnitude of which could not be determined on initial evaluation due to muscle splinting.

Primary concerns of B.S. were related to reduction in pain symptoms and improvement in jaw function. She was not particularly concerned with dental or facial esthetics. A lengthy initial discussion with the patient regarding the potential lack of any relationship between her malocclusion and pain and dysfunction symptoms was presented. The factors that possibly might contribute to her symptoms, including stress, muscle hyperactivity, parafunction, and the centric relation-centric occlusion discrepancy, were discussed.

A sequential plan for reversible treatment was offered to the patient. This included alteration of diet, home exercises, nonsteroidal inflammatory drugs, muscle relaxants, and physical therapy. The potential use of an autorepositional splint in combination with the other re-

versible treatment was suggested. A general discussion covering the potential irreversible treatment of her malocclusion involving both orthodontics and surgery, should the reversible phase result in significant pain reduction, was also completed at this time.

The patient agreed with the initial treatment plan, including splint therapy. Impressions were taken and models mounted on a semiadjustable articulator. Bite registrations were completed for both the centric occlusion and centric relation positions (Fig. 19-28, *A* and *B*). An autorepositional splint was constructed in the centric relation position (Fig. 19-28, *C*). This was delivered to the patient and was modified slightly to accommodate for distalization of the mandible over the next 4 weeks.

After a period of 4 months, during which the splint was worn full-time, the patient reported almost total resolution of pain and dysfunction symptoms. At the time of recall evaluation, there was no tenderness to the muscles of mastication, and maximum voluntary opening was 41 mm again with no joint noise. There was no tenderness to the TM joints on palpation. At this point, the patient expressed a desire to pursue orthognathic surgery. The possibility that orthodontics and surgical correction would not provide a resolution of her TM joint symptoms was again discussed in detail.

A final treatment plan was generated, which included:

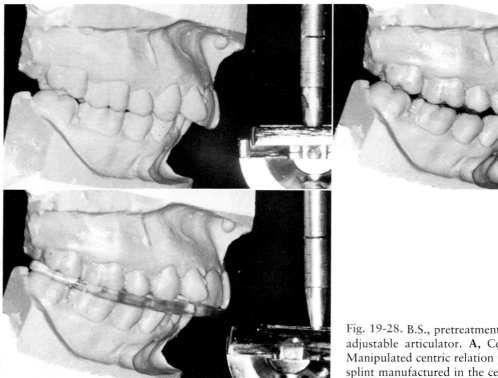

Fig. 19-28. B.S., pretreatment models mounted on a semiadjustable articulator. **A,** Centric occlusion position. **B,** Manipulated centric relation position. **C,** Autorepositional splint manufactured in the centric relation position.

Case 1—cont'd.

1. Removal of one lower incisor tooth.
2. Placement of orthodontic appliances on both arches.
3. Leveling and alignment for presurgical coordination.
4. Mandibular advancement (sagittal split osteotomy) with wire osteosynthesis and 8 weeks of maxillomandibular fixation.
5. Finishing orthodontics.
6. Physical therapy as required for jaw function rehabilitation.

The presurgical orthodontic setup was completed, and the patient returned for presurgical records. During the time of orthodontic preparation, the patient had a few episodes of muscular and TM joint pain as well as limitation of opening. However, these were not severe compared with pretreatment symptoms and were of short duration. The presurgical photographs showed facial features identical to those seen in the pretreatment photographs (Fig. 19-29, *A* and *B*). At the time the occlusal photographs were taken, it was obvious that the patient had two distinct bites and had trouble predictably functioning into either one of these positions. Fig. 19-29, *C* and *D*, shows the centric occlusion position

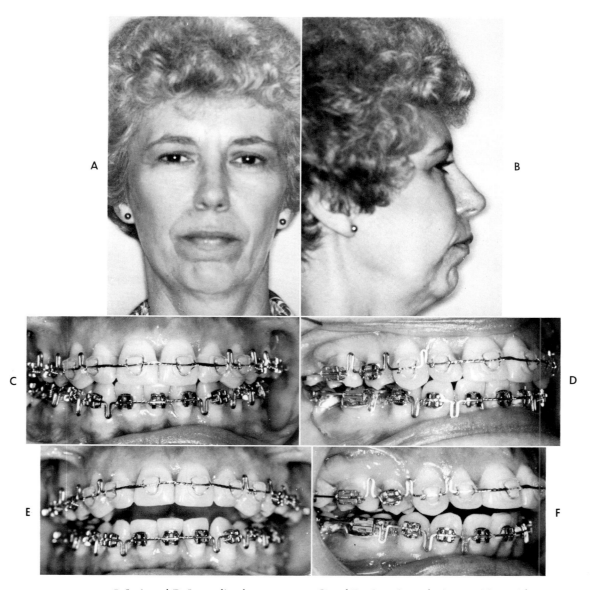

Fig. 19-29. B.S. **A** and **B**, Immediately presurgery. **C** and **D**, Centric occlusion position with the patient postured forward. **E** and **F**, Occlusal position with the patient in a more retruded centric relation position.

Continued.

Case 1—cont'd.

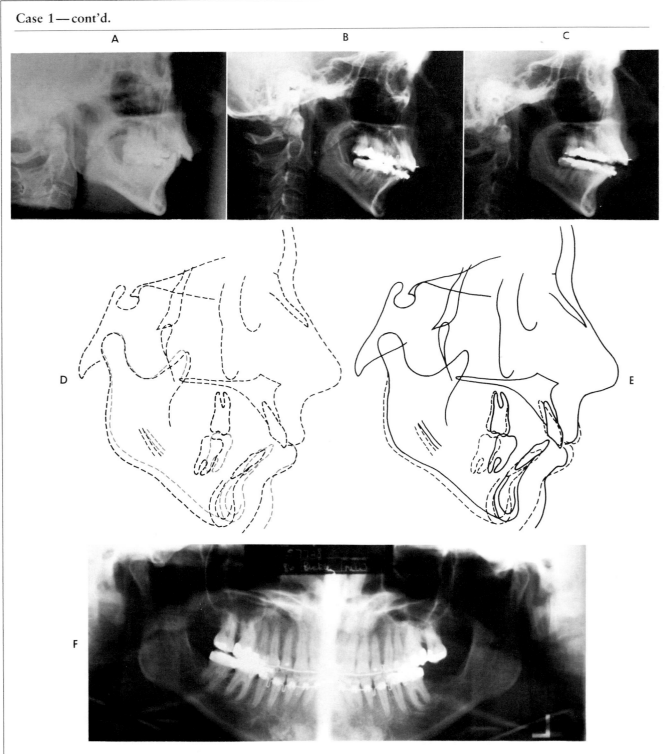

Fig. 19-30. B.S., cephalometric radiographs. **A,** Pretreatment—centric relation position. **B,** Presurgical—centric occlusion position. **C,** Presurgical repeated in the centric relation position. **D,** Superimposition of presurgical cephalometric radiographs, centric occlusion *(dashed pink)* and centric relation *(dashed black)*. **E,** Cephalometric superimposition of pretreatment *(solid line)* and presurgical *(dashed line)* centric relation. **F,** Presurgical panoramic film.

Case 1—cont'd.

obtained when the patient was asked to bite on all of her teeth. Fig. 19-29, *E* and *F*, shows the position obtained when asked to allow her jaw to "drop back" and touch her back teeth. Evaluation of the pretreatment and presurgical radiographs showed the changes in incisor positioning due to orthodontic preparation. In addition, the changes in mandibular position as a result of deprogramming of the occlusion were obvious (Fig. 19-30, *A-E*). Panorex radiographs showed normal joint anatomy presurgically (Fig. 19-30, *F*).

The bilateral sagittal ramus osteotomy advanced the mandible. Wire osteosynthesis fixed the bony segments, and the patient was placed in maxillomandibular fixation for 8 weeks. Following release of fixation, the patient was continued in light elastics with the splint in place for 2 weeks. The splint was removed and the

patient was seen immediately by the orthodontist for placement of arch wires to begin the finishing sequence (Fig. 19-31, *A-C*). A postoperative cephalometric radiograph demonstrates the mandibular advancement (Fig. 19-31, *D*).

Finishing orthodontics was completed. During the entire finishing sequence, the patient's joint symptoms and function were evaluated in detail on each visit. During this entire time, the patient remained essentially symptom-free with a continued progression to 39 mm of postsurgical voluntary opening. In the presence of a good facial and occlusal result and with the absence of TM joint and muscle symptoms, the patient was debanded (Fig. 19-32, *A-E*). Recall radiographs show good mandibular position and normal condylar architecture (Fig. 19-33).

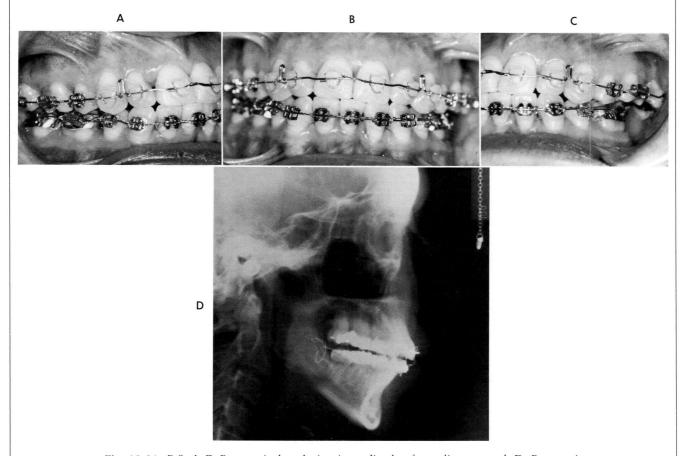

Fig. 19-31. B.S. **A-C,** Postsurgical occlusion immediately after splint removal. **D,** Postsurgical cephalometric film.

Continued.

Case 1—cont'd.

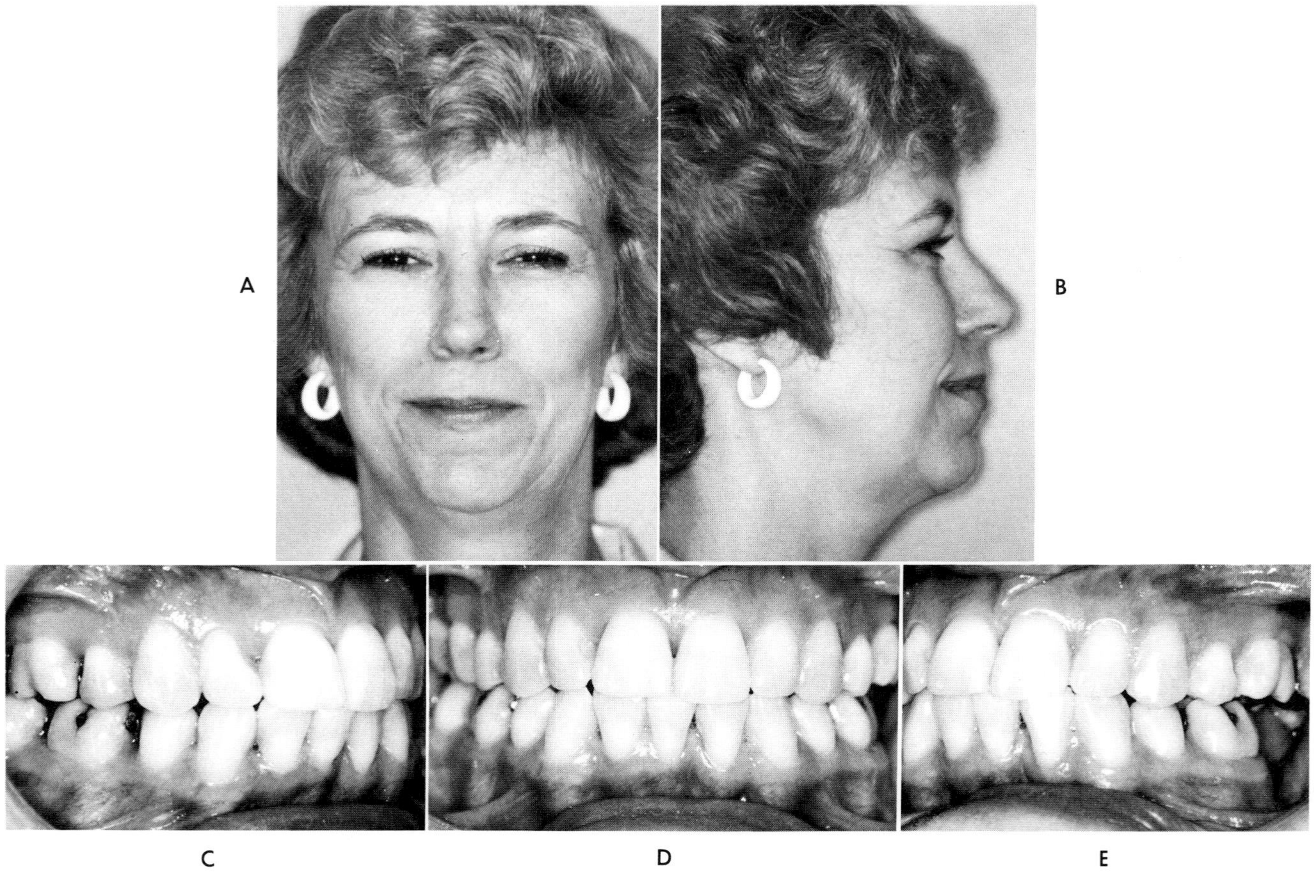

Fig. 19-32. B.S., 2-year recall.

Case 1—cont'd.

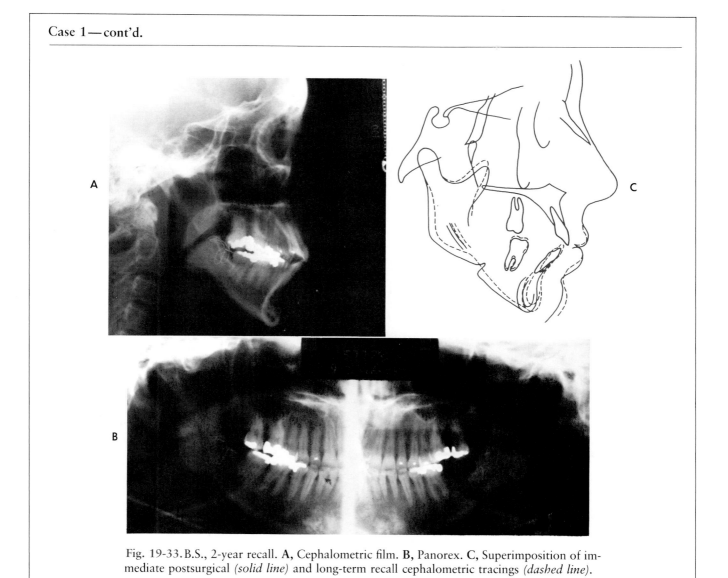

Fig. 19-33. B.S., 2-year recall. **A,** Cephalometric film. **B,** Panorex. **C,** Superimposition of immediate postsurgical *(solid line)* and long-term recall cephalometric tracings *(dashed line)*.

Case 2

K.K., a 24-year-old white male, presented for evaluation of bilateral TM joint and muscular pain. The pain in the muscles of mastication had been present for approximately 14 months. The pain symptoms had been constant throughout this time but seemed to have increased in severity in recent months. The patient noticed no TM joint noises but did describe occasional TM joint pain. He noted no limitation of opening but felt that pain in the muscle area prevented him from eating normally. He also reported some difficulty sleeping due to significant muscle pain. When questioned about any facial or dental concerns, he did describe some dissatisfaction with his facial appearance. When attempting to smile he showed no upper incisor teeth.

His previous dental history revealed evaluation by several other practitioners for TM joint problems. The patient had begun treatment prescribed by other dentists, including attempts at stress reduction with EMG biofeedback and muscle relaxation training, nonsteroidal inflammatory drugs, muscle relaxants, and splint therapy. He had one splint constructed for the lower arch. While he felt that this resulted in some reduction in discomfort, he was not totally satisfied with this splint. He sought treatment from another practitioner, who constructed a splint for the maxillary arch. Again he felt that this improved his symptoms to some degree, but results were not completely satisfactory. At one point, he attempted wearing both splints at the same time (they obviously were not made to be compatible with one another). During the time of simultaneous splint wearing, he felt that he realized the most decrease in pain symptoms. His medical history was essentially noncontributory.

Initial evaluation of the face showed an obvious short face with a Class III profile (Fig. 19-34, *A* and *B*). There was an obvious flat mandibular plane and extremely strong masseter muscles. No incisor exposure occurred at rest or smile. Palpation revealed tenderness and obvious hypertonicity in several areas of the masseter, temporalis, medial, and lateral pterygoid muscles. There was no tenderness to the TM joints on palpation. Maximum opening was 48 mm with protrusion, left and right lateral excursions, of approximately 10 mm. The occlusion was essentially Class I with some spacing anterior in both arches (Fig. 19-34, *C-E*). There was no obvious centric relation/centric occlusion discrepancy. Cephalo-

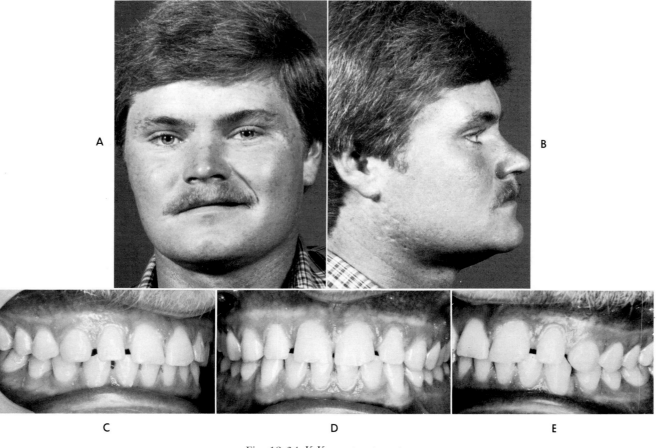

Fig. 19-34. K.K., pretreatment.

Case 2—cont'd.

metric and panoramic radiography confirmed the pretreatment clinical impression of a short-face syndrome with no obvious TM joint pathology (Fig. 19-35, *A-C*). The initial problem list for K.K. included:
1. Myofascial pain/muscle hyperactivity disorder. After careful questioning it was noted that the patient was under some stress; pain increased when stress seemed to be the greatest.
2. Vertical maxillary deficiency.
3. Anterior spacing in both arches.

A frank discussion of the role of stress, muscle hyperactivity, and pain was presented to the patient. At this time,

after mutual agreement, the patient was to be referred to a clinical psychologist for evaluation. Alteration in dietary habits and some suggestions for jaw exercises attempting to reduce jaw pain were suggested. A referral to physical therapy for EMG biofeedback and relaxation training was made at that time as well as a continuing prescription for a nonsteroidal antiinflammatory drug.

Initial reversible treatment also included splint therapy. Initially a bite opening splint was constructed that was modified over several weeks until a bite opening position was achieved at which the patient experienced no

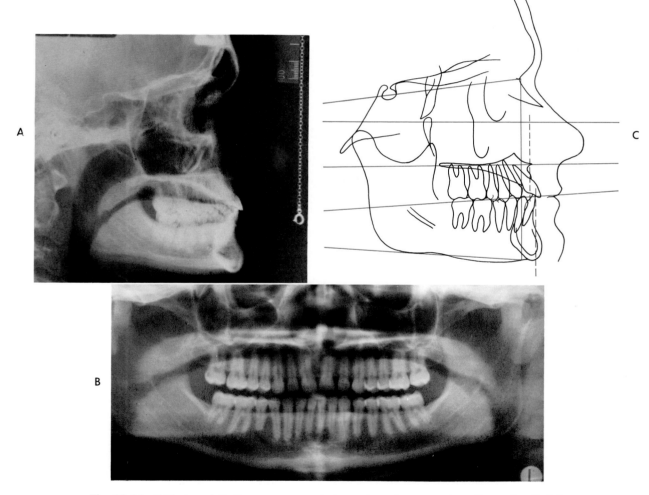

Fig. 19-35. K.K. **A** and **B**, Pretreatment cephalometric and panoramic radiographs. **C**, Initial cephalometric tracing. Note the rotated occlusal plane and the overall skeletal deep-bite pattern, with the palatal and mandibular planes nearly parallel to the true horizontal. The mandible is rotated up and forward, with maxillary incisor protrusion compensating for the Class III jaw relationship. Cephalometric measurements: N perp to A, 5 mm; N perp to Pg, 14 mm; AB difference, −3 mm; UFH, 53 mm; LFH, 59 mm; mand plane, 4 degrees; MxI to A vert, 8 mm, 40 degrees; MnI to B vert, 1 mm, 20 degrees.

Continued.

Case 2—cont'd.

significant muscle or TM joint symptoms (Fig. 19-36, *A* and *B*). The splint was worn for 6 months, during which time the patient experienced a near-complete resolution of muscle symptoms. At this point, EMG surface electrode recording was done with and without the splint to confirm our clinical impression of significant reduction in muscle activity when the vertical dimension was increased (Fig. 19-36, *C* and *D*). At this point, the patient felt strongly that he desired to pursue a more permanent treatment plan that might result in resolution of his symptoms.

The final treatment plan suggested to the patient included:
1. Placement of orthodontic appliances on the maxilla and mandible.
2. LeFort I osteotomy with vertical downgrafting of the maxilla.
3. Finishing orthodontics.
4. Final jaw rehabilitation.
At this point, the patient clearly stated that he did not want to pursue orthodontic treatment because of the expense and time involved. In this case, the treatment plan was modified, using fracture arch bars for maxillo-mandibular fixation rather than orthodontic appliances.

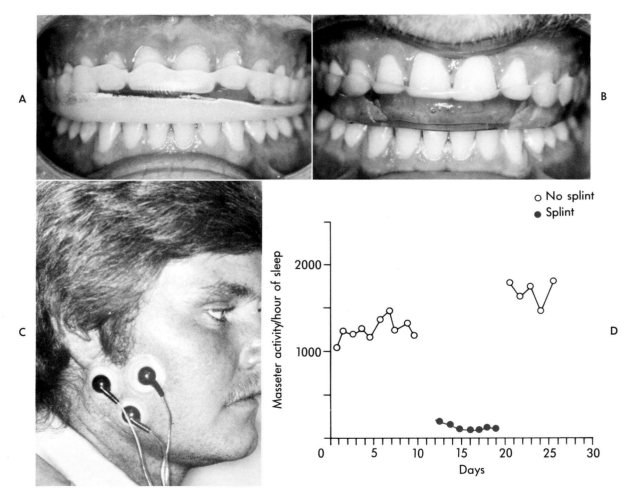

Fig. 19-36. K.K. **A,** Initial splint with increased vertical dimension. **B,** Final splint. This splint was worn full time for over 6 months. **C,** Surface electrodes for EMG recording. **D,** Diagram of masseter activity recording showing sharp reduction in this activity during the time the splint was worn.

Case 2—cont'd.

A LeFort I osteotomy with a vertical downgrafting of approximately 11 mm was performed. In addition to short-term maxillomandibular fixation and suspension wiring, stabilization at the osteotomy site was enhanced using a 45-mil stainless steel wire screwed to the zygoma and inserted into a buccal tube embedded in the occlusal splint. Maxillomandibular fixation was released at 2 weeks, and the patient was allowed to function with the maxillary splint in place for 3 months. During this time, the splint could be removed by the surgeon so that the patient could perform oral hygiene followed by reinsertion of the splint. Fig. 19-37, *B* and

C, shows the postsurgical result and magnitude of surgical change. Three months following the surgical procedure, the splint, arch bars, and stabilization wires were removed. The patient functioned predictably into his occlusal relationship, which was essentially unchanged from the pretreatment condition.

On recall evaluation, the patient had a pleasing change in facial esthetics, with adequate maxillary incisor exposed at rest and full smile (Fig. 19-38, *A* and *B*). The occlusion was essentially unchanged postsurgically (Fig. 19-38, *C-E*). Fig. 19-39 demonstrates the postsurgical to long-term follow-up change. The patient remained free of symptoms in the follow-up period.

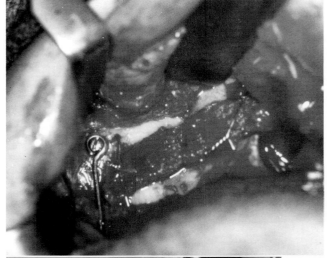

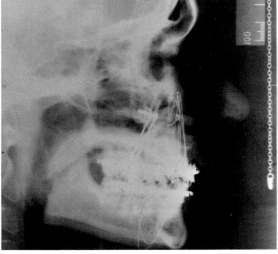

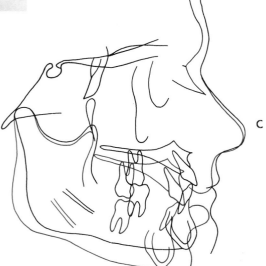

Fig. 19-37. K.K. **A,** Surgical procedure showing interpositional bone graft used to downgraft the maxilla. **B,** Immediate postsurgical cephalometric radiograph. **C,** Superimposition of pretreatment position *(solid black)* and immediate postsurgical result *(solid red).*

Continued.

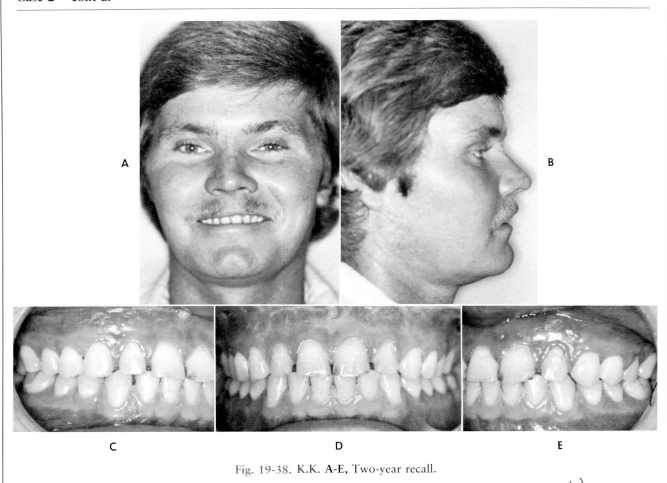

Fig. 19-38. K.K. **A-E,** Two-year recall.

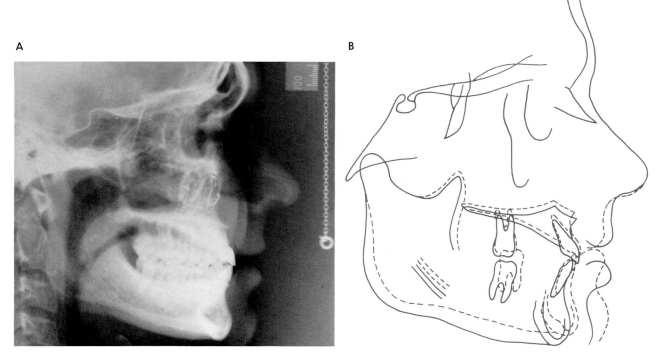

Fig. 19-39. K.K. **A,** Recall cephalometric radiograph. **B,** Superimposition of immediate post-surgical *(solid red)* and recall *(dashed red)* cephalometric tracings.

Case 3

H.M., a 52-year-old white female, was referred for evaluation of right TM joint pain with occasional muscular symptoms. She stated that she had had joint noise and pain in both TM joints for a number of years. This had become worse on the right side in the 2 to 3 months before her presentation for evaluation. The noise initially began as a clicking of both joints but recently had progressed to a persistent grinding noise in the right side. She did note some decrease in the right TM joint noise in the past 1 month. She described the pain as a dull, throbbing pain in the area of the TM joint, which was worse after extended talking or eating and at the end of the day. She also felt that she developed muscle pain in both masseter areas that seemed to be most apparent during the maximum right TM joint pain. Significant reduction in maximum opening and difficulty in chewing occurred due to the joint pain. Within the few months before treatment, she had noted what she described as a progressive change in her bite, with no contact on the left side of her mouth. Her previous dental history was significant only for multiple restorations in all areas of her mouth. Recently, she had discussed her problem with her local dentist, who explained the pathophysiology of degenerative joint disease to her and constructed a bilateral posterior coverage splint in an attempt to stabilize her occlusion. Her medical history was noncontributory, revealing no symptoms in other joints.

Initial clinical evaluation revealed no obvious dentofacial abnormality from a facial esthetics standpoint (Fig. 19-40, *A* and *B*). There was slight tenderness to the right masseter muscle and significant tenderness over the right TM joint area both posteriorly and laterally. A very mild crepitus was noted on maximum opening. Maximum voluntary opening was 31 mm, which could be stretched to 37 mm with production of significant pain in the right joint area. Evaluation of the occlusion demonstrated premature contact in the right posterior segment with a complete open bite on the left side (Fig. 19-40, *C-E*). There was significant pain on manipulation, and no CR-CO discrepancy could be demonstrated. Preoperative radiographs were taken. The most

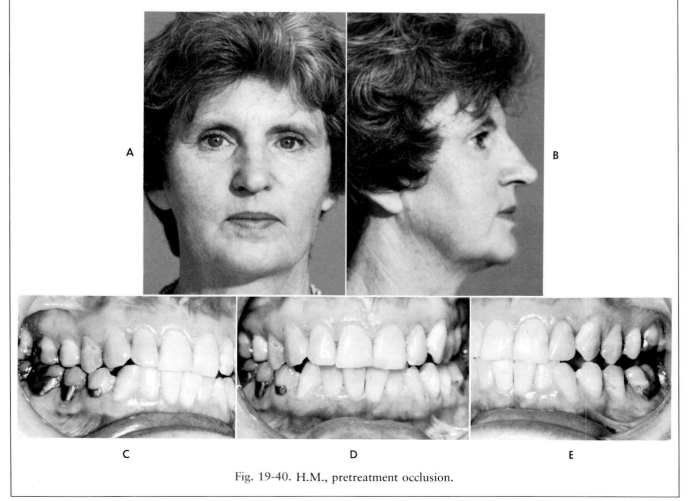

Fig. 19-40. H.M., pretreatment occlusion.

Continued.

Case 3—cont'd.

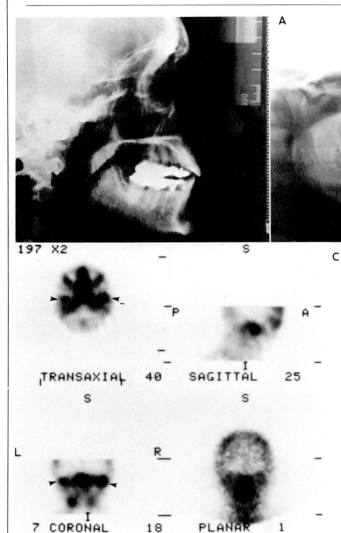

Fig. 19-41. H.M., pretreatment **A**, cephalometric and **B**, panoramic radiographs. Note the shortened condyle on the right side. **C**, Bone scans showing increase in activity in area of TM joints *(arrow)*.

significant finding on the initial films was the apparent shortening of the right condyle (Fig. 19-41, *A* and *B*). A bone scan was obtained demonstrating a marked increase in bone activity of the right joint (Fig. 19-41, *C*). The initial problem list generated for H.M. included:

1. Right TM joint pain and dysfunction (degenerative joint disease).
2. Malocclusion with premature right posterior contact and left side open bite.
3. Multiple teeth with large restorations indicated for prosthetic restoration.

The initial therapy for H.M. included placement on a nonsteroidal antiinflammatory drug (Dolobid, 500 mg b.i.d.), strict instructions for a nonchew diet, a prescription for ultrasound to be administered by a physical therapist, and adjustment of her current splint. Addition of acrylic to provide improved stabilization of both sides of the arch was completed (Fig. 19-42). Although

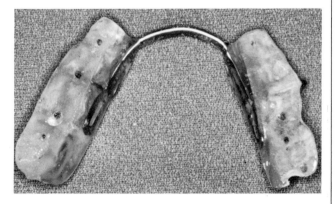

Fig. 19-42. Splint used to provide stabilization on both the left and right sides of the mandible. Although a partial covered splint is generally not preferred, the patient's preexisting splint was adjusted to accommodate the changing occlusion.

Case 3—cont'd.

a splint without full arch coverage is not perferred in our clinic, it was felt that modification of her current splint would provide reasonable occlusal contact in the initial reversible treatment phase. The most important concept regarding the initial treatment phase for H.M. was to monitor her progress during a waiting period and hope that her TM joint symptoms would subside. If no resolution of her symptoms occurred, consideration would then be given to open joint surgery.

Over a period of 4 to 5 months, the patient reported significant improvement in symptoms, with almost a complete resolution by the fifth month. At this point, the patient continued in a waiting phase for 6 additional months. In the absence of symptoms during this period, a final treatment plan was discussed with the patient. It was also emphasized at the this time that further treatment of her occlusion guaranteed elimination of the recurrence of any pain or dysfunction symptoms.

The final treatment plan for this patient included:

1. Placement of orthodontic appliances on the maxillary and mandibular arches.
2. Orthodontic alignment and leveling of the arches.
3. Bone scanning of the TM joint to evaluate activity before surgical treatment.
4. LeFort I osteotomy with superior repositioning of the right posterior segment to correct the open bite.
5. Finishing orthodontics.
6. Debanding followed by a 6-month to 1-year waiting period.
7. Final prosthetic restorations.

After initial orthodontic alignment and leveling, the patient returned for presurgical evaluation. Facial photographs showed no significant change from the pretreatment photographs (Fig. 19-43, *A* and *B*). A careful assessment was completed at this time to determine whether an unacceptable esthetic change would result from superior repositioning of the posterior maxillary segment, which would produce a cant in the maxillary alignment. Photographs of the presurgical occlusion are shown in Fig. 19-43, *C-E*. A significant worsening of the occlusal relationship had taken place as a result of further degenerative changes in the TM joint as well as the orthodontic alignment and leveling.

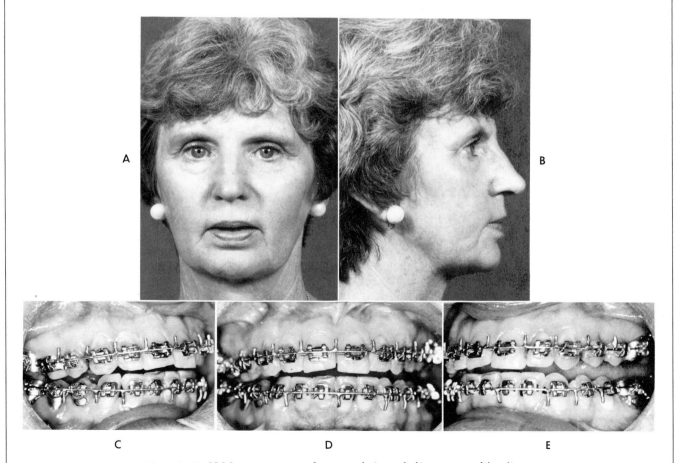

Fig. 19-43. H.M., presurgery, after completion of alignment and leveling.

Continued.

Case 3—cont'd.

Pretreatment radiographic evaluation included a cephalometric and panoramic radiograph as well as a bone scan (Fig. 19-44, *A-C*). The bone scan showed no significant activity in the area of either TM joint. The cephlometric superimposition documented presurgical orthodontic changes (Fig. 19-44, *D*).

The LeFort I osteotomy included a superior repositioning of the right posterior maxillary segment (Fig. 19-45, *A*). RIF was used, allowing the patient to function immediately postoperatively. With bone plates, function was facilitated with an interocclusal splint and light elastics

(Fig. 19-45, *B* and *C*). After a 6-week period of postsurgical function, the splint was removed (Fig. 19-45, *D*). The patient was referred immediately to the orthodontist for placement of finishing arch wires. Fig. 19-46 documents the postsurgical changes.

Orthodontic alignment and leveling was completed. A careful assessment of TM joint signs and symptoms was completed at this time. Maximum voluntary opening was 40 mm with no significant pain in the muscles of mastication or TM joints. No TM joint noise was noted. After debanding, some initial prosthetic buildup

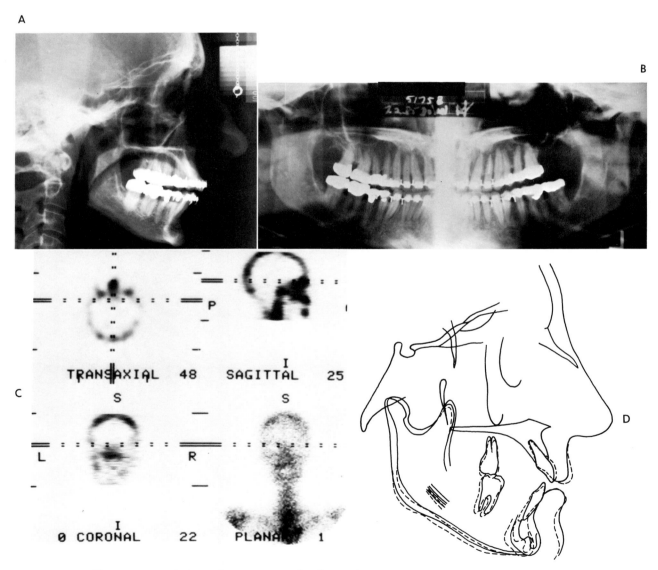

Fig. 19-44. H.M., immediate presurgical radiographs. **A,** Cephalometric film. **B,** Panorex. **C,** Bone scan. Note disappearance of significant activity in the area of the TM joints. **D,** Superimposition of pretreatment *(solid black)* and immediate presurgical *(dashed black)* cephalometric tracings.

Case 3—cont'd.

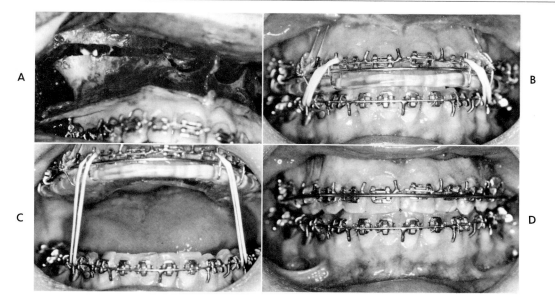

Fig. 19-45. H.M. **A,** Intraoperative photographs showing amount of superior repositioning in the right maxillary area. **B** and **C,** Immediate postsurgical functioning into the splint with use of light guiding elastics. **D,** Occlusion immediately after splint removal.

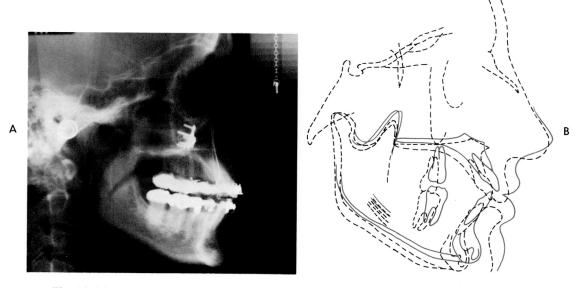

Fig. 19-46. H.M. **A,** Immediate postsurgical cephalometric radiograph. **B,** Superimposition of presurgical *(solid red)* and immediate postsurgical *(dashed black)* cephalometric tracings.

Continued.

procedures were completed, but the final prosthetic restoration was deferred for 1 year (Fig. 19-47). In the absence of TM joint symptoms during a 1-year postsurgical phase, the final prosthetic restorations were completed. Fig. 19-48, *A-E* demonstrates the final facial esthetic and occusal results, and Fig. 19-49 the final recall position, jaw anatomy, and superimposition of long-term postoperative change. The patient experienced no significant episodes of pain or limitation of TM joint function at any time after the intial resolution of symptoms in the preorthodontic phase.

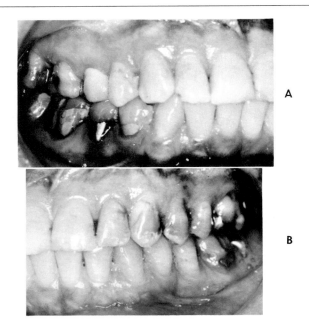

Fig. 19-47. H.M. **A** and **B,** View of occlusion after debanding. Initial buildups had all been completed at this stage, but final prosthetic restoration was deferred for 1 year.

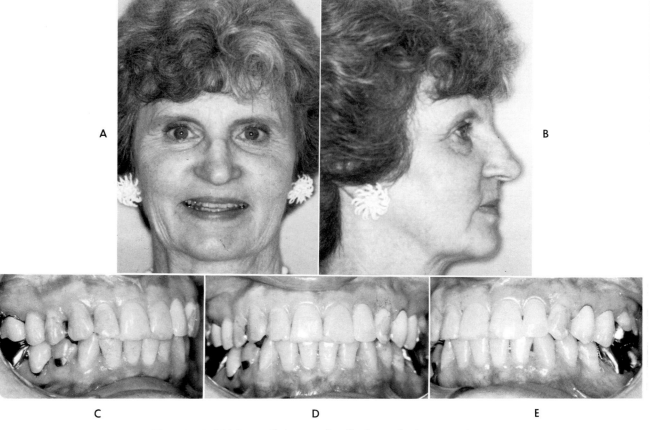

Fig. 19-48. H.M., recall 1 year after final prosthetic restoration.

Case 3—cont'd.

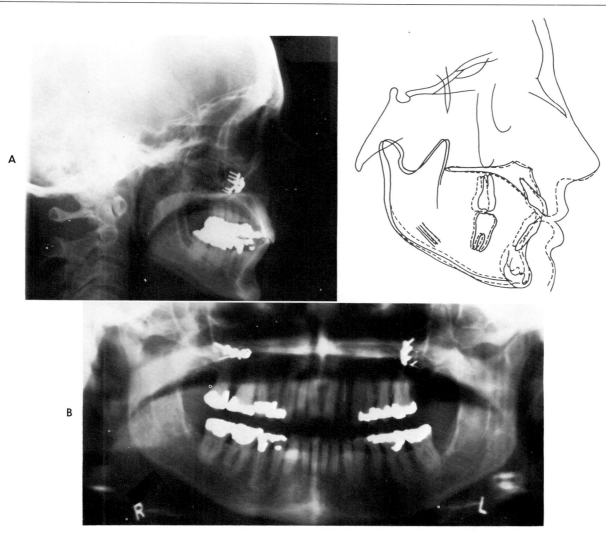

Fig. 19-49. H.M., recall radiographs. **A**, Cephalometric film. **B**, Panelipse. **C**, Superimposition of immediate postoperative *(solid red)* and recall *(dashed red)* cephalometric tracings.

REFERENCES

1. Agerberg G, Carlsson GE: Functional disorders of the masticatory system. I. Distribution of symptoms according to age and sex as judged from investigation by questionnaire, Acta Odontol Scand 30:597-613, 1972.
2. Molin C, Carlsson GE, Friling B, Hedegard B: Frequency of symptoms of mandibular dysfunction in young Swedish men, J Oral Rehabil 3:9-18, 1976.
3. Swanljung O, Rantenanen T: Functional disorders of the masticatory system in southwest Finland, Community Dent Oral Epidemiol 7:177-182, 1979.
4. Helkimo M: Epidemiological survey of dysfunction of the masticatory system, Oral Sci Rev 7:54-69, 1976.
5. Magnusson T, Carlsson GE: Recurrent headaches in relation to temporomandibular joint pain-dysfunction, Acta Odontol Scand 36:333-338, 1978.
6. Ingerslev H: Functional disturbances of the masticatory system in schoolchildren, J Dent Child 50:445-450, 1983.
7. Brandt D: Signs and symptoms of TMJ dysfunction in children. In Carlsson DS, McNamara JA, Jr, Ribbens KA (editors): Developmental aspects of temporomandibular joint disorders. Craniofacial Growth Series, Center for Human Growth and Development, monograph 16, Ann Arbor, 1985, University of Michigan Press.
8. Egermark-Eriksson I, Carlsson GE, Ingervall B: Prevalence of mandibular dysfunction and orofacial parafunction in 7, 11 and 15 year old Swedish children, Eur J Orthod 3:163-172, 1981.

9. Williamson EH: Temporomandibular dysfunction in pre-treatment adolescent patients, Am J Orthod 72:429-433, 1977.

10. de Boever JA, van den Berghe L: Longitudinal study of functional conditions in the masticatory system in Flemish children, Community Dent Oral Epidemiol 15:100-103, 1987.

11. Riolo ML, Brandt D, TenHave TR: Associations between occlusal characteristics and signs and symptoms of TMJ dysfunction in children and young adults, Am J Orthod 92:467-477, 1987.

12. Wanman A: Craniomandibular disorders in adolescents. A longitudinal study in an urban Swedish population, Swed Dent J [Suppl] 44:1-61, 1987.

13. Gazit E, Lieberman M, Eini R, et al: Prevalence of mandibular dysfunction in 10 to 18 year old Israeli school-children, J Oral Rehabil 11:307-317, 1984.

14. Rugh JD, Solberg WK: Oral health status in the United States: temporomandibular disorders, J Dent Educ 49:399-405, 1985.

15. Rugh JD, Solberg WK: The identification of stressful stimuli in natural environments using a portable biofeedback unit. Proceedings of the Biofeedback Research Society Fifth Annual Meeting, Colorado Springs, Feb. 1974.

16. Rugh JD, Solberg WK: Electromyographic studies of bruxist behavior before and during treatment, J Dent Res 54(special issue A):L-563, 1975 (abs).

17. Greene CS, Marbach JJ: Epidemiological studies of mandibular dysfunction: a critical review, J Prosthet Dent 48:184-190, 1982.

18. Egermark-Eriksson I, Carlsson GE, Magnusson T: A long term epidemiological study of the relationship between occlusal factors and mandibular dysfunction in children and adolescents, J Dent Res 66:67-71, 1987.

19. Posselt U: The temporomandibular joint and occlusion, J Prosthet Dent 25:432-438, 1971.

20. Solberg WK, Flint RT, Brantner JP: Temporomandibular joint pain and dysfunction: a clinical study of emotional and occlusal components, J Prosthet Dent 28:412-422, 1972.

21. Droukas B, Lindee C, Carlsson GE: Occlusion and mandibular dysfunction: a clinical study of patients referred for functional disturbances of the masticatory system, J Prosthet Dent 53:402-406, 1985.

22. Roberts CA, Tallents RH, Katzberg RW, et al: Comparison of internal derangements of the TMJ with occlusal findings, Oral Surg Oral Med Oral Pathol 63:645-650, 1987.

23. Clarke NG: Occlusion and myofascial pain dysfunction: is there a relationship? J Am Dent Assoc 104:443-446, 1982.

24. Seligman DA, Pullinger AG, Solberg WK: The prevalence of dental attrition and its association with factors of age, gender, occlusion and TMJ symptomatology, J Dent Res 67:1323-1333, 1988.

25. Egermark-Eriksson I, Ingervall B, Carlsson GE: The dependence of mandibular dysfunction in children on functional and morphological malocclusion, Am J Orthod 83:187-194, 1983.

26. Mohlin B, Thilander B: The importance of the relationship between malocclusion and mandibular dysfunction and some clinical application in adults, Eur J Orthod 6:192-204, 1984.

27. Mohlin B, Ingervall B, Thilander B: Relationship between malocclusion and mandibular dysfunction in Swedish men, Eur J Orthod 2:229-238, 1980.

28. Hansson T, Oberg T: Arthrosis and deviation in form in the temporomandibular joint, Acta Odontol Scand 35:167-174, 1977.

29. Solberg WK, Bibb CA, Nordstrom BB, Hansson TL: Malocclusion associated with temporomandibular joint changes in young adults at autopsy, Am J Orthod 89:326-330, 1986.

30. O'Ryan F, Epker BN: Temporomandibular joint function and morphology. Observations on the spectra or normalcy, Oral Surg Oral Med Oral Pathol 78:272-279, 1984.

31. Laskin DM, Ryan WA, Greene CS: Incidence of temporomandibular symptoms in patients with major skeletal malocclusions: a survey of oral and maxillofacial surgery training programs, Oral Surg Oral Med Oral Pathol 61:537-541, 1986.

32. Upton LG, Scott RF, Hayward JR: Major maxillo-mandibular malrelations and temporomandibular joint pain-dysfunction, J Prosthet Dent 51:686-690, 1984.

33. Proffit WR, Phillips C, Dann C IV: Who seeks surgical-orthodontic treatment? A review of patients evaluated in the UNC Dentofacial Clinic, Int J Adult Orthod Orthognath Surg [in press].

34. Sternback RA: Varieties of pain games. In Bonica JJ (editor): Advances in neurology: international symposium on pain, vol 4, New York, 1973, Raven Press.

35. Bonica JJ (editor): Advances in neurology: international symposium on pain, vol 4, New York, 1973, Raven Press.

36. Rugh JD, Solberg WK: Psychological implications in temporomandibular pain and dysfunction, Oral Sci Rev 7:3-31, 1976.

37. Lundeen TJ, Levitt SR, McKinney MW: Clinical applications of the TMJ scale, J Craniomand Pract 6:339-345, 1988.

38. Dawson PE: Evaluation, diagnosis, and treatment of occlusal problems, ed 2, St. Louis, 1989, The CV Mosby Co.

39. Blaschke DD, White SC: Radiology. In Sarnat BG, Laskin DM (editors): The temporomandibular joint. Biological diagnosis and treatment, ed 3, Springfield, Ill, 1980, Charles C Thomas, Publisher.

40. Hansson T, Oberg T: Arthrosis and deviation in form in the temporomandibular joint, Acta Odontol Scand 35:167-174, 1977.

41. Blair GS, Chalmers IM, Leggat TG, Buchanan WW: Circular tomography of the temporomandibular joint, Oral Surg Oral Med Oral Pathol 35:416-427, 1973.

42. Dolwick MF, Katzberg RW, Helms CA, Bales DJ: Arthrotomographic evaluation of the temporomandibular joint, J Oral Surg 37:793-799, 1979.

43. Katzberg RW, Dolwich MF, Helins CA, et al: Arthrotomography of the temporomandibular joint, AJR 134:995-1003, 1980.

44. Helms CA, Morrish RB, Jr, Kirlos LT, et al: Computed tomography of the temporomandibular joint: preliminary observations, Radiology 145:719-722, 1982.

45. Tucker MR, Guilford WB, Thomas PM: Versatility of CT scanning for evaluation of mandibular hypomobility, J Oral Maxillofac Surg 14:89-92, 1986.

46. Manzione JV, Katzberg RW, Tallents RH, et al: Magnetic resonance imaging of the temporomandibular joint, J Am Dent Assoc 3:398-402, 1986.

47. Katzberg RW, Bessette RW, Tallents RH, et al: Normal and abnormal temporomandibular joint: MR imaging with surface coil, Radiology 158:183-189, 1986.

48. Oesterreich FU, Jend-Rossmann I, Jend HH, Triebel HJ: Semi- quantitaive SPECT imaging for assessment of bone reaction to internal derangements of the temporomandibular joint, J Oral Maxillofac Surg 45:1022-1028, 1987.

49. Tsui BM, Gullberg GT, Edgerton ER, et al: Design in clinical utility of a fan beam collimater for SPECT imaging of the head, J Nucl Med 27:810-819, 1986.

50. Ackerman JL, Proffit WR: Treatment response as an aid in diagnosis and treatment planning, Am J Orthod 57:490-496, 1970.

51. Riggs RR, Rugh JD, Borghi W: Muscle activity of MPD and TMJ patients and non patients, J Dent Res 61:277, 1982 (abs 886).

52. Solberg WK, Clarke GT, Rugh JD: Nocturnal electromyographic evaluation of bruxism patients undergoing short term splint therapy, J Oral Rehabil 2:215-223, 1975.

53. Griffin JE, Karselis GD, Terrence C: Ultrasonic energy in physical agents for physical therapists, Springfield, 1979, Charles C Thomas, Publisher.

54. Travell JG, Simons DJ: Apros of all muscles in myofascial pain and dysfunction: the trigger point manual, Baltimore, 1983, Williams & Wilkins.

55. Kessler, RM: Friction massage in management of common muscular skeletal disorders. In Kessler RM, Hertling D (editors): Management of common musculoskeletal disorders: physical therapy principles and methods, Philadelphia, 1983, Harper & Row, Publishers, Inc.

56. Ward TG, Smith DG, Sommar M: Condylotomy for mandibular joints, Br Dent J 103:147-148, 1957.

57. Tassanen A, von Konow L: Closed condylotomy in the treatment of idiopathic and traumtic pain-dysfunction syndrome of the temporomandibular joint, Int J Oral Surg 2:102-106, 1973.

58. Finn RA, Throckmorton GS, Bell WH, Legan HL: Biomechanical considerations in the surgical correction of mandibular deficiency, J Oral Maxillofac Surg 38:257-264, 1980.

59. Proffit WR, Phillips C, Fields HW, Turvey TA: The effect of orthognathic surgery on occlusal force, J Oral Maxillofac Surg 47:457-463, 1989.

60. Wessberg GA, Diryan FS, Washburn MC, et al: Neuromuscular adaptation to surgical superior repositioning of the maxilla, J Oral Maxillofac Surg 9:117-122, 1981.

61. Van Sickels JE, Ivey Dw: Myofascial pain dysfunction: a manifestation of the short face syndrome, J Prosthet Dent 42:547-550, 1979.

62. Piecuch J, Tideman H, DeKoomen H: Short face syndrome: treatment of myofascial pain dysfunction by maxillary disimpaction, Oral Surg Oral Med Oral Pathol 49:112-116, 1980.

63. Tucker MR, Thomas PM: Temporomandibular pain and dysfunction in the orthodontic surgical patient: rationale for evaluation of treatment sequencing, Int J Adult Orthod Orthognath Surg 1:11-22, 1986.

64. Sanders B, Buoncristiani R: Diagnostic and surgical arthroscopy of the temporomandibular joint: clinical experience with 137 procedures over a two year period, J Craniomandib Disor 1:202-213, 1987.

65. Dolwick MF, Franco JE, Lemke RR, Rugh JD: Symptomology in TMJ surgical patients: a long term followup, J Dent Res 66:118, 1987 (abs 96).

66. Weinberg S, Craft J: Unilateral atrophy of the mandibular condyle after closed subcondylar osteotomy for correction of mandibular prognathism, J Oral Maxillofac Surg 38:366-368, 1980.

67. Phillips RM, Bell WH: Atrophy of mandibular condyles after sagittal ramus split osteotomy. Report of case, J Oral Maxillofac Surg 36:45-49, 1978.

68. Meyer RA: The autogenous dermal graft in temporomandibular joint disk surgery, J Oral Maxillofac Surg 46:48-56, 1988.

69. Delwick MF, Sanders B: TMJ internal deranagement and arthrosis: surgical atlas, St. Louis, 1985, The CV Mosby Co.

70. Tucker, Kennady MC, Jacoway JR: Autogenous auricular cartilage implantation following diskectomy in the primate temporomandibular joint, J Oral Maxillofac Surg 48:38-44, 1990.

71. Lindqvist C, Jokinen J, Paukku P, Tasanen A: Adaptation of autogenous costocondylar grafts used for temporomandibular joint reconstruction, J Oral Maxillofac Surg 46:465-470, 1988.

72. Kent JN, Misiek DJ, Akin RK, et al: Temporomandibular joint condylar prosthesis: a ten year report, J Oral Maxillofac Surg 41:245-254, 1983.

73. Bell WH, Gonyea W, Finn RA, et al: Muscular rehabilitation after orthognathic surgery, Oral Surg Oral Med Oral Pathol 56:229-235, 1983.

74. Glienburg RW, Laskin DM, Blaustein DI: The effects of immobilization of the primate temporomandibular joint: a histologic and histochemical study, J Oral Maxillofac Surg 40:3-8, 1982.

75. Lydiatt DD, Davis LF: The effects of immobilization on the rabbit temporomandibular joint, J Oral Maxillofac Surg 43:188-193, 1985.

76. Buckley MJ, Tulloch JFC, White RP, Jr, Tucker MR: Complications of orthognathic surgery. A comparison between wire fixation and RIF, Int J Adult Orthod Orthognath Surg 4:69-74, 1989.

77. Kundert M, Hadjfanghelou O: Condylar displacement after sagittal splitting of the mandibular rami, J Oral Maxillofac Surg 8:278, 1980.

Index